Atlas of General Surgery

Second Edition

Atlas of General Surgery

Second Edition

Selected from
Operative Surgery
Fourth Edition

Compiled by

Hugh Dudley ChM, FRCS(Ed), FRACS, FRCS
Professor of Surgery, St Mary's Hospital, London, UK

David C. Carter MD, FRCS(Ed), FRCS(Glas)
St Mungo Professor of Surgery, University of Glasgow;
Honorary Consultant Surgeon, Royal Infirmary, Glasgow, UK

R. C. G. Russell MS, FRCS
Consultant Surgeon, Middlesex Hospital, St John's Hospital for Diseases of the Skin,
and Royal National Nose, Throat and Ear Hospital, London, UK

Butterworths
London Boston Durban Singapore Sydney Toronto Wellington

First published 1981

British Library Cataloguing in Publication Data

Rob, Charles
[Rob & Smith's operative surgery. *Selections*]
Atlas of General Surgery: selected from Operative Surgery, fourth edition.–2nd ed.
1. Surgery, Operative
I. [Rob & Smith's operative surgery. *Selections*]
II. Title III. Smith, Rodney Smith, *Baron*.
IV. Dudley, Hugh V. Carter, David C. VI. Russell, R. C. G. VII. Rob and Smith atlas of general surgery
617'.9 RD32

ISBN 0-407-00377-0

Library of Congress Cataloging in Publication Data

Atlas of general surgery.

"Selected from Operative surgery, fourth edition."
Rev. ed. of: Rob and Smith atlas of general surgery. c1981.
Includes bibliographies and index.
1. Surgery, Operative. I. Dudley, Hugh A. F. (Hugh Arnold Freeman) II. Carter, David C. (David Craig) III. Russell, R. C. G. IV. Rob & Smith's operative surgery. V. Rob and Smith atlas of general surgery. [DNLM: 1. Surgery, Operative–atlases. W0 517 A8794]
RD32.A76 1986 617'.91 86-24468
ISBN 0-407-00377-0

Photoset by Butterworths Litho Preparation Department
Printed and bound by Butler & Tanner, Frome

Contributors

James T. Adams MD
Professor of Surgery, University of Rochester Medical Center, Rochester, New York, USA

John Alexander-Williams MD, ChM, FRCS, FACS
Consultant Surgeon, The General Hospital, Birmingham, UK

E. Amdrup MD, PhD
Professor of Surgery, University of Aarhus; Chief Surgeon, Surgical Gastroenterological Department L, Kommunehospitalet, Aarhus, Denmark

I. Barnett Angorn (deceased) FRCS(Ed), FRCS
Professor of Surgery, University of Natal, Durban, South Africa

John P. Blandy MA, DM, MCh, FRCS
Professor of Urology, The London Hospital Medical College; Consultant Urologist, St Peter's Hospital, London, UK

L. H. Blumgart MD, FRCS(Ed), FRCS(Glas), FRCS
Professor of Surgery and Director, Department of Surgery, Royal Postgraduate Medical School and Hammersmith Hospital, London, UK

Herbert Brendler MD
Professor, Department of Urology, The Mount Sinai Medical Center, New York, USA

Robert Britten-Jones MB, BS, FRCS, FRACS
Senior Visiting Surgeon, Royal Adelaide Hospital, South Australia

Charles G. Clark MD, ChM, FRCS, FRCS(Ed)
Professor of Surgery and Director of Surgical Unit, University College Hospital, London, UK

A. Cuschieri MD, ChM, FRCS(Ed), FRCS
Professor and Head of Department of Surgery, Ninewells Hospital and Medical School, University of Dundee, UK

J. L. Dawson MS, FRCS
Consultant Surgeon, King's College Hospital, London, UK

A. H. K. Deiraniya FRCS
Consultant Cardiothoracic Surgeon, Wythenshawe Hospital, Manchester, UK

P. Devitt MS, FRCS
Lecturer in Surgery, University of Liverpool; Honorary Senior Registrar, Royal Liverpool Hospital, Liverpool, UK

H. Brendan Devlin MA, MD, MCh, FRCS, FRCSI
Consultant Surgeon, North Tees General Hospital, Stockton on Tees, Cleveland; Associate Lecturer in Clinical Surgery, University of Newcastle Upon Tyne, UK

James A. DeWeese MD, FACS
Professor and Chairman, Division of Cardiothoracic Surgery, University of Rochester Medical Center, Rochester, New York, USA

Hugh Dudley ChM, FRCS, FRCS(Ed), FRACS
Professor of Surgery, St Mary's Hospital, London, UK

H. H. G. Eastcott MS, FRCS
Honorary Consultant Surgeon, St Mary's Hospital, London, UK

Terence A. H. English MB, BSc, MA, FRCS
Consultant Cardiothoracic Surgeon, Papworth and Addenbrooke's Hospitals, Cambridge, UK

Victor W. Fazio MB, BS, FRACS, FACS
Chairman, Department of Colon and Rectal Surgery, The Cleveland Clinic Foundation, Cleveland, Ohio; Medical Director, Rupert B. Turnbull Jr School of Enterostomal Therapy, The Cleveland Clinic Foundation, Cleveland, Ohio, USA

L. P. Fielding MB, FRCS
Chief of Surgery, St Mary's Hospital, Waterbury, Connecticut; Associate Professor of Surgery, Yale New Haven Hospital, Connecticut; Visiting Clinical Scientist, St Mary's Hospital Medical School, London, UK

Edward G. Flickinger MD
Associate Professor of General Surgery, School of Medicine, East Carolina University, Greenville, North Carolina, USA

Sir Patrick Forrest MD, ChM, DSc, FRCS, HonFACS
Regius Professor of Clinical Surgery, University of Edinburgh, UK

Geoffrey Glazer MS, FRCS, FACS
Consultant Surgeon, St Mary's Hospital, London, UK

Peter Goldstraw FRCS, FRCS(Ed)
Consultant Thoracic Surgeon, Brompton, Middlesex and University College Hospitals, London, UK

J. C. Goligher ChM(Ed), FRCS(Ed), FRCS
Consultant in General and Colorectal Surgery, Leeds; Emeritus Professor of Surgery, University of Leeds; Consulting Surgeon, St Mark's Hospital, London, UK

David Gough FRCS, FRCS(Ed), FRACS, DCH
Consultant Paediatric Surgeon, Royal Manchester Children's Hospital, Pendelbury, Manchester, UK

Roger Grace FRCS
Consultant Surgeon, The Royal Hospital, Wolverhampton, UK

J. D. Griffiths MS, FRCS
Consultant Surgeon, St Bartholomew's Hospital and the Royal Marsden Hospital, London, UK

A. A. Gunn ChM, FRCS(Ed)
Consultant Surgeon, Bangour Hospital, Broxburn, West Lothian, Scotland, UK

P. R. Hawley MS, FRCS
Consultant Surgeon, St Mark's Hospital and King Edward VII Hospital for Officers, London, UK

R. J. Heald MChir, FRCS
Consultant Surgeon, North Hampshire Group of Hospitals, Basingstoke, UK

John T. Hobbs MD, FRCS
Senior Lecturer in Surgery, University of London; Consultant Surgeon, St Mary's Hospital, London, UK

L. E. Hughes DS, FRCS, FRACS
Professor of Surgery, Welsh National School of Medicine, Cardiff, UK

P. S. Hunt MS, FRACS
Surgeon, Prince Henry's Hospital, Melbourne; Associate Professor, Monash University, Melbourne, Australia

Raymond Hurt FRCS
Thoracic Surgeon, Regional Thoracic Surgical Centre, North Middlesex Hospital, and St Bartholomew's Hospital, London, UK

R. D. Illingworth MB, FRCS
Consultant Neurosurgeon, Charing Cross and Central Middlesex Hospitals, London; Honorary Consultant Neurosurgeon, Westminster Hospital, London, UK

Thomas T. Irvin PhD, ChM, FRCS(Ed)
Consultant Surgeon, Royal Devon and Exeter Hospital (Wonford), Exeter, UK

Miles Irving MD, ChM, FRCS
Professor of Surgery and Consultant Surgeon, Hope Hospital, Salford, UK

John W. Jackson (deceased) MCh, FRCS
Formerly Consultant Thoracic Surgeon, Harefield Hospital, Middlesex, UK

George W. Johnston MCh, FRCS
Consultant Surgeon, Royal Victoria Hospital, Belfast; Honorary Lecturer in Surgery, Queen's University, Belfast, UK

A. W. Jowett FRCS
Consultant Thoracic Surgeon, The Royal Hospital, Wolverhampton, UK

Mark Killingback FRCS, FRCS(Ed), FRACS
Surgeon, Edward Wilson Colon and Rectum Unit, Sydney Hospital, Sydney, Australia

R. M. Kirk MS, FRCS
Consultant Surgeon, Royal Free Hospital, London, UK

Michael Knight MS, FRCS
Consultant Surgeon, St George's Hospital and St James' Hospital, London, UK

Sir Hugh Lockhart-Mummery KCVO, MD, MChir, FRCS
Consulting Surgeon, St Thomas' Hospital and St Mark's Hospital, London; Consultant Surgeon, King Edward VII Hospital for Officers, London, UK

Peter H. Lord MChir, FRCS
Consultant Surgeon, Wycombe General Hospital, High Wycombe, Buckinghamshire, UK

W. Scott McDougal MD
Professor and Chairman, Department of Urology, Vanderbilt University Medical Center, Nashville, Tennessee, USA

Warwick Macky OBE, MS, FRCS, FRACS
Urologist, Auckland Hospital, New Zealand

C. V. Mann MCh, FRCS
Consultant Surgeon, The London Hospital and St Mark's Hospital, London, UK

N. A. Matheson ChM, FRCS, FRCS(Ed)
Consultant Surgeon, Aberdeen General Hospitals, Aberdeen, UK

Douglas M. Millar FRCS, FRCS(Ed)
Consultant Surgeon, Essex County Hospital, Colchester, UK

Euan Milroy MB, BS, FRCS
Consultant Urologist, The Middlesex Hospital, London, UK

J. P. Mitchell CBE, TD, MS, FRCS, FRCS(Ed)
Honorary Professor of Surgery (Urology), University of Bristol, UK

C. F. Murnaghan MD, ChM, FRCS(Ed), FRCS, FRACS
Professor of Surgery, University of New South Wales; Urological Surgeon, The Prince Henry and Prince of Wales Hospitals; Consultant Urologist, the Royal Sydney Hospital, Sydney and the Royal Hospital for Women, Paddington, New South Wales, Australia

R. J. Nicholls MChir, FRCS
Consultant Surgeon, St Thomas' Hospital and St Mark's Hospital, London, UK

M. J. Notaras FRCS, FRCS(Ed)
Consultant Surgeon, Barnet General Hospital; Honorary Senior Lecturer and Consultant Surgeon, University College Hospital, London, UK

Richard G. Notley MS, FRCS
Senior Consultant Urological Surgeon, Royal Surrey County Hospital, Guildford, Surrey, UK

Marshall J. Orloff MD
Department of Surgery, School of Medicine, University of California, San Diego, USA

Sir Alan G. Parks (deceased) MCh, FRCS, FRCP
Formerly Consultant Surgeon, The London Hospital and St Mark's Hospital, London, UK

A. L. G. Peel MA, MChir, FRCS
Consultant Surgeon, North Tees General Hospital, Stockton on Tees, Cleveland, UK

John Percy FRACS, FACS
Consultant Surgeon, North Shore Medical Centre, St Leonard's, New South Wales, Australia

Malcolm O. Perry MD
Professor of Surgery, Cornell University Medical College, New York, USA

Walter J. Pories MD, FACS
Professor and Chairman, Department of Surgery, School of Medicine, East Carolina University, Greenville, North Carolina, USA

John P. Pryor MS, FRCS
Consultant Urologist, King's College and St Peter's Hospitals, London; Dean, Institute of Urology, London University, UK

John R. Richardson, Jr MD
Clinical Associate Professor of Urology, Dartmouth, Hitchcock Medical School, Hanover, New Hampshire, USA

Thomas J. Rohner, Jr MD
Professor of Surgery (Urology), Chief, Division of Urology, Pennsylvania State University College of Medicine and The Milton S. Hershey Medical Center, Hershey, Pennsylvania, USA

R. C. G. Russell MS, FRCS
Consultant Surgeon, Middlesex Hospital, St John's Hospital for Diseases of the Skin, and the Royal National Nose, Throat and Ear Hospital, London, UK

P. E. A. Savage MS, FRCS
Consultant Surgeon, Queen Mary's Hospital, Sidcup, Kent, UK

R. Shields MD, FRCS, FRCS(Ed)
Professor of Surgery, University of Liverpool; Honorary Consultant Surgeon, Royal Liverpool Hospital and Broadgreen Hospital, Liverpool, UK

John Terblanche ChM, FRCS, FCS(SA)
Professor and Head, Department of Surgery, University of Cape Town and Groote Schuur Hospital; Co-Director, Medical Research Council Liver Research Group, University of Cape Town, South Africa

A. E. Thompson MS, FRCS
Consultant Surgeon, St Thomas's Hospital, London, UK

James P. S. Thomson MS, FRCS
Consultant Surgeon and Dean of Postgraduate Studies, St Mark's Hospital, London; Consultant Surgeon, Hackney Hospital; Honorary Lecturer in Surgery, St Bartholomew's Hospital, London, UK

Ian P. Todd MS, MD(Tor), FRCS, DCH
Consulting Surgeon, St Bartholomew's Hospital, London; Consultant Surgeon, St Mark's Hospital and King Edward VII Hospital for Officers, London, UK

Christopher Wastell MS, FRCS
Consultant Surgeon, Westminster and St Stephens Hospitals, London; Professor of Surgery, Westminster Medical School, London, UK

R. B. Welbourn MA, MD(Cantab), Hon MD(Karolinska), FRCS, FCS(West Africa), Hon MRCS(Denmark)
Emeritus Professor of Surgical Endocrinology, Royal Postgraduate Medical School and Hammersmith Hospital, London, UK

Thomas Taylor White MD
Clinical Professor, Department of Surgery, University of Washington School of Medicine, Seattle, Washington, USA

J. E. A. Wickham MS, FRCS
Director of the Academic Unit, Institute of Urology, University of London; Senior Consultant Urological Surgeon, St Bartholomew's Hospital, London; Consultant Surgeon, St Peter's Hospital Group, London, UK

R. E. Williams MD, ChM, FRCS(Ed), FRCS
Consultant Urologist, The General Infirmary and St James's University Hospital, Leeds, UK

Contributing Medical Artists

Anne Barrett
Medical Illustrator, 43 Vineyard Hill Road, London SW19, UK

Daniel S. Beisel MA
Medical Illustrator, Department of Educational Resources, The Milton S. Hershey Medical Center, Hershey, Pennsylvania 17033, USA

Angela Christie MMAA
14 West End Avenue, Pinner, Middlesex HA5 1JB, UK

Michael Courtney
78 Alfred Road, Hastings TN35 5HY, UK

C. Darton

Paul Darton NDD, MAA
Medical Artist, The Middlesex Hospital Medical School, London, UK

Diane Elliott
Medical Illustrator, Photography and Illustration Service, University of Rochester, School of Medicine and Dentistry, Rochester, New York, USA

Arthur Ellis
Medical Artist, School of Medicine, University of Auckland, New Zealand

Brendan Ellis
Medical Artist, Department of Medical Illustration, Royal Victoria Hospital, Grosvenor Road, Belfast, Northern Ireland

Susan W. Evans NDD
Bargate House, Brewood, Stafford, UK

Susan Hales
41 Barnhorn Road, Cooden, Sussex, UK

Barbara Hyams
Medical Illustrator, 'Poynings', Northchurch Common, Northchurch, Berkhamstead, Herts, UK

P. G. Jack MMAA, AIMBI
Department of Teaching Media, University of Southampton, Hants, UK

Kathleen I. Jung MS, BS, AMI
The Cleveland Clinic Foundation, Cleveland, Ohio, USA

Robert N. Lane
Medical Artist, Studio 19a, Edith Grove, Chelsea, London SW10, UK

Gillian Lee FMAA
Medical Illustrator, Burnham, 15 Little Pluckets Way, Buckhurst Hill, Essex IG9 5QU, UK

Nigel Lucius DA
Department of Medical Illustration, University of Aberdeen, Scotland

Ann McNeill
Department of Clinical Surgery, The Royal Infirmary, Edinburgh, Scotland

Kevin Marks BA(Hons)
Illustrator, 53 Rookwood Avenue, Wallington, Surrey SM6 8HQ, UK

Anita Matthews BFA, AMI
Medical Illustrator, Photography and Illustration Service, University of Rochester, School of Medicine and Dentistry, Rochester, New York, USA

Richard Neave FMAA, AIMBI
Medical Artist, 89 Stamford Road, Bowden, Cheshire, UK

Gillian Oliver
Medical Illustrator, 71 Crawford Road, Hatfield, Herts AL10 0PF, UK

Oxford Illustrators
Aristotle Lane, Oxford, Oxon, UK

Mary Margaret Peel
Medical Illustrator, Veterans Administration Medical Center, Nashville, Tennessee, USA

Jean Perry AIMBI
Department of Medical Illustration, North Manchester General Hospital, Crumpsall, Manchester M8 6RB, UK

Carol J. Pienta
Medical Illustrator, Audio-Visual Services Center, School of Medicine, East Carolina University, Greenville, North Carolina, USA

Robert M. Reed
Manager of Biomedical Communications, The Cleveland Clinic Foundation, Cleveland, Ohio, USA

Franca Rubiu
Medical Artist, Department of Medical Illustration, The University of New South Wales, The Prince of Wales Hospital, Randwick, Sydney, NSW 2031, Australia

Kenneth Sanderson
Artist, The University of Liverpool, Merseyside, UK

D. D. Simmonds
Chief Medical Artist, Royal Postgraduate Medical School, London, UK

Cathy Slatter
Medical Illustrator, 16 Gravel Path, Berkhamstead, Herts, UK

Maureen M. Sheddon
Medical Artist, Ninewells Hospital and Medical School, Dundee, Scotland

P. Somerset BA
Medical Artist, Wythenshawe Hospital, Manchester, UK

Robert Wabnitz AMI
Medical Illustrator, Photography and Illustration Service, University of Rochester, School of Medicine and Dentistry, Rochester, New York, USA

Patrick Wheeler
Department of Surgery, University of Cape Town, Cape Town, South Africa

John B. Williamson
Medical Illustrator, 9 Cross Street, Holyland Common, Barnsley, South Yorkshire, UK

Philip Wilson
23 Normanhurst Road, St Paul's Cray, Orpington, Kent BR5 3AL, UK

Phyllis Wood AMI
Assistant Director, Health Science Illustration, University of Washington School of Medicine, Seattle, Washington, USA

Contents

Abdomen

Introduction

The multi-volume work which would encompass the best of modern surgical technique was conceived in the 1940s by Professor Charles Rob (then of St. Mary's and now of the Uniformed Forces Institute in the USA) and Mr. Rodney Smith (now Lord Smith of Marlow). That it was a timely and appropriate venture is clear from the fact that a second edition was required by 1968 and a third in 1977–80. A fourth edition is now being published on a continuous basis.

The very wide span of the work has had the effect that the ever-changing components of what we can term 'surgery in general' have become spread through numerous volumes. There is no harm in this but from time to time it would seem not unreasonable to draw together these scattered strands to provide a vade-mecum which, if it could not be fitted in the hip pocket, might at least have more portability than the encyclopaedic work from which it was derived. Hence this Atlas. We do not claim that it is the absolute right choice: like any anthology it will contain some things deemed unnecessary and lack other things which many would feel should be included. Nevertheless, it has been compiled, on the basis of an ad hoc consensus of opinion, from operations that have been found useful by practising surgeons.

Nearly all the material in this presentation is directly culled from the current editions of *Operative Surgery*. We have revised the sections on intestinal stapling and we are grateful to Mr. Geoffrey Glazer for his help in this regard.

As we move on through a fourth edition of the greater text, the selection of the contents for the abbreviated Atlas will doubtless change. At the moment we believe it includes much that is of the best in modern surgery and moreover provides an entry point to the larger work.

Hugh Dudley
D. C. Carter
R. C. G. Russell

Wound closure

Walter J. Pories MD, FACS
Professor and Chairman, Department of Surgery, School of Medicine,
East Carolina University, Greenville, North Carolina

Introduction

Good surgeons close wounds precisely. They recognize that careful reconstruction of the skin barrier protects against infection and deformity and that proper apposition of tissues is required for strong healing and avoidance of hernias, dehiscences and eviscerations.

Principles

Incisions

1

Good closures require proper incisions and elegant surgical techniques. The incision must be made cleanly and perpendicular to the skin.

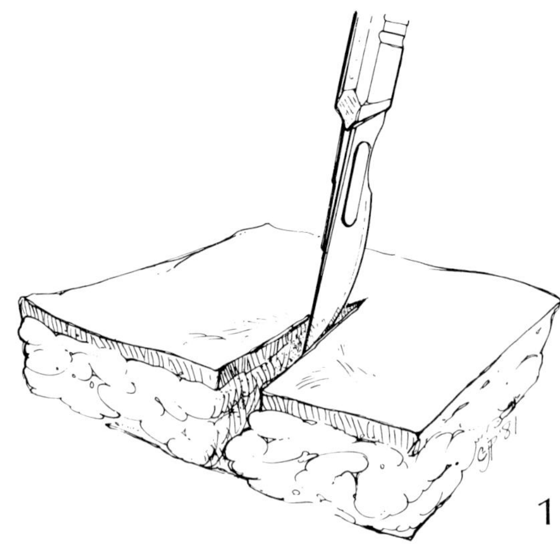

1

2

An incision which is made obliquely and in a jagged, erratic line will heal poorly, with a thick, irregular scar. Optimal incisions are easily made where the skin is taut, as on the extremities, chest and upper abdomen. Where skin is loose, as in the breast or around the navel, the skin must be stretched tight by traction as the incision is made.

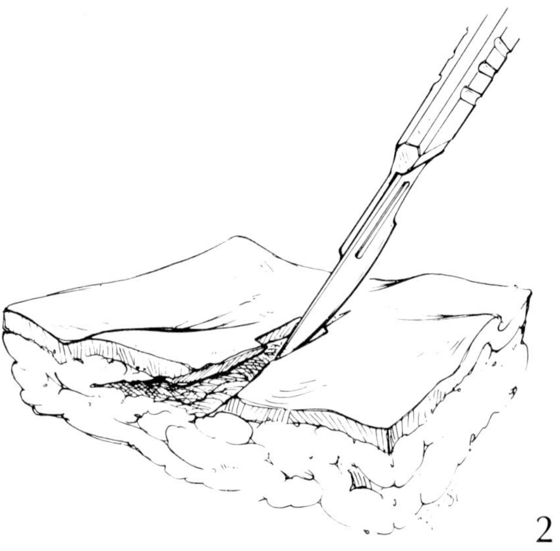

2

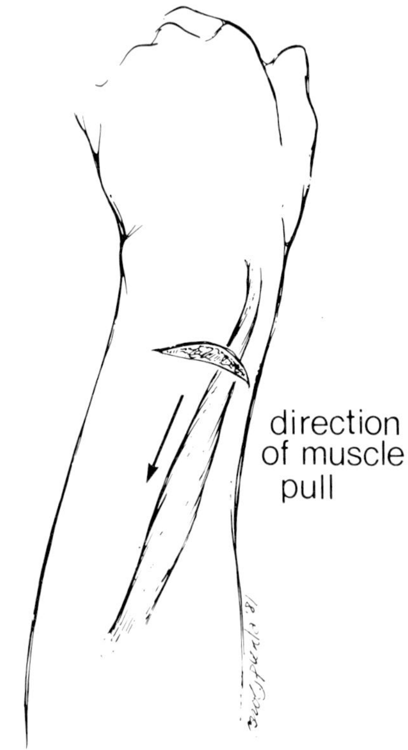

3

3

Wounds heal better if they are made parallel to wrinkle lines and across the lines of muscle pull. Frequently such wounds approximate themselves; exercise and activity aid in keeping the wound edges together.

4

Wrinkle lines occur in all parts of the body. They are readily identified by pinching the skin and subcutaneous tissues. If the part to be incised is inflamed or distorted, examination of the normal limb or the mirror-image area of the head, neck or trunk in the same manner will serve as a guide. When the breast is examined in this way, for example, it is readily apparent that the most cosmetic incisions are circumareolar or within the submammary fold.

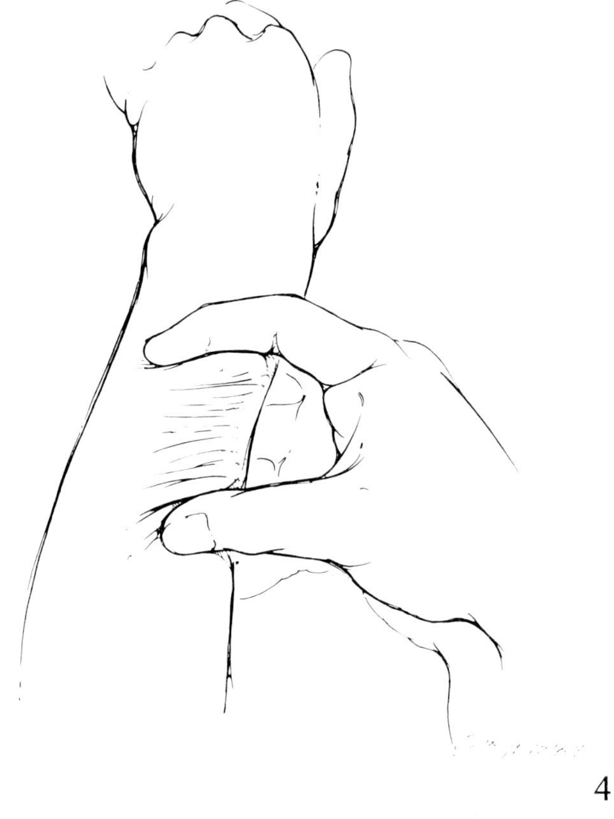

4

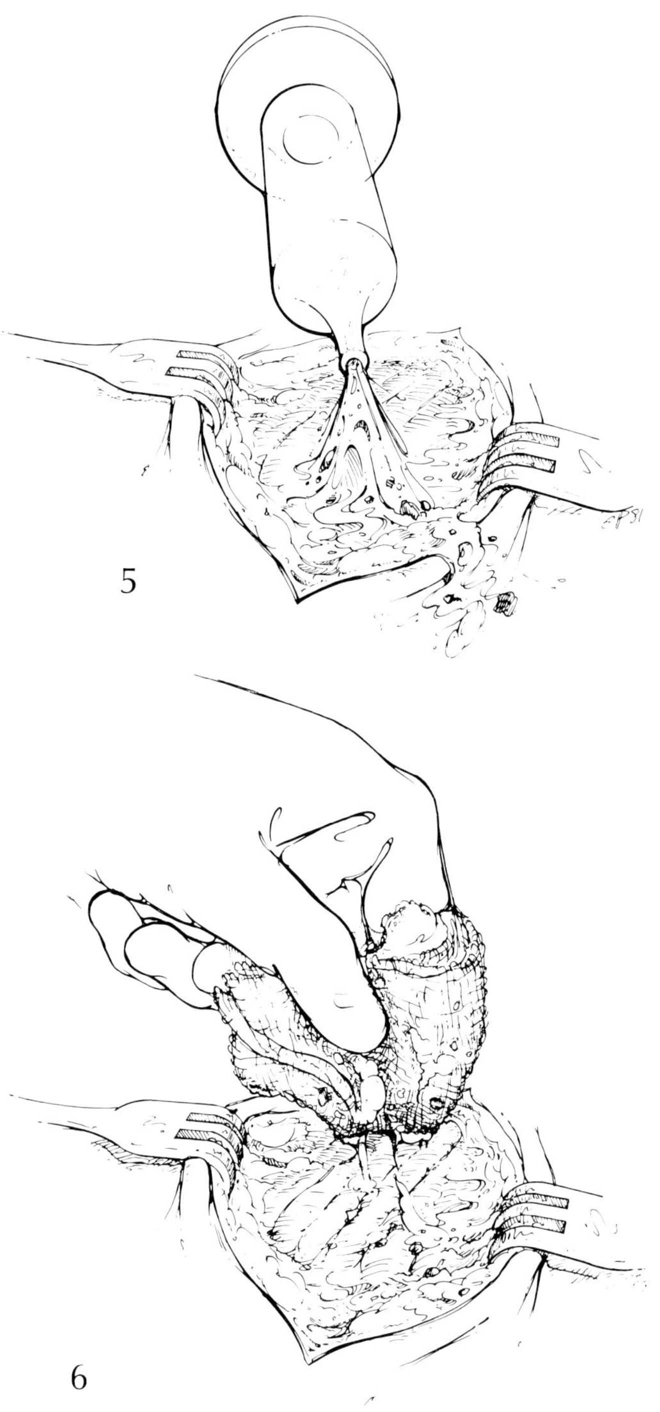

5

6

5 & 6

Irrigation

Irrigation is a mainstay of good wound closure. Washing the wound thoroughly with isotonic saline dilutes the bacterial population and removes pieces of dead fat, detritus and loose clot, each of which can serve as a nidus for infection. It is important to let the irrigation float these chunks off, or to pick them up with a sponge; simply sucking the pool of fluid just lets the fat and clots sink back down into the wound. Adding antibiotics (0.5 g kanamycin or neomycin per 1000 ml of solution) to the irrigating solution has proved helpful in contaminated cases.

Careful handling of tissues

7

Good wound closures require the approximation of normal tissues. Old scars should be excised, skin edges must not be burned by the cautery, the field should be dry, and foreign bodies, whether detritus, clot or suture material, should be kept to a minimum.

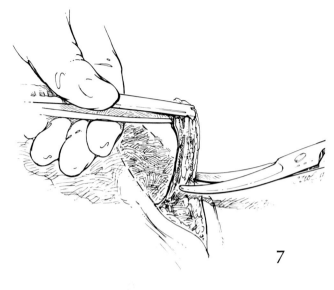

7

8

The tissues must be handled gently. Rough retraction with bruising and crushing from the carelessly placed clamp or too firmly squeezed forceps exacts a price in tissue damage, infection and ugly scarring. Wounds extending through several layers should be closed by reapproximating these layers as precisely as possible.

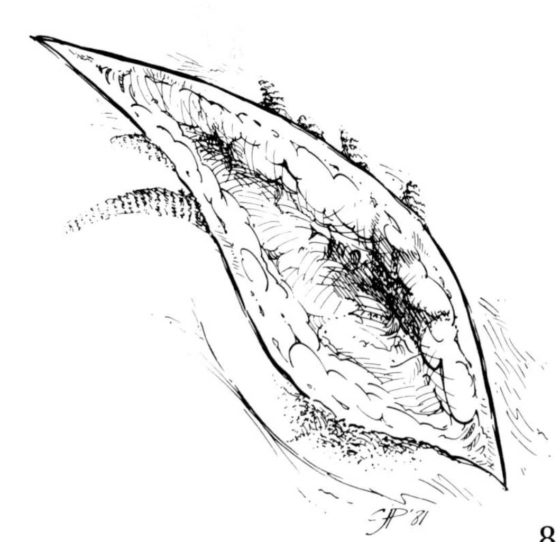

8

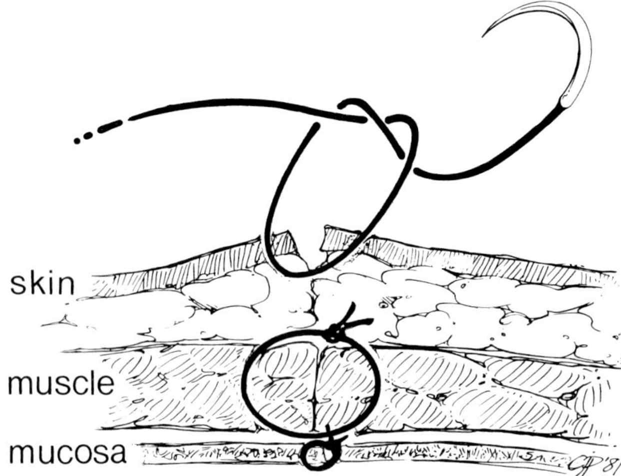

9

9

Suture technique

Sutures should approximate tissues, not strangle them. Knots should be tied gently and securely, both to avoid a noose effect and to ensure that the knots stay tied. We prefer an initial two granny knots to permit precise cinching of the knot, followed by a locking half-hitch which then squares the last knot. Other surgeons prefer three knots, with each of the latter two squaring the one preceding it. When monofilament material, which slips easily, is used, three surgeon's knots are preferable.

Types of closure

10

Primary closure

Tissues which are clean and free of infection can be approximated by primary closure. If the closure is well done, optimal healing and minimal scar formation follow.

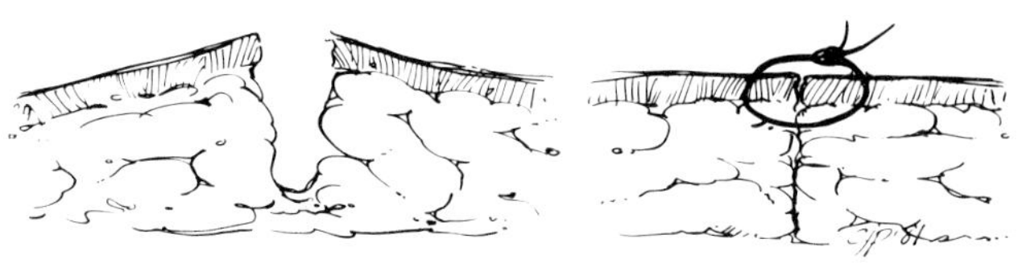

10

11

Secondary closure

Wounds allowed to granulate, either because of contamination, neglect or other reasons, are said to undergo secondary closure, or healing by second intention. The safety of this approach to infected wounds has been proven for centuries; its disadvantage is the long time required for healing and the heavy scarring which usually results.

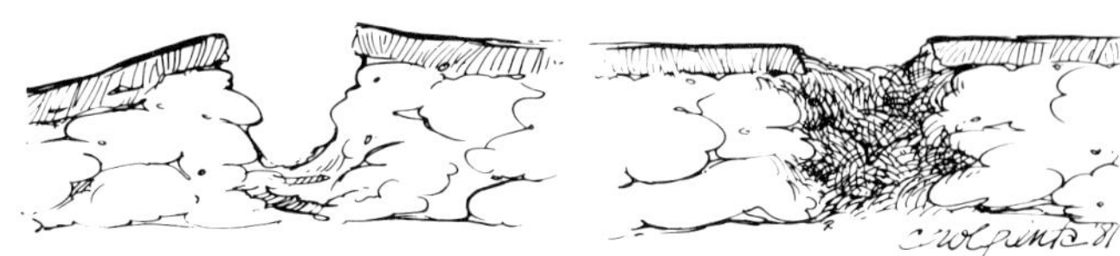

11

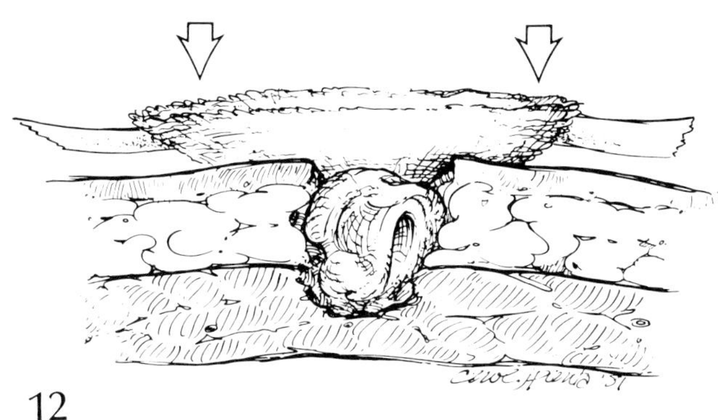

12

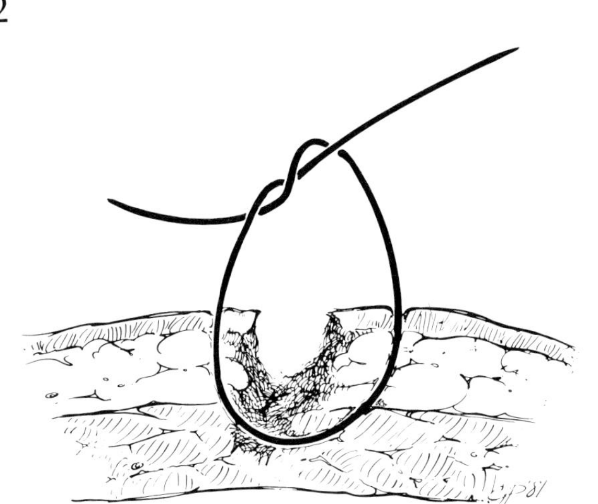

13

12 & 13

Delayed primary closure

Delayed primary closure offers the advantage of secondary closure without its disadvantages. This method is used for contaminated wounds such as those associated with emergency colon resections and war injuries. When the operation has been completed and all necrotic tissue and foreign matter have been removed, the wound is gently filled with fine mesh gauze and covered with a thick layer of gauze, secured with layers of tape to create an occlusive dressing. The dressing is not changed, unless the patient's condition worsens, for 4–5 days. At the end of that time, the dressing is removed under sterile precautions, preferably in the operating theatre. If the wound appears clean, the skin and underlying tissues can be closed securely. In most cases, the strength and cosmetic appearance of the wound will generally be as good as if the same tissues had been closed primarily after a clean operation. Delayed primary closure has saved many soldiers' lives; it is one of the major advances contributed by war surgery.

SELECTED SKIN CLOSURES

14

The *interrupted suture* remains the 'gold standard' for wound closure. If the sutures are precisely placed at the same level and the skin is gently reapproximated, optimal healing will take place, with minimal scar. For the best cosmetic result, in facial incisions or lacerations, for example, the sutures should be 1 mm apart and 1 mm from either edge; in other less noticeable areas, the stitches are usually 1 cm apart.

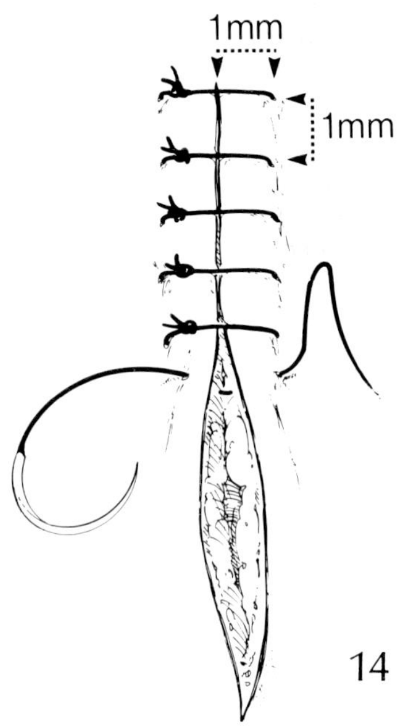

14

15

The *mattress suture* is most useful in areas where the skin is loose and overlap is likely to occur, as in the necks of aged patients, and for the beginning surgeon who has problems handling the over-and-over interrupted suture.

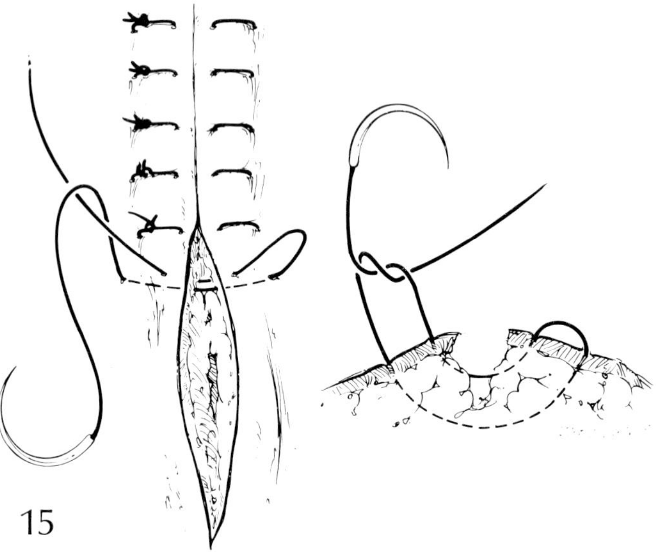

15

16

The *continuous overhand suture* is a rapid and efficient closure, but it is easily drawn too tight and tends to overlap. It is most useful where the skin is thick, as in the chest or back, or where rapid closure is desirable.

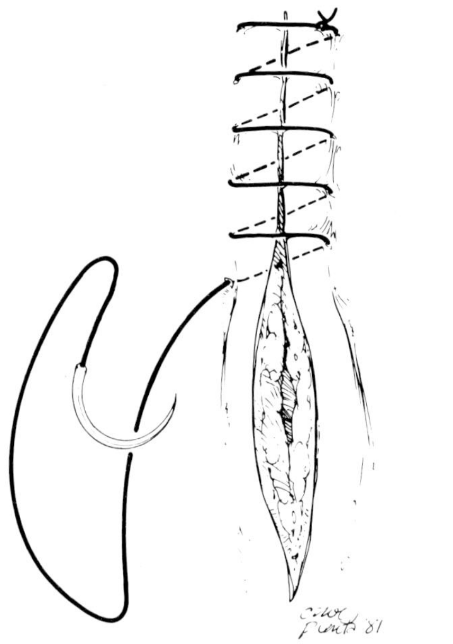

16

17

The *continuous mattress suture* is a useful and effective closure without the tendency of the ordinary suture to overlap.

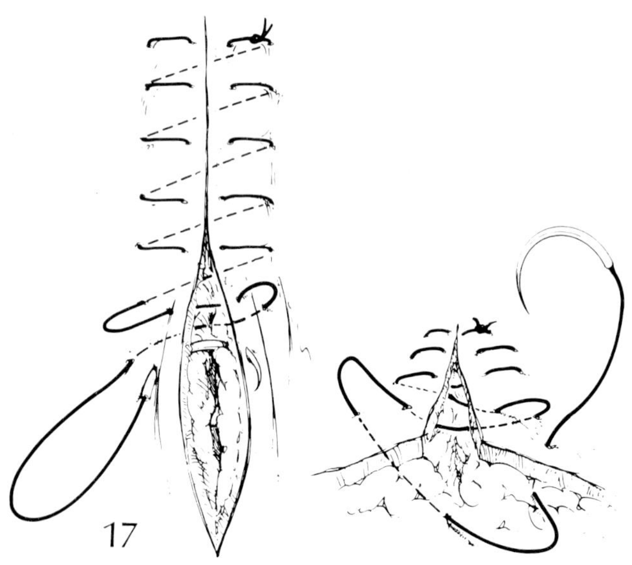

17

The *subcuticular suture* is a demanding stitch, but it has many rewards. It avoids the 'railroad-track' scars which follow most other closures, eliminates often arduous suture removal (especially in children), and provides precise approximation of epidermal tissues. This stitch can be done as a pullout suture with 3/0 monofilament nylon (Ethilon) or polypropylene (Prolene) or with a buried absorbable suture, such as 4/0 polyglactin 901 (Vicryl).

18–22

The *buried subcuticular suture* is begun with a stitch near the far edge of the wound; the needle is then brought out precisely at the corner to begin the suture line. The needle picks up about 1 mm of dermis just below the level of the epidermis, in progressive stepwise fashion along the length of the wound. The stitch can be ended by bringing it out at right angles to the wound or by tying a small slipknot in the end of the suture. The suture line is then painted with a skin adhesive, such as tincture of benzoin, and stabilized with a half-inch strip (Steri-strip) or a piece of paper tape. Tension is maintained on the suture until the paper strip has been placed; it can then be cut off flush with the skin.

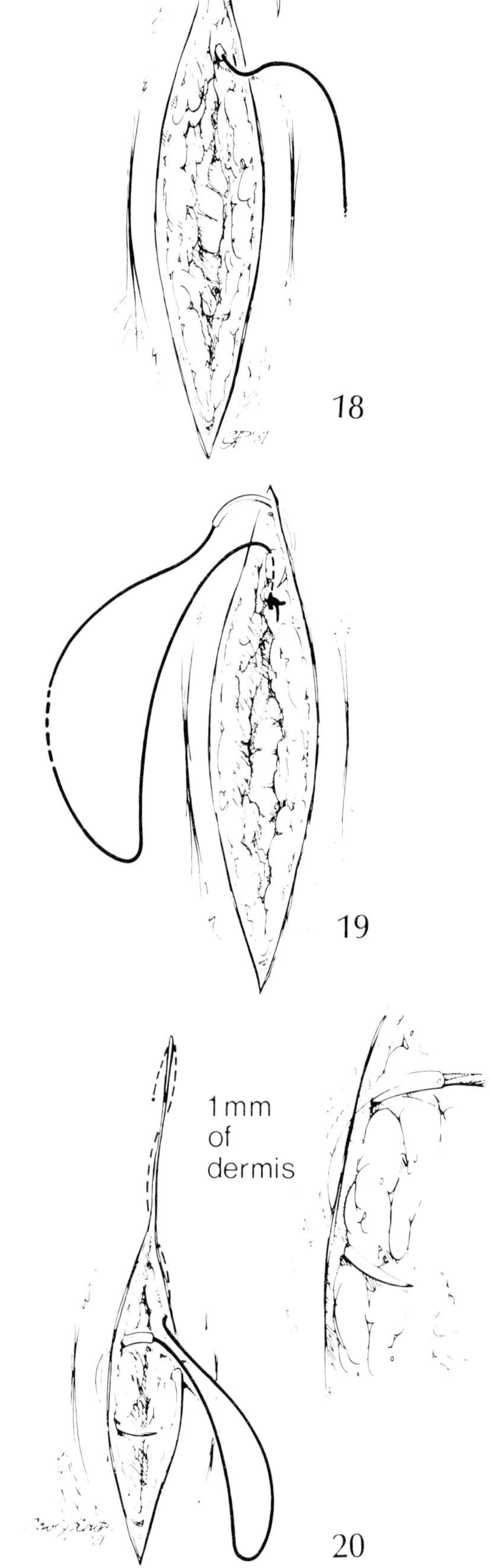

18

19

22

21

20

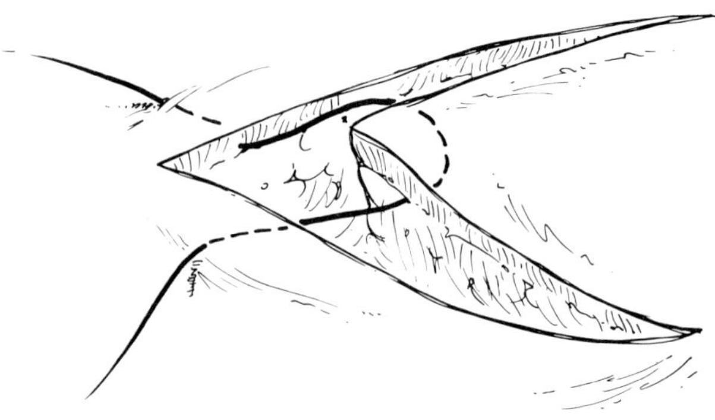

23

23, 24 & 25

The *corner stitch* is useful for the repair of jagged lacerations, for Z-plasties, and for the approximation of T incisions. The suture picks up the corner just below the epidermis, guides it precisely into the adjoining tissues and avoids the problem of necrosis of tissue in the angle that is sometimes caused by strangulating interrupted sutures.

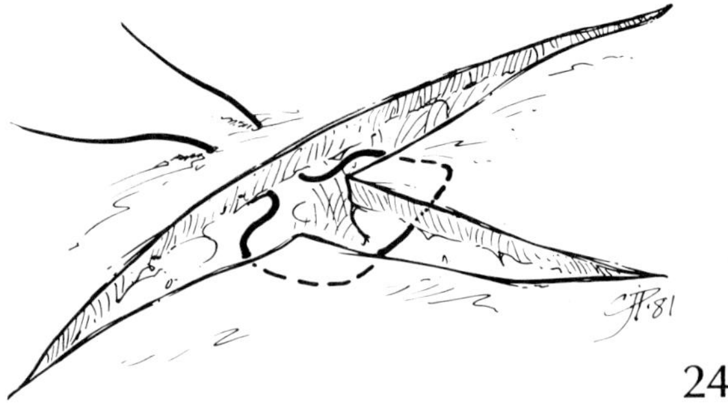

24

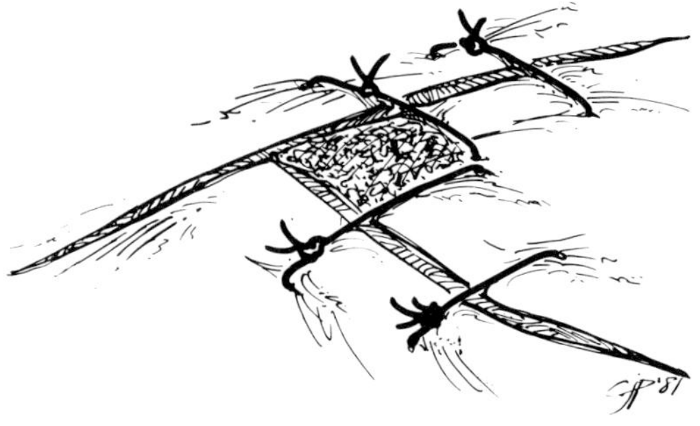

25

NEW SKIN CLOSURES

Tradition dies hard and at the time of writing most wounds are still closed with sutures. Many descriptions will be found throughout this book and its companion volumes. However, new techniques, some based on old ideas, are now taking hold.

26a–e

Clips and staplers

The old Michel clip (*a*) has the merits of simplicity and cheapness, but it is sometimes difficult to avoid the edges turning in. Newer devices are disposable and have a magazine of many staples (*b*). For the insertion of both clips and staples the wound edges must be held up beyond the point of application (*a* and *b*) though with the automatic device and sufficient hands, a slight eversion may be practised (*c*). Clips and staples are easily removed, usually with purpose-designed forceps (*d* and *e*).

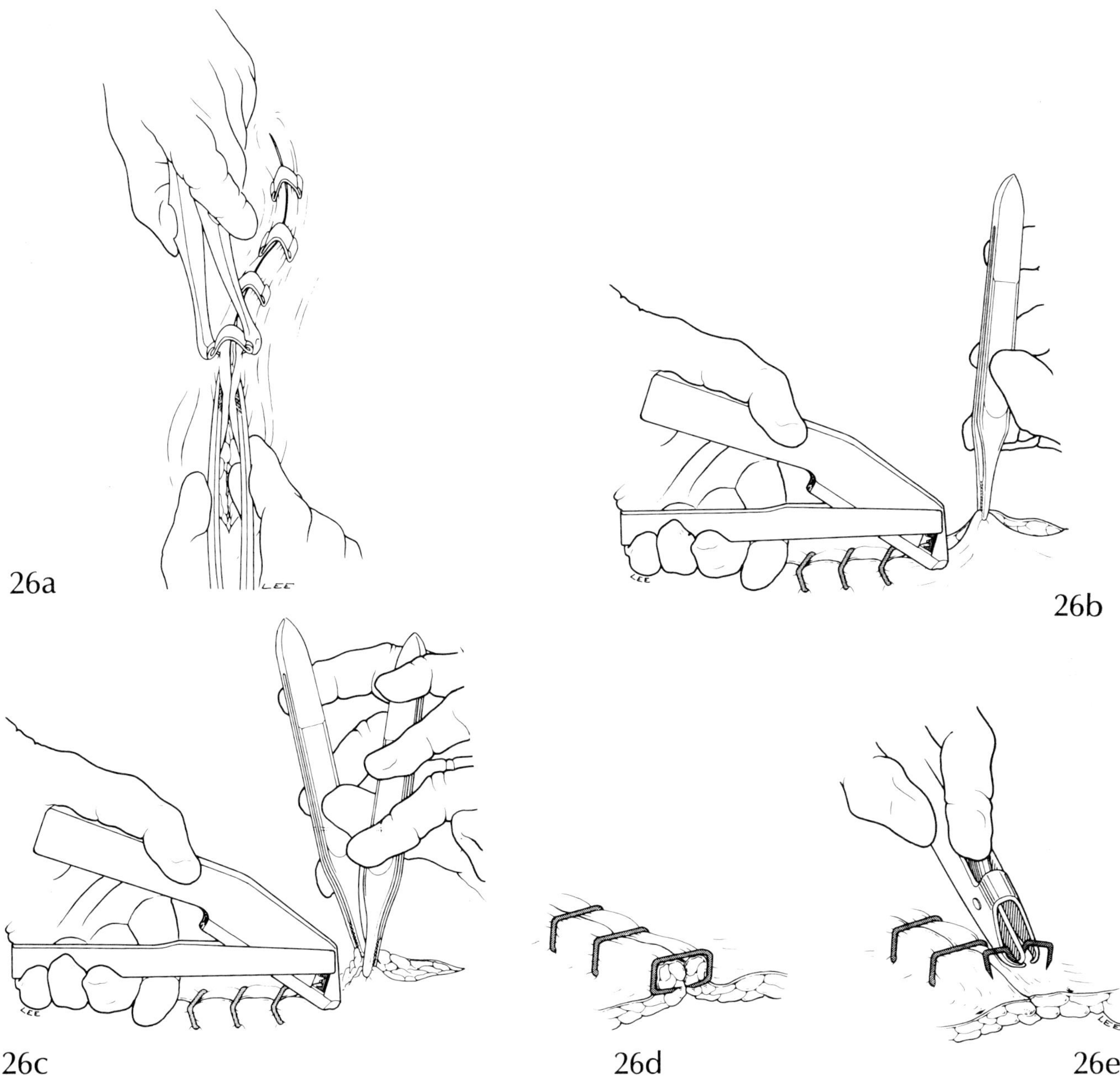

26a

26b

26c

26d

26e

27–30

Tape

Microporous adhesive tape (Steri-strip; Ethistrip) or, more recently, microporous film (Op-Site) may be laid across the wound. The cosmetic result is excellent. For this purpose it is essential that the wound edges are quite dry. A light spray of quick drying but sticky material (e.g. tincture of benzoin or collodion) may be used with advantage to aid adhesion.

In all these techniques of coaptation a sub- or intradermal stitch should be used to reduce distractive forces at the line of incision.

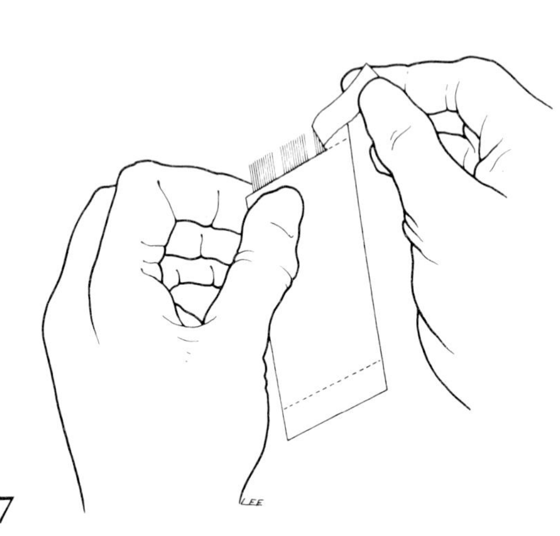

27

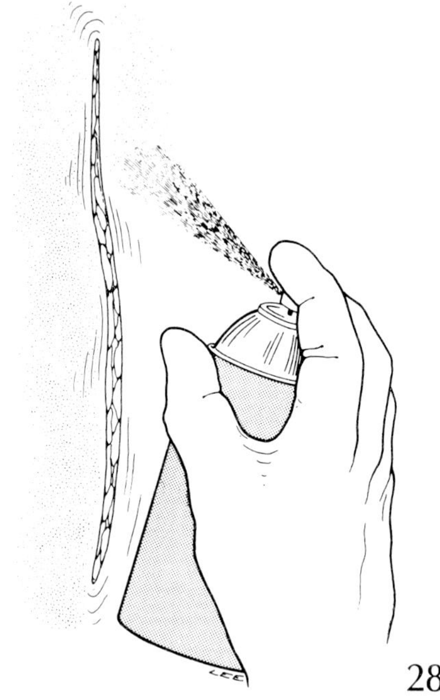

28

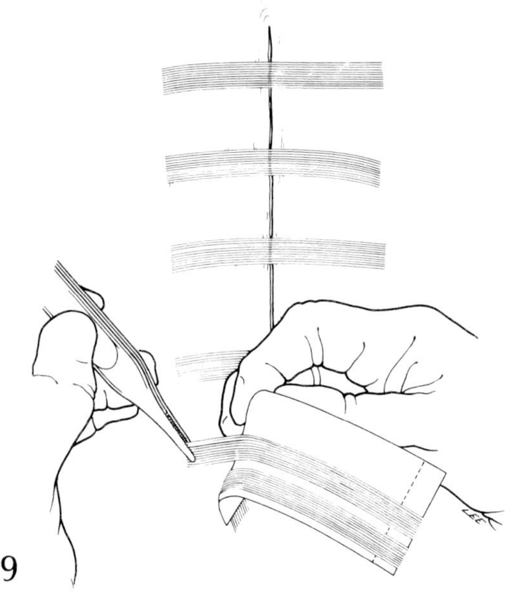

29

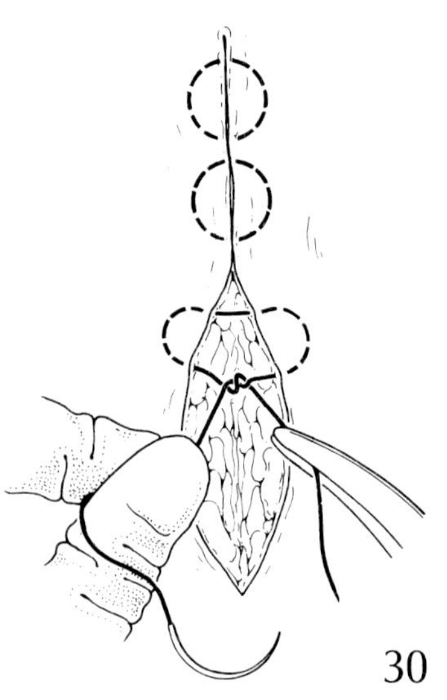

30

Further reading

Aston, S. J. The choice of suture material for skin closure. Journal of Dermatological Surgery 1976; 2: 57–61

Conn, J., Oyasu, R., Welsh, M., Beal, J. M. Vicryl (polyglactin 910) synthetic absorbablè sutures. American Journal of Surgery 1974; 128(1): 19–23

Devenev, C. W., Dunphy, J. E., Heppenstall, R. B., et al. Wound management in selected tissues. In: Hunt, T. K., Dunphy, J. E., eds. Fundamentals of wound management in surgery, p. 456. New York: Appleton-Century-Crofts, 1979

Edlich, R. F., Rodeheaver, G. T., Thacker, J. G., Edgerton, M. Technical factors in wound management. In: Hunt, T. K., Dunphy, J. E., eds. Fundamentals of wound management in surgery, p. 364. New York: Appleton-Century-Crofts, 1979

Horton, C. E., Adamson, J. E., Mladick, R. A., Carraway, J. H. Vicryl synthetic absorbable sutures. American Surgeon 1974; 40: 729–731

Laufman, H., Rubel, T. Synthetic absorbable sutures. Surgery Gynecology and Obstetrics 1977; 145: 597–608

Martyn, J. W. Clinical experience with a synthetic absorbable surgical suture. Surgery Gynecology and Obstetrics 1975; 140: 747–748

Postlethwait, R. W., Smith, B. M. A new synthetic absorbable suture. Surgery Gynecology and Obstetrics 1975; 140: 377–380

Van Winkle, W., Hastings, J. C., Barker, E., Hines, D., Nichols, W. Effect of suture materials on healing skin wounds. Surgery Gynecology and Obstetrics 1975; 140: 7–12

Principles of small grafts and flaps

Edward G. Flickinger MD
Associate Professor of General Surgery, School of Medicine,
East Carolina University, Greenville, North Carolina

Introduction

A well healed wound, the hallmark of a successful surgical endeavour, combines restoration of structural integrity and unencumbered function with an acceptable appearance. The surgeon works toward this desirable goal by gentle handling of tissues, careful debridement, meticulous haemostasis and a layered wound closure that is free of tension. When deficiencies in function and appearance might result from primary wound closure, it should be avoided. Clinical judgement will direct the surgeon to alternative measures in such situations.

Additional skills required for management of the moderately complex wounds frequently encountered in general surgery include grafting of autologous skin and use of small local skin flaps. Skin grafts and flaps are useful adjuncts to basic wound care when the surgeon combines a thorough grasp of their underlying principles with a precise application of their technique. Both methods may be practised in the clinician's office, in the emergency department or in standard operating suites, without any expensive, sophisticated instruments. Type, size and location of the wound will determine the best place to operate and whether local or general anaesthesia is appropriate.

The patient can benefit in terms of reduced pain, shorter treatment time and less anxiety, if the surgeon uses skin grafts and small local flaps with foresight. This chapter will cover the techniques of those skin grafts and flaps which are a useful part of every surgeon's armamentarium.

Skin grafts

1

Free autologous skin grafts are classified according to thickness. A graft of epidermis and superficial dermis containing dermal appendages is a partial or split-thickness graft. The donor site for such a graft will heal spontaneously, by re-epithelialization, much as an abrasion heals. A graft including all layers of skin is a full-thickness graft, and the donor site for such a graft must undergo partial-thickness skin grafting or primary reapproximation when possible. Generally speaking, the thinner a free skin graft is, the more likely it is to take, possibly at the expense of wound contracture. Conversely, the thicker the graft, the less predictable is its take; but if a thick graft is successful, contracture will be minimal.

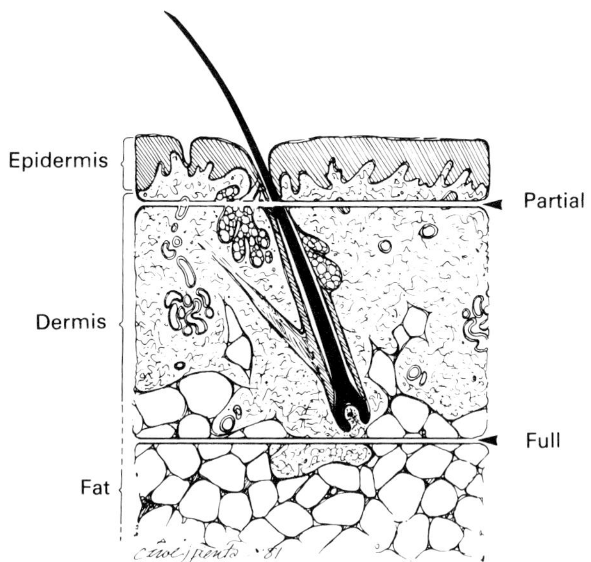

1

When a wound requires grafting, the surgeon must decide upon the appropriate thickness of the graft, both for immediate coverage and for long-term functional and cosmetic result.

Free skin grafts should be avoided in grossly contaminated or previously irradiated wounds. Similarly, grafting is contraindicated over areas of exposed tendon, cartilage or bone. The probability that the graft will take may be improved by careful surgical technique, maintenance of stability of the recipient bed and graft apposition, and control of infection, particularly streptococcal infection.

The techniques of partial-thickness and full-thickness skin grafts will be presented in detail.

PARTIAL-THICKNESS SKIN GRAFTS

Partial-thickness skin grafts are appropriate for situations in which maximum take is the primary consideration. Thin partial-thickness grafts may take even though the recipient bed is less than ideal. Such grafts may also be useful when a minimum of donor skin is available, such as in a large surface area burn. Frequent recourse to the common donor site is possible when this approach is used. A case that seems likely to progress to wound contracture over a period of time would better be treated by some method other than a partial-thickness skin graft.

Instruments

2

Dermatomes are finely calibrated instruments used for obtaining skin grafts of varying partial thickness. The Braithwaite and Watson knives operate manually, whereas the Brown dermatome requires electrical or compressed-air power to provide the necessary reciprocating blade action. Simple dial adjustments alter graft thickness by 0.001 inch increments. Both techniques can be rapidly mastered. Preference for one instrument over the other is a personal choice, although the size of graft needed may be influential. The Brown dermatome easily harvests uniform long skin strips up to 7.5 cm (3 inches) in width, while the Braithwaite or the Watson knife may produce narrow, irregular pieces unless skilfully used. Naturally the blades of either instrument must be sharp for best results.

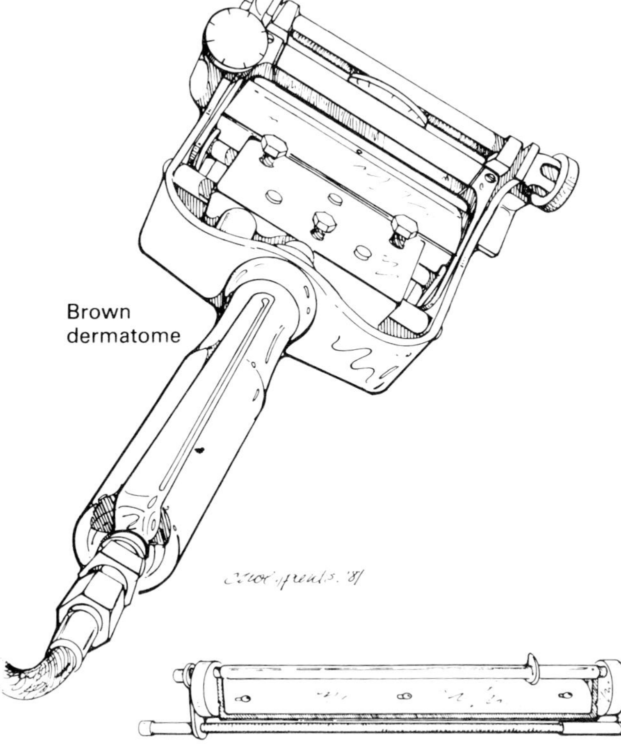

2

Graft procurement

Careful selection of the donor site is imperative. A flat or minimally contoured surface, with skin colour and texture resembling that surrounding the wound is best. Care must be taken to match glabrous skin grafts to appropriate sites, hairy grafts to defects in hairy areas. A further consideration in choice of donor site may be the size of the wound to be covered. Finally, the defect remaining after harvesting of the graft should not further handicap the patient.

3

Common donor sites for partial-thickness skin grafts are the anterolateral aspects of thighs and flanks.

Once a site has been chosen, local hair should be clipped or shaven and the area thoroughly cleansed. It may be desirable to use cleansing agents that will not discolour the skin (PHisoHex, saline rather than povidone-iodine) during the graft harvest.

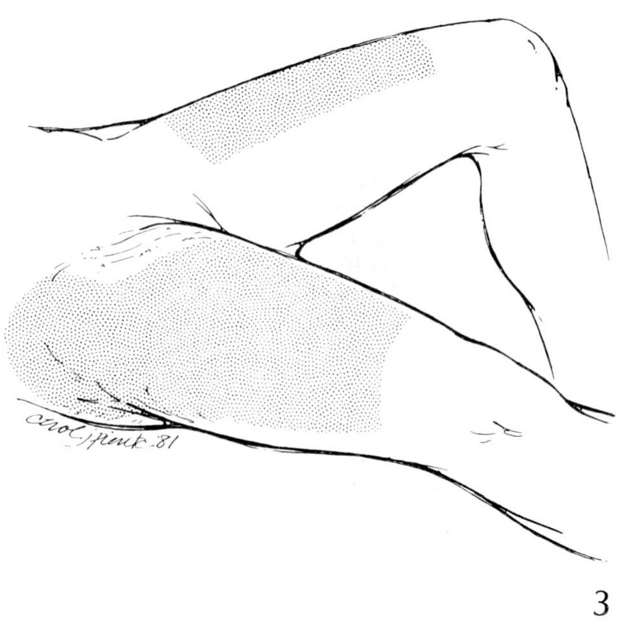

3

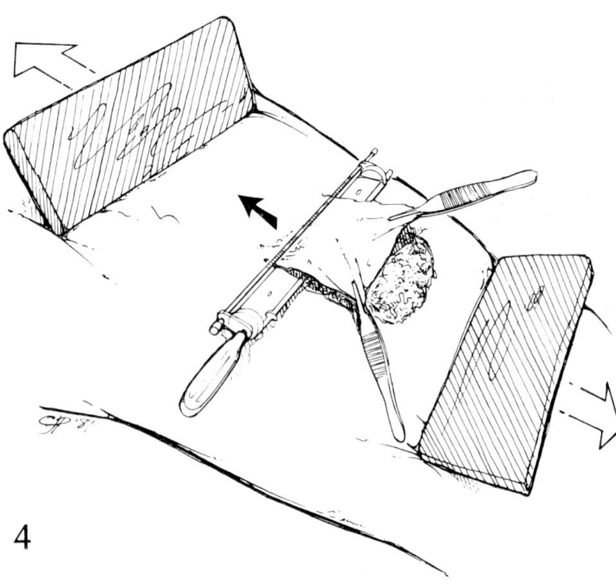

4

4

The entire donor site is painted with mineral oil to provide lubrication during the procedure. Wooden skin boards are then used to flatten the skin at the proposed donor site and adjusted as needed to facilitate graft harvest.

5

Braithwaite knife and Brown dermatome harvest skin grafts by controlled advance of the reciprocating blade. Both instruments are applied firmly to the skin during the procedure; it is impossible to cut too deeply into the dermis because of inherent safety features of the instruments. Irregularities in graft thickness will occur when the pressure is uneven. Once the desired graft has been obtained, it may either be applied directly to the wound or stored briefly in saline-soaked gauze. If surplus skin has been obtained, it should be reapplied to the donor site or stored in a skin bank, if such a facility exists. The donor site is then covered with either fine mesh gauze or Xeroform and a protective dressing.

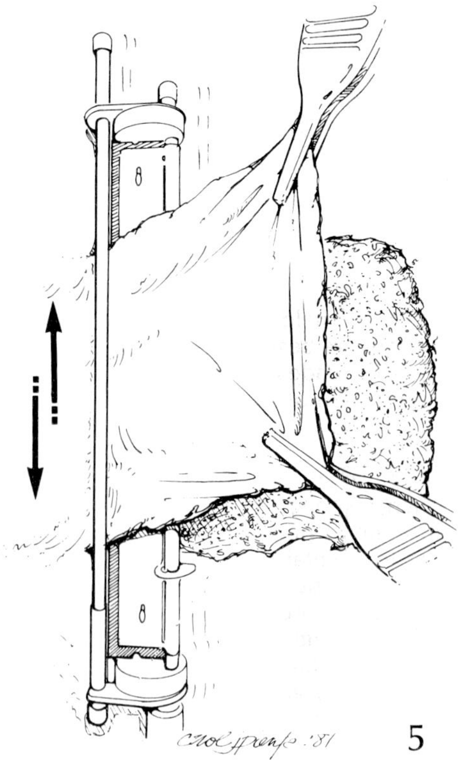

5

Graft application

6

Before direct application of the partial-thickness graft, the wound should be cleansed gently and debrided if necessary. Any areas of hypertrophic granulation tissue should be smoothed in order to obtain a uniform bed on which the graft will lie. If the graft is to be meshed, to cover a larger surface area, this is done immediately before application.

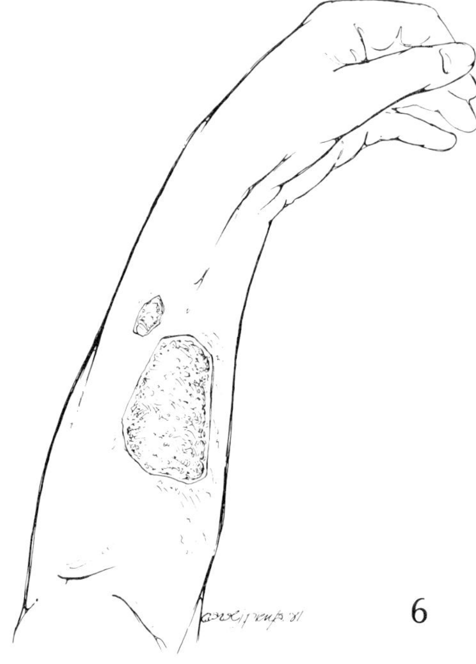

6

7

The graft is then positioned to cover the wound, with care to maintain direct graft–wound apposition.

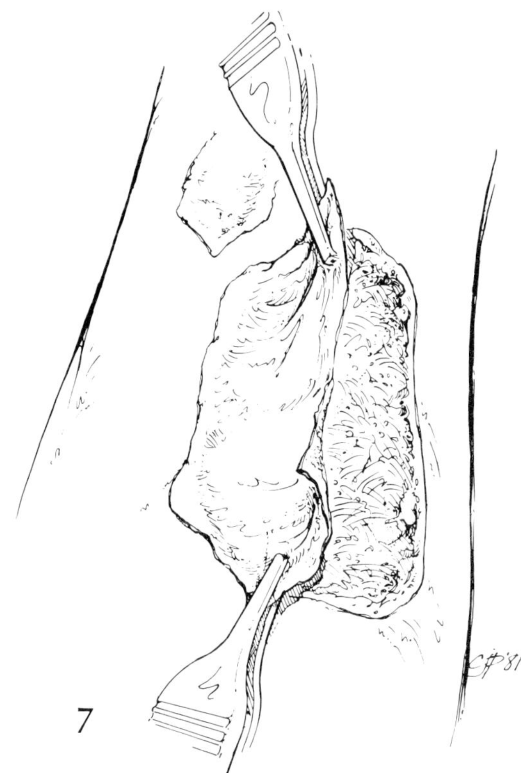

7

8

Small grafts can be held in position with adhesive strips, while larger ones are best secured by fine sutures. Several small cuts may be made into the graft to provide drainage for any accumulation of serum or blood.

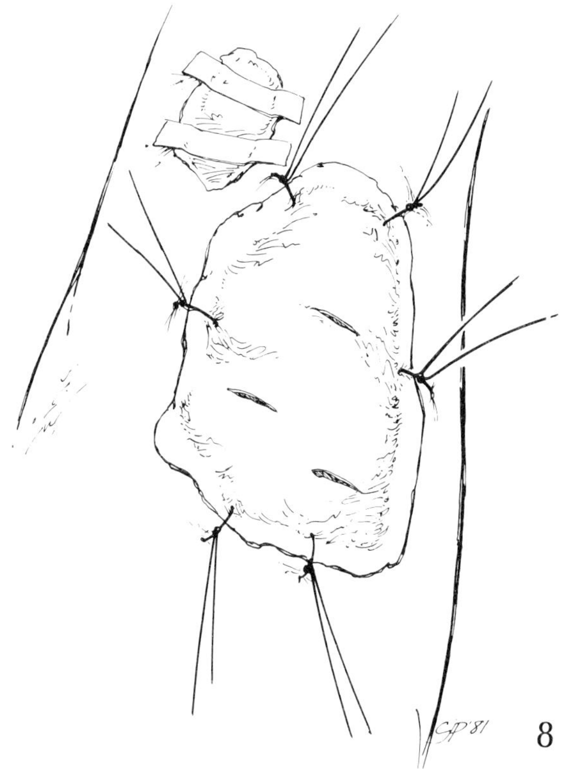

8

Fine-mesh gauze or Xeroform is applied as a topical dressing. Then, depending upon the size and location of the wound, either a pressure dressing or a cotton stent may be used to maintain direct graft–wound contact. At times it may even be necessary to enclose a grafted extremity in a cast to prevent motion between the wound and the graft. The original dressing is maintained for 5–7 days, during which time the graft will take. When the dressing is removed, great care should be taken not to disrupt the healing process. Any problems will usually be apparent at the time of the first dressing change.

PINCH GRAFTS

9

Pinch grafts may occasionally be useful in sites where, over time, partial-thickness grafts are likely to break down because of predictable wear and tear. Certain wounds of the hands and feet and those over bony prominences are suitable for pinch grafting.

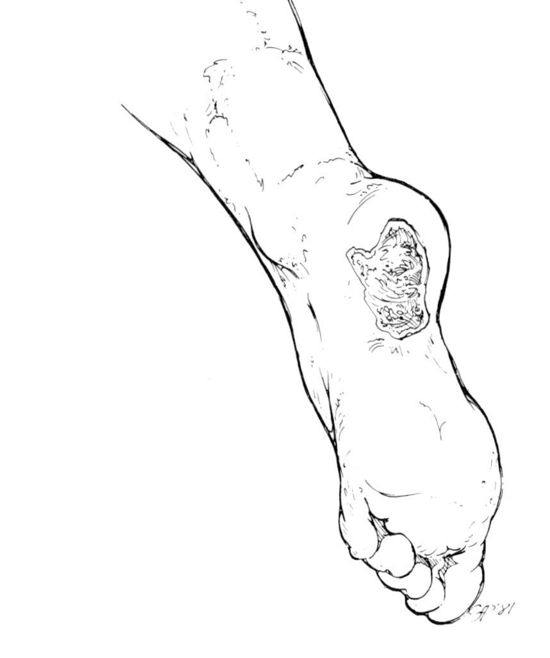

9

10

Pinch grafts are small discs of skin (approximately 1 cm in diameter) with both partial- and full-thickness elements. The thicker elements provide better protection against local trauma, while the partial-thickness elements provide a better chance of take and a margin for re-epithelialization. This form of grafting is no longer as popular as previously, but its principles and techniques may occasionally be useful.

The advantage of pinch grafting is that it can be performed under local anaesthesia by those with minimal experience in other forms of grafting. Its main disadvantage is the final pebbled appearance of both the donor and the grafted sites.

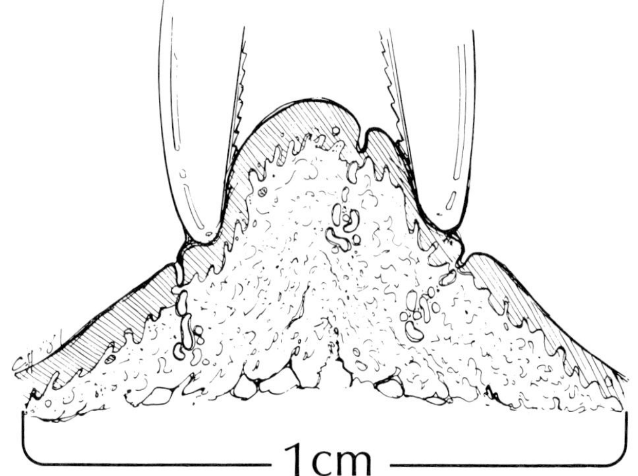

10

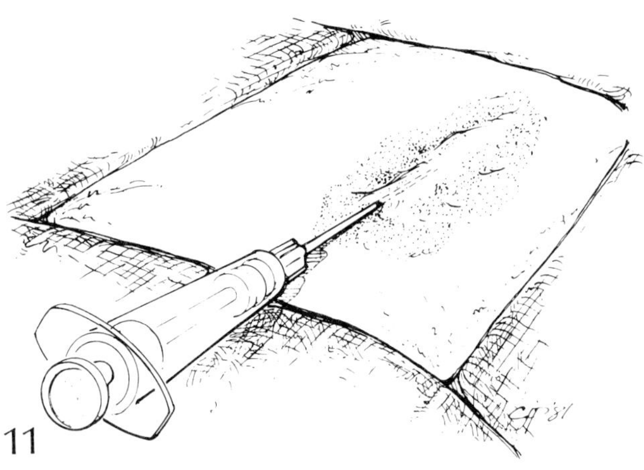

11

Graft procurement

11

The defect requiring grafting will dictate the surface area of skin to be prepared for harvest. The local hair should be trimmed away and the skin cleansed. A local anaesthetic agent is then administered subcutaneously by a fine-gauge needle in an area sufficient for providing the desired number of pinch grafts to be harvested.

12

After satisfactory anaesthesia has been obtained, a small mound of skin is elevated by the tip of a straight needle or fine forceps. A standard scalpel blade is then used to excise a disc of skin measuring approximately 1 cm in diameter. In this fashion, multiple grafts are obtained. The donor site is then dressed sterilely to allow for healing by granulation and re-epithelialization.

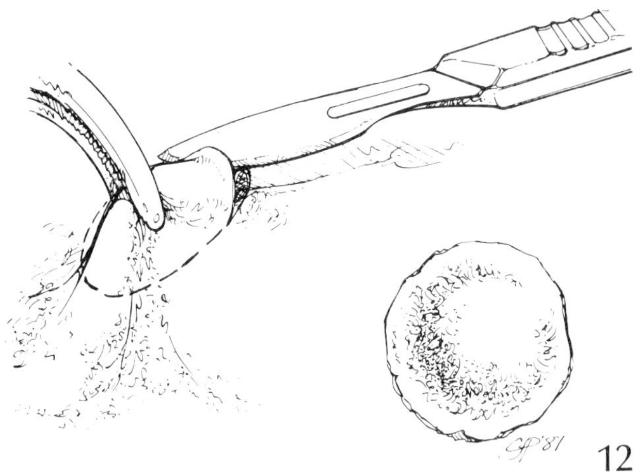

12

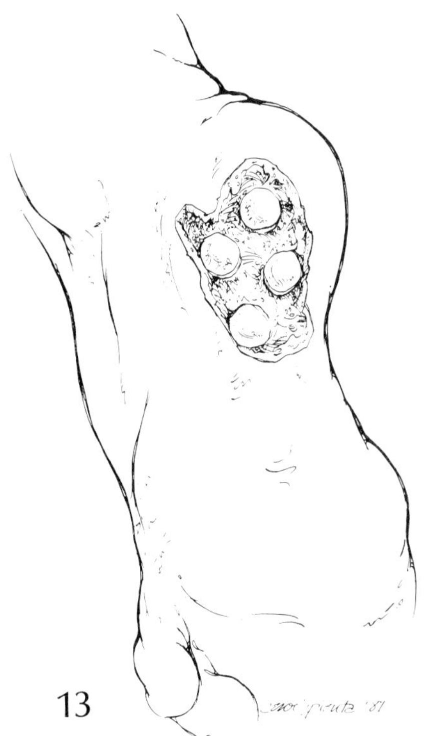

13

13

Graft application

The wound is prepared for receiving the graft by gentle cleansing and minor debridement when necessary. The pinch grafts are applied to the wound, allowing about 1 cm between graft margins. Fine-mesh gauze or Xeroform, together with a sterile dressing, protects the grafts during the healing phase. About 5 days are required for graft take.

FULL-THICKNESS SKIN GRAFTS

Full-thickness skin grafts are recommended for small wounds of the face and neck where cosmesis is a crucial consideration. Appropriate colour, texture, contour and durability can be achieved with minimal contraction in a well executed full-thickness graft.

Because its rate of take is less predictable, a full-thickness graft should be applied only when the wound exhibits either a fresh or a rich granulating surface conducive to healing.

14

The lesion is excised with an appropriate margin, with the long axis of the wound aligned with the wrinkle lines for the best cosmetic result.

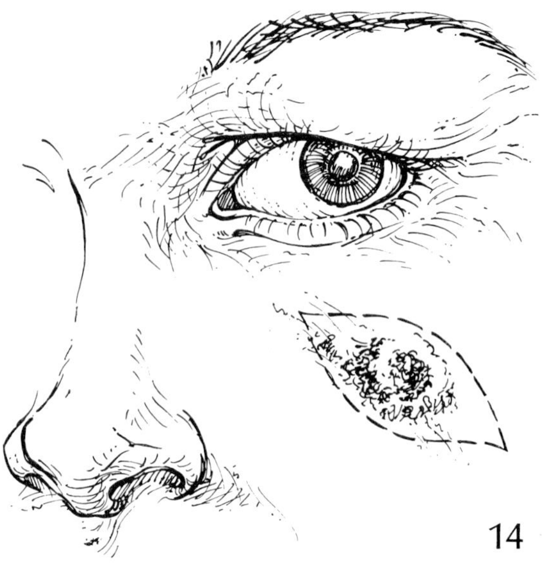

14

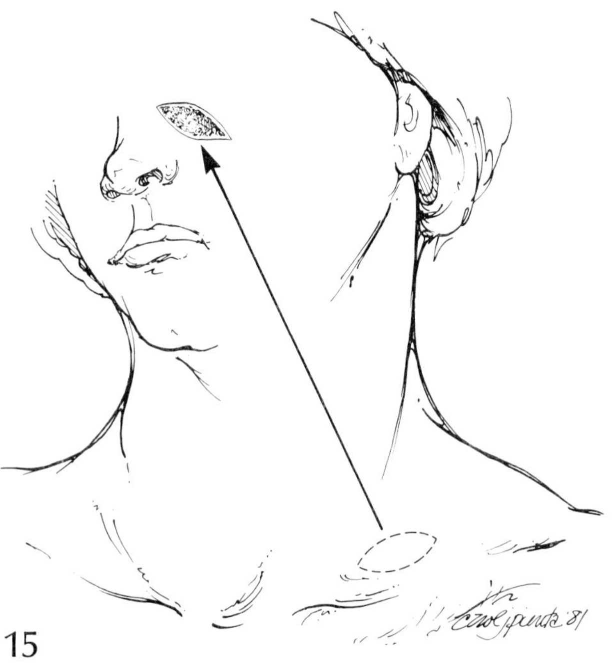

15

Graft procurement

15

The final appearance of a grafted wound of the face or neck is critical; thus the donor skin should be similar in colour and texture to that of the face and neck. The groin and supraclavicular area of the neck are frequently chosen sites. Occasionally the anterior and lateral chest may serve.

After an appropriate site has been selected, the hair is clipped and the skin cleansed as in other grafting procedures. The surgeon should measure the wound carefully, transcribing its exact dimensions to the donor site. The proposed graft is then outlined by a marking pen.

16

The graft is excised at the interface of dermis and subcutaneous fat, with special care being taken to protect the graft edges from unnecessary trauma.

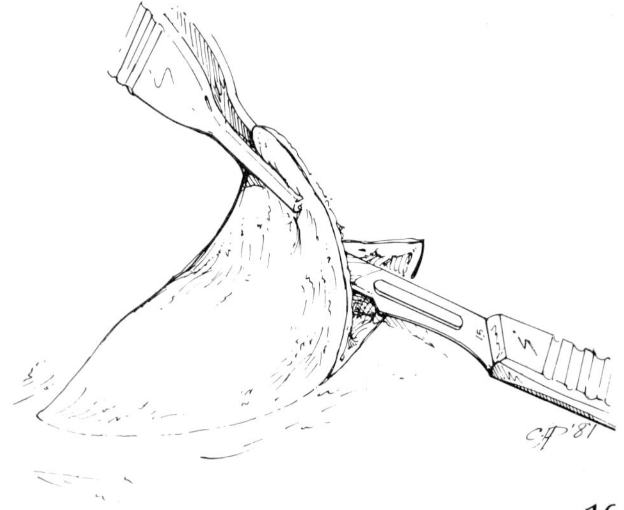

16

17

Before graft application, all residual fat adherent to the dermal surface should be meticulously scraped off with the edge of a scalpel blade to assure the best chance of graft take.

18

The donor site is closed by approximation of the edges.

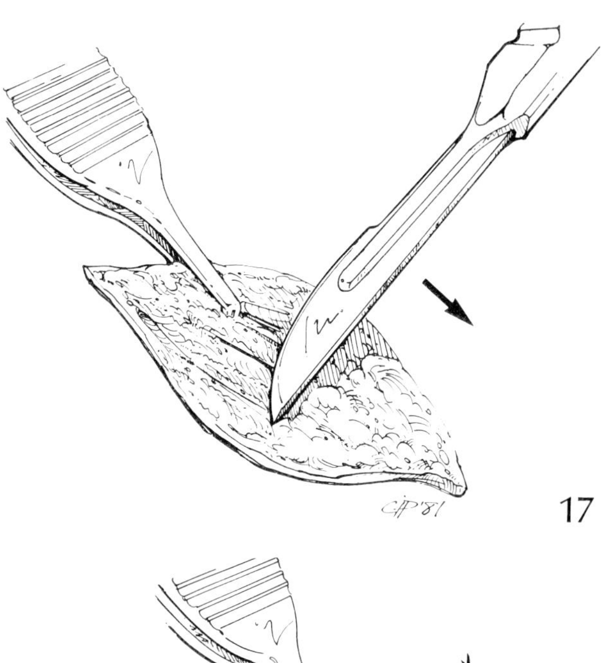

17

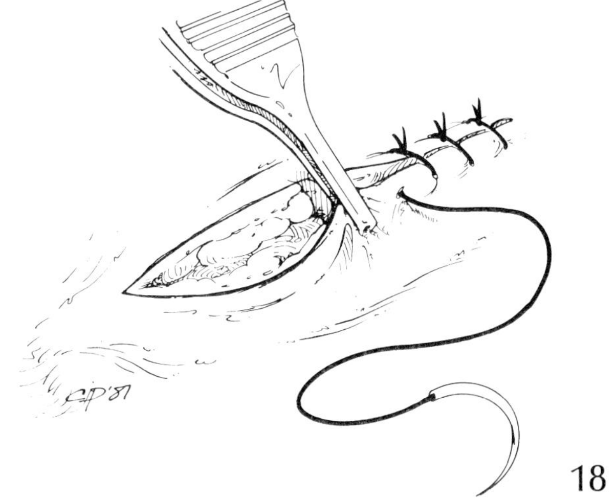

18

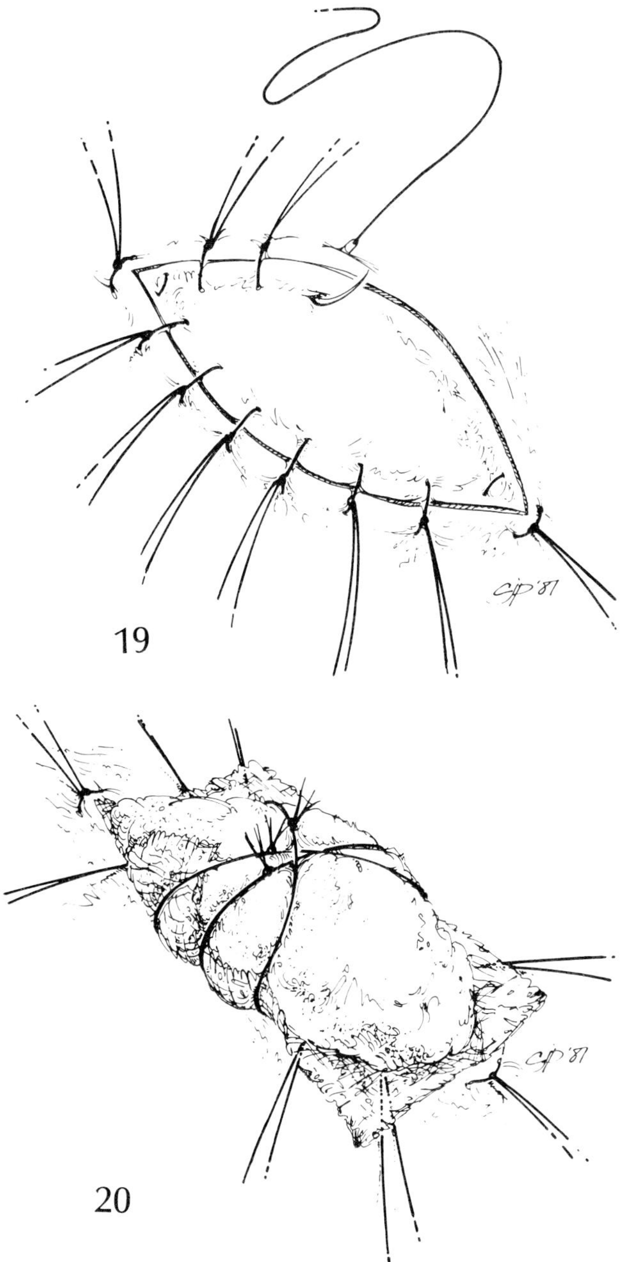

19

20

Graft application

19

The full-thickness graft is placed directly upon the clean wound and anchored in place with fine sutures.

20

It is usually desirable to tie these sutures over Xeroform and a cotton stent to provide continuous graft–wound apposition. Five to seven days will be required for the graft to take securely.

Local skin flaps

General surgeons frequently face wounds involving full-thickness loss of skin and exposed tendon, bone or cartilage. These may be managed best by reorienting nearby skin flaps of like colour and texture. Such wounds include avulsion injuries or excision sites, the edges of which cannot be approximated primarily without undue tension or an unsatisfactory final appearance. Other wounds requiring local flaps include lacerations through and perpendicular to natural skin folds or across joints. Primary closure of such defects could produce an undesirable cosmetic result or functional impairment. Proper management of these cases requires a working knowledge of advancement flaps, rotation flaps and Z-plasty.

A great deal of forethought in designing a skin flap, combined with meticulous technique, is essential for successful healing. Well vascularized and redundant skin adjacent to the wound is desirable if local flaps are to be used. When redundancy is lacking, a secondary donor defect is often the price paid for satisfactory coverage of the primary wound. Such a defect, when covered by a partial-thickness skin graft, should not be cosmetically undesirable or functionally limited.

ADVANCEMENT FLAPS

21, 22 & 23

Local undermining

The simplest form of advancement flap technique involves local undermining of skin edges to allow approximation without tension.

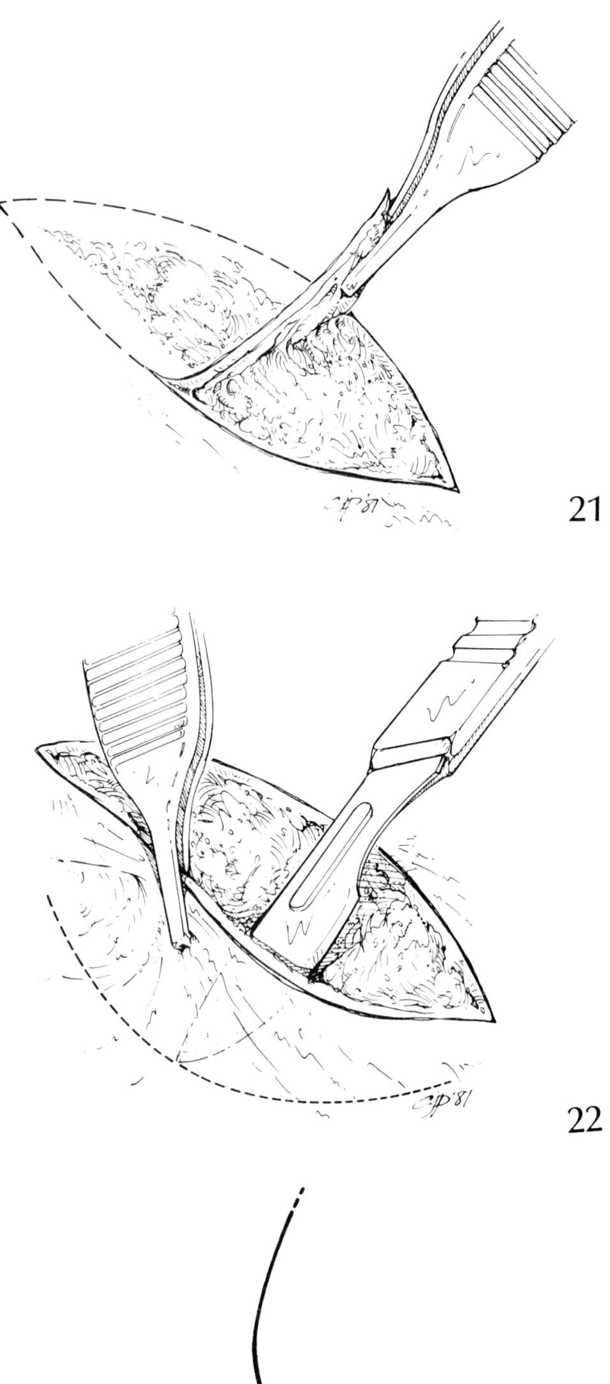

21

22

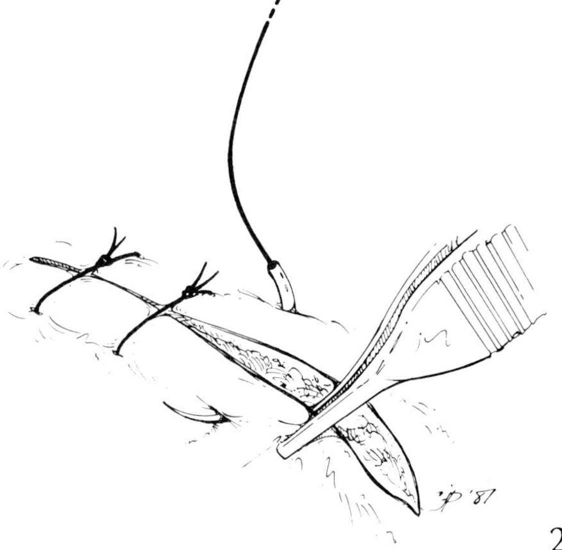

23

Utilization of adjacent skin

24

When simple undermining is insufficient for satisfactory closure, an advancement flap can be designed, utilizing adjacent lax and vascularized skin. The dimensions of the flap are ultimately limited by the blood supply derived from the base of the flap. While vascularity varies in different parts of the body, one should avoid flap length-to-width ratios exceeding 2:1.

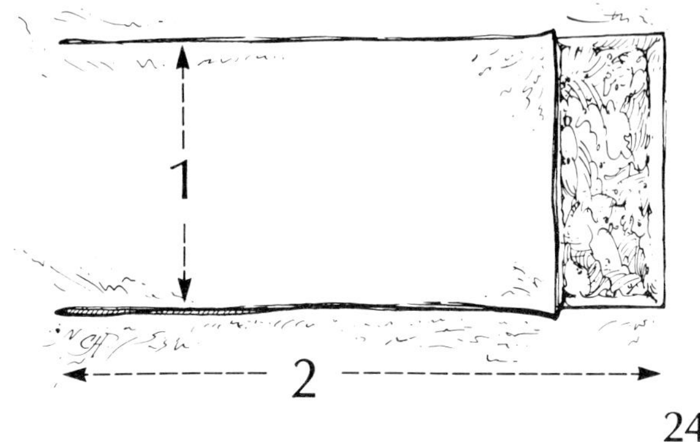

24

25

The lesion is excised, with a rectangular margin to accommodate the flap. The flap edges are incised and the skin undermined through fat.

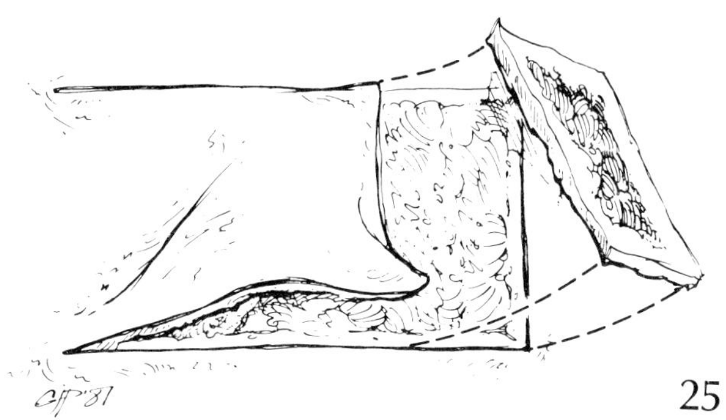

25

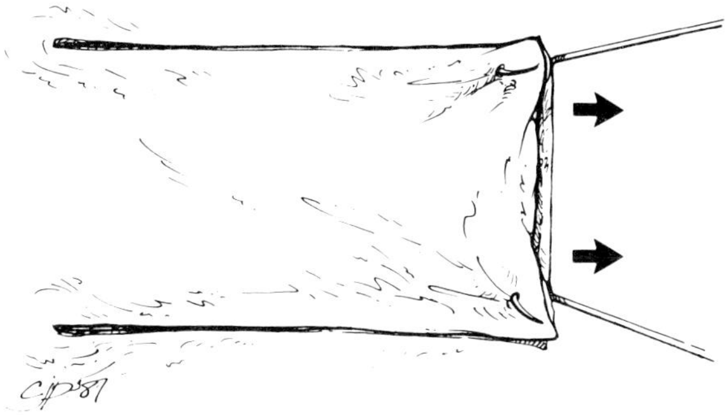

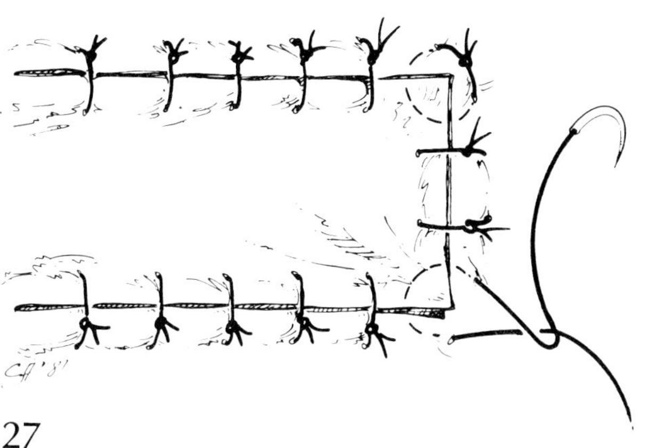

26

26

Gentle handling of the flap with fine skin hooks is essential for preventing necrosis along the margins.

27

27

The flap is advanced to cover the primary wound and sutured into place. This is what one generally hopes for but rarely achieves without excessive tension or an unsightly 'dog-ear'.

Excision of dog-ear

28 & 29

As suturing progresses toward the base of the flap, a dog-ear on one side or both may become apparent. In this event, an incision should be made at right angles to the flap; the triangle so formed is undermined and excised.

30

The flap may then be sutured securely into place. Even with this modification, the practical application of advancement flaps may be limited, because suture line tension cannot be totally avoided.

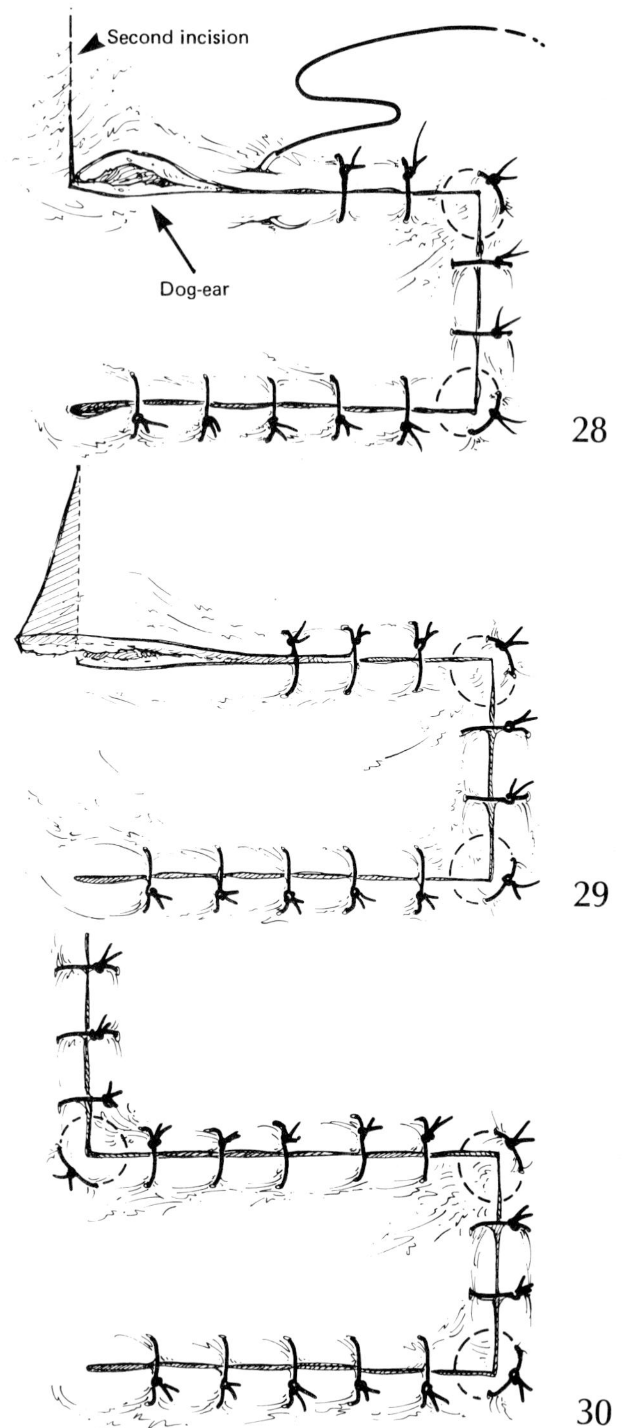

28

29

30

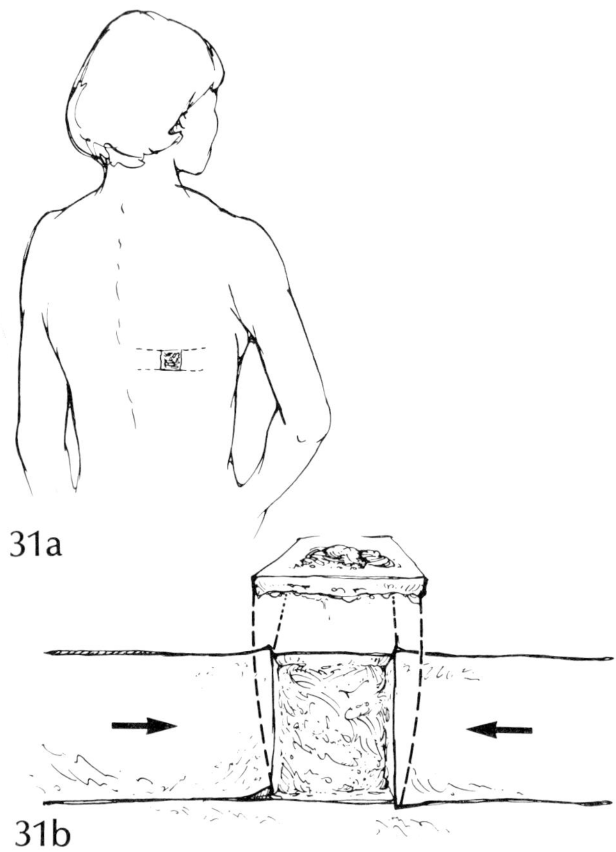

31a

31b

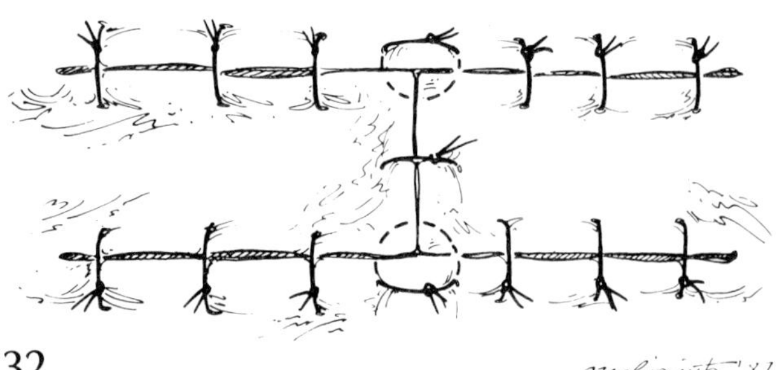

32

31 & 32

Wide excision

A modification of the advancement flap technique can be used in closing large defects of the back created by widely excising a lesion, such as a malignant melanoma. The so-called 'bra-strap closure' is completed by creating bilateral advancement flaps with medial approximation of one flap to the other.

ROTATION FLAP

33a & b

A rotation flap is applicable for covering triangular defects. The apex of the triangle defines the base of the proposed flap to be rotated over the defect. Before any incision is made, the proposed flap should be accurately measured and drawn out to ensure appropriate dimensions. The base of the triangular defect is continued radially to inscribe the flap margins. The defect itself is a segment of the inscribed arc.

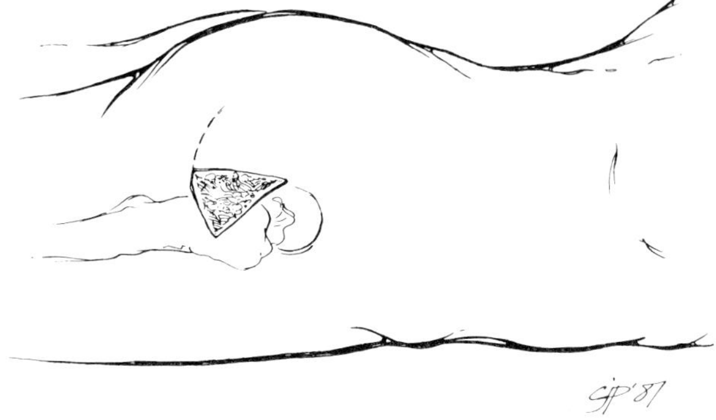

33a

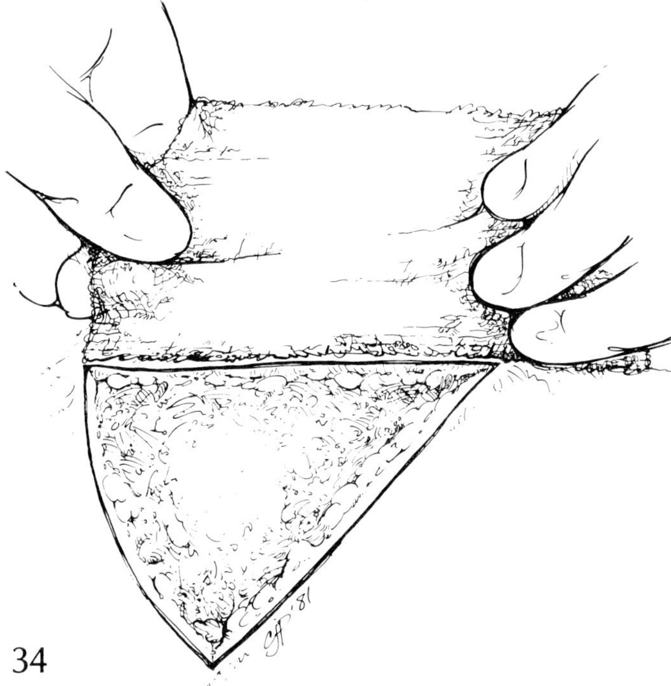

34

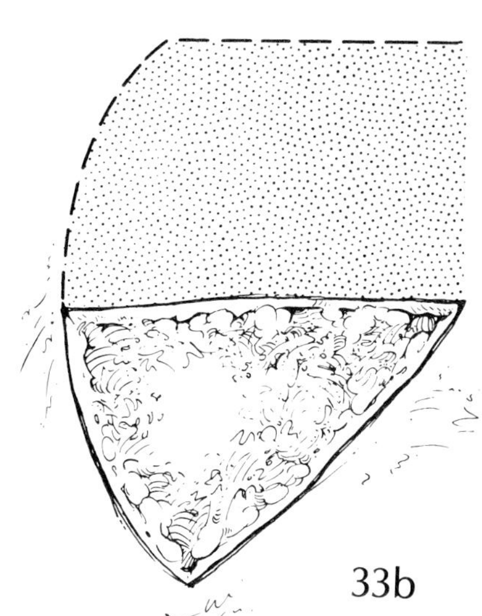

33b

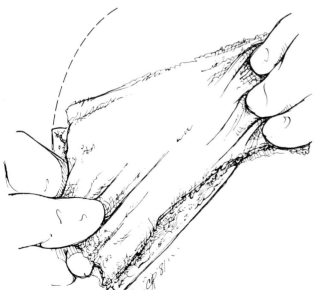

34 & 35

The flap's adequacy may be confirmed by using a mock-up of a strip of cloth with dimensions the same as those of the proposed flap, rotated over the defect as a trial. The flap's base must be sufficiently wide to provide adequate vascularity once the flap is developed.

35

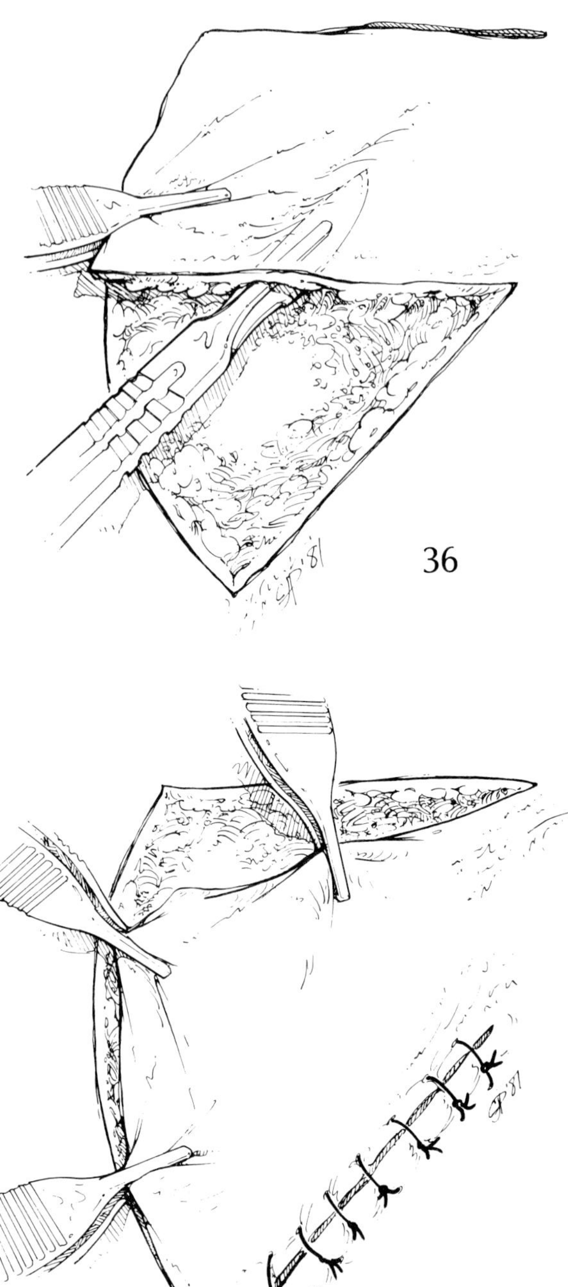

36

37

36 & 37

The flap is finally rotated over the primary defect and sutured into place by redistributing the tension. If excessive tension develops at the suture line, grafting may be necessary to close the secondary defect.

Proper planning and meticulous surgical technique can spell the difference between failure and success. Sound principles must never be bypassed for the sake of merely closing the wound. A flap with marginal vascularity under tension is doomed from the start.

Z-PLASTY

38

A Z-plasty involves transposition of two triangular skin flaps which functionally lengthen a wound while redistributing tension across it. Although a Z-plasty is usually employed as a secondary procedure to revise an unsightly scar or release a contracture across a natural skin crease, it may be used in the primary closure of certain wounds. By using a Z-plasty as a primary mode of wound care, a laceration is broken up into several components, many of which can be neatly camouflaged in natural skin creases. This technique is particularly useful in dealing with certain lacerations of the face or ones which traverse joint creases. Forethought in designing an appropriate Z-plasty can frequently ensure a pleasing cosmetic result while maintaining function.

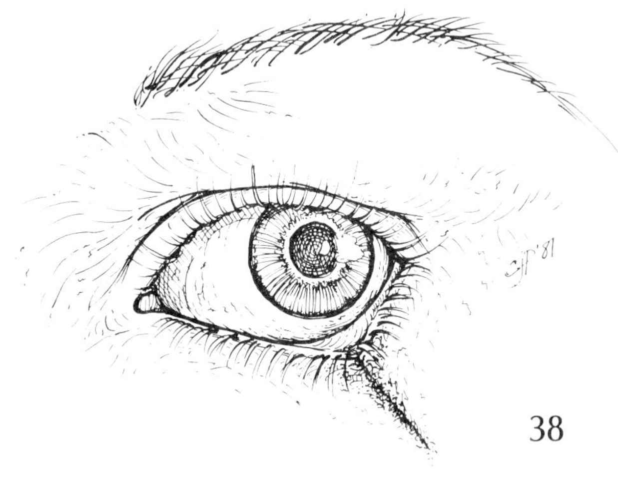

38

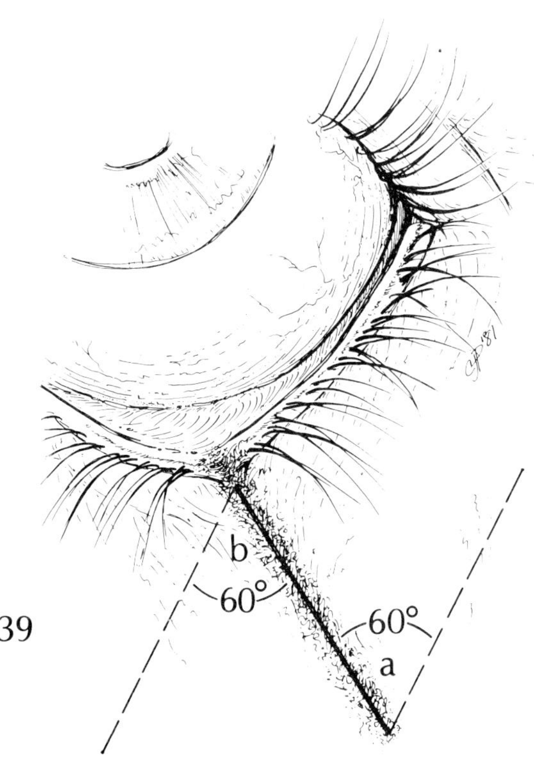

39

39

A Z-plasty is performed only after it has been carefully mapped out. The central aspect of the Z represents the primary laceration or the scar to be revised. The two limbs of the Z are parallel lines that intersect the central portion at a 60° angle. In constructing the Z, all segments should be of equal length to provide maximum wound lengthening.

40

After the procedure has been clearly thought out, the appropriate incisions are made and flaps developed.

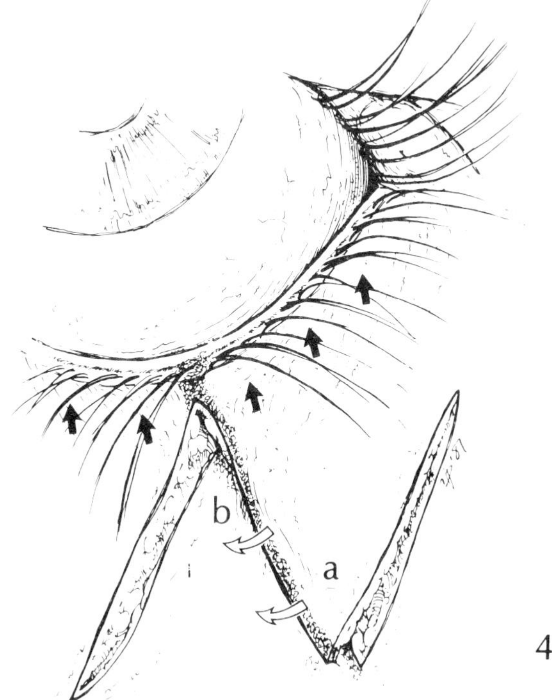

40

41 & 42

The two newly constructed triangular skin flaps are then transposed and sutured in place.

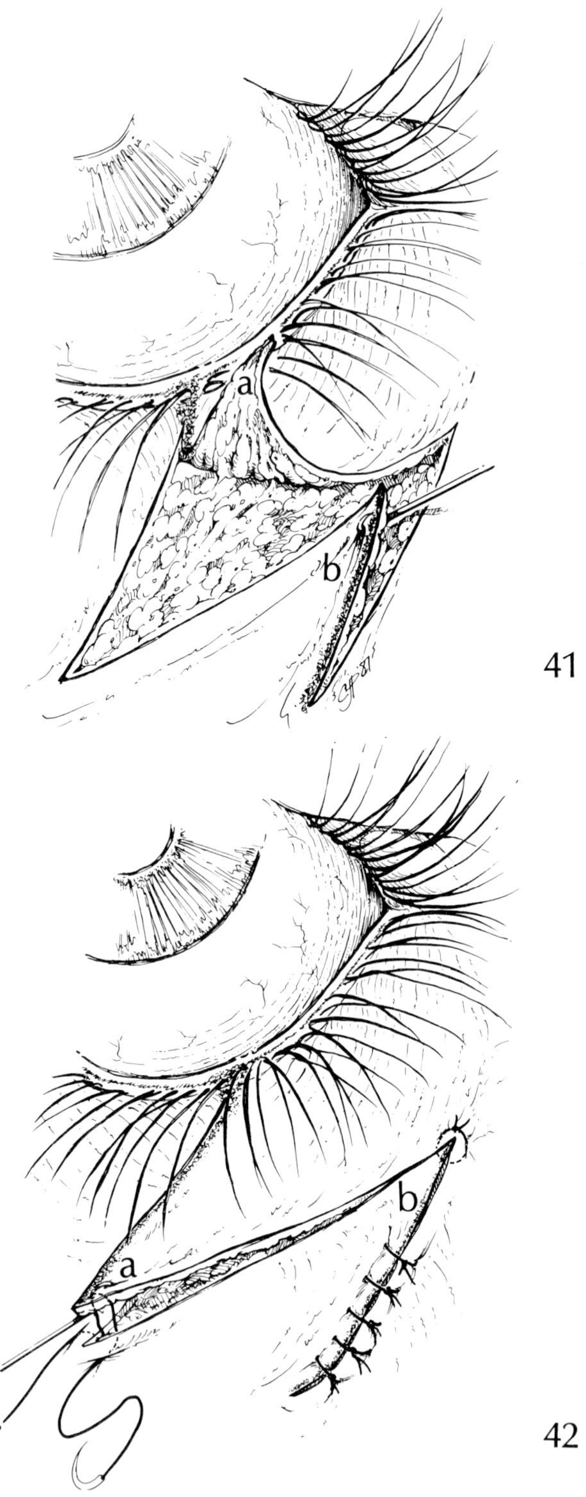

41

42

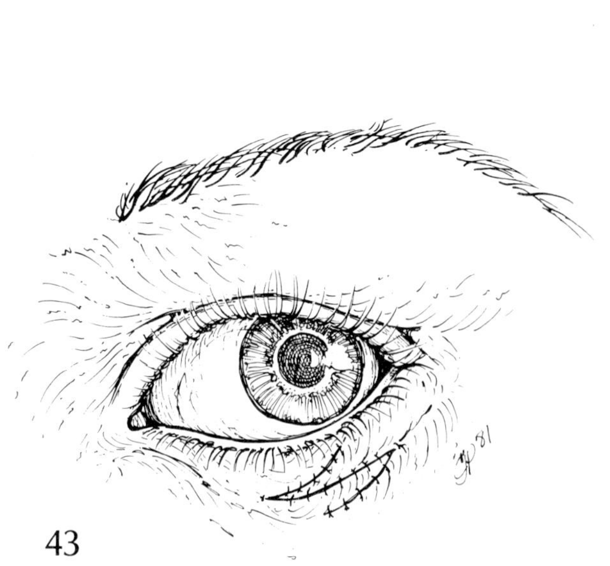

43

43

This series of manoeuvres creates a new Z, the central portion of which lies perpendicular to the original defect. Ischaemia and necrosis of wound margins, particularly of the tips of the skin flaps, represent potential complications, best avoided by meticulous surgical technique throughout.

Biopsy of specific tissues

R. C. G. Russell MS, FRCS
Consultant Surgeon, St John's Hospital for Diseases of the Skin and The Middlesex Hospital, London

Introduction

Biopsy of specific tissues is usually undertaken by the surgeon because a lump, whose nature is unknown, is present, or because a tissue diagnosis is required in a patient who is ill from a known or unknown cause. A biopsy cannot be performed without thoughts about a differential diagnosis because the tissue being removed for examination may not give the information sought, or the tissue being removed may not be the appropriate material for the group of conditions under consideration. In addition, it is important to be clear what examinations are required on the specimen to be removed and to have arranged these beforehand with due attention to the needs of the pathologist.

Many patients upon whom biopsies are required are unwell; careful consideration must therefore be given to the choice of anaesthesia – local, regional block or general anaesthesia. Because of the poor condition of many of these patients, it is useful to decide if further biopsies might be necessary to establish the diagnosis, and to carry these out, especially if they are uncomfortable (e.g. a bone marrow biopsy), under the same anaesthetic. It cannot be too strongly emphasized that these patients require a full assessment before the biopsy.

The cross-reference in this chapter refers to *Operative Surgery: General Principles, Breast and Extracranial Endocrines, 4th Edition*

Lymph node biopsy (see *also* chapter on 'Managing the surgical operative specimen,' pp. 70–76)

This procedure is performed to elucidate the cause of enlarged nodes, the extent of a disease process or to determine the nature of a general illness in which there may or may not be lymphadenopathy. The biopsy must not impede future surgical procedures, nor compromise the clearance of a cancer. Other methods of achieving the diagnosis should have been excluded, e.g. laryngoscopy for a laryngeal carcinoma with cervical node metastases. On occasion, the surgeon is presented with a patient who has multiple nodes: in this case, the biopsy should be taken away from the site of any infection, the axilla or neck being preferable to the groin, and a site where discrete nodes can be removed is chosen rather than a biopsy of a matted mass of lymphoid tissue. When the lymph nodes are only just enlarged, lymph nodes from several sites may have to be removed before a satisfactory diagnosis can be made; a firm node is usually a better prospect than a rubbery or diffuse node. At all times glands draining areas affected by an eczematous skin eruption should be avoided as these present particular histological difficulties. Whenever possible several nodes should be removed from the one site, and all nodes should be removed without damage to the capsule as this aids histological examination.

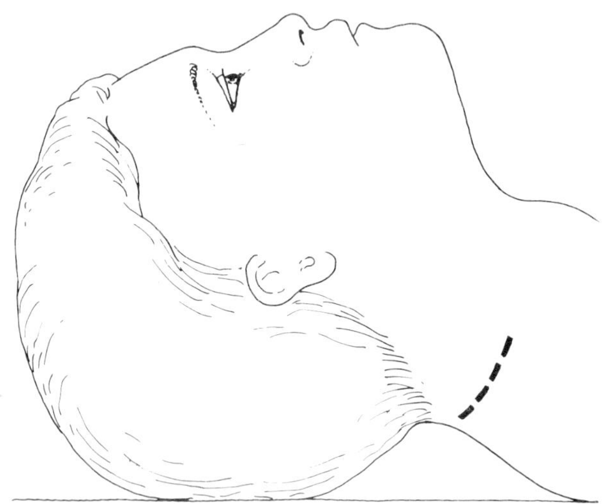

1

1

The incision

The line of incision should be planned to follow a suitable skin crease, which is usually apparent at sites where lymph nodes are commonly situated. To decrease bleeding, it is useful to inject adrenaline 1:200000 beneath the line of the planned incision and around the nodes which are about to be removed. The incision should be twice the length of the node which is to be excised or longer if it is deep in the axilla.

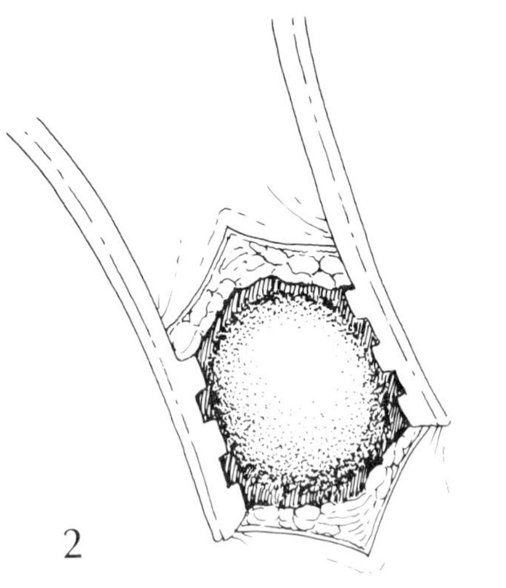

2

2

Exposure of node

The skin, fat and superficial fascia or platysma in the neck are divided to reveal a potential space in which the superficial nodes lie. A self-retaining retractor is inserted to hold back the deep fascia, so exposing the node or nodes.

3

Dissection of node

By blunt dissection the node can be exposed, leaving the vascular attachments intact. These vessels are now grasped with dissecting forceps and cauterized. By holding the vessel and surrounding fascia the lymph node can be enucleated without damage to the capsule. Haemostasis should proceed as the node is mobilized because haemorrhage obscures dissection and can be difficult to control once the node has been removed.

3

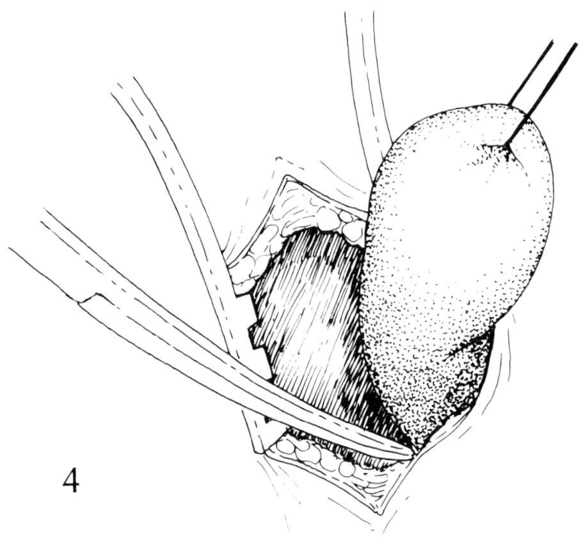
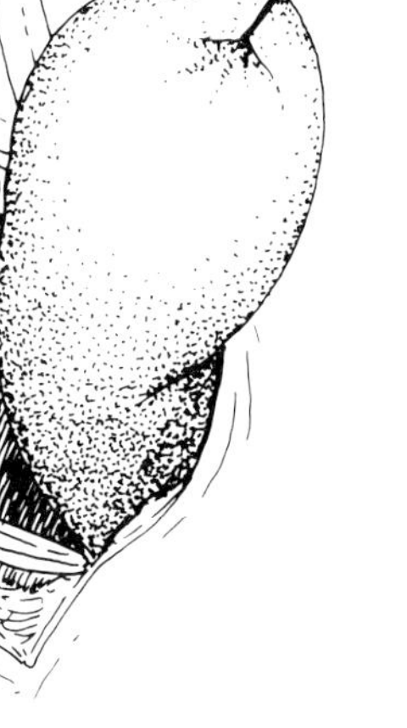

4

4

Exploration for further nodes

Once the main node has been removed the wound is explored for further nodes. Usually two or three adjacent lymph nodes can be enucleated through the same incision.

5

Closure of wound

The fascia is closed with interrupted sutures and the skin by a subcuticular polypropylene suture. The wound is supported by skin tapes. Drainage is unnecessary unless a large mass has been removed.

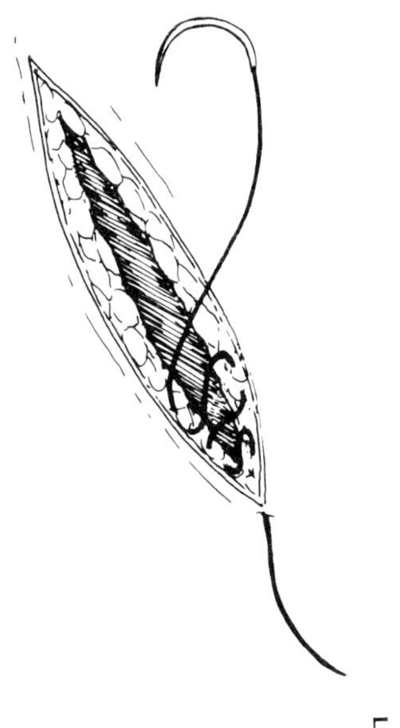

5

Biopsy of an artery

The commonest artery for biopsy is the temporal artery in order to confirm or refute the diagnosis of temporal arteritis. By definition the artery is prominent and easily palpable so that identification is not a problem. Local anaesthesia is quite adequate for this procedure.

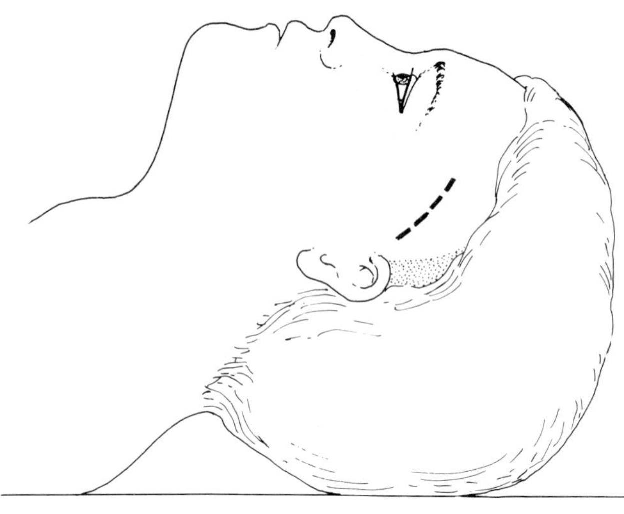

6

6

The incision

After preparation of the skin and before injection of local anaesthetic the line of the vessel is marked. If the affected vessel runs close to the hairline, then the incision can be hidden in the hairline, otherwise the skin crease nearest the line of the vessel is chosen.

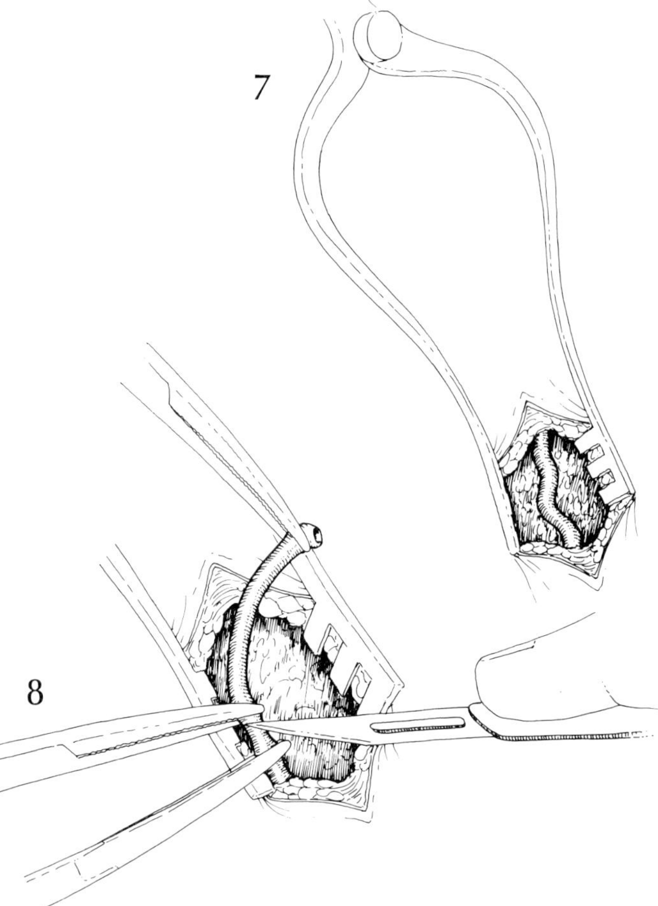

7

8

7 & 8

Dissection of artery

The incision is extended down to the temporal muscle on which the artery lies. A small self-retaining retractor is inserted. The vessel should be dissected out, starting proximally and avoiding handling the vessel. When the proximal end has been mobilized, two mosquito forceps are applied to the artery, which is divided. The proximal end is tied, while the distal end is mobilized for 2 cm before clamping and tying the distal end. Cautery should be avoided until the vessel is removed.

9

Closure

Two or three sutures are inserted in the fascia, and the skin is closed with a subcuticular polypropylene stitch, which is supported by skin tapes.

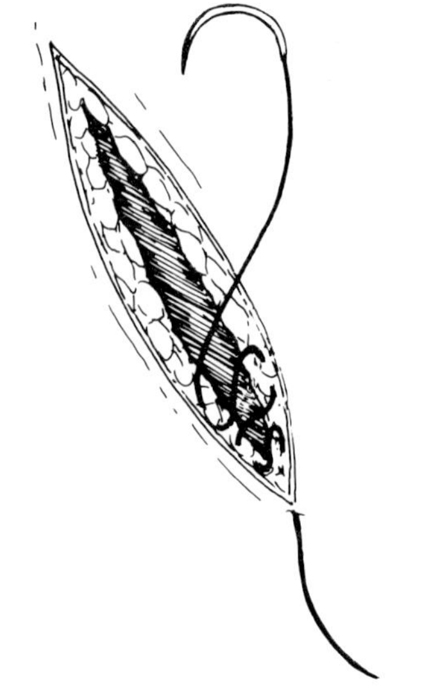

9

Muscle biopsy

The usual reason for a muscle biopsy is to confirm or refute the presence of dermatomyositis. A muscle affected early and commonly in this condition is the deltoid muscle. This muscle is suitable for biopsy under a local anaesthetic. The skin can be affected in dermatomyositis, and thus a skin biopsy should be performed at the same time.

10

The incision

After the injection of local anaesthetic beneath the skin and around the surface of the deltoid, a vertical elliptical incision is made and an ellipse of skin excised.

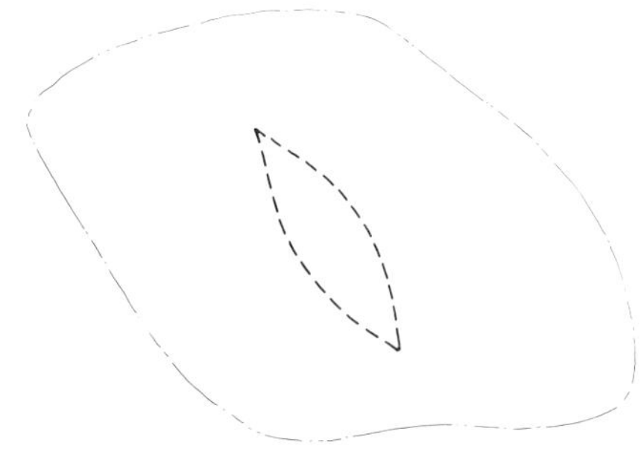

10

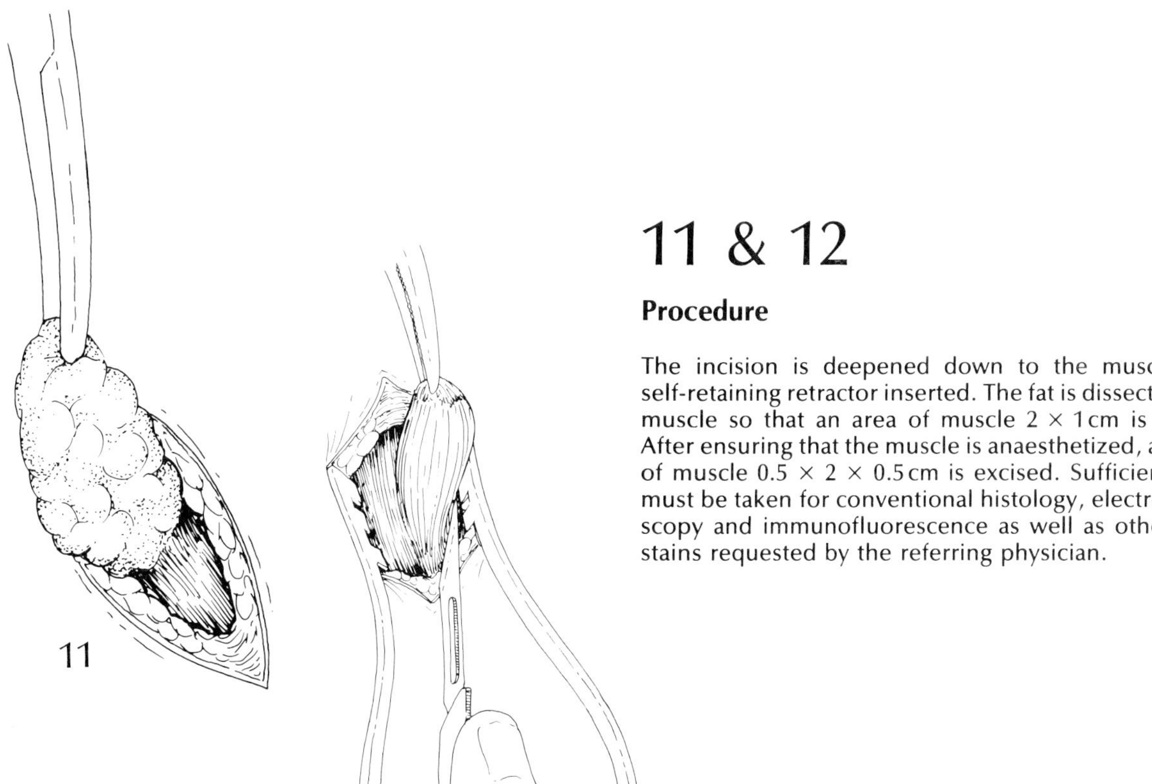

11

12

11 & 12

Procedure

The incision is deepened down to the muscle and a self-retaining retractor inserted. The fat is dissected off the muscle so that an area of muscle 2 × 1 cm is exposed. After ensuring that the muscle is anaesthetized, a segment of muscle 0.5 × 2 × 0.5 cm is excised. Sufficient muscle must be taken for conventional histology, electron microscopy and immunofluorescence as well as other special stains requested by the referring physician.

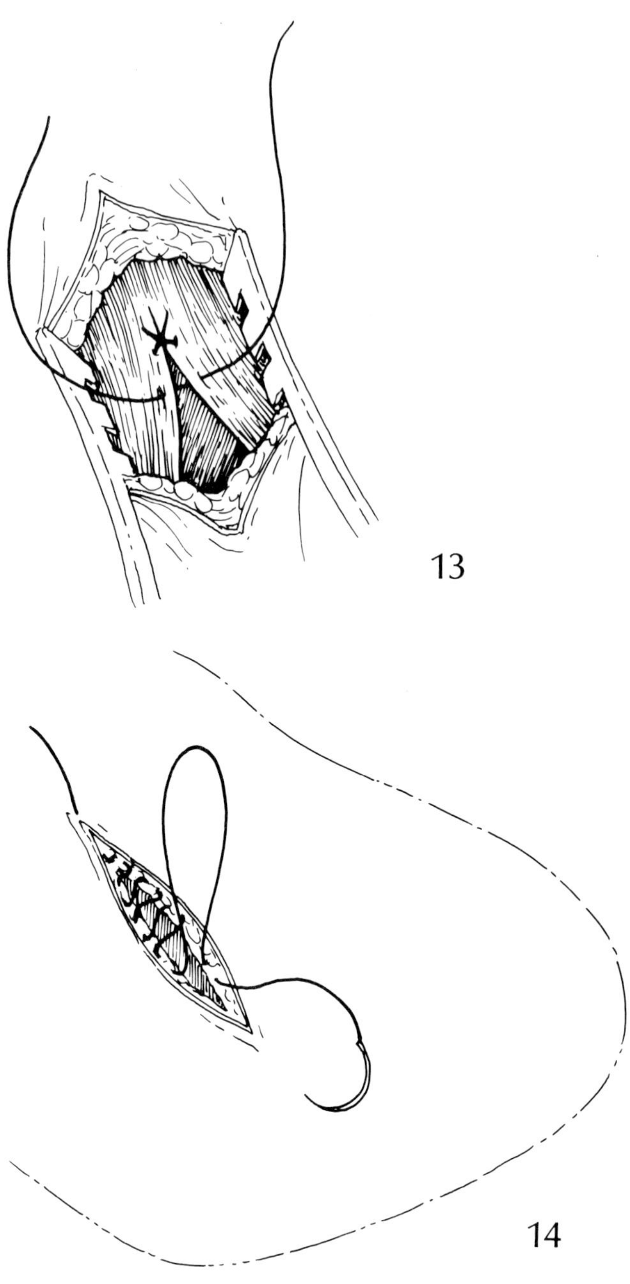

13 & 14

Closure

The muscle is closed with an interrupted suture, as is the fat. The skin is closed with a subcuticular polypropylene stitch and the wound is supported by skin tapes.

Nerve biopsy

A nerve biopsy is a rare request. Before undertaking such a biopsy the surgeon must be cognisant of the exact requirements of the physician, the type of nerve required and the techniques to be used for examination of the specimen. Once these criteria have been determined the selected nerve segment can usually be removed quite satisfactorily under a local anaesthetic. Care must be taken during the dissection not to handle the nerve, and cautery near the nerve should be avoided.

Postoperative care

No special care is required following these procedures. The main complication to be encountered is infection. The sutures should not be removed early as many patients requiring biopsies are ill, and the wounds may heal less well than usual.

Surgical access in pulmonary operations

Peter Goldstraw FRCS, FRCS(Ed)
Consultant Thoracic Surgeon, Brompton Hospital, Middlesex Hospital and University College Hospital, London, UK

Introduction

A wide spectrum of surgical pathology may affect the lungs and other organs of the chest. With a sound knowledge of anatomy and an appreciation of the exposure required the surgeon may tailor the site and extent of his incision. There is, therefore, no 'standard' thoracotomy incision. Commonly used incisions include the following.

Choice of incision

The lateral thoracotomy incision is shown in detail in *Illustrations 10–21*. The patient lies in the lateral position and the incision passes between two ribs, dividing all the attachments of one rib to the other. Depending on individual preference the patient may be inclined backwards and the incision carried further anteriorly (the anterolateral approach) or placed in the prone position and the incision carried more posteriorly (the posterolateral approach). In either event the incision between the ribs is total and access is gained by the bucket-handle movement of the ribs above separating from those below. There is little justification now for the removal of the rib, particularly in children where such a manoeuvre encourages the later development of scoliosis.

The lateral thoracotomy incision provides excellent exposure of the whole of the ipsilateral lung and its hilum, the mediastinum and diaphragm. In the left chest this incision exposes the lower oesophagus and descending aorta, while on the right access is given to the whole of the intrathoracic oesophagus.

Median sternotomy has been greatly popularized by cardiac surgeons. It may be used to resect anterior mediastinal tumours and affords access to both pleural spaces, permitting bilateral pleurectomy or limited procedures on the lungs to remove bilateral bullae or metastases. A limited upper sternotomy is adequate for thymectomy and gives access to the trachea as far inferiorly as the carina. As an extension to a cervical incision this approach is occasionally necessary for the removal of a large retrosternal goitre.

The cross-references in this chapter refer to *Operative Surgery: Alimentary Tract and Abdominal Wall, Volume 2, 4th Edition*

MEDIAN STERNOTOMY

1

The patient is positioned supine, with a sandbag placed transversely beneath the shoulders to elevate the manubrium and hence render the sternum horizontal. A vertical skin incision is made from the suprasternal notch to the tip of the xiphoid.

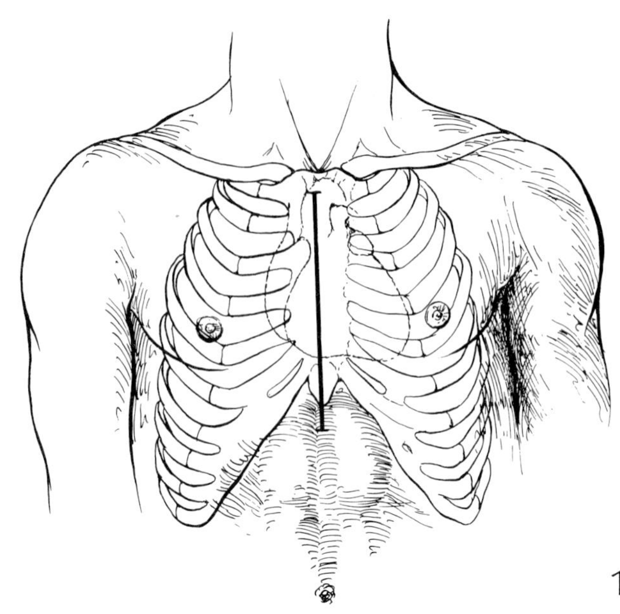

1

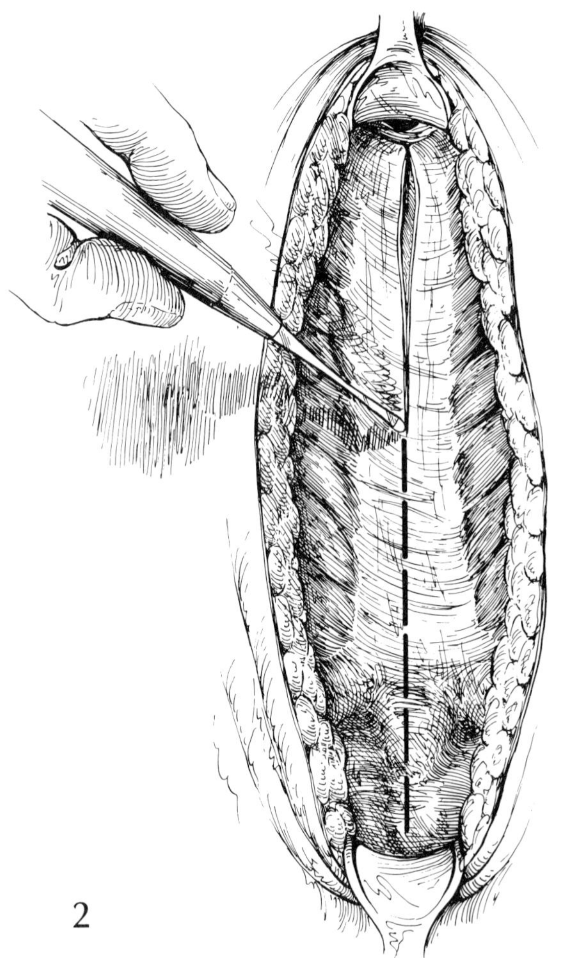

2

2

Diathermy is used to make a vertical incision in the periosteum of the sternum, taking care to remain in the midline. The transverse suprasternal ligament is divided and a finger insinuated into the superior mediastinum. At the lower margins of the incision the xiphoid process is divided vertically and a finger may then be insinuated into the retrosternal space. This finger may then strip the pleura to each side.

3

Using a vertical sternotome the sternum is divided longitudinally. If the anaesthetist allows the lungs to deflate during this manoeuvre, there is less chance that the pleura will be opened inadvertently.

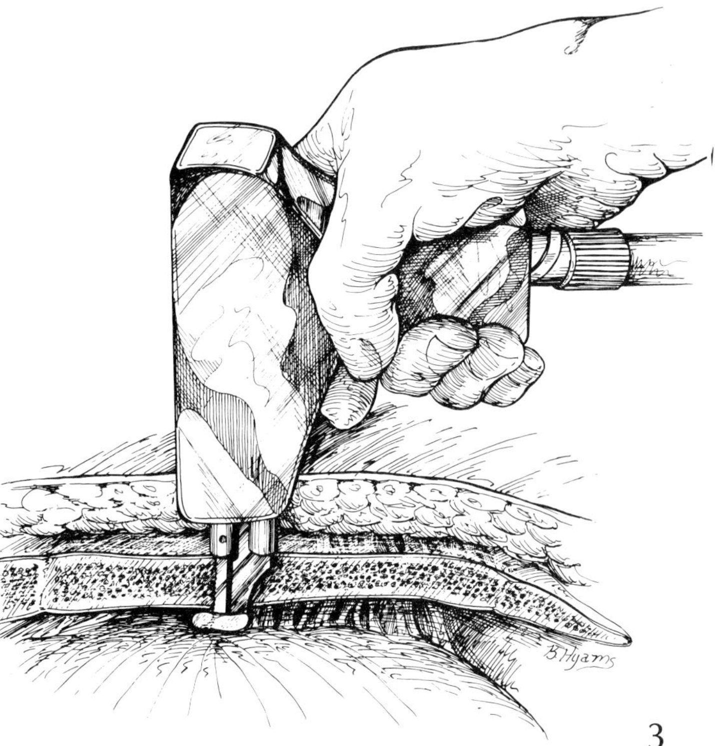

3

4

4

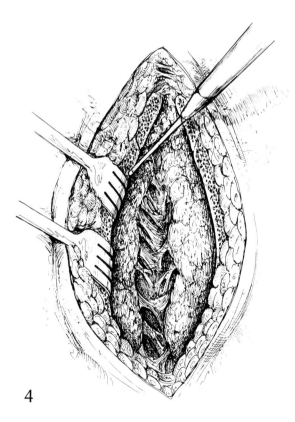

The sternal margins are elevated using retractors. Diathermy is used to control bleeding from the periosteal surfaces. Any bleeding from the cancellous bone may be controlled with small quantities of bone wax. This procedure is then repeated by the assistant for the opposite sternal margin. A parallel-sided, geared retractor can then be inserted to spread the sternal edges.

Closure

The sternal margins should be firmly approximated using interrupted wire sutures. The pectoralis muscles are approximated in the midline and skin closed.

The cosmetic appearance of this operation may be considerably improved if a transverse submammary skin incision is utilized. This approach has been popularized by Professor A. G. Brom of Leiden. It requires considerably more dissection to elevate the skin flaps to the sternal notch, but access is unhindered.

COMBINED THORACOLAPAROTOMY

Thoracic incisions may be continued into the abdomen, and this may be necessary to resect residual tumour in the lungs, mediastinum or abdomen.

The median sternotomy extended as a midline laparotomy allows limited access to both lungs and pleural spaces and the lymph node chain along the abdominal aorta and pelvic brim.

5 & 6

The left thoracolaparotomy incision, along the eighth or ninth rib, crosses the costal margin, divides the diaphragm circumferentially and may then pass obliquely to the linea alba or extend as a paramedian laparotomy. This incision gives good access to the lower oesophagus, stomach and spleen and in addition is used to resect tumour deposits in the left lung, mediastinum and abdomen. It affords good access to the nodes behind the crura of the diaphragm – a common site for lymph node metastases ascending from the abdomen and testes.

The right thoracolaparotomy incision mirrors that on the left. The liver is dislocated laterally with the hepatic veins. We have used this incision to resect residual tumour deposits in the right lung, main carinal nodes, liver and para-aortic chain.

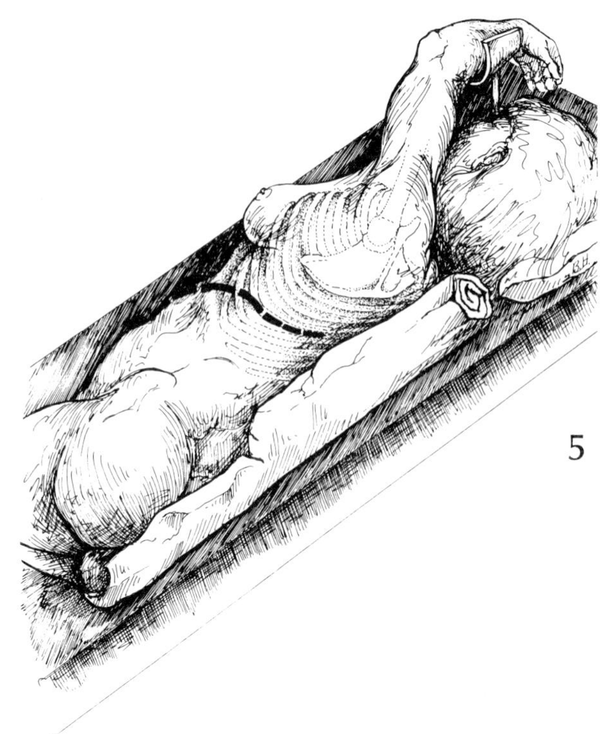

5

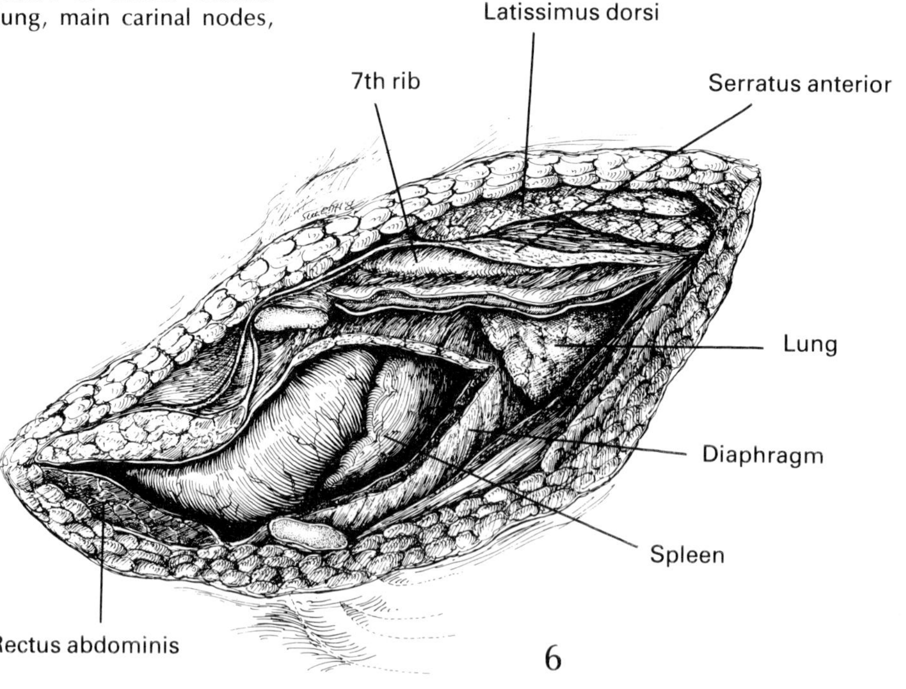

6

7 & 8

TRANSVERSE BILATERAL THORACOTOMY

This incision, once popular for cardiac operations, is now rarely used. It entails division of the serratus anterior and pectoralis muscles on each side, entering the pleural spaces through the fifth or sixth interspace, and completing the incision by transverse division of the sternum with sacrifice of both internal mammary arteries. It is a painful incision but allows more extensive exposure of the lungs, particularly the posterior aspect of the lower lobes.

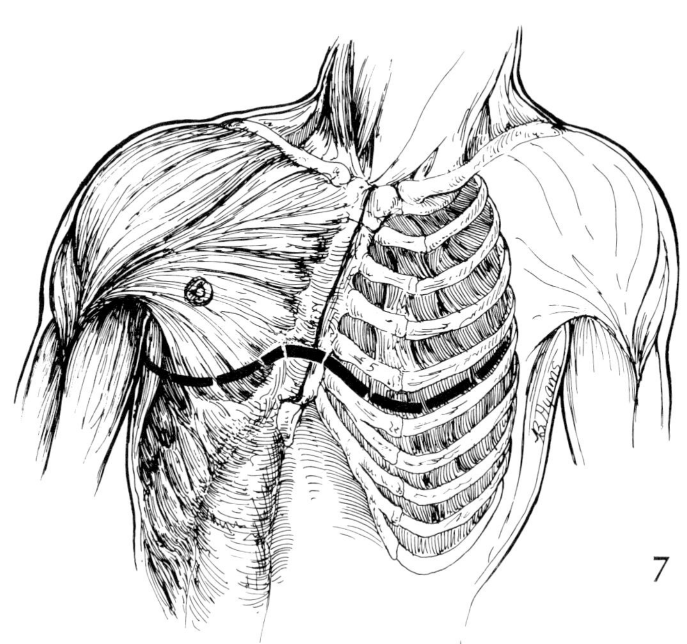

7

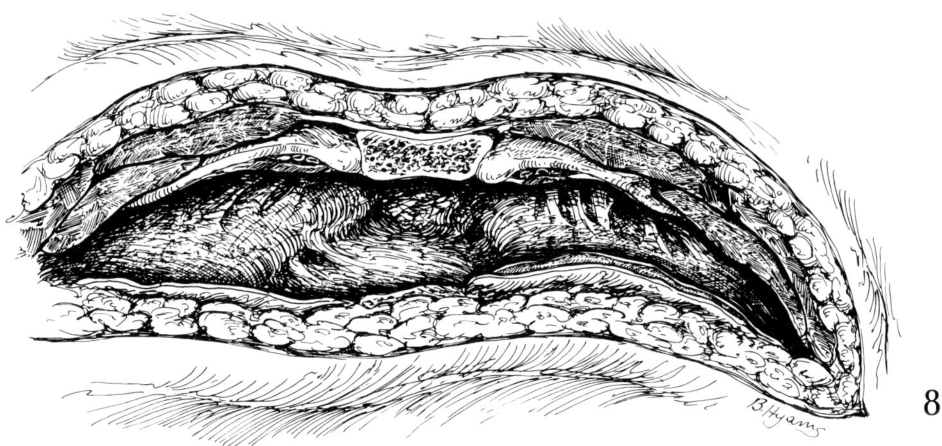

8

LIMITED INCISIONS

Short transverse intercostal incisions may be made anteriorly through the second interspace to biopsy anterior mediastinal masses. On the left this anterior mediastinotomy is a valuable staging procedure when assessing upper lobe tumours. Similar limited incisions anteriorly through the fifth interspace allow biopsy of the lung and pleura, and on the left also permit biopsy and fenestration of the pericardium.

Preoperative

Preoperative preparation

Intensive physiotherapy of a high order is essential following any operation on the lungs. All patients will therefore benefit from a short period in which to practise the manoeuvres their physiotherapists will be utilizing after surgery. Those patients producing large volumes of sputum can be considerably improved but will require several days of intensive physiotherapy aided by antibiotics and antispasmodics as appropriate. The length of preoperative preparation required depends not only upon the extent of the proposed resection but also upon the severity of the underlying lung disease. Those patients with severe chronic conditions producing large volumes of sputum may require prolonged treatment to create the optimum conditions even if only minor surgery is proposed.

In most hospitals the operative site is shaved the day before surgery. This allows time for the superficial abrasions to become colonized by bacteria and may predispose to wound sepsis. Depilatory creams are expensive and can cause irritation. We have found the best compromise to be shaving of the operative field in theatre after the induction of anaesthesia.

Anaesthesia

9a–d

After the induction of anaesthesia, bronchoscopy is recommended as a final check on the situation and to permit bronchial toilet. It will often provide useful information for the anaesthetist, aiding the positioning of the double-lumen tube. A double-lumen endobronchial tube greatly facilitates exposure within the chest, and avoids conflict between anaesthetist and surgeon. Correct positioning of a Robertshaw tube is shown in (*a*) and (*d*), while (*b*) and (*c*) show some common malpositions.

It will be appreciated that the right-sided tube is the more difficult to position, and hence its use is reserved for operations requiring division of the left bronchial tree. For all other operations a left-sided tube (*d*) is to be preferred irrespective of the side of the thoracotomy. An improperly positioned double-lumen tube does not protect the contralateral lung and may hamper exposure. The surgeon must thus be prepared to accept an endotracheal tube if his anaesthetist cannot confidently position the endobronchial tube. After intubation, monitoring lines and intravenous drips are inserted as necessary. For most major resections a peripheral drip and central venous catheter are desirable.

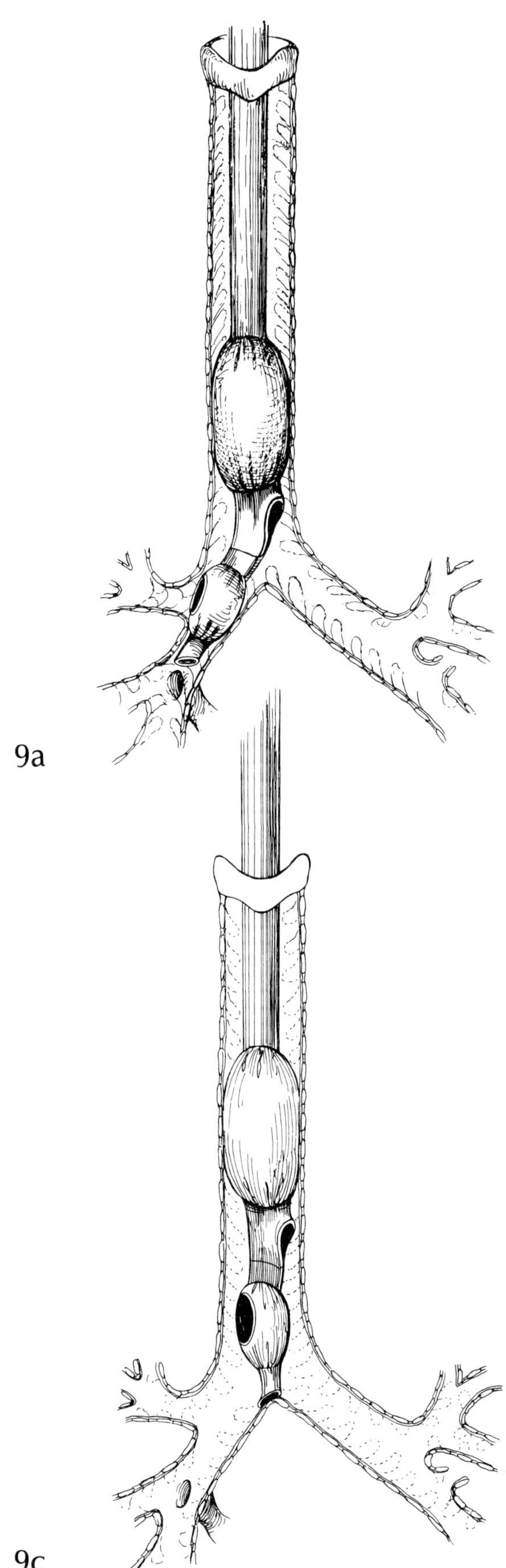

9a

9c

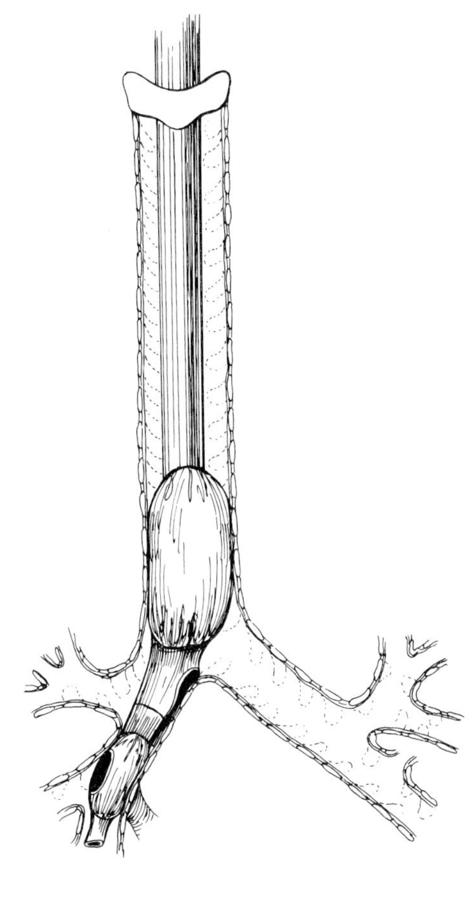

9b

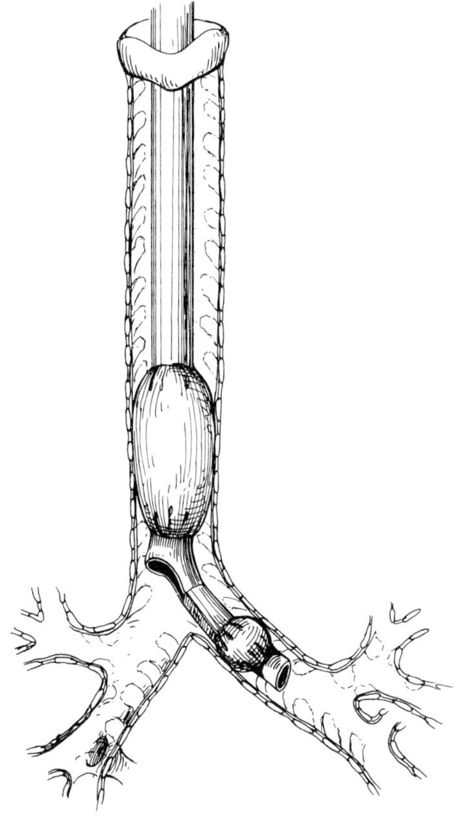

9d

Lateral thoracotomy

10

Position of patient

The patient is secured in the full lateral position. This may be achieved with a pillow and sandbags, but is facilitated by a support bag containing small polystyrene beads which becomes a firm mould when air is evacuated. The bottom leg is flexed and the uppermost knee supported on a pillow. The upper arm rests on a support.

It is at this stage that we undertake shaving of the operative site. The skin is then prepared with an alcohol-based antiseptic containing iodine or chlorhexidine. Care should be taken not to spill excessive spirit over the patient and diathermy plate. Conventional draping with sheets and a transparent adhesive incise drape is adequate. We prefer to spray the operative field and surrounding area with an adhesive aerosol, and to use a single large sheet of 150 gauge transparent polythene. This forms the incise drape and dispenses with the need for additional sheets. The diathermy quiver and sucker are held in place using thin adhesive strips. This simple method has the advantage of giving clear vision of all drips, catheters and anaesthetic tubes and is far cheaper than commercially available incise drapes.

The skin incision commences 3 cm beneath the nipple and extends in a gentle arc 2 cm below the angle of the scapula, to end midway between the spinous processes and the posterior border of the scapula. In the female the position of the breast must be noted and the mobile position of the nipple is misleading. The incision is inevitably made lower and is best started lateral to the breast.

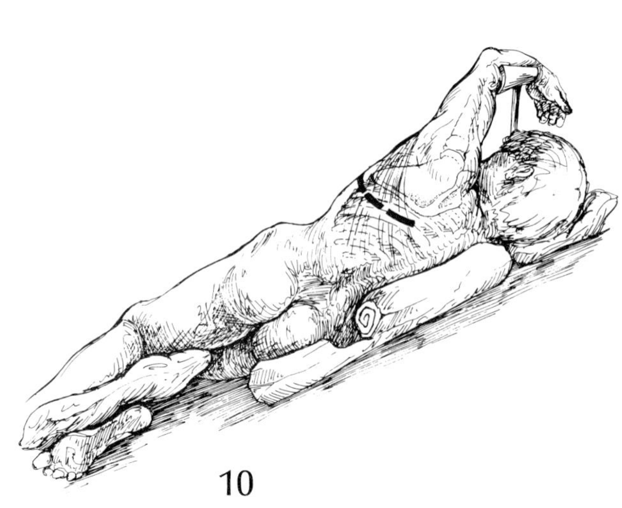

10

11

The incision is carried deeper using the diathermy spatula. Lattisimus dorsi is transected towards the lower margin of the incision since the lower segment is inevitably denervated. The fascia posterior to serratus anterior continues as a firm sheet onto the posterior border of the scapula. The incision through this fascia is carried inferiorly along the posterior edge of serratus anterior. This muscle is then divided towards the lower part of the incision from its posterior margin anteriorly until the belly arising from the desired rib is encountered. The ribs are counted from above, the highest palpable rib being the second. The first rib is obscured by scalenus posterior except over a short segment near the vertebrae.

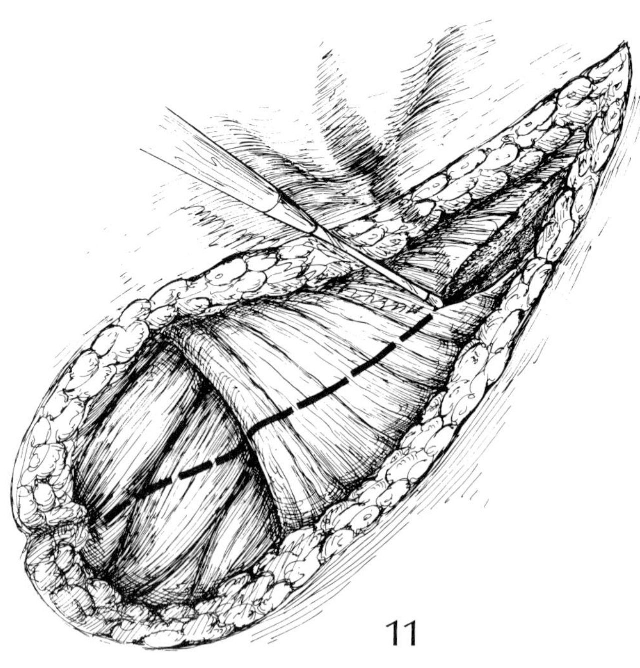

11

12

An incision through the bed of the fifth or sixth rib will give access to the pulmonary hilum; the fifth rib is used for upper lobectomy, the sixth for lower and middle lobectomy, and either may be used for pneumonectomy.

The belly of serratus anterior arising from the chosen rib is cut from the upper border of the rib and the diathermy is used to score the lateral aspect of the periosteum, extending posteriorly until the border of the erector spinae is encountered and notched.

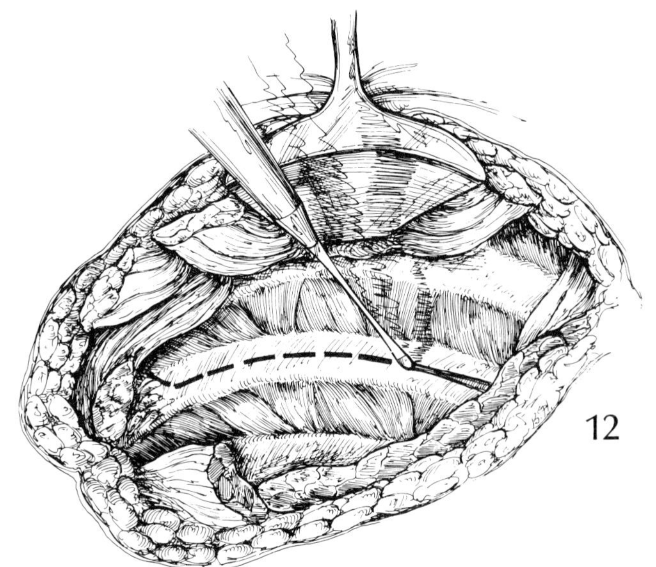

12

13

The edge of a raspatory is inserted into this notch and drawn along the upper surface of the rib. For this first stroke the handle of the raspatory is kept flat against the chest wall and the blade lifts the periosteum from the rib. A second stroke in the same direction, keeping the handle of the raspatory vertical, exposes the parietal pleura. The inferior border of the rib is then exposed at the posterior angle.

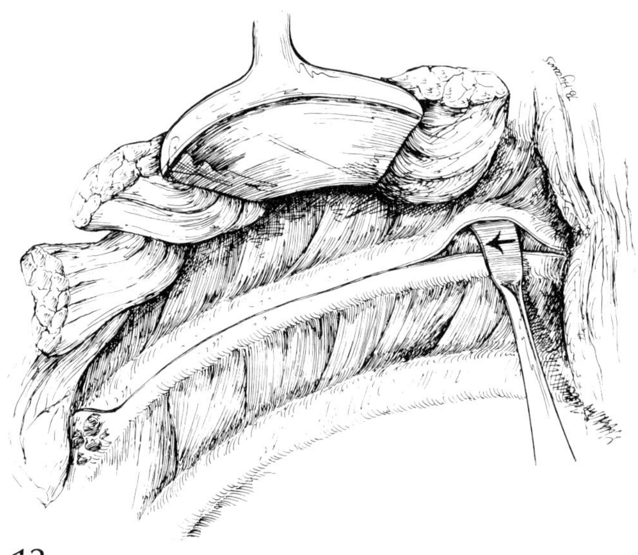

13

14

Using a costotome 1 cm of the posterior angle of the rib may be excised. This manoeuvre adds little to the exposure, but decreases tension on the posterior attachments of the rib, reducing the frequency of severe post-thoracotomy pain.

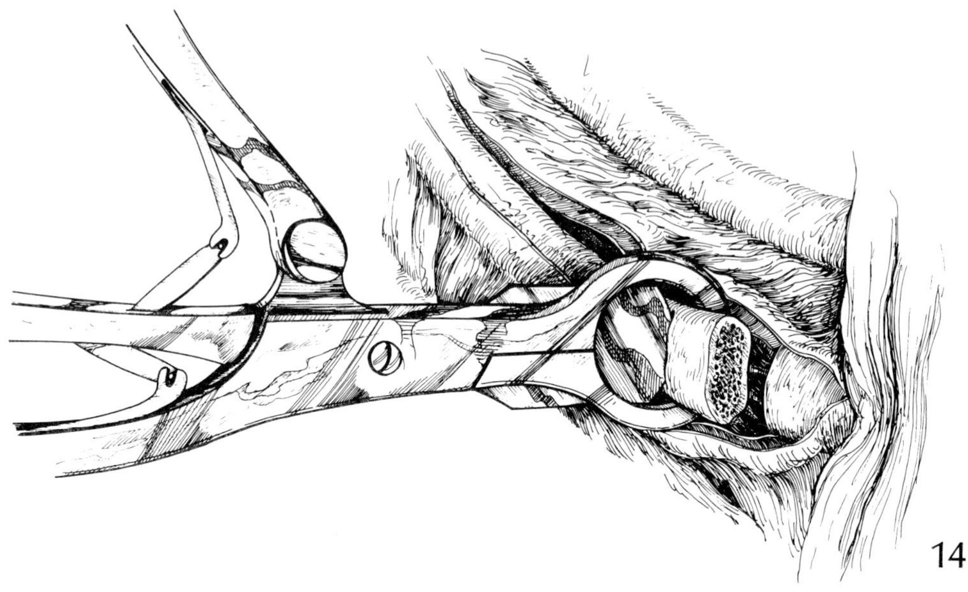

14

15

The pleura is incised where adhesions are least likely.

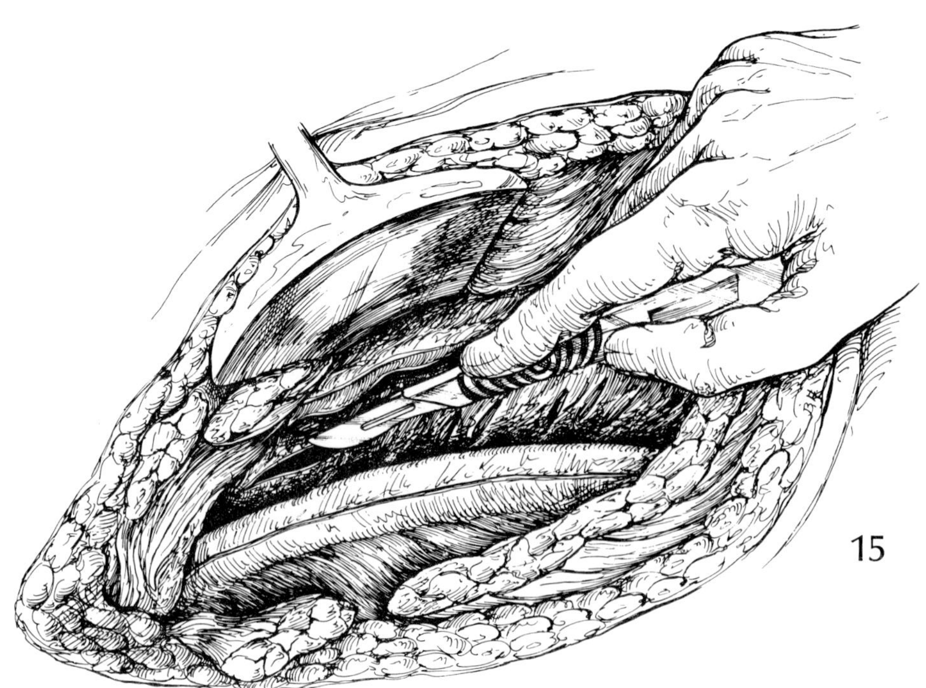

15

16

If the pleural space is free the pleura is split the length of the incision and two Price-Thomas retractors inserted. It is often helpful to have a deeper blade on the upper arm of each retractor to allow for the extra depth imposed by the scapula. Progressive steady retraction will then provide adequate exposure for the majority of intra-thoracic procedures. A headlight is a great asset in the dark recesses of the thoracic cavity.

17

If adhesions are encountered a Tudor-Edwards retractor is used to gently separate the rib margins and a Roberts forcep is used to evert the pleura. Sharp dissection is then undertaken to clear a sufficient area to allow safe introduction of the Price-Thomas retractors.

Should the tumour involve the pleura over the incision or dense inflammatory adhesions make access difficult an extrapleural mobilization aids access. This is a bloody plane and the pleural space should be re-entered once free of the troublesome area.

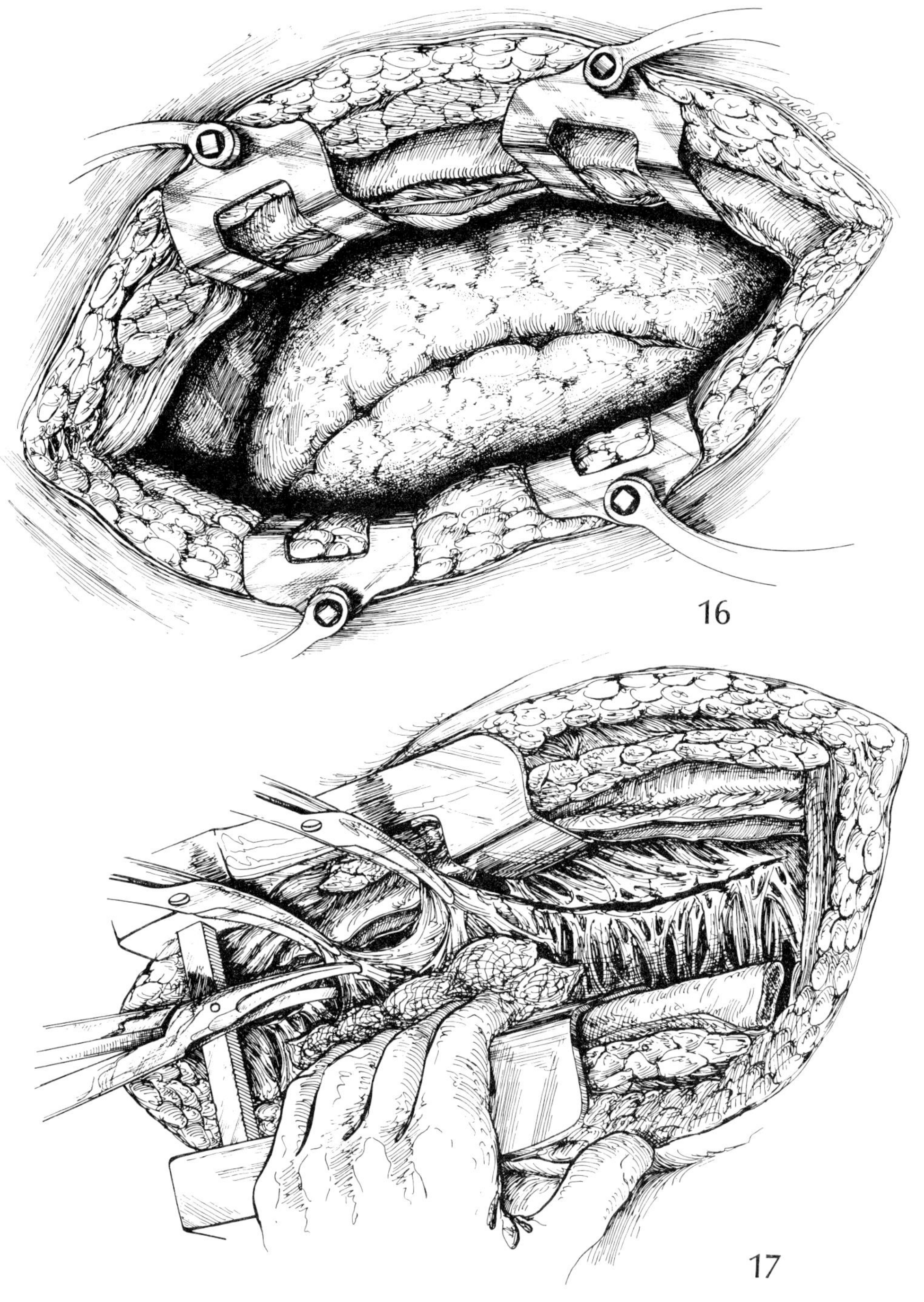

16

17

18

If it is necessary to resect a portion of chest wall over the upper lobe the incision can be extended posteriorly and superiorly midway between spinous processes and the posterior border of the scapula to the vertebra prominens.

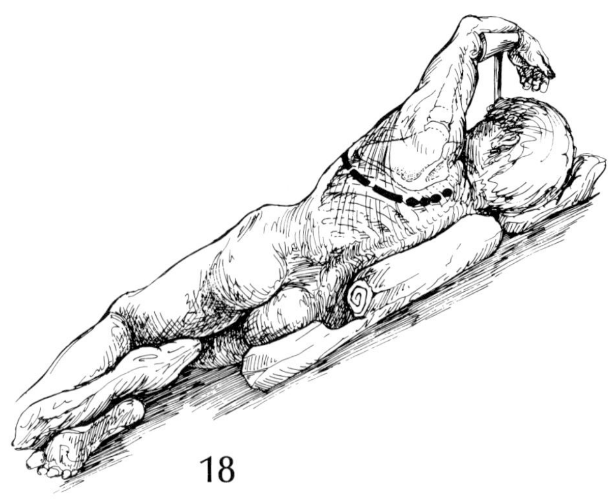

18

19

The underlying muscles – trapezius, the rhomboids and serratus posterior superior – are divided near their origins from the spine through their aponeuroses. This extension allows forward displacement of the scapula and gives access to the first rib. It may be necessary to divide the costal components of serratus anterior and scalenus posterior to expose the second, third and fourth ribs anteriorly.

19

To mobilize and deliver a large bulky tumour it may be necessary to divide one or two ribs above, below, or both above and below the incision. One centimetre of each rib is excised from the posterior angle to prevent painful clicking of the ribs postoperatively. The intervening intercostal bundles may have to be divided and both ends of the vessels transfixed.

20

If particular difficulty is encountered mobilizing over the apex or in the costodiaphragmatic recess a second thoracotomy may be performed utilizing the existing incision through skin and muscle. The muscles are retracted to expose a rib two or three places away from the original incision and the pleural space is entered as before.

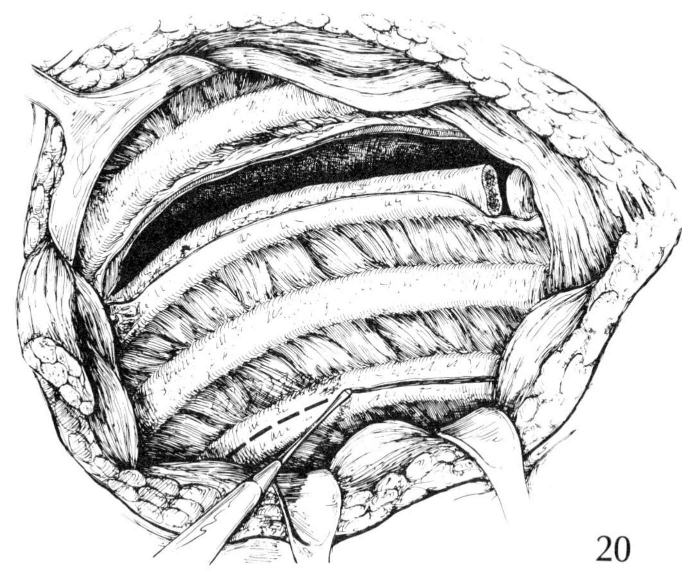

20

Chest drainage

After pneumonectomy a drain is unnecessary unless bleeding is expected. If a drain is omitted then air should be aspirated from the pneumonectomy space after chest closure, when the patient is supine and extubated. Aspiration continues until the mediastinum is drawn to the operative side, allowing optimum expansion of the remaining lung. Mediastinal shift is assessed by tracheal displacement and the slight negative pressure necessary on aspiration. If excessive mediastinal shift is induced venous inflow may be hindered with a rise in jugular venous pressure and a fall in cardiac output. It is preferable to err on the side of caution and to be prepared to aspirate the pneumonectomy space again in the ward once a chest X-ray is available. Nursing staff must be warned that in the absence of a drain greater vigilance is necessary to detect unexpected bleeding into the pneumonectomy space (*see* chapter on 'Resection of the lung', pp. 149–177.

For most intrathoracic procedures a single chest drain is inserted through a low stab incision. A stiff plastic catheter with a radiopaque line is preferable, and if a further basal hole is cut in the radiopaque line this catheter will function as an apical and a basal drain. If air leak is anticipated, as after lobectomy, two such drains are positioned, one anteriorly and one posteriorly, each connected to a separate underwater seal bottle.

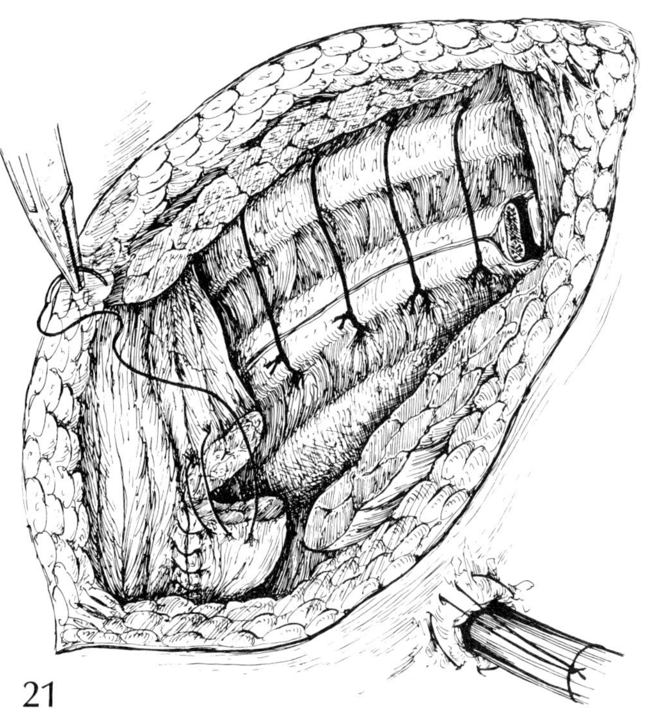

21

21

Closure

The ribs are approximated using five or six sutures, passing above the upper rib and below the lower one. These pericostal sutures should be of a strong braided material capable of sliding knots. Then progressive tightening of these sutures will draw the ribs together without the need for a brutal rib approximator. The sutures are tightened and the knots completed, taking care to lay the knots square to prevent later slackening.

Gentle pressure by the anaesthetist upon the shoulder then slides the scapula into its anatomical position and the muscles are sutured in layers using continuous absorbable sutures such as polyglycolic acid polymers. A continuous subcutaneous and subcuticular suture of similar material completes the closure giving a pleasant cosmetic result.

At the termination of the anaesthetic, a suction bronchoscopy is valuable where excessive sputum was present prior to surgery, especially in patients with limited pulmonary reserve. This must be skilled and expeditious.

Postoperative care

Drainage

Negative pressure applied to the drainage bottles will speed expansion of the remaining lung, tamponading any air or blood leak and promoting rapid obliteration of the pleural space. Suction of 15–20 mmHg may be delivered by a pump or wall suction capable of dealing with a large volume air leak and with suitable safety controls to prevent excessive vacuum. A large volume displacement pump such as the Vernon-Thompson or Clements pump is suitable, but the Roberts pump is obstructive if air leak is vigorous. Suction should never be applied to the chest drain in the pneumonectomy space.

Pain relief

Adequate pain relief is essential if the patient is to cooperate with the physiotherapist and yet any respiratory depression must be avoided. The use of the cryoprobe is gaining popularity but requires special equipment and expertise. An intravenous infusion of pethidine has proved safe, reliable and most effective in practice. Pethidine 2 mg/kg body weight is inserted into 100 ml of 5 per cent dextrose and 10–20 ml/hour are infused via a control mechanism such as an Ivac pump. The rate of infusion is varied by the nursing staff to provide satisfactory pain relief, but to leave the patient alert and cooperative. The rate may be increased temporarily just before and during physiotherapy.

Complications

Sputum retention

This is the commonest problem after pulmonary resection and if not recognized and treated quickly leads to retention pneumonia, hypoxaemia and the need for mechanical ventilation. The problem should be anticipated when extensive resections are performed on patients with limited pulmonary reserve, especially if additional predisposing factors such as chest wall resection or resection of the phrenic or recurrent laryngeal nerves have been necessary. Management consists of vigorous physiotherapy with adequate analgesia, but unless this succeeds rapidly suction bronchoscopy is advisable. Tracheostomy should be performed if the problem recurs or is expected to recur. Broad-spectrum antibiotics are useful but are of secondary importance.

Arrhythmias

Supraventricular tachycardias, most commonly atrial fibrillation, may occur at any time after thoracotomy, but most commonly occur 2–5 days after surgery. Such a complication is more prevalent after complicated operations, especially if the pericardium has been opened; it may also occur during a postoperative recovery complicated by sputum retention. Such a complication is often anticipated and the patient digitalized prophylactically.

Additional complications such as haemothorax or bronchopleural fistula are now rare and should be treated by reoperation (*see* chapter on 'Bronchopleural fistula after pneumonectomy and lobectomy, pp. 204–209). Dehiscence of the thoracotomy wound has not occurred in our practice using this method of closure.

Surgical access to the heart and great vessels

Terence A. H. English, MB, BSc, MA, FRCS
Consultant Cardiothoracic Surgeon, Papworth and Addenbrooke's Hospitals, Cambridge, UK

Introduction

Satisfactory exposure of the operative field is the key to accurate anatomical dissection and safe surgical repair. Provision of optimum exposure is dependent on correct positioning of the patient on the operating table and on making the most appropriate incision for the operation to be performed.

Positioning the patient on the operating table

After induction of anaesthesia it is the responsibility of the surgeon to ensure that the patient is positioned correctly on the operating table. Different operations demand different routes of surgical access but the general principles relating to patient positioning are common to all situations and include the following:

1. All pressure areas, including the vertex of the head, must be adequately protected.
2. No metallic parts of the operating table, or its fixtures, should be in direct contact with the patient.
3. Electrical leads and catheters should not be kinked, nor allowed to cross under pressure areas.
4. The patient should be properly earthed. This is especially important in cardiac surgical patients who are often connected to a variety of electrical apparatus.
5. Unless a midline incision is used, the patient should be placed towards the edge of the operating table nearest the surgeon.
6. The patient's position must be stable on the table, thereby allowing the table to be rotated through its longitudinal or transverse axis if necessary. Such stability is achieved by a combination of pelvic and arm supports, supplemented by firm broad strapping.

The cross-reference in this chapter refers to *Operative Surgery: Cardiac Surgery, 4th Edition*

Median sternotomy

Indications

This is the standard incision for most open intracardiac operations and is an excellent incision. It can be made rapidly through a relatively bloodless field and gives good exposure to all aspects of the heart. The aorta and right atrium are readily accessible so that, in an emergency, arterial and venous cannulation for bypass can be accomplished with the minimum of delay.

The incision is simple to make and close and, providing the divided edges of the sternum are securely approximated, it is relatively painless and heals well.

1

Position of patient and preparation

The patient is placed supine on the operating table, and after induction of anaesthesia ECG electrodes are applied, an electrocautery pad is placed beneath the buttocks and a urinary catheter is inserted and attached to a plastic measuring bag suspended from the operating table.

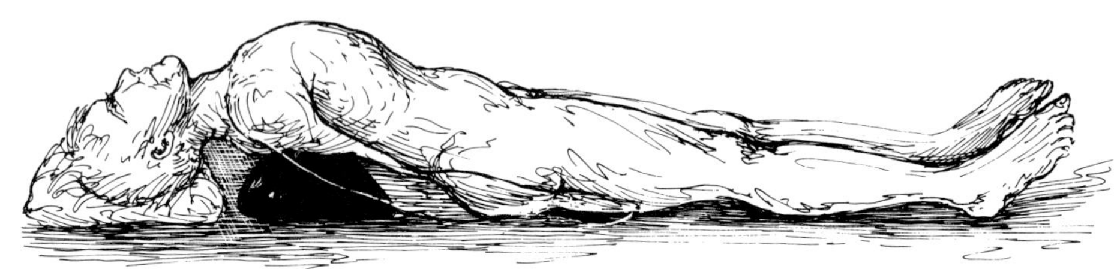

1

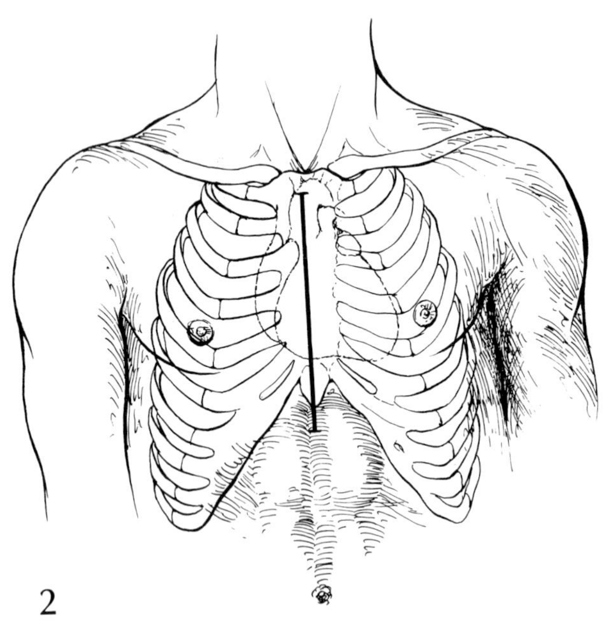

2

2

Incision

After preparation of the skin and the application of sterile drapes, a vertical skin incision is made from 2 cm below the suprasternal notch to 4 cm below the xiphisternum (Figure 1). It is important to divide the sternum precisely in the midline and this is facilitated by identifying the attachment of the linea alba to the xiphisternum below and the middle of the suprasternal notch above.

3

These two points are then joined by an electrocautery incision which is carried down to the sternal periosteum and acts as a marker for subsequent division of the sternum by the saw.

After gentle finger dissection deep to the upper manubrium between the two sternal heads of the sternomastoid muscle the suprasternal ligament is divided by electrocautery. Inferiorly the linea alba is incised throughout the length of the skin incision, taking care to preserve the underlying peritoneum, after which the xiphisternum is divided by scissors. A transverse vein running superficial to the sternoxiphisternal junction usually requires coagulation.

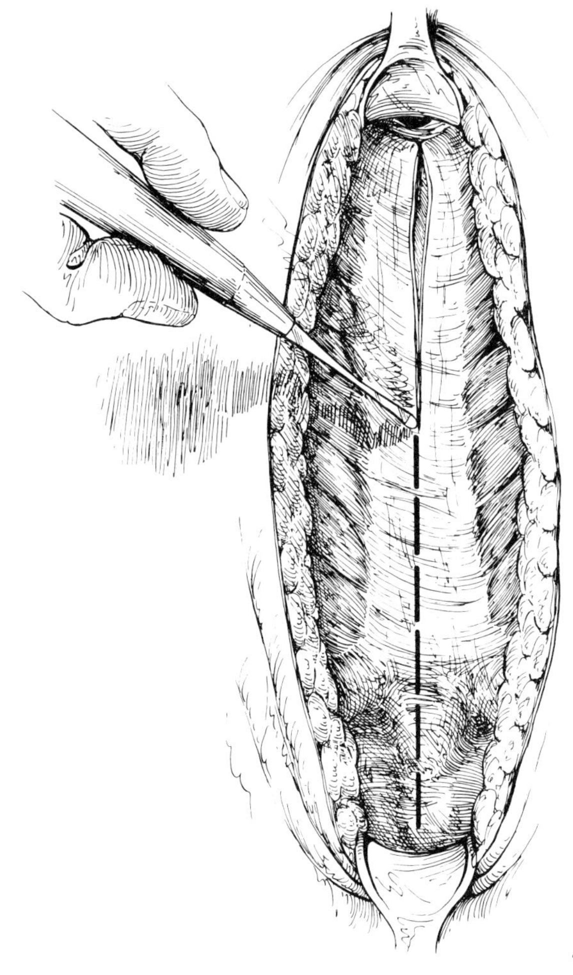

3

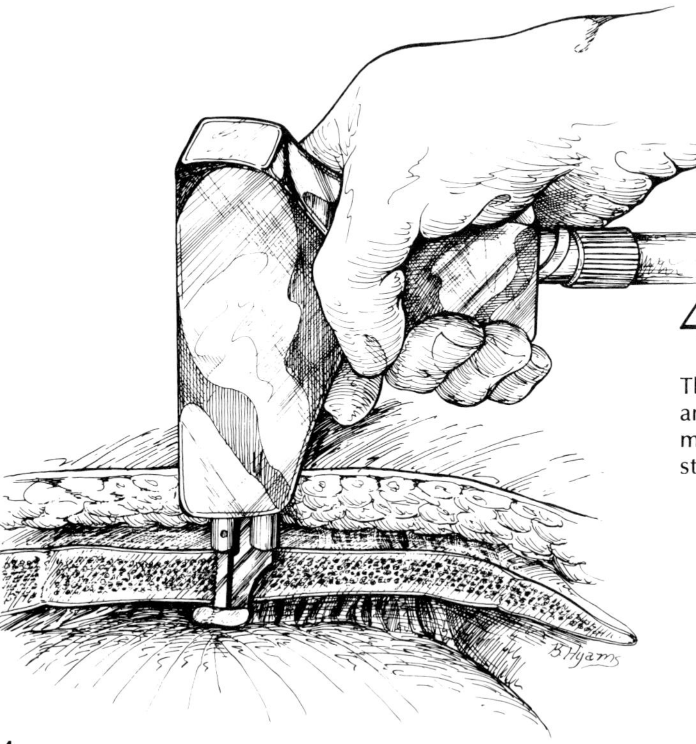

4

4

The sternum and manubrium are then divided cleanly with an oscillating saw. Various types of saws are available, the most suitable of which include a guard to protect structures deep to the sternum from damage.

5

The sternal edges are individually retracted and the periosteum cauterized on both sides from below upwards as far as the manubriosternal joint. A small retractor (Tuffier) is then inserted below and the suprasternal ligament divided with scissors. This allows haemostasis to be effected for the upper part of the incision; small amounts of bone wax are applied where necessary.

6

The left innominate vein is identified in the mediastinal fat in the upper part of the incision. This allows accurate definition of the thymus gland, or its remnant, which is separated into its two lobes. If an additional central venous line is required, the innominate vein may be cannulated via a small purse-string suture at this stage and the catheter advanced into the superior vena cava. One of the pleural reflections, usually the right, often extends across the midline and, if so, it is gently mobilized off the pericardium by a combination of blunt and sharp dissection.

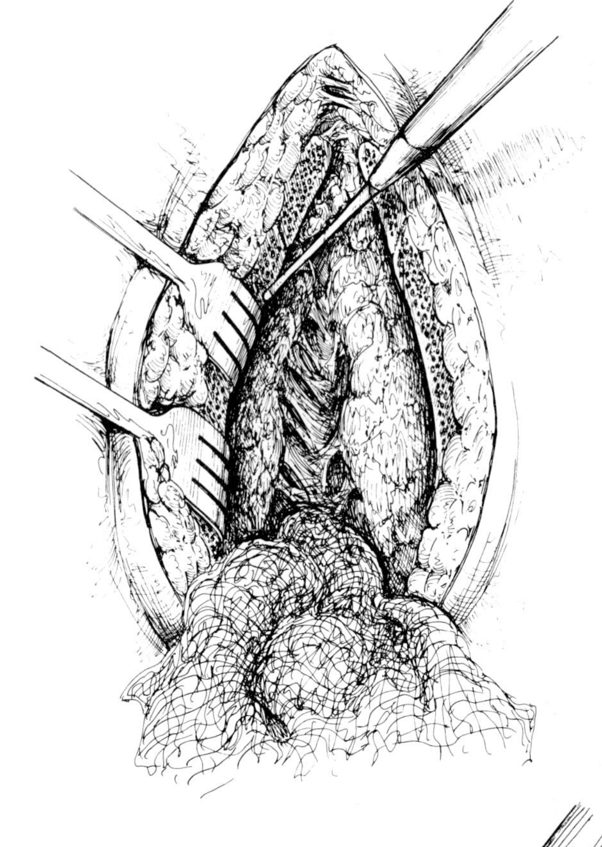

5

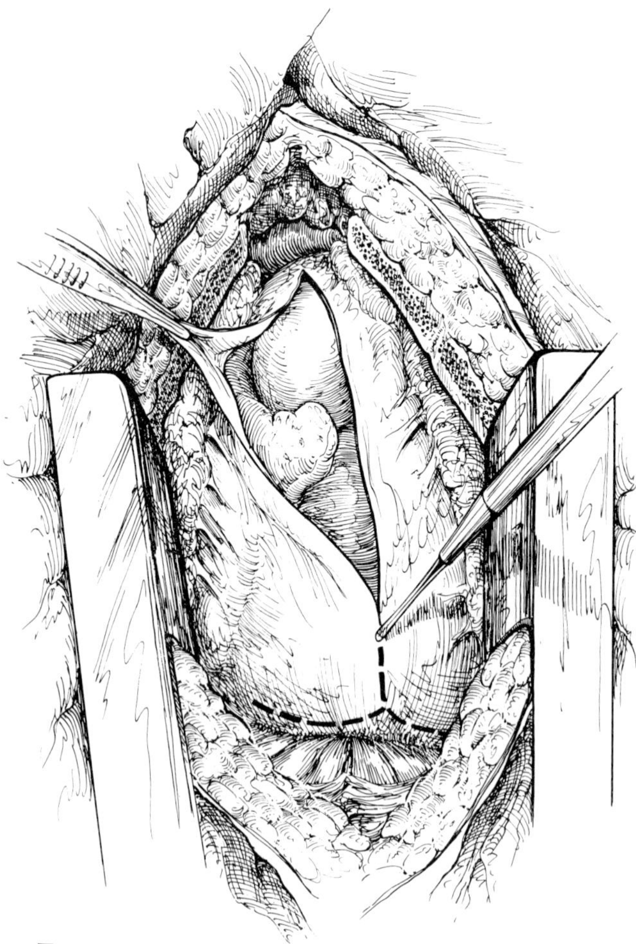

7

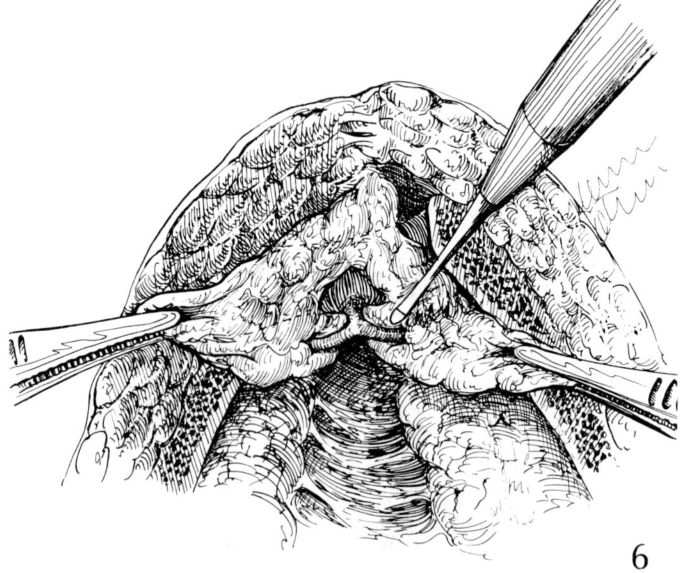

6

7

The pericardium is now exposed throughout its length and is divided by a gentle curved incision slightly to the left of the midline. The upper part of this incision extends as far as the pericardial reflection on to the aorta. The small retractor is removed and, after wound towels have been placed over the divided margins of the sternum, a large sternal retractor is introduced.

8

Increased mobilization is gained in the lower part of the wound by incising the pericardium laterally at its reflection with the diaphragm. The retractor may now be opened to the desired extent and the incision completed by suturing the upper cut edges of the pericardium to the wound towels.

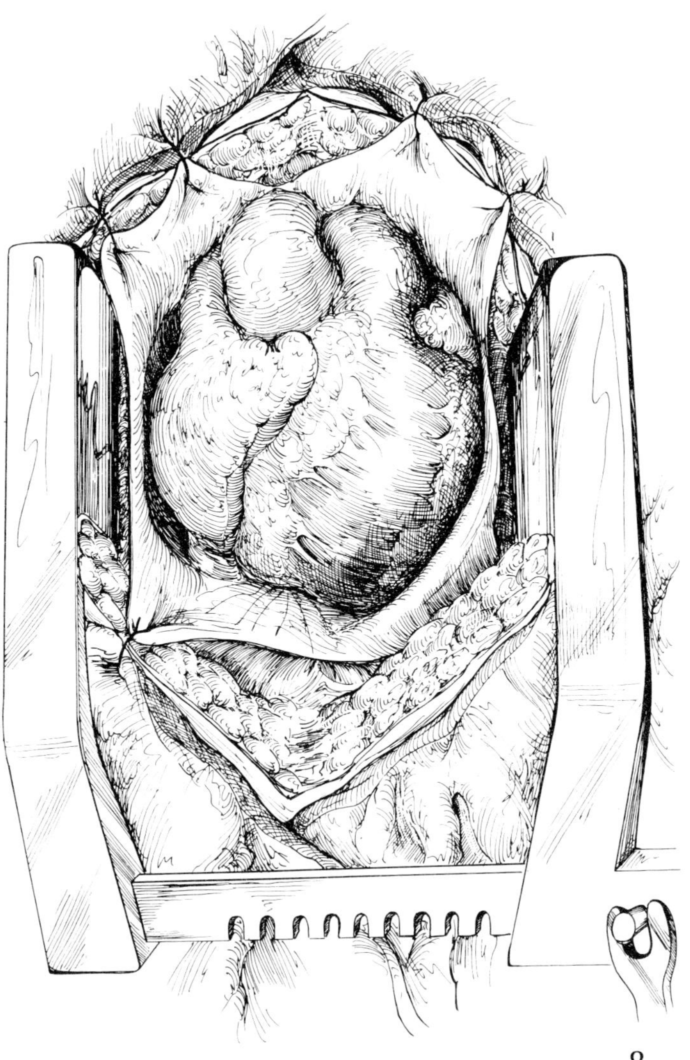

8

9

The heart having been exposed, preparations for cardiopulmonary bypass are completed by passing tapes around the aorta and, where relevant, both venae cavae. If the haemodynamic state is unstable, the latter is deferred until bypass has been commenced. A fine Teflon catheter may now be placed in the left atrium via the right superior pulmonary vein for pressure monitoring, and diagnostic pressures can be measured in the relevant cardiac chambers and great vessels. Further management, including heparinization and cannulation of the heart, is described in the chapter on 'Cardiopulmonary bypass and circulatory support', pp. 51–64.

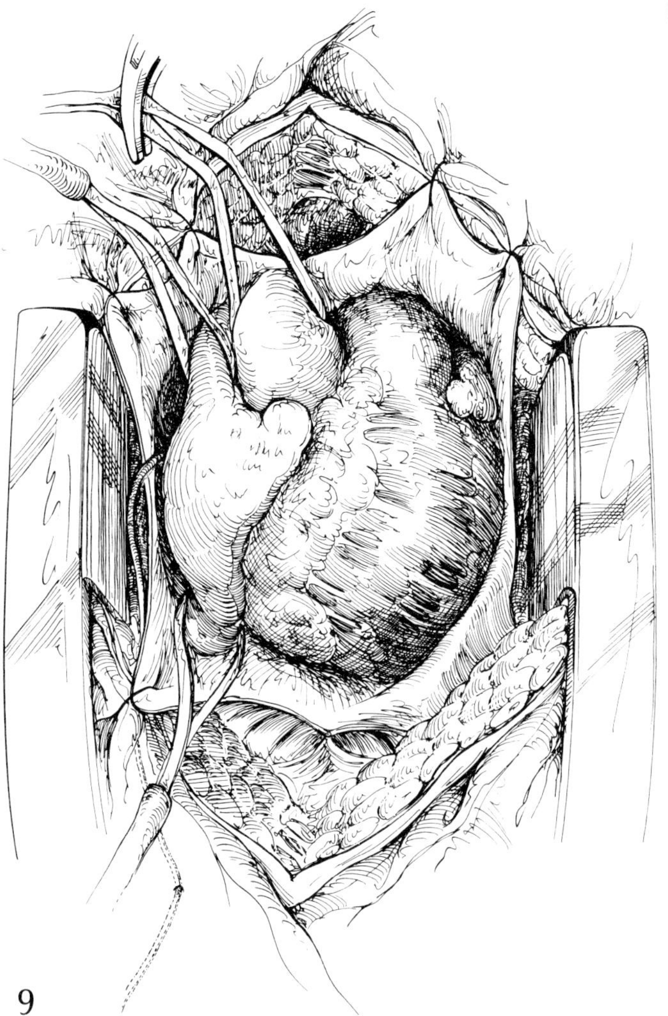

9

10, 11 & 12

Closure of a median sternotomy incision is performed with interrupted wire sutures placed through the sternum. It is probably unnecessary to close the pericardium. Two drains are usually inserted.

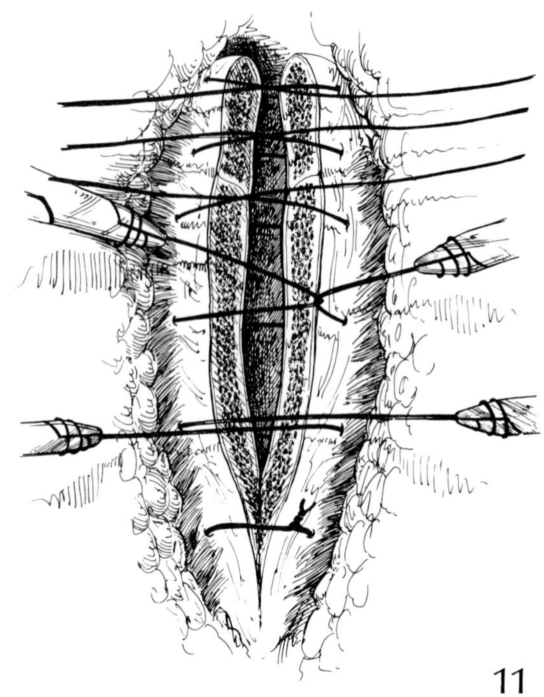

11

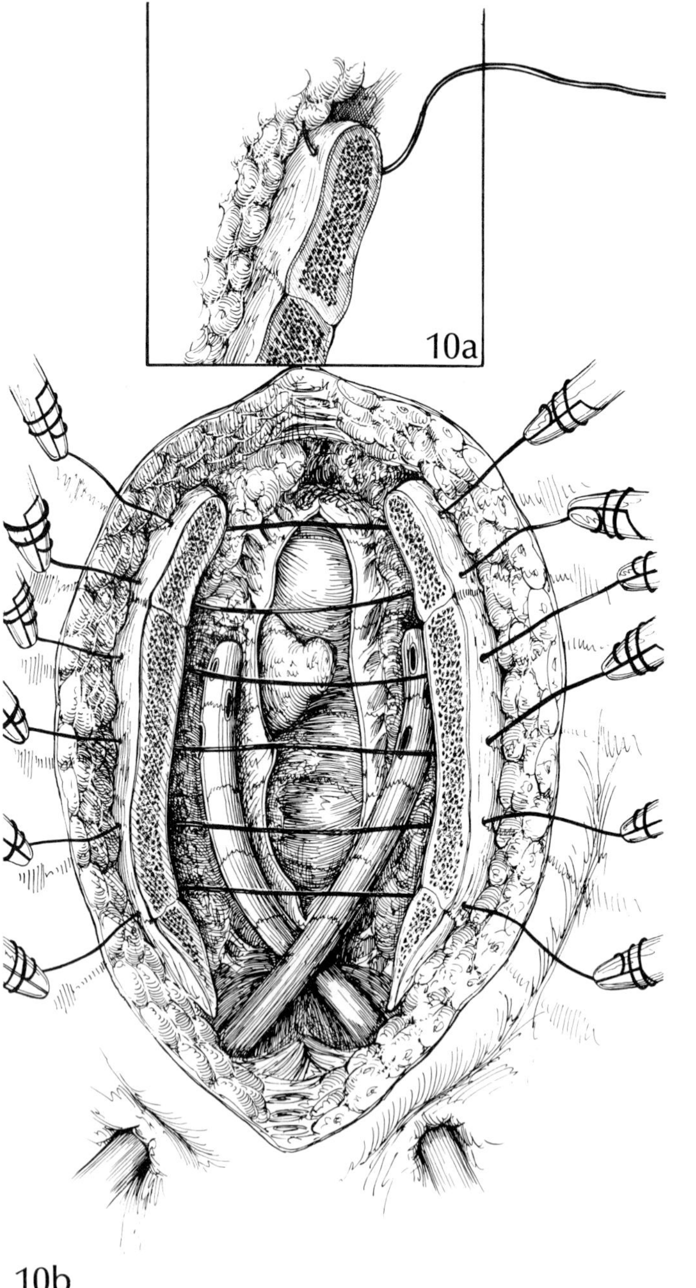

10b

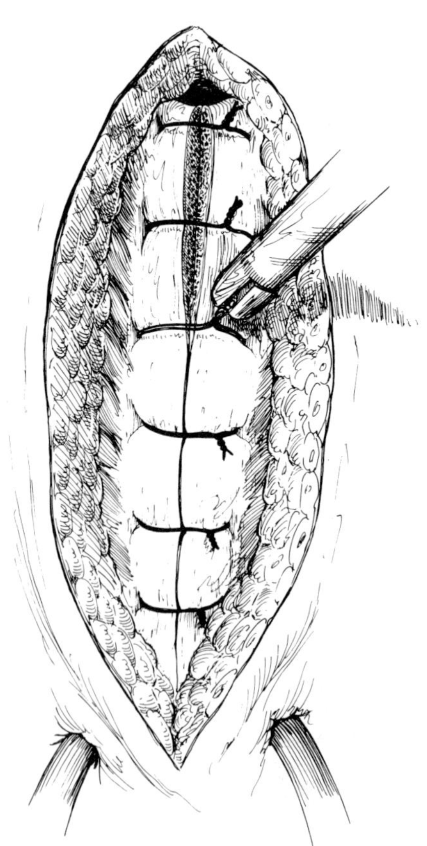

12

Posterolateral thoracotomy

Indications

This is the best incision for surgical procedures on structures in the central and posterior mediastinum. These include operations for:

1. Persistent ductus arteriosus;
2. Coarctation of the aorta;
3. Creation of systemic-pulmonary anastomoses;
4. Aneurysms and traumatic ruptures of the descending thoracic aorta.

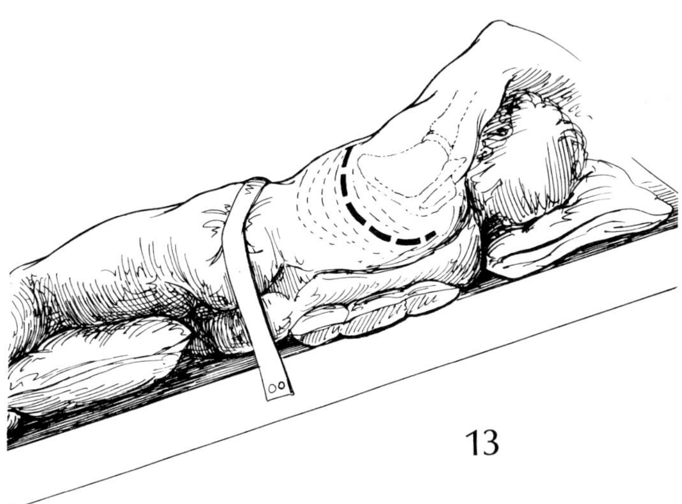

13

13

Position of patient

A stable full lateral position is required. This usually necessitates both a pelvic support and an anterior chest support. The back of the patient is placed adjacent to the edge of the operating table and the relevant scapula is elevated and abducted on the chest wall so as to give maximum access to the rib cage. This is obtained by holding the upper arm in abduction above the head and elevating the shoulder when positioning the patient on the table.

Skin incision

The skin incision is related to the extent and the level of thoracotomy that is planned. Most cardiac operations involving the arch and upper descending thoracic aorta are best performed through the lower border of the fourth rib. For closure of a persistent ductus arteriosus in an infant or child, a limited posterior thoracotomy will generally suffice, whereas a much fuller lateral incision is indicated for repair of coarctation of the aorta in an adult.

The incision commences anteriorly at the level of the mid-axillary (or mid-clavicular) line and extends posteriorly around the chest to a finger's breadth below the inferior angle of the scapula. From there it curves upwards to a point level with the spine of the scapula and midway between the spinous processes and the vertebral border of the scapula (*see Illustration 13*). The incision is then deepened vertically through the subcutaneous fat.

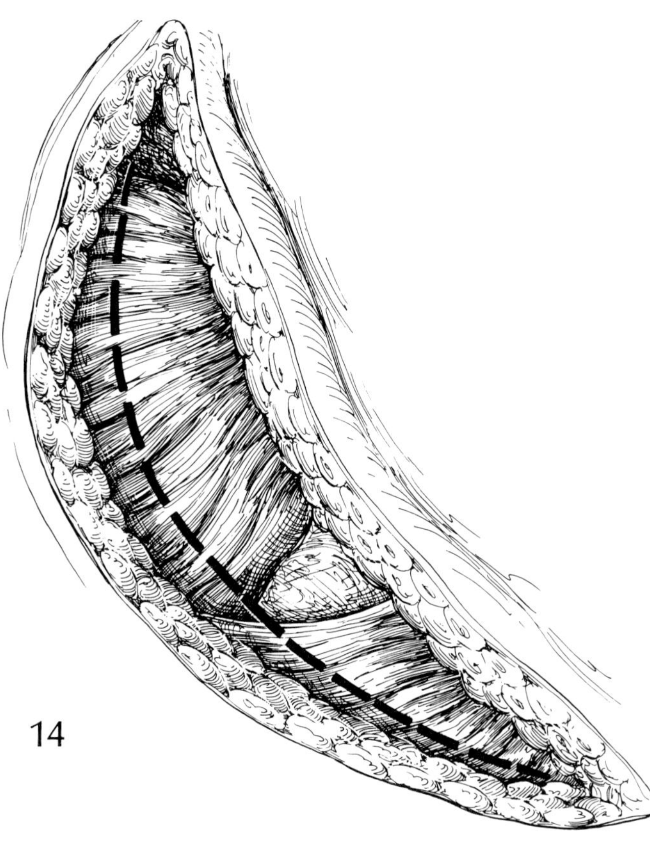

14

Muscle layer

For practical purposes two muscle layers are encountered:

1. Latissimus dorsi and trapezius;
2. Serratus and rhomboid major.

14

The anterior border of latissimus dorsi is located and the muscle divided throughout its length as low as possible, in the line of the skin incision. Electrocautery is used for this division. Posteriorly the muscular plane extends as a fascial layer to join the lower border of trapezius muscle, which itself is then divided as far as the upper margins of the skin incision.

15

In the centre of the wound the ribs and intercostal layer are now only covered by a further fascial layer which is incised. Posterosuperiorly this fascia is continuous with rhomboid major, the lower part of which is divided.

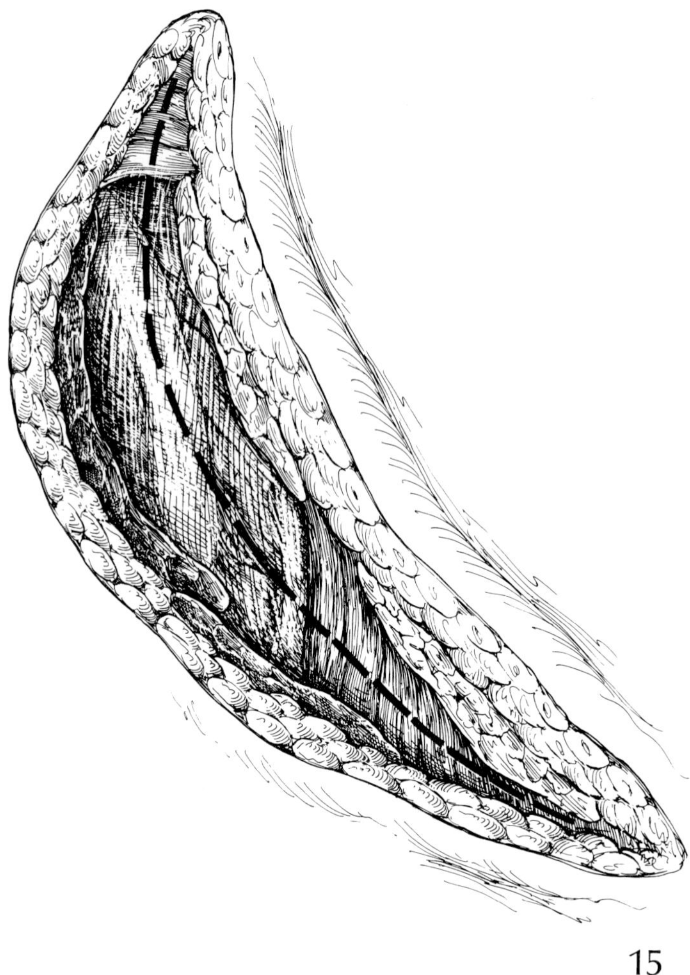

15

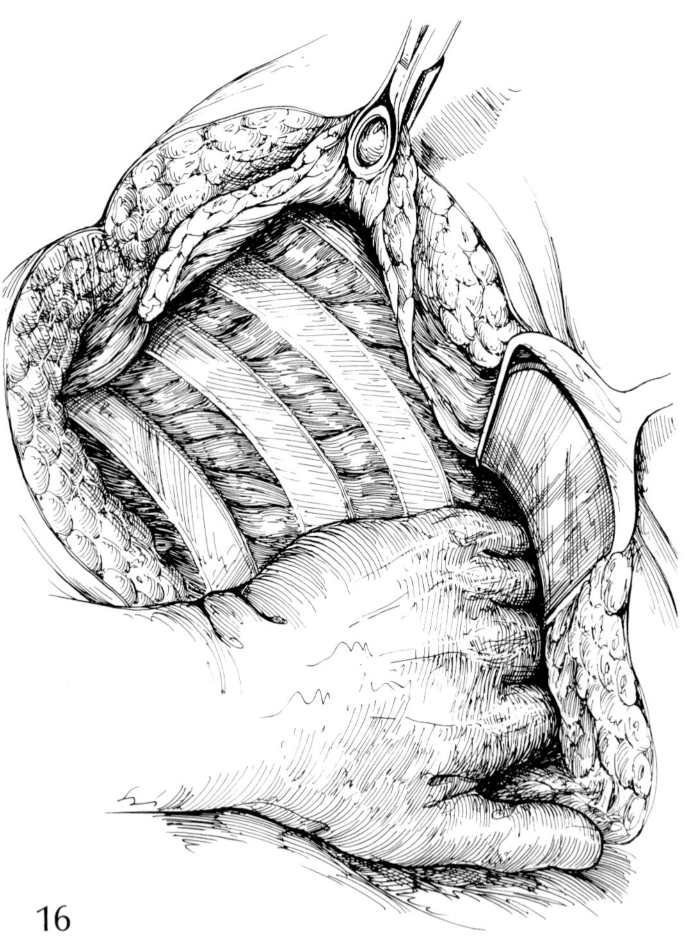

16

16

At this stage the selected rib should be identified by elevating the scapula with a retractor and introducing a hand into the avascular plane between it and the intercostal layer, keeping as close to the vertebral column as possible. The ribs can then be counted downwards, either from the first rib (which may be difficult to feel in adults), or from the third rib, which usually produces a natural step in the chest wall curvature, thereby allowing its identification.

17

The anterolateral part of the rib cage is covered by serratus anterior and, if additional exposure is required, the lower four digitations arising from the fifth, sixth, seventh and eighth ribs may be divided or detached from their costal origins. (These four digitations converge on the inferior angle of the scapula.) The incision on to the selected rib can then be continued anteriorly beneath skin and subcutaneous tissue, thereby exposing most of the length of the chosen rib, except posteriorly where it is covered by the erector spinae muscle mass.

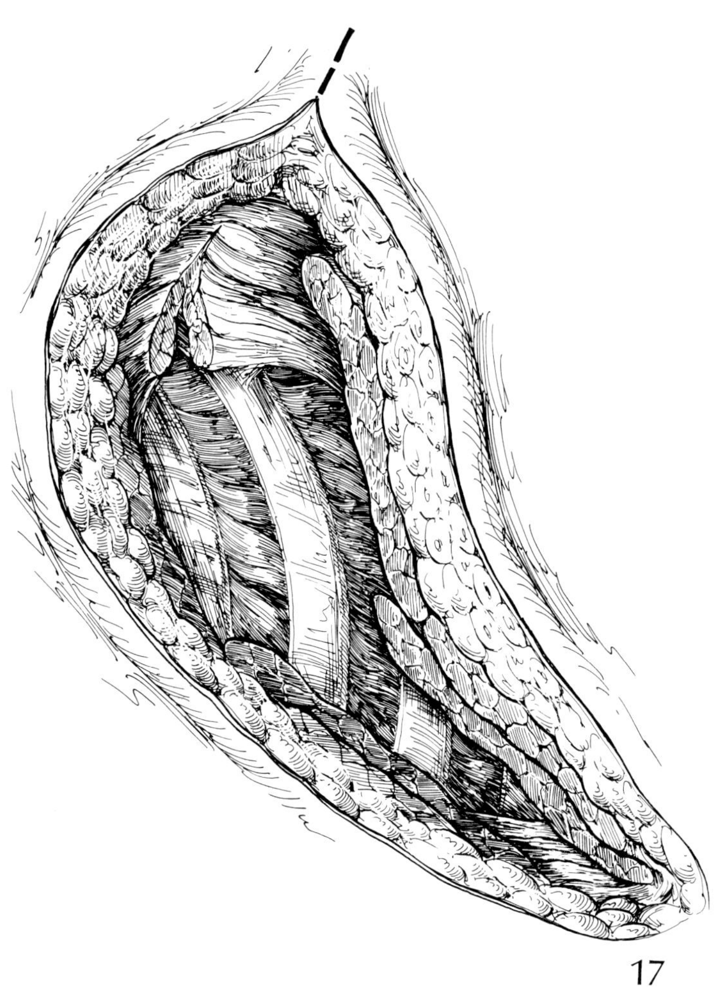

17

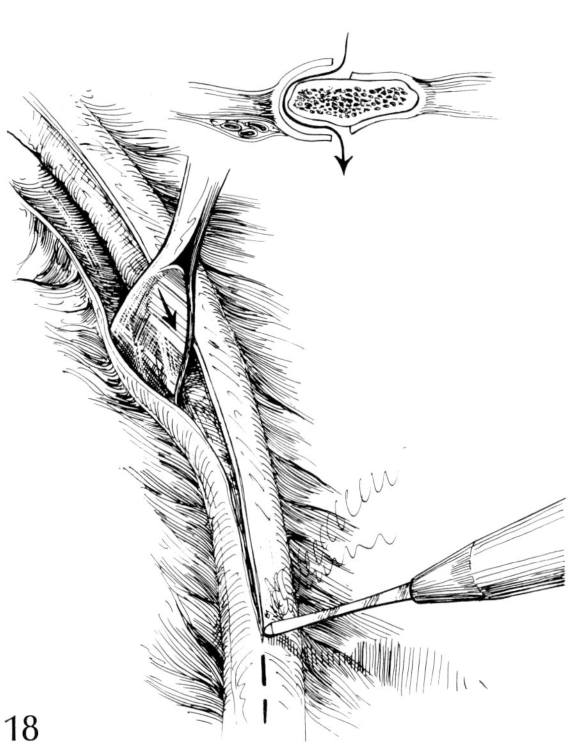

18

Intercostal layer

18

Entry into the chest cavity is gained by elevating the periosteum from the lower border of the rib and then incising the avascular plane forming the bed of the rib.

19a & b

Resection of a rib is now seldom necessary. Spreading the ribs for thoracotomy involves an extreme exaggeration of the natural rib movements and places an abnormal degree of strain on the anterior and posterior hinge mechanisms. It is important therefore to free the rib adequately so that its natural 'bucket-handle' movement can be made use of. Anteriorly this is accomplished by elevating the periosteum from the rib as far as possible and posteriorly by detaching and retracting the erector spinae muscles from the posterior end of the rib and then dividing the costotransverse ligament between it and the rib below with a Semb's chisel. (This may not be necessary in young children.) If proper mobility is ensured in this way and if the ribs are spread intermittently and progressively, it is rare to cause rib fractures.

If, however, access in the adult remains limited owing to increased ligamentous rigidity, resection of a short portion of the posterior part of the rib is sometimes necessary. This is performed by elevating the periosteum circumferentially from that part of the rib lying beneath the erector spinae muscles and then resecting a 2 cm length subperiosteally using a Tudor Edwards costotome.

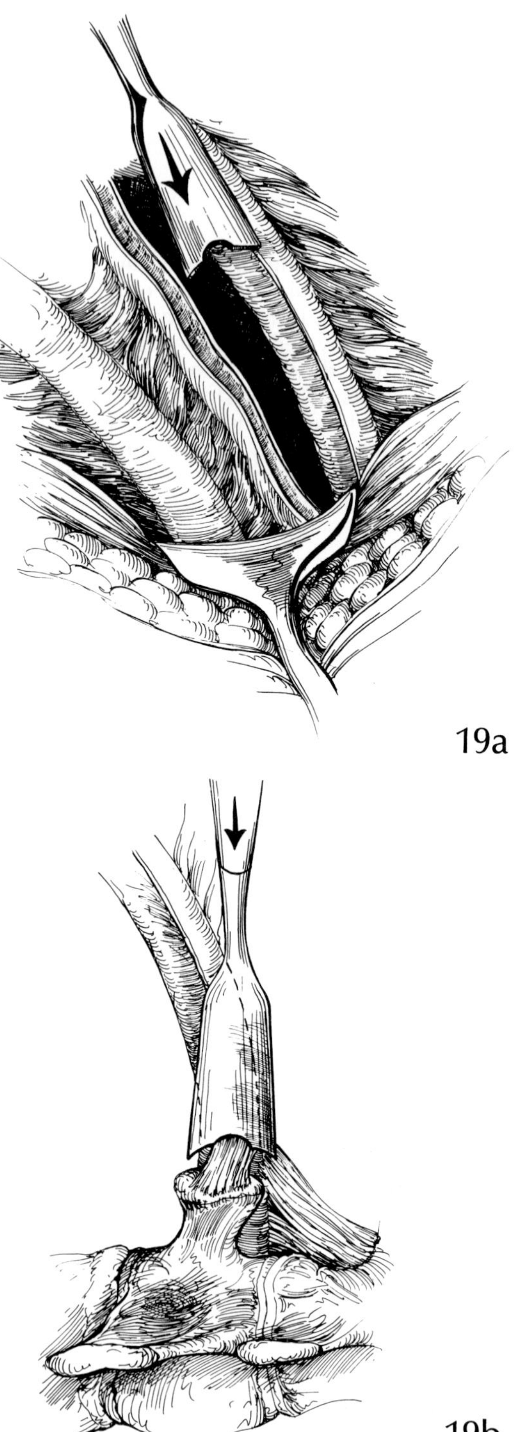

19a

19b

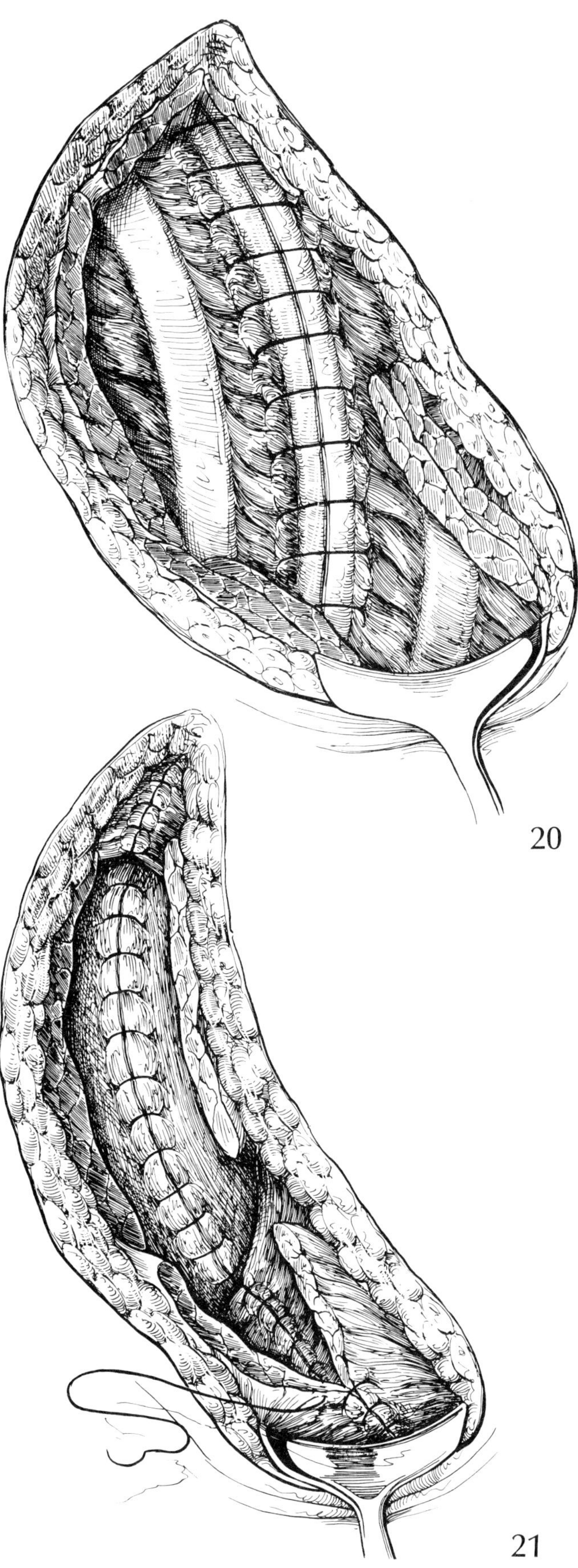

20

21

20 & 21

During closure, the muscles are approximated in the same three layers using continuous non-absorbable suture throughout.

Anterolateral thoracotomy

Indications

On the left this incision gives satisfactory exposure of the left atrial appendage, pulmonary artery and left ventricular apex. It is therefore an appropriate incision for closed mitral valvotomy and for banding of the pulmonary artery. On the right it provides good access to the right atrium and both venae cavae and has been used for intra-atrial correction of transposition of the great arteries, and for closure of atrial septal defects. Right anterolateral thoracotomy has also been advocated by some for mitral valve repair but median sternotomy is now always preferable.

22

Position of patient

The patient is placed in an oblique lateral position on the operating table, incorporating a sandbag behind the sacrum and dispensing with the pelvic support. The arm that is uppermost is supported by appropriate strapping, thereby preventing the thorax from rotating too far posteriorly.

Skin incision

For closed mitral valvotomy it is important that the chest be entered via the lower border of the fifth rib. The fifth costal cartilage whould be identified by counting down from the second costal cartilage, which is identified by manubriosternal junction (angle of Louis), and clearly marked at its junction with the sternum. This is best done before the skin is prepared and drapes applied and allows the fifth rib to be identified with certainty during the subsequent procedures. The skin incision commences anteriorly over the previously marked costal cartilage and curves inferiorly along the inframammary skin crease and then posteriorly in a horizontal direction to end 2 cm below the inferior angle of the scapula. The incision is then deepened through the subcutaneous fat.

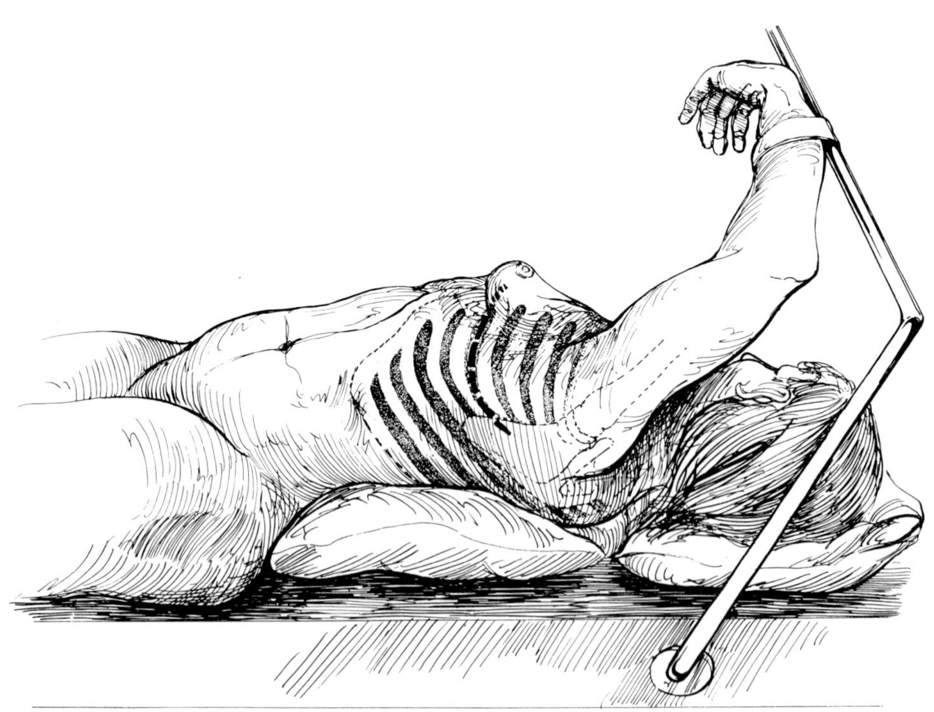

22

Muscles

23

The anterior border of latissimus dorsi is exposed posteriorly and in adult males this part of the muscle is divided in the line of the skin incision. Division of the muscle is usually not necessary in women and children.

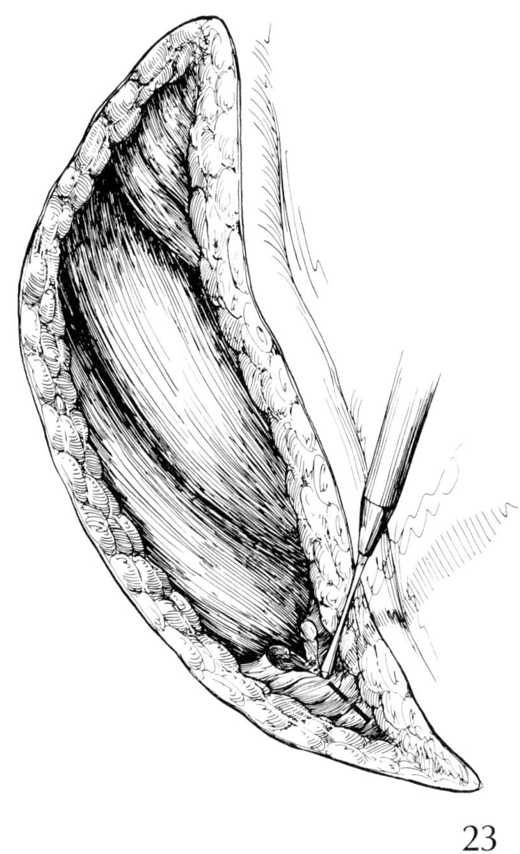

23

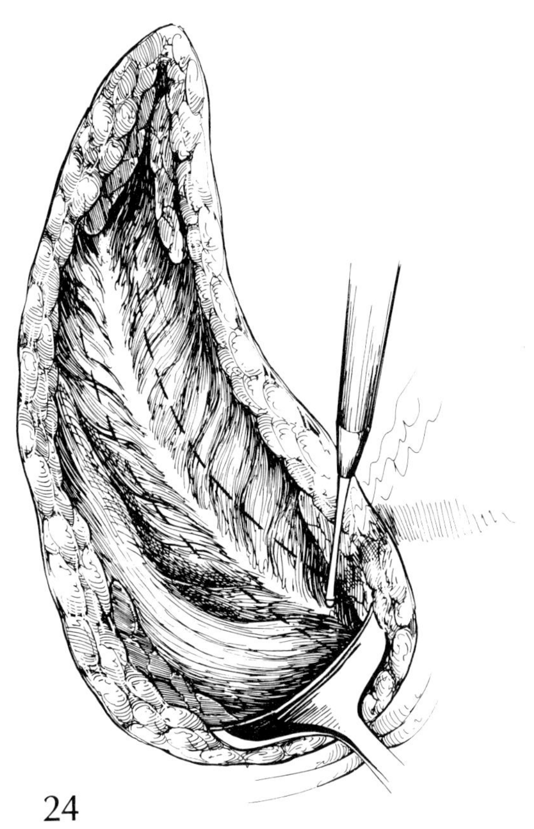

24

24

Anteriorly, fibres of the pectoralis major and rectus abdominis muscles are divided by electrocautery along the line of the fifth costal cartilage. In women that part of the breast overlying the fifth rib needs to be elevated as the dissection proceeds laterally. When the digitation of serratus anterior into the fifth rib is encountered, it is split longitudinally in the line of the muscle fibres, which coincides with the line of the rib.

This muscle split is extended posteriorly as far as the nerve to serratus anterior, which runs down on the external surface of the muscle and must be preserved. A hand is then inserted through this opening into the natural tissue plane deep to serratus anterior and the muscle split extended by manual separation of the fibres.

Intercostal layer

25

A scapula retractor is now inserted and the scapula elevated and retracted posteriorly. Division of the periosteum with electrocautery proceeds posteriorly as far as can be visualized and the periosteum is elevated from the inferior surface of the rib. The chest cavity is then entered through the exposed periosteal rib bed. Anteriorly the perichondrium is more difficult to elevate cleanly from the underlying cartilage but care here allows more satisfactory closure later.

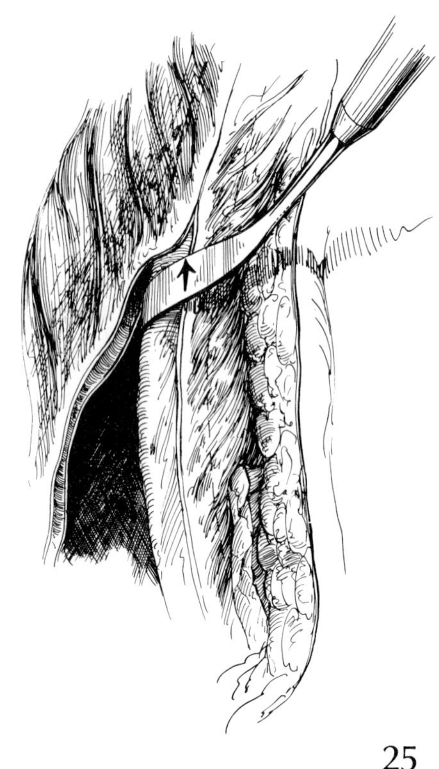

25

26

As the costal cartilage is retracted upwards, the internal mammary vessels are identified anteriorly and divided after suture-ligation. This allows free costosternal subluxation, which is preferable to fracture at the costosternal junction. A Price-Thomas rib-spreader is then introduced with the hinge mechanism posteriorly and the ribs gently spread apart. If access is adequate, this can usually be improved by extending the detachment of the intercostal layer from the lower border of the rib posteriorly, thereby increasing hinge mobilization.

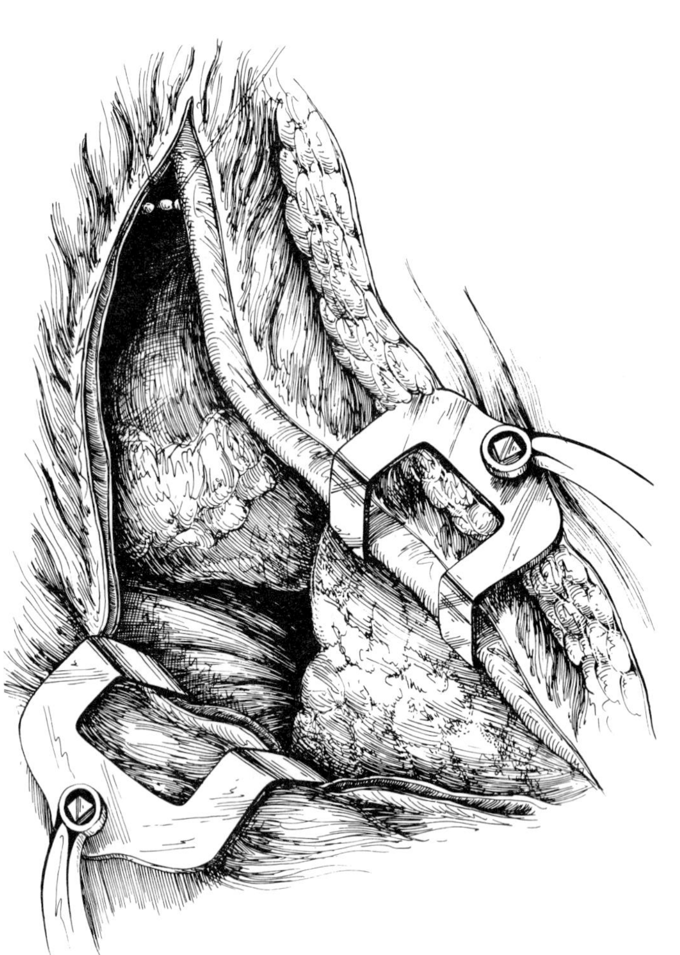

26

27 & 28

Closure is effected by approximation of the intercostal and muscle layers with continuous monofilament sutures. It will be noted that the incision is a relatively avascular one compared with posterolateral thoracotomy. Other advantages include its stability and a reduced incidence of post-thoracotomy wound pain.

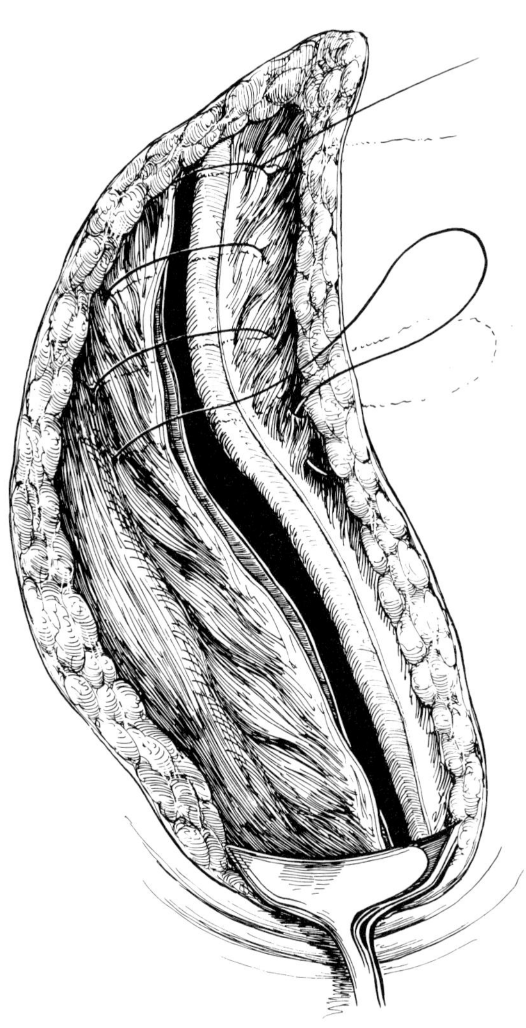

27

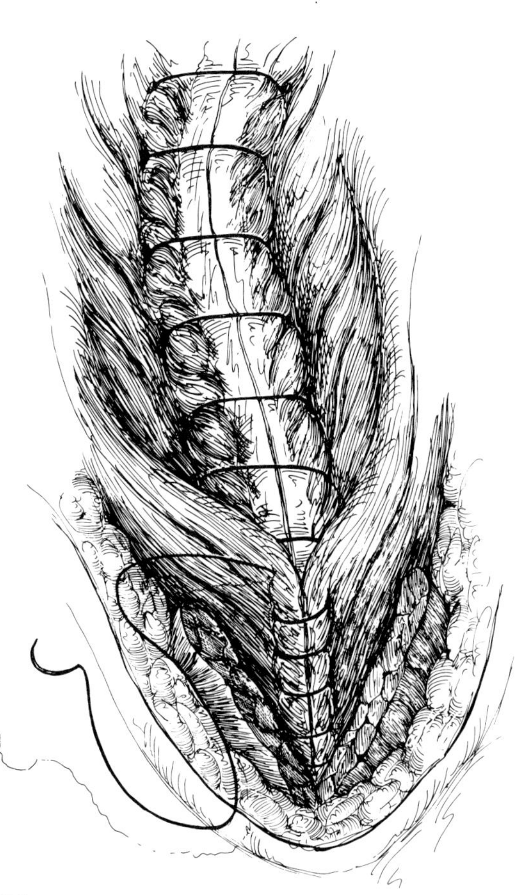

28

Resection of lung

Raymond Hurt FRCS
Thoracic Surgeon, Regional Thoracic Surgical Centre, North Middlesex Hospital, Edmonton, London and St Bartholomew's Hospital, London, UK

TYPES OF RESECTION

Resection of lung may be by pneumonectomy, lobectomy (which may be combined with a segment of an adjacent lobe), segmental resection or wedge resection. The type of resection will depend on the pathology and extent of the disease. In some cases a resection of part of the chest wall may be required and it may be necessary to stabilize the resulting deficit by a prosthesis of Marlex mesh or tantalum gauze. In other cases a bronchoplastic procedure with 'sleeve' resection of the main bronchus will enable a lobectomy rather than a pneumonectomy to be carried out.

Indications for resection

Carcinoma

In Europe and the United States about 90 per cent of lung resections are carried out for carcinoma. Resection is the treatment of choice for this disease, including small cell carcinoma[1,2] (although some authorities would exclude tumours of small cell histology), provided that:

1. the patient is fit enough to undergo operation;
2. there is no evidence of spread of the growth outside the chest;
3. there is no clinical or investigatory evidence of inoperability.

Unfortunately only about one-third of patients in whom a diagnosis of carcinoma is made are found to be suitable for operation.

Resection for carcinoma may be by standard pneumonectomy (simple extrapericardial), extended pneumonectomy (radical intrapericardial), lobectomy or segmental resection. Pneumonectomy might seem to be the only logical operation for carcinoma of the lung but as many of these patients also have chronic bronchitis this operation is often unfortunately very disabling and many are never able to resume work, especially if they are over the age of 55 years. Because of this, lobectomy and, much less often, segmental resection are both carried out and both have provided excellent results in terms of cure rate as well as quality of life[3]. Lobectomy for peripheral carcinoma is as effective in curing the patient as pneumonectomy – and carries a lower operative mortality[4,5]. Segmental resection for small peripheral carcinoma in the elderly has also provided satisfactory results[6]. Lobectomy is sometimes combined with a segmental resection of an adjacent lobe, e.g. upper lobectomy with resection of the apical segment of the lower lobe, or lower lobectomy with resection of the lingular segment of the left upper lobe or the posterior segment of the upper lobe. It is often only possible to make the final decision at operation. In the three years 1975–1977 a total of 451 resections for carcinoma of the bronchus were undertaken by the author and his senior colleague – of these, 204 were pneumonectomies, 228 lobectomies and 19 segmental resections.

Benign tumours

Benign tumours such as carcinoid or hamartoma may be treated by local bronchial resection or enucleation unless they occlude a bronchus and cause distal infection or bronchiectasis, in which case a lobectomy or pneumonectomy will be necessary.

Unless indicated otherwise the cross-references in this chapter refer to *Operative Surgery: Thoracic Surgery, 4th Edition*

Bronchiectasis

The extent of the bronchiectasis must be assessed by complete bronchograms of both lungs so that the segmental involvement can be accurately defined. Surgical treatment should excise all the affected segments or lobes, and it is therefore essential that the disease is well localized and not scattered throughout both lungs. Removal of the affected area may be by pneumonectomy, lobectomy or segmental resection. If pneumonectomy is contemplated the contralateral lung must be normal. Bilateral lobectomy or segmental resection may also be undertaken. In patients with bilateral disease resection is contraindicated if more than seven to eight segments are involved.

Chronic infection

If the infection cannot be controlled by prolonged courses of an appropriate antibiotic, a lobectomy or even pneumonectomy will be necessary. In these cases hilar dissection is likely to be very difficult and this may make a more limited resection impossible.

Tuberculosis

Modern antituberculosis drugs have revolutionized the treatment of tuberculous but operation may still be required in patients who have developed drug resistance, who continue to be sputum-positive or who have non-tuberculous infection distal to a bronchostenosis. The assessment of these patients for surgery is often very difficult and the indications for operation controversial.

Secondary carcinoma

Secondary deposits in the lung from carcinoma and sarcoma occur frequently. They are usually multiple but may occur singly; if so, they should be excised, provided there is no evidence of any other metastases and the primary tumour has been treated two or more years previously.

Preoperative

Assessment

The preoperative assessment of patients undergoing lung resection is vitally important. Unfortunately there are no definite standards to establish whether a patient is sufficiently fit to tolerate operation and many factors must be taken into account. For example, whereas an obese bronchitic middle-aged patient may not survive a lung resection, a relatively thin man of 75 years or more may tolerate the procedure very well if not bronchitic. The clinical assessment must take into account the following:

1. *Chronic bronchitis* A long history of bronchitis always indicates a greatly increased risk for a patient undergoing lung resection, whether a lobectomy or pneumonectomy. Even if he survives the operation he may be left a respiratory cripple, especially after a pneumonectomy.
2. *Bronchospasm* This also indicates a greatly increased risk, though to some extent it may be controlled by antispasmodic drugs and steroids. However, patients with significant bronchospasm will usually not tolerate a lung resection. In a few patients the bronchospasm may be associated with the lesion for which operation is required (e.g. unilateral due to benign bronchial tumour or bilateral due to tracheal tumour) and will itself be relieved by operation. But this is very different from the bilateral bronchospasm so often associated with chronic bronchitis.
3. *Clinical examination* The chest movements and configuration of the chest must be assessed by clinical examination. Patients with a 'barrel-shaped' chest (large anteroposterior diameter) often suffer from chronic bronchitis and emphysema, and this will be confirmed by the radiological absence of lung markings and a depressed diaphragm. Excessive obesity also increases the operative risk.
4. *Lung function studies* It is customary to undertake extensive lung function studies in patients considered for lung resection[7]. However, although these tests provide valuable confirmatory evidence of impaired lung function, they are often very difficult to interpret and do not replace the simple tests of asking the patient how short of breath he is on exercise and of walking with him up two flights of stairs.

Preparation of the patient

This is of vital importance and 2–3 days of intensive preoperative treatment will often shorten the patient's stay in hospital by 2–3 weeks – and may even be life-saving. The aims of treatment are:

1. reduction of bronchial infection by the appropriate antibiotic and postural drainage if necessary;
2. reduction of bronchospasm by antispasmodic drugs such as ephedrine or salbutamol (Ventolin), together with steroids if necessary;
3. correction of anaemia; and
4. instruction in deep breathing exercises by the physiotherapist.

Surgical anatomy

1

Bronchopulmonary segments

The two lungs are basically very similar, despite the fact that on the right side there are three lobes and on the left two. The classification of the bronchopulmonary segments adopted by the Thoracic Society of Great Britain[8] is as follows.

Right lung

Upper lobe:	(*1*) apical, (*2*) posterior, (*3*) anterior.
Middle lobe:	(*4*) lateral, (*5*) medial.
Lower lobe:	(*6*) apical, (*7*) medial basal (cardiac), (*8*) anterior basal, (*9*) lateral basal, (*10*) posterior basal.

Left lung

Upper lobe:	(*1*) apical, (*2*) posterior, (*3*) anterior, (*4*) superior division of lingula, (*5*) inferior division of lingula.
Lower lobe:	(*6*) apical, (*8*) anterior basal, (*9*) lateral basal, (*10*) posterior basal. (N.B. Segment 7 is omitted in the left lung).

Each lung has an *upper lobe,* which is divided into anterior, apical and posterior segments. On the right side these segmental bronchi branch as a trifurcation, but on the left side there is usually an apicoposterior stem bronchus and a separate anterior segmental bronchus.

The right *middle lobe* lies anteriorly and is a branch of the intermediate bronchus. In the left lung, however, the middle lobe is represented by the lingular segment, the first segmental bronchus of the left upper lobe which passes anteriorly and inferiorly.

The *lower lobe* on each side is composed of three basal segments, together with an apical lower segment lying posteriorly, which in the right lung arises immediately opposite the middle lobe. In the right lower lobe there is, in addition, a medially placed cardiac segment arising between the apical lower lobe bronchus and the basal divisions.

The portion of bronchus between the right upper lobe and the middle lobe is described as the intermediate bronchus.

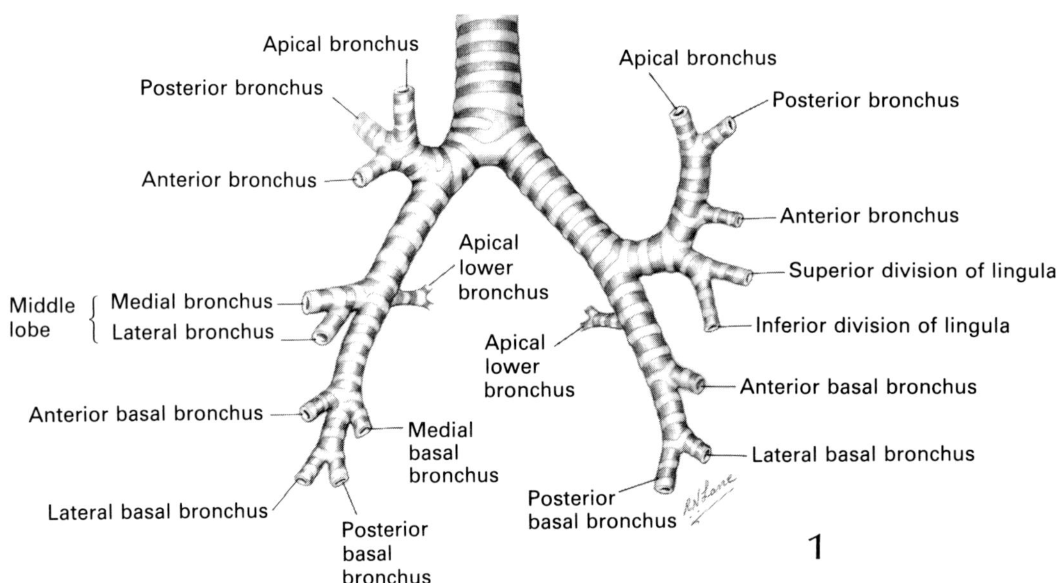

1

2 & 3

Pulmonary vasculature

Each segment functions as an individual unit and has its own bronchus, artery and vein. The segmental arteries run very close to the bronchi, usually on their superior or lateral aspect, whereas the *segmental veins* run between the segments from which they receive tributaries. The segments are held together by loose connective tissue and no bronchi or arteries cross the intersegmental plane. The *pulmonary arterial branches* are closely related to the corresponding bronchi. These usually follow a regular pattern[9], but variations are common and they must always be carefully dissected and identified during lobar or segmental resection.

The lung has a systemic as well as a pulmonary blood supply, and will survive ligation of a main pulmonary artery. The *bronchial arteries* arise from the descending thoracic aorta or upper intercostal arteries and run along the corresponding bronchi. They become very much dilated in any long-standing condition associated with chronic infection (e.g. bronchiectasis). The bronchial veins drain into the systemic and pulmonary circulations.

The following anatomical points must be borne in mind when resecting lung.

1. The origin of the right upper lobe is *very* close to the carina. Indeed, at bronchoscopy the right upper lobe orifice and the carina appear to be almost the same distance from the upper jaw.
2. The middle lobe and the apical segment of the right lower lobe arise from the intermediate bronchus immediately opposite each other. This is of importance in right lower lobectomy.
3. The middle lobe vein drains into the right superior vein and when performing a right upper lobectomy it is most important to preserve this vein.

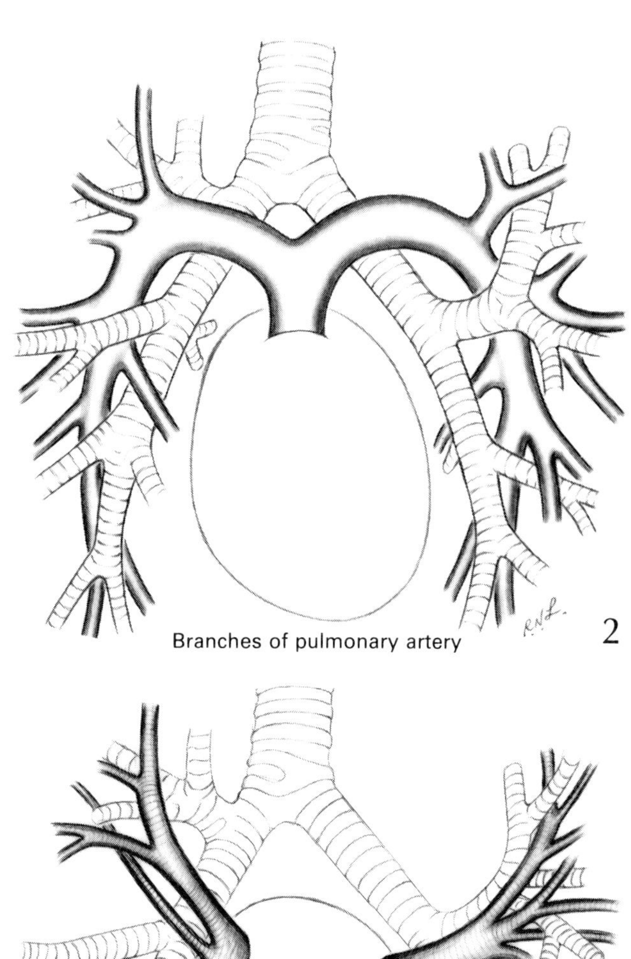

Branches of pulmonary artery 2

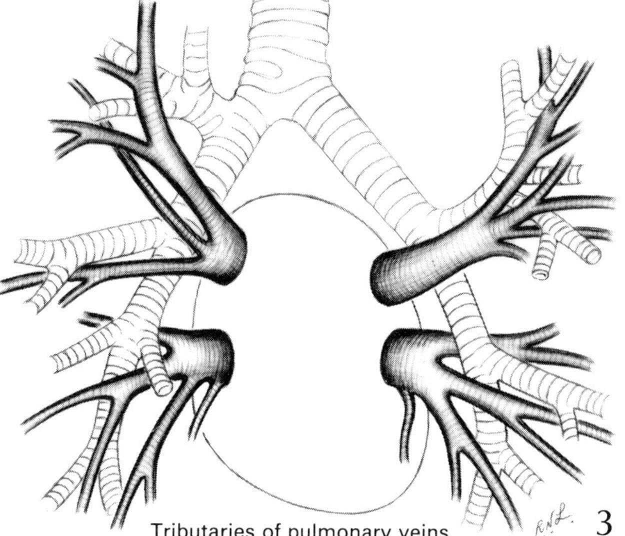

Tributaries of pulmonary veins 3

Surgical approach

A posterolateral thoracotomy through the bed of the fifth rib provides the best exposure for all lung resections and allows the hilum to be approached from both in front and behind, which is extremely useful if the growth is advanced and the dissection difficult. The 'face-down' position is no longer necessary or advisable now that a wide range of effective antibiotics is available for preoperative preparation – it precludes access to the pulmonary vessels from in front, makes the operation unnecessarily difficult and makes early ligation of the superior pulmonary vein in carcinoma resections impossible.

Sequence of dissection

In all cases of resection for carcinoma it is advisable first to divide the vein draining the affected lobe in order to prevent tumour embolization during manipulation of the lung. Thereafter it does not matter in which order the hilar structures are divided, though if there is an excessive amount of sputum or haemoptysis it is preferable at least to clamp, if not actually divide, the bronchus first. With all due respect to modern anaesthetic technique, it is not possible or wise to rely on control of bronchial secretions by the anaesthetist, however expert he may be in positioning the various types of endobronchial tubes or blockers. Except in such cases it is usually convenient to divide the bronchus last.

Division of the main pulmonary artery and veins

The dissection and control of the pulmonary vessels during lung resection is often very difficult, mainly because *both* arteries and veins are very fragile and tear easily. The O'Shaugnessy right angled clamp and the Crafoord uncovered curved coarctation clamp are suitably rounded at their ends and are very useful and safe instruments for the hilar dissection.

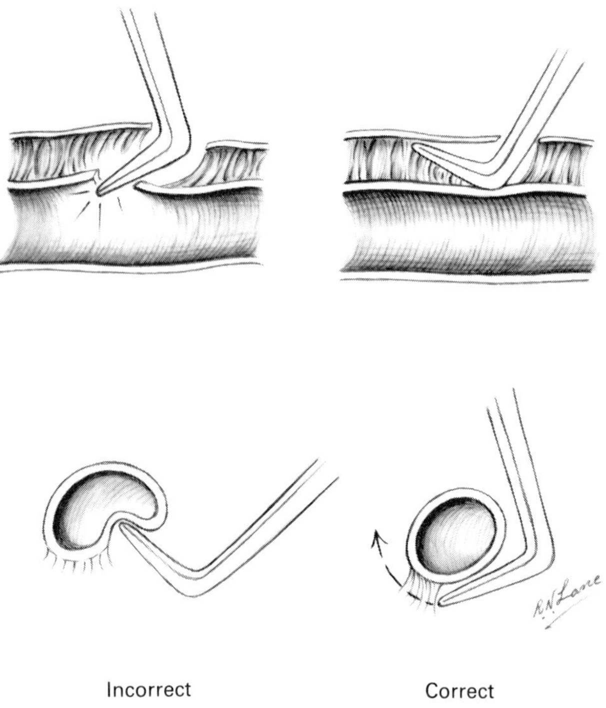

4

The pulmonary artery and veins, together with their branches and tributaries, are all enclosed in a sheath of fascia. This fascia must be deliberately picked up with fine-toothed forceps (Stille's forceps are ideal) and cut with scissors. It will then be very much easier, and certainly very much safer, to isolate and divide the vessel. The two proximal ligatures should be tied so that they overlap. There should be a cuff at least 1 cm long distal to the two ligatures – if this is not possible then it is wise to apply a Satinsky clamp and suture the divided vessel with a continuous 4/0 Mersilene suture. A transfixion suture may cause problems and is not required if an adequate cuff of vessel is available or if a Satinsky clamp is used. The ligature material must be reasonably thick – a thin ligature may cut through the vessel. No. 1 Mersilene is suitable. The distal ligatures may be multiple ligatures on the branches or tributaries of the vessel rather than on the main vessel itself. Alternatively, if there is insufficient length of vessel for a distal ligature, a clamp may be used distally and the vessel divided with a knife flush with the clamp. It is most important to make sure that the assistant relaxes on the lung retraction at the moment when the ligatures are being tied.

Dissection of lobar pulmonary arteries and veins

5

When ligating an arterial branch of the pulmonary artery it is important to avoid 'tenting up' of the main vessel and subsequent slipping of the ligature (slightly exaggerated in this illustration).

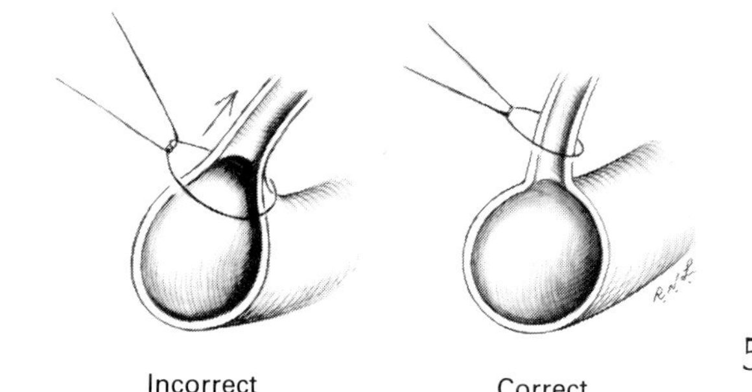

5

6

It is sometimes difficult to mobilize an arterial branch completely before its ligature, and the method illustrated usually overcomes this problem.

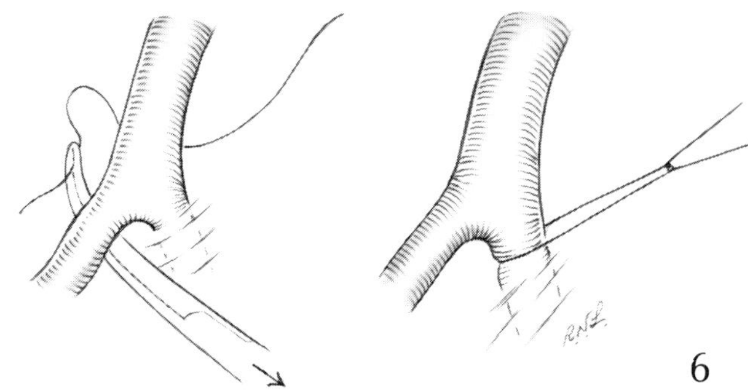
6

Closure of bronchus

There are several acceptable methods for closure of the bronchus, none of which completely avoids the complication of a bronchopleural fistula. The American automatic stapler (Auto Suture Model TA 30) is being increasingly used (*see* chapter on 'Use of stapler in lung surgery', pp. 185–188 and appears to be a quick and safe (though expensive) moethod of bronchial closure.

7

A long bronchial stump is an important contributory factor in the formation of a bronchopleural fistula. It must therefore be avoided and the bronchus divided close to the trachea or adjacent lobar bronchus.

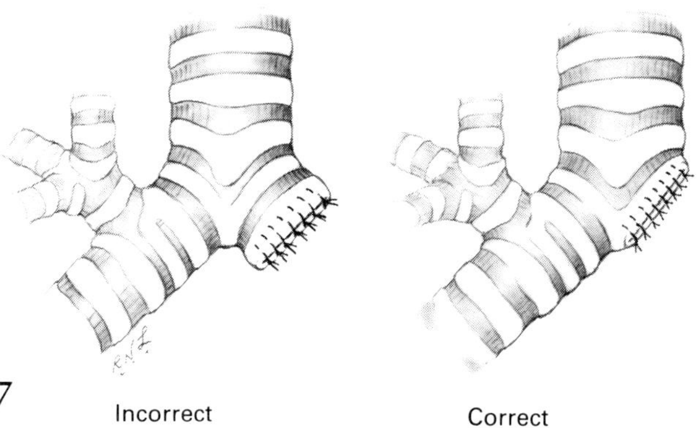

7

8

The author's preferred technique is to use the Brock non-crushing clamp with the handles towards the patient's head so that the membranous (posterior) wall of the bronchus is brought against the concavity of the C-shaped cartilage. Care must be taken not to place the clamp too proximal as the opposite main bronchus may be narrowed or the anaesthetist's tube compressed and subsequently caught in the sutures. The bronchus is divided with a long-handled angled knife and the stump closed with interrupted figure-of-eight No. 2 SWG stainless steel wire sutures on atraumatic needles about 1.5 mm apart so that the proximal loop is inserted under the blades of the clamp. For a left pneumonectomy the needles should be curved, but for all other resections straight needles are easier to use. The clamp is slipped out of the suture loops after first separating the blades, and the sutures are then tied. It is important to cut the bronchial sutures short to avoid the danger of the ends of the wire suture perforating adjacent structures, e.g. the oesophagus after a right pneumonectomy or the pulmonary artery after a left pneumonectomy. It is best to tie three knots and to cut flush with the third knot. Airtight closure may be confirmed by pouring saline on to the stump and requesting the anaesthetist to apply gentle pressure.

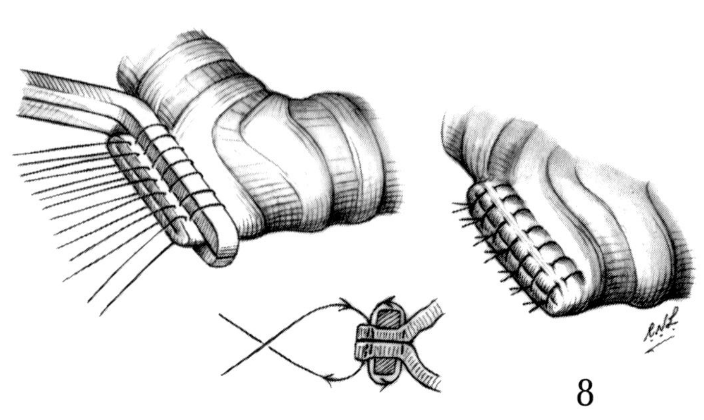

8

9

Open technique

A clamp is placed on the bronchus distally, and the bronchus is incised, divided and then closed with interrupted 3/0 Ethibond non-absorbable sutures on an atraumatic needle. These may be simple sutures or figure-of-eight sutures (as in this illustration). The membranous posterior wall of the bronchus is very thin and great care must be taken when tying the sutures. Anaesthesia is by a cuffed tube into the opposite lung so there is no escape of anaesthetic gases while the bronchus is open.

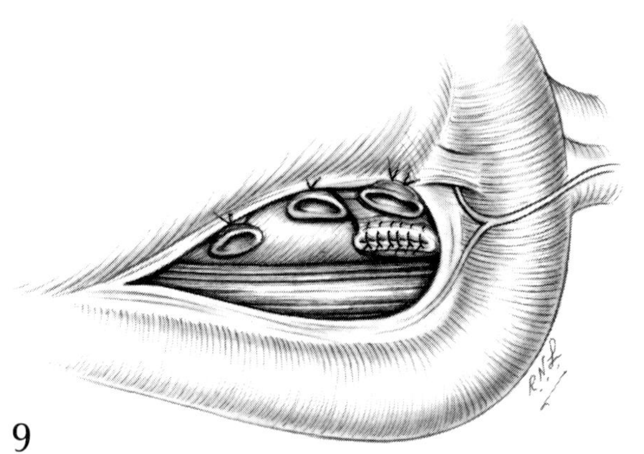

9

The operations

PNEUMONECTOMY

This may be a *standard pneumonectomy,* with division of the pulmonary vessels outside the pericardium and removal of carinal, paratracheal, pretracheal and para-oesophageal lymph nodes if they appear to be involved, or an 'extended' *radical pneumonectomy,* with division of the vessels inside the pericardium and removal of all the involved lymphatic glands described above. This extended operation must of necessity be more limited on the left than on the right because of the interposition of the aortic arch. Operability is decided by vision and palpation, though a final decision may not be possible until the pericardium has been opened and a hilar dissection attempted. Mediastinal lymph node involvement must be assessed and a decision made whether to open the pericardium in order to divide the pulmonary artery and veins. The liver should be palpated for possible secondary deposits and if necessary the diaphragm opened.

All of the following indicate that the tumour is inoperable.

1. Inability to separate the tumour from the aorta or superior vena cava.
2. Inability to separate the tumour from the lower end of the trachea.
3. Spread of growth along the pulmonary veins and to the left atrium so that the vein cannot be divided, even by 'pinching up' a portion of atrial wall.
4. Spread of growth along the pulmonary artery to such an extent that it cannot be divided even proximal to the obliterated ductus arteriosus on the left side or medial to the superior vena cava on the right side.
5. Inability to separate the tumour from vertebral bodies.
6. Involvement of oesophageal mucosa – if the growth involves only the muscle it may still be removable.

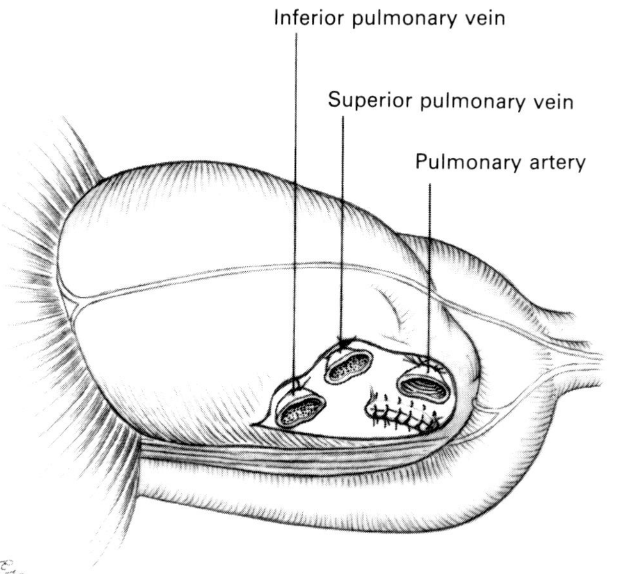

10

Left standard pneumonectomy (extra pericardial)

10

The left main bronchus is just below and behind the pulmonary artery, the superior pulmonary vein is immediately below the pulmonary artery and in front of the bronchus, and below them both is the inferior pulmonary vein.

Exposure

11

The periosteum is stripped from the upper border of the fifth rib, the rib bed is incised and the pleural cavity opened. The apex of the lung is mobilized and drawn downwards so that the aortic arch and hilum are clearly seen. If the lung is very adherent to the chest wall an extrapleural strip should be carried out over the adherent area, and care must be taken to avoid damage to the aorta and its branches posteriorly and superiorly or the internal mammary artery or phrenic nerve anteriorly.

The superior or inferior pulmonary vein is divided first, depending on the position of the tumour.

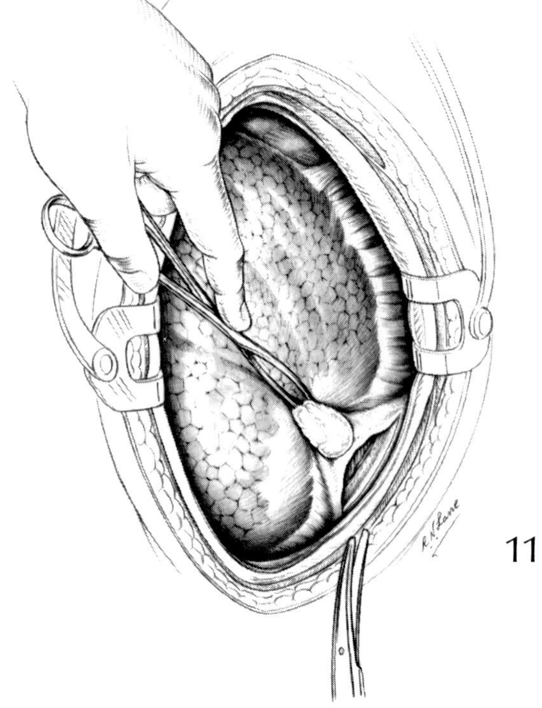

11

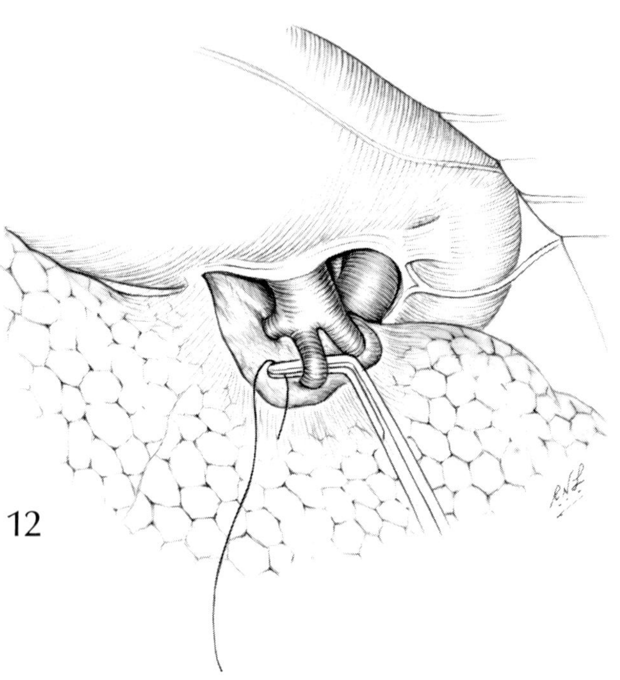

12

12

The *superior pulmonary vein* is approached from in front and the lung retracted backwards. The pleura and adventitia around the vein are incised and the vein is separated from the artery which is situated posteriorly. The vein is then divided between two proximal ligatures and another distal ligature or clamp, or as shown in this illustration, in which the tributaries are ligated separately.

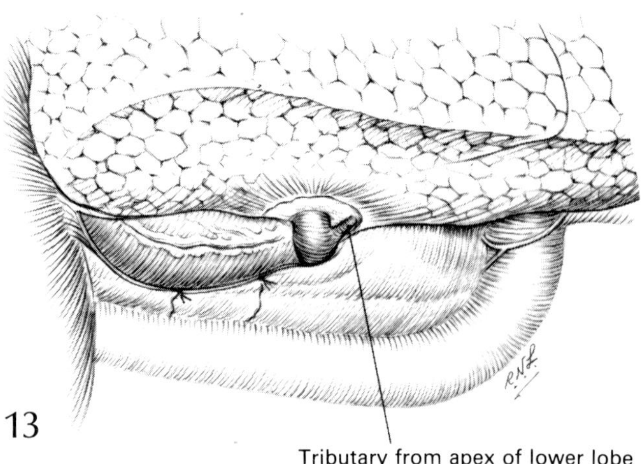

13

13

The *inferior pulmonary vein* is exposed by retracting the lower lobe upwards and forwards so that the vein is approached from behind. This is usually easier than approaching it from in front. The pulmonary ligament is divided (it often contains a small artery which requires ligation) and the dissection is carried up between its two layers until the inferior pulmonary vein is reached. Immediately below the vein there is often a lymphatic gland (of Brock) to mark its position. The adventitia around the vein is incised, and the vein is isolated and then divided between two No. 1 silk ligatures proximally and a clamp or another ligature distally, ensuring that an adequate cuff of vein remains. The vein may be approached from in front or behind, or a combination of both. Not infrequently the tributary from the apex of the lower lobe enters the pericardium separately from the main vein to join it *inside* the pericardium. This requires separate ligation and division. In this illustration it joins the inferior vein outside the pericardium.

14

The *pulmonary artery* is next isolated and divided between double proximal ligatures and another ligature or clamp placed distally. A Crafoord clamp or finger is passed from above downwards behind the artery and between the artery and the main bronchus. Some firm tissue (fold of pericardium over the vestigeal vein of Marshall) must be divided on the inferior aspect of the artery before the clamp can be passed round completely. The artery is divided between double proximal ligatures and another ligature or clamp placed distally.

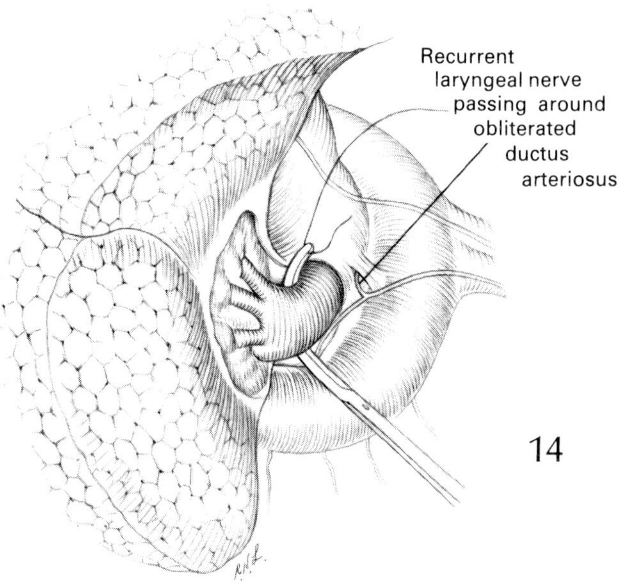

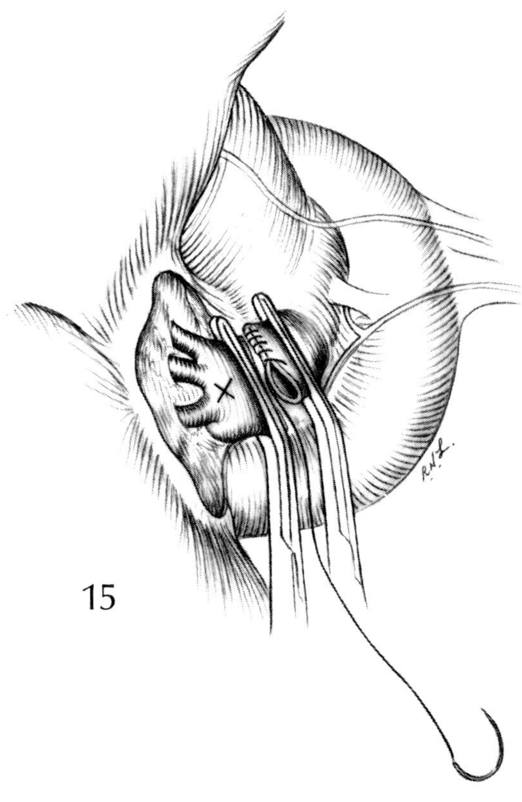

15

If an adequate cuff of pulmonary artery is not obtained the artery should be clamped and sutured with a continuous suture. In this illustration there is sufficient length of artery to permit the application of a distal clamp or ligature. But if tumour is situated over the area marked with a X then the proximal end of the artery will need to be sutured.

16

Finally, the bronchus must be defined. The surrounding adventitious tissue containing bronchial arteries and pulmonary branches of the vagus must be divided between clamps. Care must be taken to preserve the recurrent laryngeal nerve as it hooks around the obliterated ductus. The bronchus must be divided flush with the carina and is closed over a non-crushing clamp or by an 'open' technique, or with an automatic stapler, as already described. The bronchial stump retracts into the mediastinum under the aortic arch.

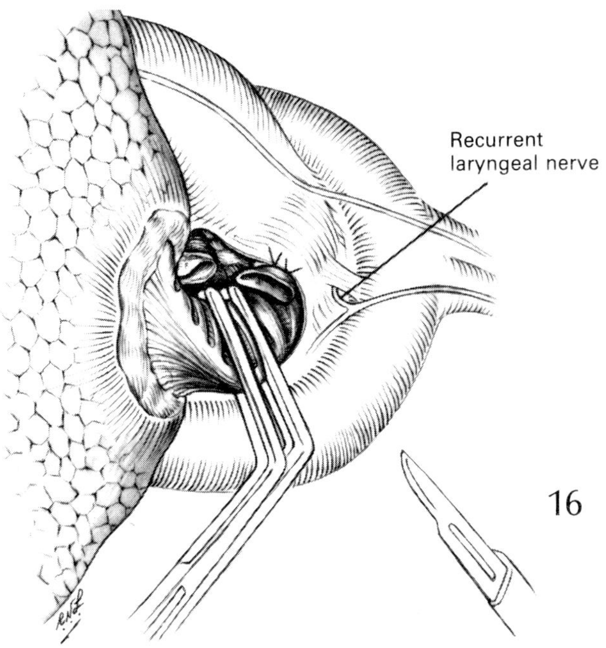

Left extended pneumonectomy (intrapericardial)

If the growth is extensive, with considerable mediastinal lymph node enlargement, an early decision must be made whether to open the pericardium. If so it is opened around the whole lung root, both anteriorly and posteriorly. It is preferable to retract the phrenic nerve anteriorly and not divide it so as to avoid paradoxical movement of the diaphragm and consequent difficulty in expectoration in the postoperative period. The situation of the growth, however, may make divison of the nerve necessary.

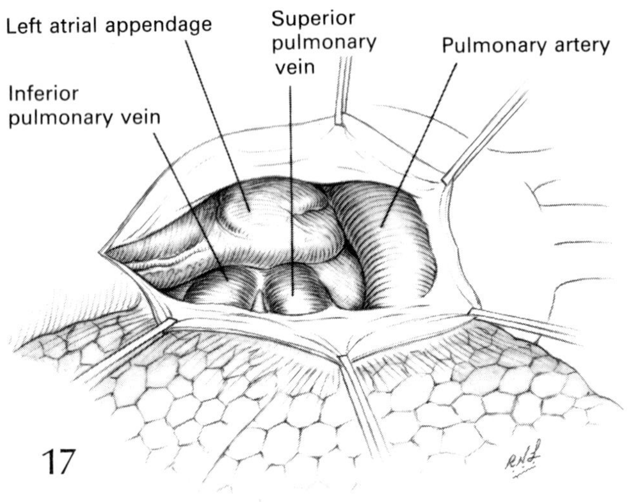

17

17

The lung is retracted posteriorly, the pericardium opened anterior to the superior pulmonary vein and the incision extended superiorly towards the pulmonary artery and inferiorly towards the pulmonary ligament. The superior vein is divided between two proximal ligatures and a distal clamp. If necessary a Satinsky clamp can be placed on the left atrial wall, the vein clamped distally and divided, and the atrial wall then closed with a continuous 3/0 Mersilene suture. The inferior vein is divided separately in a similar way.

It may be preferable to divide the common pulmonary vein rather than the superior and inferior vein separately, in which case a Satinsky clamp should be placed on the common vein or atrial wall and the vessel closed with a continuous suture, as shown in *Illustration 26*.

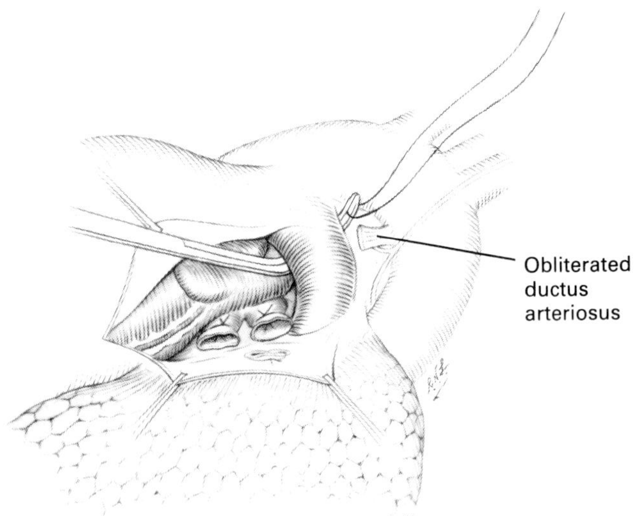

18

18

The pulmonary artery is generally divided distal to the obliterated ductus arteriosus (*see Illustration 14*) but it is sometimes necessary to divide the obliterated ductus in order to obtain an adequate cuff on the pulmonary artery. The artery is shown being doubly ligated but if there is insufficient cuff the ligatures are very likely to 'roll off' the divided pulmonary artery because of continued pulsation and in such a case the artery must be closed with a continuous 4/0 Mersilene suture.

19

The dissection is continued to expose the oesophagus posteriorly and care must be taken not to damage it on the medial side of the main bronchus or in the region of the inferior pulmonary vein. A small portion of oesophageal muscle may be removed, provided the mucosa is preserved. The vagus may need to be divided, preferably distal to the recurrent laryngeal nerve, though if there are numerous involved glands in the subaortic fossa the vagus may have to be divided above the aortic arch and the recurrent laryngeal nerve sacrificed.

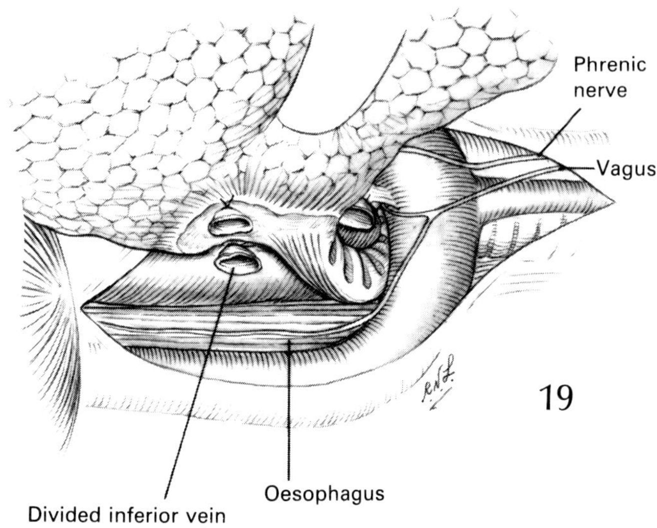

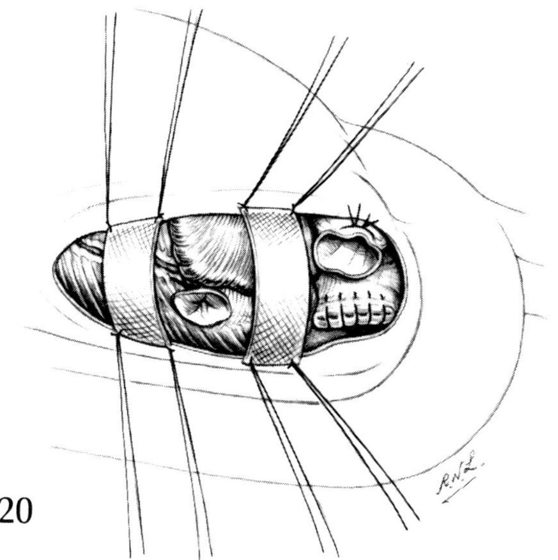

20

Management of pericardium

The pericardium should not be closed – indeed this would only rarely be possible. If any bleeding occurs it is much better for the blood to drain into the pleural cavity rather than to remain within a sutured pericardium and possibly cause cardiac compression from tamponade. If the pericardial defect is large the serious and usually fatal complication of herniation of the heart may occur – this should be prevented by suturing 1 cm wide Teflon strips to the edge of the pericardium across the defect.

Right standard pneumonectomy (extrapericardial)

21

The pulmonary artery is immediately in front of the bronchus, with the superior pulmonary vein just below and a little in front, and the inferior pulmonary vein lower still.

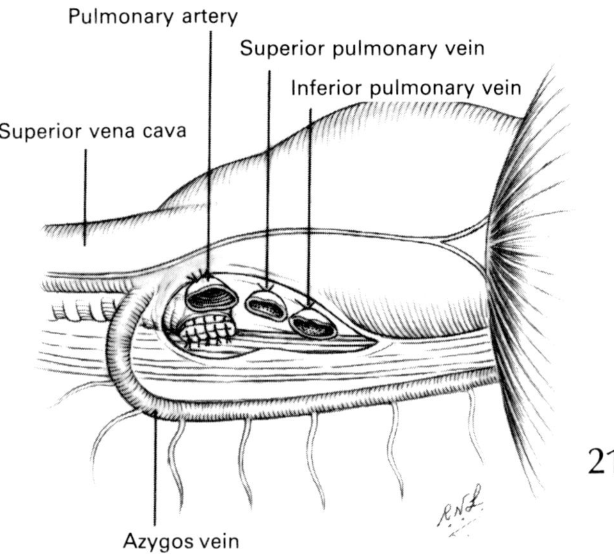

21

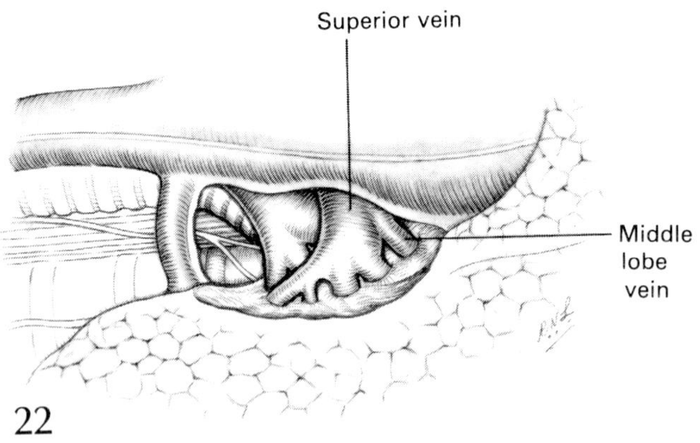

22

22

The *superior pulmonary vein* is exposed by retracting the lung backwards, when the vein will be seen entering the pericardium. The overlying pleura is divided before isolation, ligation and division of the vein and its tributaries. The most inferior tributary drains the middle lobe.

23

The *inferior pulmonary vein* is exposed by retracting the lung anteriorly and dividing the pulmonary ligament between clamps (there is often a small artery in the ligament which requires ligation). The dissection is carried up between its layers until the inferior vein is reached. Immediately below the vein there is often a lymphatic gland (of Brock) – this will aid its identification. The adventitia around the vein is incised, and the vein isolated and then divided between two No.1 silk ligatures proximally and a clamp or another ligature distally, ensuring that an adequate cuff remains. The vein may be approached from in front or behind, or a combination of both. Not infrequently the tributary from the apex of the lower lobe enters the pericardium separately from the main vein to join it *inside* the pericardium. It will require separate ligation and division. In this illustration it joins the inferior vein outside the pericardium.

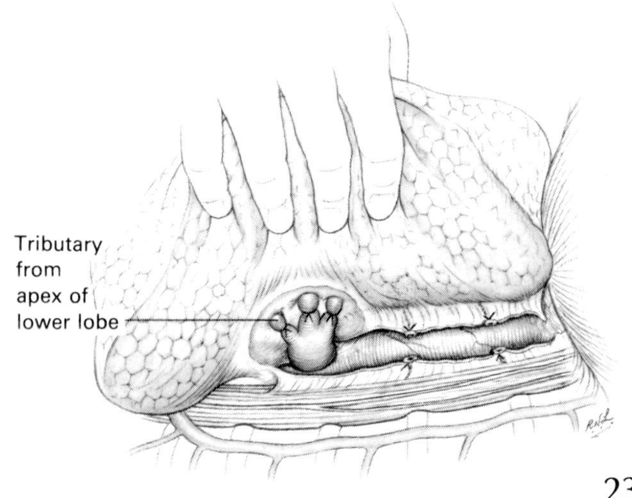

23

24

The *pulmonary artery* must next be divided – and the previous division of the superior pulmonary vein makes this easier. There is a condensation of tissue between the superior vena cava and pulmonary artery (shown by the dotted line) which should be deliberately cut with scissors. This frees a considerable *additional length* of pulmonary artery. It is then very easy to encircle the artery; this is carried out most safely by the right index finger from below upwards. The artery is divided between double ligatures placed proximally and a clamp or ligature distally. In this illustration the inferior and superior veins are shown undivided.

Finally the bronchus is divided flush with the carina (*see Illustrations 7–9*).

The lung is removed, together with the subcarinal lymph nodes.

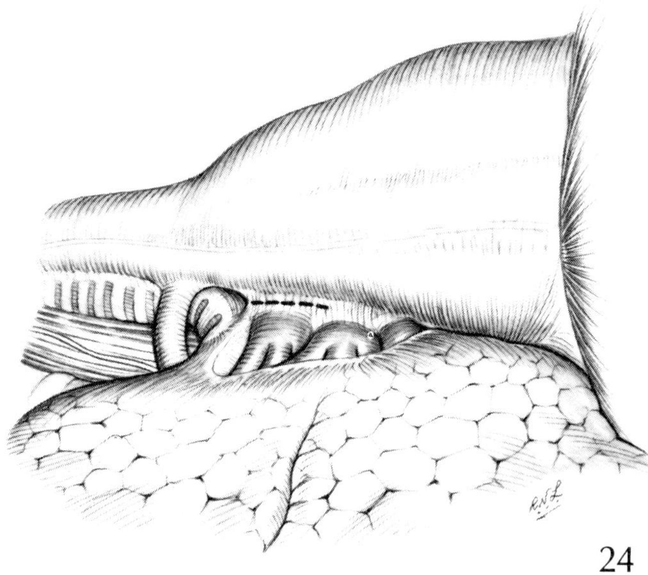

24

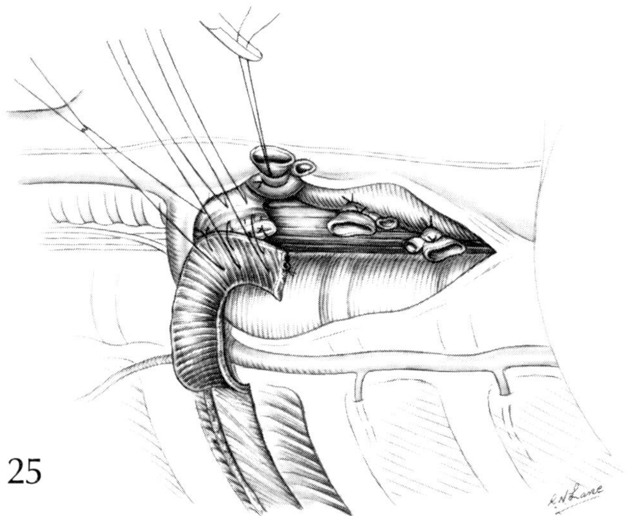

25

25

A bronchopleural fistula is almost unknown after left pneumonectomy but unfortunately occurs in a number of cases after right pneumonectomy, however careful the technique and even though care is taken to avoid a long bronchial stump. It is most likely to occur in those cases of advanced carcinoma in which there has been extensive excision of enlarged paratracheal glands and consequent impairment of blood supply to the sutured bronchus.

It is sometimes possible to cover the bronchial stump with adjacent pleura. A pedicled intercostal muscle bundle, with careful preservation of its blood supply, is recommended by some surgeons and is shown in this illustration. A second row of sutures is placed between the posterior border of the muscle bundle and the posterior edge of the sutured bronchus.

Right extended pneumonectomy (intrapericardial)

26

The lung is retracted posteriorly, the pericardium opened anterior to the superior pulmonary vein and the incision extended superiorly over the pulmonary artery towards the superior vena cava and inferiorly towards the pulmonary ligament. The veins are divided between two proximal ligatures and a distal clamp. The inferior vein is often best approached from below and behind (*see Illustration 13*). In some cases the growth will be so close to the atrium that it will be necessary, as in this illustration, to divide the common vein between a Satinsky clamp placed on the wall of the left atrium and two clamps (not shown) on the distal ends of the veins. The atrial wall is then closed with a continuous 3/0 Mersilene suture.

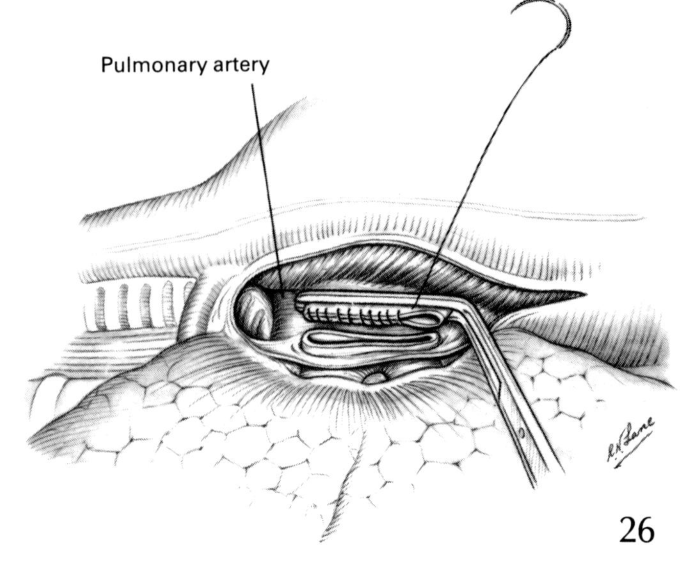

26

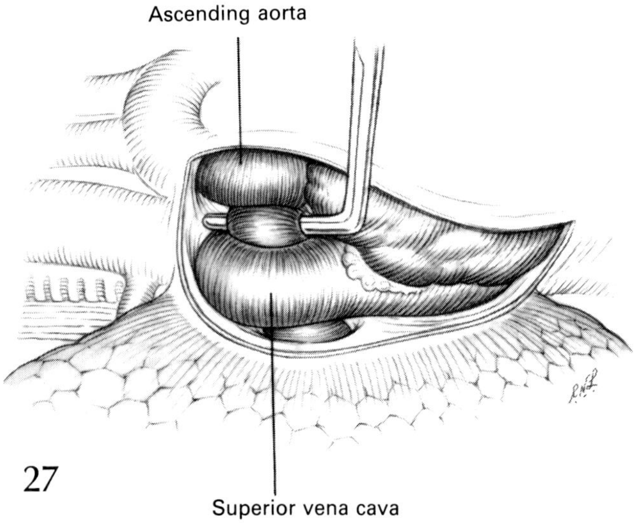

27

27

The right pulmonary artery is usually isolated and divided as shown in *Illustration 24*. It is possible, however, to ligate it *medial* to the superior vena cava and this may be necessary because of the extent of the growth. If the pulmonary artery is torn during its initial dissection, it may occasionally be life-saving. The superior vena cava is retracted laterally, horizontal incisions are made in the pericardium immediately above and below the pulmonary artery, and an O'Shaugnessy clamp can then be gently passed around the artery.

28

Once the artery and veins have been divided and the lung has been retracted anteriorly, the azygos vein is divided and the areolar tissue containing the paratracheal and pretracheal lymph nodes is removed completely, exposing the side of the trachea, the superior vena cava and the ascending aorta. The dissection is carried from the oesophagus behind to the internal mammary artery in front. The oesophagus is exposed posterior to the lung root and any lymph nodes are excised with the lung. The vagus nerve may need to be divided.

The main bronchus is then isolated and divided as already described.

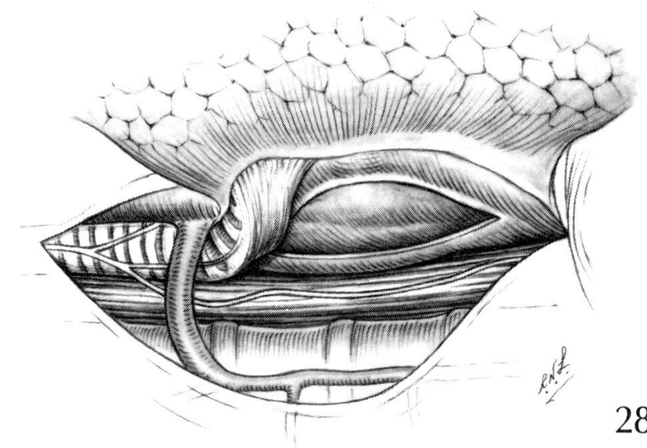

28

Drainage after pneumonectomy

There is a surprising difference of opinion amongst thoracic surgeons concerning the advisability of draining the pleural space after pneumonectomy, and at a recent meeting of the Society of Thoracic and Cardiovascular Surgeons of Great Britain and Ireland members were equally divided in their views. It is the author's opinion that a basal intercostal tube connected to an underwater seal should always be inserted after a pneumonectomy. This tube should be clamped but be released every hour for one minute only and the drainage noted. Suction must *never* be applied as this would lead to too much mediastinal displacement and cause hypotension by impairing venous return to the heart. The tube is removed after 24 hours. If this routine is used any postoperative haemorrhage will be obvious – this complication is not always easily diagnosed after pneumonectomy and patients who have not had a drain in place are known to have died without the cause being recognized. There is no risk of infection if the tube is removed after 24 hours and, moreover, the need for postoperative aspiration is avoided.

If the space is not drained the intrapleural pressure should be adjusted to a slightly negative level at the end of the operation by an intercostal catheter inserted through the third space anteriorly. This is then connected to an underwater seal and left in place until the patient has been placed on his back. It is then removed.

LOBECTOMY

Indications

Lobectomy is indicated in carcinoma of the bronchus if:

1. the growth is relatively peripheral and confined to one lobe (or middle and right lower lobe) – in the case of an upper lobe growth, especially on the right, it is possible to obtain almost as good a clearance of lymphatic glands as by pneumonectomy.
2. the patient is considered unfit for pneumonectomy because of age or impaired lung function.

The final decision whether to carry out a lobectomy or pneumonectomy must remain until the operation because the growth may be more extensive than anticipated.

Lobectomy is also carried out for bronchiectasis, lung abscess, benign tumours and other miscellaneous conditions.

Anatomy

The subsequent illustrations depict the anatomy of the vessels commonly found but there are many variations in the bronchovascular pattern, and these have been admirably described by Boyden[9]. All lung resections are 'voyages of discovery' with certain well-defined landmarks. Abnormal positions of the arterial and venous branches and tributaries are often encountered and it is always necessary to be prepared for this. It is most important to expose the hilar vessels adequately before any actual division is made in order to be sure which vessels lead to and from the part of the lung to be removed.

In all cases of lobectomy or segmental resection it is wise to request the anaesthetist to inflate the lung after the bronchus has been clamped and *before* it is divided to ensure that the proposed division is not too proximal – a mistake surprisingly easy to make.

Upper lobectomy is a more difficult operation than lower lobectomy because of the more complex arrangement of the upper lobe arterial branches as they leave the main arterial trunk and the close proximity of the superior pulmonary vein to the main pulmonary artery to the lower lobe (the 'upper lobectomy trap'). This artery lies immediately posterior to the vein, and damage to the artery will jeopardise the preservation of the lower lobe. The pulmonary vein, which lies in front of the hilum, should be divided first in cases of carcinoma, opening the pericardium if necessary.

Right upper lobectomy

29

The lobe is retracted posteriorly to expose the venous drainage. It is most important to preserve the middle lobe vein, which drains into the superior vein. The division of the veins to the upper lobe must therefore be distal to the middle lobe vein, which must first be identified. Division of these veins will expose the apical and anterior segmental arteries. These are divided. The posterior segmental artery to the upper lobe arises lower down below the upper lobe bronchus and often *quite close* to the middle lobe artery. It may not easily be visible until the bronchus has been divided. It is not visible in this illustration in which the veins to the upper lobe would usually have been divided *before* the arterial branches are ligated.

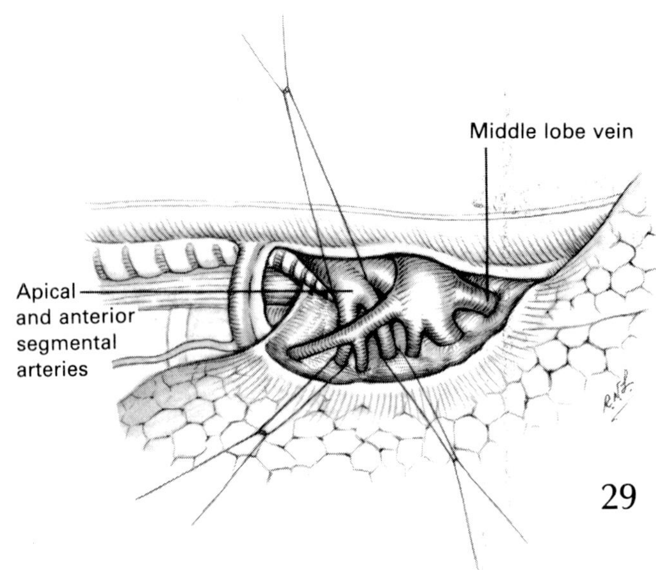

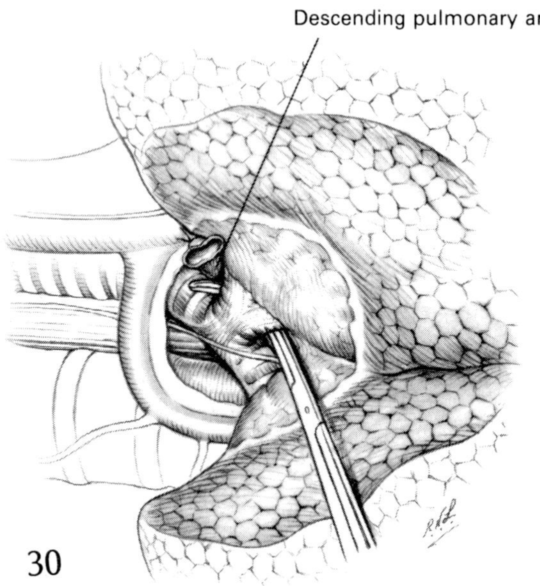

30

The lobe is retracted forwards to expose the upper lobe bronchus. Only two of the segmental divisions are visible. The margins of the bronchus are defined, the adventitia containing bronchial arteries is divided between clamps and the upper lobe bronchus is clamped with a non-crushing clamp. Note that the descending pulmonary artery is immediately anterior to the upper lobe bronchus.

31

The bronchus is divided close to the main bronchus but not so close that the lumen is narrowed. This is most important to prevent postoperative lower lobe collapse. The bronchial stump is closed as described under pneumonectomy, or with simple interrupted 2/0 Ethibond (Ethicon) sutures on a 25 mm half-circle eyeless needle. The *posterior segmental* arterial branch to the upper lobe is not visible – it is deep to the blades of the distal bronchial clamp and will become visible when traction is applied to this clamp.

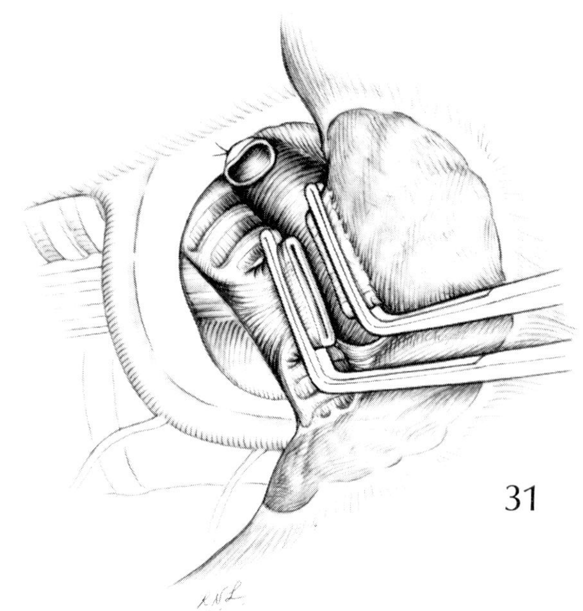

31

32

32

The hilar structures have now all been divided but the lobe may not yet be completely free – it may still be partially attached to the apex of the lower lobe and there may also be an incomplete fissure or no fissure between the upper and middle lobes. Any attachment to the apex of the lower lobe is managed by division of lung tissue between clamps. The apex of the lower lobe is closed with a continuous suture over the clamp. The lobe is then separated from the middle lobe by traction on the divided upper lobe bronchus and gentle blunt dissection with the index finger in the relatively avascular interlobar plane, as in segmental resection (*see Illustration 45*) commencing at the hilum and working towards the periphery. Inflation of the lung by the anaesthetist will help in the identification of the correct plane. Small air leaks and bleeding points are controlled by ligation. Finally the pulmonary ligament should be divided so as to allow the lower lobe to swing upwards to fill the upper part of the chest.

Left upper lobectomy

33

After division of the superior pulmonary vein (*see Illustration 12*) the lobe is retracted anteriorly to expose the arterial branches, of which there are three to five. These branches are divided separately. The lingular artery often arises from a basal branch to the lower lobe (as in this illustration) and not from the main artery itself. The division must therefore not be too proximal. The arterial branch to the apex of the lower lobe is visible *proximal* to the lingular branch.

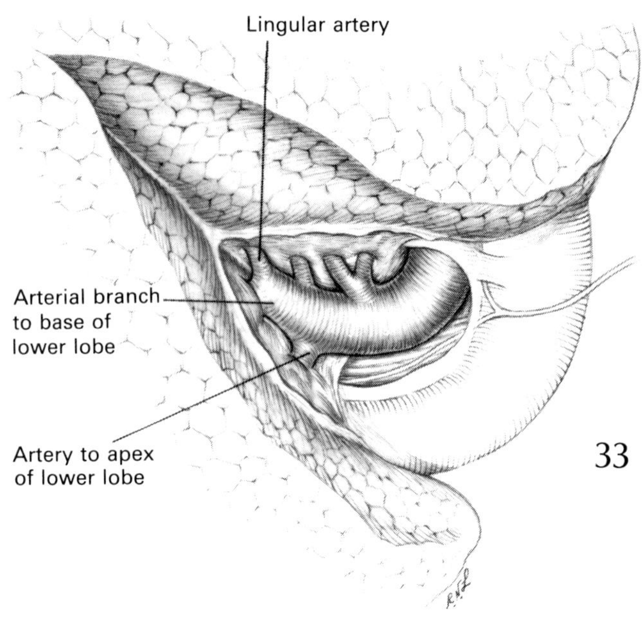

33

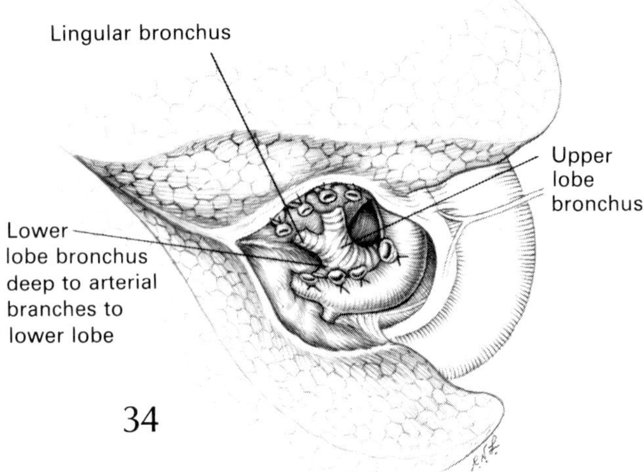

34

34

The artery to the lower lobe is retracted posteriorly to expose the upper lobe bronchus. The margins are defined, the adventitia containing bronchial arteries is divided between clamps and the upper lobe bronchus is clamped with a non-crushing clamp. The bronchus is divided and closed as described for right upper lobectomy. Any attachment to the apex of the lower lobe is managed by division of lung tissue between clamps. The apex of the lower lobe is then closed with a continuous suture over the clamp (*see Illustration 32*). Finally the pulmonary ligament should be divided to allow the lower lobe to swing upwards to fill the upper part of the chest.

Right lower lobectomy

The inferior vein should be divided first in resection for bronchial carcinoma. The lower lobe is retracted upwards and the pulmonary ligament divided between clamps. The vein is divided outside or inside the pericardium, as appropriate (*see Illustration 23*). The fissure between the two lobes should be exposed and developed if necessary to reveal the arterial branches to the lower lobe, which are situated in the depths of the fissure immediately overlying the bronchus. All the branches must be displayed before any division is carried out.

35

Care must be taken to preserve the right middle lobe artery, which arises opposite the artery to the apex of the lower lobe. There may be two branches. The arteries to the apex of the lower lobe and the basal segments must all be divided separately.

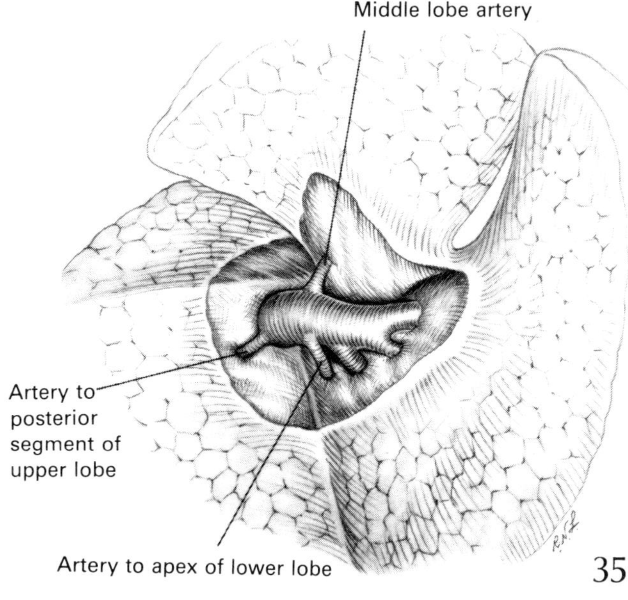

35

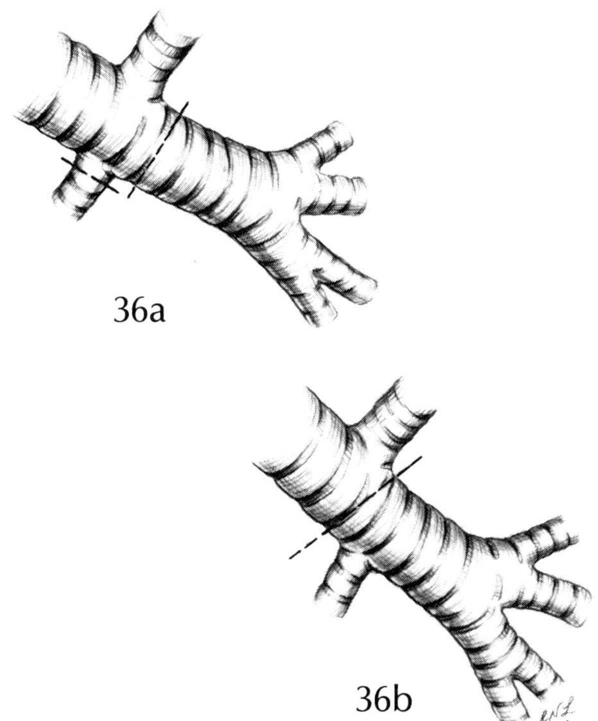
36a
36b

36a & b

The bronchus to the middle lobe must be preserved and not narrowed – it usually arises opposite the bronchus to the apical segment of the lower lobe. It is usually necessary to divide the apical lower segmental bronchus and the lower lobe bronchus separately (*a*). If the middle lobe bronchus is more proximal than usual this separate division may not be necessary (*b*).

If there is an incomplete fissure between the apex of the lower lobe and the upper lobe, the separation is as described for upper lobectomy (*see Illustration 32*).

Left lower lobectomy

37

The inferior vein and arterial branches to the lower lobe are divided as described for right lower lobectomy. Care must be taken to preserve the lingular artery, which may arise from a basal branch artery or from the main artery. It is never possible to ligate the artery to the lower lobe as a single trunk.

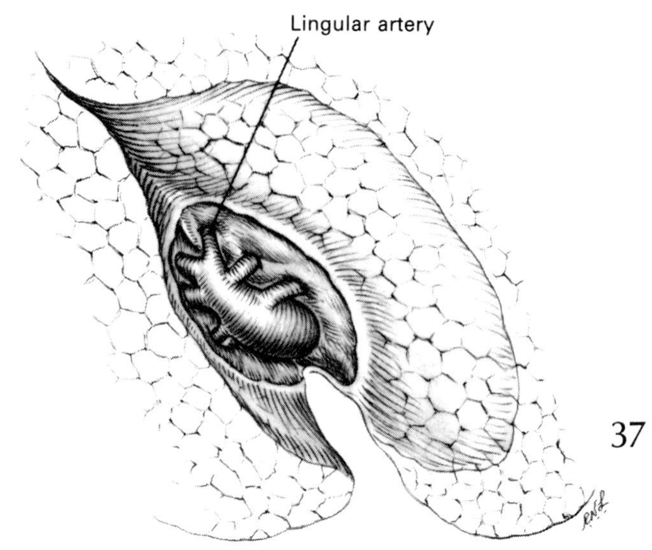

37

38

The bronchus is defined by dividing the peribronchial tissue containing the bronchial arteries. The pulmonary artery is retracted anteriorly so that the upper lobe bronchus is identified. This identification of the upper lobe is important to prevent narrowing of the upper lobe bronchus by too proximal application of the bronchus clamp or even division of the main bronchus itself. The lower lobe bronchus is then clamped and divided close to the upper lobe, taking care not to narrow the origin of the upper lobe bronchus. The bronchial stump is closed as in upper lobectomy. A suture line flush with the upper lobe is important – a long stump is the usual cause of a bronchopleural fistula.

If there is an incomplete fissure between the apex of the lower lobe and the upper lobe, the lobe is separated as described for upper lobectomy.

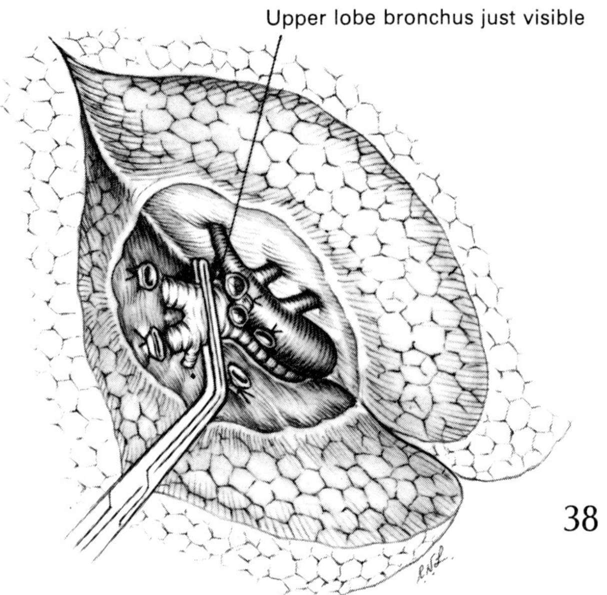

38

Middle lobectomy

The middle lobe is retracted posteriorly to expose the origin of the middle lobe vein, which is divided between ligatures close to its entry into the superior vein (*see Illustration 29*). The lobe is then retracted anteriorly, and the oblique and horizontal fissures between the upper, middle and lower lobes are developed to expose the arterial branches to the middle and lower lobes. The middle lobe is supplied by one or two arteries which pass anteriorly from the right main pulmonary artery opposite or just proximal to the branch to the apex of the lower lobe (*see Illustration 35*). The middle lobe artery is divided between ligatures and the middle lobe bronchus can then be seen and defined. It is divided and closed as in upper or lower lobectomy. The middle lobe can now be removed by traction on the middle lobe bronchus and gentle dissection with the index finger in the plane between the middle and upper lobes (see chapter on 'Segmental resection', pp. 85–88 in this chapter). Inflation of the upper lobe by the anaesthetist will help to define the correct plane. Small air leaks and bleeding points are controlled by ligatures.

Right lower and middle lobectomy

A right lower and middle lobectomy is frequently required for a carcinoma of the lower lobe which has extended to involve the middle lobe bronchus. It may also be required for bronchiectasis, which not infrequently involves both lobes. The technique for the venous and arterial ligation is as described for middle lobectomy and right lower lobectomy. The bronchial dissection is similar to a left lower lobectomy, i.e. the right upper lobe must be visualized before the bronchus clamp is applied so as to avoid a long bronchial stump or a narrowed right upper lobe bronchus.

SLEEVE RESECTION

Upper lobectomy with 'sleeve' resection of the main bronchus is a most valuable procedure in cases in which the growth involves the actual origin of the upper lobe bronchus at its junction with the main bronchus and where a standard upper lobectomy would not provide a complete removal of the growth. In these cases a 'sleeve' of main bronchus is removed with the upper lobe and the two ends of the main bronchus are re-anastomosed. This technique may be used for the left or right upper lobe, though it is technically more difficult on the left side because of the proximity of the aortic arch. The lymphatic drainage area can be removed as completely as by pneumonectomy. The technique is most valuable in older patients, or in younger patients with diminished respiratory reserve, in that it allows the tumour to be removed while preserving the right lower and middle lobes or left lower lobe. If necessary the resection may be extended to include a 'sleeve' of the main pulmonary artery. The final decision concerning the possibility of 'sleeve' resection must be taken at thoracotomy. The technique is best reserved for squamous carcinoma or for innocent tumours. It should not be used for anaplastic carcinoma.

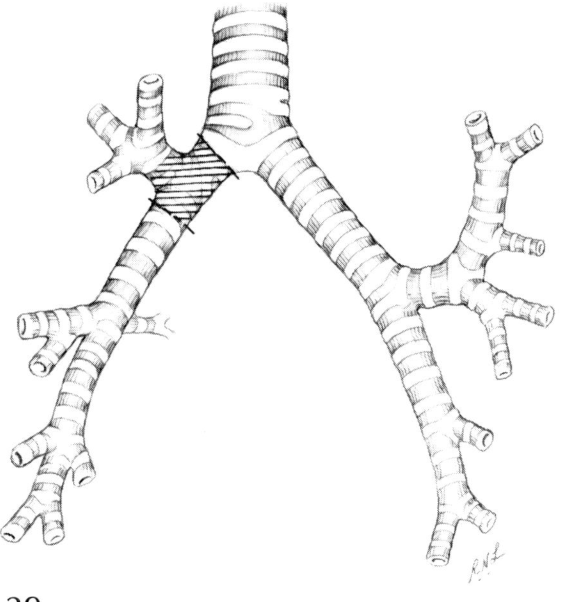

39

Right upper lobectomy with sleeve resection of main bronchus

39

Anaesthesia into the opposite lung must be by double-lumen tube. If the tumour is localized and it is decided that this technique can be carried out, the venous and arterial dissection is performed as already described. The shaded area represents the extent of resection of the main bronchus for a carcinoma at the origin of the right upper lobe bronchus. A standard right upper lobectomy could not be carried out as the site of division of the bronchus would be through tumour.

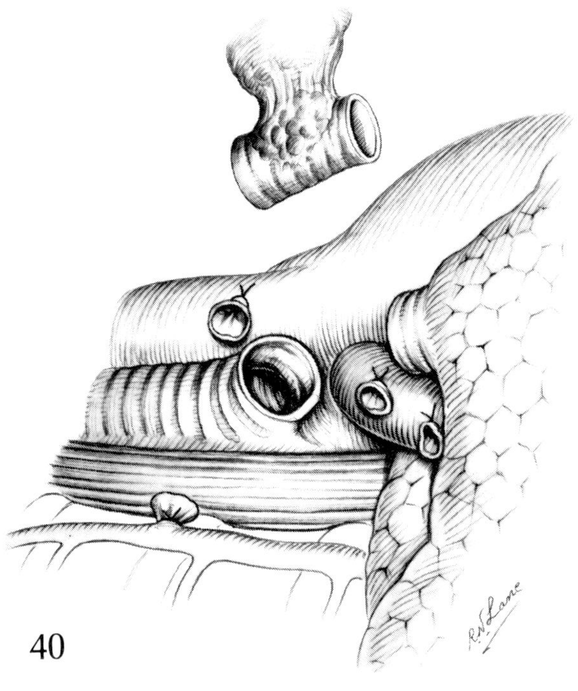

40

40

The arterial and venous dissection has already been completed. The azygos vein is divided. The pulmonary artery is separated by gentle finger dissection from the bronchus. A cylinder of main bronchus up to about 2.5 cm in length is isolated by division of the main bronchus proximally and distally. The proximal end of the bronchus may be left open but the distal portion should be temporarily occluded with ribbon gauze to prevent the entry of blood. The upper lobectomy may then be completed as already described. The lower and middle lobes must be mobilized by division of the pulmonary ligament.

41a & b

The two ends of the bronchus are anastomosed with interrupted 3/0 Ethibond on an atraumatic needle, with the knots on the outside of the bronchus. The sutures should be about 2 mm apart. Any discrepancy in size of the two portions of the bronchus can generally be overcome by placing the sutures closer together on the distal bronchus or by cutting the distal bronchus obliquely to increase its diameter. If this does not suffice, a wedge of main bronchus may be resected and a repair carried out as illustrated. Before final closure the lower lobe should be aspirated by a fine catheter. Airtight closure is easily obtained and the lower and middle lobes are readily inflated by the anaesthetist. A flap of pleura should be placed between the bronchus and pulmonary artery in order to prevent the rare but well-recognized late complication of secondary haemorrhage from the pulmonary artery.

Perhaps rather surprisingly there are no special immediate postoperative problems after this operation. The main late complication is a stricture at the site of the anastomosis, but the incidence of this is not high.

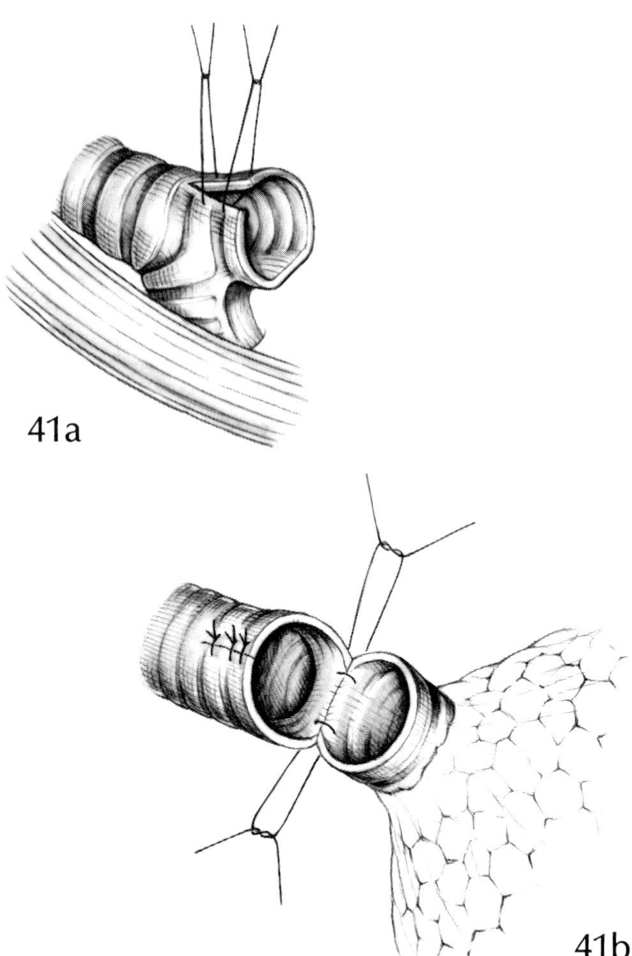

41a

41b

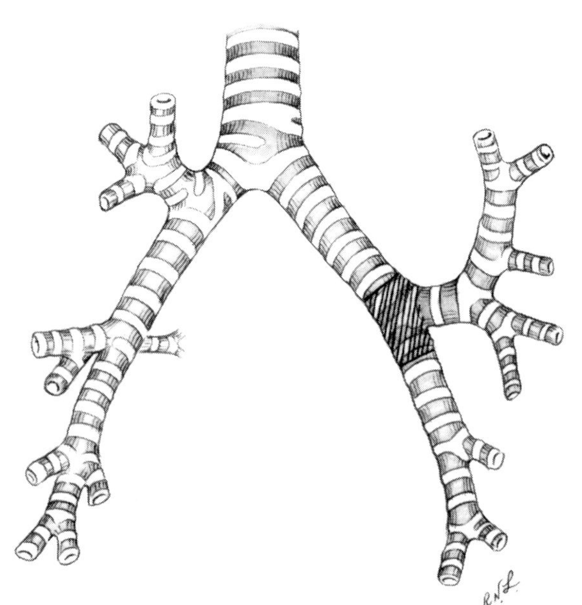

42

Left upper lobectomy with sleeve resection of main bronchus

42

The shaded area represents the extent of resection of the main bronchus for a carcinoma at the origin of the left upper lobe bronchus. The bronchial anastomosis is considerably more difficult on the left side because of the position of the aorta, but this may be retracted most efficiently by Cummings' shaped aortic retractor (G.U. Manufacturing Co. Ltd).

SEGMENTAL RESECTION OF LUNG

Any segment of the lung may be resected, though in the case of carcinoma it is the lingula or apical segment of the lower lobe that is most commonly removed[10], especially in the case of a localized peripheral tumour in an elderly patient with poor respiratory function. Other conditions requiring segmental resection are bronchiectasis, innocent tumours and congenital abnormalities.

General principles of segmental resection

Each bronchopulmonary segment has its own individual artery and bronchus. The vein runs *between* the segments in the intersegmental plane, receiving tributaries from both adjacent segments. When a segment is to be resected the appropriate segmental artery and bronchus are divided at the hilum. A clamp is then placed on the distal end of the bronchus. The segment can be separated from the adjacent lung by traction on this bronchus and gentle dissection with the index finger from the hilum outwards in the relatively avascular intersegmental plane. The correct plane is shown by the line of the intersegmental vein, which must remain in place undisturbed. Its tributaries from the segment to be removed are divided. Inflation of the remainder of the lung by increased endotracheal pressure will assist in defining the correct line of separation.

There is only minimal air leak from the damaged alveoli and these soon seal off with swab pressure. Very little, if any, lung suture is required. The raw surface of the lung should not be oversewn, as any attempt to do this will only increase the air leak. The bronchial stump is closed by an 'open' technique with two or three simple stainless steel or Ethiflex sutures.

Excision of apical and posterior segments of left upper lobe (apicoposterior segmental resection)

These two segments are a frequent site for tuberculosis and before the advent of modern antituberculous chemotherapy apicoposterior segmentectomy was a commonly performed operation. Although now rarely performed, it will be described in detail to show the principles of segmental resection.

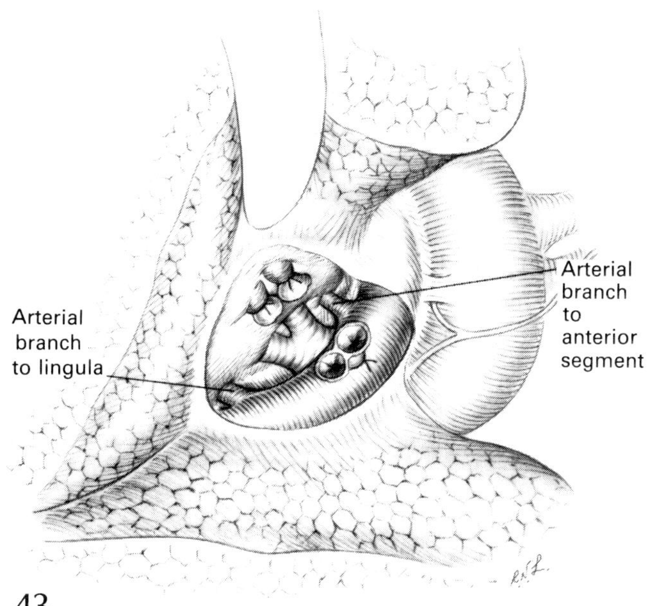

43

43

The lung is approached from above and behind, as in left upper lobectomy. The pulmonary artery and its branches are exposed. The most proximal branch supplies the anterior segment. The next two branches have been identified as those supplying the segments to be removed and have therefore been divided. The fourth (undivided) branch can be seen passing inferiorly to the lingula.

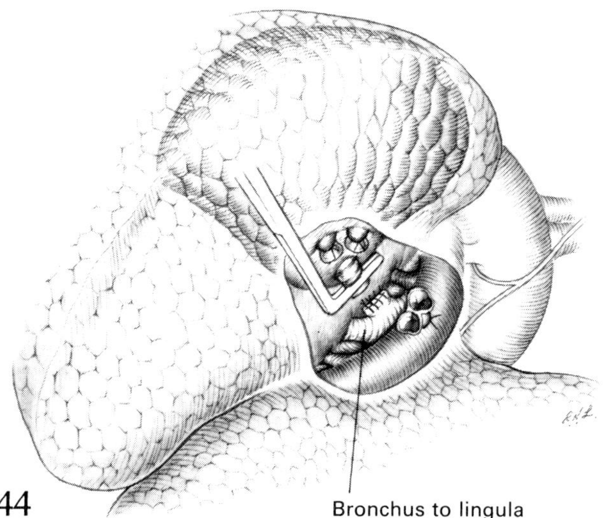

44

44

The apical and posterior segmental bronchi usually arise from a single branch of the left upper lobe (*see Illustration 1*). This must be identified first by palpation and then by dissection deep to the divided arteries. It is advisable to confirm its identity by clamping the bronchus with a non-crushing clamp and requesting the anaesthetist to inflate the lung. The lack of aeration will usually be obvious, though transsegmental 'air drift' may make this less clear. Once the bronchus has been identified, it is clamped distally, divided, and closed by an 'open' technique with simple interrupted sutures. It is important to appreciate the close proximity of the anterior segmental bronchus, which is easily damaged if the apicoposterior bronchus is divided too close to its origin. In this illustration the anterior segmental bronchus is deep to the sutured bronchus and not visible.

45

Once the arterial branches and bronchus have been divided, the correct plane for separation is identified by gentle traction on the bronchus clamp, possibly assisted by the anaesthetist applying gentle positive pressure. The separation is further assisted by gentle sideways movement of the pulp of the index finger. The correct plane is indicated by the intersegmental vein, which should remain undisturbed on the raw surface of the segment which is not being removed.

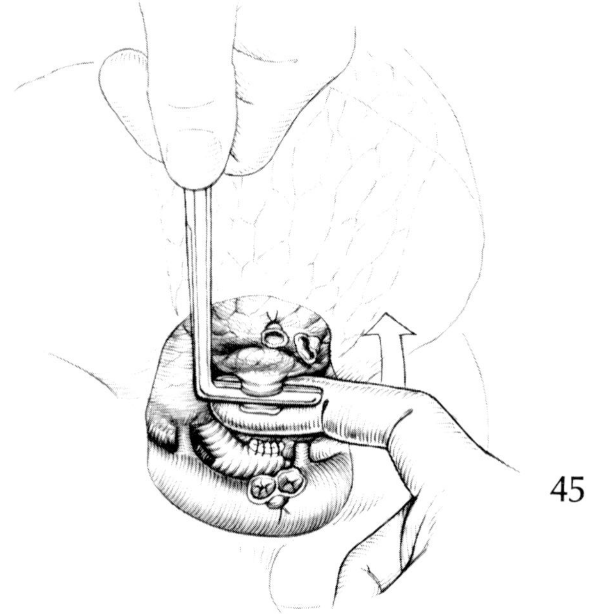

45

46

The separation is further helped by placing the hand under the segments to be removed and applying traction on the bronchus while at the same time applying gentle finger pressure to the plane of cleavage, making sure to leave the intersegmental vein intact. A few tributaries of the intersegmental vein require ligation and division.

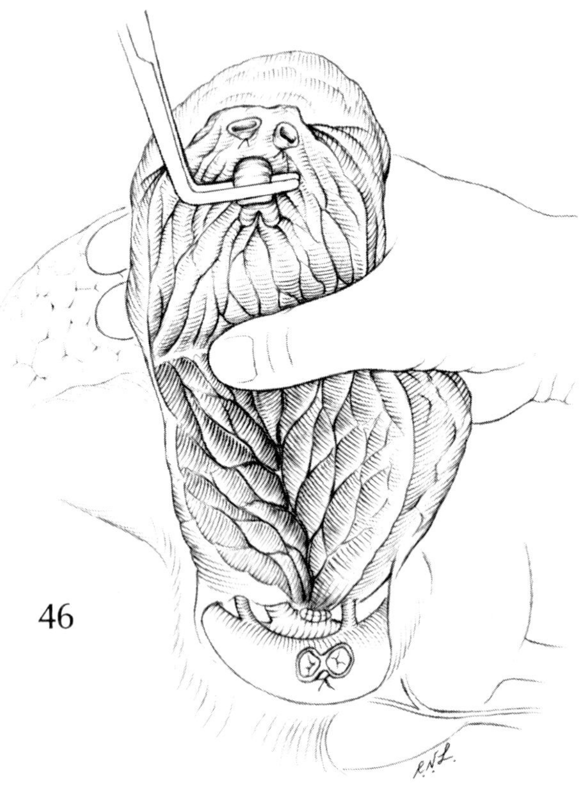

46

47

The segments being removed are now held only by the visceral pleura, which should be cut with scissors. Bubbles show the site of a small air leak from the remainder of the upper lobe – this will cease with pressure from a swab.

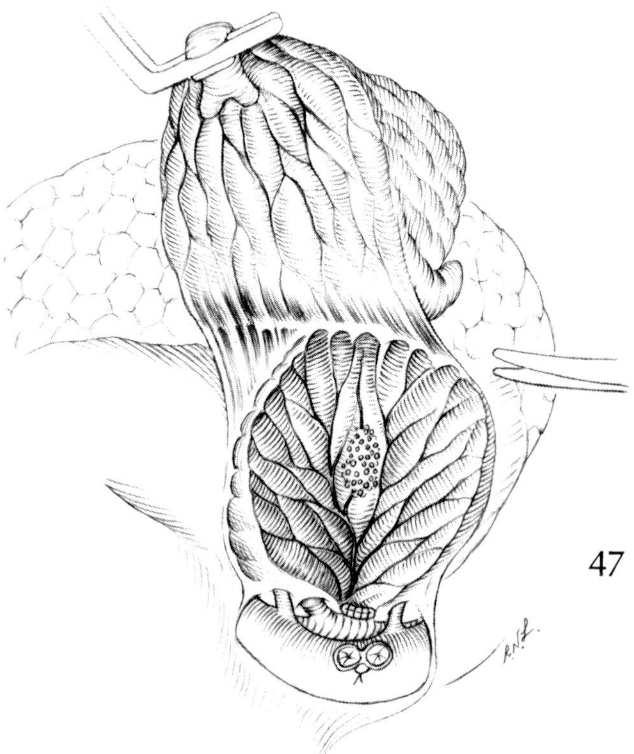

47

48

Sometimes an air leak from a bronchiole will require suture. The anaesthetist should inflate the lung fully to test for any other air leaks, but unless these are very large they will usually close during the first 48 hours after operation by the raw surface of the segment adhering to the parietal pleura or adjacent lung. It is unwise to suture the edges of the raw surface of the lung together as this will inevitably cause *increased* air leak.

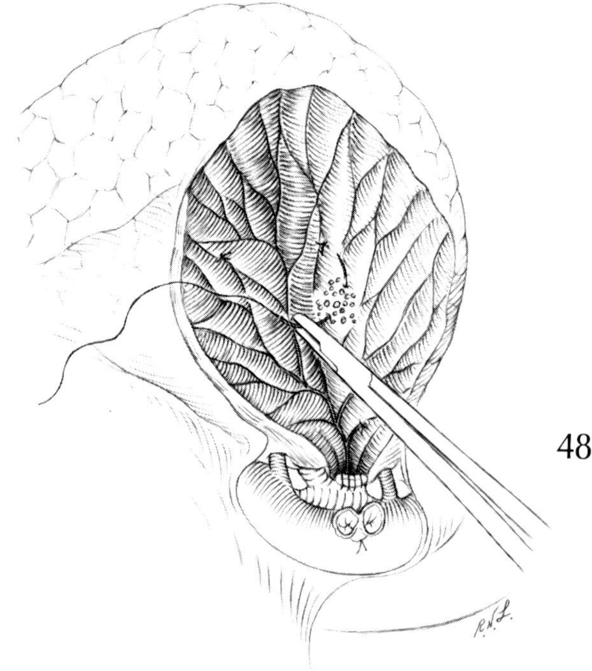

48

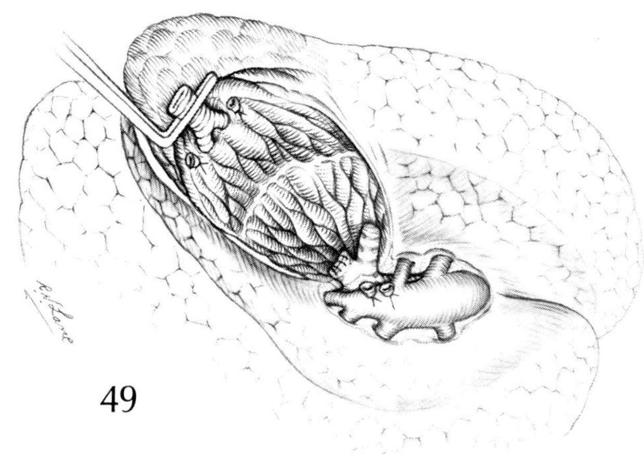

49

49

Lingulectomy

The lingular vein (situated anteriorly) is divided before the lingular artery and the origin of the lingular bronchus is then defined. It is the first inferior branch of the upper lobe bronchus (*see Illustration 1*). The lingular bronchus is divided and traction on the distal end, combined with finger dissection in the intersegmental plane, will complete the segmentectomy. In this illustration two arterial branches to the lingula are shown and have been divided.

50

Removal of apical segment of left lower lobe

The segmental vein is situated posteriorly (*see Illustration 13*). It usually drains into the inferior vein but may enter the pericardium separately. The artery is approached through the oblique fissure and divided (it has immediately divided into two branches in this illustration). The segmental bronchus will be seen immediately underneath. This too is divided and the segmentectomy completed as previously described.

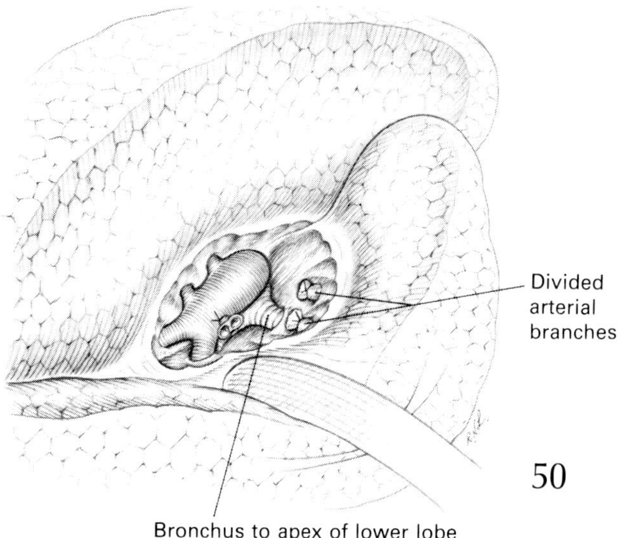

50

51

Removal of posterior segment of right upper lobe

The upper lobe bronchus is approached from behind after separating the upper and lower lobes. Its posterior division is identified by palpation and then by dissection. In this illustration, in which only the posterior and anterior segmental branches of the upper lobe bronchus are visible, a clamp has been passed under the posterior segmental bronchus. The posterior segmental artery arises as the most distal of the upper lobe branches of the main pulmonary artery, often quite close to the middle lobe artery. It has already been divided.

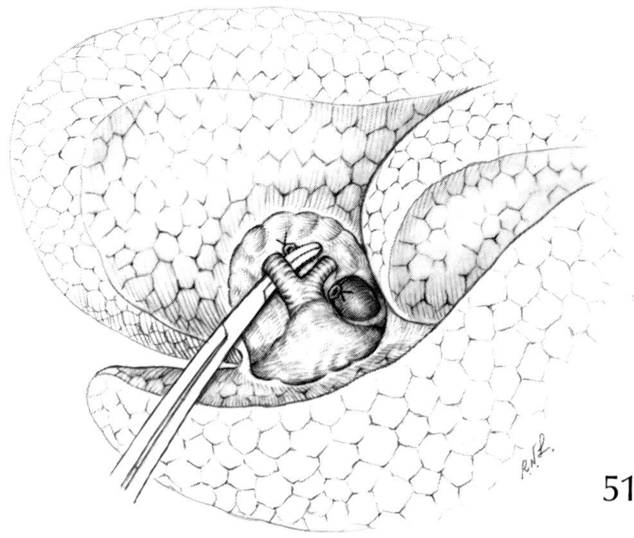

51

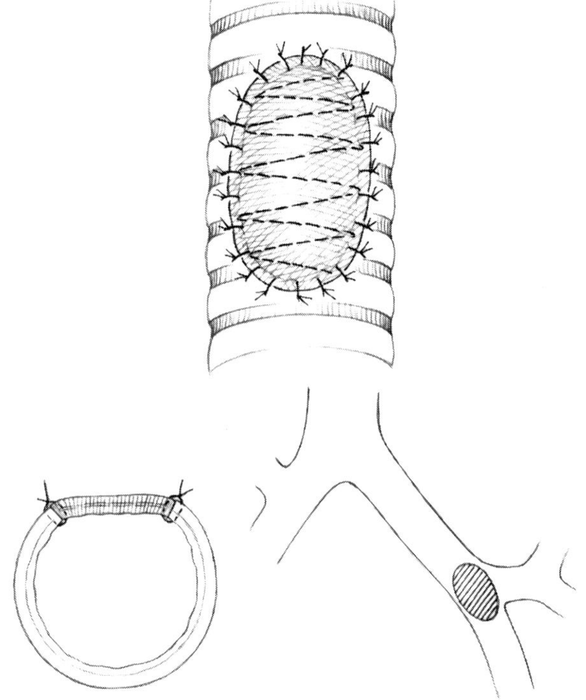

52

52

Gebauer skin graft

The use of a Gebauer skin graft[11], first described for the treatment of tuberculous strictures of the trachea and bronchi in 1950, is a valuable bronchoplastic technique for the local resection of benign bronchial tumours. The graft is full thickness skin and is taken from the edge of the thoracotomy wound. Fatty tissue is removed from the posterior surface and the graft is cut slightly larger than the defect in the bronchus to be closed. This is important as otherwise stenosis will occur later. The graft is strengthened by a lattice work of No.2 SWG stainless steel wire through its thickness and then sutured in place with interrupted 3/0 Mersilene sutures, with the epidermis inside. These grafts regain a blood supply and remain as viable tissue. The adjacent bronchial epithelium grows over the inner surface of the graft and the hair follicles gradually disappear.

Postoperative care

After lobectomy or segmental resection it is most important to obtain early expansion of the remainder of the lung. It is also vital to prevent tracheobronchial infection and its sequelae by enthusiastic and efficient physiotherapy. The following measures are important.

1. *Expectoration* must be actively encouraged, verbally as well as by manual support of the chest on the side of operation. If the sputum is thick and tenacious, 4-hourly inhalations of menthol, Friar's Balsam, or in severe cases tyloxapol (Alevaire), are advisable. A mucolytic agent such as bromhexine hydrochloride (Bisolvon) is also very useful.
2. *Analgesics* will relieve thoracotomy pain and increase the effectiveness of expectoration. But excessive analgesia must be avoided as this will reduce the cough reflex and lead to sputum retention and lobar collapse.
3. *Postural drainage ('tipping')* should be carried out for one-half to one hour three times daily immediately after inhalations, or more often if expectoration of sputum is inadequate.
4. *Antibiotic cover* is generally given for 10 days, as so often patients undergoing lung resection have associated chronic bronchitis. The sputum must be sent for bacteriological examination and the antibiotic changed if necessary. Chloramphenicol is often life-saving in elderly patients.
5. *Ambulation* is encouraged and the patient should be allowed out of bed on the second or third day, even though chest drainage tubes are still in place.
6. *Chest tube management* will depend on postoperative progress. The apical and basal drainage tubes drain air and blood-stained fluid respectively. They are both connected to suction via underwater drainage bottles. They should remain in place for a varying number of days, depending on the amount of drainage and the radiographic appearances.

Complications

1. *Sputum retention.* Collapse-consolidation of a lobe or lung, together with diffuse bronchopneumonia, will occur if expectoration of sputum is inadequate. This will lead to respiratory insufficiency and general weakness, which in turn will cause increased difficulty in expectoration. Bronchoscopy must be carried out, and if this has to be repeated frequently a tracheostomy will be necessary. A recent innovation is a minitracheostomy in which a small suction tube is inserted through the cricothyroid membrane[12].
2. *Atrial fibrillation.* Many patients over the age of 50 years will develop atrial fibrillation during the first 10 days after lung resection, especially if the pericardium has been opened. If the heart rate is fast, a shock-like condition may occur. The irregularity should be confirmed by electrocardiography and requires urgent digitalization.
3. *Bronchospasm.* This is best treated by ephedrine, salbutamol (Ventolin) or hydrocortisone.
4. *Surgical emphysema.* Surgical emphysema will occur if the drainage tubes become kinked or blocked or if the air leak from the raw surface of the lung is greater than the suction pump can handle. The tube must either be made patent or replaced by a new tube, or the sucker must be removed to allow the free escape of air through the bottle.
5. *Haemorrhage.* If this is severe, the chest must be reopened to secure haemostasis.

Late complications

Empyema after lobectomy or segmentectomy

The diagnosis will be suspected by the onset of fever and radiological evidence of increased fluid, aspiration of which will reveal its purulent nature. The empyema should be drained by rib resection. An empyema may be associated with a bronchopleural fistula. This should be suspected if the patient is expectorating blood-stained purulent sputum and may be confirmed by the injection of methylene blue into the empyema and its subsequent appearance in the sputum. The fistula will usually close spontaneously once the empyema is drained and the lung expands.

Post-pneumonectomy empyema

This complication may or may not be associated with a bronchopleural fistula. If there is no fistula an attempt should be made to sterilize the empyema cavity by daily aspiration and instillation of the appropriate antibiotic. The initial aspiration should be through a thoracoscope in order to remove all infected fluid and fibrin. After 14 days the interval between aspirations can be increased, provided the fluid remains sterile. Frequently, however, a permanent rib resection drainage is required as it may be impossible to sterilize the cavity. In some cases a thoracotomy and evacuation of the pneumonectomy space will result in permanent sterility of the space. After several months it may be wise to obliterate the pneumonectomy space by an extensive lateral thoracoplasty.

If associated with a bronchopleural fistula, the empyema should be drained by rib resection followed about 6 months later, when the infection has subsided and if the patient is fit enough, by a lateral thoracoplasty (with preservation of the first rib) together with a modified Roberts' flap operation in which the decostalized chest wall is sutured on to the open bronchial stump. Complete healing usually occurs within a few weeks.

Post-pneumonectomy bronchopleural fistula

This complication is extremely serious and very often requires permanent tube or stoma drainage of the pneumonectomy space, and may even lead to death. The pneumonectomy space may or may not be infected. The fistula almost always occurs on the right side, usually in those cases in which the blood supply to the bronchial stump has been reduced by the removal of enlarged paratracheal lymph nodes. Most often a fistula occurs 7–21 days after operation but it may occur after several months.

The sudden expectoration of blood-stained sputum, exacerbated by the patient lying towards the contralateral side and dramatically relieved by the patient lying on the pneumonectomy side, is diagnostic of this complication. The development of a fistula is a surgical emergency and it is vital for the patient to be instructed to lie on the pneumonectomy side until the pleural space is evacuated, either by intercostal tube or thoracoscopic suction. If the diagnosis is in doubt, methylene blue should be injected into the pneumonectomy space – its appearance in the sputum will be diagnostic.

The management of the fistula depends on whether the pleural fluid is sterile. In addition, bronchoscopy should be performed if the fistula has occurred late in order to exclude recurrence of the carcinoma. *If the fluid is sterile* the bronchus should be resutured. As the patient will be in the lateral position, it is most important to prevent aspiration of fluid into the remaining lung. It is dangerous to rely on a cuffed endobronchial tube to prevent this happening, however expert and persuasive the anaesthetist. The only safe procedure is to aspirate the pneumonectomy space dry through a thoracoscope immediately before thoracotomy in the operating theatre, with the patient in the sitting position. This will prevent any possibility of aspiration of fluid and a consequent inhalation pneumonitis in the remaining lung.

The pneumonectomy space is opened, fibrin and blood clot are removed and the fistula is identified. The bronchial stump must be mobilized and closed as described in the chapter on 'Bronchopleural fistula', pp. 204–209.

If the fluid is infected an attempt to resuture the bronchus will almost inevitably fail. In addition the thoracotomy wound itself will become infected. The empyema should initially be drained by rib resection. About 6 months later, when the infection has subsided, an extensive lateral thoracoplasty (with preservation of the first rib) should be performed, together with a modified Roberts' flap operation in which the decostalized portion of chest wall is sutured on to the open bronchial stump. In many cases complete healing of the fistula will eventually occur.

If a recurrence of carcinoma at the bronchial stump is the cause of the fistula, treatment can only be palliative and directed towards the prevention of aspiration of infected pleural fluid into the contralateral lung. A rib resection drainage should be carried out. Radiotherapy is not advisable.

References

1. Levison, V. What is the best treatment for early operable small cell carcinoma of the bronchus? Thorax 1980; 35: 721–724
2. Shore, D. F. E. and Paneth, M. Survival after resection of small cell carcinoma of the bronchus. Thorax 1980; 35: 819–822
3. Bates, M. Surgical treatment of bronchial carcinoma. Annals of the Royal College of Surgeons 1981: 63: 164–167
4. Belcher, J. R. Lobectomy for bronchial carcinoma. Lancet 1959; 2: 639–642
5. Flavell, G. Conservatism in surgical treatment of bronchial carcinoma – a review of 826 personal operations. British Medical Journal 1962; 1: 284–287
6. Bates, M. Segmental resection for bronchial carcinoma. Thorax 1975; 30: 235
7. Saunders, K. B. The assessment of respiratory function. British Journal of Hospital Medicine 1975; 14: 228–238
8. Thoracic Society of Great Britain. The nomenclature of broncho-pulmonary anatomy. Thorax 1950; 5: 222–228
9. Boyden, E. A. Segmental anatomy of the lungs: a study of the patterns of the segmental bronchi and related pulmonary vessels. New York: McGraw-Hill, 1955
10. Le Roux, B. T. Management of bronchial carcinoma by segmental resection. Thorax 1972; 27: 70–74
11. Gebauer, P. W. Reconstructive surgery of the trachea and bronchi: late results with dermal grafts. Journal of Thoracic Surgery 1951; 22: 568–584
12. Matthews, H. R. and Hopkinson, R. B. Treatment of sputum retention by minitracheotomy. British Journal of Surgery 1984; 71: 147–150

Surgical treatment of achalasia of the cardia

Diffuse oesophageal spasm ('corkscrew oesophagus') and periphrenic diverticulum

A. W. Jowett FRCS
Consultant Thoracic Surgeon, The Royal Hospital, Wolverhampton, UK

ACHALASIA OF THE CARDIA

Preoperative

Diagnosis

Though barium swallow examination usually confirms clinical suspicion, manometric tests should be performed to demonstrate the motility disorder; these are essential in mild or early cases.

Oesophagoscopy should be carried out to exclude a carcinoma, either one involving the cardia and mimicking the X-ray appearance of achalasia or one which has already developed in the dilated oesophagus above. In all but the mildest cases the oesophagus contains a large volume of secretions and decomposing food. Rigid rather than fibreoptic endoscopy allows this to be cleared with large-bore suction. Washing out is often necessary. Anaesthetic induction should be in the semi-sitting position to reduce overspill risks, and, for the same reason, the cuff of the endotracheal tube should be inflated except at the moment of introduction of the rigid oesophagoscope. The oesophageal mucosa is often inflamed. The cardia is usually further from the incisor teeth than normal for the patient's size. However, if long enough, the oesophagoscope can usually be passed into the stomach without encountering much resistance or requiring dilatation, especially if a small bougie is used to indicate the forward direction to be followed.

Indications

Surgery is indicated in all cases except when the general condition and especially when respiratory function is poor and cannot be adequately improved. In these, daily self-bouginage using a Hurst mercury bougie may be considered. Older endoscopic procedures aimed at rupturing the circular muscle at the cardia, using instruments such as Plummer's hydrostatic bag or the Henning dilator, cannot be recommended. Newer instruments for forceful dilatation which can be introduced using a fibreoptic instrument without general anaesthesia have still not been fully assessed but may prove to have a place in a few high-risk patients.

Heller's myotomy is, however, the treatment for all uncomplicated cases but must always be accompanied by a definitive hiatus hernia repair to prevent the risk of subsequent complications from gastro-oesophageal reflux. In cases with gross megaoesophagus or where, for some other reason, a previous Heller's operation has failed, partial or total excision of the thoracic oesophagus should be considered. Direct anastomosis between the dilated oesophagus and the fundus of the stomach must never be contemplated as this must always result in severe reflux.

The cross-reference in this chapter refers to *Operative Surgery: Thoracic Surgery, 4th Edition*

HELLER'S MYOTOMY

The operation consists of complete division of the circular muscle at the oesophagogastric junction.

The length of this division must always be adequate. Below, it should extend for a short distance onto the stomach, and above, it should be continued until no more hypertrophied muscle is encountered. In cases which show little muscle hypertrophy, the myotomy should extend for at least 7 cm up the oesophagus.

A thoracic, thoracoabdominal or entirely abdominal approach can be used. For the majority of cases, the operator should select the approach normally preferred for repair of the hiatus. However, the exposure obtained by thoracotomy is the most satisfactory and always allows upward extension of the myotomy if necessary. In the rare case of achalasia associated with an elevated cardia the thoracic approach is essential.

Preoperative preparation

Even in cases with little oesophageal dilatation, careful clinical and radiological assessment should be made to estimate the degree of 'overspill pneumonitis'. When the oesophagus is large and oesophagoscopy reveals much debris, this should be cleared completely, washing out if necessary. Following this, the patient should be allowed a fluid diet only and must not be allowed to sleep flat. Physiotherapy and appropriate antibiotic treatment may be required for some time before the pneumonitis is adequately controlled.

The operation

Care should again be exercised during the anaesthetic induction. Oesophagoscopy is performed to clean the oesophagus thoroughly.

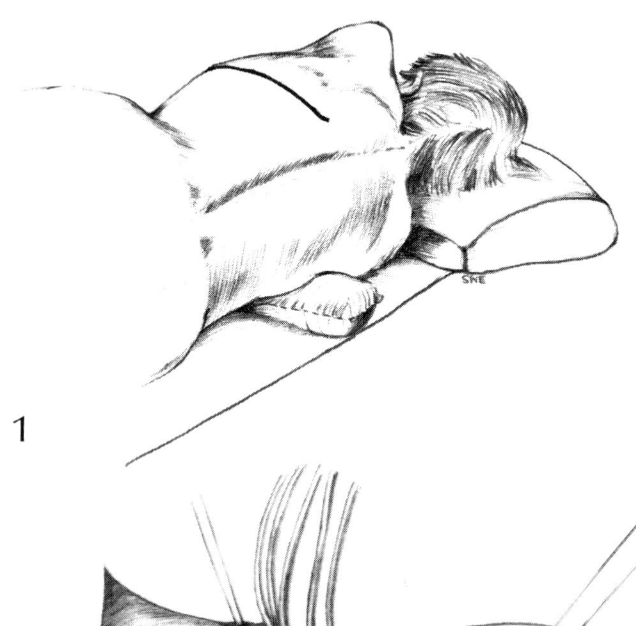

1

1

For the thoracic approach, the patient is allowed to roll about 15° forwards from a true lateral position. This allows good exposure from a higher and therefore less painful thoracotomy. A sandbag is placed under the lower ribs.

2

2

Exposure of lower end of the oesophagus

The thorax has been opened by stripping the periosteum from the upper border of the left seventh rib. The pleura over the lower oesophagus is incised vertically and carefully dissected to form flaps for subsequent reconstitution.

3

Mobilization of oesophagus, cardia and upper stomach

Dissecting with care to avoid the adjacent right pleura, the oesophagus is lifted out of its bed and a tape passed round it. Further dissection around the hiatal margin allows the cardia and some stomach to be pulled up into view. Any fat in this area is carefully removed and the vessels always present just below the cardia are identified, ligated and divided to allow access in the line of the proposed myotomy.

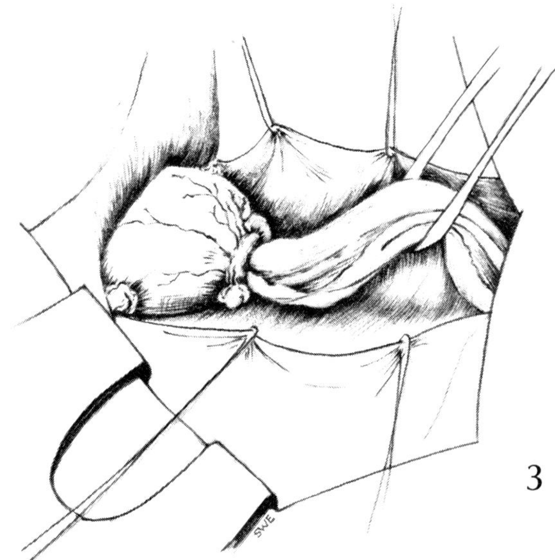

3

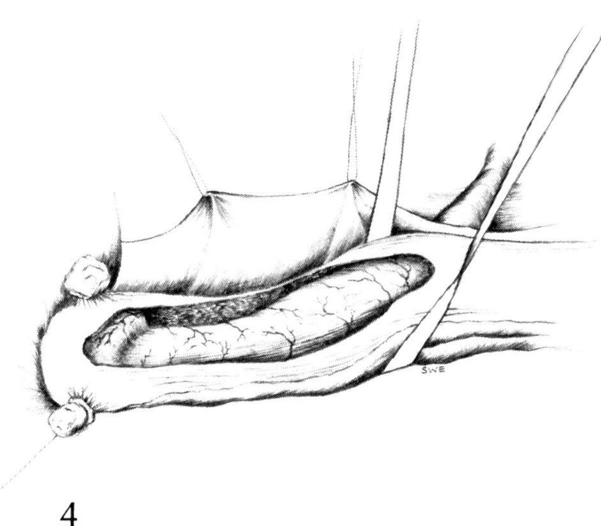

4

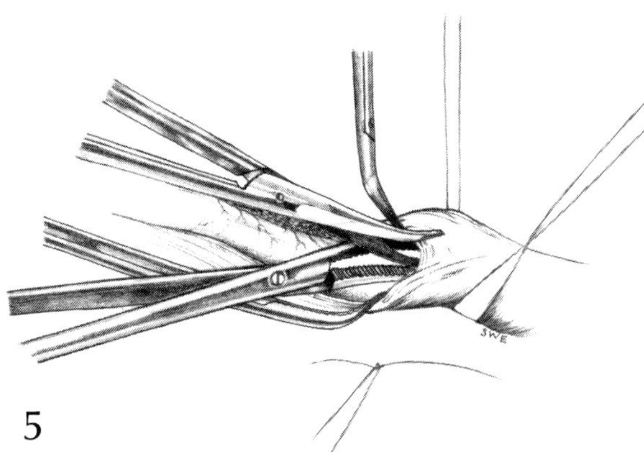

5

4 & 5

Division of the muscle

The incision along the line of the oesophagus, avoiding the vagal nerves, should be started some distance above the oesophagogastric junction. It is deepened until the mucosa is exposed. The submucosal venous plexus is a guide to this plane. At this stage diathermy must be avoided because of the risk of mucosal damage. Once identified, this plane is followed downwards across the junction onto stomach for a short distance. Here, at the oesophagogastric junction, the risk of opening the mucosa is greatest. The incision is then extended upwards on the oesophagus until the circular muscle no longer appears hypertrophied. Unless circular muscle hypertrophy is obviously extending higher than this, upward myotomy can be stopped at the level of the inferior pulmonary vein.

Holding up the cut muscle edges with forceps, a third pair of forceps can be used to extend the plane between the mucosa and the circular muscle and this facilitates safe muscle division. The use of scissors rather than a knife decreases the risk of mucosal damage.

It is unwise to have an oesophageal tube *in situ* during the myotomy as this may also increase the risk of opening the mucosa. However, a tube gently introduced at this stage by the anaesthetist will demonstrate the finest fibres of any residual circular muscle requiring division. Accidental perforation of the mucosa is immediately obvious and should be carefully repaired using fine interrupted sutures, and the postoperative regimen will require modification.

HIATUS HERNIA REPAIR

A formal hiatus hernia procedure will guard against reflux complications and does not appear to impede oesophageal emptying. The thoracic approach for Heller's myotomy described allows a Belsey type of operation (see chapter on 'Thoracic repair of hiatus hernia', pp. 286–291) to be performed which has the additional possibility of placing the cardia well below the hiatus. This helps to correct the often sigmoid deformity of the usually elongated oesophagus which will further assist oesophageal emptying. However, because the myotomy lays bare the mucosa on the front of the oesophagus, only the medial and lateral pairs of mattress sutures can be inserted.

Reconstitution of the pleura

The pleural flaps are approximated with interrupted sutures. A single intercostal tube is inserted and the sandbag removed before closure of the chest.

Postoperative care

Prevention of chest complications

Because of chronic lung damage from overspill, special care needs to be taken. Certainly if it was considered necessary during the preoperative preparation, appropriate antibiotic cover should be continued after surgery. The intercostal tube can usually be removed on the day following operation.

Resumption of feeding

Oral fluids can normally be started on the day following operation. However, if the mucosa has been damaged and repaired, antibiotics should be given, the intercostal tube should be kept in for longer and oral intake delayed until mucosal integrity has been checked radiographically on the fifth to seventh day.

Follow-up

Though swallowing is greatly improved after Heller's myotomy it must be remembered that achalasia is a disease which affects more of the oesophagus than just the cardia. Oesophageal motility remains abnormal and a megaoesophagus does not return to normal size.

Also, it appears that an adequate Heller's operation does not overcome the predisposition of achalasia patients to develop oesophageal carcinoma later. Even with diligent and extended follow-up a carcinoma developing in a megaoesophagus is almost always inoperable by the time symptoms suggest investigation.

DIFFUSE OESOPHAGEAL SPASM ('Corkscrew oesophagus')

Diagnosis

Barium swallow examination suggests the condition and frequently also demonstrates the presence of a hiatus hernia with gastro-oesophageal reflux. Manometric studies in a specialist unit and other oesophageal function studies are essential before considering surgical intervention.

Surgical treatment

This should be considered only when the symptoms are very severe and do not respond to a strict medical hiatus hernia regimen. Some cases may benefit from repair of the hiatus hernia. In others an extended Heller's myotomy is indicated. The upward extent of muscle division is indicated by the manometric test findings. The technique is similar to that described for the standard myotomy and, again, an efficient repair of the hiatus must be carried out.

PERIPHRENIC DIVERTICULUM

Should the symptoms from a periphrenic diverticulum of the oesophagus indicate the need for surgical intervention, simple excision of the diverticulum alone is liable to be followed by breakdown of the suture line. A Heller's myotomy at the cardia should always be carried out to prevent this complication.

Further reading

Harley, H. R. S. Achalasia of the Cardia. Bristol: John Wright, 1978

Pulsion intubation of the oesophagus

I. Barnett Angorn FRCS(Ed), FRCS
Professor of Surgery, University of Natal, Durban, South Africa

Introduction

Peroral pulsion intubation is used almost exclusively for the palliation of dysphagia due to malignant obstruction of the oesophagus and cardia. The technique is preferable to traction intubation which requires laparotomy and gastrotomy with an increase in morbidity and a prolongation of hospital stay. Pulsion intubation permits correction of protein–energy malnutrition with minimal dietary modification, and relief can be obtained from the sequelae of pulmonary aspiration or oesophagorespiratory fistula.

Preoperative

Indications

Pulsion intubation to relieve dysphagia may be required:

1. In neoplastic strictures of the oesophagus, usually squamous carcinoma in the following circumstances.
   (*a*) Medical contraindications to surgery or radiotherapy.
   (*b*) Clinically detectable organ invasion or distant dissemination.
   (*c*) Dysphagia due to tumour recurrence following surgery or radiotherapy.
   (*d*) Malignant strictures longer than 6 cm involving the upper thoracic oesophagus (20–32 cm from the incisor teeth). These tumours are invariably unresectable.
   (*e*) Demonstrable oesophagotracheal or oesophagobronchial fistula.
   (*f*) Unresectability established at laparotomy or thoracotomy.
   (*g*) The development of an anastomotic stricture following surgery or a fibrous stricture following radiotherapy.
2. Where unresectable tumours of the stomach invade the cardia and lower oesophagus.
3. Where the oesophagus is compressed or invaded by intrathoracic tumours.
4. In patients with benign oesophageal strictures, where surgery is contraindicated and repeated dilatation is hazardous or ineffective.

Contraindications

Failure of the cricopharyngeal sphincter to close over the proximal end of the tube causes gagging and will preclude intubation of high lesions.

Intubation in the presence of jaw fixity, ankylosis of the cervical spine or thoracic spinal deformity can be facilitated by using the fibreoptic endoscope and a flexible introducer.

Preparation of patient

Anteroposterior and lateral chest X-rays (1.8 m films) followering a barium swallow will indicate the level of obstruction, the length of the stricture and the alignment of the oesophageal axis. Dentures should be removed and loose teeth extracted. Food and fluids are withheld for 12 h before intubation. Fluid contents are aspirated and food residues removed by oesophageal wash-outs.

Equipment

Both the rigid and flexible oesophagoscope should be available. The 35 cm rigid Negus oesophagoscope allows adequate biopsy and dilatation of lesions of the upper thoracic oesophagus.

The flexible instrument is preferred for lesions of the distal oesophagus and cardia. Introduction of a guide-wire into the stomach via the biopsy channel under direct visual or radiological control permits safer dilatation of distal strictures.

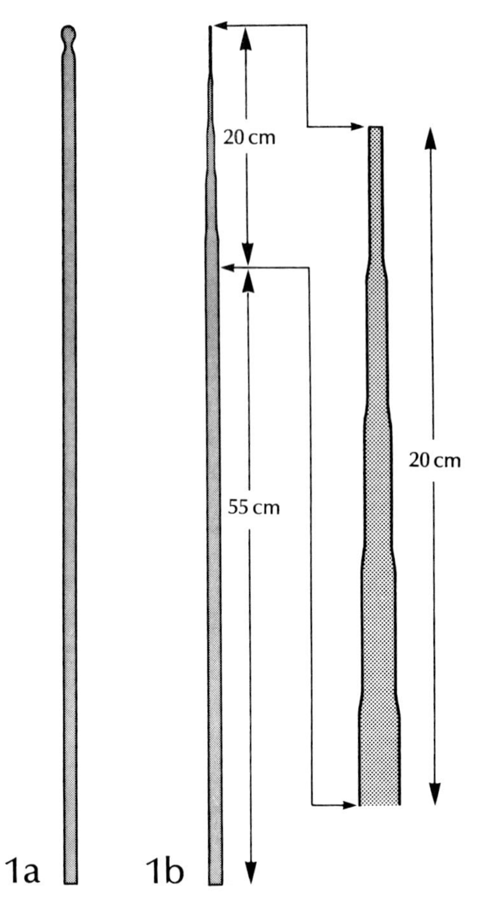

1a & b

Bougies

Graduated neoplex oesophageal bougies (*a*) can be passed via the rigid oesophagoscope for dilatation under vision.

Alternatively the solid but flexible Celestin dilator (*b*) can be passed over a guide-wire. Each dilator is 75 cm long with a central channel. The dilating complex is 20 cm long and has an external diameter covering the range of either 4–12 mm (in 2 mm steps) or 4–18 mm (first step of 8 mm, followed by 2 mm steps).

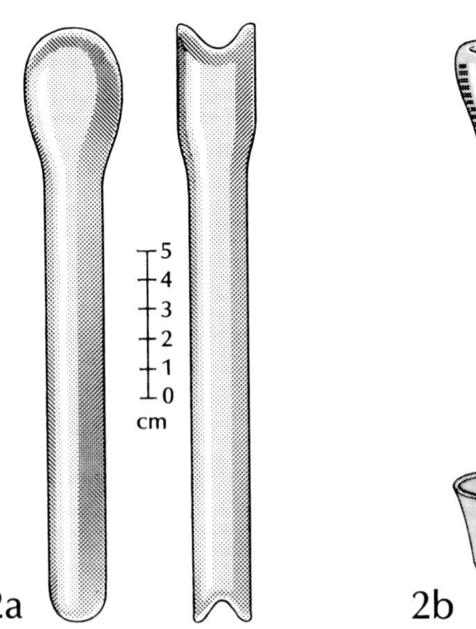

2a & b

Tubes

The Procter-Livingstone tube (*a*) is preferred. It is an armoured soft latex rubber tube with an internal diameter of 12 mm and an outer diameter of 18 mm. The proximal end is expanded to fit snugly above the tumour and prevent food passing between the tube and the oesophageal wall. Three lengths are available: 10 cm, 15 cm and 19 cm. An attractive alternative is the Celestin pulsion tube (*b*) with a distally sited flange to prevent cephalad displacement. This tube can be inserted with a special balloon introducer stiffened by the use of a mandril.

3

Position of patient

The patient lies supine on the operating table, the head supported on a grommet ring. The table break permits flexion and extension of the cervical spine.

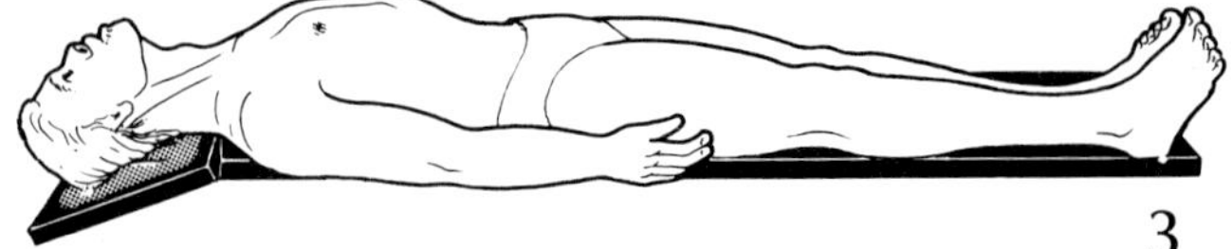

Anaesthesia

General anaesthesia using a high dose Fentanyl technique allows rapid induction and reversal of anaesthesia. An endotracheal tube should be inserted after preliminary bronchoscopy.

The operation

Endoscopy

Bronchoscopy is first performed to identify compression of the tracheobronchial tree, tumour invasion or the presence of a fistula. Tracheobronchial secretions are aspirated. The well lubricated oesophagoscope is then advanced under direct vision as far as the stricture, from which biopsies are taken.

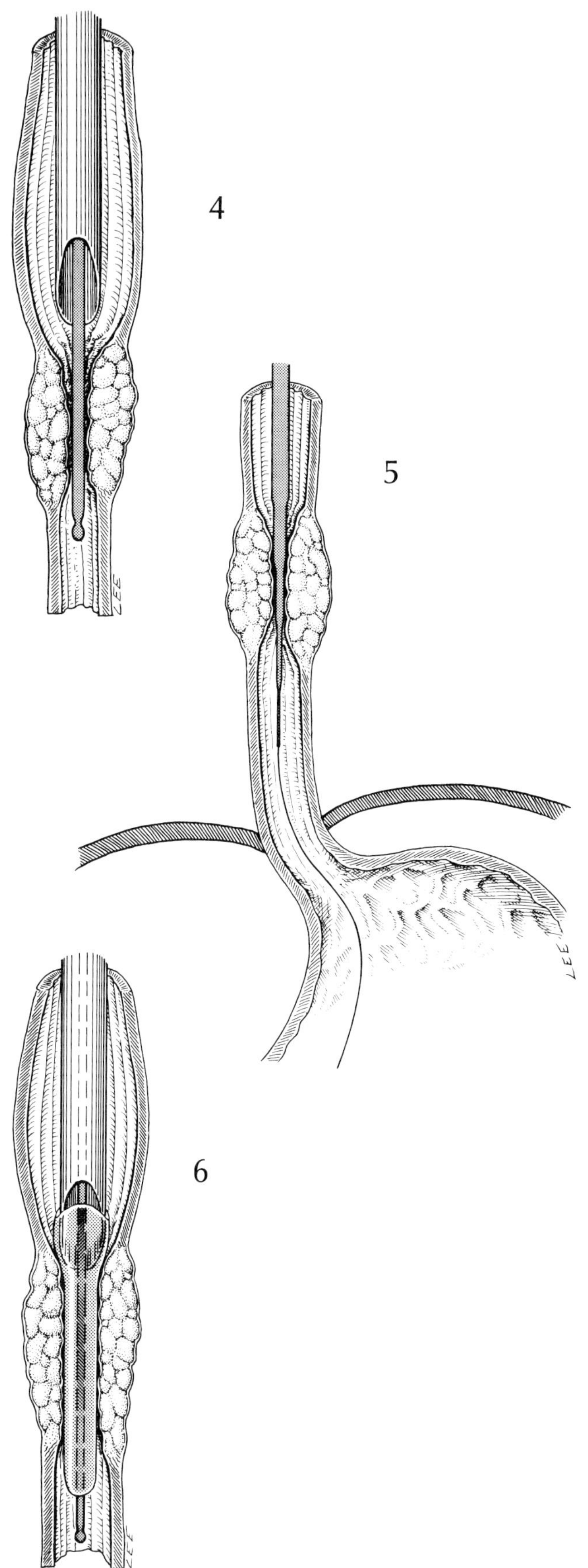

4

Stricture dilatation using the rigid oesophagoscope

Dilatation is achieved by the sequential passage of graduated bougies to 40 Fr gauge. To avoid perforation of the oesophagus or stomach, the bougie should only traverse the length of the stricture. Longitudinal rupture of a tumour during dilatation does not increase morbidity as the tube effectively tamponades any mural defect.

5

Stricture dilatation using the flexible endoscope

An Eder–Puestow guide wire is passed through the stricture via the biopsy channel of the endoscope. A generous length of wire should be advanced into the stomach to avoid withdrawal during removal of the dilator. After withdrawal of the endoscope the Celestin dilator is threaded over the guide wire until the maximum diameter of the dilating complex traverses the stricture. The wire is firmly held by an assistant to prevent curling or displacement.

6

Intubation

A 20 Fr gauge bougie is passed through the dilated stricture and left *in situ*. A lubricated tube of appropriate length is inserted over the bougie, through the stricture, using the rigid oesophagoscope as a 'pusher'. The expanded proximal end of the tube rests on the upper shoulder of the stricture. The bougie and oesophagoscope are removed after verifying that the tube is correctly sited.

Postoperative care

Patients must be nursed in the semi-sitting position and carefully observed, particularly for evidence of respiratory obstruction, aspiration pneumonia and oesophageal perforation.

Routine contrast studies will confirm the position and patency of the tube. In the absence of complications oral feeding can be begun immediately.

Complications

Haemorrhage

Major haemorrhage is uncommon, and usually ceases spontaneously. Fatal haemorrhage is associated with aortic disruption.

7

Oesophageal perforation

Perforation occurs during bouginage either at the junction of normal oesophagus and the upper end of the tumour or near the cardia where the oesophagus deviates to the left. The tube may project through the perforation into the mediastinum. Emergncy treatment should include oesophageal bypass.

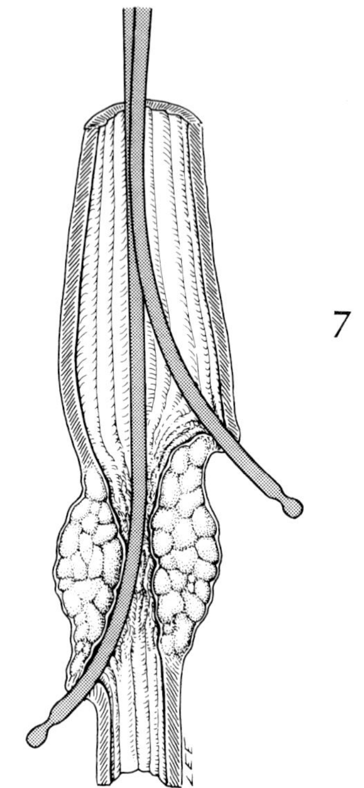

7

Tube migration

Proximal migration is commoner than distal migration. Patients complain of dysphagia and contrast studies confirm the diagnosis. Tube removal and replacement is well tolerated.

Tube obstruction

Tube obstruction can result from food impaction, tube migration or failure of a short tube completely to traverse the stricture. Oesophagoscopy and contrast studies will aid in identifying the nature of the obstruction.

Respiratory

Intubation of bulky tumours may produce tracheal compression, necessitating removal of the tube for the relief of respiratory obstruction.

Bronchial aspiration should be treated by bronchoscopic suction. Atelectasis and bronchopneumonia may follow, requiring physiotherapy and antimicrobial agents.

Further reading

Atkinson, M., Ferguson, R., Parker, G. C. Tube introducer and modified Celestin tube for use in palliative intubation of oesophagogastric neoplasms at fibreoptic endoscopy. Gut 1978; 19: 669–671

Celestin, L. R., Campbell, W. B. A new and safe system for oesophageal dilatation. Lancet 1981; 1: 74–75

Hegarty, M. M., Angorn, I. B., Bryer, J. V., Henderson, B. J., Le Roux, B. T., Logan, A. Pulsion intubation for palliation of carcinoma of the oesophagus. British Journal of Surgery 1977; 64: 160–165

Operations for carcinoma of the thoracic oesophagus and cardia

John W. Jackson MCh, FRCS
Formerly Consultant Thoracic Surgeon, Harefield Hospital, Harefield Middlesex, UK

Preoperative

Indications and preparation

Age alone is not a bar to surgery for these lesions; the majority of patients are in the seventh decade and a number are over 80 years of age.

Increasing dysphagia at first to solids and then subsequently to soft foods and finally fluids leads to weight loss, inanition and dehydration.

The tumour is locally invasive and may extend beyond the normal confines of the oesophagus and stomach to become adherent to adjacent structures in the chest and abdomen. Lymph nodes are frequently involved but do not preclude a worthwhile resection; in the presence of liver or peritoneal metastases resection is of very doubtful value and alternative palliative procedures should be considered.

The prime aim of operation should be to remove the ulcerating fungating growth that lies in direct communication with the mouth and to restore swallowing. If at the same time a satisfactory cancer excision is obtained it should be regarded as a bonus. A mortality of 10 per cent is surgically acceptable and the extension of life by 1 or 2 years a real benefit to an elderly person. Operation has to be a once only procedure – there is seldom time for staged operations at this age. If dysphagia is complete operation should be carried out as soon as anaemia and dehydration have been corrected.

A careful clinical examination is essential to exclude other contraindications to radical surgery, e.g. metastases to the neck glands, liver and peritoneum. A rectal examination is carried out to exclude pelvic metastases and to assess the prostate. Severe constipation, often made worse by recent barium studies, may need attention so as to avoid faecal impaction in the postoperative period.

The cross-references in this chapter refers to *Operative Surgery: Thoracic Surgery, 4th Edition*

Investigations

Radiology

Diagnosis is established by barium swallow; if possible the distal oesophagus, stomach and cardia should be outlined in the examination. A chest X-ray is necessary to exclude carcinoma of the bronchus – the next most common cause of dysphagia – and to detect any pneumonic change due to spill from the oesophagus to the trachea. Mediastinal widening due to glands or tumour should also be looked for. Sometimes a tumour at the cardia may produce a filling defect in the fundus air bubble. If there is no fundus bubble dysphagia is absolute, but the presence of air indicates that there is a passageway.

Oesophagoscopy

Oesophagoscopy is essential to determine the level and extent of the lesion. Froth, food and other residue should be removed. Sometimes it may be possible to pass the instrument beyond the lesion into the distal oesophagus, affording temporary relief of dysphagia. Several biopsies should always be taken and the distance of the proximal and distal level of the tumour from the upper incisor teeth should be recorded. If it is not possible to get past the lesion with the oesophagoscope cautious attempts at dilatation may be made with a Moloney bougie. Perforation is an indication for emergency surgery.

Bronchoscopy

Bronchoscopy is carried out in every case to exclude primary carcinoma of the bronchus or direct or indirect involvement of the bronchial tree by the oesophageal growth. The distance of the carina from the upper incisor teeth at the time of bronchoscopy is always recorded and compared with the upper and lower level of the lesion in the oesophagus. If there is the least doubt about the appearances of the bronchial mucosa a biopsy is taken. While the patient is relaxed under the anaesthetic the abdomen should be palpated to feel for and exclude any mass in the stomach, liver secondaries, ascites or a barium-loaded bowel.

Preoperative treatment

It may be possible to improve the patient's swallowing temporarily by removing impacted food or fungating tumour at the time of oesophagoscopy. Usually dehydration and electrolytic imbalance need to be corrected by intravenous therapy. Anaemia should be corrected by blood transfusion. With intravenous alimentation there is rarely any need for a feeding gastrostomy or jejunostomy. It is usually better to proceed to surgery.

Simple dental treatment should be carried out during this period – scaling and the removal of loose teeth which might be dislodged at operation. Oral candidiasis is common and antifungal agents may be required.

Chest infection, often associated with oesophageal spill-over, may call for a period of treatment with physiotherapy and antibiotics.

Generally these patients do not benefit by having their operations deferred.

The operations

The oesophagus may be replaced by stomach, colon or small intestine. If the growth is confined to the oesophagus the author uses stomach and if the cardia and lower oesophagus are involved jejunum is preferred. An upper partial gastrectomy with oesophagogastric anastomosis may be justified in the elderly if the stomach is not grossly involved or where metastases indicate a poor prognosis. The procedure will restore swallowing and rid the patient of the alimentary part of his tumour. The use of colon is described in the chapter on 'Colon replacement of the oesophagus', pp. 355–369).

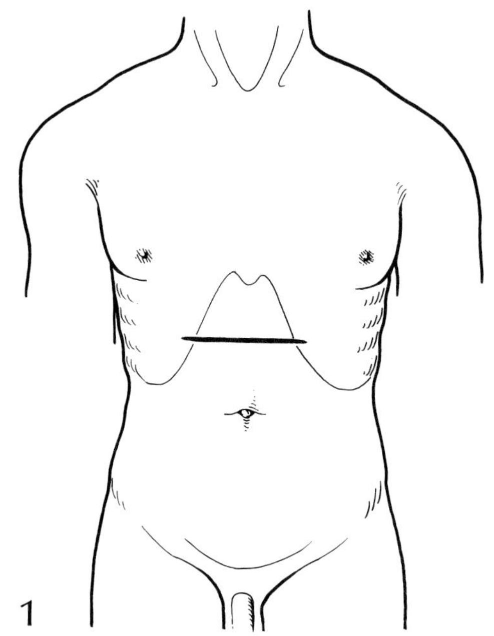

1

OESOPHAGECTOMY WITH GASTRIC REPLACEMENT (IVOR LEWIS)

Anaesthesia

The patient is anaesthetized and a double lumen tube inserted so that the right lung can be excluded from the circuit for part of the operation.

An intravenous drip, using a central venous pressure line, is set up. The bladder is catheterized and the catheter left in for 24–48 h. Urinary output is recorded half hourly during the operation and at regular intervals in the post-operative period.

Stage 1: Abdominal

1

The incision

With the patient supine laparotomy is made using an upper midline incision or a transverse incision midway between the xiphoid process and umbilicus, dividing the rectus muscles. This affords good access to the pylorus and to the spleen and cardia.

The abdomen is explored to exclude metastases or other disease. If growth is palpable at the cardia a left-sided approach may be preferred and the incision can be extended into the chest along the eighth rib. Alternatively, the abdomen can be closed (after mobilization of the stomach) and the patient turned, with resection and anastomosis through a left thoracotomy.

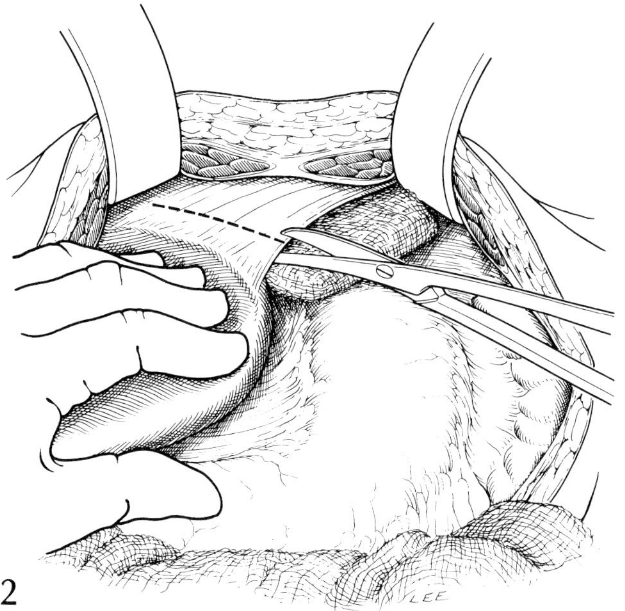

2

2

Division of the left triangular ligament should be carried out at an early stage. The ligament is brought into view by placing a swab or pack behind it before dividing it with scissors. The left lobe of the liver may now be retracted downwards so as to reveal the oesophageal hiatus.

3

The stomach, omentum and transverse colon are delivered into the wound. An opening is made in the gastrocolic omentum on the greater curve below the short gastric vessels, so as to gain access to the lesser sac. The gastrocolic omentum is divided or separated from the colon, preserving the right gastroepiploic arch. The short gastric and left gastric vessels are divided using forceps and ligature or the Auto Suture LDS instrument. It is important not to tie or clip too close to the greater curve of the stomach. The spleen is not removed as a set part of the operation but if it is in the way or bleeds it should be removed. The gastrohepatic omentum is opened and frequently carries a sizeable hepatic branch from the left gastric artery, which may be divided provided there is an adequate main hepatic artery. The right gastric vessels are preserved and the left gastric pedicle is cleared from above and from behind within the lesser sac; the artery and vein are tied separately close to the coeliac axis. Any enlarged glands are removed and sent for histological examination. The oesophageal hiatus is defined by sharp dissection. The phreno-oesophageal ligament is divided and the oesophagus mobilized above and below the hiatus. It is not necessary to enlarge the hiatus. The mediastinum is explored through the hiatus using finger and swabs. Pyloroplasty is only carried out if the pylorus is small or scarred. A patulous pylorus or overzealous pyloroplasty may induce biliary reflux to the gastric remnant and cause oesophagitis above the oesophagogastric anastomosis postoperatively.

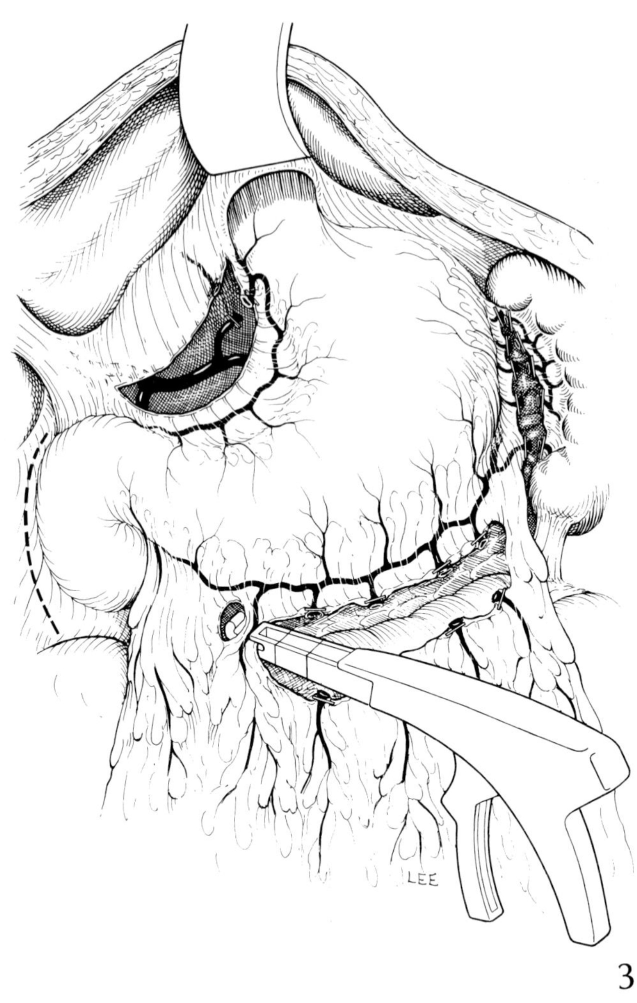

3

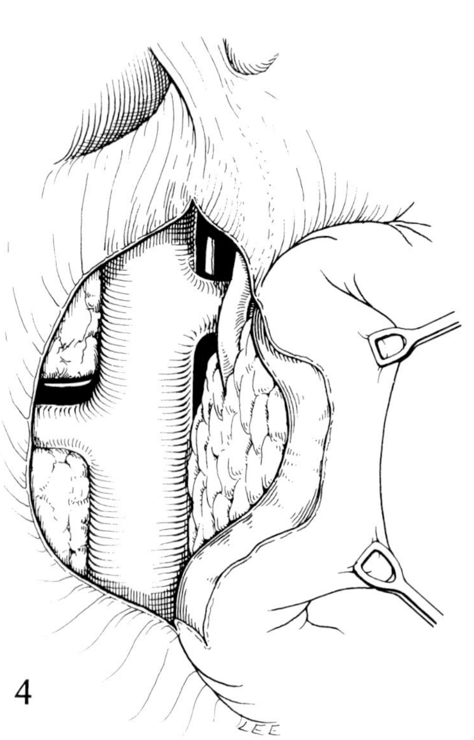

4

4

The peritoneum lateral to the duodenum may be divided to improve mobilization of the pylorus and if extra length is required it may also help to mobilize the duodenum and the head of the pancreas.

When haemostasis is satisfactory the viscera are replaced and the abdomen closed.

Stage II: Thoracic

Anaesthesia

If a double lumen endotracheal tube has been inserted at the time of induction it is a distinct advantage to exclude the right lung from the anaesthetic circuit for at least part of this stage of the operation.

5

Position of patient and incision

The patient is turned on to the left side and secured to the table. A right thoracotomy is carried out along the upper border of the sixth rib.

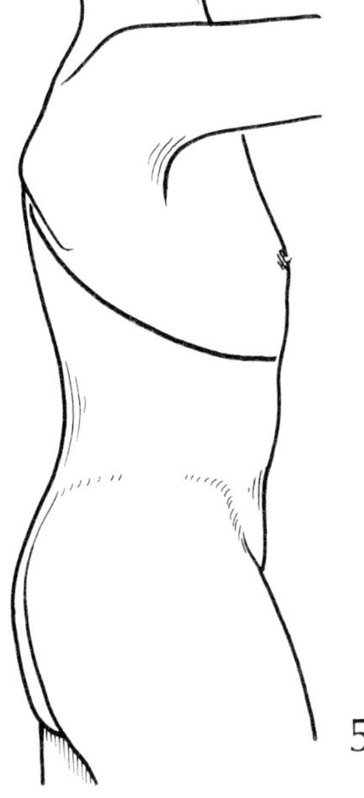

5

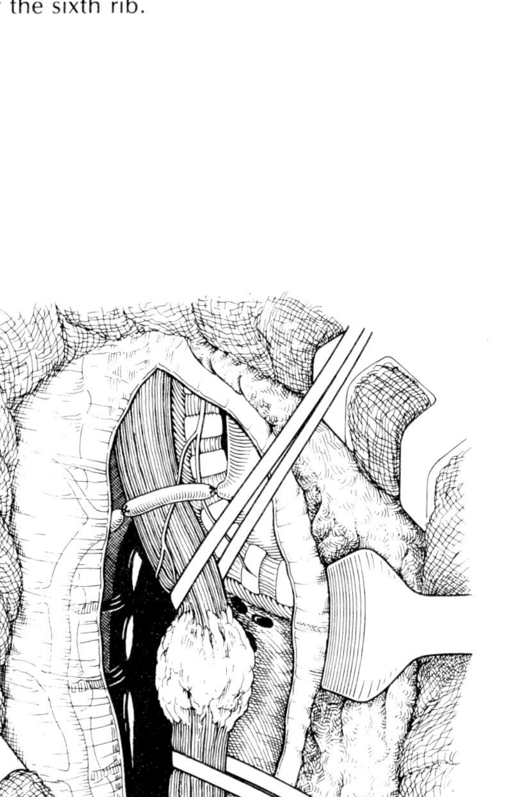

6

6

The lung is freed to the hilum, retracted anteriorly and allowed to collapse. The lesion in the oesophagus is inspected and palpated. The azygos vein is ligated and divided and the mediastinal pleura opened along the length of the oesophagus.

Tapes are passed around the oesophagus above and below the tumour. Using sharp dissection in front of the oesophagus the pericardium, lower trachea and both main bronchi are separated from the oesophagus taking the subcarinal and mediastinal lymph nodes with the oesophagus. A plane is then opened posteriorly between the oesophagus and the spine and aorta. The tumour may be densely adherent to any one of these structures as if by direct extension, and it must be separated by a process of sharp dissection, stealth and persuasion. Clean and intact mobilization is not always possible. Occasionally the oesophageal lumen is entered but it is essential to avoid the disaster of entering the aorta or the tracheobronchial tree. The thoracic duct may be seen or divided inadvertently, resulting in the escape of chyle into the mediastinum. The divided ends must be sought, and tied, clipped or oversewn. Otherwise it should be removed along with any associated lymph nodes. One or two sizeable vessels from the aorta may need to be ligated or secured with a suture.

7

As soon as the oesophagus and its tumour are free in the mediastinum the stomach is delivered into the chest through the oesophageal hiatus; its initial presentation is noted so as to avoid subsequent rotation – the greater curve should lie towards the mediastinum. The pylorus may present through the hiatus. The upper oesophagus is mobilized to the base of the neck.

A Petz clamp or other stapling instrument is applied obliquely across the stomach below the cardia, preserving the lateral part of the fundus.

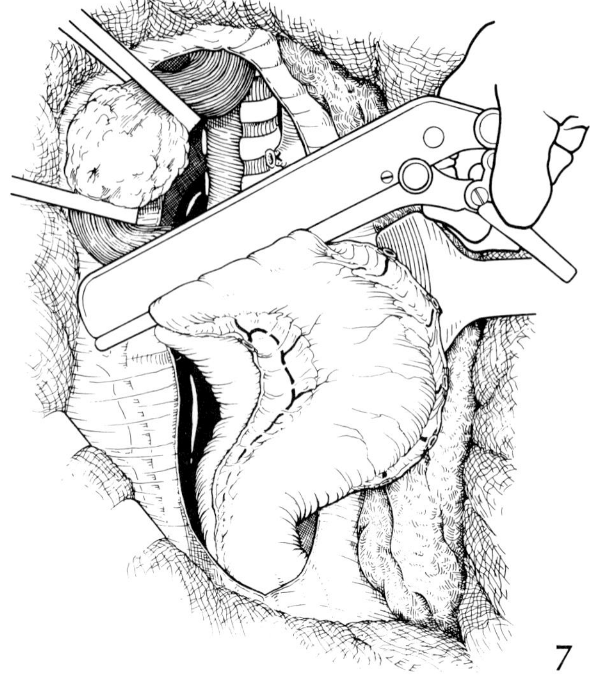

7

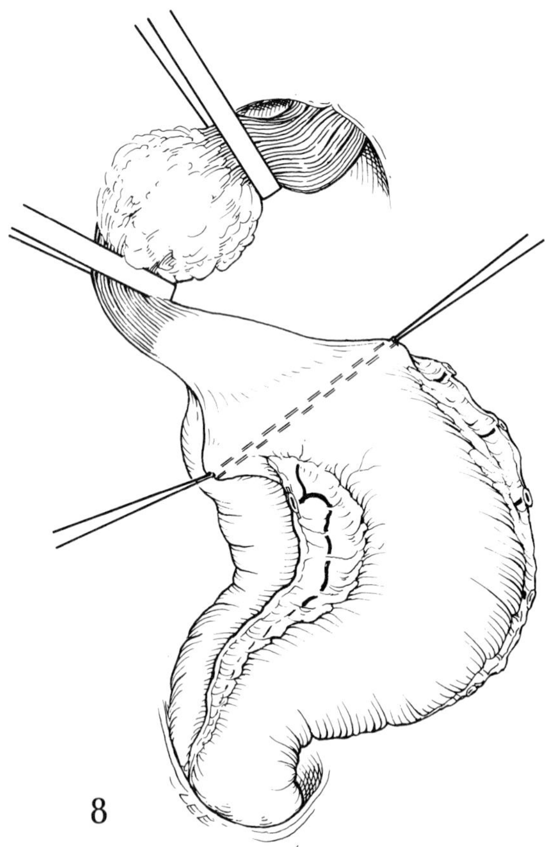

8

8

The stomach is divided with diathermy or a knife between the rows of staples.

9

The stapled stomach edge is oversewn with a continuous suture of 2/0 chromic catgut. The suture is tied and the ends held in forceps.

9

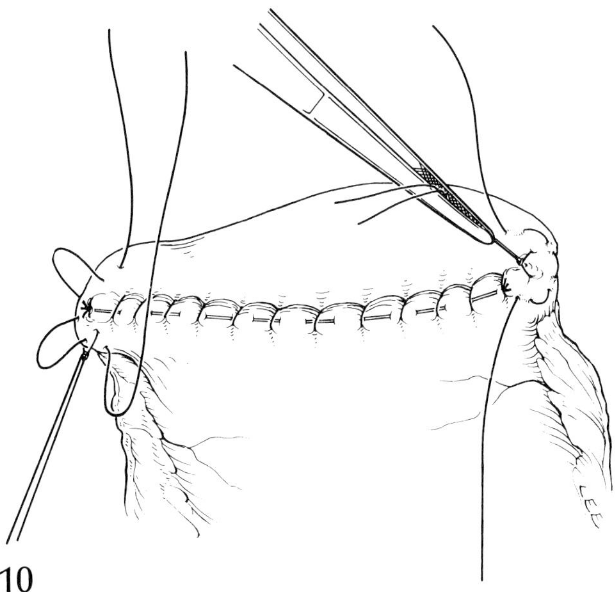

10

10

The TA 90 Auto Suture instrument inserts two rows of overlapping staples in close approximation and these do not need to be oversewn, but the line of staples should be invaginated by a continuous Lembert suture of chromic catgut so as to ensure serosal apposition and prevent contact and contamination of the mediastinum by the divided mucosa.

Several seromuscular bites (4 or 5) of a non-absorbable suture (3/0 linen) encircle the ends of the catgut suture (or staple) line in an open horseshoe formation.

11

The catgut knot and the end of the catgut suture line are invaginated and the linen suture tied as the catgut is cut close to its knot.

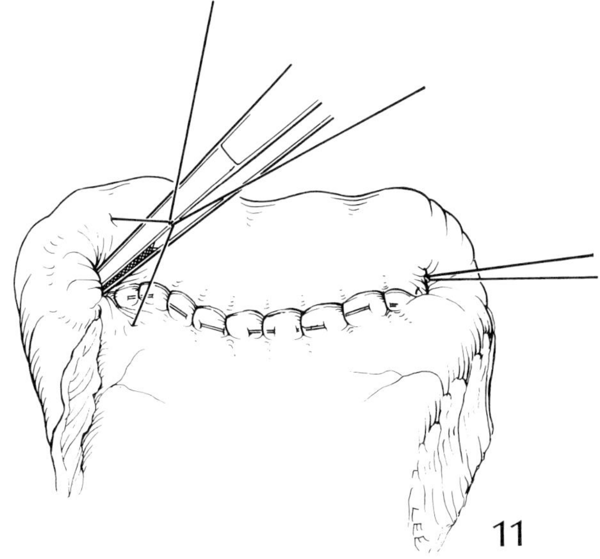

11

12

Interrupted seromuscular mattress stitches of linen are now placed over the intervening segment.

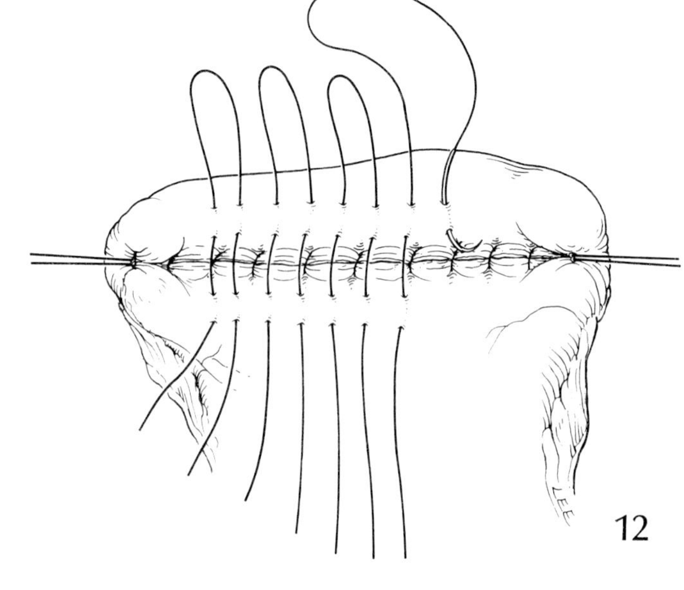

12

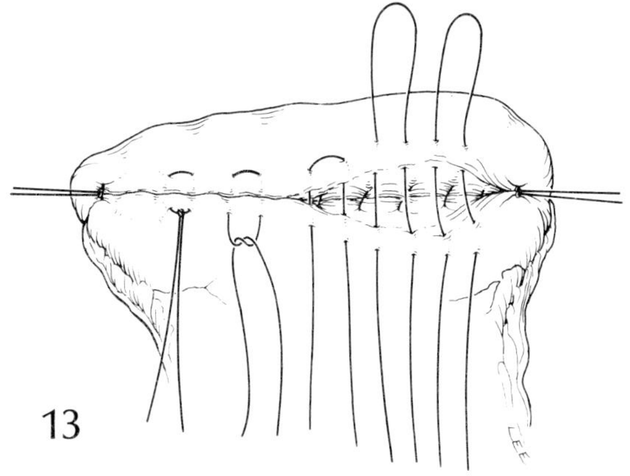

13

13 & 14

The sutures are tied and serosal apposition is secured over the whole length of the suture line.

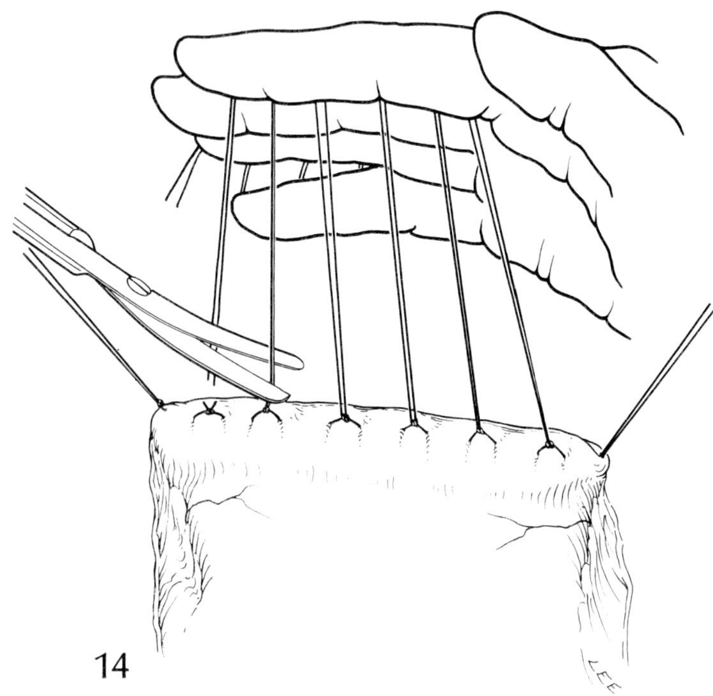

14

15

The stomach is laid in the oesophageal bed and its highest point, usually the fundus, should reach the root of the neck – indeed if the oesophageal tumour is high, anastomosis can be effected in the neck by a separate cervical incision after the chest is closed (*see* chapter on 'Colon replacement of the oesophagus', pp. 355–369).

A site is chosen near the fundus of the stomach for anastomosis with the oesophagus. It should be away from the suture line closing the upper end of the stomach so as to avoid leaving a bridge of ischaemic tissue.

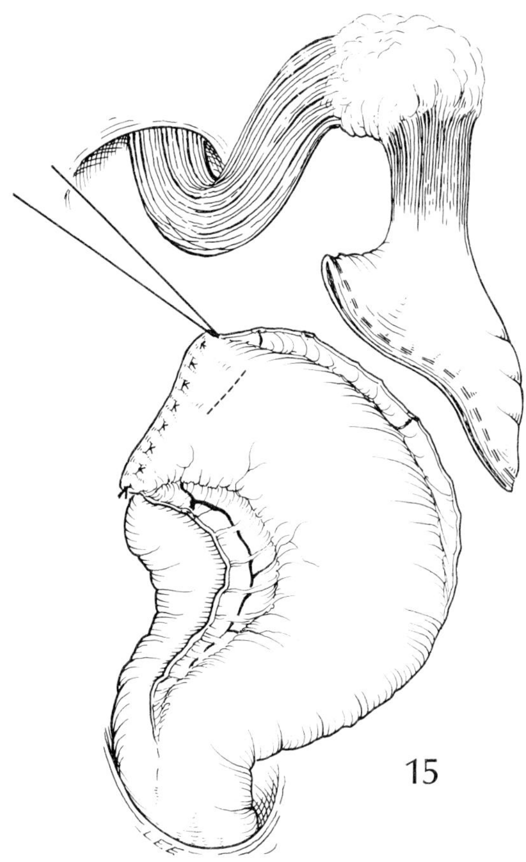
15

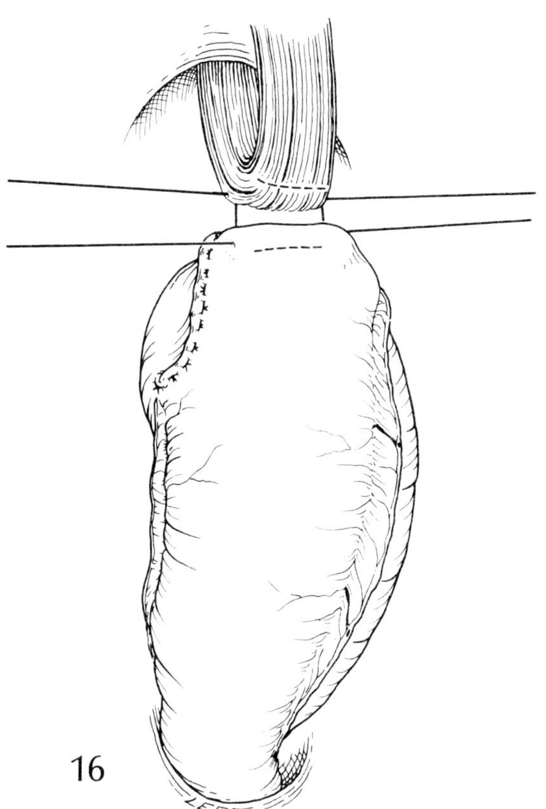
16

16

Two seromuscular (3/0 linen) stitches are placed between the oesophagus above the proposed site of section and on either side of the place chosen for the gastric stoma.

17

Four or five seromuscular stitches are inserted between these to bring the oesophagus and stomach together without tension or tearing. The outer stitches are clipped or preserved, the inner cut.

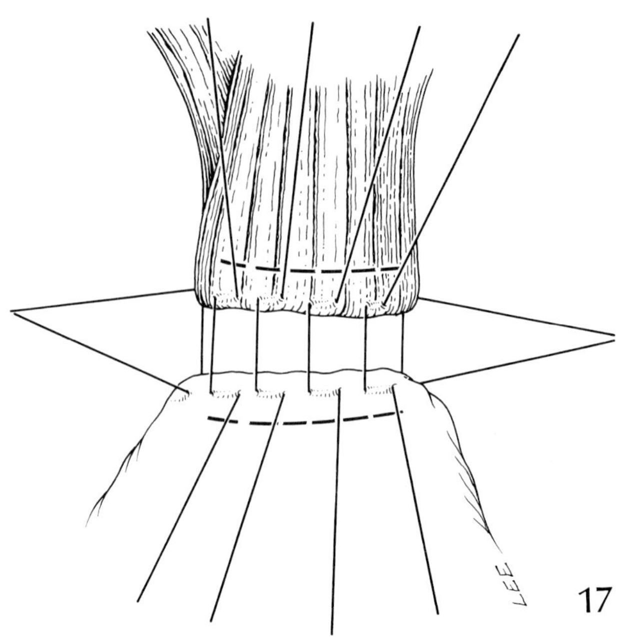

17

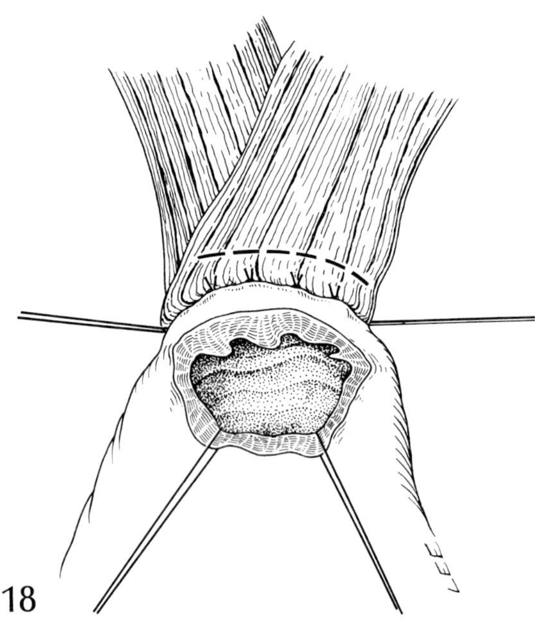

18

18

The stomach is opened with scissors or diathermy along the line chosen for the stoma and excess gastric contents removed with gentle suction. Haemostasis is secured. Two 3/0 Ethibond stay sutures are placed in the free edge of the stomach opening so as to divide it into three equal parts and held in mosquito forceps.

19

The oseophagus is divided with a knife at a point level with the stoma. Free bleeding should occur and clamps are not used here. A clamp may be applied to the distal oesophagus to avoid spillage. The specimen is removed.

Two stay sutures of 3/0 Ethibond are inserted on the free edge of the divided oesophagus to match those on the stomach and are held in mosquito forceps. These hold the oesophagus and the gastric stoma open.

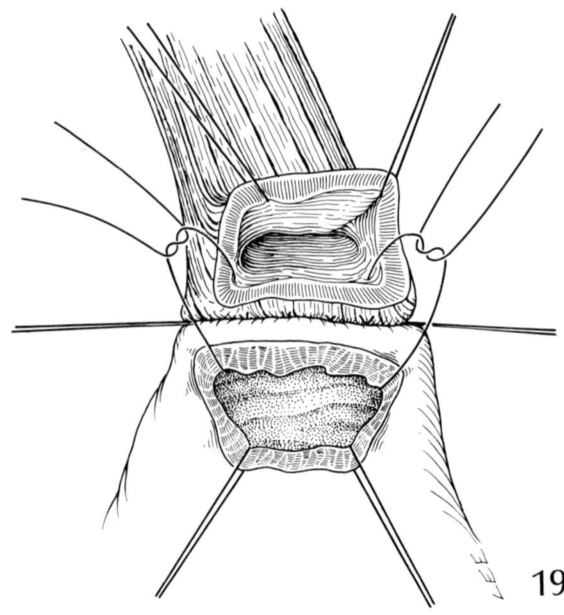

19

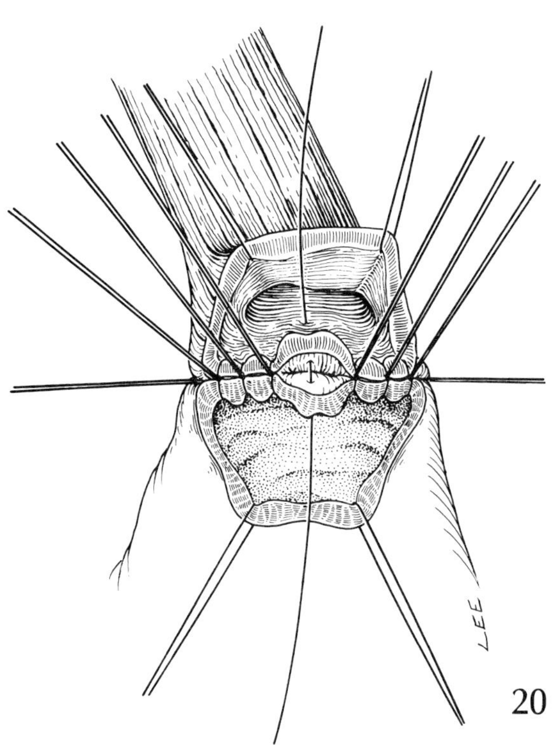

20

A row of interrupted, all-layers stitches is applied between the stomach and oesophagus posteriorly. The knots are tied on the mucosa.

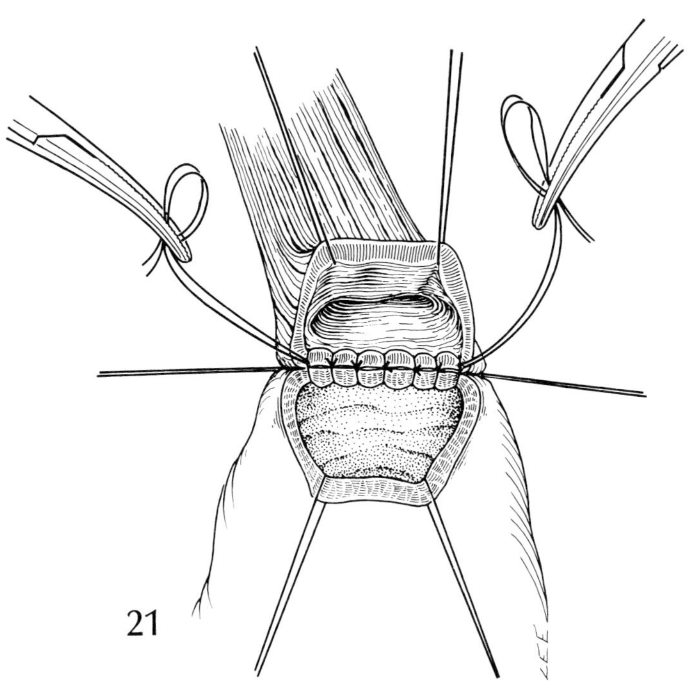

21

The end stitches are preserved and held in forceps with a loop for easy identification, and the remainder are cut.

22

A nasogastric tube with a radiopaque marker line is passed down the oesophagus by the anaesthetist to the anastomosis and its tip advanced through the stomach towards the pylorus so that it lies near the pylorus with the side-holes in the stomach to prevent distension of the elongated tube-like stomach.

Closure of the front row of the anastomosis commences at each angle using a series of interrupted Connell all-layers stitches. Each stitch starts and finishes on the outside of the stomach or oesophagus with a loop on the mucosa so as to invert the mucosa.

When tied, the knots of this row are outside the lumen of the anastomosis.

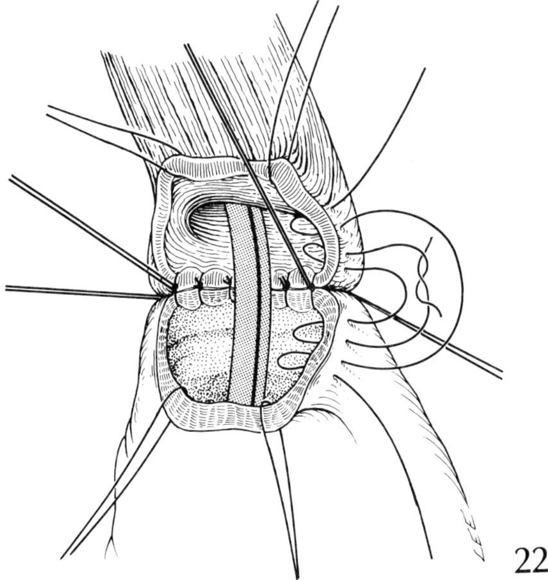

23

After two or three of these stitches have been placed near each angle the internal angle stitches held in *Illustration 21* are cut and the 3/0 Ethibond stay sutures removed. Further Connell stitches close the middle third. The stitches clipped and preserved in *Illustration 17* are retained.

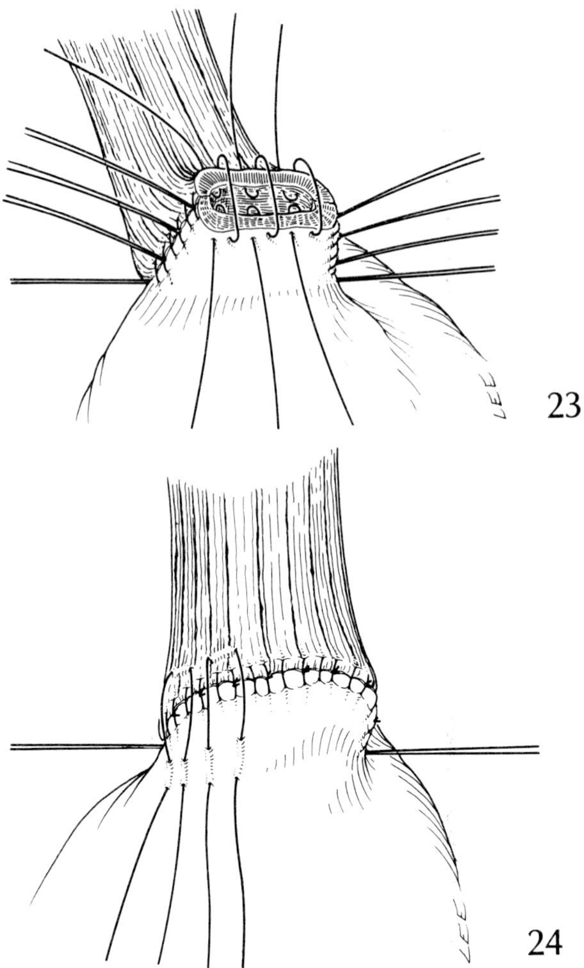

23

24

24

A row of interrupted seromuscular stitches, two bites on the stomach and one transversely on the oesophagus, so as to pick up its outer longitudinal muscle, draws a cuff of stomach up over the previous layer and hides it from sight.

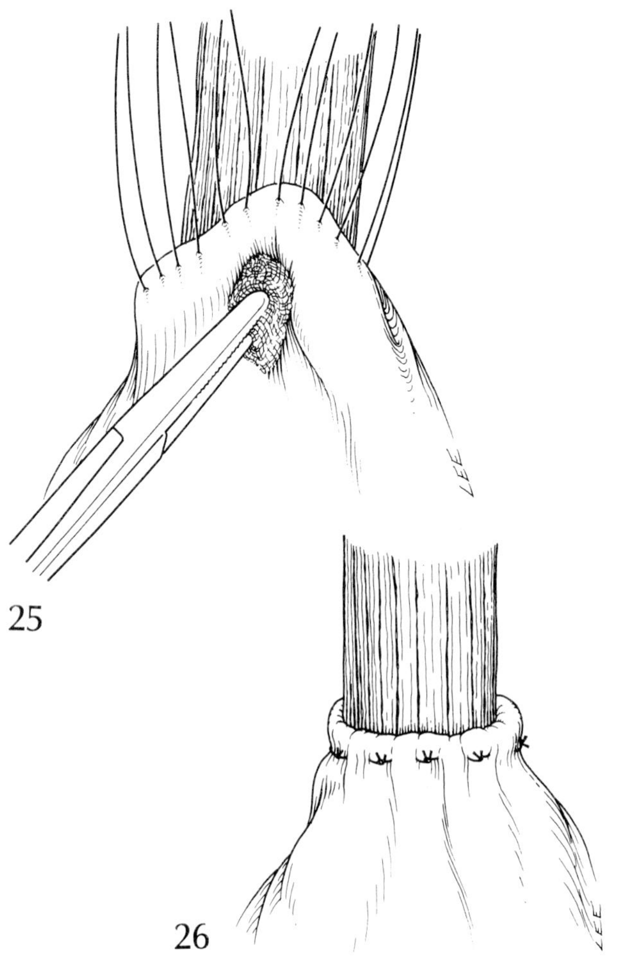

25

26

25

When tying these stitches the stomach is eased up over the oesophagus with a swab or pledget to avoid tension and promote inversion.

26

The anastomosis is now complete. Additional stitches are rarely indicated.

There should be no tension, and any redundant stomach in the chest may be returned to the abdomen. The anastomosis and the tube of stomach take their place in the mediastinum in the bed of the excised oesophagus.

The pleura is loosely closed over the anastomosis.

A basal intercostal drain (36 Fr) is inserted posteriorly to drain the costodiaphragmatic sulcus; its tip may be fixed in position by a catgut stitch. It should not encroach on the stomach or anastomosis. A separate mediastinal drain (32 Fr) may be placed at the same time if there is uncertainty about the viability of the stomach or the anastomosis or fear of a chylous leak. The tip is positioned and secured with a loop of catgut.

The lung is now reinflated and the chest closed.

TOTAL GASTRECTOMY WITH JEJUNAL REPLACEMENT, ROUX-EN-Y

The aim of this operation is to remove the entire stomach and as much as possible of the oesophagus above the tumour (10–12 cm) along with the left gastric glands, sometimes taking spleen and pancreas back to the portal vein.

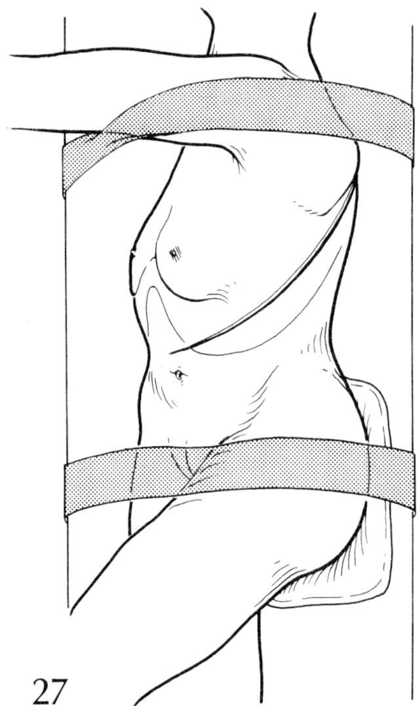

27

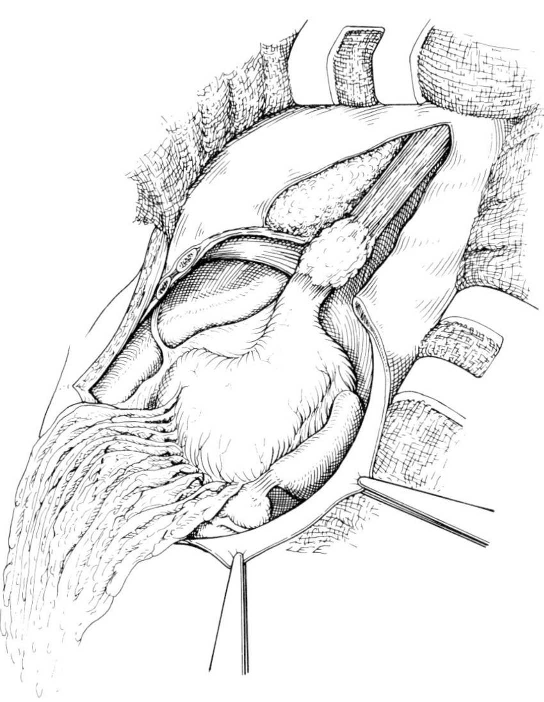

28

Anaesthesia

The patient is anaesthetized and a double lumen tube inserted so that the left lung can be excluded from the anaesthetic circuit for part of the operation.

An intravenous drip, using a central venous pressure line, is set up. The bladder is catheterized and the catheter left in for 24–48 h. Urinary output is recorded half hourly during the operation and at regular intervals in the post-operative period.

Position of patient and incision

27

The patient is secured on the operating table in a semi-lateral position with the pelvis at 45° and the chest nearly vertical to facilitate access to the chest and the abdomen.

The full incision extends from the midline anteriorly between the xiphoid and the umbilicus obliquely across the costal margin and along the seventh or eighth ribs, to the interval between the tip of the scapula and the spine.

The abdomen is opened first between the midline and the costal margin, dividing the left rectus muscle. The extent and operability of the lesion are assessed. Free fluid, peritoneal seedlings, liver and pelvic metastases indicate that a palliative procedure is all that can be achieved. Fixation near the hiatus or involvement of coeliac axis glands are unfavourable signs but need not constitute a bar to resection and a trial mobilization may be deemed worthwhile.

Once it has been decided to proceed, the skin incision is continued over the costal margin, dividing the latissimus dorsi and serratus muscles as far as the trapezius. The periosteum on the entire length of the upper border of the seventh or eighth rib is stripped, the pleura opened and a chest spreader inserted. The costal margin is cut and the musculophrenic vessels secured.

28

The diaphragm is divided circumferentially, leaving a short cuff attached to the rib cage. The anaesthetist allows the left lung to become deflated and retracted forwards so as to expose the oesophagus. The pulmonary ligament is divided and the mediastinal pleura opened along the oesophagus which is now separated from the back of the pericardium anteriorly and the aorta posteriorly. Several large aortic oesophageal vessels may require ligation. The thoracic duct is not so frequently seen from this side but may require ligation. The oesophagus is mobilized with as much fat and as many glands as possible to the level of the aortic arch and the left main bronchus. If the right pleural cavity is opened the pleura must be repaired, otherwise bowel might herniate into the right chest.

29

The lienorenal ligament is divided and the perinephric space entered so as to mobilize the spleen. A decision must now be made whether to preserve or remove the spleen, bearing in mind the possible benefits with respect to cancer clearance against the possible problem of post-splenectomy sepsis. If the spleen has to be removed the splenic artery and veins are dissected out, tied and divided. Otherwise the short gastric vessels are divided, preserving the spleen. The stomach and omentum are now separated from the colon as far as the pylorus, usually in an avascular plane (*see* p. 000). Lesser sac adhesions are divided and mobilization completed from the pylorus to the hiatus. Sometimes the oesophagus may be mobilized without dividing the hiatus. If the tumour is adherent at the hiatus the diaphragm should be divided to this point and the lesion mobilized by including part of the muscle of the hiatus and crura. The left gastric vessels are cleared and divided close to the coeliac axis. The gastrohepatic omentum is divided, taking care to ligate the hepatic branch of the left gastric artery.

If the tumour is adherent to the tail of the pancreas but the lesion is otherwise operable, the tail of the pancreas should be mobilized with the spleen and the splenic vessels and divided close to the superior mesenteric vein (*see* p. 000). The splenic and left gastric arteries are ligated flush with the coeliac axis.

The pancreas is transected, the pancreatic duct (or ducts) ligated and the raw surface excluded from the peritoneal cavity. If in doubt a drain should be left in. Partial pancreatectomy increases the morbidity of the operation and should only be carried out if the pancreas is invaded by tumour.

Before dividing the pylorus, the right gastric and gastroepiploic vessels and closing the duodenum, it is wise first to prepare the jejunum for the Roux-en-Y reconstruction. Occasionally a suitable length of jejunum cannot be obtained and a decision will then have to be made as to whether to interpose a segment of colon between the oesophagus and the duodenum (*see* chapter on 'Colon replacement of the oesophagus', pp. 000–000) or to fashion a tube from the greater curve of stomach.

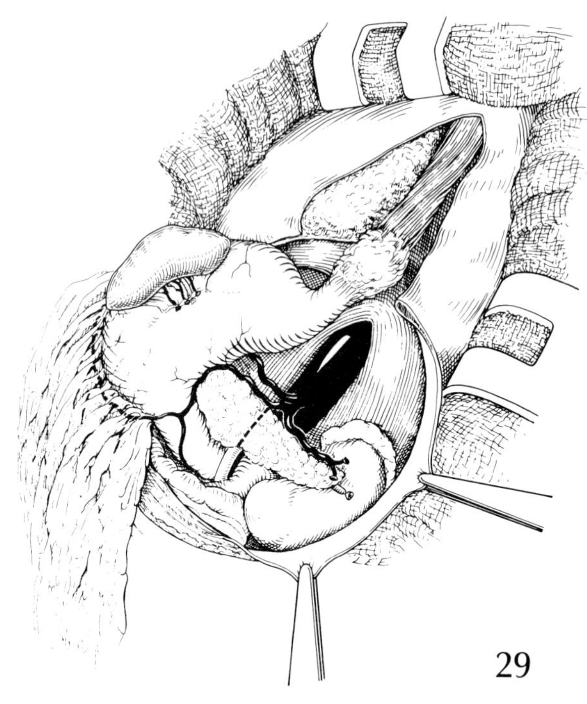

29

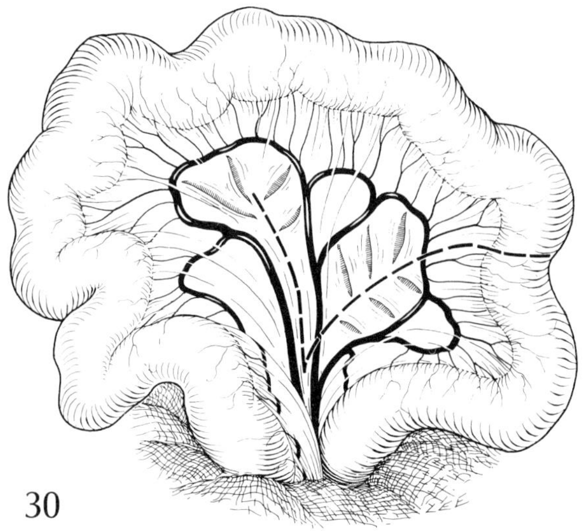

30

30

The jejunum below the duodenojejunal flexure is inspected and a loop selected where the mesentery is beginning to lengthen and the vascular pattern becomes more easily discernible. The vessels in the mesentery may be more readily displayed by turning off the room and overhead lights and transilluminating it with a beam from a horizontal spot lamp. From the proposed point of division the arteries and veins are tied and divided individually so as to preserve the vascular arcades to a length of distal jejunum. The pulsations close to the bowel are observed as each major vessel is clamped. With patience and by making radial slits on either side of the mesentery a loop 25–30 cm long is made available. The small bowel is then divided between non-crushing clamps and the ends covered and returned to the abdomen while the oesophagogastric excision is completed.

31

The right gastric and gastroepiploic vessels are now secured and the pylorus mobilized as far as the duodenum. The duodenum is divided between Payrs crushing clamps (or with the TA 30 or GIA Auto Suture instruments).

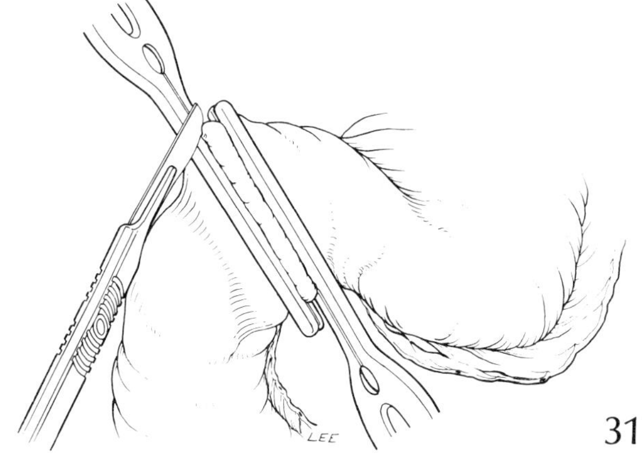

31

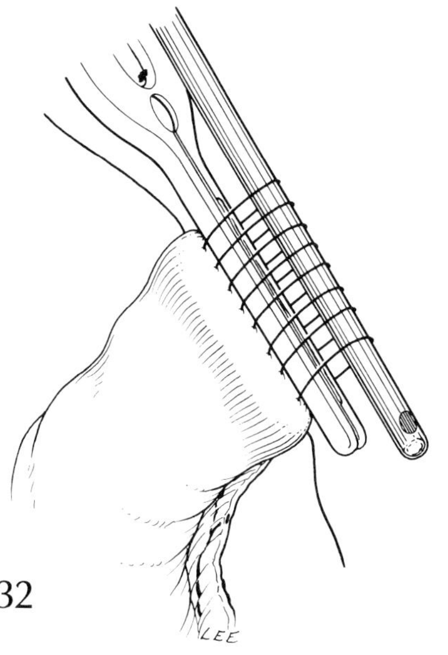

32

32

If a Payrs clamp is used the crushed duodenal stump must be oversewn with catgut. A metal rod (usually the sucker tube) placed over the Payrs clamp helps to form a series of open loops which facilitate removal of the Payrs clamp.

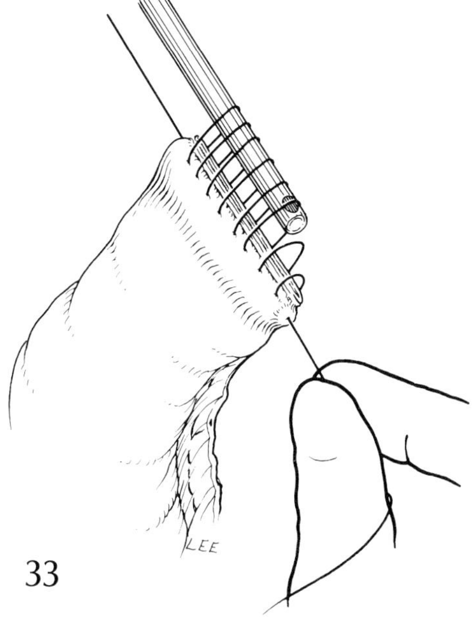

33

33

On removal of the clamp the sucker tube is withdrawn as the loops are tightened.

The sutured (or stapled) stump is then invaginated as follows.

34

A four-bite seromuscular horse-shoe suture is placed at each corner and tied.

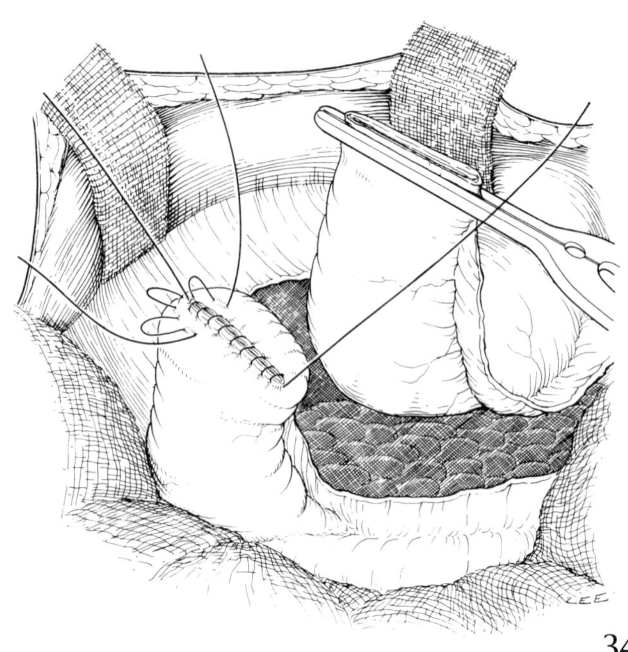

34

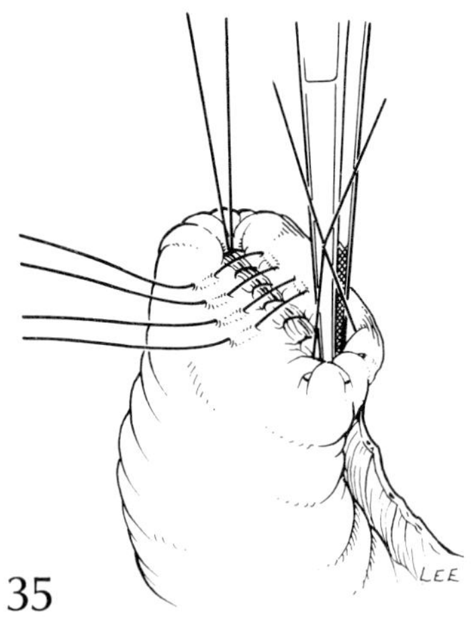

35

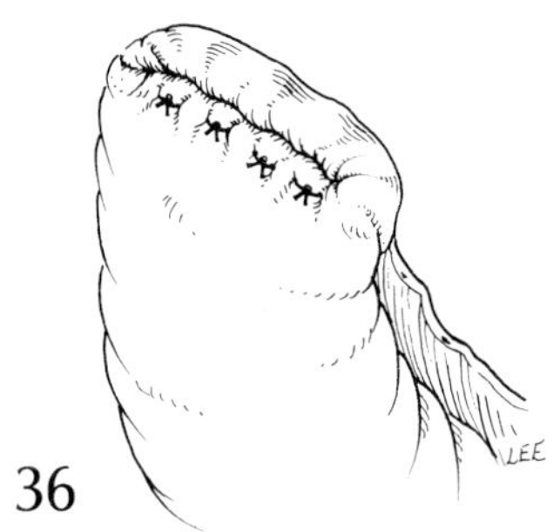

36

35 & 36

Three or four interrupted seromuscular sutures are now placed over the intervening segment.

The entire stomach tumour and lower oesophagus, and if necessary the spleen and tail of the pancreas, are now free. The oesophagus is mobilized in the mediastinum to above the level of the inferior pulmonary vein and sometimes to the aortic arch. The distal jejunum is drawn up posteriorly through the transverse mesocolon and the oesophageal hiatus to lie in the oesophageal bed.

End-to-end anastomosis is effected between the oesophagus and the jejunum below the aortic arch by the method described for oesophagogastric anastomosis (*see Illustrations 16–26*). Occasionally it may be necessary to shorten the jejunal loop because of redundancy or uncertainty about the blood supply to the end. If extra length is required an end-to-side anastomosis may provide an extra 3–4 cm.

A nasogastric tube is passed from the mouth down the upper oesophagus across the anastomosis as previously described.

37

The tip of the nasogastric tube is located below the opening in the mesocolon at the site of the end-to-side jejunojejunal anastomosis which is now effected using the same principles as in oesophagogastric anastomosis. This completes the Roux-en-Y. The mediastinal pleura is repaired and the jejunum and the anastomosis buried in the mediastinum. The oesophageal hiatus and the opening in the mesocolon are closed around the jejunal segment and the free edges of the mesentery are attached to the peritoneum so as to prevent internal herniation.

The diaphragm and costal margin are repaired with non-absorbable sutures. The chest is drained and the abdomen and chest wall closed.

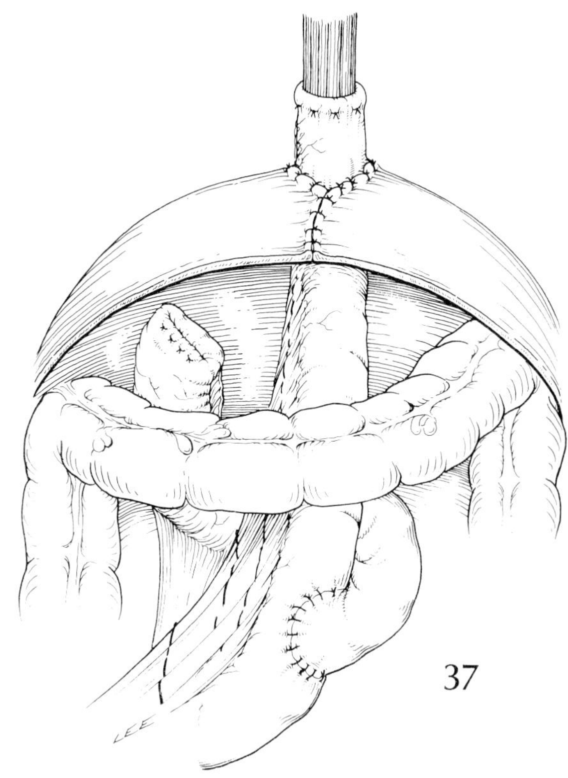

37

Postoperative care and complications

Blood transfusion is continued to match the estimated blood loss. During the operation the patient may lose imperceptibly a considerable volume of fluid from the exposed viscera in the chest and abdomen and this must be replaced intravenously. Central venous pressure should be recorded and maintained at 10–14 cmH_2O. Haemoconcentration must be avoided. A steady flow of urine is a satisfactory index of adequate fluid replacement.

Antibiotics are administered if indicated.

The nasogastric tube is allowed to siphon into a bag and may be aspirated occasionally. As soon as bowel sounds return, oral feeding is begun with sips of water, tea or ice cream and progressively increased. Warm and cold feeds each stimulate peristalsis.

The chest drain is removed as soon as drainage is minimal and the chest X-ray satisfactory, and often before commencing feeding. It is not left longer 'just in case of a leak at the anastomosis'.

Leaks from the anastomosis become less common with experience. They should be suspected when there is undue pain or fever or if a pleural effusion develops and they must be confirmed by Gastrografin swallow as immediate resuture is the only hope of salvation. Some surgeons insist on a satisfactory Gastrografin swallow before commencing oral feeding.

Barium studies are necessary if dysphagia develops postoperatively: sometimes the anastomosis will need dilatation and this may have to be repeated but usually an adequate diet maintains a satisfactory lumen. If dysphagia returns or persists after 3 months local recurrence is probable.

When a total gastrectomy has been carried out macrocytic anaemia may eventually develop and it is wise to commence injections of vitamin B12 while the patient is in hospital and advise that they be repeated monthly.

Postgastrectomy dumping may occasionally be experienced. If so, the patient is advised to take extra nourishment between the three main meals of the day; a lump of sugar or a piece of chocolate may reverse early symptoms.

An alteration in bowel habit – more frequent stools – is common and a fatty stool may be experienced after the Roux-en-Y operation, but this usually settles. Diarrhoea may be controlled by codeine phosphate tablets 30 mg hourly until the diarrhoea stops and then less frequently; but first, and always, a rectal examination should be performed to exclude spurious diarrhoea due to impacted faeces or barium.

Further reading

Jackson, J. W., Cooper, D. K. C., Guvendik, L., Reece-Smith, H. The surgical management of malignant tumours of the oesophagus and cardia: a review of the results in 292 patients treated over a 15 year period (1961–75). British Journal of Surgery 1979; 66: 98–104

McKeown, K. C. Trends in oesophageal resection for carcinoma, with special reference to total oesophagectomy. Annals of the Royal College of Surgeons of England 1972; 51: 213–239

Ong, G. B. Unresectable carcinoma of the oesophagus. Annals of the Royal College of Surgeons of England 1975; 56: 3–14

Nissen's fundoplication

A. H. K. Deiraniya FRCS
Consultant Cardiothoracic Surgeon, Wythenshawe Hospital, Manchester, UK

Introduction

Recognition of the role played by reflux in the causation of symptoms and pathological changes in patients with sliding hiatus hernia diverted attention away from the anatomical aspects of surgical repair of the hernia and emphasized the primary importance of the antireflux component of the operation.

Nissen's fundoplication[1,2] is most effective in abolishing reflux at the gastro-oesophageal junction, irrespective of whether it is carried out above or below the diaphragm. The success of intrathoracic fundoplication in controlling reflux undermined the long-held surgical belief that the presence of an intra-abdominal segment of the oesophagus was essential to gastro-oesophageal competence.

It is now well established that the vast majority of peptic strictures of the oesophagus can be managed successfully without the necessity for oesophageal resection and replacement once reflux at the gastro-oesophageal junction is abolished. Fundoplication alone, or in combination with a Collis gastroplasty[3], is now frequently used in the management of patients with peptic strictures of the oesophagus. A stricture that is easily dilatable endoscopically or retrogradely at operation will resolve in the vast majority of cases with fundoplication alone. Fibrous strictures associated with a short oesophagus require the addition of a Collis gastroplasty as in the combined Collis-Belsey operation pioneered by Pearson (*see* volume on *Cardiothoracic Surgery*, 3rd ed., p. 439), or preferably by the combined Collis-Nissen fundoplication. Fundoplication plays a dual role in the combined operation: it prevents reflux and provides added cover to potential sites of leakage.

The likelihood of reflux oesophagitis and its sequelae developing in patients following local resection of the oesophagus and gastro-oesophageal anastomosis or Heller's myotomy is considerably reduced by the addition of fundoplication.

Extensive mobilization of the oesophagus under direct vision allows the reduction of the cardia below the diaphragm in the vast majority of patients with sliding hiatus hernia and reflux. However, there remain a small number of patients in whom reduction is impossible owing to gross shortening of the oesophagus. The technical simplicity and reliability of the intrathoracic Nissen wrap in controlling reflux in this small group of patients led to its use by surgeons as an alternative to the more major operation of resection and/or replacement. However, in some patients the intrathoracic fundoplication is liable to the potentially lethal complication of rupture into the pleural cavity, pericardium or bronchial tree. Accordingly, intrathoracic fundoplication should be reserved for elderly and frail patients with severe reflux symptoms in whom the cardia cannot be placed below the diaphragm. A gastroplasty and intra-abdominal fundoplication is recommended for the remaining patients in that group.

History of operation

The first fundoplication was performed by Nissen in 1936[1] as an added protection against leakage from an oesophagogastric suture line in the course of a limited oesophageal resection for benign disease in a young man. The lower oesophagus was implanted into the anterior wall of the stomach, in the same fashion as the rubber tube is implanted in a Witzel's gastrostomy. The patient was noted to be free from reflux symptoms 16 years later, an observation which led Nissen to recognize the crucial role played by the gastric wrap-round in reflux control. In 1955 he added fundoplication to anterior gastropexy (Nissen I), then his operation of choice for sliding hiatus hernia. Shortly afterwards the combined operation was superseded by fundoplication alone (Nissen II)[2]. The operation soon gained widespread acceptance in Europe and America. Nissen performed the operation through a left subcostal incision and stated the aims of the operation as the elimination of the hernia, reduction of the cardia below the diaphragm, reconstruction of the oesophagogastric angle and the re-establishment of a valvular mechanism at the cardia.

Preoperative

Preoperative investigations

A thorough evaluation of the clinical and laboratory data as well as the results of radiological and endoscopic examination is essential for accurate diagnosis and management. The importance of ascertaining that symptoms are not due to other conditions cannot be overstated. The presence of associated diseases of the gall bladder, stomach or duodenum should be remembered and their contribution to the overall clinical picture assessed. Barium examination of the oesophagus, stomach and duodenum is routine in all cases and gives essential information concerning oesophageal motility and length and the reducibility or fixation of the hiatus hernia as well as its type. Furthermore, radiological studies will reveal the presence and location of a stricture and demonstrate the presence of gross gastro-oesophageal reflux and any associated lesions in the stomach or duodenum. A preoperative oesophagoscopy is mandatory as it will reveal the extent and severity of oesophagitis and allow dilatation and biopsy of stricture, as well as biopsy of any other suspicious area of oesophageal mucosa. Routine biopsy of grossly 'inflamed' oesophageal mucosa occasionally reveals unsuspected neoplasia and is recommended.

Indications for operation

The chief indication for operative treatment is the presence of severe symptoms of reflux unresponsive to medical treatment. Other indications for operative intervention are severe oesophagitis at oesophagoscopy, dysphagia due to stricture formation, bleeding, whether acute or chronic, and aspiration pneumonitis. All patients with paraoesophageal hiatus hernia who are acceptable operative risks should be advised to undergo operation in view of the unacceptably high risk of major complications associated with this type of hernia. The operation is inappropriate in patients with oesophageal motility disorders.

The operation

The operation can be performed using either an abdominal or transthoracic approach. The abdominal route may have some merit in patients with coexistent abdominal pathology. The thoracic approach is indicated in obese patients, in recurrent herniation, in patients with panoesophagitis and oesophageal shortening and where a suspicion of malignancy exists. Extensive oesophageal mobilization can be performed under direct vision using the thoracic approach, thus making it possible in the vast majority of patients to replace the gastro-oesophageal junction below the diaphragm without undue tension. Our preferred approach to be described later is thoraco-abdominal. This provides good access to both the chest and the upper abdomen, making it possible to carry out lower oesophageal and upper gastric resection with considerable ease. However, access to the duodenum and gall bladder through this incision is limited and can be improved by extending the incision across the costal margin into the left upper quadrant of the abdomen.

Anaesthesia

After induction, a double-lumen endotracheal tube is introduced. While the patient is still in the supine position a 40–50 Fr Maloney dilator is introduced into the upper oesophagus. The patient is then placed in the lateral decubitus position.

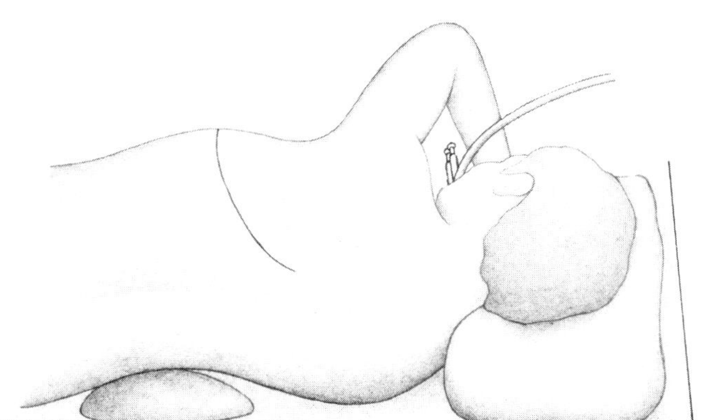

1

1

The incision

A standard posterolateral thoracotomy incision is made along the line of the eighth rib. The periosteum is incised with a fine diathermy needle from the sacrospinalis muscle at the back to the cartilage in front. The periosteum is stripped off the upper border using a curved raspatory and a small segment of the back end of the rib under the sacrospinalis muscle is removed with a costotome. The pleural cavity is entered by incising the rib bed. A Finochietto chest spreader is inserted and gradually opened to provide wide exposure. The anaesthetist is asked to deflate the left lung.

Mobilization of the oesophagus and hernia and diaphragmatic incision

2

The inferior pulmonary ligament is divided until the inferior pulmonary vein comes into view. The lung is retracted forwards and upwards. The posteromedial pleura overlying the oesophagus is incised. The oesophagus, with the vagus nerves attached to its wall, is encircled with a nylon tape and elevated from its bed by gentle traction. The lower oesophagus is mobilized upwards and downwards, dividing the oesophageal arterial branches between ligatures and carefully preserving the vagus nerves. The extent of the oesophageal mobilization necessary to effect reduction without tension depends on the presence or absence of perioesophagitis and the size of the hiatal hernia. Mobilization up to the level of the aortic arch is likely to be necessary in the presence of perioesophagitis and a large hernia. The oesophagus is mobilized downwards to the hernia or phreno-oesophageal ligament if no hernia is present. At the diaphragmatic level the crural fibres of the hiatal margin are displayed. The diaphragm is incised circumferentially through the muscular part, about 5 cm from its costal attachment, for a distance of 15 cm. The incision lies anterior to the phrenic nerve as it enters the diaphragm and extends backwards to well beyond the lateral extent of the spleen. It is important not to divide the diaphragm too close to the chest wall as it will make subsequent closure difficult. This type of incision preserves the nerve supply to the diaphragm and gives excellent access to the upper abdomen.

Two fingers of the left hand are passed through the incision in the diaphragm up through the hiatus to act as a guide while the phreno-oesophageal ligament and peritoneal reflection in front and on each side of the hernia are divided. Complete freeing of the cardia is achieved by division of the remaining connections posteriorly between clamps, as these contain significant arterial branches of the phrenic and gastric arteries. The fat pad overlying the gastro-oesophageal junction is completely removed as far laterally as the vagus nerves. The nylon tape round the oesophagus is passed through the hiatus into the abdomen.

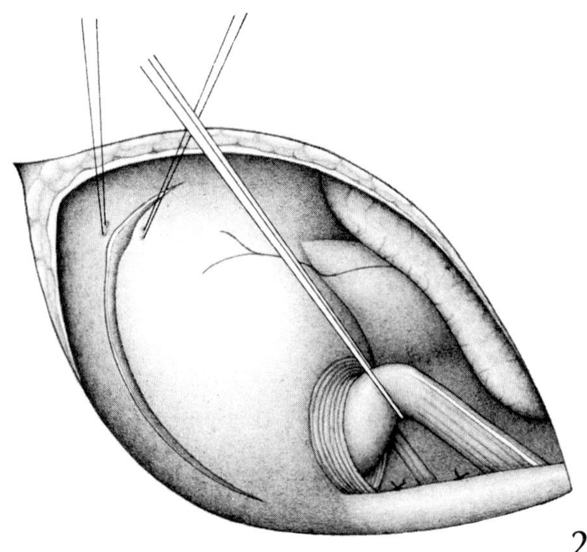

2

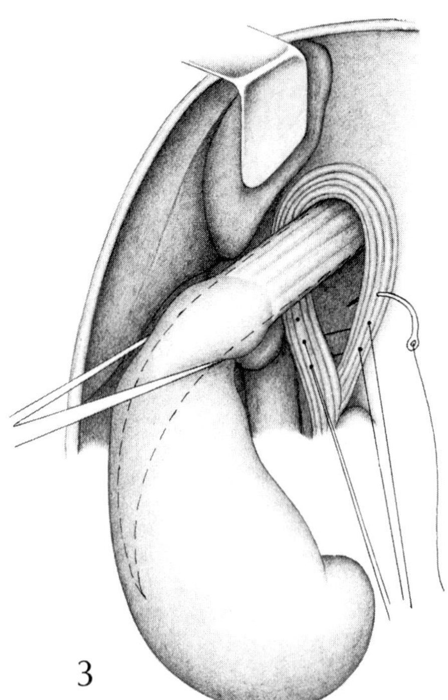

3

3

Exposure of hiatal region and oesophagus from abdomen

The left triangular ligament is divided, taking care not to injure the inferior phrenic vein. The left lobe of the liver is retracted to the right. The upper part of the gastrohepatic omentum is divided between ligatures. This will bring into view the caudate lobe of the liver and, lying alongside it on the left, the right limb of the right crus of the diaphragm. The proximity of the inferior vena cava to this structure must be remembered. It lies immediately posterolateral to the right margin of the hiatus and can be injured if excessively deep bites are taken in the right limb of the crus.

The widened hiatus can now be narrowed using interrupted No. 1 silk sutures on a 45 mm atraumatic needle, taking generous, full-thickness bites of both margins of the hiatus and including the peritoneum. Before these sutures are tied the Maloney bougie, which had been previously introduced into the upper oesophagus, is passed into the stomach and the sutures tied sufficiently tightly to approximate the crura. Excessive tension while tying these sutures will result in strangulation of the crural muscle and cutting out of sutures. The reconstructed hiatus should have enough room to accommodate the oesophagus, with the indwelling bougie, and the tip of the index finger; otherwise, troublesome postoperative dysphagia may occur.

4

Fundoplication: stage 1

The fundus and the upper third of the greater curvature are completely mobilized by division of the vasa brevia, taking special care not to injure the spleen or to include any of the stomach wall in the ligatures. Any adhesions to the posterior wall of the proximal half of the stomach should be divided. After mobilization is complete the fundus is pushed, from the patient's left to right, behind and around the posterior wall of the terminal oesophagus until the edge of the fundal fold appears on the right side of the oesophagus. The edge of the fold is held in this position with Duval tissue forceps. Further gentle traction on the Duval forceps, aided by pushing with the surgeon's right hand, ensures that a good fold of fundus lies to the right of the oesophagus. At the conclusion of this manoeuvre there should be two stomach pouches, one on either side of the oesophagus.

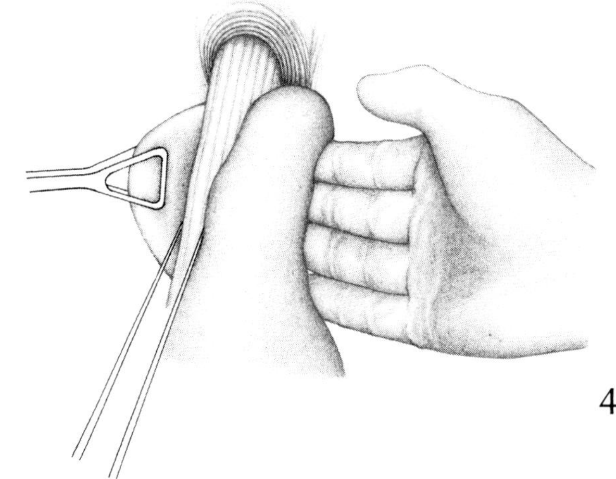

4

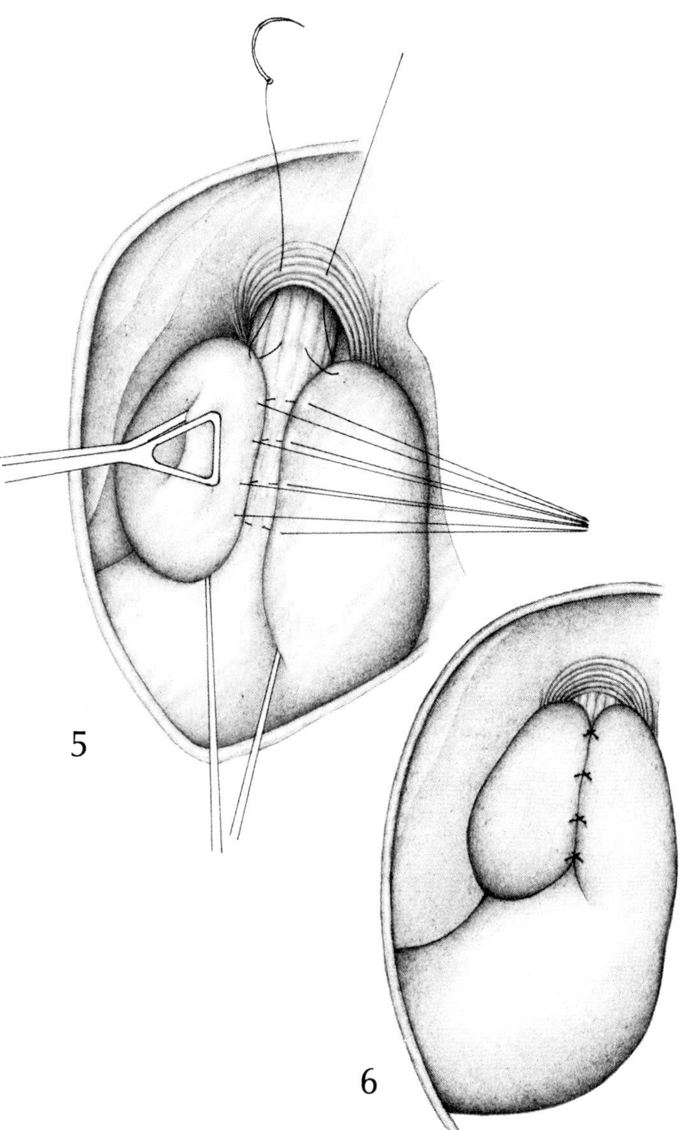

5

6

5 & 6

Fundoplication: stage 2

The pouches are brought together in front of the oesophagus by four or five interrupted 2/0 silk sutures, inserted at 1 cm intervals. The sutures pick up the seromuscular layer of the stomach pouch on either side and the muscle layer of the oesophagus in the middle. Extra care is taken to avoid penetration into the lumen of the oesophagus or stomach. (Fatalities have followed careless placement of these sutures.) All the sutures are put in before they are tied. The first and uppermost suture is a mattressed suture which passes first through the hiatal margins, then through one side of the stomach, the oesophagus, the other side of the fundus and then back through the hiatus. When all sutures have been placed they are tightened, while a finger is placed beneath the fundal cuff thus formed and alongside the oesophagus with its indwelling bougie to ensure that the calibre of the oesophageal lumen and space for expansion during swallowing is not compromised. Should the fundal wrap prove to be tight, the sutures are repositioned; otherwise they are tied with a bougie in position. Too tight a fundoplication will produce dysphagia and too lax a wrap will not restore competence. The Maloney bougie is now removed.

7

Closure of the diaphragm

Meticulous closure of the diaphragm is essential to prevent herniation. The diaphragm is closed with interrupted, figure-of-eight, silk sutures, placed so that every stitch takes up, in addition to muscle, the peritoneum and the diaphragmatic pleura. The chest is closed, leaving a basal drainage tube connected to an underwater seal.

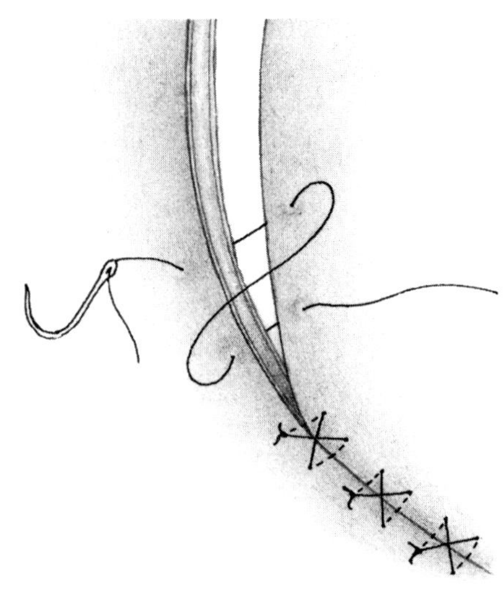

7

Postoperative care

Physiotherapy, instituted preoperatively, is continued in the postoperative period to prevent pulmonary atelectasis from sputum retention. The chest tube is usually removed within 24 hours, after a chest film has confirmed satisfactory expansion of the lungs. We have found the use of a nasogastric tube unnecessary. Fluids are commenced on the return of peristalsis, usually within 48 hours. In the early postoperative phase carbonated drinks are discouraged as they may produce gastric distension. The oral intake is progressively increased and patients are usually able to tolerate a normal diet within a week of operation. Transient dysphagia due to oedema at the cardia is encountered in a few patients. Venous thrombosis and pulmonary embolism pose a constant threat to patients after hiatus hernia repair, particularly if a concomitant splenectomy is necessitated by inadvertent injury of the spleen. Prophylactic measures, including early ambulation and minidose heparin anticoagulation, are advisable.

References

1. Nissen, R. Die Transpleurale Resektion der Kardia. Deutsche Zeitschrift für Chirurgie 1937; 249: 311–316

2. Nissen, R., Rossetti, M. Surgery of the cardia ventriculi. Ciba Symposium 1963; 11: 195–223

3. Orringer, M. B., Sloan, H. Combined Collis-Nissen reconstruction of the oesophagogastric junction. Annals of Thoracic Surgery 1978; 25: 16–21

Further reading

Mansour, K. A., Burton, H. G., Miller, J. I., Hatcher, C. R. Complications of intra-thoracic Nissen fundoplication. Annals of Thoracic Surgery 1981; 32: 173–178

Nicholson, D. A., Nohl-Oser, H. C. Hiatus hernia. a comparison between two methods of fundoplication by evaluation of the long-term results. Journal of Thoracic and Cardiovascular Surgery 1976; 72: 938–943

Rossetti, M. Allgöwer, M. Fundoplication for treatment of hiatal hernia. Progress in Surgery 1973; 12: 1–21

Abdominal repair of oesophageal hiatus hernia

R. C. G. Russell MS, FRCS
Consultant Surgeon, The Middlesex Hospital, London

Preoperative

Introduction

The sphincter mechanism at the lower end of the oesophagus normally prevents reflux of gastric contents into the oesophagus on bending, lying or even hanging upside down, and yet allows regurgitation when vomiting is needed to evacuate a distended, disturbed or irritated stomach. The mechanism of this sphincter remains a subject of debate. It probably represents a complex combination of factors, several of which may be destroyed without the efficiency of its action. These factors include, from within the oesophagus outwards, a plug-like action of the mucosal folds at the cardia, a physiological sphincter at the lower end of the oesophagus, a valve-like effect of the obliquity of the oesophagogastric junction, a diaphragmatic sling which maintains the normal position of the cardia, and the positive intra-abdominal pressure which squeezes the walls of the intra-abdominal part of the oesophagus together. The relative importance of these factors is unknown, but it seems that the physiological lower oesophageal sphincter is probably pre-eminent, thus accounting for the asymptomatic patient with an intrathoracic stomach. In the clinical assessment of a patient it is not the hernia on which attention should be focused, but rather the symptoms and their severity. Reflux of gastric contents into the oesophagus produces retrosternal pain which may radiate into the epigastrium, the chest, the jaws and even the arms. It occurs especially on lying down, bending over or when the intra-abdominal pressure is raised by straining. It may be associated with belching, excessive salivation and reflux of acid contents into the mouth. Dysphagia is present in up to 40 per cent of patients and its presence is unrelated to the length of history. Other symptoms include regurgitation, vomiting, nausea and back pain.

Reflux of acid into the lower oesophagus leads to oesophagitis, ulceration, stricture formation and even perforation. The presence of these complications can best be assessed by fibreoptic oesophagoscopy with biopsy of the inflamed or ulcerated areas to exclude the presence of carcinoma which may be the cause of the dysphagia in an otherwise symptomless hiatus hernia. The severity of the oesophagitis bears little relationship to the severity of the symptoms and is not an indicator of whether medical or surgical treatment should be advised.

A barium examination is important in the assessment of the hernia to determine whether it is of the rolling (or paraoesophageal; about 1 per cent of all hiatus hernias) or the sliding variety. During the study an assessment should be made of whether the oesophagogastric junction is fixed or mobile. Manometry of the oesophagogastric junction is of little value in the management of the patient, but it can help the surgeon in quantifying whether a surgical procedure is adequate. No surgical procedure should be considered unless the surgeon is satisfied that the symptoms are caused by the hernia and, if doubt exists, operative treatment should not be contemplated until all other causes have been excluded and a positive acid perfusion test obtained.

Indications

(*1*) The most common indication is a failure of medical management to control the symptoms. Such medical management must have been supervised, and should include a prolonged trial with the histamine H_2 antagonist, cimetidine. (*2*) Bleeding occurring on more than one occasion or, more rarely, an iron-deficiency anaemia when all other causes have been excluded. (*3*) Oesophagitis with an oesophageal ulcer or a fibrous stricture which is causing dysphagia. (*4*) Paraoesophageal hernia.

Preparation

The surgeon must decide whether the hernia is to be repaired by a transabdominal or a transthoracic approach. If a transabdominal approach is undertaken it is crucial that the hernia can be reduced to a subdiaphragmatic position. Thus a hernia which on a barium examination is shown to be fixed above the diaphragm with the presence of an oesophageal ulcer and severe oesophagitis on oesophagoscopy is unlikely to be easily reduced by a transabdominal approach. On the other hand, an oesophagogastric junction which reduces easily in the upright position during the barium meal examination is ideal for the transabdominal approach. Between these extremes there are times when careful judgement is necessary to decide whether an abdominal or thoracic approach should be employed; when the hernia is being repaired for the second time a thoracic approach is preferable especially if there has been much oesophageal dissection on the first occasion. In making this decision the surgeon must remember that unless the hernia is perfectly reduced the repair will fail. The advantage of the abdominal approach is that it allows examination of the rest of the abdominal cavity and enables the surgeon to anchor the oesophagogastric junction in an intra-abdominal position.

A nasogastric tube should not be passed preoperatively in order to minimize the chance of acid reflux. The patient is prepared for upper abdominal surgery in the normal way and the procedure performed under general anaesthesia with muscle relaxation. The patient is placed supine with the operating table tilted towards the surgeon, and the head raised.

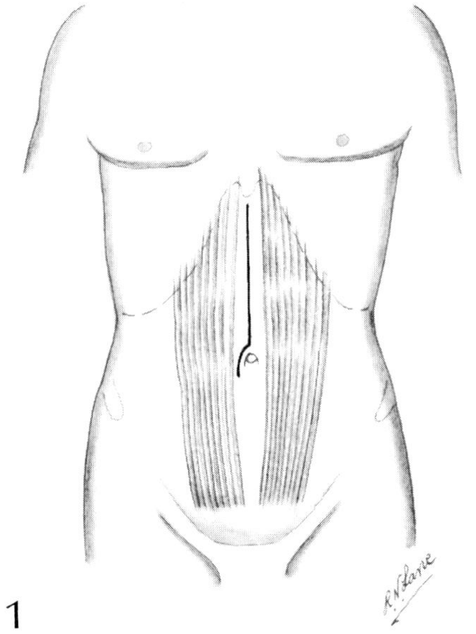

1

The operation

1

The incision

An upper midline or left paramedian incision extending from the xiphisternum to the umbilicus, or just below in an obese patient, offers the best exposure.

2

Mobilization of left lobe of liver

The left lobe of the liver is grasped with one hand and retracted inferiorly. Under direct vision, the left triangular ligament, which is now on the stretch, is divided with scissors. The mobilized left lobe is displaced downward and inward on itself and, covered with a gauze pad, is retracted medially. This exposes the cardia of the stomach and the oesophageal hiatus.

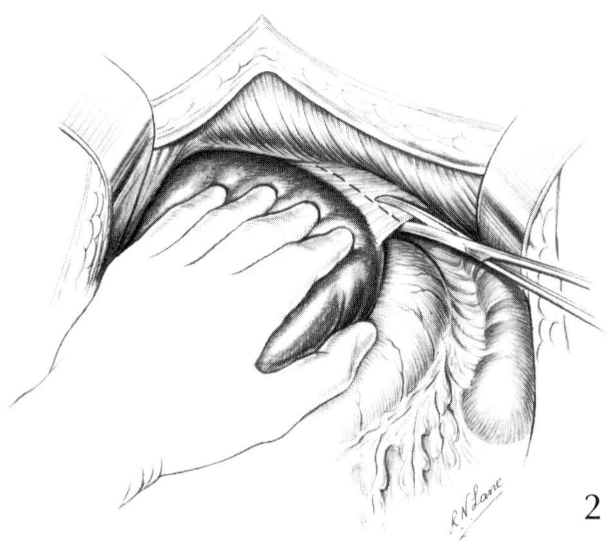

2

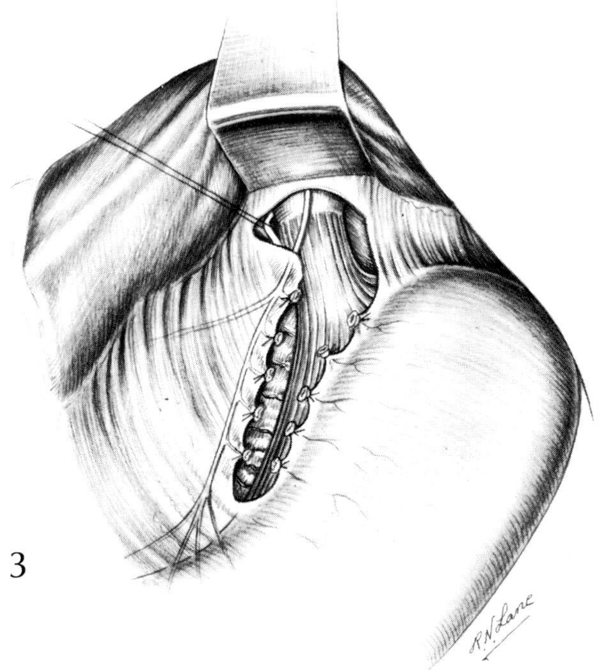

3

3

Exposure of oesophagogastric junction

Because fixation of the oesophagogastric junction to the preaortic fascia is an important step in the performance of this procedure, clear exposure of the junction without damage to the vagus nerves, other than to the fundus of the stomach, is necessary. This is best achieved by dissecting the lesser curve of the stomach as in proximal gastric vagotomy. The dissection should be started 2 cm above the incisura angularis and continued upward until the oesophagogastric junction is clearly exposed. This dissection is aided by the injection of a solution of 1:200 000 adrenaline between the peritoneal layers of the lesser omentum in order to separate the anterior and posterior leaves of the peritoneum and reduce bleeding.

4

Reduction of hernia

The dissection of the lesser curve is continued upwards onto the anterior surface of the oesophagus dividing the phreno-oesophageal ligament on the front of the oesophagus. Downward traction on the oesophagogastric junction will complete the reduction of the hernia and enable a sling to be passed around the oesophagus. The stomach, oesophagogastric junction and lower oesophagus can now be retracted away from the posterior abdominal wall so that 6 cm of oesophagus and 10 cm of stomach are free of peritoneal attachments.

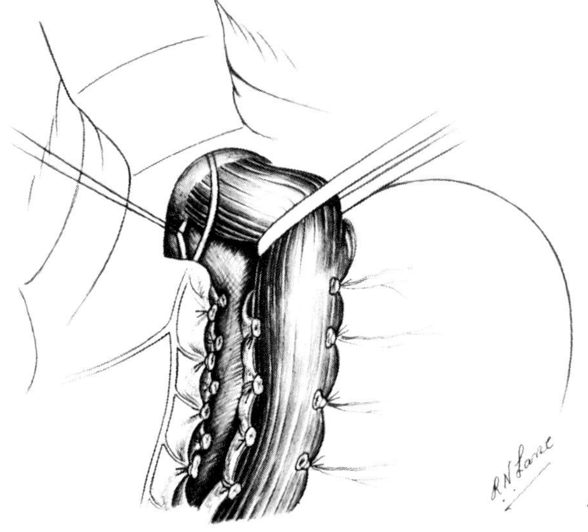

4

5

Exposure of preaortic fascia

With the oesophagus retracted away from the posterior abdominal wall, the hiatus and the left and right crura are exposed. The aorta is exposed through the preaortic fascia at the level of the hiatus. The left index finger is passed into the plane between the aorta and preaortic fascia behind the dense fibres of the median arcuate ligament to the base of the coeliac artery.

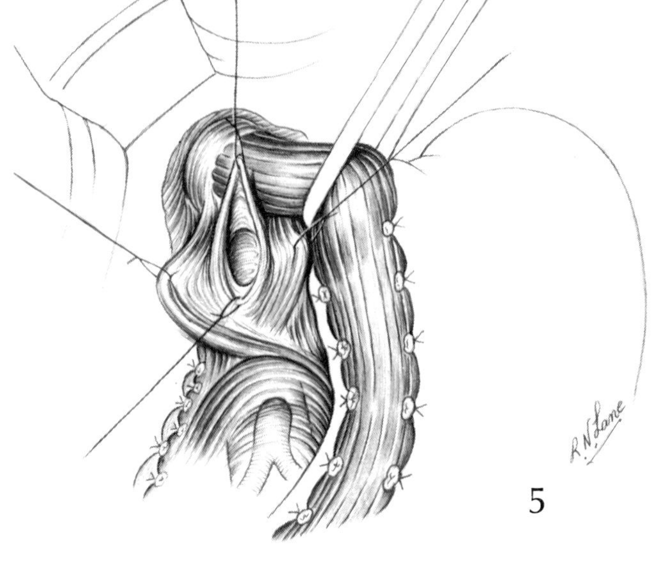

5

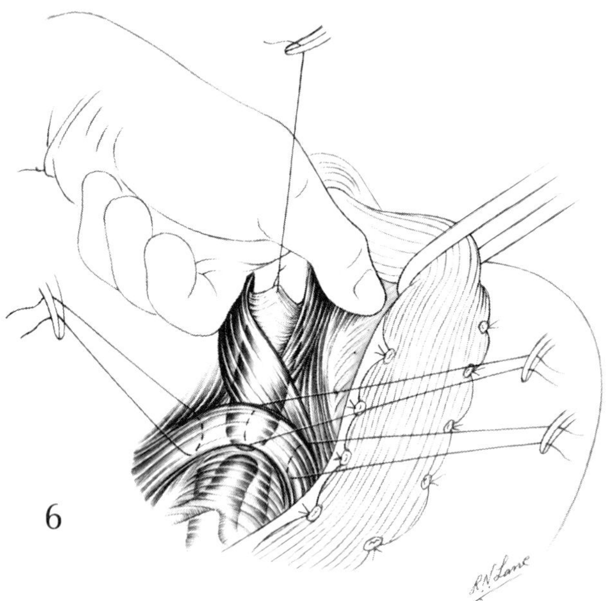

6

6

Placement of sutures

With the finger behind the preaortic fascia and the median arcuate ligament, three sutures of 1/0 braided polyamide (Nuralon) are passed through the full thickness of the fascia and ligament and left untied with the needles attached.

7

Approximation of crura

The crura are approximated by three or four sutures of 1/0 braided polyamide (Nuralon), allowing, after tying the final suture, one finger to slide easily through the reconstructed hiatus. Care must be taken to avoid damage to the anterior or posterior vagus nerve.

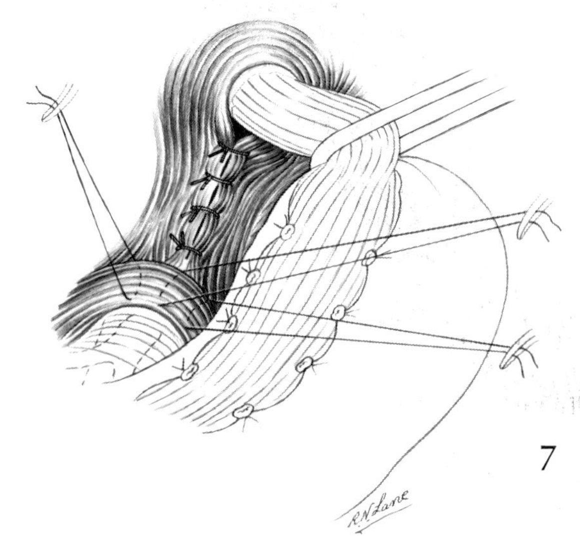

7

8

Reconstruction of oesophagogastric angle

The fundus of the stomach behind the oesophagus is grasped by two pairs of tissue-holding forceps and sutured by interrupted 3/0 braided Polyamide sutures to the exposed oesophageal wall over a length of 4 cm with the lowest suture at the oesophagogastric junction. In a similar manner the anterior wall of the fundus of the stomach is sutured to the anterior right lateral wall of the oesophagus, leaving 1 cm of oesophagus exposed. The plication should be loose so that the oesophagus is not compressed; this can be ensured by performing the partial plication over a mercury bougie in the oesophagus. The three sutures in the median arcuate ligament are placed through the serosa of the stomach at 1 cm intervals above, at and below the oesophagogastric junction and tied, so anchoring the junction to the posterior abdominal wall.

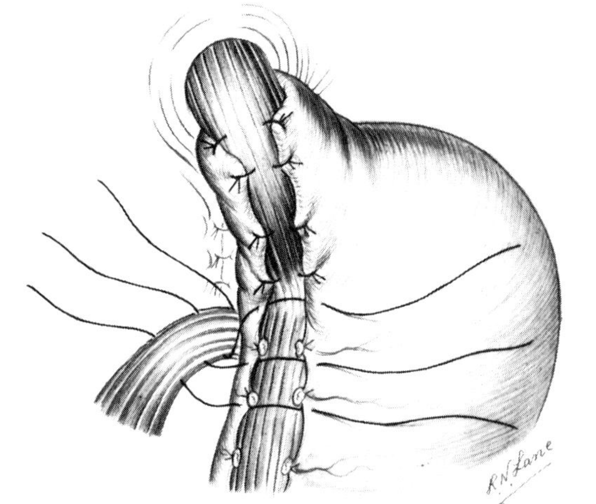

8

9

Fixation of stomach to diaphragm

The line of sutures on the anterior aspect of the oesophagus is continued upwards so that the anterior wall of the oesophagus is covered by the fundus of the stomach. The fundus is finally sutured to the undersurface of the diaphragm with three or four interrupted sutures.

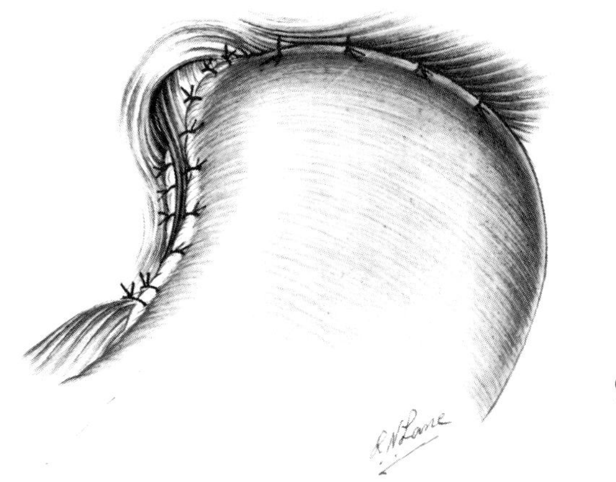

9

Postoperative care and complications

Aftercare follows a standard routine of nothing by mouth and intravenous fluids until there is a resumption of normal peristaltic activity, after which liquids and then solid food is offered. Early complications specific to the repair include surgical trauma to the spleen or oesophagus, resulting respectively in haemorrhage or perforation. Care must be taken during the operation to avoid injury to the organs by adequate mobilization of the oesophagogastric junction especially posteriorly and around the fundus of the stomach. Any injury to the spleen should be treated by splenectomy, and damage to the oesophagus managed by patching with the fundus of the stomach, followed by the abstinence from all fluids until a Gastrografin swallow confirms the absence of a fistula. Before the patient leaves hospital a barium meal or oesophageal manometry, if available, should be undertaken to confirm the satisfactory nature of the repair.

The major short-term complication is dysphagia which usually responds to a single dilatation while the major long-term complication is recurrence. The recurrence rate varies considerably but this type of repair should give a less than 5 per cent chance of recurrence.

Further reading

Earlam, R. Clinical tests of oesophageal function. London: Crosby, Lockwood Staples, 1976

Hill, L. D. Progress in the surgical management of hiatal hernia. World Journal of Surgery 1977; 1: 425–438

Vansant, J. H., Baker, J. W., Ross, D. G. Modification of the Hill technique for repair of hiatal hernia. Surgery, Gynecology and Obstetrics 1976; 143: 637–642

Access to the abdomen and lower chest

Hugh Dudley ChM, FRCS, FRCS(Ed.), FRACS
Professor of Surgery, St Mary's Hospital, London

Introduction

Use and wont have simplified methods of access so that only a few incisions are now commonly used. Furthermore, their choice has become so much a matter of surgical intuition that to restate principles is almost superfluous. However, the following apply.

Vertical incisions, median or paramedian (of adequate length), provide speed of access and ease of closure and the possibility of exploration of all four quadrants by extension. Access to lateral structures is poor unless they can be mobilized on a pedicle that is of midline origin (e.g. a vascular mesentery). Access to the lateral subdiaphragmatic area is also not good.

Transverse and oblique incisions are usually more tedious to make, cause a somewhat greater loss of blood and, except in the infant where the subdiaphragmatic and pelvic hollows are very shallow, do not give as good access at the extremities of the abdominal cavity. The exception to the last statement is a properly placed 'roof top' incision for access to the liver and biliary tree on the right and to the spleen on the left.

Transverse and oblique incisions have a better reputation for freedom from disruption. This may be spurious because (*1*) they are made in circumstances when disruption is unlikely and (*2*) the quoted incidence of wound disruption for vertical incisions is almost certainly too high.

1

Entry into the abdomen

Most surgeons use the knife for traversing the layers of the abdominal wall. Cutting diathermy is unsatisfactory on fat and, in muscles such as the rectus, vessels tend to spring back before they are sealed. However, some surgeons prefer it. In using the knife, it is useful to clear soft tissue away with the flat of the blade so as to expose a generous width of aponeurosis or linea alba. The skin should be held on the stretch.

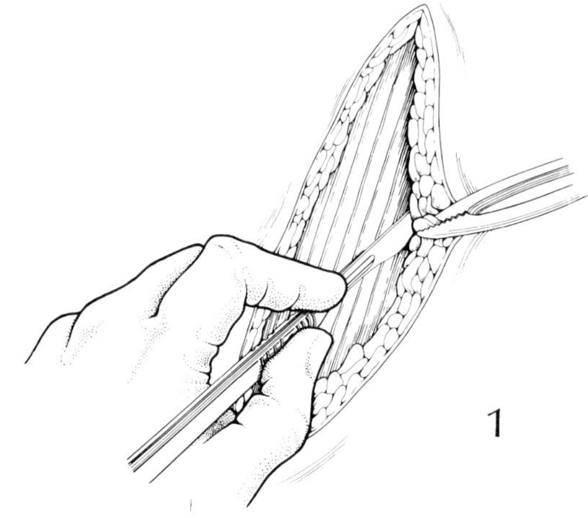

1

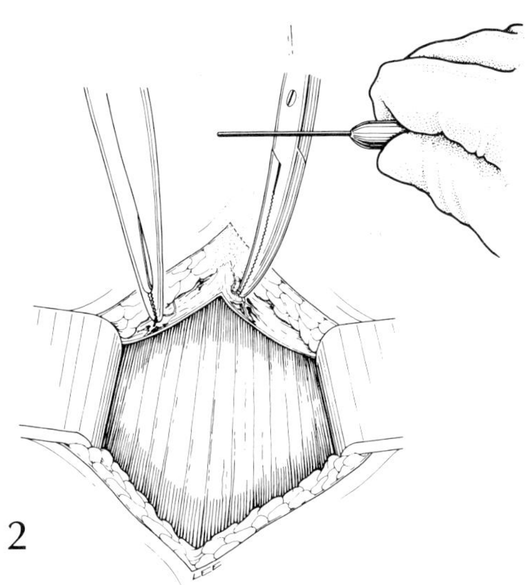

2

2

Haemostasis

Haemostasis in the skin and subcutaneous tissue is obtained by the method of the surgeon's choice. Application of artery forceps everts the wound edges, so making identification of the deeper layers easier. Each may then be touched with a diathermy point. Alternatively, an insulated diathermy forceps may be used both to pick up and coagulate. Fine ties of synthetic absorbable material may be substituted for diathermy but this is a more tedious technique.

Re-entry

Caution should be observed on re-entry in two respects.

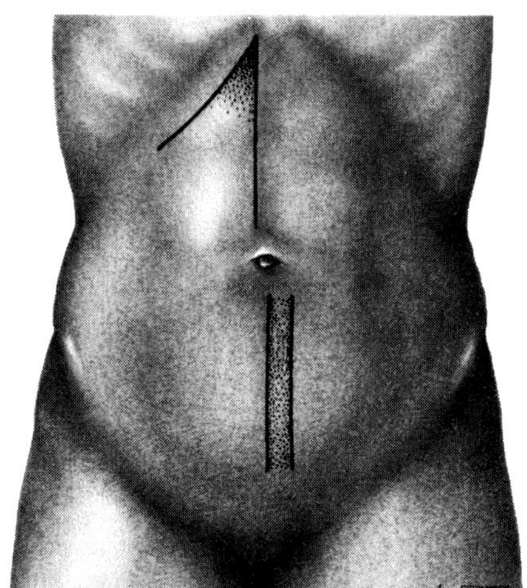

3

3

First 'tram lines' or the oblique confluence of two incisions should be avoided because there is a small but real risk of skin necrosis in the areas shown.

4

Second, damage to underlying adherent structures should be avoided at all costs. This is best achieved by entering if possible at a point away from the original incision by extending it in the appropriate direction for a short distance and by adopting the technique shown.

The deepest identifiable layer of the abdominal wall is turned back and with the exposed contents stretched by the hand sharp dissection is made delicately with the knife. At a variable distance from the wound, in all but the most unfavourable circumstances, free peritoneal cavity is encountered and it is then possible to dissect off the remaining adhesions with greater rapidity and safety.

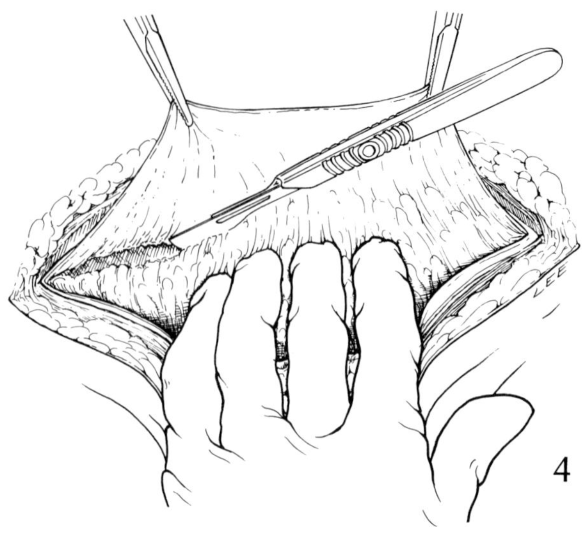

4

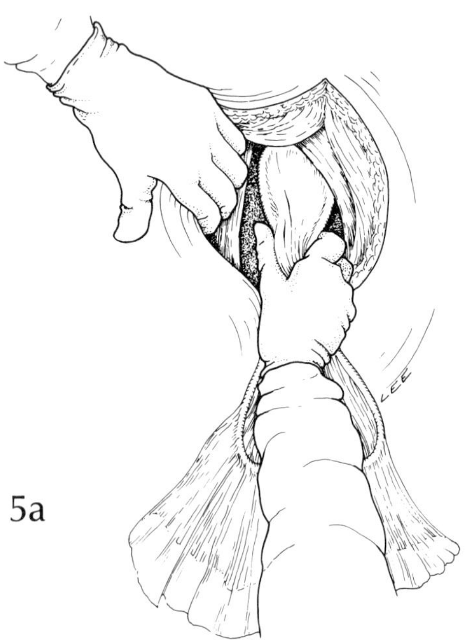

5a

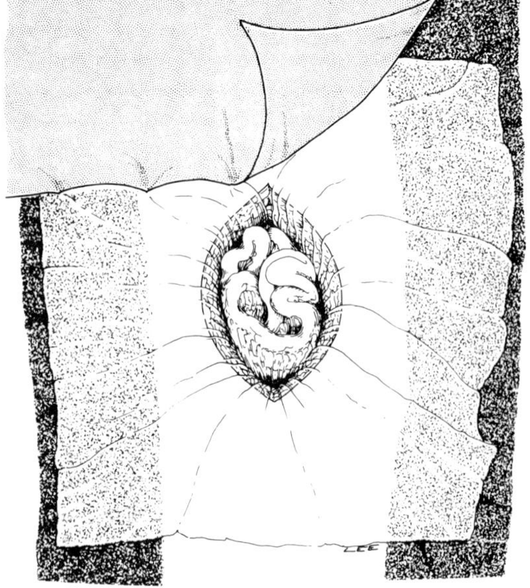

5b

5a & b

Wound protection

Opinions have differed about the value of protecting the wound from contamination (principally from organisms which originate in the operating field). Current evidence[1] supports the view that an impermeable barrier which excludes the wound completely, as distinct from towels which merely exclude the skin, is useful and the author recommends it. The protector is mounted on a flexible plastic ring which is held in the hand as shown (*a*). When insertion is complete the edges are secured with clips so converting a slit into an oval (*b*).

Drainage

6 & 7

Abdominal cavity drainage should, without exception, be through a separate stab incision. Tubes – connected to a closed system – are much to be preferred to gauze, rubber strip or collapsible soft tubing ('Penrose drain'). They should be secured by one of the methods shown.

Wound drainage is best done with suction drains inserted through separate stab incisions and is especially indicated if the abdominal wall is fat. A feeling that a drain is necessary in the wound itself is an indication to leave that wound open. (*See also* the chapter on 'Wound drainage' in the *General Principles, Breast and Extracranial Endocrines* volume.)

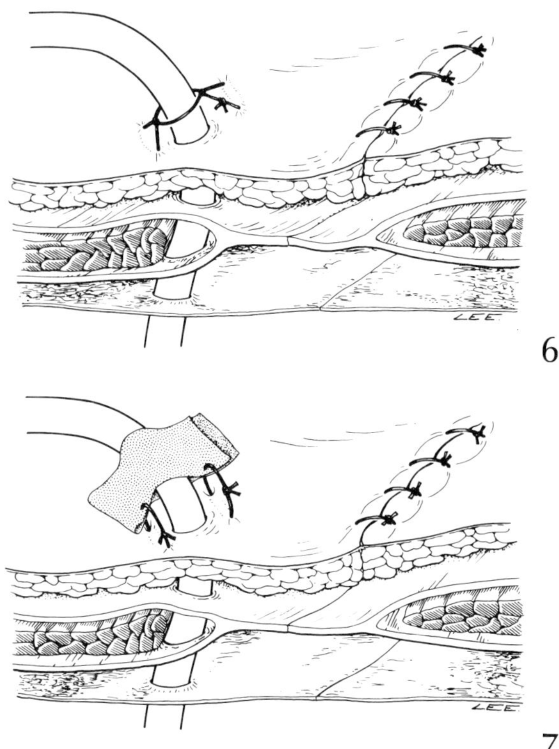

6

7

Closure

Closure of all abdominal incisions has been greatly simplified by the realization that nearly all heal by forming a block of fibrous tissue; that disruption is overwhelmingly a mechanical problem[2,3]; and that proper distribution of forces by the use of large bites of relatively heavy non-absorbable material is a virtual guarantee against difficulty. There are now many published series, the first being that of Jones[4], to attest to the efficacy of this technique though it has not completely eliminated incisional hernia[5].

8a, b & c

Monofilament nylon (1 metric) or stainless steel (28 s.w.g.) (not polypropylene) is passed through all layers deep to the skin at least 1 cm away from the wound edge at intervals of 0.5 cm (*a* and *b*). Peritoneum is included but if there is difficulty it need not be. Knots are tied as shown (*c*).

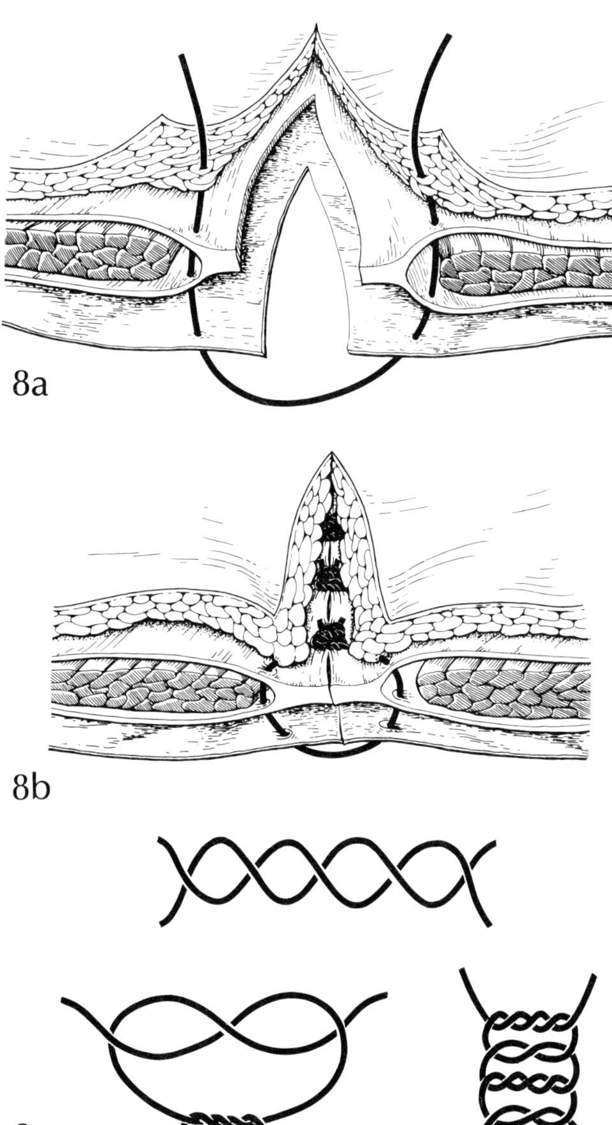

8a

8b

8c

9a–d

A continuous technique may also be used but the abdominal wall must not be dragged together and the stitch should be at least four and preferably six times the wound length. For this technique a doubled 1 metric stitch is looped at one end of the wound and the usual large bites taken (*a* and *b*). The closure is finished by using the loop of the last stitch to make a double knot (*c* and *d*).

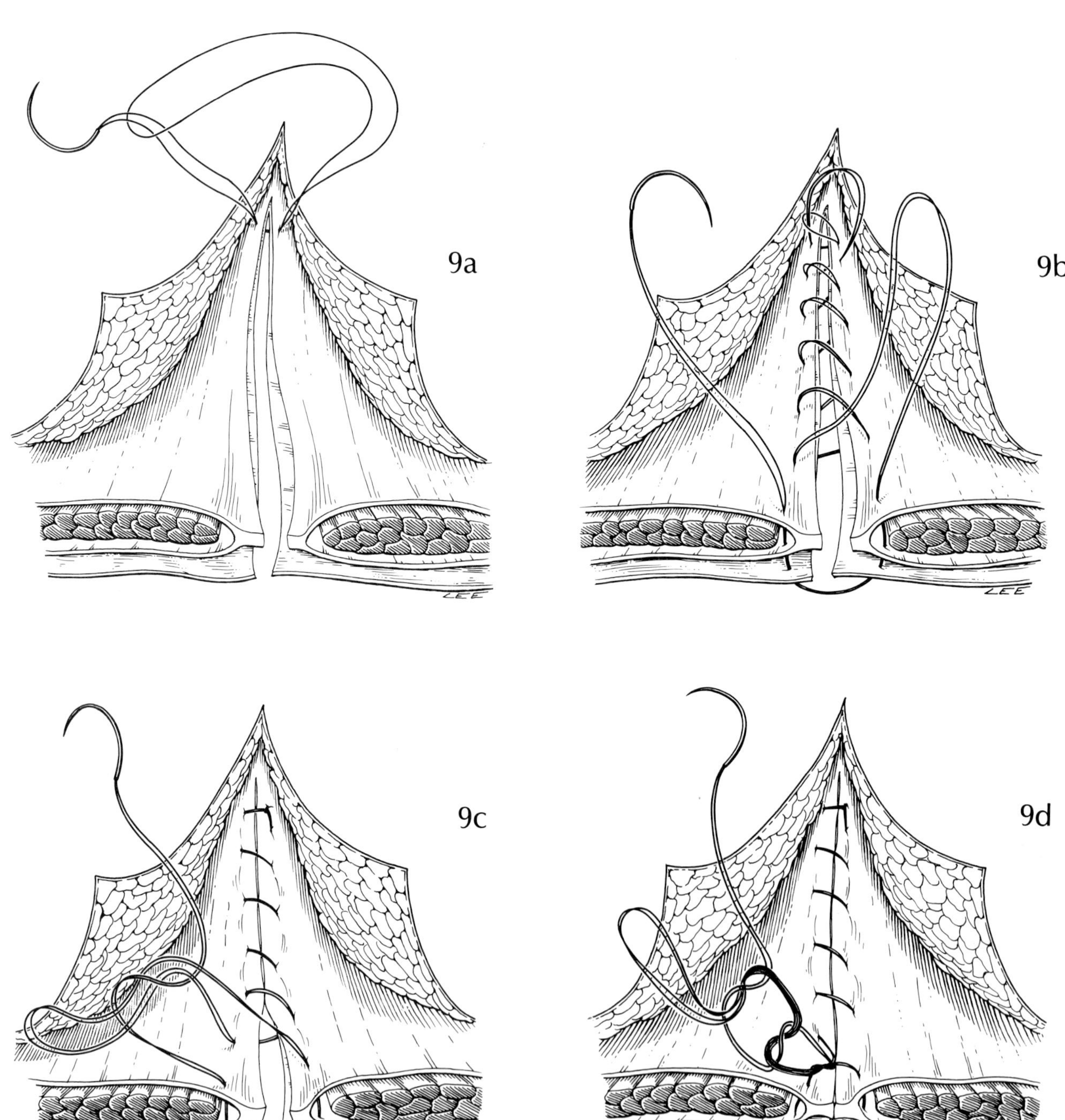

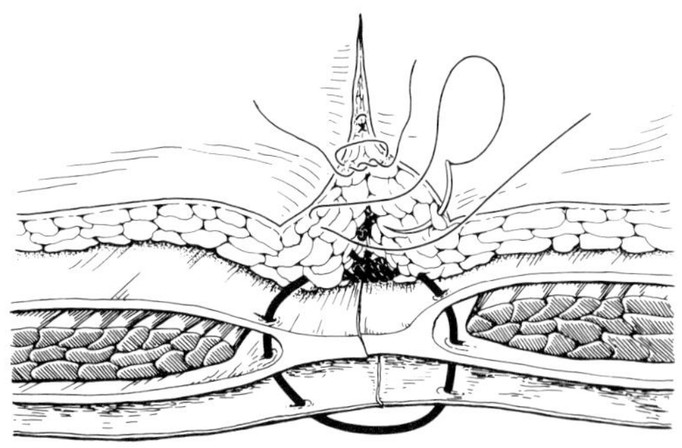

10a

10a & b

The subcutaneous layers are obliterated with interrupted sutures; and to ensure accurate apposition of the skin edge, particularly for the vertical incision which may otherwise be somewhat unsightly, a deep dermal inverted suture may be used (*a*). (Alternatively, with the technique of mass closure it is feasible to leave a potentially infected laparotomy wound open for delayed primary closure by suture or tape.) The skin is closed with fine monofilament sutures or clips. For unequivocally clean transverse or oblique incisions a continuous intradermal (subcuticular) stitch (*b*) gives the best cosmetic result and may be either of synthetic absorbable material or fine monofilament in which case Denis Browne's technique is used.

Mass closure may be used in all abdominal incisions except those made by splitting muscles along different lines, e.g. grid-iron incision for appendicectomy or lumbar sympathectomy.

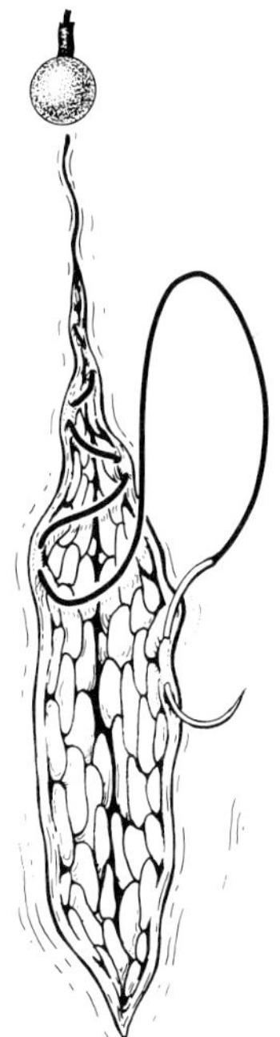

10b

Particular incisions

Midline

EPIGASTRIC INCISION

11

A suitable incision for most surgery in the supracolic compartment. If the operation is on the stomach or duodenum it is wise *not* to extend the incision beyond the umbilicus because this will only lead to annoying protrusion of the colon. Upwards extension is described below. Unless the incision is extended beyond the umbilicus it is usually unsuitable for (*1*) wide laparotomy, (*2*) biliary tract surgery or (*3*) the removal of an enlarged spleen. Slightly more laterally placed incisions are preferable for all these purposes.

The knife passes through the stretched skin and subcutaneous tissues down to but not at this stage through the linea alba. The fat is carefully dissected off this structure about 1 cm to either side by using the flat of the knife (*see Illustration 1*). This not only permits easy identification of the exact midline but also provides room for the mass closure already described.

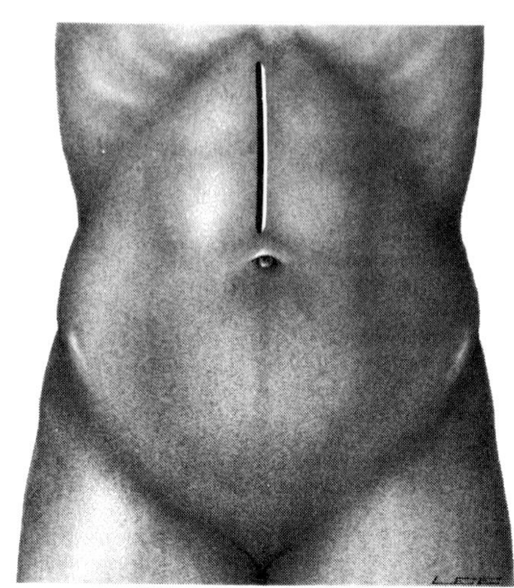

11

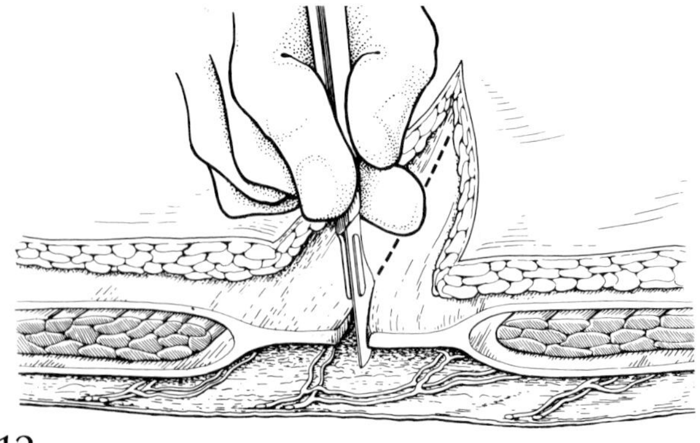

12

12

The linea alba is next incised in the line of the incision to expose the extraperitoneal fat and underlying diaphenous peritoneum. A few vessels course across this.

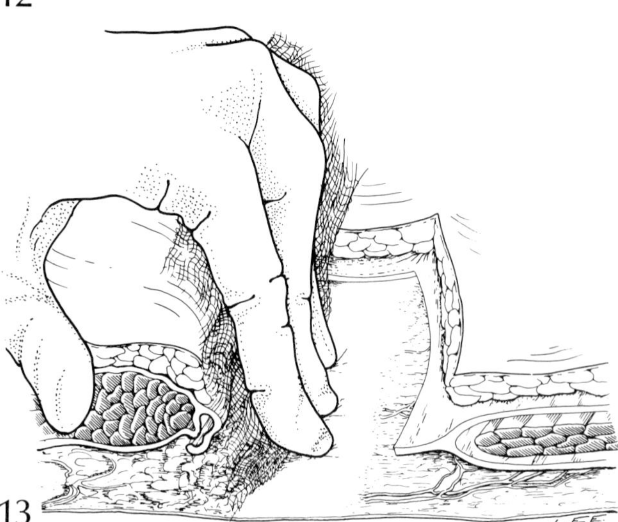

13

13

Most of the fat and vessels may be displaced laterally by blunt gauze dissection. Any remaining vessels are coagulated.

14

The peritoneum is picked up and incised with the knife at about the junction of the middle and lower thirds of the wound, then split with scissors.

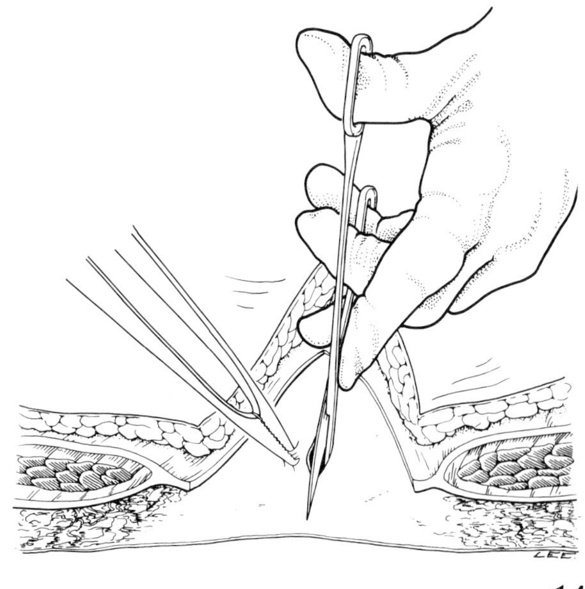

14

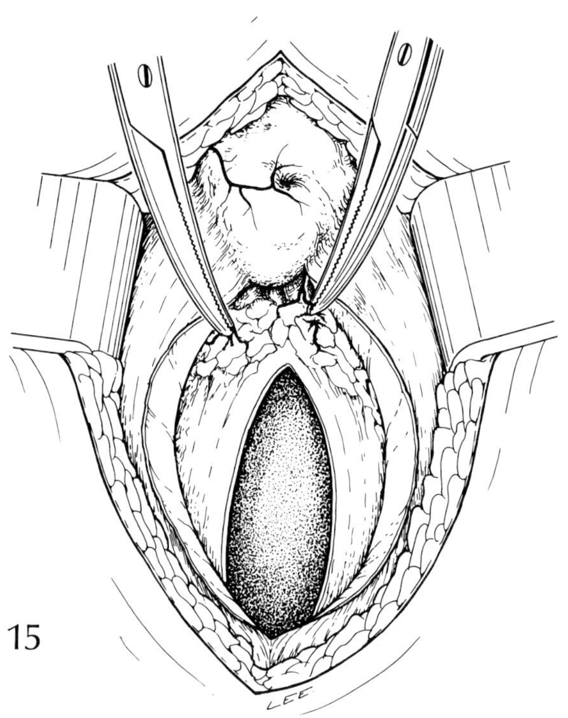

15

15

At the upper end of the peritoneal incision more fat is often encountered and a further vessel must be coagulated.

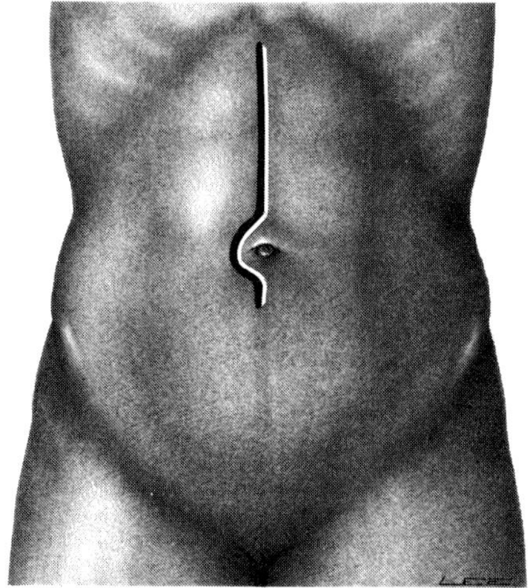

16

Extension

16

Downwards

The umbilicus is skirted to right or left and the incision continues in the linea. It is sometimes difficult to avoid entering one or other rectus sheath but this is of no consequence.

17a & b

Upwards

Either through or to one or other side of the xiphoid is possible and the choice depends on the additional exposure required and the shape of this cartilagenous structure. If through, the xiphoid can often be cut with a heavy pair of scissors (*a*); alternatively double-action bone shears are used (*b*). If to the side, a terminal branch of the internal mammary will always be encountered and should be deliberately sought to avoid troublesome bleeding. It is more easily coagulated than ligated (*a*).

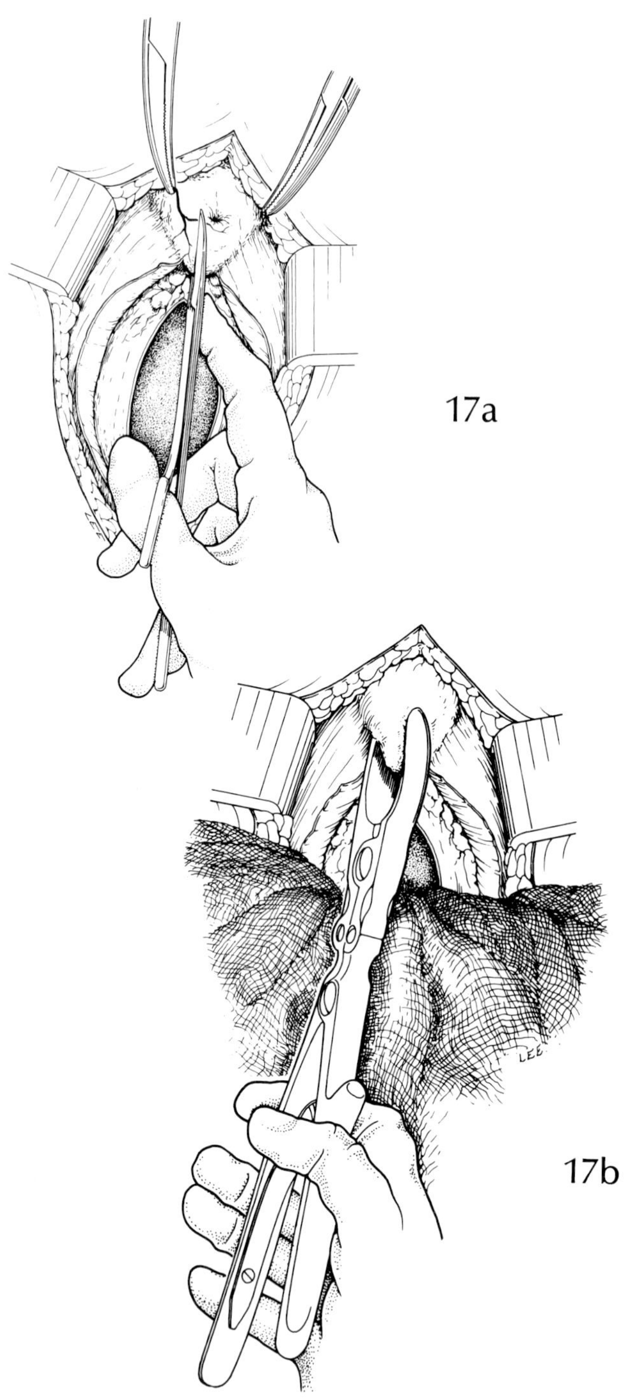

17a

17b

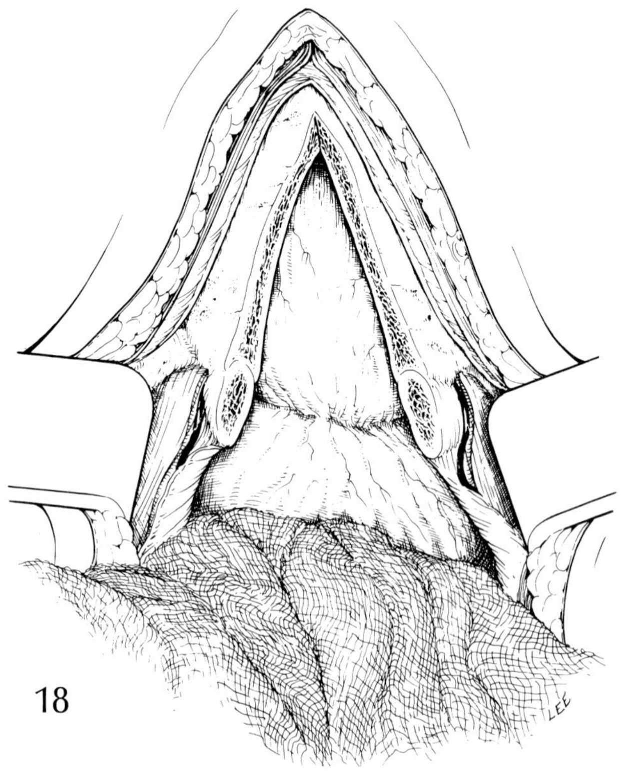

18

18

For very extensive exposure it is effective to split the lower third of the sternum with a power saw.

Closure

The single-layer closure already described should be used.

SUBUMBILICAL MIDLINE INCISION

This incision has enjoyed a poor reputation for disruption but this probably reflects inadequate methods of closure. It has only a small place in abdominal as distinct from gynaecological surgery, but may be occasionally required as an extension for wide exposure or exploration (e.g. surgery of the aorta). It is made and closed in a similar manner to the upper midline incision. As with the upper end of this, at the lower end of the subumbilical incision, the parietal peritoneum moves away posteriorly over the dome of the bladder. Care must be taken not to damage the latter.

Paramedian

The major virtue this has over a midline incision is that it gives slightly better access to one or other side of the abdomen. The apparent additional virtue of having the rectus muscle intervening between the incision in the anterior and posterior sheaths is largely offset by the transverse lie of the fibres in both these layers (*but see* lateral paramedian *below*). Security comes, as in the midline incision, from the method of closure. It follows that there is little to be gained by the use of a rectus-displacing incision and that, if one is employed, the closure sutures should also displace the rectus to get a firm deep bite in the anterior and posterior sheaths at least 1 cm back from the cut edge (*see Illustration 22*).

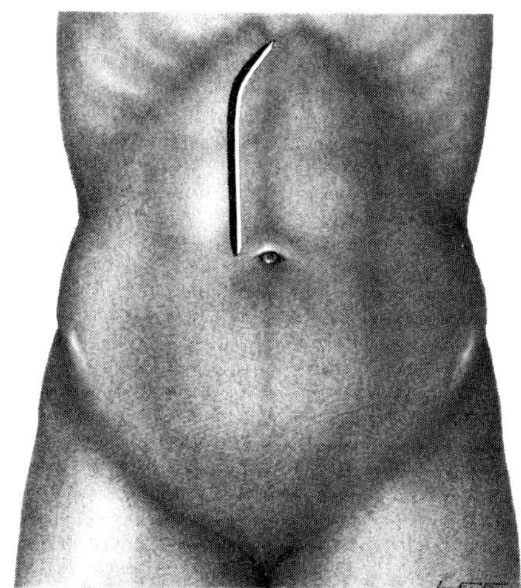

19a

19a & b

The technique is the same in the upper and lower abdomen with two exceptions: (*a*) at the upper end of the supraumbilical incision additional room may be gained by angling the incision medially (Mayo-Robson extension); (*b*) below a point midway between the umbilicus and symphysis pubis the posterior rectus sheath is deficient. Closure is then dependent entirely on effective suturing of the anterior sheath.

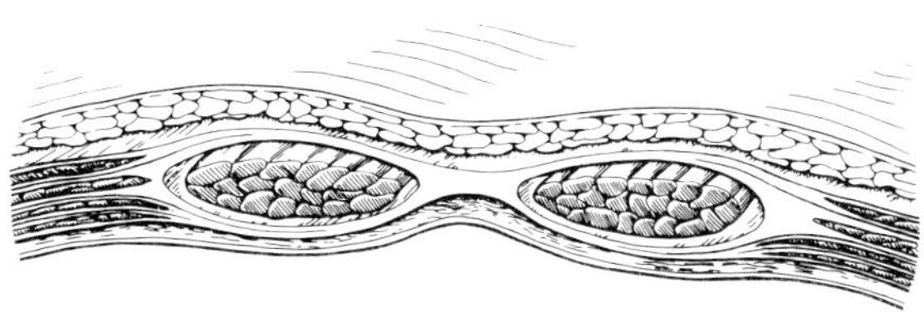

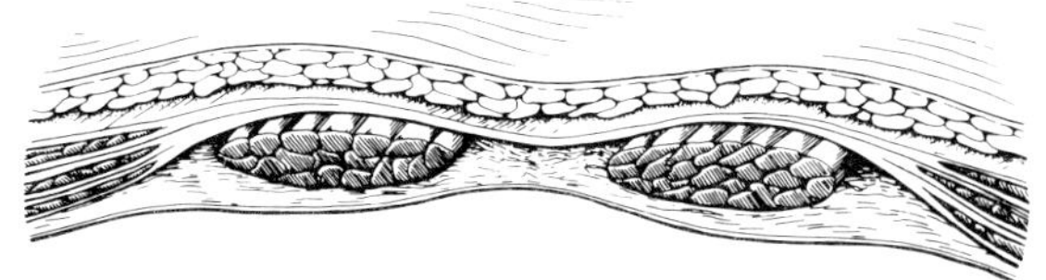

19b

Reflection of the rectus

20

If this is desired, tendinous intersections must be freed in the upper abdomen. The anterior rectus sheath is cleared as for the linea alba in a midline incision and incised vertically. The medial cut edge is seized with forceps and lifted vertically. The tendinous intersections are adherent to and blended with this layer and must be freed by sharp dissection. One or more blood vessels need to be dealt with in each intersection. The rectus may then be retracted laterally and the posterior rectus sheath and peritoneum incised together. In the right upper abdomen this brings the operator down to the right of the falciform ligament which may have to be divided if exposure is required to the left of the midline.

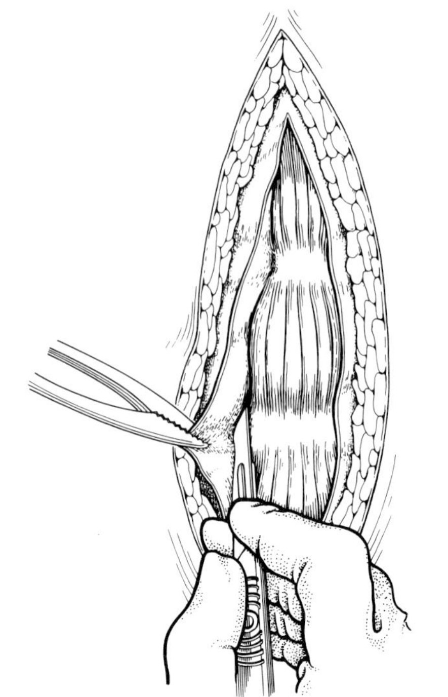

20

21

Transrectus incision

Alternatively, and in the author's view preferably, the rectus muscle is incised longitudinally no more than 1 cm from its medial border. Bleeding is encountered from vessels in the muscular belly laterally but is easily controlled by coagulation or by fine over-and-over sutures.

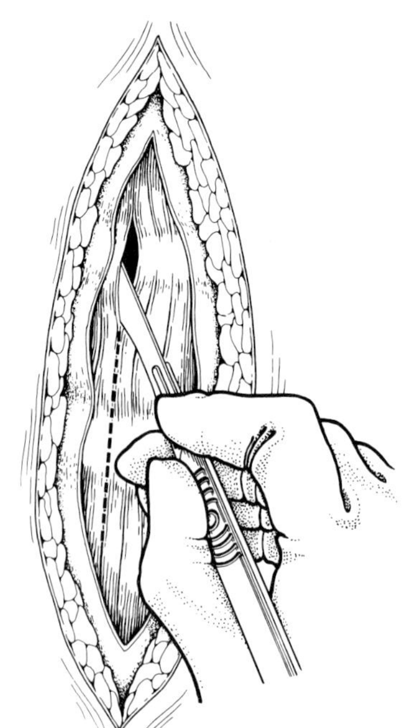

21

22

Closure

Using the mass closure principle, sutures are inserted through the adjacent linea alba and peritoneum medially and through both layers of the rectus sheath laterally. The lateral muscle is displaced away by the needle. In a rectus-splitting incision the narrow medial strip of muscle is included in the stitch. Problems have not been encountered with this technique.

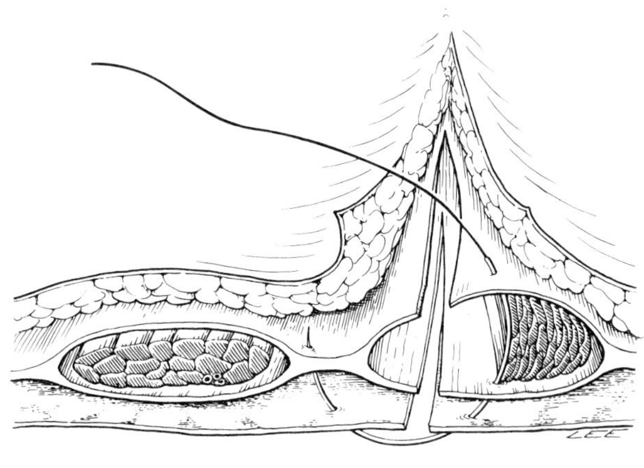

22

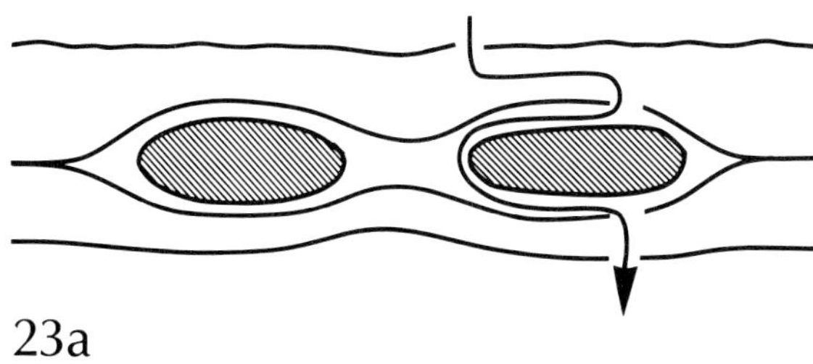

23a

23a & b

A more laterally placed variant of the rectus-displacing incision has recently been described – the lateral rectus incision[4]. The pathway of the incision is shown in (*a*). The wide flaps of sheath so fashioned (*b*) can be coapted with standard small-bite continuous or interrupted technique and, according to its inventors, using any conventional suture material. As high an immunity from disruption as that for mass-closed midline incisions has been achieved and the incidence of hernia may be less.

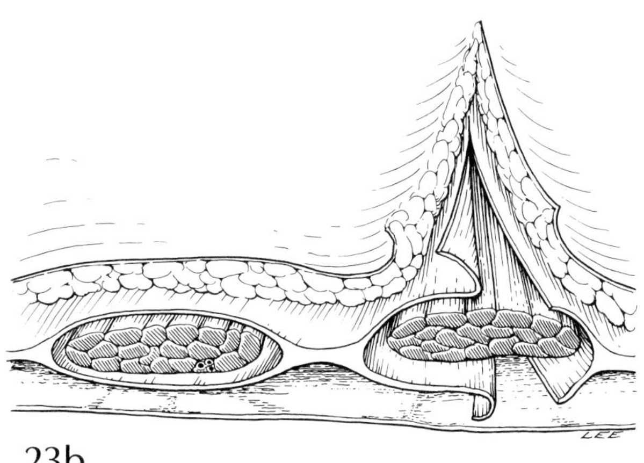

23b

Kocher's incision

24a & b

The skin incision is 2.5 cm below the costal margin and parallel to it (*a*). The medial end is at the midline so that as the cut is deepened it penetrates the rectus sheath and divides the vertical fibres of the rectus (*b*). Branches of the superior epigastric artery and occasionally the vessel itself are encountered here and must be dealt with by ligature or diathermy. More laterally, the flat muscles are divided in the line of the incision and one or at the most two segmental nerves, often with their accompanying vessels, must be divided. However, every effort should be made to preserve nerves placed laterally in the wound. The incision is deepened through all layers to open the peritoneum. Extension across the midline and down the other costal margin may be used to provide generous exposure of the upper abdominal viscera (*see Illustration 26*). Closure is by the interrupted mass technique already described or in layers using non-absorbable sutures.

Kocher's incision gives good access to the biliary tract, the liver and, on the left, to the spleen. However, for free access to the whole of the biliary apparatus and particularly to explore the head of the pancreas and the papilla, the author prefers a long right paramedian incision, which must be extended well below the umbilicus so that its lateral edge can be sufficiently retracted.

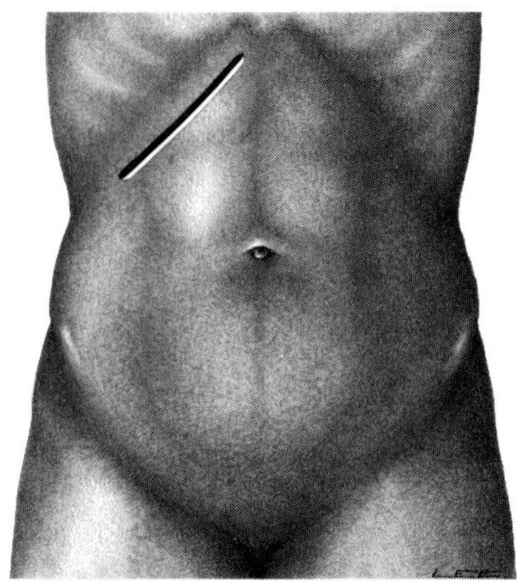

24a

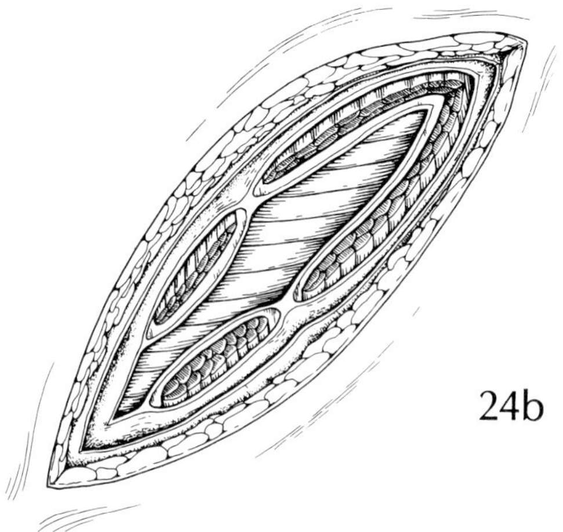

24b

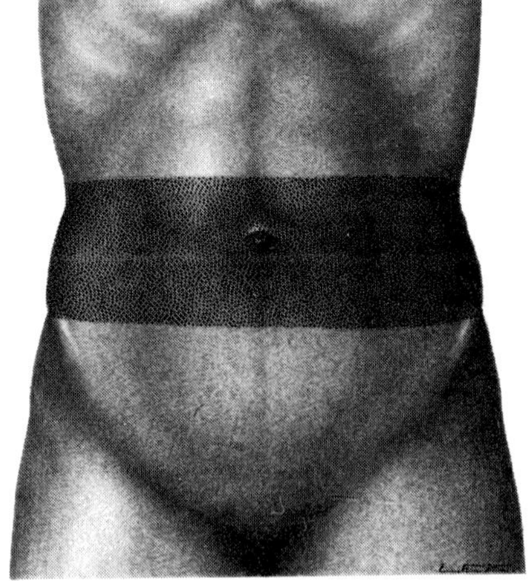

25

Transverse muscle-cutting incisions

25

A muscle-cutting incision to expose intraperitoneal structures may be made anywhere in the zone shown and may divide either or both rectus muscles. Such incisions give good exposure for right or transverse colectomy. They may be closed in one layer or layer-by-layer and are unlikely to disrupt.

26

An increasingly popular incision for difficult upper abdominal surgery (e.g. hepatic resection, bile duct strictures and the like) is the 'roof top' approach first extensively employed for bilateral adrenalectomy from the front. It is essentially a double Kocher's though, particularly in those with a broad costal margin, its inclination is more horizontal. Otherwise the technique of making and closing the incision is as that for Kocher's incision.

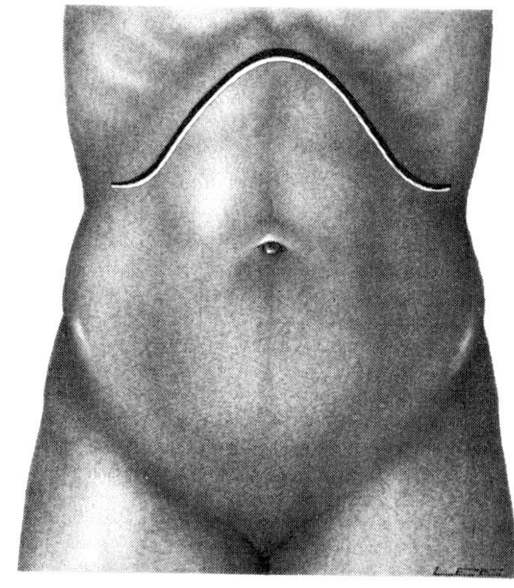

26

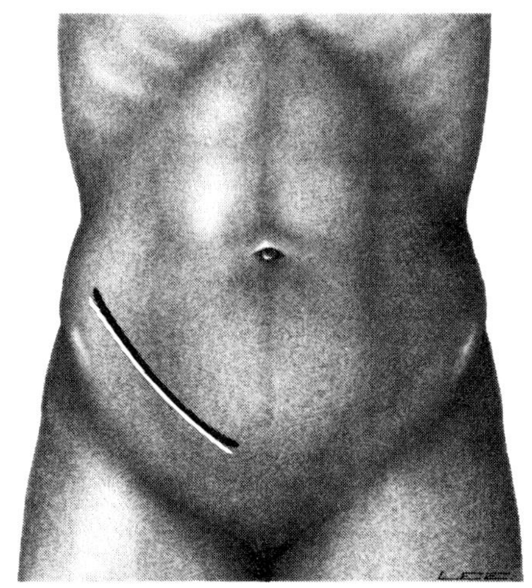

27

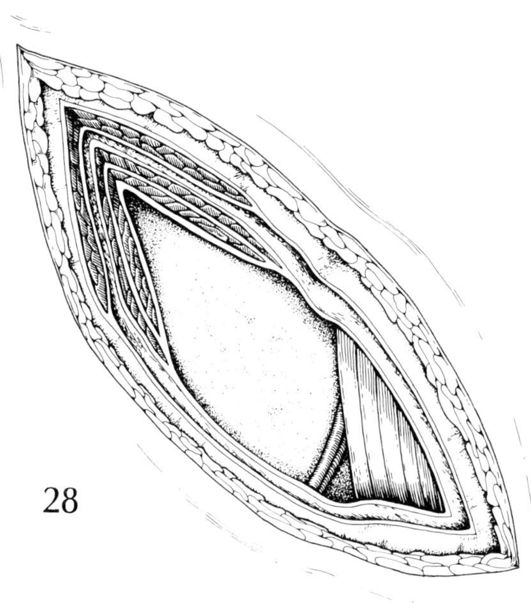

28

27 & 28

A slightly more oblique, open curved, muscle-cutting incision may be made in either iliac fossa, that on the right being usually known as Rutherford Morrison's incision though it was probably first used by Astley Cooper. This gives good access to a difficult inflamed appendix. Sigmoid colectomy may also be done on the left side but access to the rectum is less satisfactory than through a left lower paramedian incision.

SYMPATHETIC CHAIN AND OTHER RETROPERITONEAL STRUCTURES

29

Good access can also be obtained to the lumbar sympathetic chain through a muscle-cutting incision which runs forward from the tip of the twelfth rib to the lateral border of the rectus sheath with the patient tilted 30° to the opposite side. A high-muscle-splitting incision is less satisfactory.

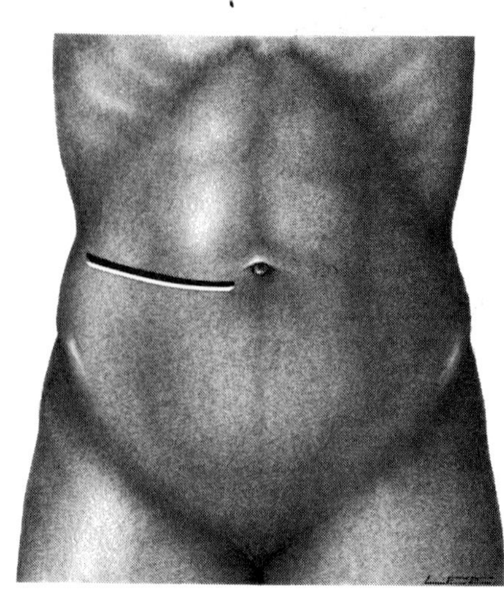

29

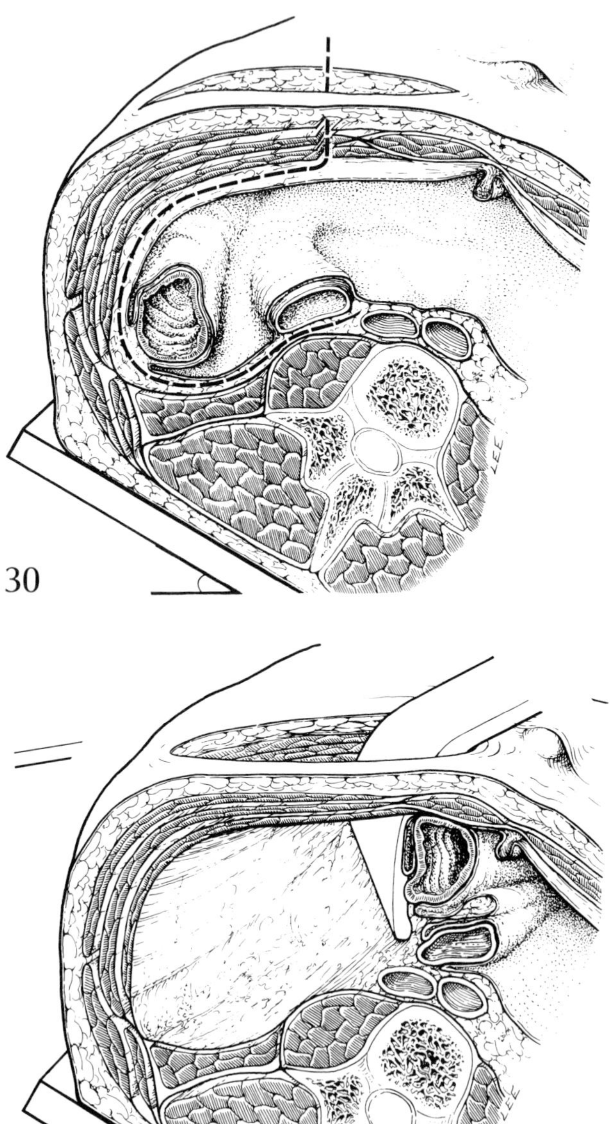

30

31

30 & 31

All muscular layers are divided down to the peritoneum; care should be taken not to open this because air within the sac interferes with the dissection. The plane of dissection follows the line shown and crosses the surface of the psoas muscle to the anterolateral aspect of the lumbar bodies. The ureter may also be found in a slightly anterior plane.

Muscle-splitting incisions

A muscle-splitting incision may be substituted for the muscle cut described in *Illustrations 27* and *28*, but the exposure is more limited.

GRIDIRON INCISION

32

The skin incision is centred on a point just lateral to the surface marking of the appendix – the junction of middle and outer thirds of a line joining the umbilicus to the anterosuperior iliac spine. The cut in the skin may be transverse, which is cosmetically more acceptable, or parallel to the line of the iliac crest, which gives a better exposure and is more easily converted into a Rutherford Morrison incision should occasion demand.

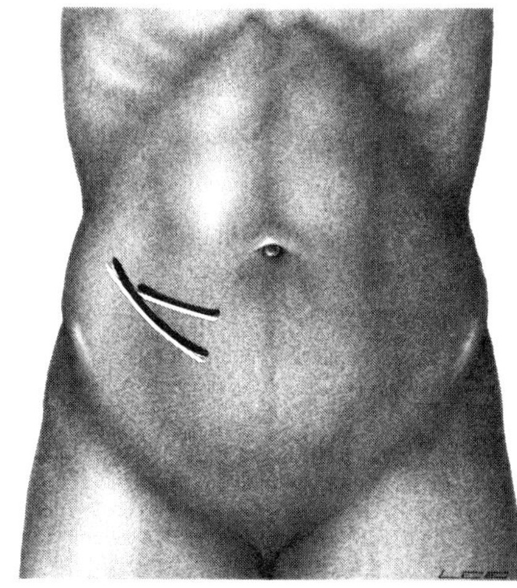

32

33

The external oblique is split in the line of its fibres to expose the underlying internal oblique and transversus muscles which at this level in the abdomen are almost in the same line. The rectus sheath should be visible medially.

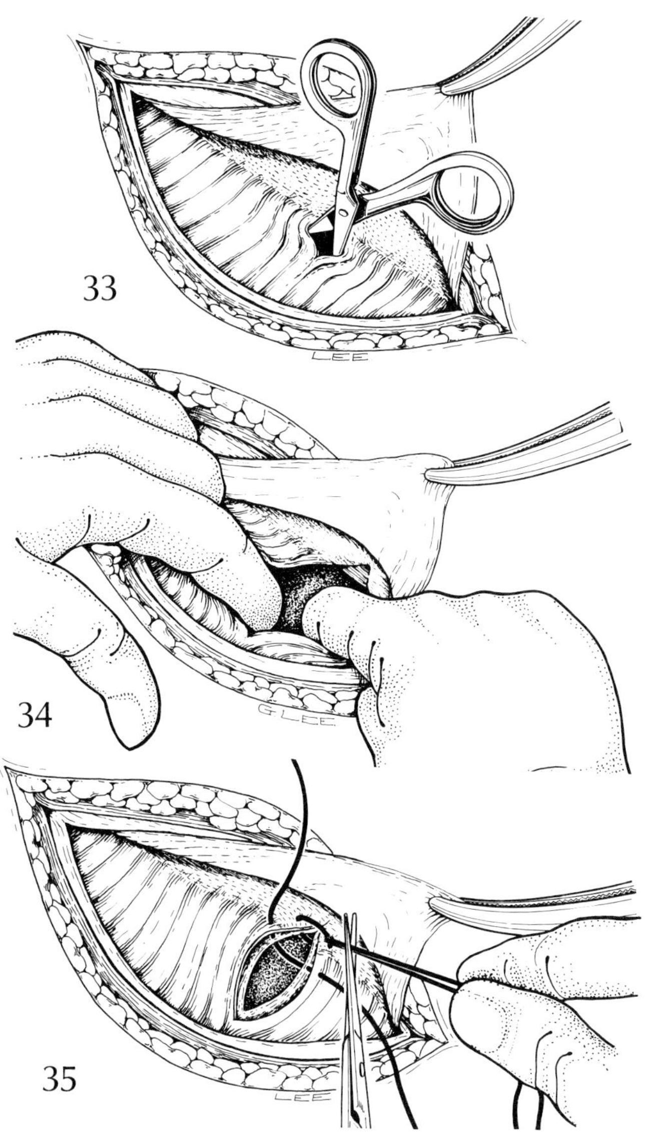

33

34

35

34

The deep muscle fibres are split transversely to reveal the peritoneum which may without detriment be opened in the same line. Additional exposure is obtained harmlessly by incising the rectus sheath.

35

Closure of the incision is conventionally in three layers – peritoneum, deep muscles and external oblique aponeurosis. However, the first two may be closed together.

A gridiron incision may, if there is severe contamination, be left open down to the peritoneum. It will usually heal well without further intervention.

PFANNENSTIEL INCISION

This incision is the one now most extensively used for surgery of the female pelvic organs and for the operations on the bladder and prostate.

36 & 37

The skin incision is parallel to the suprapubic crease and just below the hair line. The anterior rectus sheaths are divided in the same line and this cut may be extended laterally to split the flat muscles if more exposure is required. The sheath is then reflected upwards, one or two small vessels on its undersurface frequently requiring coagulation. The recti can now be separated in the midline and retracted laterally. The preperitoneal (transverse) fascia is exposed and dissection may then proceed in this plane or the peritoneum may be opened.

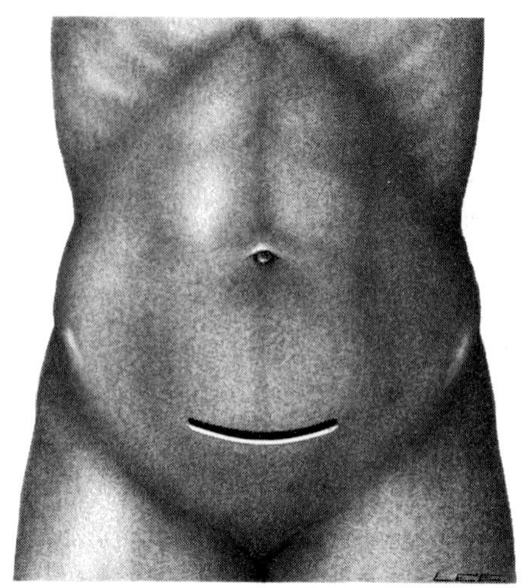

36

Closure

The peritoneum, if opened, is closed with a running stitch. The recti fall together and the anterior sheath is approximated with either continuous or interrupted sutures according to the surgeon's preference.

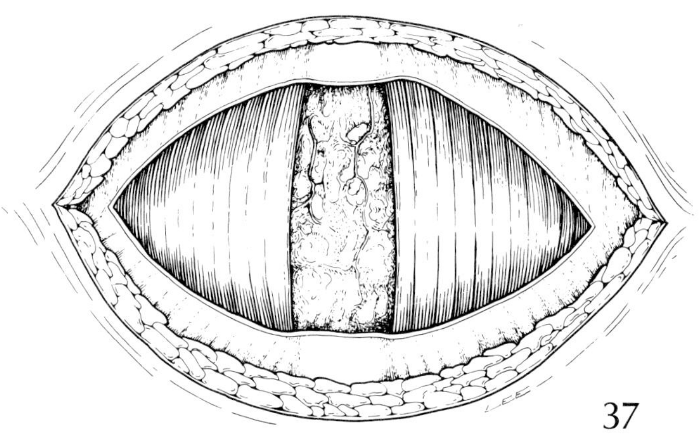

37

38

THORACOABDOMINAL INCISION

38

The abdominal structures under cover of the rib cage may be exposed more easily by opening the chest as well as the abdomen. A useful general purpose incision runs in the line of the eighth or ninth rib from the lower border of the scapula across the costal margin and towards the umbilicus. As shown, the patient is turned two-thirds of the way on to the opposite side; a greater tilt is not recommended because it leads to difficulty in exposing the abdominal viscera.

39

The layers of the chest and abdomen are related as follows.

External oblique – continuous over both
Internal oblique – in the line of the rib
Transverse – interdigitates with the diaphragm.

Therefore, as the incision is deepened these structures are encountered seriatim. The rib may be either resected subperiosteally, mobilized so that entry may take place on the deep aspect of the periosteum or alternatively an intercostal space may be used. For ease and firm closure the first is recommended for the occasional operator. Entry into the chest and the deeper layers of the abdomen exposes transversus and diaphragm with a bridge overlying them formed by the costal cartilages. A short length of costal cartilage is excised.

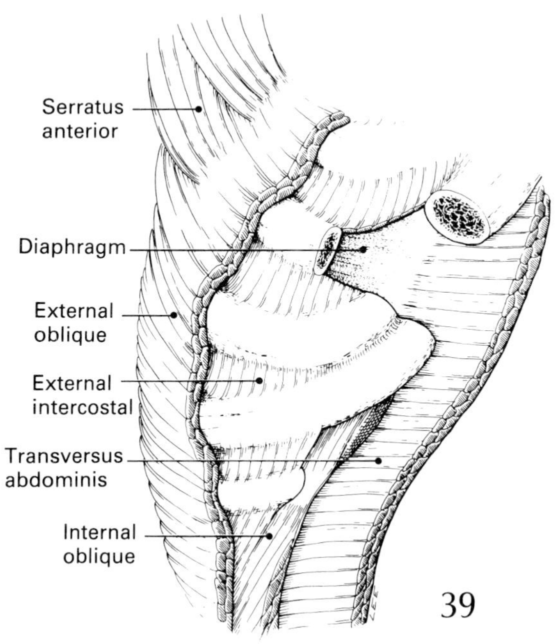

39

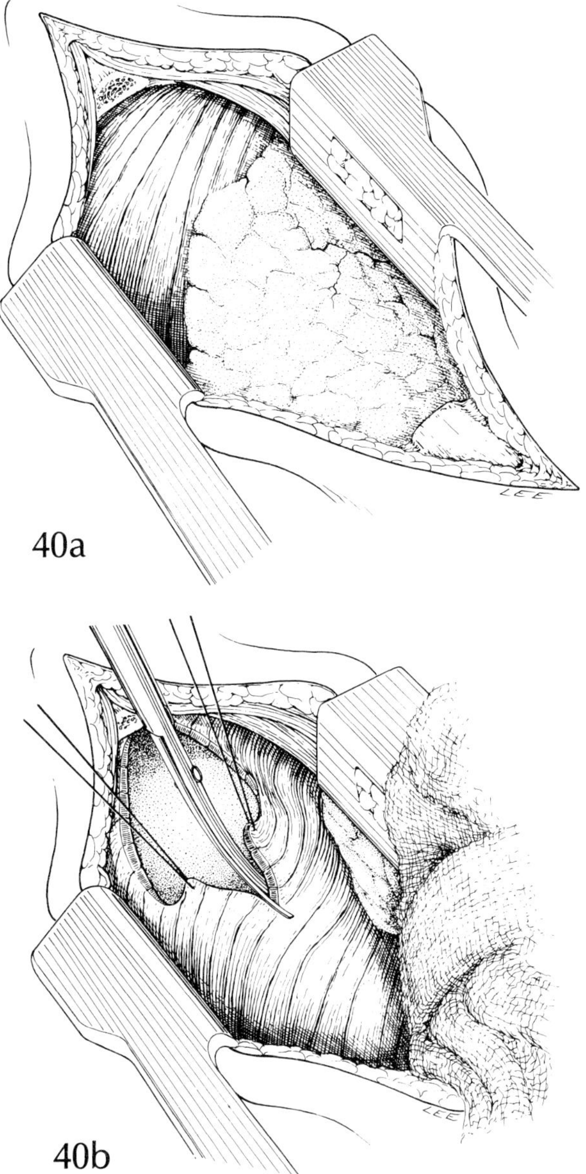

40a

40b

40a, b & c

Alternatively the incision may be limited to the chest but the diaphragm incised in the same line. The left side is shown. The transversus and underlying peritoneum are split and a self-retaining retractor (Finochietto) inserted into the chest and slowly opened (*a*). This places the diaphragm on the stretch and permits its incision (*b*). For tumours at the cardia which may have invaded muscle, a radial split is appropriate in the diaphragm (*c*); for all other purposes the diaphragmatic innervation should be preserved by making a peripheral incision 1.4–2 cm inside the line of attachment to ribs.

The small vessels which are always encountered should be under-run with fine sutures which can then be used to hold up the cut edge. By turning the flap of diaphragm one way or the other, chest and abdomen may be freely seen. Closure of the diaphragm is by interrupted non-absorbable sutures and that of the abdominal wall either in layers or by the one-layer technique described for the abdomen.

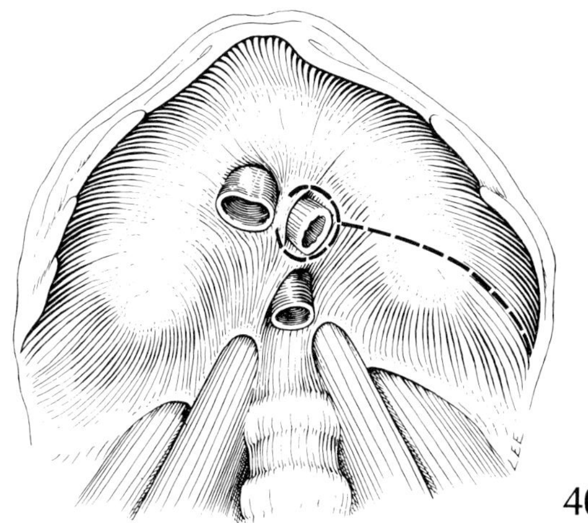

40c

Management of the septic and complicated abdomen – polypropylene mesh closure

In peritonitis, progressive abdominal distension occurs which tends to disrupt the wound. Furthermore, there is often a need for re-entry to clear out residual inter-mesenteric, pelvic or subphrenic abscesses. For these purposes techniques have been developed to permit both 'give' in the abdominal wall without necrosis from cutting out of sutures and easy re-entry. Though there have been many variants considered, the simplest technique is to insert a patch of polypropylene mesh[6,7].

Once peritoneal toilet is complete and decompression has been achieved (*see* p. 153) in this volume, the anaesthetist provides complete relaxation. The gap that then exists is measured and an oblong of polypropylene cut to one and a half times its size.

41 & 42

The polypropylene is stitched 1.5–2 cm under the peritoneal edge with interrupted 1 polypropylene sutures.

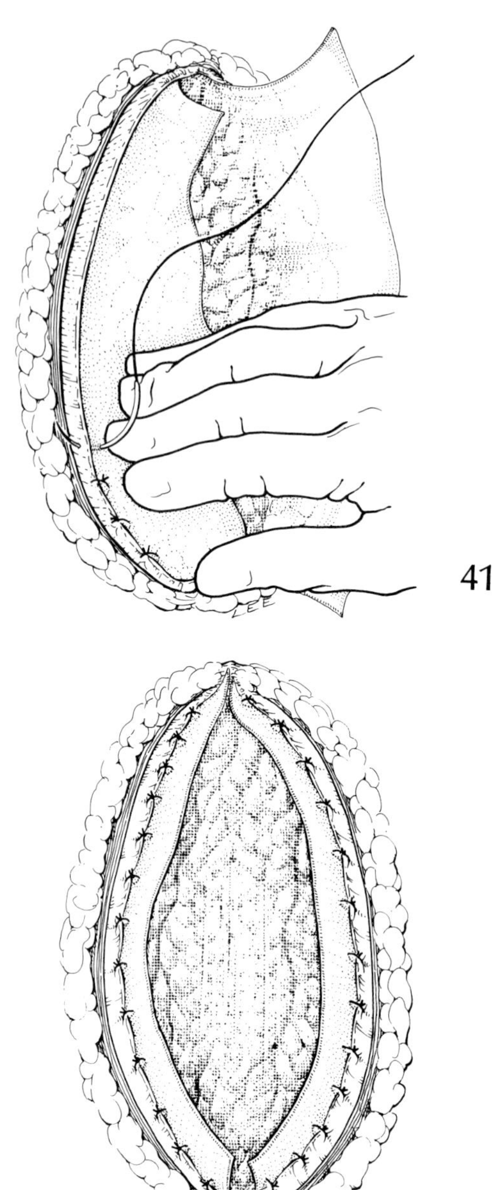

41

42

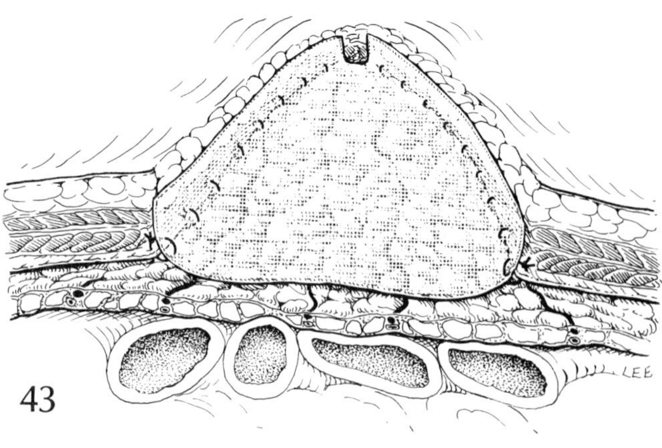

43

43

If possible, omentum is positioned deep to the mesh.

44

Suction drains are laid across the mesh to scavenge exudate for the first 48 h.

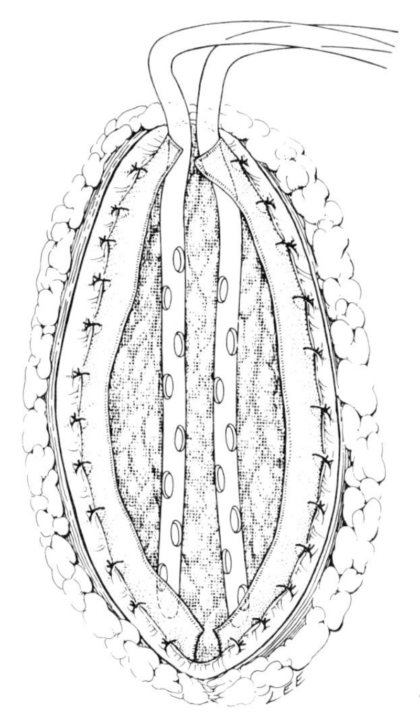

44

45

Gauze dressings are then applied and changed as necessary.

In most circumstances a fibrinous membrane forms, granulation tissue replaces this and the wound heals by second intention or may be skin grafted, though a delayed flap closure is preferable. Persistent sepsis may require removal but an incisional hernia will almost inevitably result.

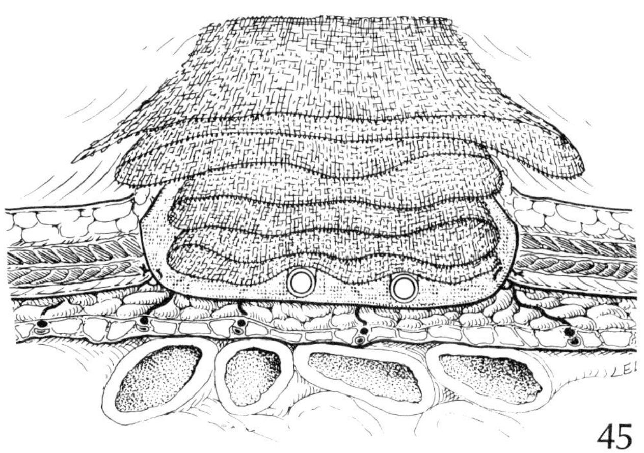

45

References

1. Raahave, D. Bacterial densities in operation wounds. Copenhagen, Arhus and Odense: FADL's Forlag, 1979
2. Dudley, H. A. F. Single layer closure of the abdominal wall. A theoretical and experimental analysis. British Journal of Surgery 1970; 57: 664–667
3. Jenkins, T. P. N. The burst abdominal wound: a mechanical approach. British Journal of Surgery 1976; 63: 873–876
4. Jones, T. E., Newell, E. T. Brubaker, R. E. The use of alloy steel wire in the closure of abdominal wounds. Surgery, Gynecology and Obstetrics 1941; 72: 1056–1059
5. Bucknall, T. E., Cox, P. J., Ellis, H. Burst abdomen and incisional hernia: a prospective study of 1129 major laparotomies. British Medical Journal 1982; 284: 931–933
6. Stone, H. H., Fabian, T. C., Turkleson, M. L., Jurkiewicz, M. J. Management of acute full-thickness losses of the abdominal wall. Annals of Surgery 1981; 193: 612–618
7. Voyles, C. R., Richardson, J. D., Bland, K. I., Tobin, G. R., Flint, I. M., Polk, H. C. Emergency abdominal wall reconstruction with polypropylene mesh. Short-term benefits versus long-term complications. Annals of Surgery 1981; 194: 219–223

Exploratory laparotomy

R. M. Kirk MS, FRCS
Consultant Surgeon, Royal Free Hospital, London

Preoperative

Indications

Every abdominal operation is an exploration. Whenever possible the opportunity should be taken to explore the whole abdomen. In this way familiarity is acquired with the appearance and feel of normal structures so that abnormalities can be recognized or confidently excluded. Occasionally important incidental findings are discovered and an alternative diagnosis may be made when an unsuspected lesion proves to be the cause of symptoms[1]. In no circumstances is exploration a substitute for careful clinical assessment, appropriate laboratory tests, endoscopy, radiology and modern imaging techniques. Laparotomy provides access within the abdomen but to the exterior only of organs, while many diseases occur within the hollow viscera.

In spite of careful investigation the cause of a persistent pyrexia may remain obscure and laparotomy is very occasionally indicated. The cause of jaundice, producing equivocal clinical and biochemical findings, is now virtually always elucidated using percutaneous liver biopsy and cholangiography, endoscopic retrograde cholangiography, laparoscopy and imaging techniques. Laparotomy is now reserved for the assessment of the extent of disease and correction of mechanical obstruction. Chronic dyspepsia associated with equivocal radiological features was formerly a frequent indication for abdominal exploration – the surgeon could easily convince himself of ulcer scarring and petechial haemorrhages. Any sequelae were attributed to the side-effects of the operation carried out to 'cure' the supposed ulcer. It would now be considered unethical to explore the abdomen before performing endoscopy.

A small residue of patients remain who have incapacitating chronic or recurring abdominal symptoms for which no cause can be found in spite of assiduous investigation, often augmented by medical and psychiatric consultations. Some of these patients are given, as a last resort, an exploratory laparotomy which should be on the understanding that if no abnormality is found, no procedure will be undertaken. The harvest of pathological lesions is usually small[2] but reassurance of the patient that serious disease has been excluded frequently has a marked and long-lasting placebo effect[1]. Such an exploration is best performed by an experienced and deliberate surgeon.

Contraindications

Complete abdominal exploration cannot be safely performed through small incisions especially sited for local procedures. If an abscess is encountered abdominal exploration should be abandoned or postponed whenever possible to avoid disseminating the infection. If generalized malignant disease is discovered, and is not producing or threatening to produce mechanical complications, the abdomen should be closed after a biopsy specimen has been taken. If dense generalized adhesions are discovered at an operation for a specific procedure, the whole abdomen should not be explored unless the patient has suffered mechanical complications from the adhesions.

The operation

The incisions

In adults vertical incisions allow more complete abdominal exploration. Transverse incisions provide good access to the abdomen in infants under the age of 18–24 months.

Supracolic compartment

1

The liver should be felt and a plan made to remove a biopsy specimen if any abnormality is found. The gall bladder is felt, especially the most dependent part where stones collect. The structures in the free edge of the lesser omentum are palpated to exclude stones in the common bile duct, tumours or enlarged glands, and to confirm normal hepatic arterial pulsation. A hand should now be passed over the spleen to estimate its size and detect any adhesions which immobilize it. The undersurface of the diaphragm should be felt, together with the oesophageal hiatus. A hiatus hernia is confirmed by sliding the gastric cardia or fundus into the chest. The body of the stomach should be both inspected and felt, particularly along the lesser curvature, for scars, tumours or rigidity of the wall suggestive of infiltration. The interior of the stomach may be inspected for potential biopsy through a longitudinal gastrotomy in the centre of the anterior wall, which is then closed. The size of the pyloric muscular ring is no measure of the pyloroduodenal canal. An adequate lumen is best confirmed by ensuring that the anterior gastric and duodenal walls can be invaginated with the index finger through the pyloric ring. The duodenal bulb should be inspected and palpated to detect a peptic ulcer or scar. In an emergency the interior of the duodenal bulb may be inspected through a longitudinal gastroduodenotomy which is subsequently closed transversely as a Heineke-Mikulicz pyloroplasty, but this irrevocably destroys the pylorus. The duodenal bulb can be examined by passing a speculum or retractors or best of all a cytoscope through a small distal gastrotomy which is subsequently closed without damaging the pylorus.

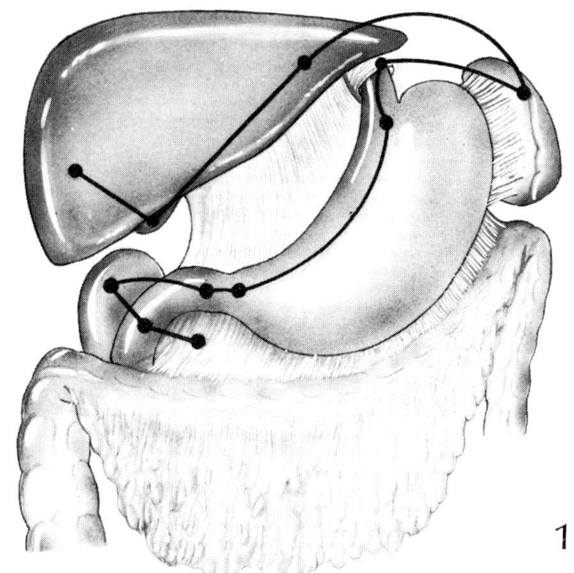

1

2

The right kidney, duodenal loop and pancreatic head are now palpated. If necessary the peritoneal floor of the foramen of Winslow may be split, allowing the finger to be insinuated posteriorly. Alternatively, Kocher's manoeuvre may be performed to mobilize the duodenal loop and pancreatic head.

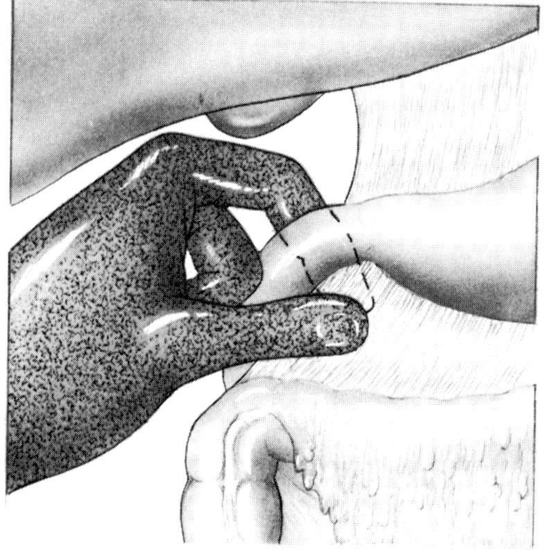

2

3

Infracolic compartment

The greater omentum, transverse colon and mesocolon are now drawn upwards out of the abdomen. The left kidney, body and tail of the pancreas, and the root of the mesentery are palpated, together with the aorta and inferior mesenteric artery. The small bowel is picked up at the duodenojejunal junction and passed through the fingers so that it is examined throughout its length. The appendix, caecum and colon are examined, to reach the rectum. The uterus, tubes and ovaries are felt in the female, the prostate gland and seminal vesicles in the male. The bladder, ureters, iliac vessels and hernial orifices are now examined.

The dorsum of the examining hand detects abnormalities of the anterior and lateral abdominal wall, but if disease is suspected the supinated hand should be inserted.

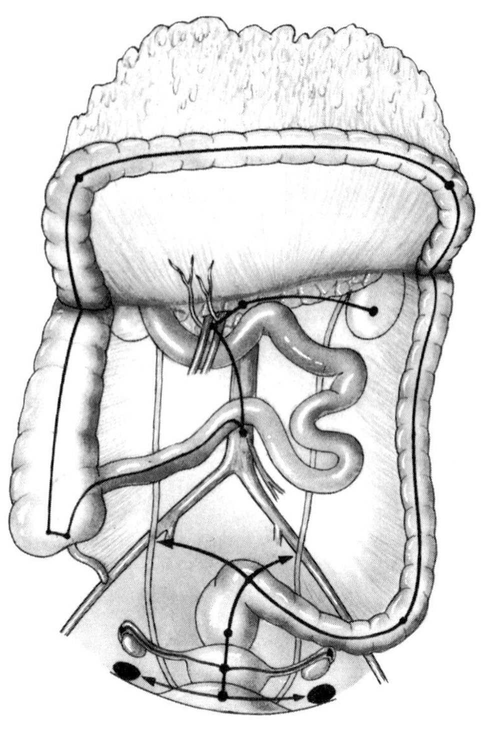

3

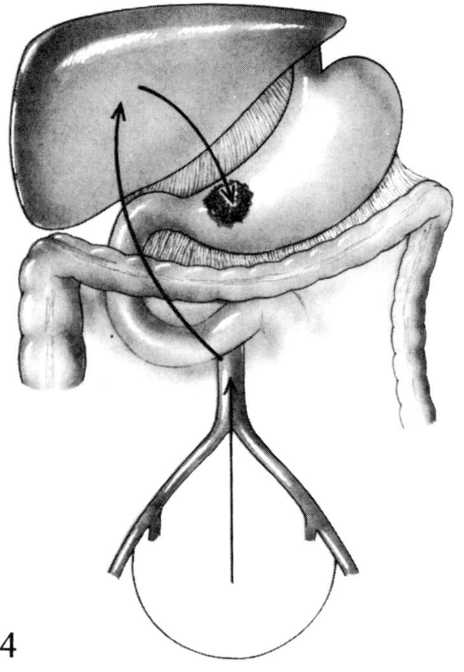

4

4

Laparotomy for suspected neoplasia

The technique of exploration should be modified so that the suspected primary site is handled last of all. The most distant area is felt and the surgeon works towards the suspect site, examining on the way the pelvic floor and parietal peritoneum for evidence of transperitoneal seedlings. The para-aortic glands, the liver and regional glands are searched for evidence of metastases. Only now is the suspected primary site examined.

Laparotomy for complications after recent operation

The abdomen should be opened carefully through the previous incision. Viscera may be adherent to the undersurface of the wound. The site of the previous operation should be carefully examined after fully displaying it. When the cause of complication is corrected the whole abdomen should be thoroughly explored to detect any feature that was missed at the first operation or that has subsequently developed.

5

Laparotomy for peritonitis

As the abdomen is entered, free air, reaction fluid, pus or leaked visceral content may be encountered. A specimen of fluid should be taken for microscopical and bacteriological examination. The primary site of secondary peritonitis is most likely to be appendicitis, a perforated peptic ulcer, cholecystitis, colonic diverticulitis, or salpingitis. A primary cause should always be carefully sought because treatment of the secondary effects alone is rarely curative.

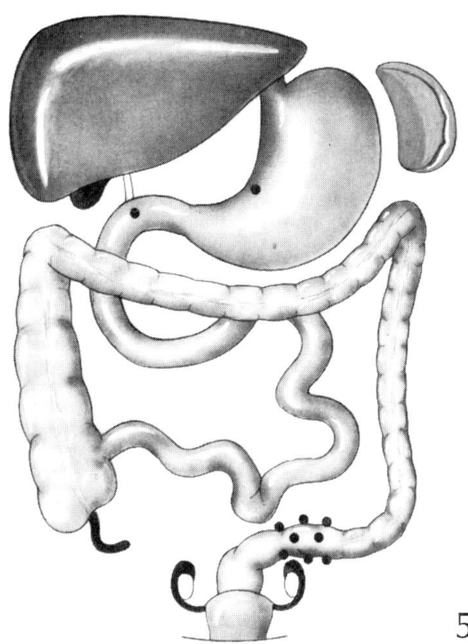

5

Laparotomy following abdominal trauma

The whole abdomen should be displayed and prepared so that any penetrating injuries may be probed and subsequently excised after following the tracks within the abdomen. Laparotomy should be converted to thoracoabdominal exploration if penetrating chest wounds exist, or if laparotomy reveals diaphragmatic injuries, severe damage to the superior surface of the liver, or injuries to the major vessels as they pass through the diaphragm. One should particularly check for signs of retroperitoneal damage.

Laparotomy for gastrointestinal bleeding *(see also* P. 261 in this volume)

The site of bleeding must be sought before proceeding to exploratory laparotomy. Fibreoptic oesophagogastroduodenoscopy is mandatory. Expertly performed barium meal radiology and arteriography are sometimes helpful. Sigmoidoscopy should always be performed and in appropriate circumstances colonoscopy if there is any possibility that the bleeding could be from the large bowel. Very bright blood may reach the anus from the large bowel. If the source of bleeding still cannot be isolated before laparotomy then the fibreoptic endoscope is taken to the operating theatre so that it can be passed into the stomach and beyond under guidance by the surgeon during the operation.

It is assumed that so far as possible lost blood has been replaced and fresh sources are available. At operation a thorough systematic abdominal exploration is performed, not only of the main gastrointestinal tract but of the other organs since blood may reach the main gastrointestinal tract from lesions outside it. If there has been recent severe bleeding, clot may be felt in the stomach, small bowel or colon. Liquid blood appears bluish when seen through the bowel wall – but then, so do most fluids.

If the cause remains obscure the gastroscope may be passed with the help of the anaesthetist, and oesophagogastroduodenoscopy is repeated. If necessary the tip of the instrument can be guided into the upper jejunum by the operator. Overinflation of the exposed viscera must be avoided. The surgeon may undertake the endoscopy himself; he may wrap the head of the instrument in sterile towels while the anaesthetist withdraws or advances the tube under direction, or he may dispense with sterility and change gown and gloves at the end of the examination. It may be necessary to exchange the endoscope for a large-bore tube to wash out the stomach with tap water at 37°C if it is full of old blood clot.

An endoscope may be unavailable or the diagnosis following endoscopy may still be in doubt. A longitudinal gastrotomy, placed midway between the greater and lesser curvatures, allows the interior of the stomach to be inspected directly using large retractors. Anterior duodenotomy may be carried proximally into the stomach to allow bleeding from a distal gastric or duodenal ulcer, or lesion at the ampulla of Vater, to be excluded. Satisfactory endoscopy of the small bowel is not easy to perform but may be attempted using a sterile sigmoidoscope introduced through one or more enterotomies. The bowel is drawn onto the shaft of the endoscope like a concertina. Colonoscopy is best accomplished by passing the fibreoptic instrument per anum.

If the cause of bleeding is discovered it can be dealt with. If it is not discovered after an assiduous search, a 'blind' procedure such as gastrectomy is contraindicated. This merely complicates the diagnosis, removes the only part of the bowel that can be satisfactorily and directly examined internally, and prejudices the patient's recovery. It is better to close the abdomen and determine to reinvestigate, and if necessary to re-explore the abdomen, if bleeding recurs.

Laparotomy for intestinal obstruction

Full clinical assessment, erect and supine radiographs of the abdomen, and sigmoidoscopy will probably have indicated the suspected site of obstruction. When the abdomen is opened distended coils of bowel often hinder exploration. It was formerly advised that the caecum should be examined to discover whether or not it is distended. Preferably the distended loops should be lifted out in moist warm towels and supported by the assistant in order to provide free abdominal access. Dilated bowel is followed distally until the obstruction is reached. The whole length of bowel is examined now or later to exclude the possibility of multiple obstructions.

Recurrent obstruction is dealt with in the same manner, but occasionally the peritoneal space is almost totally obliterated, the obstructive site is obvious and appears to be solitary. It is sometimes best to compromise by dealing with the obstruction, eschew complete exploration and determine to reopen the abdomen if the condition does not resolve.

Neonatal obstruction offers special problems and the diagnosis should already be fairly certainly established by clinical and radiological assessment. For general use a supraumbilical transverse incision is satisfactory.

References

1. Kirk, R. M. Exploration of the abdomen. Annals of the Royal College of Surgeons of England 1976; 58: 452–456

2. Scott, P. J., Hill, R. S., Lo Su Fook, A., Bensley, K. E. Benefits and hazards of laparotomy for medical patients. Lancet 1970; 2: 941–946

Laparotomy for intestinal obstruction – general principles

N. A. Matheson ChM, FRCS, FRCS(Ed.)
Consultant Surgeon, Aberdeen General Hospitals

Diagnosis

When the intestine is acutely obstructed definite symptoms and signs follow. These comprise abdominal pain, borborygmi, vomiting, constipation and distension. The presence and prominence of each is dependent on the site, completeness and duration of obstruction but, in combination, they usually result in a characteristic presentation and a straightforward diagnosis.

In high small bowel obstruction vomiting occurs early and is prominent whereas pain and distension are absent. In low small bowel obstruction pain and borborygmi are salient whereas vomiting and distension occur later and to a milder degree. In distal colonic obstruction distension is the cardinal feature whereas pain occurs late and vomiting may be absent. In acute intestinal obstruction these differences, taken together with the patient's past and present history and the findings on examination, usually lead to a firm diagnosis and also make it possible in most instances to differentiate small bowel from colonic obstruction.

Erect and supine X-ray films of the abdomen are reliable in confirming or refuting the clinical diagnosis. However, the paucity of X-ray signs in high jejunal obstruction or when the small bowel content is wholly fluid should not be forgotten. In addition, colonic fluid levels resulting simply from liquid colonic content, as in diarrhoea or after an enema, are not necessarily indicative of colonic obstruction. As well as serving to confirm a diagnosis of intestinal obstruction, abdominal X-rays will usually enable small bowel obstruction to be differentiated from large bowel obstruction and may show the cause of the obstruction as, for example, in gallstone ileus or in caecal or sigmoid volvulus. Finally, when gas is seen to extend to the rectum despite colonic distension the X-ray evidence may refute a clinical diagnosis of mechanical colon obstruction and suggest an abnormality of colonic motility. The descriptive term 'pseudo-obstruction' has been applied to such instances in some of which it is possible to establish the underlying cause but most of which are unexplained. The X-ray features are important in drawing attention to the desirability of avoiding operation. Every patient in whom a clinical diagnosis of distal colonic obstruction has been made should be examined with a sigmoidoscope and a very strong case can also be made for the invariable use of an emergency contrast study (Gastrografin enema) before deciding on the need for operation.

Indications for operation

In small bowel obstruction there is always a risk of vascular strangulation with subsequent intestinal necrosis. Though the order of the risk varies with the nature of the obstruction, it is sufficiently frequent and a sufficiently serious threat to survival that it must constantly be kept in mind. Further, though signs of peritonitis are indicative of strangulation, these may be absent and it is emphasized that strangulation cannot be reliably diagnosed clinically except at a late stage. The hazard of strangulation, together with the mechanical nature of small bowel obstruction, is good reason to support the general principle that this condition should be treated by urgent operation, a policy that has the additional advantages of establishing the diagnosis and effecting immediate relief.

There are some exceptions to the rule. Small bowel obstruction occurring within days of an abdominal operation may be managed – at least initially – without reoperation. This more evasive approach in the special case of postoperative intestinal obstruction appears illogical and unsatisfactory but is justified by the desirability of avoiding the obvious hazards of a second abdominal exploration during recovery from the first. Aside from anaesthetic risks such a sequence is destructive to morale. Of technical hazards, the most important by far is the risk of accidental intestinal perforation at a recently made anastomosis or elsewhere. The disastrous consequences that so often follow such an error are a powerful deterrent to re-exploration in the postoperative period. In addition, the possibilty that the obstruction may be in part, the result of abnormal postoperative autonomic function and therefore potentially reversible is also often taken to justify a policy of non-interference.

Effective management without operation largely depends on efficient gastrointestinal decompression. Peroral intestinal tubes of the Miller-Abbot or Cantor types are difficult to pass and are seldom used in the United Kingdom. Instead, a nasogastric tube is relied on to decompress not only the stomach but also the small bowel. In addition, strangulation even if less frequent in postoperative intestinal obstruction is still a hazard that is particular difficult to detect clinically. Finally, the development of intestinal obstruction after an abdominal operation may be secondary to a serious intraperitoneal abnormality, most often sepsis, that is best managed actively. Non-operative management is therefore fundamentally unsatisfactory in this situation as it is in other types of intestinal obstruction.

In the individual patient, however, when the risks of re-exploration are weighed against those of avoiding it, non-operative management is more often than not justified. If embarked upon, its limitations must be clearly understood and a deadline should be set on the proposed duration of its use. All too often in these situations day after day slips past without good evidence of relief of the obstruction while the patient insidiously loses ground and ultimately, when the inevitability of reoperation is patently obvious, the threat to survival has become serious. Thus, it is a sound discipline to set a deadline at the outset of non-operative management beyond which it will not be continued in the absence of clear evidence that the obstruction has been relieved. Such a deadline should usually be at 48 or 72 h at which time, in the face of persisting obstruction, reoperation should not be shirked despite the risks, the difficulties and the natural reluctance to accept the possibility that the initial procedure has been technically imperfect.

A precisely limited period of non-operative care may also be justified in patients presenting *de novo* with intestinal obstruction in whom, because of other disease, the risks of anaesthesia and operation outweigh those of conservative treatment. Few patients fall into this class.

In large bowel obstruction non-operative management is appropriate in the infrequent situation where obstruction is the result of faecal impaction. If colonic motility is normal, constipation is an unusual cause of a colonic obstruction sufficient to produce typical clinical and radiological features and is seen almost exclusively in elderly patients. Colonic obstruction should never lightly be attributed to such a cause but where it seems possible attempts to relieve it manually and by enemas are justified. A similar policy is appropriate in adults with Hirschsprung's disease, or with other less well defined abnormalities of colonic motility grouped together as pseudo-Hirschsprung's disease, who present with colonic obstruction as a result of faecal impaction. It is also theoretically appropriate if a confident preoperative diagnosis of pseudo-obstruction can be made on the basis of evidence from plain X-rays, sigmoidoscopy and emergency distal colonic contrast studies. However, the diagnosis is often not made until operation and when colonic distention is marked operation may be the only effective means of combating the risk of caecal perforation.

Conservative management with sigmoidoscopic decompression is usually dramatically effective in patients with sigmoid volvulus but recurrence is likely.

Otherwise, colonic obstruction is an indication for urgent operation.

Preoperative

The loss of extracellular fluid, by vomiting into the lumen of the distended bowel and into the peritoneal cavity as a result of strangulation, varies with the degree and duration of obstruction. Its extent may be judged from the history, the patient's general appearance, the tissue turgor, the state of the peripheral circulation and the degree of peripheral venous filling. The required volume of intravenous sodium and water together with potassium for replacement is a matter of guesswork, but replacement should be rapid and it should seldom be necessary to delay operation for more than 4–6 h to permit restoration of extracellular fluid volume towards normal.

During intravenous replacement of water and electrolyte losses, a vented nasogastric tube, with continuous suction, helps to relieve the discomfort of vomiting and empties the stomach in preparation for anaesthesia.

The operation

The incision

In obstruction caused by an external hernia the incision is placed in relation to the hernia. In inguinal and femoral herniae a preperitoneal approach gives good exposure for intestinal resection when necessary. Otherwise a longitudinal incision gives the best extensible exposure. The skin component is placed 1–2 cm to either side of the umbilicus. Its length and vertical placement in relation to the umbilicus is influenced by the confidence with which the operative procedure can be predicted beforehand. In the frequent case of uncertainty the incision may be sited with its midpoint at the umbilicus and can if necessary be extended in either direction. The subcutaneous fat is incised obliquely to gain the linea alba and the abdominal wall is incised in the midline. Midline incisions are rapidly made with minimal tissue trauma and give unrivalled access from xiphoid to pelvis if necessary. The possible criticism that midline incisions are prone to dehiscence and herniation is answered by the use of a mass closure technique (*see* p. 129 in this volume).

The peritoneum should be incised with care lest a tensely distended, thin-walled loop of underlying bowel be accidentally opened, a mistake difficult to correct and potentially fatal. In addition, a sudden release of intraperitoneal pressure with abrupt evisceration and loss of the splint provided by the abdominal wall may result in spontaneous rupture of the attenuated and devitalized caecal wall in a late, closed loop colonic obstruction. The peritoneum should, therefore, be opened carefully and distended bowel kept within by the assistant's hand until the incision is complete. Pressure is then gradually released, allowing the abdominal contents to spill out gradually and gently.

Establishing the diagnosis

More often than not, clinical assessment together with X-ray appearances will have made possible preoperative differentiation between small and large bowel obstruction. However, particularly with caecal tumours with ileocaecal incompetence, the appearances may be those of distal small bowel obstruction. Whether or not the distinction is clear beforehand, the differentiation between small and large bowel obstruction is the first step in the operation. Collapsed small bowel and distended colon makes colonic obstruction in the presence of a competent ileocaecal valve obvious. If the ileocaecal valve is incompetent, distended small bowel loops may be associated with colonic obstruction, but gross jejunal distension is a feature of small bowel obstruction. The differentiation is therefore often made at first sight but may be confirmed or established by palpating the caecum. It is self-evident that caecal distension is a feature of large bowel obstruction and that a flaccid collapsed caecum confirms the presence of small bowel obstruction.

The second step in the operation is to establish the cause. In small bowel obstruction this is best done by complete evisceration of the distended loops, after which the site where distension ceases abruptly and collapsed bowel follows may be obvious. This is particularly so in intrinsic small bowel obstruction, the result for example of stricture, tumour or obturation by food or gallstone. If, however, the obstruction is the result of adhesion or involvement of the small bowel in an inflammatory or neoplastic process deep in the pelvis, the diagnosis may not be clear because complete evisceration from the pelvis is not possible and grossly distended loops obscure the view. In these circumstances it is best to decompress the small bowel by retrograde stripping (*see* below) after which the nature of the obstruction is much more easily determined. On occasion, small bowel decompression results in release of the obstruction after which the cause may be difficult to pinpoint but this is of no disadvantage to the patient.

In large bowel obstruction finding the site is straightforward except in patients with pseudo-obstruction or ill understood defects in colonic propulsion. When caecal distension has been confirmed the transverse colon is readily examined in the upper part of the wound. When it is collapsed the diagnosis of obstruction between caecum and transverse colon – nearly always because of carcinoma – is simple. When the transverse colon is distended, the small bowel is eviscerated and the left colon examined visibly and by palpation. Collapsed descending colon leads to the diagnosis of obstruction at the splenic flexure whereas distended descending colon indicates obstruction in the sigmoid colon or rectum. It is seldom necessary to decompress the colon to make a diagnosis although the manoeuvre may play a very useful part in management.

Intestinal decompression

Though it has not been shown that decompression of the distended intestine speeds its functional recovery, it has practical value in reducing the lumen and content of the bowel when an anastomosis is proposed, in facilitating abdominal closure and in reducing diaphragmatic splinting. In some cases of distal small bowel obstruction the diagnosis can be more easily established.

Until recently, decompression of the distended small bowel by the insertion of rigid or flexible appliances through a distal ileal enterotomy was popular. However, the risks of contamination are great and during the past 10 years the technique of retrograde stripping, which is simple, safe and effective, has come to replace invasive methods. Retrograde stripping depends on the observation that intestinal content can regularly be emptied back into the stomach to be removed by aspiration through a wide-bore stomach tube. Alternatively, the tube may be guided into the third or fourth part of the duodenum, but this additional manoeuvre is not necessary. If the degree of distension is moderate stripping may begin distally at the site of obstruction.

1

The bowel is held lightly in the fingers of the left hand and the index and middle fingers of the right hand are applied across it, rather like an occlusion clamp.

The pressure applied is just sufficient to prevent escape of intestinal content and the bowel is decompressed by progressive stripping through the fingers of the right hand. As the proximal jejunum becomes increasingly distended there may be a temporary delay in the passage of fluid through the duodenojejunal flexure and the pylorus. If so, firm pressure over the first part of the jejunum will ensure rapid and continued emptying into the stomach. If this manoeuvre is necessary the column of accumulated fluid should not be allowed to escape on release of the stripping fingers but should be held in place by the assistant who applies his fingers across the bowel in a similar way. If distension is pronounced the jejunum should be emptied first before attempting to strip the whole small intestine. Retrograde stripping of the small intestine can usually be accomplished rapidly and when properly done does not involve excessive handling of the bowel.

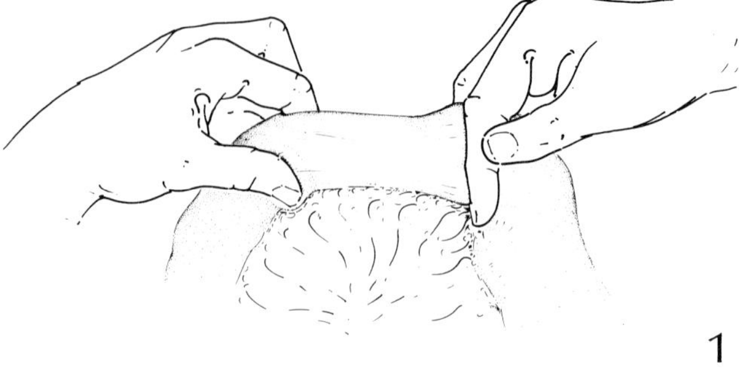

1

Decompression need not be an invariable part of the operative management of small bowel obstruction; its need is judged on the degree of distension and to some extent on the nature of the procedure required to relieve the obstruction.

In large bowel obstruction it may not be necessary to decompress the distended right colon that is about to be resected by hemicolectomy, although if distension is gross the decompressed colon is more easily and more safely handled during mobilization. In addition, even if a loop or end colostomy is proposed, colonic decompression will often facilitate the operation.

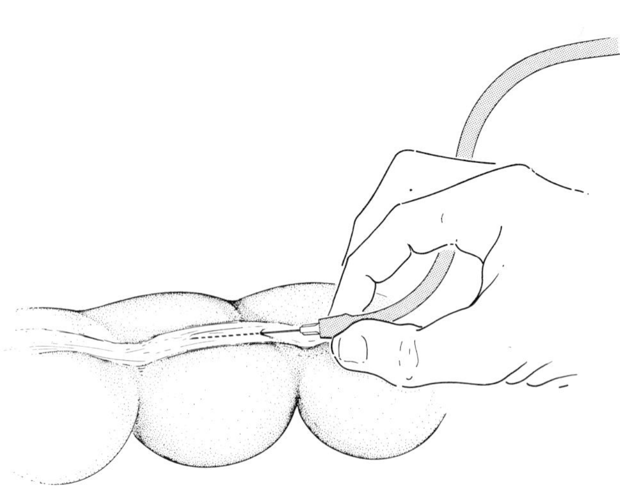

2

2

It is often forgotten that the intraluminal content in colonic distension is very largely gaseous and may therefore be readily removed through a fine-bore needle. There is no place for colotomy and the insertion of a wide-bore tube, flexible or otherwise; contamination is the inevitable result. Similarly, distal ileal enterotomy with the passage of a tube through the ileocaecal valve is inadvisable. The large bowel may be readily decompressed at any site although most easily in the transverse colon by the insertion of a standard intravenous needle (21 gauge) connected to a short length of latex tubing and thence to a source of suction. Pressure is applied in the flanks to drive gas into the transverse colon. The serosa is pierced over a taenia coli and the needle advanced in the intramuscular plane for 1.5–2 cm before dipping down through the mucosa into the lumen.

As gas is aspirated, distended colon elsewhere is compressed to refill the emptying transverse colon. The oblique course of the needle puncture and its small size prevent subsequent leakage and a purse-string suture is not necessary. On withdrawal, the needle and the whole length of suction tubing to which it is attached is carefully discarded without contact with gloves, instruments or drapes, and the puncture site is wiped with an antiseptic solution such as acriflavine. Needle aspiration may be repeated at other sites if necessary but this is not usually the case.

General principles in definitive management

The relief of acute small bowel obstruction is generally straightforward. An adhesive band is simply dealt with and intrinsic lesions are hardly more difficult to manage. Bolus obstruction is relieved by milking the mass of food into the caecum or by removing the responsible gallstone by enterotomy proximal to the site of impaction. Less frequent causes such as tumours and strictures are managed by immediate resection with end-to-end anastomosis. More difficult is the situation where loops of small bowel are matted in the pelvis, densely adherent to a source of chronic sepsis, diverticular disease, tubo-ovarian sepsis or Crohn's disease, or to a neoplastic process – rectal, ovarian or uterine. Only gentle fingertip dissection and pinching beyond the edge of the bowel will enable such loops to be delivered without perforation. Furthermore, experienced judgement may be necessary to tell whether the basic process is inflammatory or neoplastic and whether the small bowel loops may be safely dissected off it.

Postoperative small bowel obstruction also presents a situation where disaster is a frequent sequel to careless operative management particularly if 2–3 weeks have elapsed since the original operation. The old incision should be reopened with great care because loops of small bowel may be adherent to the abdominal wall and are all too easily damaged during incision of the peritoneum. Once the peritoneum has been opened the appearances may be those of several small bowel loops matted both together and to the parietal peritoneum as a result of dense fibrofibrinous adhesions. In this situation, finger dissection is the only safe way of slowly and patiently delivering one loop from another and from adjacent viscera until the whole length of small bowel lies completely free. Patients with recurrent small bowel obstruction present a similar problem, ofen with widespread adhesions, but such adhesions are fibrous and require sharp dissection for their division. Extreme care is essential to avoid damaging the bowel.

In occasional patients with complicated recurrent small bowel obstruction there may be indications for operative small bowel intubation as described by Munro and Jones[1]. An elongated PVC balloon catheter 3 m (10 ft) long and of 18 Ch. gauge with additional side-holes in the distal half is led through a stab incision in the left flank and inserted through a jejunostomy encircled with a purse-string suture of 2/0 chromic catgut. The tube is fed down the small bowel by traction on the inflated balloon until its tip lies in the terminal ileum. The balloon is deflated and may be manipulated through the ileocaecal valve after which it is reinflated to prevent retraction. It is important to fix the site of jejunostomy to the parietal peritoneum at the site of puncture using a few fine catgut sutures so that the risk of peritoneal contamination on withdrawal of the tube 10 or more days later is prevented. The value of the long intestinal tube depends, first, on its splinting effect; the bowel with its contained tube assumes a series of gentle curves without acute kinks thereby lessening the risk of further recurrent obstruction. Second, the tube ensures efficient decompression after operation.

In large bowel obstruction, which is most often caused by cancer, the type of operation undertaken and its outcome is largely influenced by the experience and competence of the operator. Obstructing tumours of the right colon and proximal transverse colon are treated by resection with ileotransverse anastomosis. Right-sided tumours are seldom inoperable even when the duodenum is involved and recourse to a bypass procedure should rarely be contemplated. Tumours of the mid or distal transverse colon up to and including the region of the splenic flexure are best dealt with by extended right hemicolectomy. Obstructing tumours of the left colon are traditionally managed by transverse loop colostomy in the first instance but the advantages of immediate resection are now widely accepted. However, after emergency left colon resection in the presence of unprepared bowel or peritoneal contamination, immediate anastomosis should be avoided in favour of an end-colostomy and mucous fistula or end-colostomy and rectal stump closure (Hartmann's procedure), which have the over-riding merit of safety. Such procedures do, however, carry the disadvantage of subjecting the patient to a subsequent and possibly difficult reconstruction from which some default. The ideal combination of emergency resection with immediate anastomosis, though it demands the highest standards of judgement and technique, may soon become orthodox if intraoperative colonic irrigation as described by Dudley, Radcliffe and McGeehan[2] fulfils its promise to make a hitherto hazardous combination safe.

References

1. Munro, A. M., Jones, P. F. Operative intubation in the treatment of complicated small bowel obstruction. British Journal of Surgery 1978; 65: 123–127

2. Dudley, H. A. F., Radcliffe, A. G., McGeehan, D. Intra-operative irrigation of the colon to permit primary anastomosis. British Journal of Surgery 1980; 67: 80–81

Intestinal anastomosis

Thomas T. Irvin PhD, ChM, FRCS(Ed.)
Consultant Surgeon, Royal Devon and Exeter Hospital (Wonford), Exeter, Devon

Introduction

Most operations on the gastrointestinal tract involve the suture or anastomosis of the gut, and it is this aspect of the surgery of the alimentary canal that is associated with dangerous complications. The breakdown of a suture line or anastomosis may result in peritonitis, faecal fistulation and serious or fatal septic complications.

Safety in gastrointestinal surgery may thus depend to a large extent on the technical expertise of the surgeon in his performance of the intestinal anastomosis. This expertise is acquired with practice but a gastrointestinal operation involves a series of exercises in surgical judgement, and it is only by attention to many details that safety is achieved in such surgery.

In this chapter the general principles and techniques of anastomoses in gastrointestinal surgery are described.

General principles

Several well established general principles of surgical technique apply to the management of all sutured wounds, including intestinal anastomoses. Other aspects of wound management, such as suture technique, have special features in gastrointestinal surgery, and several factors unrelated to surgical technique may affect the healing of intestinal anastomoses.

TECHNICAL PRINCIPLES

Access and exposure

Like most surgical procedures intestinal anastomoses become difficult if the surgical access and exposure are unsatisfactory. This may result from inadequate anaesthesia and muscle relaxation, poor assistance, an inappropriate surgical incision or one of inadequate length, and imperfect illumination of the operative field. Poor access for an anastomosis may also result from inadequate mobilization of the viscera and this is likely to occur in the surgery of anatomically fixed and deeply placed viscera such as the oesophagus, colon and rectum.

The surgeon should never have to struggle with an anastomosis because of limited access. When difficulty is encountered the problem should be carefully assessed and an attempt must be made to improve the exposure. If the difficulty seems insurmountable it may be prudent to consider an alternative procedure which avoids an anastomosis.

Blood supply

A poor blood supply is inimical to the healing of all wounds and the preparation for an anastomosis must be meticulous to avoid disturbance of the blood supply to the cut ends of the gut. The only absolute criterion of an adequate blood supply is the presence of free arterial bleeding from the cut edges of the bowel. The absence of visible or palpable arterial pulsation in the mesenteric vessels is not necessarily of significance but blanching or cyanosis of the cut edges of the bowel and the presence of a dark, venous type of bleeding are signs of an inadequate blood supply.

The blood supply to an anastomosis may be compromised in several ways: undue tension on the suture line resulting from inadequate mobilization of the viscera; devascularization of the bowel during mobilization or preparation for the anastomosis; strangulation of the tissues by tightly knotted sutures; and the excessive use of diathermy coagulation in achieving haemostasis in the cut ends of the bowel.

Before commencing an anastomosis the surgeon should ensure that the ends of the bowel can be easily apposed and, if the ends can be made to overlap, it can be safely assumed that there will be no undue tension on the suture line. Haemostasis in the cut edges of the bowel may be achieved either by the individual ligation of vessels or by the use of diathermy coagulation. The latter method has the disadvantage that it may result in a greater degree of tissue necrosis at the suture line but it is certainly a less tedious technique than the ligature of vessels and, in practice, little tissue damage will result if the use of diathermy is limited to controlling only the major bleeding points. Minor oozing should be ignored but significant arterial bleeding should be checked as there is a tendency for the bleeding vessels to retract within the tissues and produce unpleasant haematomas.

In performing an anastomosis some surgeons place non-crushing occlusion clamps across the bowel to avoid soiling of the operative field with intestinal contents. It is important, however, that these clamps are applied lightly and never across the mesentery of the intestine for fear of damaging the blood supply to the anastomosis. The author avoids the use of these clamps in oesophageal anastomoses because the blood supply to the cut end of the oesophagus is entirely dependent on intramural blood flow, which will be at least temporarily interrupted by occlusion clamps. Soiling of the operative field is seldom a problem in oesophageal anastomoses.

Suture technique

The basic principles of intestinal suture were established more than 100 years ago and have undergone little modification. Secure healing of an anastomosis is dependent on accurate apposition of the serosal or the outer surfaces of the bowel and this is achieved by the use of a suture technique which inverts the cut edges of the gut. The principle of inversion in gastrointestinal anastomoses has been challenged by Ravitch *et al.*[1] who claimed that everting techniques of suture gave satisfactory results in intestinal anastomoses in experimental animals. This has not been the experience of others, however, and clinical studies of everting anastomoses in the colon have shown that the everting method results in a high incidence of anastomotic dehiscence and that it is manifestly inferior to the traditional inverting technique[2].

The vast majority of surgeons use an open method of intestinal anastomosis. 'Aseptic' or closed techniques of anastomosis achieved some popularity in the earlier part of this century owing to the belief that the breakdown of anastomoses resulted from the bacterial contamination of the peritoneum which occurred during the construction of the open type of anastomosis. Several ingenious techniques of 'aseptic' anastomosis were devised but they were not generally accompanied by a reduction in the incidence of anastomotic dehiscence and most surgeons now rely on the simpler, open methods of anastomosis.

One aspect of the technique of intestinal suture which has remained the subject of some controversy is the use of one or two layers of sutures in anastomoses. The two-layer inverting suture technique was devised by Czerny and is the method used by the majority of surgeons. Halsted and Cushing recommended the use of one layer of sutures in intestinal anastomoses and it has been suggested that the single layer of sutures results in less ischaemia and tissue necrosis, and less narrowing of the intestinal lumen than the two-layer method. In practice, however, narrowing of the bowel lumen is hardly ever a clinical problem with the two-layer inverting method of suture, and there is no convincing evidence that single-layer techniques are inherently more sound than the standard two-layer method of intestinal anastomosis. Studies in experimental animals and randomized clinical trials have not established any consistent difference between one- and two-layer methods of suture[3–7], and the excellent results of single-layer anastomoses reported by some surgeons[8] may be due to the expertise of the surgeon rather than the method of anastomosis (*see* p. 161 in this chapter).

Like many surgeons the author uses both single-layer and two-layer methods of anastomosis in gastrointestinal surgery: a two-layer method is used for anastomoses in the oesophagus, stomach, duodenum and small intestine; and a single-layer technique is used in the colon and rectum. In each instance the choice of suture method is based on the knowledge that the method gives satisfactory results in the author's hands rather than on scientific evidence of its value. However, the clinical studies of Everett[7] and Matheson and Irving[8] provide persuasive evidence that the single-layer suture technique is the method of choice in anastomoses involving the extraperitoneal rectum. A single-layer suture technique is certainly a much simpler technical exercise than the two-layer method in very low rectal anastomoses and the author recommends its use.

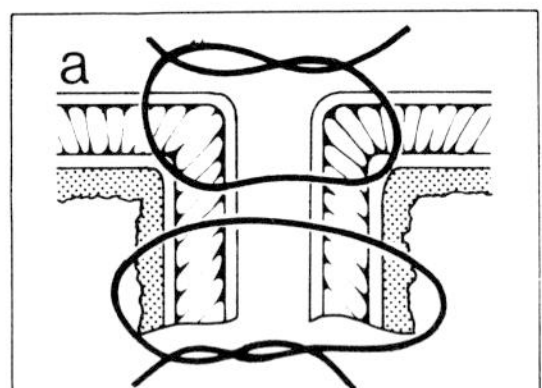

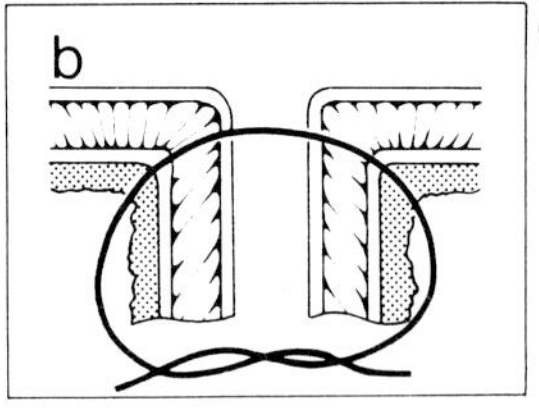

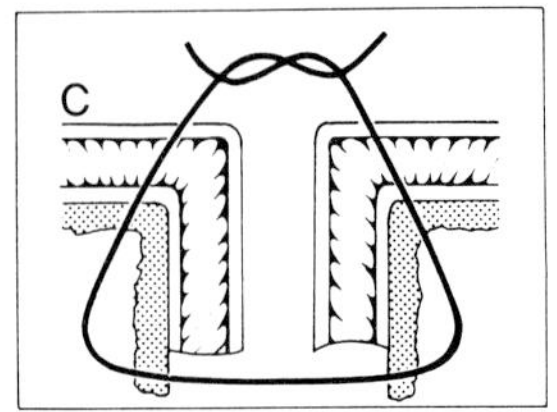

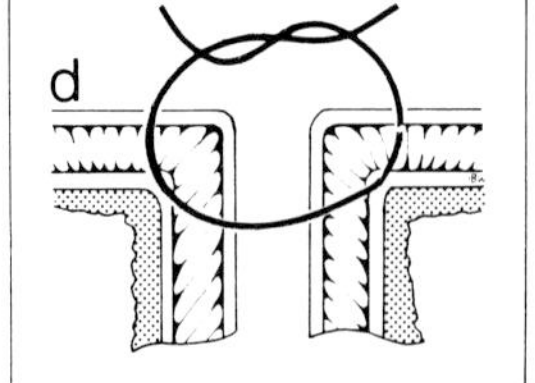

1

1a–d

Standard sutures

The standard two-layer anastomosis (*a*) consists of an inner layer of sutures incorporating the full thickness of the bowel wall and an outer layer of sutures inserted through all layers except mucosa. This second layer is frequently referred to as a *seromuscular stitch* but it should in fact include the collagenous submucosal layer of the bowel because more superficial sutures have a tendency to cut out. Single-layer techniques of suture are shown in (*b*), (*c*) and (*d*). In (*b*) the suture is inserted from the mucosal aspect of the bowel through the full thickness of the bowel wall and inversion of the anastomosis results when the suture is tied. The Gambee stitch (*c*) is inserted through all layers of the bowel wall and it is passed twice through the mucosa on each side of the anastomosis to secure mucosal inversion. The Gambee suture technique thus results in minimal inversion of the cut edges of the bowel and it is a popular suture technique in the operation of Heineke-Mikulicz pyloroplasty. In (*d*) the suture is a submucosal stitch inserted from the serosal aspect of the bowel, as in the outer layer of a two-layer anastomosis.

Suture materials

A variety of absorbable and non-absorbable suture materials is used in the anastomosis of the intestine. Experimental studies have suggested that anastomoses made with absorbable sutures are weaker than those made with non-absorbable materials during the early phase of healing but the difference is slight and probably of no clinical significance[9]. In practice, two-layer anastomoses are made with an inner layer of absorbable sutures and an outer layer of non-absorbable sutures, and single-layer anastomoses are usually made with non-absorbable materials.

Chromic catgut is the most popular absorbable suture material, and there is no convincing evidence that other materials such as polyglycolic acid and polyglactin are superior to catgut for intestinal suture. Various non-absorbable suture materials are used including silk, linen, polypropylene and synthetic polyesters. The presence of non-absorbable suture material on the mucosal aspect of the gut provokes a significant foreign body reaction and granuloma formation is not uncommon. This is of little practical significance in anastomoses in the small and large intestine but the presence of non-absorbable sutures in the gastric mucosa may result in ulceration and clinical symptoms. There are theoretical advantages in the use of monofilament non-absorbable materials such as stainless steel wire, nylon or polypropylene in that these materials may cause less tissue reaction than braided sutures, but the difference in the intestine appears to be relatively minor[10] and the monofilament sutures have inferior handling qualities. Most surgeons, including the author, prefer braided suture materials.

The size or gauge of the suture material used in anastomosis of the intestine is not standard but most surgeons use 00 or 000 sutures in adult surgery. The use of smaller, ultrafine suture materials in adults is probably misguided as there is a tendency for these sutures to cut through the bowel wall.

FACTORS AFFECTING THE HEALING OF ANASTOMOSES

Anastomoses of the stomach, duodenum and small intestine seldom give rise to complications. Dehiscence is chiefly a problem in anastomoses involving the oesophagus, colon and rectum. Multiple factors may be implicated in anastomotic dehiscence including poor surgical technique, lack of judgement, and various local and systemic abnormalities in the patient. Recent work by Fielding *et al.*[11] has suggested that surgeon-related variables are of much greater importance than local or systemic patient-related variables in the pathogenesis of anastomotic dehiscence.

Local factors

Sepsis

Clinical and experimental studies have shown that peritoneal sepsis has an adverse effect on the healing of anastomoses[12], and the problem arises chiefly in the surgery of the large intestine. A significant incidence of anastomotic dehiscence is encountered when a primary anastomosis of the colon is performed in the management of perforated diverticulitis or carcinoma and in traumatic injuries of the left colon. Experimental studies have shown that infection causes a reduction in collagen synthesis and increased lysis of collagen in colonic anastomoses[13, 14].

The surgeon should avoid an anastomosis in the presence of established peritoneal sepsis and the bowel should be exteriorized as a colostomy or ileostomy. Alimentary continuity can be safely re-established at a later date as an elective procedure.

Postoperative peritoneal sepsis and anastomotic complications may result when significant faecal contamination or soiling of the peritoneum occurs during surgery. In some cases, as in the surgery of advanced tumours of the large intestine, some degree of soiling may be unavoidable but it should always be regarded as a serious complication. When gross faecal soiling occurs in conjunction with other local factors which may propagate peritoneal infection, such as residual tumour, an extensive retroperitoneal dissection or traumatic injuries to other viscera, it is often advisable to avoid an anastomosis and exteriorize the bowel as a colostomy or ileostomy.

Mechanical state of the bowel

Faecal loading of the colon has an adverse effect on the healing of colonic or rectal anastomoses[15]. The mechanical state of the bowel is a factor which may determine the success or failure of anastomoses in the left colon or rectum, and it is a major factor in the high incidence of dehiscence which follows primary anastomosis of the left colon in operations for acute obstruction.

2

In elective colonic surgery, thorough mechanical preparation of the bowel is an integral factor in the safe conduct of colonic and rectal anastomoses. Techniques of whole-gut irrigation[16] are increasingly replacing the traditional methods of bowel preparation by purging and enemas. In the method used by the author, the patient is given 4 litres of normal saline by nasogastric tube every hour until the rectal effluent is clear. The procedure is usually completed within 3h and excellent preparation of the bowel is achieved.

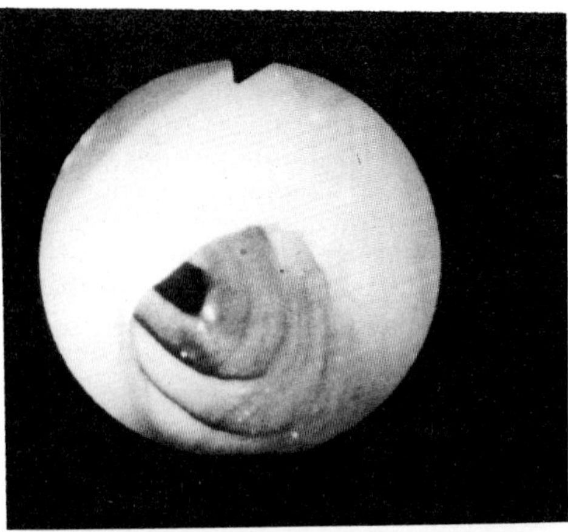

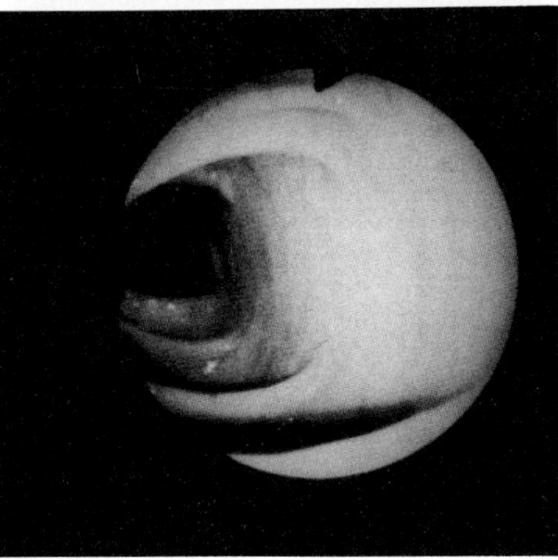

2

Colonoscopic photographs showing the appearance of the colonic lumen after whole-gut irrigation

Surprisingly, the bacterial content of the colon remains high despite such preparation[17] and it is now customary to use antimicrobial agents to reduce the infectivity of the colonic contents. There is no convincing evidence that prophylactic antimicrobial therapy prevents anastomotic dehiscence but it results in a reduction in the incidence of abdominal wound infection following intestinal surgery[18], and it seems likely that the septic complications of anastomotic dehiscence may be less severe when the bowel is prepared with antibiotics[19]. Most oral antibiotic regimens that are effective in sterilizing the intestinal contents have the potential disadvantage that they may cause a clostridial pseudomembranous colitis. However, the short-term use of sytemic antibiotics is less likely to lead to this complication and systemic therapy appears to be more effective in the prevention of postoperative sepsis in colonic surgery[20].

Mechanical preparation of the bowel may be ineffective when there is some degree of colonic obstruction and the safest policy in such cases is to avoid a primary anastomosis after bowel resection. Dudley, Radcliffe and McGeehan[21] have described an ingenious method of intraoperative colonic irrigation followed by primary anastomosis in such cases but the method requires further evaluation. Primary anastomosis should also be avoided in emergency operations for acute obstruction of the left colon. An immediate bowel resection is probably the treatment of choice for obstructing carcinoma of the left colon rather than the traditional policy of preliminary colostomy and staged resection[22], but a primary anastomosis is best avoided and the safest policy is to exteriorize the proximal cut end of the bowel as a colostomy. Alimentary continuity can be re-established at a second operation.

Drains

The use of peritoneal drains is regarded by many surgeons as a necessary feature of the management of anastomoses, particularly in the surgery of the colon and rectum. Many protagonists of the use of drains claim that they safeguard the patient against anastomotic leakage by permitting the development of an enterocutaneous fistula when anastomotic dehiscence occurs rather than a diffusing faecal peritonitis. However, the value of drainage is by no means established and experimental studies have suggested that peritoneal drains may actually increase the incidence of anastomotic dehiscence[23].

The author uses peritoneal drains for the purpose of removing any blood or serum after operations involving significant dissection and mobilization of the viscera, and in operations complicated by significant faecal contamination. The drains are not deliberately placed in the vicinity of anastomoses and they are removed after 48 h.

Faecal diversion

A proximal loop colostomy or a caecostomy may be used for the temporary protection of anastomoses in the left colon or rectum. These procedures are usually reserved for 'high-risk' anastomoses such as the very low colorectal anastomosis or an anastomosis made in the presence of unfavourable local conditions. There is no evidence that proximal faecal diversion prevents anastomotic dehiscence but it does appear that the septic complications of dehiscence may be less serious when the faecal stream has been diverted[24].

Systemic factors

The precise role of systemic abnormalities in the pathogenesis of anastomotic dehiscence has not been clearly defined but it seems probable that such factors are of much less significance than local factors or surgeon-related variables. The systemic factors which do appear to exert an unfavourable effect on anastomotic healing include advanced malignancy, malnutrition and colorectal operations resulting in excessive blood loss[12, 15].

Severe malnutrition results in reduced collagen synthesis and impaired healing of colonic anastomoses[25]. Experimental studies in small animals have suggested that the effects of malnutrition on intestinal healing are rapidly reversed by the provision of energy and amino acids[26] but clinical studies have not confirmed that short-term nutritional support has significant practical value in patients undergoing gastrointestinal surgery[27, 28].

Several factors may be responsible for the relationship between intraoperative blood loss and the healing of anastomoses. Traumatic or bloody operations on the colon in experimental animals result in peritoneal sepsis and, as a consequence, an increased incidence of anastomotic dehiscence[29]. This factor may partly account for the high incidence of anastomotic dehiscence in patients with advanced malignant disease since this seems to be largely a complication of extensive operations for the removal of fixed tumours[15]. Hypovolaemia and tissue hypoxia resulting from intraoperative blood loss may also have adverse effects on the healing of anastomoses. Gilmour *et al.*[30] found that a 10 per cent reduction in the blood volume of the dog was accompanied by a 28 per cent reduction in colonic blood flow and oxygen availability, and these changes were only slowly reversed by correction of the blood volume deficit.

Surgeon-related variables

The significance of patient-related variables or the local and systemic factors affecting anastomotic integrity was examined by Schrock, Deveney and Dunphy in 1700 large bowel anastomoses performed at the University of California, San Francisco[12]. Clinical evidence of anastomotic leakage occurred in 1.7 per cent of patients who were judged to have no adverse local or systemic factors whereas 6.7 per cent of patients, in whom one or more adverse factors were present, developed this complication. However, a recent study by Fielding *et al.*[11] has suggested that surgeon-related variables may be of much greater significance in the pathogenesis of anastomotic dehiscence. In a study of 1466 large bowel anastomoses performed by 84 surgeons in 23 hospitals in the United Kingdom the incidence of anastomotic dehiscence experienced by different surgeons ranged from 0.5 per cent to more than 30 per cent. These results cannot be accounted for by differences in patient population and the inevitable conclusion from these observations is that some surgeons perform remarkably badly in the clinical management of intestinal anastomoses. The factors which account for these bad performances are obscure: they may be failures of judgement; failures of surgical technique; or a combination of these factors. What is certain, however, is that such complications and failures need not happen, and that they can be reduced to a minimal level by attention to the principles and technical aspects of intestinal anastomosis described in this chapter.

The anastomoses

Anastomoses may be made end-to-end, end-to-side or side-to-side, but generally the method used in any operation is fairly standard. In this section, the indications for the use of the different types of anastomosis and the techniques of intestinal suture will be described.

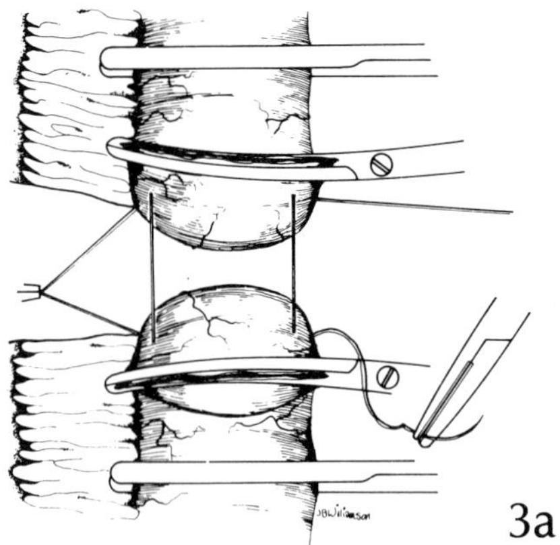

3a

END-TO-END ANASTOMOSIS

Small bowel anastomosis

3a, b & c

Insertion of posterior outer layer of sutures

The divided ends of the bowel are held in crushing clamps, and light occlusion clamps are applied across the bowel, care being taken to avoid the application of these clamps across the mesentery. The two-layer inverting anastomosis begins with the insertion of the outer layer of interrupted submucosal sutures on the posterior aspect of the anastomosis (*a* and *b*). Non-absorbable sutures of silk or other braided material are used, and they are inserted first at the mesenteric and antimesenteric borders of the intestine. The sutures are tied when this layer is complete and the crushing clamps can then be amputated (*c*), thus opening the bowel lumen.

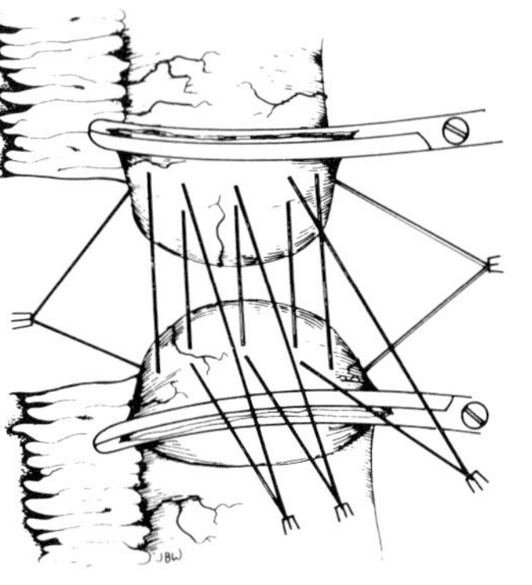

3b

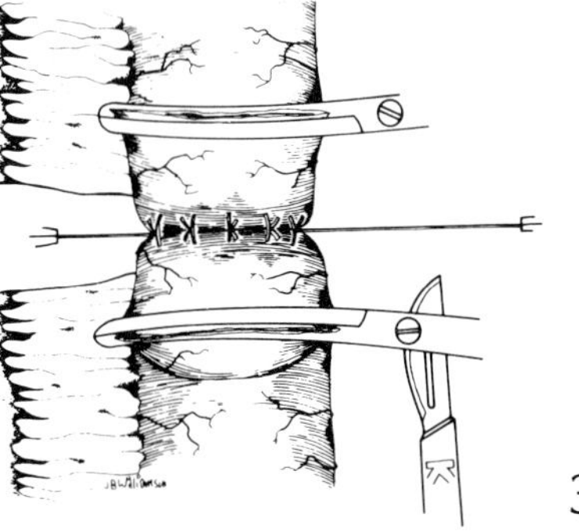

3c

4a–g

Inner layer of sutures

A continuous chromic catgut suture is used for the inner layer of the anastomosis, which begins at the antimesenteric end. The suture is inserted through all layers of the bowel wall and tied on the serosal aspect (*a*). A forceps is applied to the short end of the suture which will be used again on completion of this layer. A continuous over-and-over suture technique is used for the posterior aspect of the anastomosis, care being taken to include all coats of the bowel wall (*b*). The mesenteric corner of the anastomosis is securely invaginated by the use of the Connell suture technique (*c*); inversion of the edges of the bowel is achieved when the suture is pulled tight (*d*). The anterior aspect of the inner layer of the anastomosis may be completed with an over-and-over suture technique but a continuous Connell technique is generally preferred (*e*). The mucosa and edges of the bowel on the antimesenteric aspect are invaginated as the last Connell stitch is pulled tight (*f*), and the suture is tied to its other end (*g*).

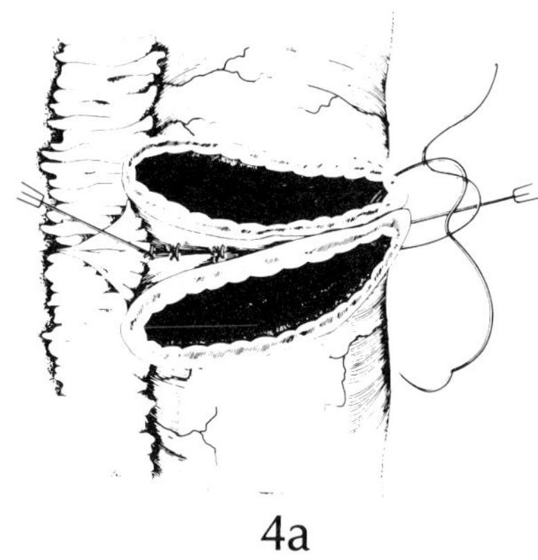

4a

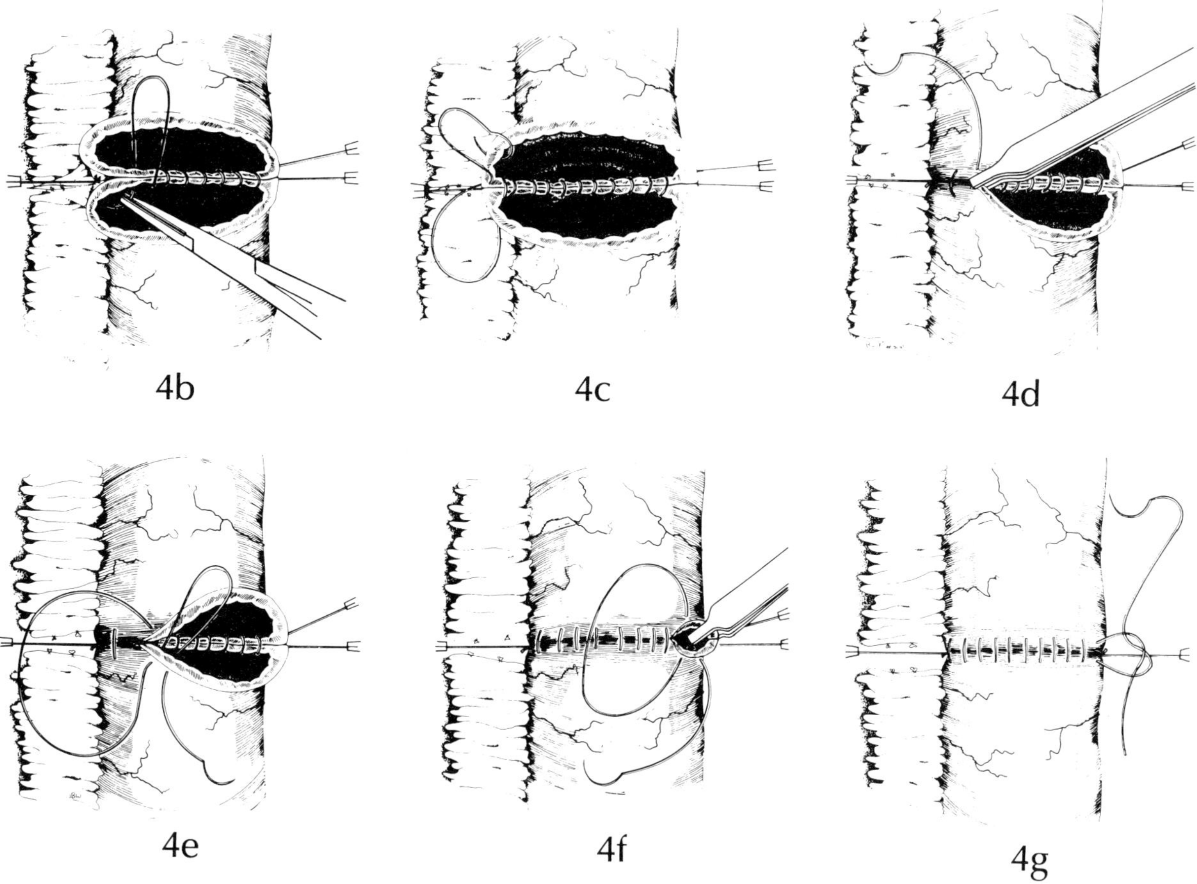

4b 4c 4d 4e 4f 4g

5a & b

Insertion of anterior outer layer of sutures

Interrupted, non-absorbable, submucosal sutures are then inserted on the anterior aspect of the bowel (*a*) and the anastomosis is completed (*b*).

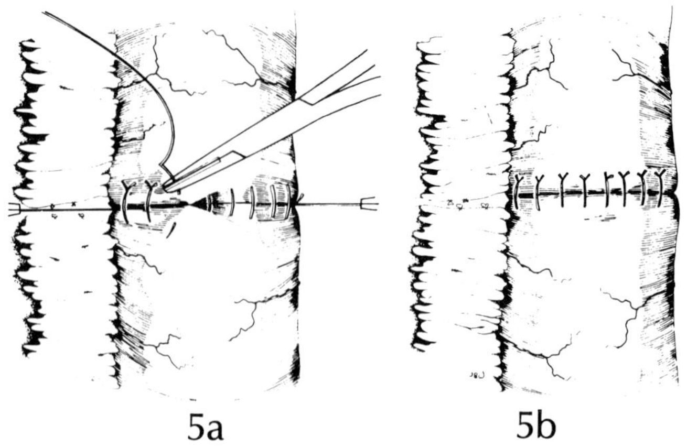

5a 5b

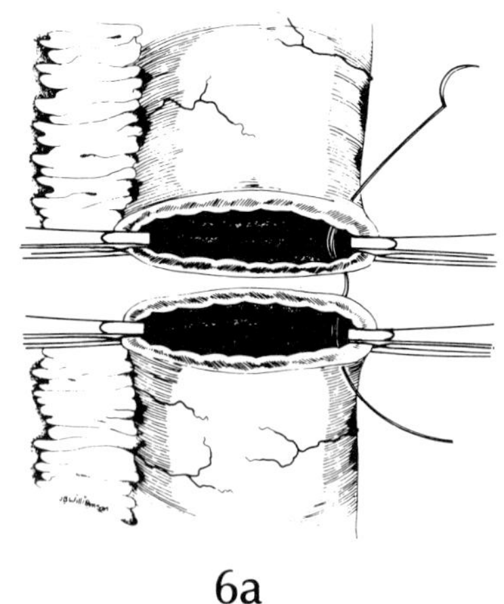

6a

6a–d

Anastomosis beginning with inner layer of sutures

Some surgeons prefer to begin the two-layer anastomosis with the insertion of the inner layer of catgut (*a* and *b*). When this layer is complete, the outer layer of sutures is inserted on the anterior aspect of the anastomosis and the anastomosis is then rotated (*c*) so that the outer layer can be completed on the posterior aspect (*d*). This method is apt to prove unsatisfactory in obese subjects when the mesentery is fat-laden because after completion of the inner layer, insertion of the outer layer of sutures on the posterior aspect of the anastomosis is difficult to achieve with precision when the mesenteric fat encroaches on the bowel wall.

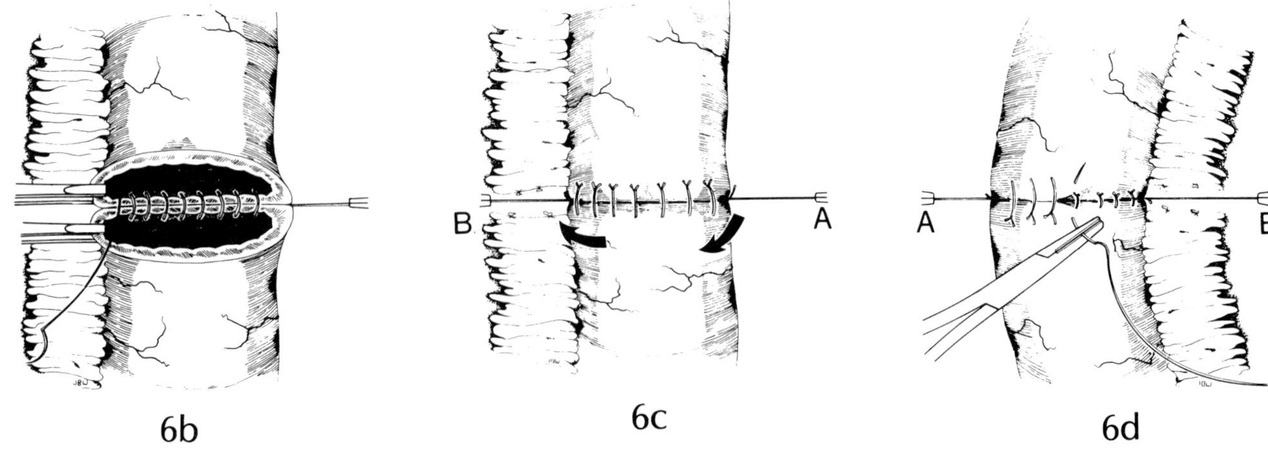

6b 6c 6d

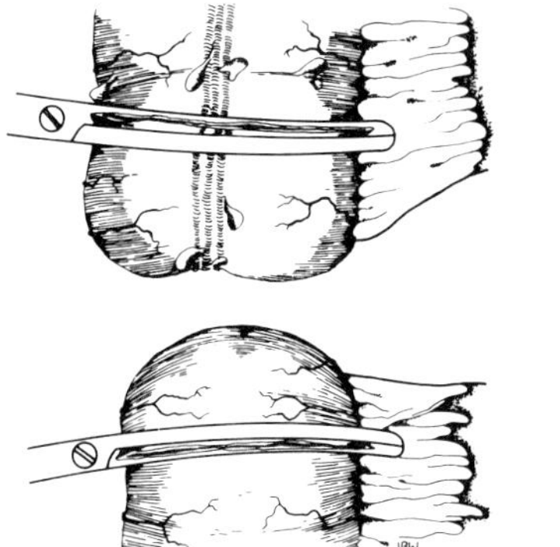

7a

Ileocolic anastomosis

7a–d

Correction for unequal ends of bowel

An end-to-end anastomosis is possible even when there is considerable disparity in the size of the two ends of bowel. This situation may arise in anastomosis of the ileum to the colon after right hemicolectomy or in operations for small bowel obstruction (*a*). The problem is solved by widening the orifice of the smaller lumen: the outer layer of submucosal sutures is inserted in an oblique fashion away from the cut edge of the bowel on the antimesenteric aspect in the end of smaller calibre (*b*); and the open end of the bowel is widened by cutting along the antimesenteric border (*c* and *d*).

Most problems of disparity can be solved in this way but some surgeons prefer to use an end-to-side technique of anastomosis in these circumstances.

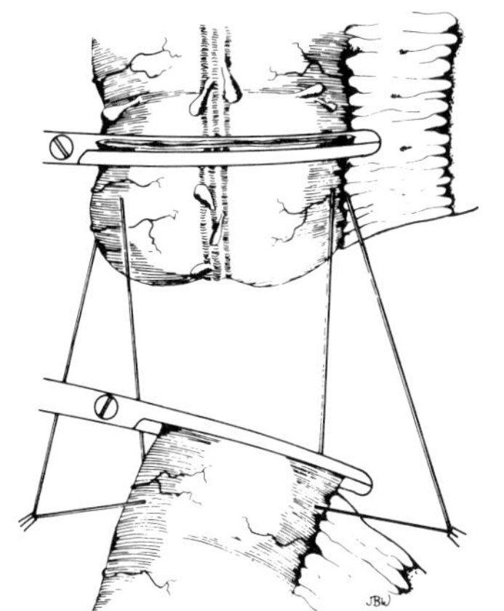

7b

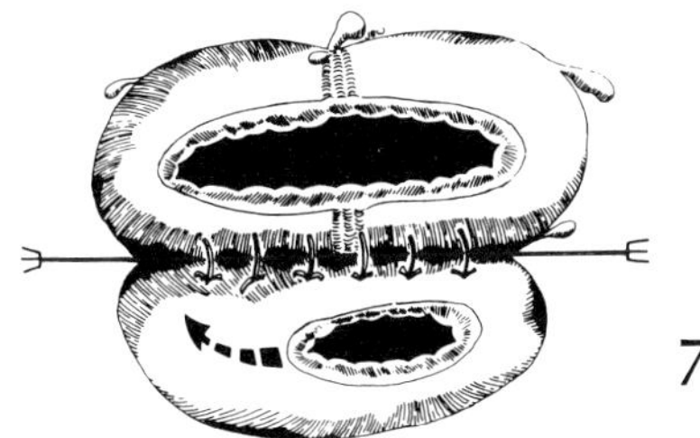

7c

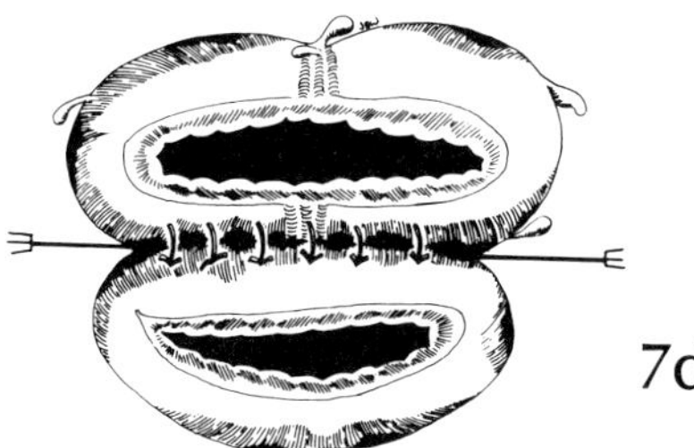

7d

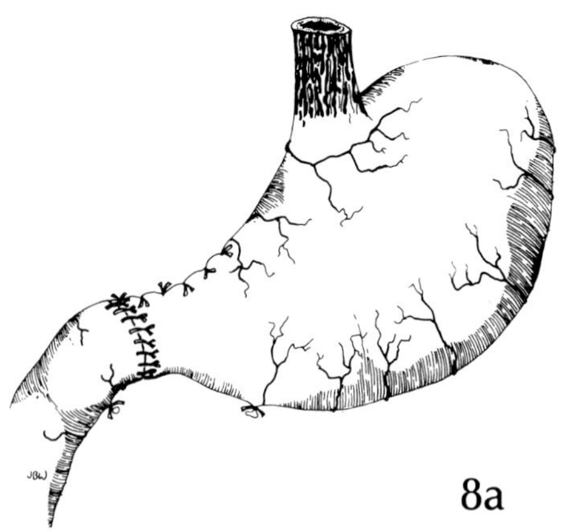

8a

8a, b & c

Gastroduodenal anastomosis

The most common end-to-end anastomosis involving the stomach is the Billroth I gastroduodenal anastomosis (*a*). Care should be taken with regard to haemostasis in this operation for the stomach is endowed with a rich blood supply and serious postoperative bleeding from the suture line may occur if haemostasis is not meticulous. The Connell suture technique is not haemostatic but a suitable method in this operation is the 'loop on the serosa' technique (*b* and *c*). This technique provides effective haemostasis and adequate inversion of the cut edges of the bowel.

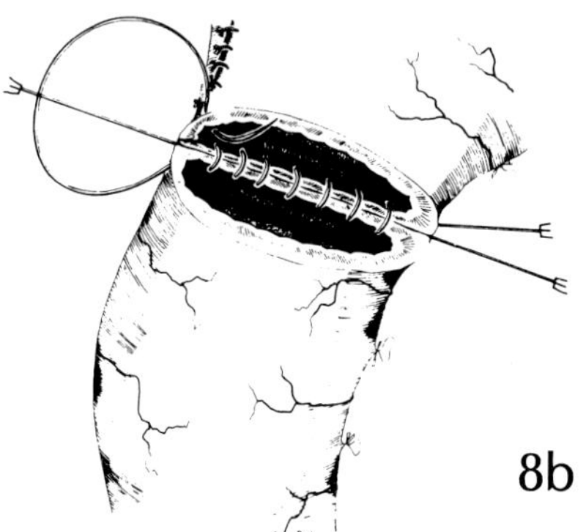

8b

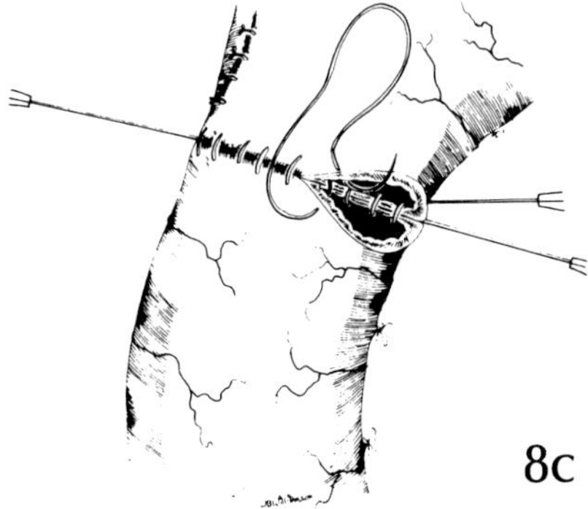

8c

Colorectal anastomosis

9a–d

Two-layer method

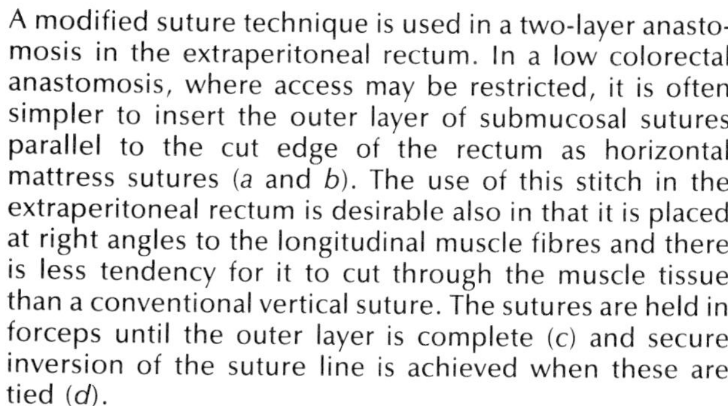

A modified suture technique is used in a two-layer anastomosis in the extraperitoneal rectum. In a low colorectal anastomosis, where access may be restricted, it is often simpler to insert the outer layer of submucosal sutures parallel to the cut edge of the rectum as horizontal mattress sutures (*a* and *b*). The use of this stitch in the extraperitoneal rectum is desirable also in that it is placed at right angles to the longitudinal muscle fibres and there is less tendency for it to cut through the muscle tissue than a conventional vertical suture. The sutures are held in forceps until the outer layer is complete (*c*) and secure inversion of the suture line is achieved when these are tied (*d*).

A similar technique is recommended in two-layer oesophageal anastomoses.

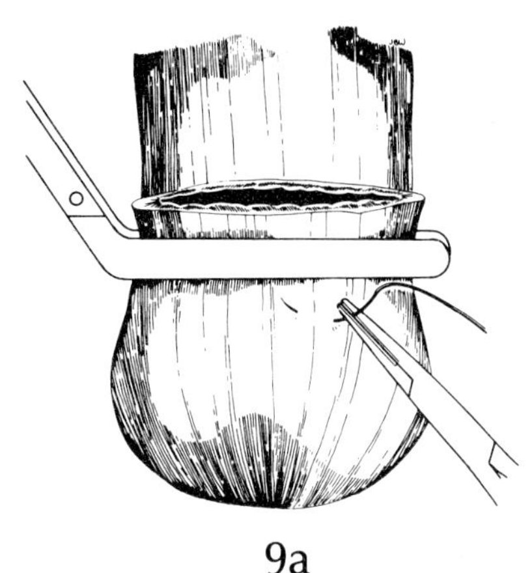

9a

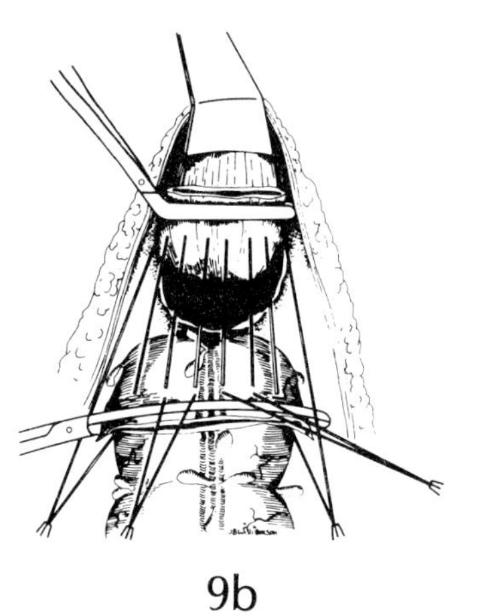

9b

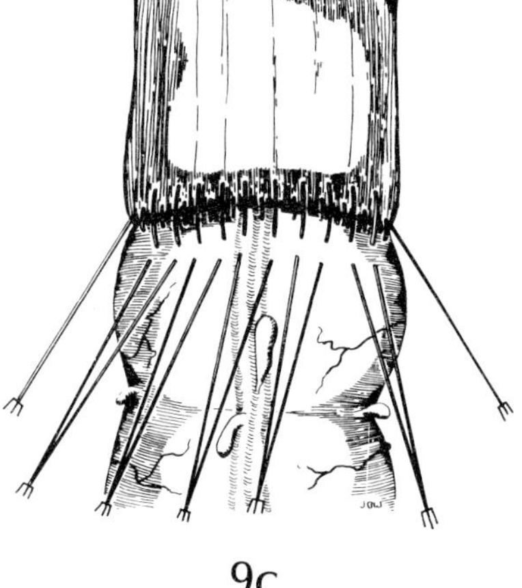

9c

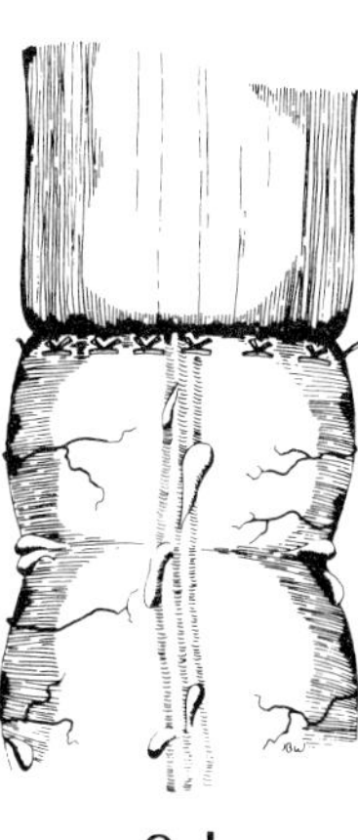

9d

10a–e

Single-layer method

A single-layer technique of anastomosis is an alternative, simpler and more satisfactory method for low rectal anastomoses. The author uses a braided suture material such as silk, and the anastomosis begins with the insertion of the mesenteric and antimesenteric sutures through all layers of the bowel wall (*a*). The posterior layer of the anastomosis consists of a series of through-and-through sutures incorporating all layers of the bowel wall. These sutures are held in forceps and tied when the layer is complete (*b*). The interval between each suture in the posterior layer should be relatively small; otherwise there is a tendency for eversion of the mucosa to occur when the sutures are tied. The anterior layer of the anastomosis is made with a similar series of full-thickness sutures, knotted on the mucosa (*c*). A small gap in the suture line finally remains in the centre of the anterior layer and this is closed with a submucosal suture inserted parallel to the edge of the suture line (*d*).

An alternative method of construction of the anterior layer is to use a series of submucosal mattress sutures (e), as in the outer layer of a two-layer rectal anastomosis.

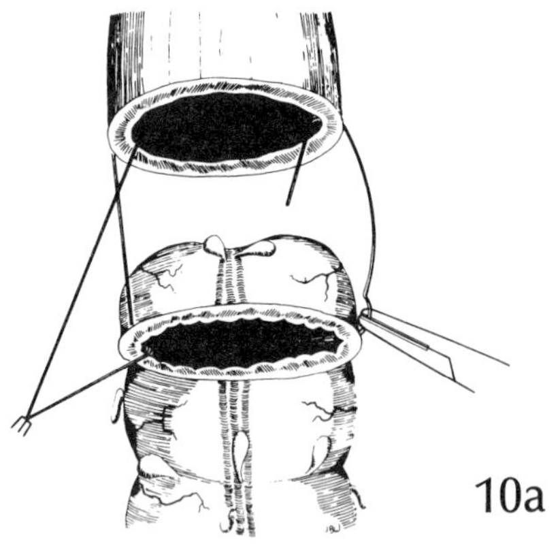

10a

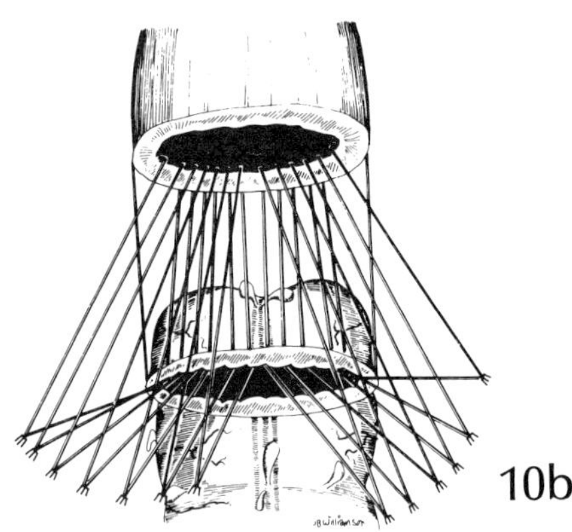

10b

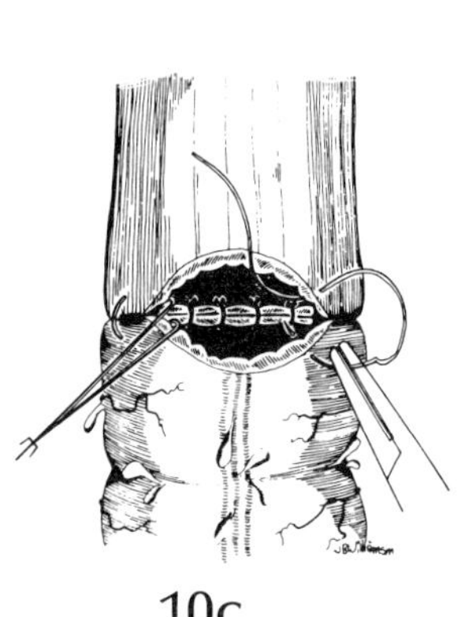

10c

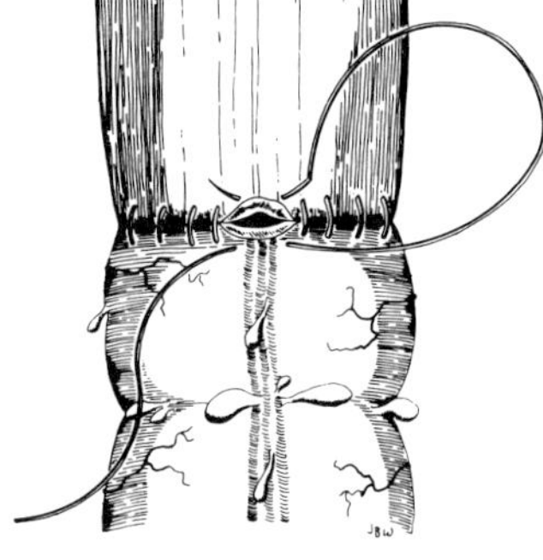

10d

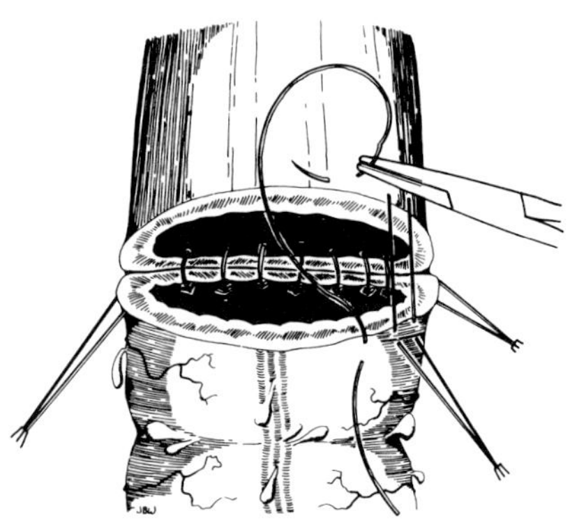

10e

END-TO-SIDE ANASTOMOSIS

This method has a number of applications in gastrointestinal surgery, particularly in the surgery of the oesophagus and stomach.

11a–h

Technique for closure of end of bowel

Some surgeons use the end-to-side method in anastomosis of the small or large intestine when a significant disparity exists between two ends of bowel. This applies particularly in the operations of right hemicolectomy and subtotal colectomy, though an end-to-end anastomosis can be achieved in these circumstances as shown in *Illustrations 7a–d*.

When an end-to-side anastomosis of the small or large intestine is performed, one end of the bowel must be closed. A two-layer inverting suture technique is used. The bowel is held in a crushing clamp and a chromic catgut suture mounted on a straight needle is inserted through all layer of the bowel wall at the antimesenteric border (*a*). The suture is knotted and the first layer begins as a continuous horizontal mattress suture (*b* and *c*). The crushing clamp is removed as the suture is again knotted at the mesenteric border of the intestine. The suture is then returned towards the antimesenteric end as a continuous over-and-over stitch incorporating all layers of the bowel wall (*d* and *e*) and it is finally knotted at the antimesenteric end (*f*). Interrupted, submucosal sutures of silk or other braided material are then inserted (*g*) and the end of the bowel is securely invaginated (*h*).

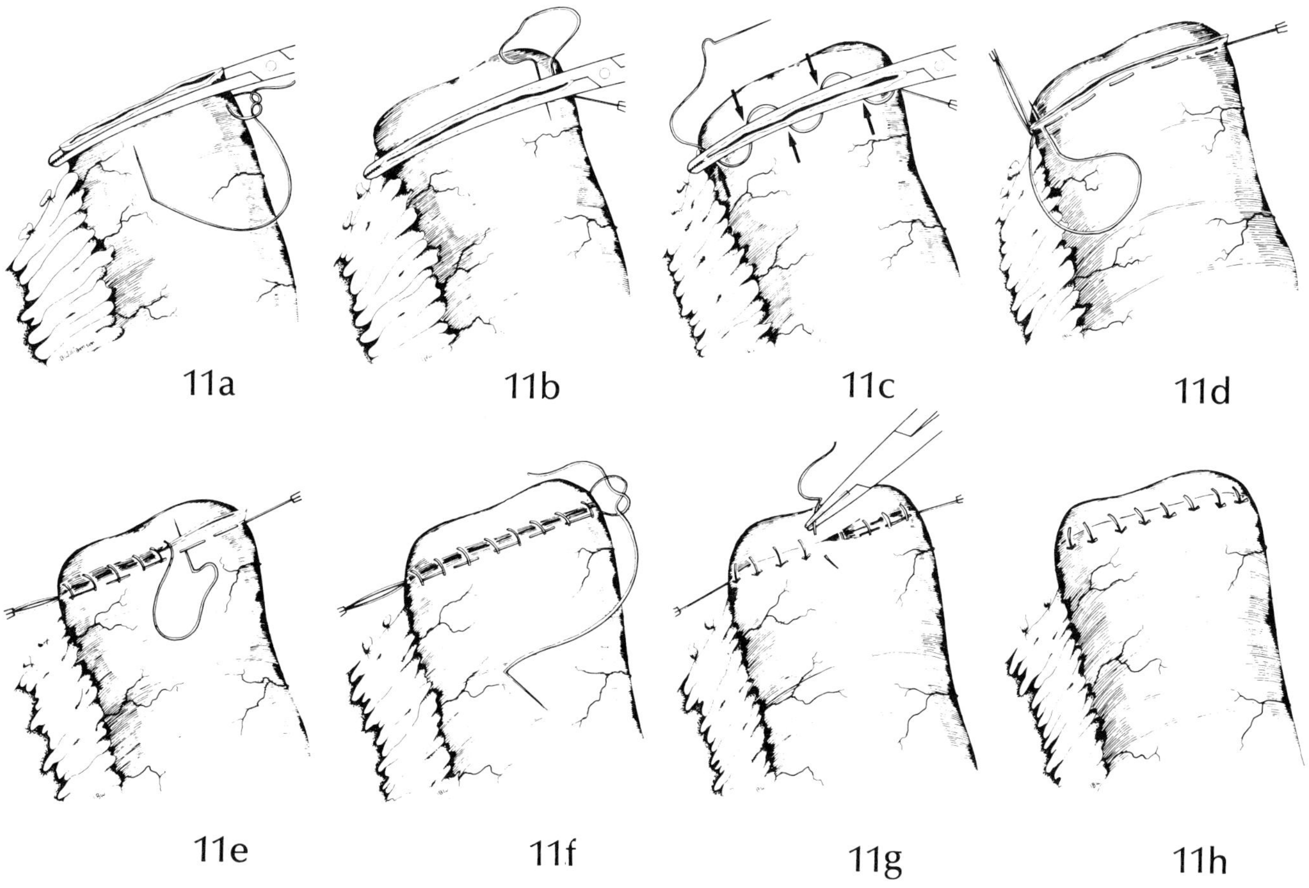

11a 11b 11c 11d

11e 11f 11g 11h

12a–d

Ileocolic anastomosis

In end-to-side reconstruction following the operation of right hemicolectomy, the end of the colon is closed and the end of the ileum is anastomosed to the side of the colon, using a standard two-layer inverting technique (*a*, *b* and *c*).

A similar technique is used by Baker in colorectal anastomoses. The side of the colon is anastomosed to the end of the rectal stump (*d*). The author seldom uses this method in colorectal anastomosis but finds it useful in anastomosis of the caecum to the rectum and in anastomosis of the ileum to the rectum after the operation of subtotal colectomy if there is a marked disparity in the size of the ileum and rectum.

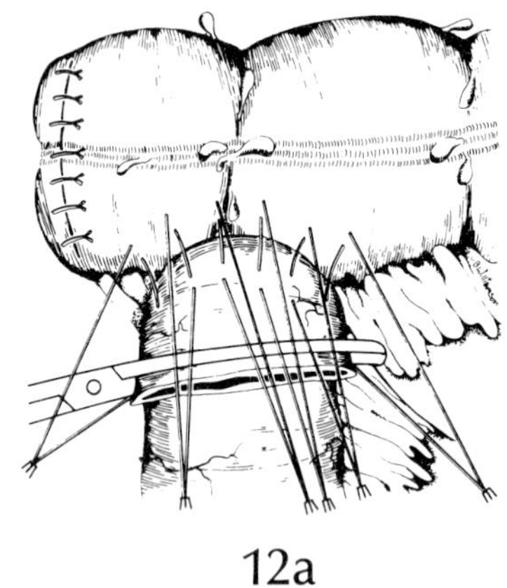

12a

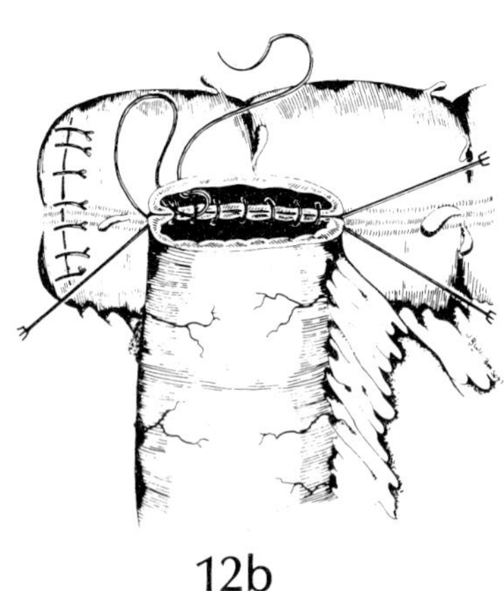

12b

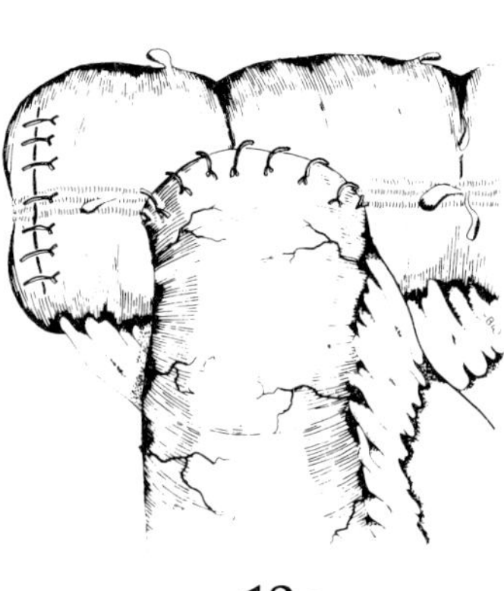

12c

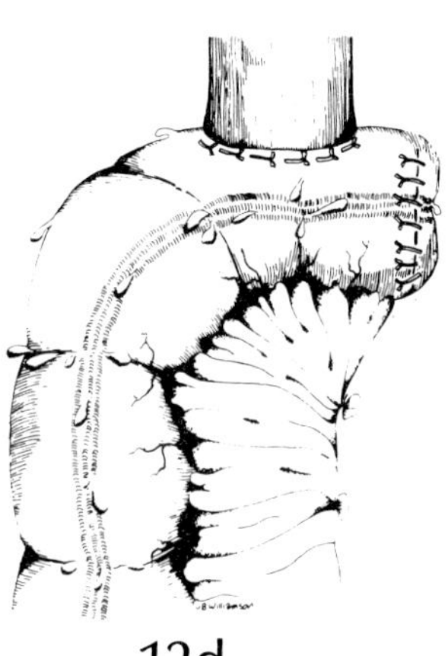

12d

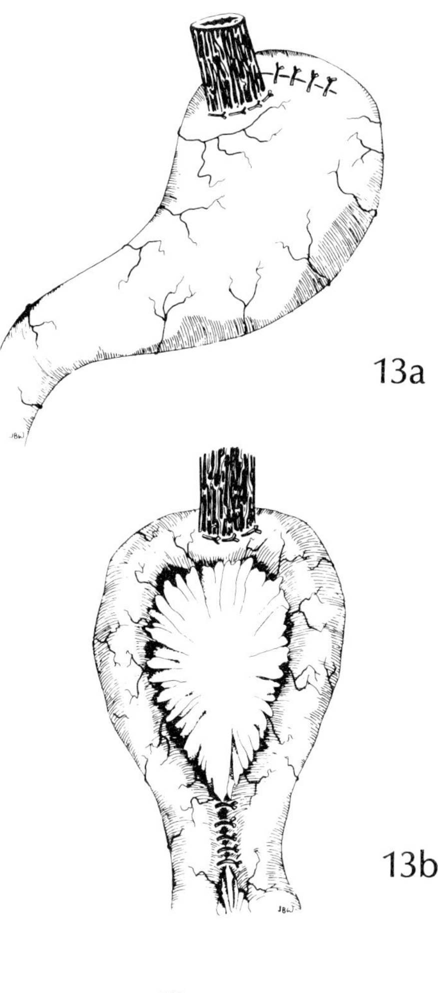

13a

13b

13a, b & c

Oesophagogastric and oesophagojejunal anastomoses

In the operation of oesophagogastrectomy (*a*), the proximal end of the gastric remnant is closed using the technique shown in *Illustrations 11a–h*, and the end of the oesophagus is anastomosed to the front of the stomach. A two-layer suture technique is used and in all oesophageal anastomoses the outer layer is made with horizontal mattress sutures inserted parallel to the cut end of the oesophagus. These sutures have less tendency to cut through the oesophageal muscle than vertical sutures and the suture technique is thus identical to that shown in low rectal anastomoses (*see Illustrations 9a–d*).

After total gastrectomy the end of the oesophagus is anastomosed to the side of the jejunum using the same two-layer suture technique. A defunctioned loop of jejunum may be used (*b*) or a Roux-en-Y type of reconstruction (*c*).

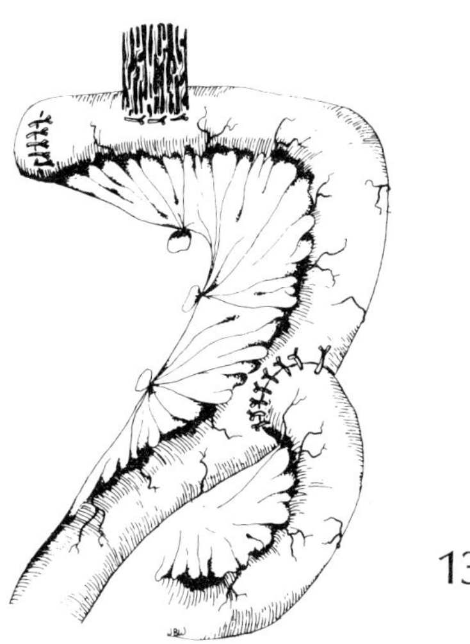

13c

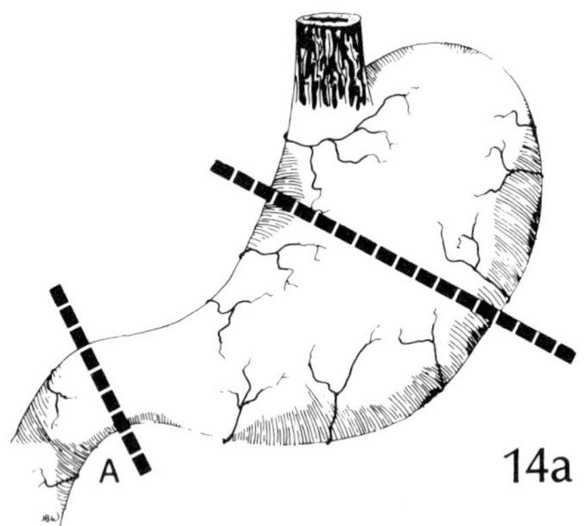

14a–d

Gastrojejunal anastomosis

In the operation of partial gastrectomy (*a*) the gastric remnant may be anastomosed end-to-side to the jejunum. The construction of this anastomosis is simplified by the use of Lane's twin occlusion clamps (*b*). A two-layer inverting suture technique is used (*c* and *d*) and many surgeons use a double layer of continuous catgut in this anastomosis. Because of the rich blood supply of the stomach, significant postoperative bleeding may occur from the suture line unless a haemostatic suture technique is used. For this reason a 'loop on the serosa' technique should be used for the inner layer of the anastomosis (*c*). The use of a non-haemostatic suture technique, such as Connell stitch, is permissible only if occlusion clamps are avoided and the bleeding vessels in the suture line can be individually secured.

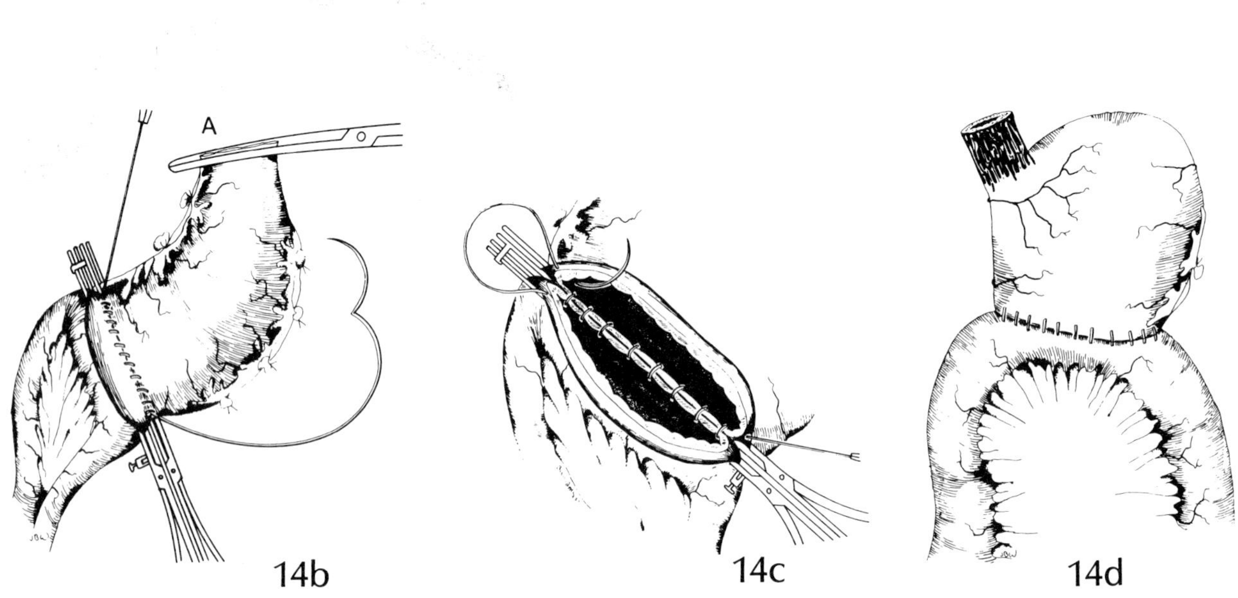

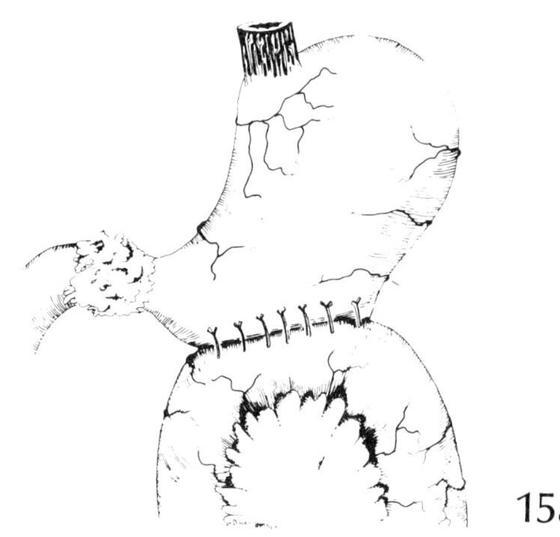

15a

SIDE-TO-SIDE ANASTOMOSIS

This method is used in gastric surgery to provide drainage of the stomach after vagotomy or to relieve gastric outlet obstruction. Its function elsewhere in the alimentary tract is chiefly in bypassing intestinal or biliary obstructions, often as a purely palliative measure in malignant disease.

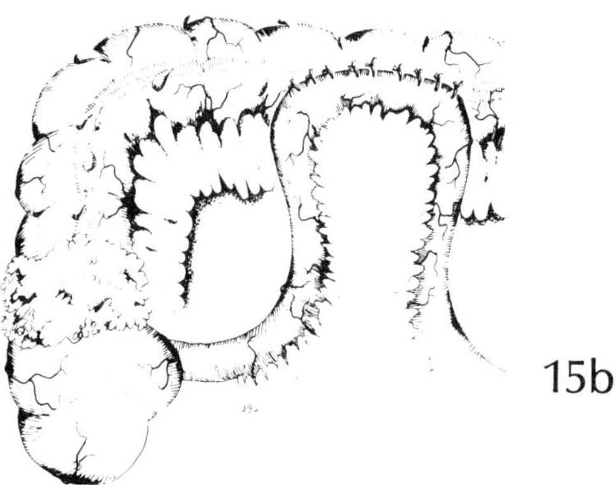

15b

15a, b & c

Bypass procedures

In the palliation of obstructive complications arising from irremovable neoplasms a two-layer inverting anastomosis is used: for neoplasms of the distal stomach a gastrojejunostomy is performed (*a*); anastomosis of the terminal ileum to the transverse colon is performed for obstructions of the right colon (*b*); and in obstructions of the common bile duct the fundus of the gall bladder is anastomosed to a defunctioned loop of jejunum (*c*).

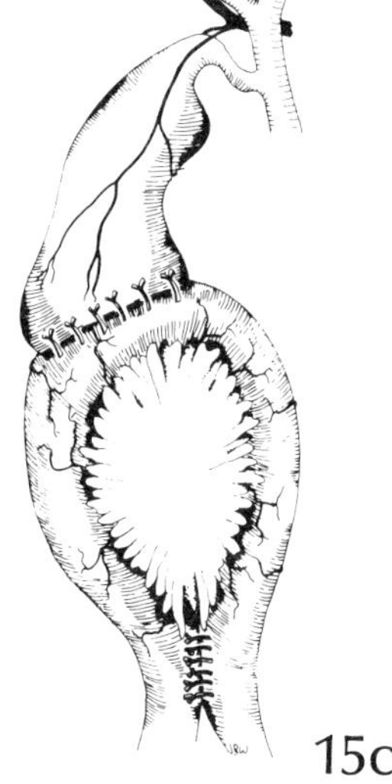

15c

Postoperative care

The postoperative management of anastomoses in the gastrointestinal tract is chiefly concerned with the restoration of normal alimentary function, and the early detection and control of complications.

A period of alimentary motor dysfunction inevitably follows anastomosis of the intestine and may or may not be apparent clinically. In some cases the early introduction of oral intake in the postoperative period is poorly tolerated. Vomiting may occur because of delayed gastric emptying; intestinal distension and vomiting may take place after anastomosis of the small or large intestine. Distension of the bowel at the suture line is undesirable on the theoretical grounds that it may cause tissue ischaemia and an increased risk of anastomotic leakage, but there is little clinical evidence to support this thesis and there is no standard regimen for the postoperative management of oral intake.

16a & b

The author does not routinely use nasogastric tubes but has a cautious attitude towards the introduction of oral intake after anastomosis of the intestine. After gastric resection, gastric emptying is assessed radiologically with Gastrografin on the first postoperative day and oral intake is permitted only if satisfactory emptying is present (*a*). Oral intake after oesophagogastric resections is not permitted for at least 5 days and then only after a Gastrografin swallow has shown that there is no leakage at the suture line (*b*). Oral intake after anastomosis of the small or large intestine is withheld until the patient has passed flatus, which is usually about the fourth postoperative day.

Intolerance of oral intake and ileus may indicate that anastomotic dehiscence has occurred. Other signs of dehiscence such as peritonitis, fistulation and systemic evidence of sepsis depend on the site of the anastomosis, the extent of the dehiscence and the nature of the intestinal contents. Dehiscence is a complication which occurs during the first few days after surgery when the integrity and strength of the anastomosis are largely dependent on the intestinal sutures, and clinical features of dehiscence seldom arise *de novo* after the first postoperative week.

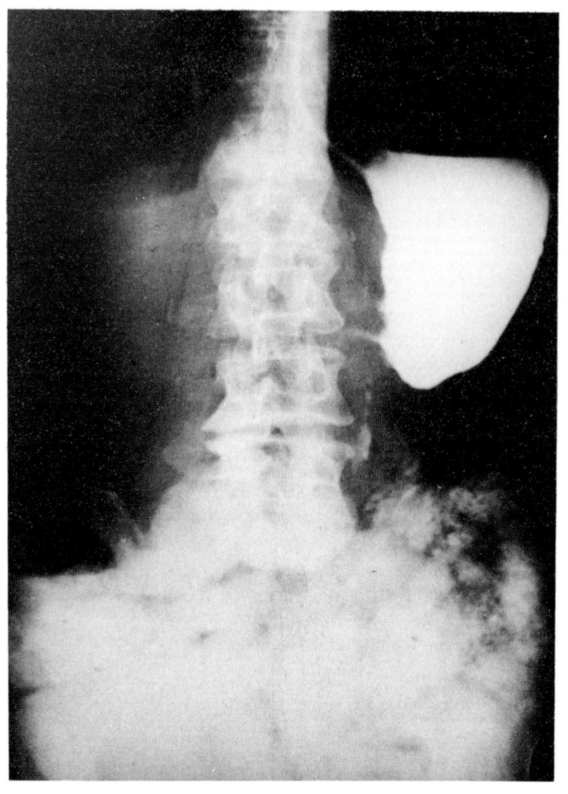

16a

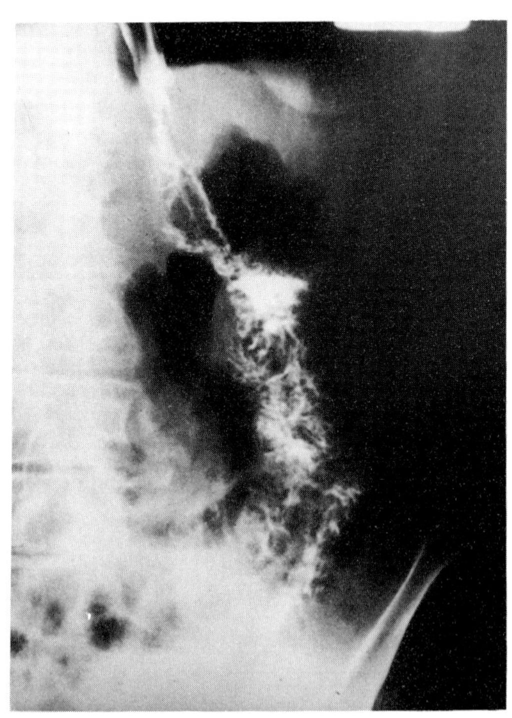

16b

References

1. Ravitch, M. M., Canalis, F., Weinshelbaum, A., McCormick, J. Studies in intestinal healing. III Observations on everting intestinal anastomoses. Annals of Surgery 1967; 166: 670–680

2. Goligher, J. C., Morris, C., McAdam, W. A. F., De Dombal, F. T., Johnston, D. A controlled trial of inverting versus everting intestinal suture in clinical large bowel surgery. British Journal of Surgery 1970; 57: 817–822

3. McAdams, A. J., Meikle, A. G., Taylor, J. O. One layer or two layer colonic anastomoses. American Journal of Surgery 1970; 120: 546-550

4. Irvin, T. T., Edwards, J. P. Comparison of single-layer inverting, two-layer inverting and everting anastomoses in the rabbit colon. British Journal of Surgery 1973; 60: 453-457

5. Irvin, T. T., Goligher, J. C., Johnson, D. A randomised prospective clinical trial of single-layer and two-layer inverting intestinal anastomoses. British Journal of Surgery 1973; 60: 457–460

6. Goligher, J. C., Lee, P. W. G., Simpkins, K. C., Lintott, D. J. A controlled comparison of one- and two-layer techniques of suture for high and low colorectal anastomoses. British Journal of Surgery 1977; 64: 609–614

7. Everett, W. G. A comparison of one-layer and two-layer techniques for colorectal anastomosis. British Journal of Surgery 1975; 62: 135–140

8. Matheson, N. A., Irving, A. D. Single layer anastomosis after rectosigmoid resection. British Journal of Surgery 1975; 62: 239–242

9. Hastings, J. C., Van Winkle, W., Barker, E., Hines, D., Nichols, W. The effect of suture materials on healing wounds of the stomach and colon. Surgery, Gynecology and Obstetrics 1975; 140: 701–707

10. Fontaine, C. J.., Dudley, H. A. F. Assessment of suture materials for intestinal use by an extramucosal implant technique and a quantitative histological evaluation. British Journal of Surgery 1978; 65: 288–290

11. Fielding, L. P., Stewart-Brown, S., Blesovsky, L., Kearney, G. Anastomotic integrity after operations for large-bowel cancer: a multicentre study. British Medical Journal 1980; 281: 411–414

12. Schrock, T. R., Deveney, C. W., Dunphy, J. E. Factors contributing to leakage of colonic anastomoses. Annals of Surgery 1973; 177: 513–518

13. Irvin, T. T. Collagen metabolism in infected colonic anastomoses. Surgery, Gynecology and Obstetrics 1976; 143: 220–224

14. Hunt, T. K., Hawley, P. R., Hale, J., Goodson, W., Thakral, K. K. Colon repair: the collagenous equilibrium. In: Hunt, T. K., ed. Wound healing and wound infection: theory and surgical practice. New York: Appleton-Century-Crofts, 1980: 153

15. Irvin, T. T., Goligher, J. C. Aetiology of disruption of intestinal anastomoses. British Journal of Surgery 1973; 60: 461–464

16. Crapp, A. R., Powis, S. J. A., Tillotson, P., Cooke, W. T., Alexander-Williams, J. Preparation of the bowel by whole-gut irrigation. Lancet 1975; 2: 1239–1240

17. Arabi, Y., Dimock, F., Burdon, D. W., Alexander-Williams, J., Keighley, M. R. B. Influence of bowel preparation and antimicrobials on colonic microflora. British Journal of Surgery 1978; 65: 555–559

18. Eykyn, S. J., Jackson, B. T., Lockhard-Mummery, H. E., Phillips, E. Prophylactic peroperative intravenous metronidazole in elective colorectal surgery. Lancet 1979; 2: 761–764

19. Matheson, D. M., Arabi, Y., Baxter-Smith, D., Alexander-Williams, J., Keighley, M. R. B. Randomized multicentre trial of oral bowel preparation and antimicrobials for elective colorectal operations. British Journal of Surgery 1978; 65: 597–600

20. Keighley, M. R. B., Arabi, Y., Alexander-Williams, J., Youngs, D., Burdon, D. W. Comparison between systemic and oral antimicrobial prophylaxis in colorectal surgery. Lancet 1979; 1: 894–897

21. Dudley, H. A. F., Radcliffe, A. G., McGeehan, D. Intraoperative irrigation of the colon to permit primary anastomosis. British Journal of Surgery 1980; 67: 80–81

22. Fielding, L. P., Stewart-Brown, S., Blesovsky, L. Large-bowel obstruction caused by cancer: a prospective study. British Medical Journal 1979; 2: 515–517

23. Manz, C. W., La Tendresse, C., Sako, Y. The detrimental effects of drains on colonic anastomoses. An experimental study. Diseases of the Colon and Rectum 1970; 13: 17–25

24. Goldstein, M., Duff, J. H. Reconsideration of colostomy in elective left colon resection. Surgery, Gynecology and Obstetrics 1972; 134: 593–594

25. Irvin, T. T., Hunt, T. K. Effect of malnutrition on colonic healing. Annals of Surgery 1974; 180: 765–772

26. Daly, J. M., Steiger, E., Vars, H. M., Dudrick, S. J. Postoperative oral and intravenous nutrition. Annals of Surgery 1974; 180: 709–715

27. Sagar, S., Harland, P., Shields, R. Early postoperative feeding with elemental diet. British Medical Journal 1979; 1: 293–295

28. Yeung, C. K., Young, G. A., Hackett, A. F., Hill, G. L. Fine needle catheter jejunostomy: an assessment of a new method of nutritional support after major gastro-intestinal surgery. British Journal of Surgery 1979; 66: 727–732

29. Irvin, T. T., Hunt, T. K. Pathogenesis and prevention of disruption of colonic anastomoses in traumatised rats. British Journal of Surgery 1974; 61: 437–439

30. Gilmour, D. G., Aitkenhead, A. R., Hothersall, A. P., Ledingham, I. McA. The effect of hypovolaemia on colonic blood flow in the dog. British Journal of Surgery 1980; 67: 82–84

End-to-end anastomosis using circular stapling devices

R. J. Heald MChir, FRCS
Consultant Surgeon, North Hampshire Group of Hospitals, Basingstoke

Introduction

The circular stapling 'guns' provide a quick and convenient alternative to manual anastomosis anywhere in the gastrointestinal tract. They are of major importance, however, when one of the bowel ends is relatively inaccessible. Thus their use has extended downwards by 5 cm or more the level at which many surgeons will undertake anastomosis on the anorectum. Not only may this reduce the need for abdominoperineal excision, but it facilitates total removal of the mesorectum which may be important in the control of rectal cancer.

The stapling devices also increase the number of anastomoses onto the oesophagus that can be achieved through an abdominal incision and the height of anastomosis possible through a left thoracotomy.

The surgeon's aim is a union in which the rings of inverted tissue are not crushed but viable and held in apposition by a perfect circle of staples. Thus the purse-string must draw in to the instrument only sufficient tissue to achieve this; an excess may result in extrusion of part of the circumference with a consequent primary defect or later necrosis of the ring of tissue and perhaps a late leak or a stricture. It is important, therefore, to take care in inserting the purse-string if the anorectal end is large or thick, and the oesophagus also requires special gentleness because of its tendency to split. Removal of the gun from any site is done with the anastomosis supported by a hand so that the tool slips out cleanly without damage.

The basic stapled anastomosis

The bowel ends

About 1–2 cm of bowel end must be cleaned of mesentery – this will later be cut off with the purse-string as the so-called 'doughnut'.

1

The purse-string

It is essential that both mucosa and either muscularis mucosae or a small piece of muscularis propria be included. It is also important that the stiches are not too widely placed – 5 mm is ideal. Suture material of 0 Prolene or nylon is suitable, and 00 will suffice when the bowel end is not bulky.

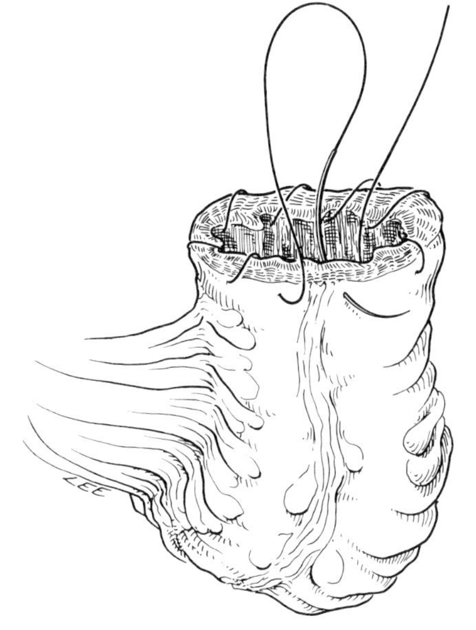

1

2

The purse-string instrument

This makes insertion very quick and simple. It is quite unsuitable low down in the pelvis, however, and is unable to cope with a bulky muscle tube. The bowel is best cut with scissors as a 'flush slice' with the knife may cut loose some of the 'bites' of the purse-string.

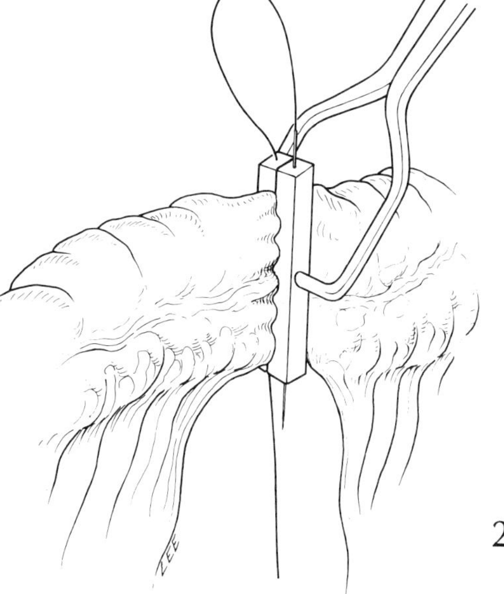

2

Use of the instrument

The SPTU Russian gun requires special attention to (*1*) correct loading of perfect staples, (*2*) sharp knife and new washer, (*3*) assembly of the instrument which must have no slack in the shaft. The EEA cartridge must be loaded with the safety catch applied or the cartridge may be wasted. The nuts at each end must be tightened and the gap checked to be around 2 mm when it is screwed right home.

With both the SPTU and the Ethicon ILS it is important that the surgeon familiarize himself with the graduated turning screw and its relationship to the gap width – a gap of between 1.5 and 2.5 mm is vital to proper function. Too much crushing may lead to necrosis and too wide a gap to a failure of the knife to cut through or of the staples to turn over.

The weapon must be lubricated liberally with blood or K-Y jelly, particularly inside the anvil.

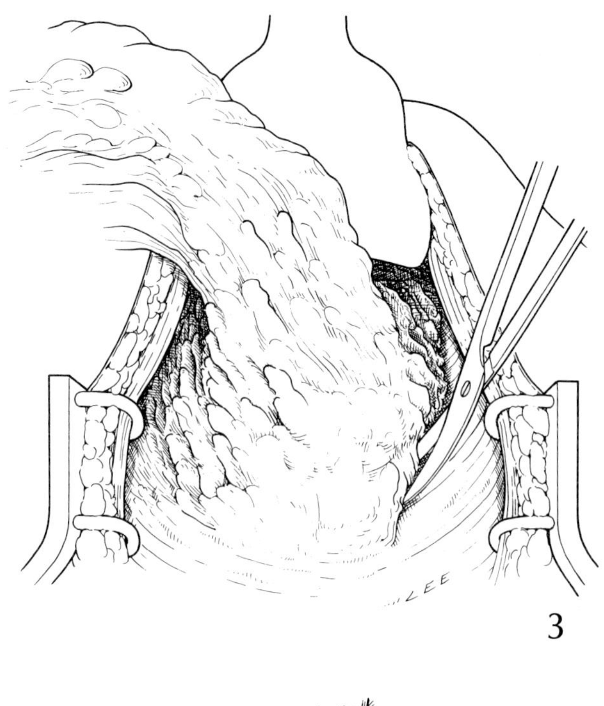

3

Specific operations

LOW ANTERIOR RESECTION OF THE RECTUM

3 & 4

Preparation of the rectal stump

Preparation and purse-stringing of the rectal end calls for great care. It is rendered easier if the plane around and behind the mesorectum is followed with sharp dissection under direct vision right down to the pelvic floor. The middle rectal vessels occasionally require ligation but little other bleeding will be encountered provided the mesorectal tissues are cut away from the levators and not entered. A clean plane around the rectal muscle is thus established without undue difficulty and excessive 'turn-in' to the gun is avoided.

The clamp and the wash-out

The rectum is now cross-clamped with a right-angled clamp beyond the tumour. In the higher tumours 5–6 cm can be left above the levators by peeling up the mesorectal tissues at the back and removing them with the specimen. If the rectum is bulky or the preparation poor, a second and opposite clamp will prevent spillage. The distal end is now washed clean from below either with water or an antitumour solution.

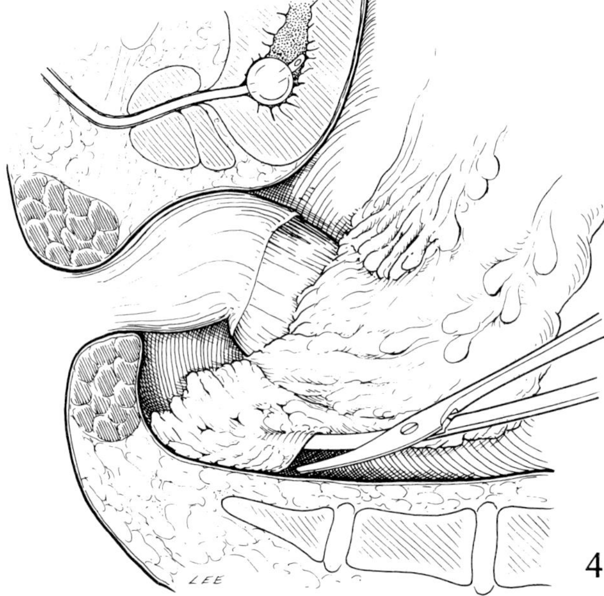

4

5

Distorting the anatomy for a low anastomosis

A St Mark's retractor is used to draw the vesicles or vagina forwards and downwards whilst the rectal wall is drawn up into the wound by the clamp. The anterior layer is incised distal to the clamp and a 0 Prolene stitch inserted 'over and over'.

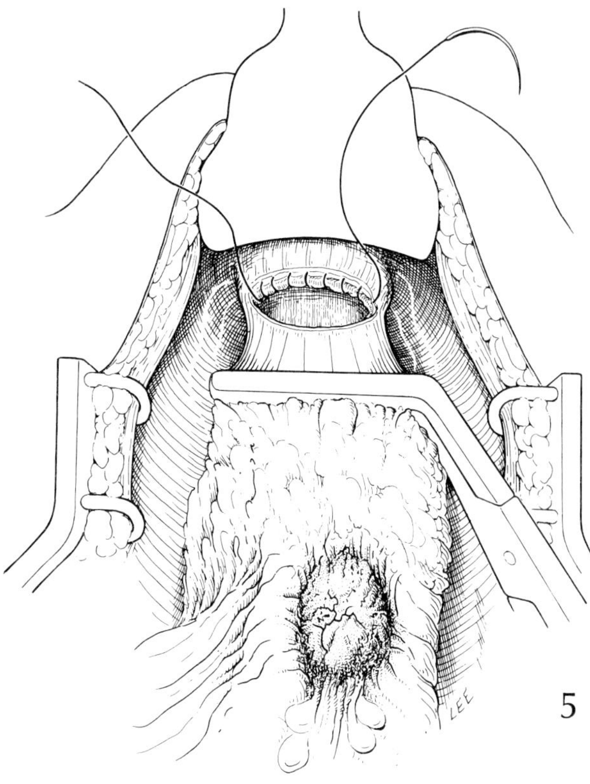

5

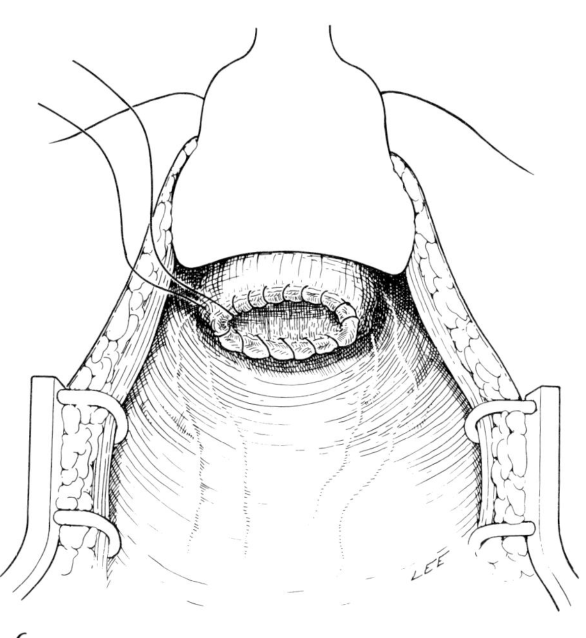

6

6

The lower purse-string

The stitch should incorporate only mucosa and the edge of the muscularis mucosae circumferentially, the latter being visible as a thin white line in the submucosa. A 5 mm gap between bites is appropriate. The posterior layer is now cut with scissors and the purse-string completed.

7

Inserting the gun

The anus is gently dilated to enable the open gun to be inserted. The distal purse-string is tightened and the thickness of the periphery of the bowel checked by feeling the cartridge through the muscle. If the purse-string has been correctly placed there should be no difficulty in feeling the edge around its whole circumference.

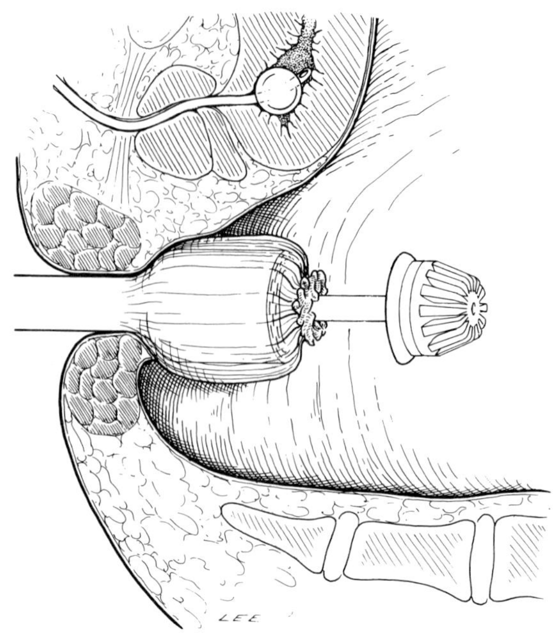

7

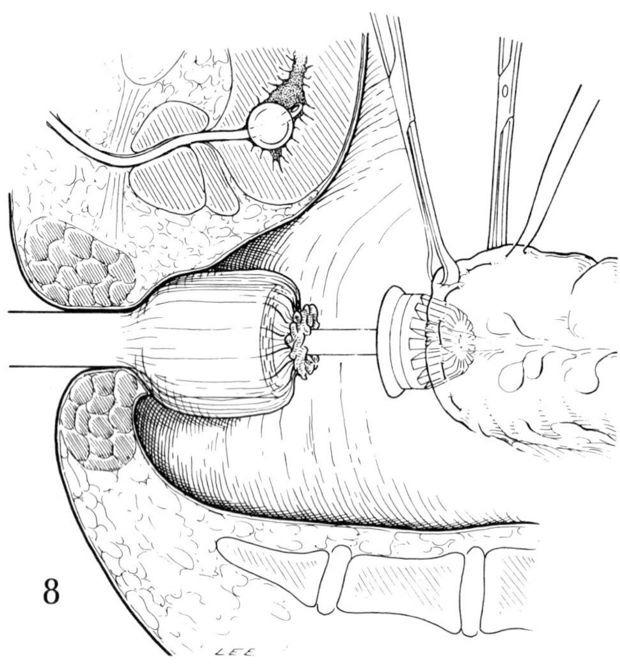

8

8

The proximal purse-string

The proximal end, possibly after gentle dilatation, is slipped over the anvil by two or three Babcock or Allis forceps. The purse-string must be slack at this stage and is tightened only when the whole circumference has passed the anvil.

9

Closing the gap

One operator protects the gap from catching pieces of fat or mesentery; the other winds the closing wheel rather slowly as the ends are squeezed together.

If the rectal end is rather bulky it may be necessary to have a slightly wider gap of around 2.5 mm or perhaps even 3.0 mm.

Firing

The handle is now firmly closed and a satisfactory 'crunch' will indicate proper function.

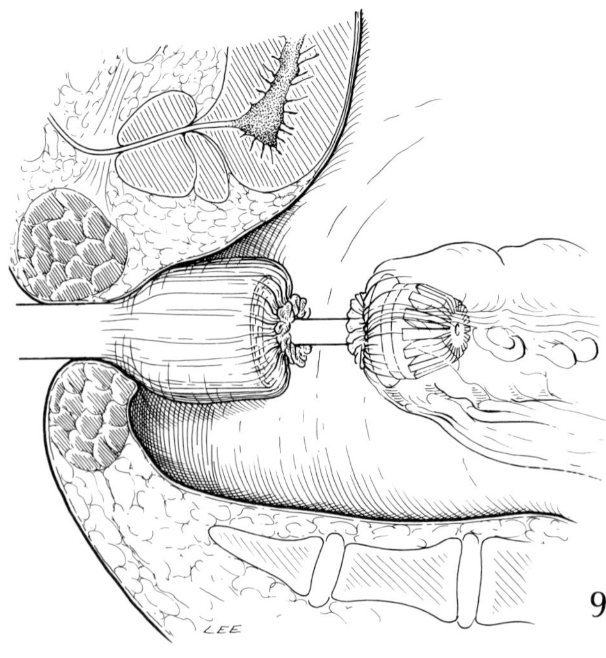

9

10

Withdrawal

It is important to withdraw the gun gently whilst the gap is opened and the whole weapon is rotated. Sometimes the mucosa may be caught slightly in the washer and this can thus be torn off without undue disruption of the anastomosis. A hand should support it through the abdomen.

11

Checking the anastomosis

There should be two complete rings of bowel end and two purse-strings. The latter should be cut to check that the actual bowel is a complete circle.

Coloured fluid such as Betadyne (iodine) solution can now be injected through the anus to check that the anastomosis is intact.

Drainage

After a wide pelvic clearance for cancer, the large space is likely to collect haematoma which may later drain through the anastomosis and lead to a late leak. An effective drainage system which will not block with clot is therefore essential: the Shirley sump drain is suitable or a wide soft silicone tube connected to a sterile bag.

Is a protecting transverse colostomy necessary?

Certainly this is the safest routine if there has been any defect or problem. It is also the safest course of action if the anastomosis lies within 6 cm of the anal verge where there may be an inherent risk of leakage. At this level urgency and even incontinence may occur in the early postoperative weeks, and it is often kinder to defer this period until the patient has recovered from the main operation.

Pitfalls

Failure of surgeon to prepare bowel ends

Cause Bulky rectal end; difficulty with purse-string low down; segments of bowel circumference missed; thick bites of muscle taken. These difficulties can lead to extrusion of part of the circumference when the gun is closed or to longitudinal splits in the rectal side of the anastomosis. The surgeon will detect the resulting defect because the lower doughnut will be incomplete or a leak will be apparent at the time of the wash-out.

Action If the anastomosis has only a localized defect it can usually be repaired with a suture and protected with a loop transverse colostomy plus a distal limb wash-out.

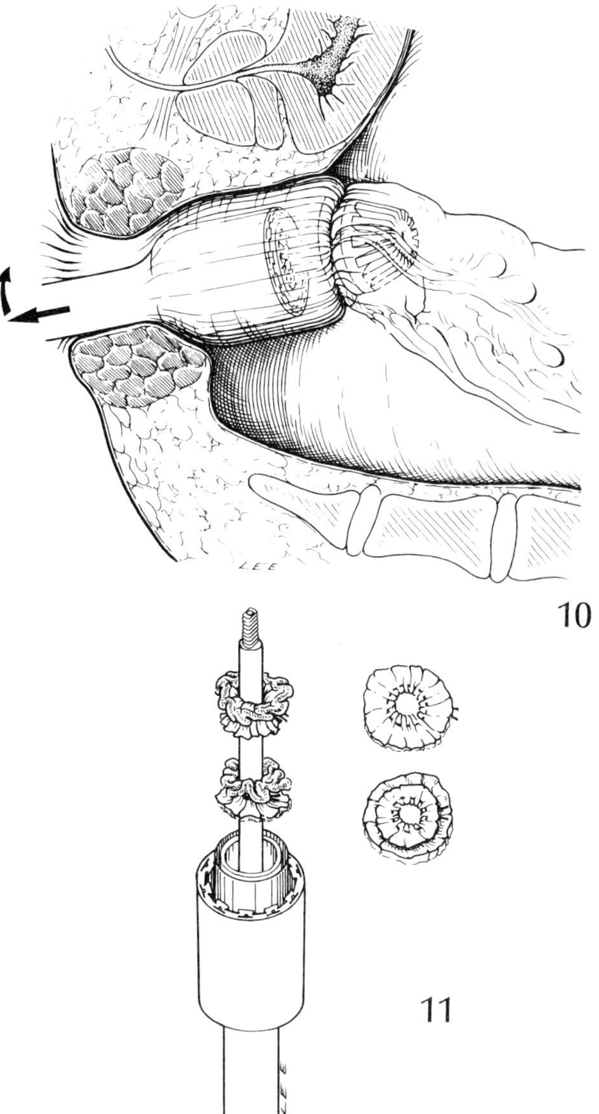

10

11

Failure of the gun

This may occur as a result of faulty loading (SPTU), worn washer or knife (SPTU), worn shaft (SPTU) or a faulty cartridge (EEA). The consequence will be that the gun cannot be withdrawn from the patient.

1. If the anastomosis appears satisfactory it may be possible to cut the 'doughnuts' free with a knife under direct vision. This will require full opening of the gun plus downward traction to intussuscept the anastomosis to an accessible point. With the SPTU it is possible to unscrew the handle completely, dismantle it and reassemble it without the staple cartridge but with the knife to create a pure 'cutting gun'.
2. If the anastomosis has also failed it is sensible to cut only the upper purse-string and to remove the anvil before withdrawing the gun. In this way the rectal purse-string and rectal stump are preserved for a 'second shot'. Before this is attempted all stray staples should be carefully picked out as they may obstruct closure.

ANASTOMOSIS AFTER OESOPHAGOGASTRECTOMY

12

If the stomach is to be used there is a choice of sites for the shaft to penetrate: the upper end of the lesser curve closure and the fundus. No actual purse-string is necessary provided a tiny hole is made for the shaft and the anvil is screwed on after it has been positioned. A pyloroplasty provides an ideal enterotomy for introduction of the instrument.

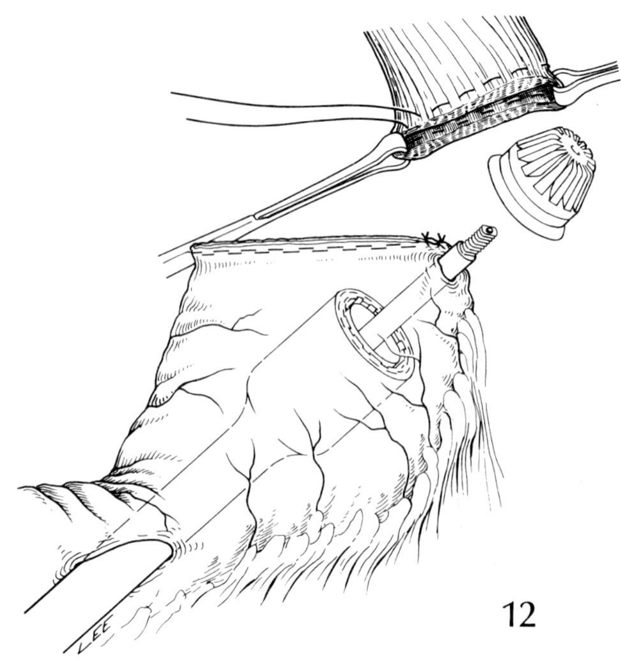

12

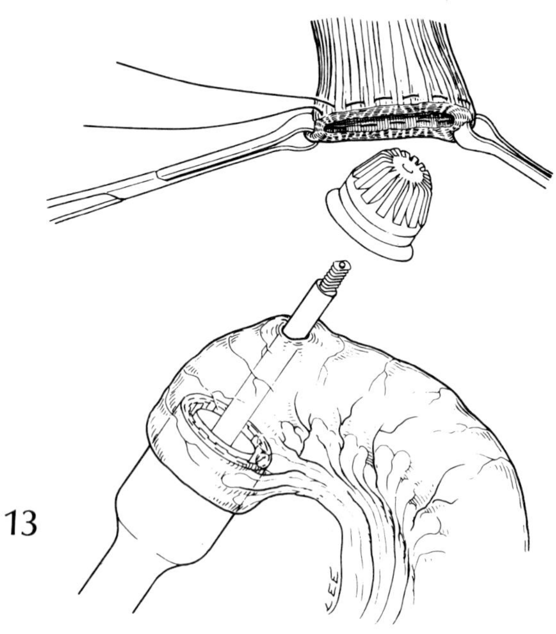

13

13 & 14

If the jejunum is to be used it is probably easier to introduce the instrument in a retrograde fashion through the end to a suitable point for oesophagojejunostomy end-to-side.

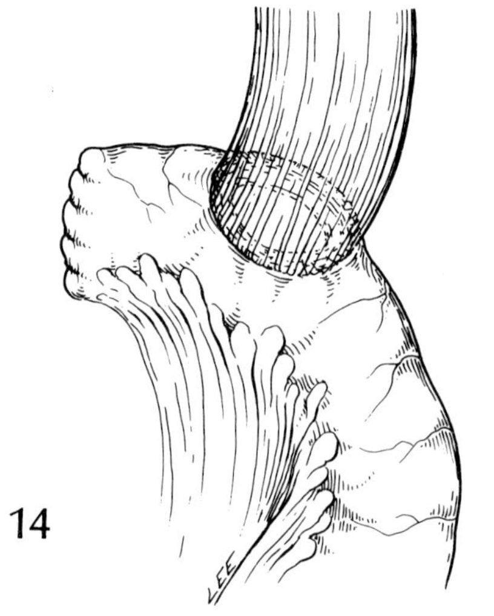

14

15 & 16

'Wrap around' and safety stitches

Whilst the gun is in position ready to be fired, 4–6 seromuscular sutures can be used to draw up stomach or jejunum as an antireflux and safety device. The gun can be drawn down and rotated to facilitate the insertion of the posterior stitches.

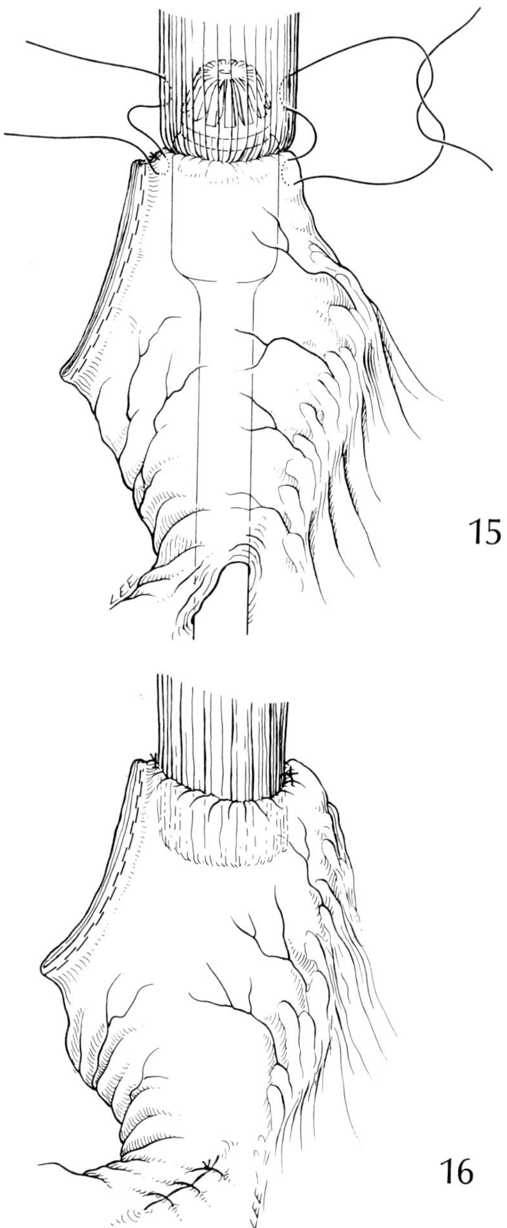

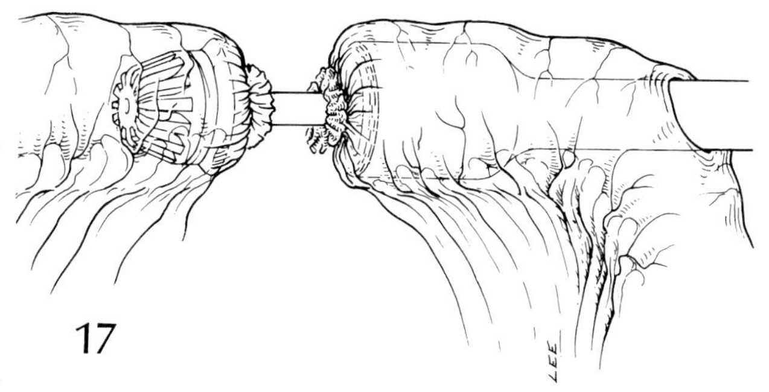

17

USE WITHIN THE ABDOMEN AT VARIOUS SITES

If there is no readily accessible orifice such as the anus or a pyloroplasty a small enterotomy must be made a few centimetres from the end to be stapled.

Staplers

Geoffrey Glazer MS, FRCS, FACS
Consultant Surgeon, St Mary's Hospital, London, W2, UK (**General**)

H. A. S. Dudley ChM, FRCS Ed, FRACS, FRCS
Professor of Surgery, St Mary's Hospital, London, W2, UK (**Linear stapling**)

General considerations in gastrointestinal tract stapling

The application of stapling devices in gastrointestinal surgery has reached a stage where most classical operations can be performed exclusively with these instruments. New techniques and applications are being regularly reported together with modifications in stapler design. The ease of application of linear staplers may lull the unwary into a false sense of security. There is a learning curve in their use and their relative simplicity does not mean that the surgical principles governing dissection, haemostasis, tissue viability and sepsis can be ignored. Consideration must also be given to the training of juniors and many would feel that the traditional techniques of hand suturing should not be lost to a new generation of surgeons. The costing arguments regarding hand-sewn versus stapled procedures are complex. But it would appear reasonable to expect reduction in the incidence of complications or a reduced period of patient hospitalization in order to offset the high cost of using several staplers in the course of an operation. However, evidence on complication rates would suggest little difference between hand-sewn and stapled procedures, and hospitalization periods are governed by so many factors that comparisons are difficult to make.

Instruments

TA

These instruments place a double row of everting (mucosa–mucosa) staggered staples 30, 55 or 90 mm long. There are two staple sizes, 3.5 mm and 4.8 mm. In addition the TA 30V (vascular) has a special cartridge for closely spaced fine staples useful in closing major blood vessels.

In both the disposable and non-disposable instrument a simple lever compresses the cartridge against the anvil and at the same time a tissue retention pin aligns the cartridge and anvil.

A recent technical development is an approximating lever which allows a half-ratchet closure of the staples, thus permitting more careful positioning of the bowel. This instrument has a longer shaft and has been designed for the 30, 55 and 90 mm staplers.

The roticulator is a new design for the 55 mm stapler and allows the ratchet head to both rotate and angulate. This stapler, which is supplied with the standard 3.5 mm or 4.8 mm staples, is useful where access in the abdomen is restricted.

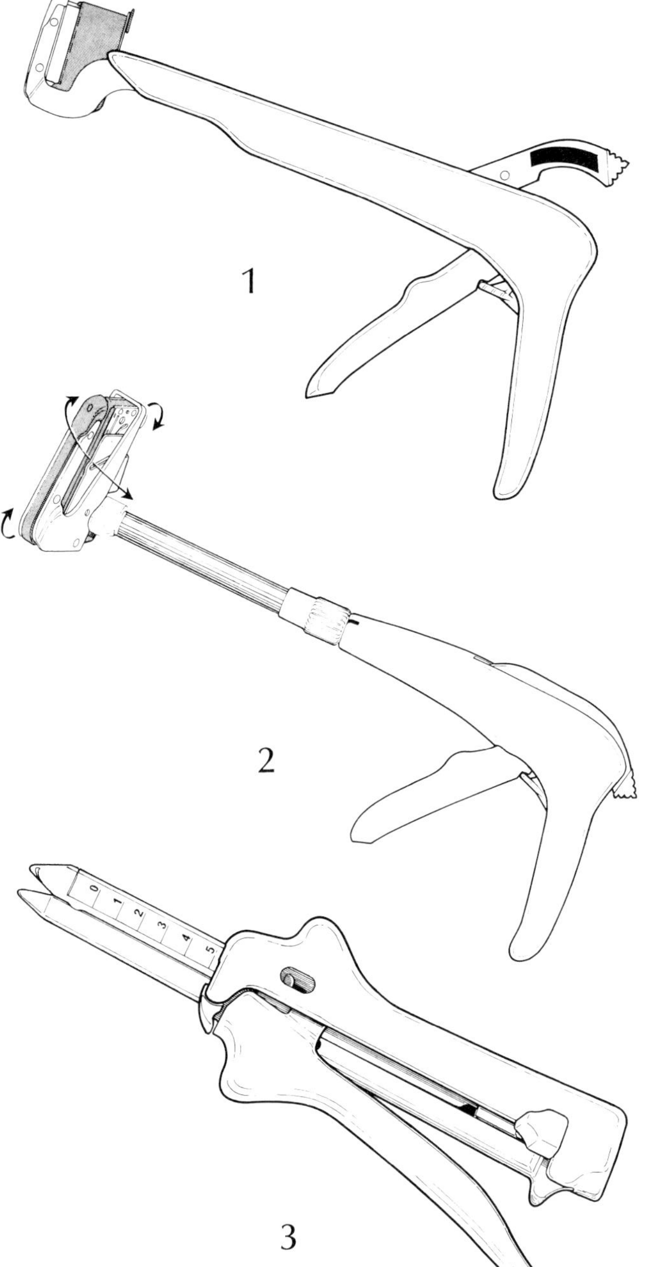

1

The TA30 linear stapler with approximating lever in the half ratchet position. The tissue retention pin is approximated but the staples are not fully closed which allows accurate tissue positioning.

2

A TA55 roticulator showing direction of movement of the head in two planes.

GIA

The GIA instrument places its staples in two double staggered rows; when applied a knife blade simultaneously divides the tissue between the two pairs of staggered rows of staples which are 3.85 mm in size. The jaws of the GIA are approximated at the same distance right to the tip of the instrument, which assures that all staples are closed to the same degree along the tissue line.

The SGIA is essentially the same instrument which places four staggered rows of staples simultaneously but without cutting between them.

3

The GIA instrument.

Practical problems with linear staplers

Mechanical

Mechanical failure is uncommon with disposable instruments.

Technical

Apart from tissue thickness mentioned below, failures can occur if a segment of bowel slips out through the jaws of the stapling instrument as it is compressed. The new half-ratchet position with the approximating lever will help in the correct placement of bowel; the position should always be checked before the stapler is fired and the bowel held in place by the use of stay-sutures or holding forceps.

Mucosal apposition and blood supply

Stapling of gut results in a mucosa-to-mucosa everted anastomosis. The staple line is safe because it is not ischaemic. The staples close in the shape of a B and the extent of the closure is dependant on tissue thickness. Blood may ooze through tissue enclosed by the stapler and on occasions vessels may bleed if they pass between the staplers. On some occasions bleeding can be quite heavy particularly when staplers are used in vascular organs such as the stomach or upper jejunum; oversewing of a GIA suture line is recommended in such situations. Control of bleeding vessels should be effected by fine sutures.

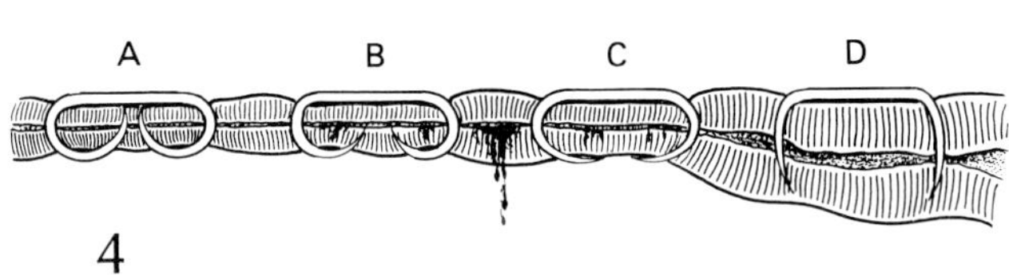

4

4

This shows the effect of tissue size on final staple configuration. Staple D will not hold as the tissue is too thick. Bleeding of the staple line is illustrated with oozing through and spurting between the staples.

Methods of controlling haemorrhage from a stapled tissue

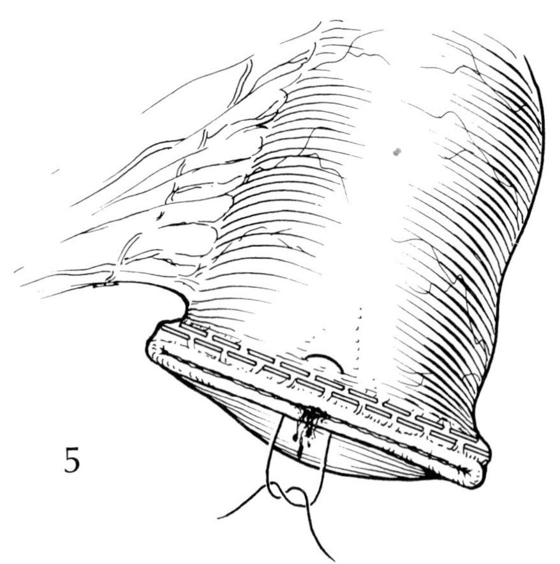

5

5

A spurting vessel is shown after linear stapling of small bowel. Control is effected by a fine mattress suture placed distal to the staple line.

6

A suture proximal to the staple line may be employed if there is insufficient tissue distal to the staples.

Multiple through and through sutures should be avoided in this position as this can cause ischaemia of the staple line.

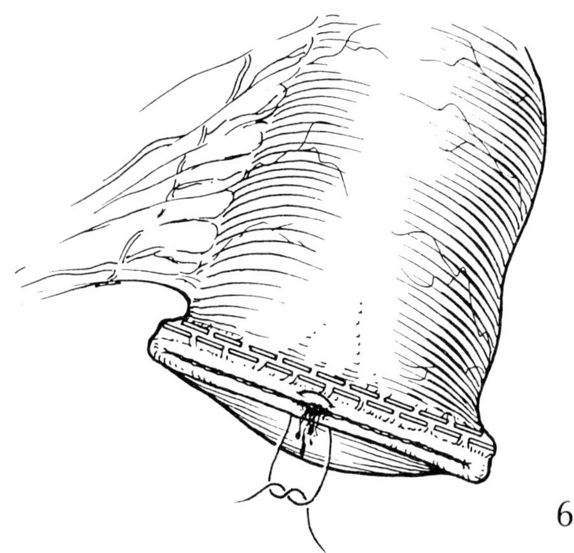

6

Tissue thickness

The 4.8 mm staples compress tissues to a thickness of 2.0 mm; 3.5 mm staples compress tissue to a thickness of 1.5 mm whilst the GIA stapler with disposable cartridge results in tissue compression to 1.75 mm. The TA instruments have an audible click when properly closed; absence of this indicates that the tissue is too thick and the instrument should not be used. The application of staplers to over-thick tissues may result in failure and breakdown of the staple line or serosal tears alongside the staples.

7

A serosal tear is shown after inappropriate closure of the duodenum; a 'repair' is effected by a running sero-muscular suture which buries both staple line and tear.

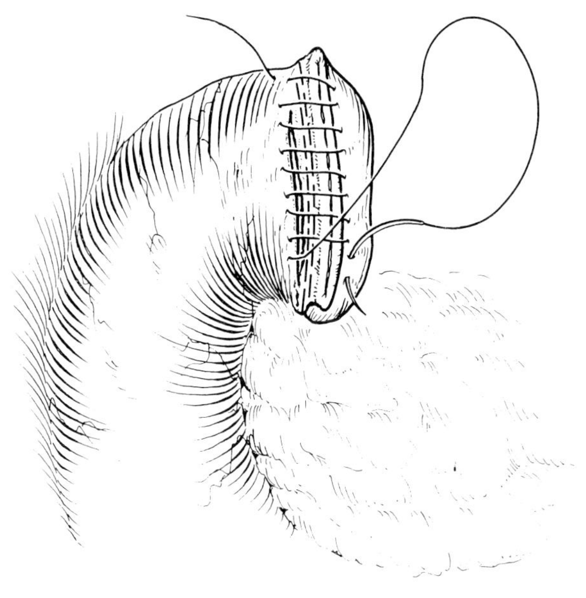

7

Applications of linear staplers

It is not proposed to illustrate here all the potential areas of use of linear staplers but rather to outline some of the situations where they may be applied. In some operations staplers are virtually mandatory (i.e. gastroplasty) whilst in others they may facilitate the procedure by allowing better control of bleeding in vascular organs (i.e. gastrotomy) or bowel leakage and sepsis (i.e. Meckel's diverticulectomy or right hemicolectomy in obstruction). Staplers may speed up the operating time, particularly when multiple bowel closures and anastomoses are required (i.e. total gastrectomy with Roux-en-Y oesophago-jejunal anastomosis). The TA roticulator can be used in certain situations where there is difficulty in obtaining access (i.e. low anterior resection prior to EEA circular stapling).

Gastroplasty

The operation of gastroplasty has been facilitated by the use of linear staplers. Various modifications of the technique have been described.

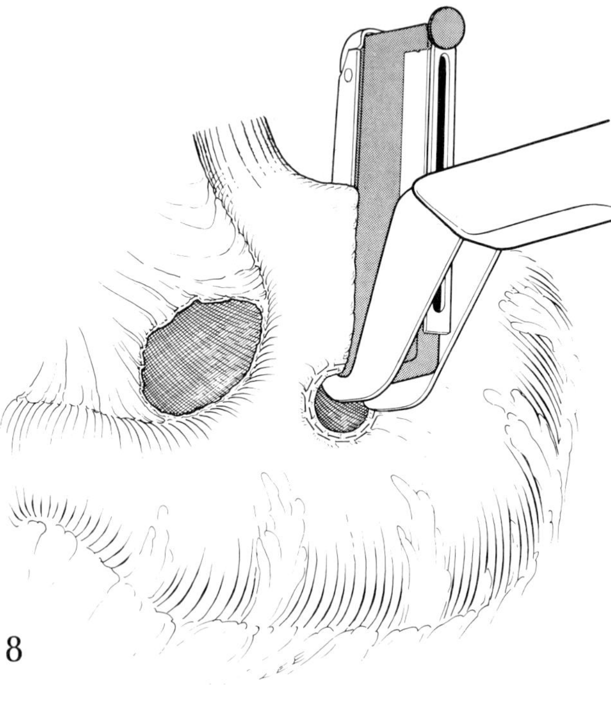

8

Vertical gastroplasty

8

The EEA inline stapling device has been used to create a circular anastomosis between the anterior and posterior walls of the stomach near the lesser curve approximately 5 cm below the oesophagogastric junction. A TA90 (4.8 mm) stapler is used to create a 5 cm long vertical stapled line. The procedure is repeated with a second application of the TA90.

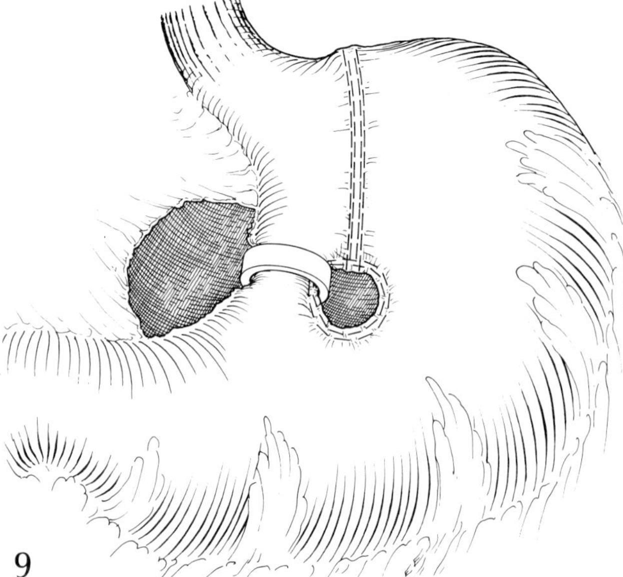

9

9

This illustration shows the final configuration of the gastroplasty showing the double row of staples and the construction of the stoma.

Meckels diverticulectomy

10

The diverticulectomy is performed with a TA instrument (30 or 55 mm) applied transversely across the base of the diverticulum. The final appearances are shown in the insert; there should be no narrowing of the bowel lumen.

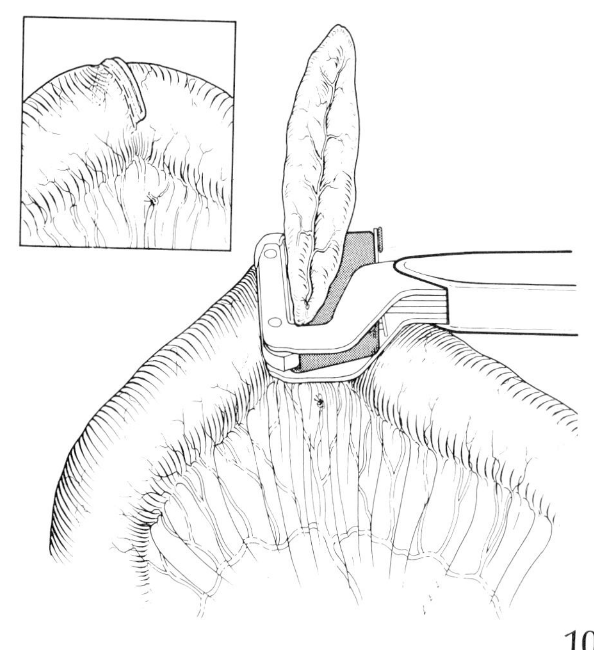

10

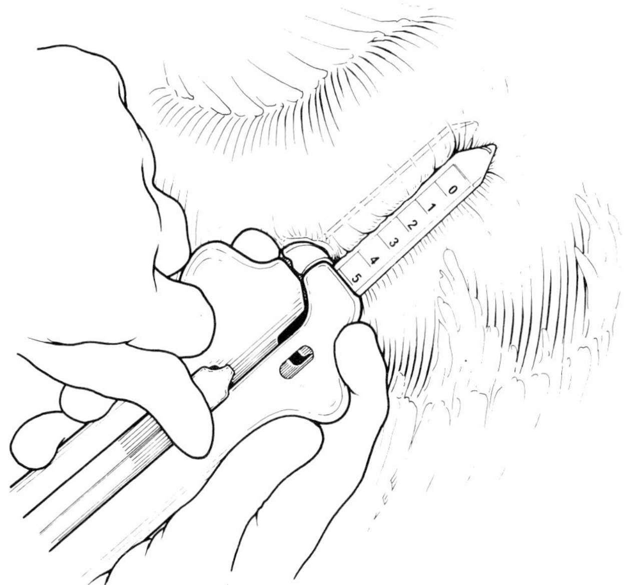

11

Gastrotomy

11

A small stab wound has been made in the anterior wall of the stomach with a scalpel or diathermy. One arm of the GIA is inserted into the gastric lumen in the direction desired and the outer arm applied to the serosal surface. The instrument is then fired as shown.

12

A 5 cm incision has been made in the anterior wall of the stomach lined by two rows of staggered staples. Haemorrhage from the edge is usually small and can be controlled if necessary by the application of small individual sutures. An extension of the gastrotomy can be achieved by another application of a GIA instrument in either direction along the long axis of the stomach.

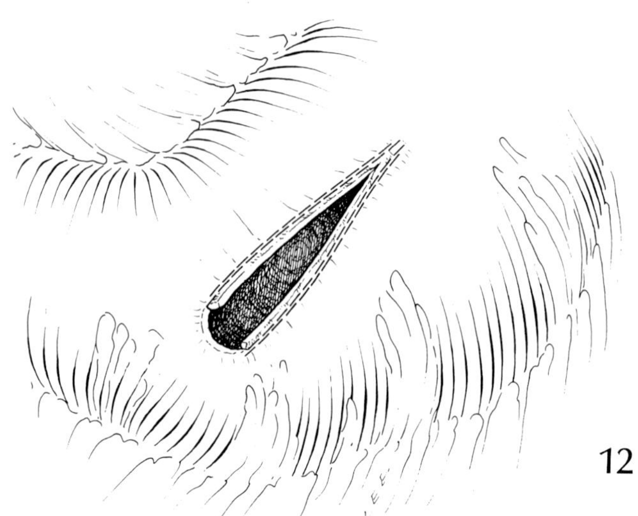

12

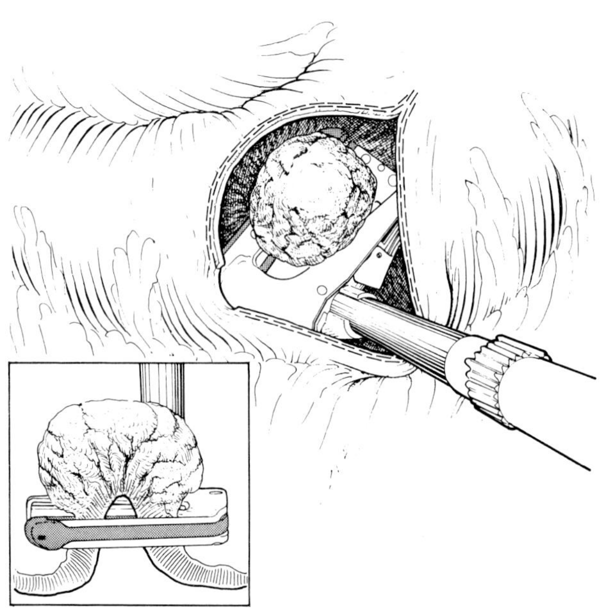

13

13

Excision of lesions of the stomach such as a leiomyoma can be achieved by a TA stapler placed across the base of the tumour. The roticulator is particularly useful in the situation illustrated with a posterior wall lesion. Complete clearance of the tumour must be obtained (inset).

14

The posterior wall of the stomach is left neatly closed. Oversewing is not generally necessary.

The anterior gastrotomy can be closed by a TA stapler. Stay sutures (or tissue holding forceps) should be used to maintain the alignment of the stomach in the stapler. The previous gastrotomy staples are then excised.

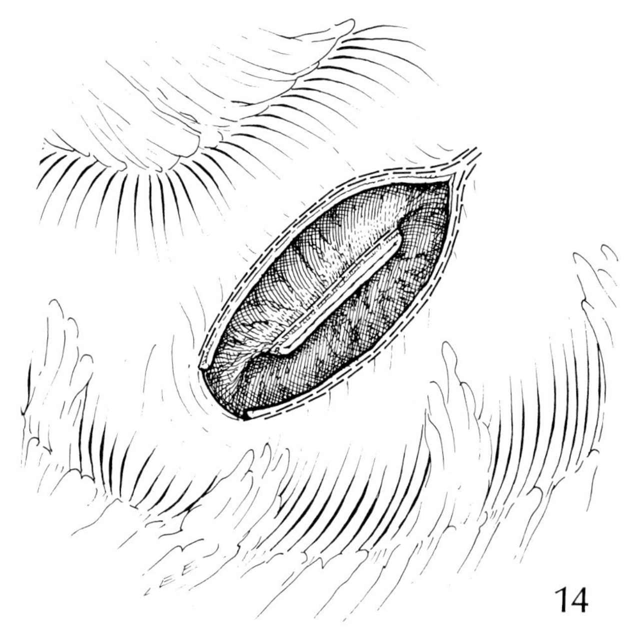

14

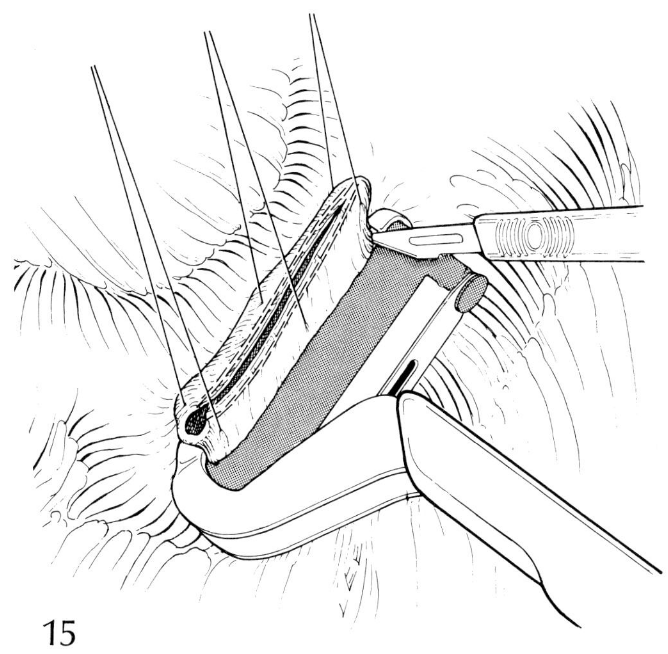

15

15

In the performance of a proximal gastrectomy for an oesophageal lesion a TA90 can be applied across the stomach for a rapid and haemostatic closure.

Bowel anastomosis

Several techniques have been evolved for the anastomosis of bowel using linear staplers. Some examples are illustrated.

16a & b

In the performance of a side-to-side anastomosis (here ileocolic) the ends of the bowel have been closed with a TA instrument (or GIA which would require oversewing) and the bowel resected. A GIA instrument is used to anastomose the bowel and entry holes for the instrument are constructed by excising the adjacent corners of the previous stapled bowel ends. The position of the two stay sutures is important; the distal suture is placed anteriorly 6 cm below the entry point (which will be just beyond the tip of the GIA instrument) and the proximal suture is placed posteriorly near the entry points of the GIA to assist by upward traction the introduction of the instrument.

The GIA has been inserted with one arm in each bowel lumen. Traction is maintained on the stay sutures. The instrument is then fired and withdrawn. The internal stoma is inspected through the entry holes for bleeding.

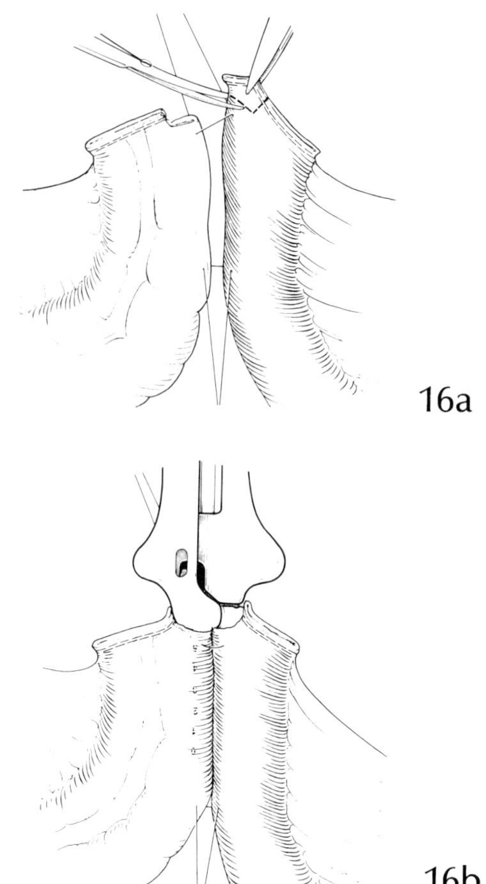

16a

16b

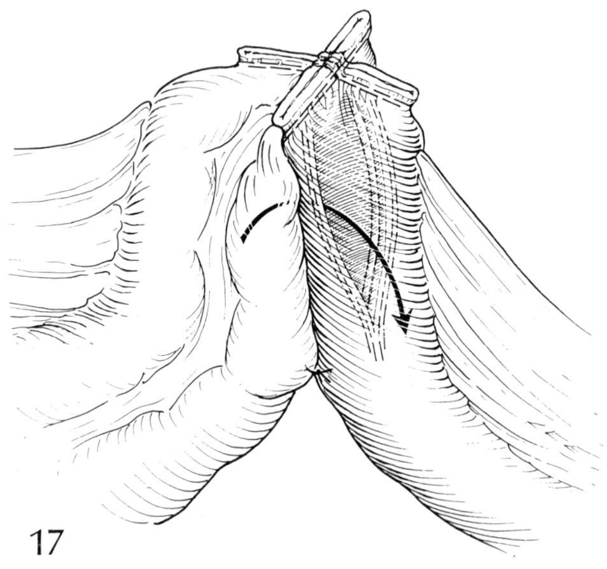

17

17

The entry holes are closed transversely using a TA stapler. This prevents narrowing of the stoma. Stapling across the previous stapling line is safe. Seromuscular buttress sutures are placed at the apex of the stoma to prevent distraction.

18

A method of performing a closed resection and small bowel anastomosis is illustrated. The bowel has been mobilized by division of the mesentery and distal occluding clamps placed. Entry holes have been made in the adjacent sides of the two small bowel loops. A stay suture has been inserted 6 cm distal to the entry holes to maintain apposition of the bowel.

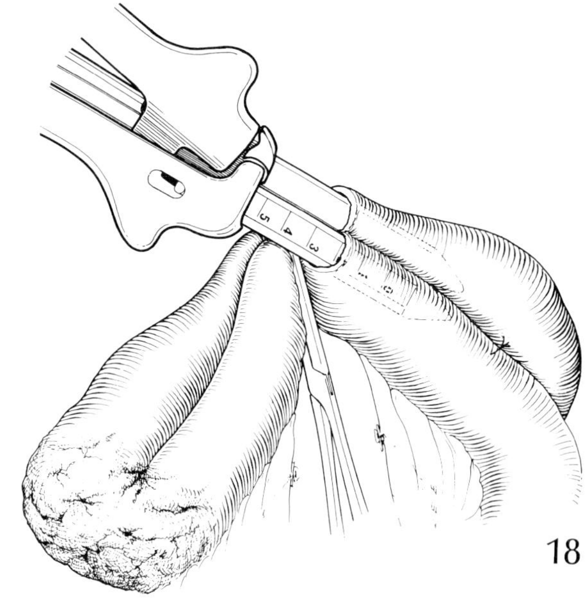

18

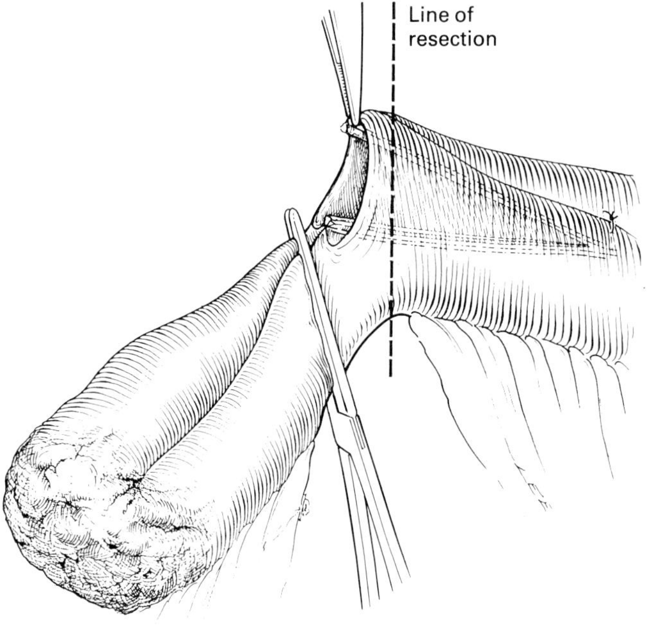

19a

19b

19a & b

The GIA has been fired and an internal stoma created. This can be inspected for bleeding through the entry holes. The line of resection is shown (*a*) and a transverse stapler is applied to complete the resection. The final side-to-side anastomosis is demonstrated (*b*).

Some applications of the TA55 roticulator

20

In the closure of the duodenum a standard TA stapler can be used but sometimes this is difficult to apply because of inadequate access. The roticulator facilitates the approach to the duodenum.

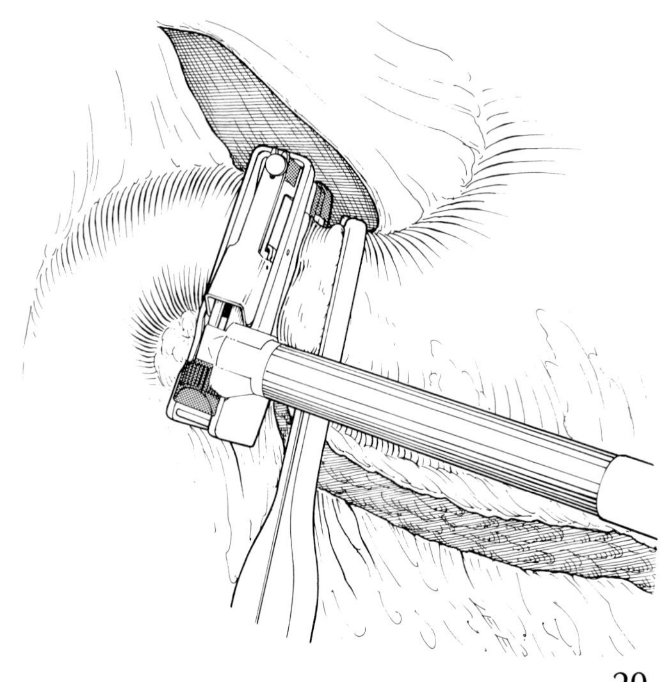

20

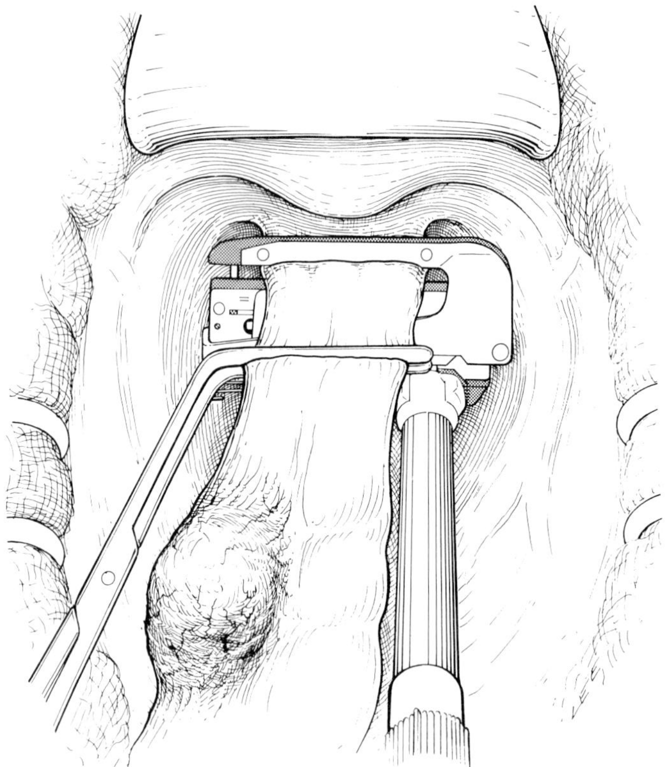

21

21

The application of a purse-string suture on the lower bowel edge can often be difficult to achieve with a circular stapler. However, the moveable head of the roticulator has proved particularly useful in gaining access where the pelvis is narrow. Thus a linear stapler can be used to close the bowel and the EEA is then introduced through the anus and fired across the linear staples.

End-to-end stapling

End-to-end stapling has its principal application at the two ends of the gastrointestinal tract: for oesophagogastric or oesophagojejunal anastomosis after resection of either stomach or oesophagus at the upper end; and for restorative resection of the rectum at the lower end. Contrary to popular opinion I do not think that in the latter situation it has extended the ability to make restoration at a lower level in the pelvis. It may have made it marginally easier but I must emphasise that stapling is as demanding as suturing and the chances of disaster just as great. The average and the best results of the two techniques are about the same and the choice between them is very much for the individual. There is now also a considerable choice of devices made by different commercial firms. It is an absolute essential of successful use of the instrument that the operator becomes thoroughly familiar with the mechanics of his chosen tool. For this reason only general principles are dealt with here.

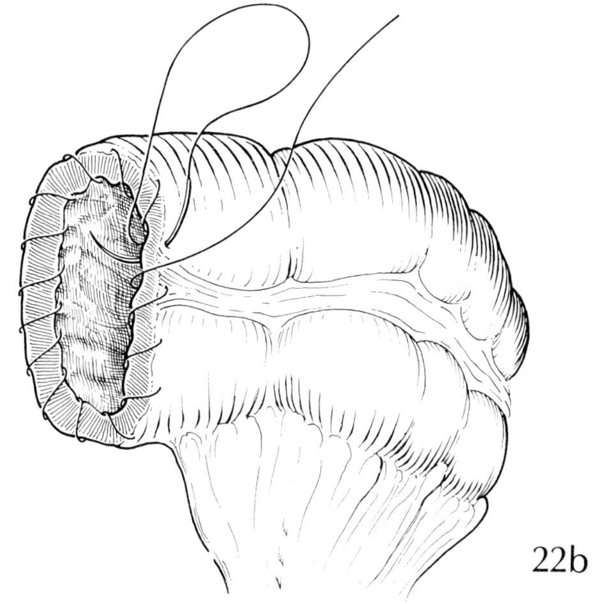

22b

Unmodified end-to-end anastomosis with linear stapler

22a–d

Purse string

Either an 'in and out' technique or an 'over and over' (whip stitch) may be used; I prefer the latter (*a and b*). In both it is important to take a small bite of the mucosa to avoid an untidy bunch of tissue after the suture has been tied (*c*). Similarly the suture must be accurately and evenly placed to avoid a gap (*d*) which can be squeezed even further open as the stapler comes together so creating a split in the staple line. The suture used for the purse string must run smoothly: 2/0 prolene is satisfactory and has the advantage of considerable strength so that there is little risk of breakage. At least four throws should be used.

There are commercial devices available for inserting the stitch using a straight needle but these are not recommended.

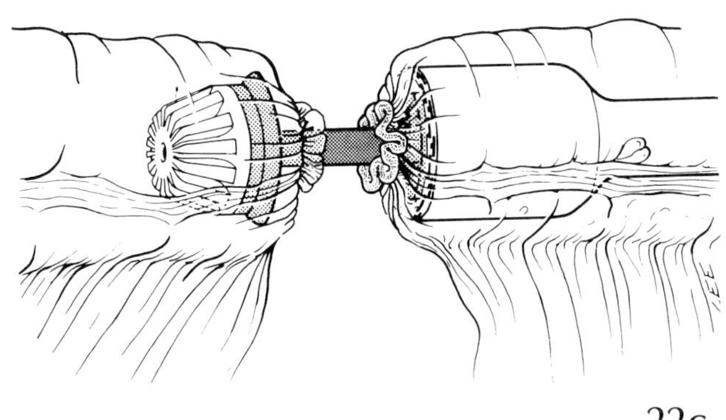

22c

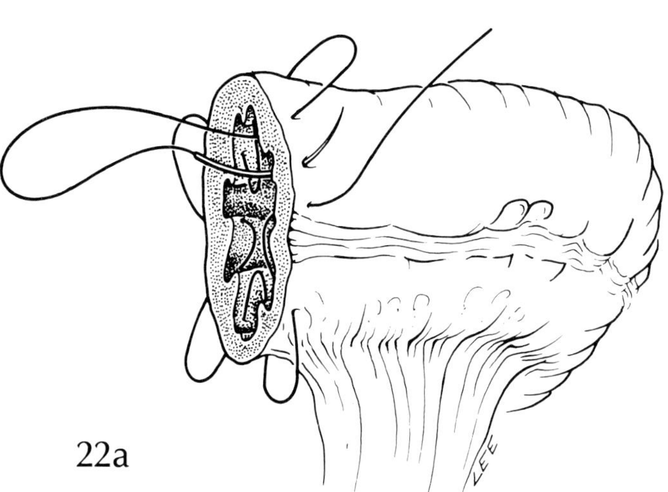

22a

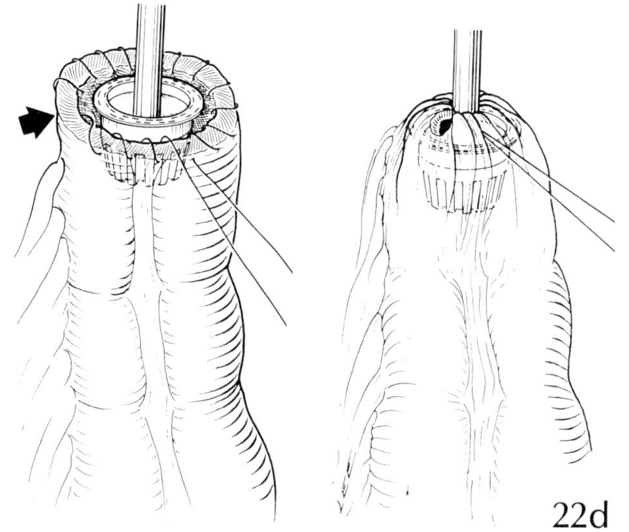

22d

Closing and discharging the stapler

23

Apposition is now achieved by screwing the stapler cartridge and anvil together. Judging the tension is quite difficult and there is no substitute for clinical experience of the sense of resistance met with as the stapler is tightened. More errors are made at this stage than at any other and it is very necessary to re-emphasise that the surgeon must fully understand his instrument. The stapler is now discharged.

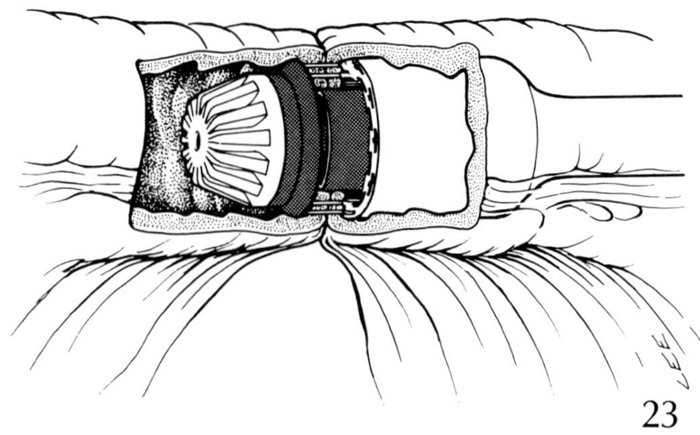

23

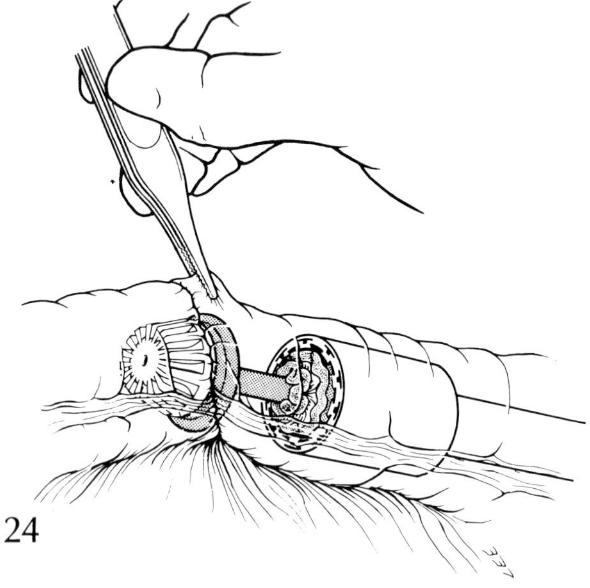

24

24

The anvil and cartridge are next separated by unscrewing the instrument for a convenient distance – usually 2–4 cm – which permits the whole instrument to be angled slightly with respect to the bowel lumen, so permitting easy disengagement.

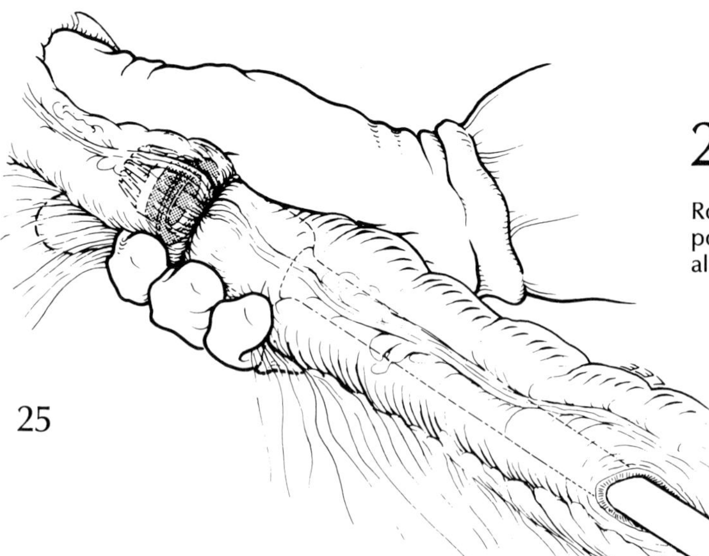

25

25

Rotation of the instrument on its long axis while, if possible, holding the anastomosis in the palm of the hand also helps to slide the head clear of the staple line.

Evaluation

26

The two cores are then removed from the stapler and carefully dissected, first with the purse string still *in situ*, and then after it has been cut in order to establish that they are anatomically complete.

Finally if the lumen is accessible, 50 ml of 1 per cent solution of methylene blue may be injected into it quickly via a nasogastric tube in the oesophagus or a Foley balloon catheter in the rectum. Alternatively, in the pelvis it is possible to fill the cavity with saline and inject 50–100 ml of air and inspect the staple line for bubbles.

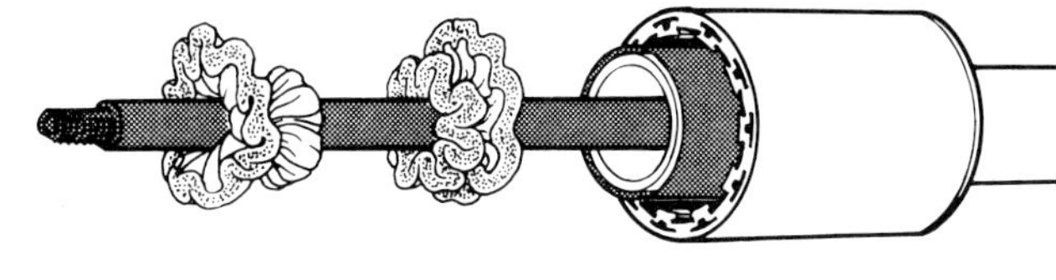

26

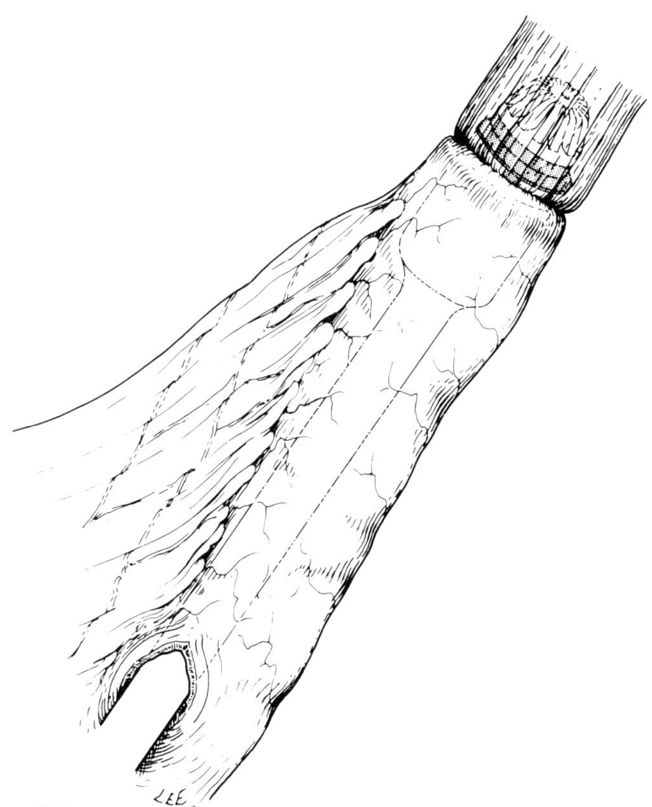

27

Special circumstances

Oesophagojejunostomy

27

Provided that the jejunal loop lies satisfactorily for end-to-end anastomosis the stapler may be inserted through the site for the subsequent jejunojejunostomy.

28, 29 & 30

In some instances the jejunal loop is bent over and then it is preferable to use end-to-side anastomosis. The technique is illustrated in 29, 30 and 31. The open proximal end of the jejunum through which the stapler has been passed can be closed either with sutures or the linear stapler (see above).

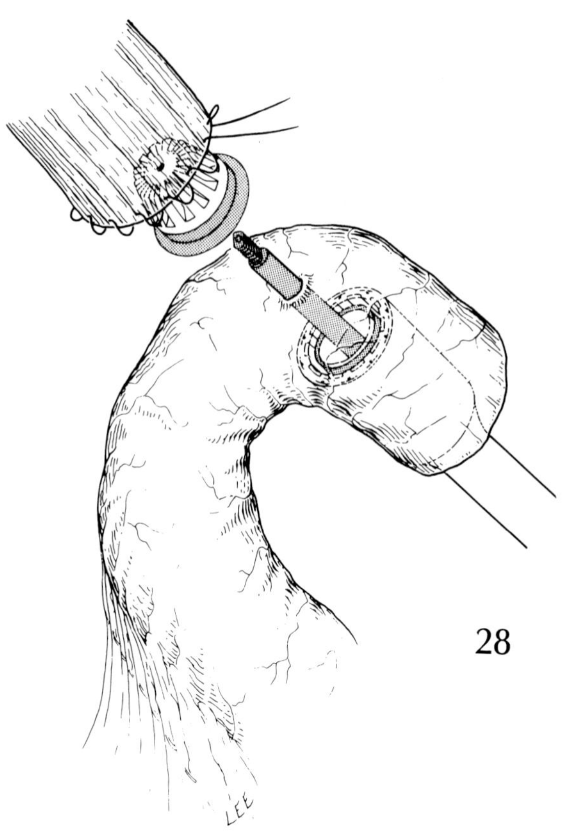

28

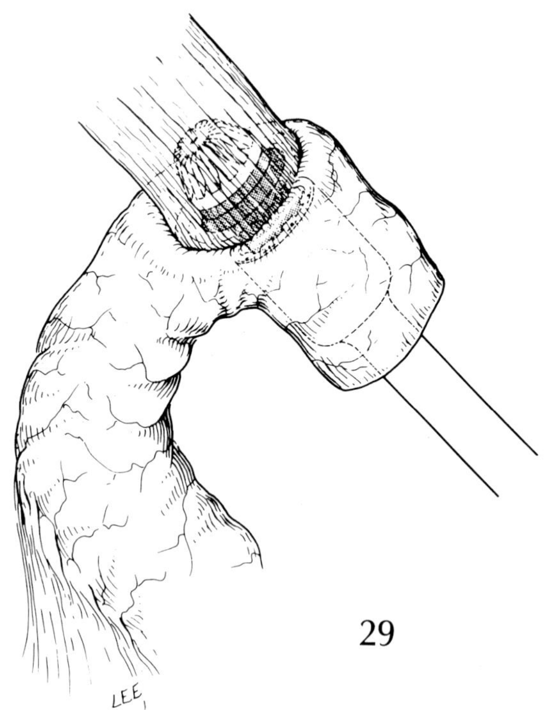

29

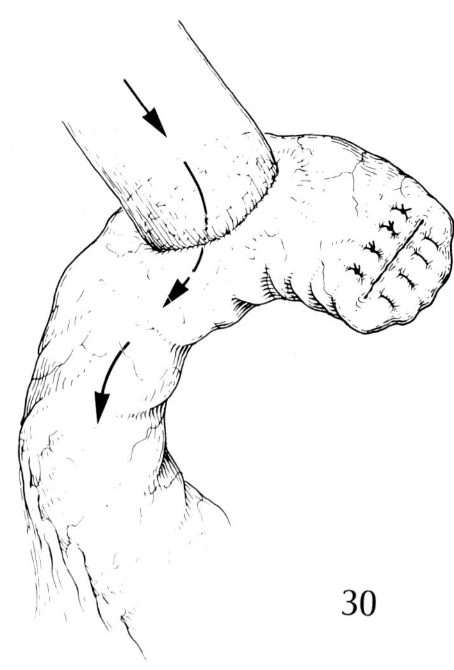

30

Reconnection after Hartmann's procedure

A similar technique is used.

31

The rectum is dissected just sufficiently to separate it from the vagina in the female or the prostate in the male.

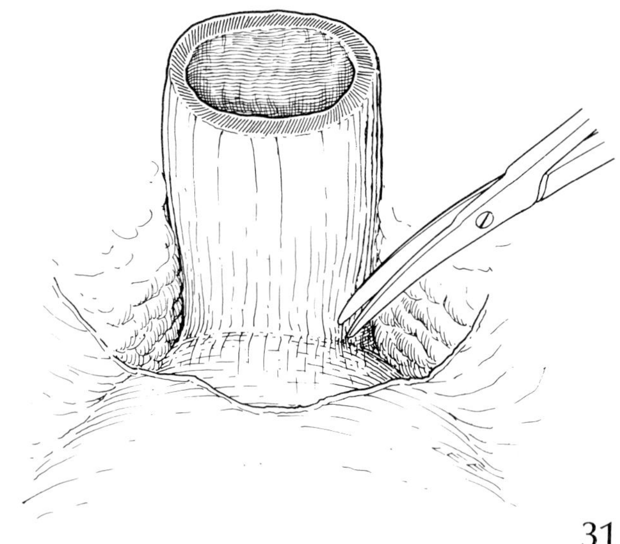

31

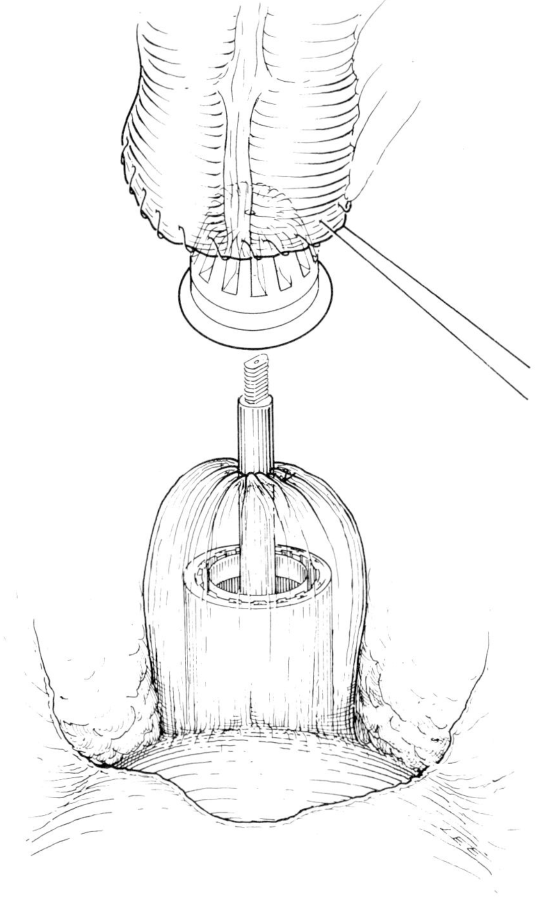

32

32

The spindle is then thrust through the apex of the rectal stump, a proximal purse string inserted and the stapler closed and discharged as for oesophagojejunal anastomosis.

Some surgeons will use a similar technique for primary left sided reconstruction after low resection in order to avoid the difficult placement of the distal purse string. The rectal stump is closed with a linear stapler and end-to-end reconstruction achieved by the technique described (see above).

Truncal and selective vagotomy, pyloroplasty and gastrojejunostomy

Christopher Wastell MS, FRCS
Consultant Surgeon, Westminster and St Stephens Hospitals, London and
Professor of Surgery, Westminster Medical School, London

Introduction

Truncal vagotomy

This procedure when combined with either pyloroplasty or gastrojejunostomy has achieved a considerable reputation because of its simplicity. It remains the most common operation employed in the United Kingdom for patients with an uncomplicated chronic duodenal ulcer. But it should be remembered that although the long-term metabolic effects are less, the symptomatic results are little better than those of partial gastrectomy[1], and this is an argument in favour of either selective or proximal gastric vagotomy where appropriate.

There are nevertheless indications for its use. These include for technical reasons: patients with cirrhosis in whom the left lobe of the liver is so rigid as to make adequate exposure and therefore safe dissection of the region of the hiatus impossible; previous splenectomy when either selective vagotomy or proximal gastric vagotomy (also known as highly selective vagotomy), both of which require division of the left gastric artery, may result in devascularization of the proximal stomach. Finally, there are occasions, such as when operating on a patient bleeding from the gastroduodenal artery, when speed is essential and therefore the simpler truncal vagotomy is preferable.

Selective vagotomy

Where gastric drainage has to be employed, for example with pyloric stenosis, stenosing ulcer of the second part of the duodenum, bleeding duodenal ulcer or following pylorotomy for inspection of the mucosa of the stomach and duodenum, selective vagotomy is to be preferred to the truncal operation. There is some evidence to suggest that the more detailed dissection involved results in a higher rate of complete vagotomy. In addition, *severe* episodic diarrhoea is rare after this procedure.

Pyloroplasy

Many varieties of pyloroplasty have been described, but the one in this section is based on that originally described by Finney[2]. It is theoretically an advantage to maintain the normal route for gastric chyme so that the intestinal endocrine organ is activated in the correct sequence and mixing with digestive enzymes occurs at the appropriate times. Iron deficient anaemia and bilious vomiting are not as frequent after pyloroplasty as they are after gastrojejunostomy. However, there are occasions when a pyloroplasty is not possible for technical reasons, usually because of a very severe duodenal ulcer producing considerable inflammatory distortion.

Gastrojejunostomy

This is always possible, even with the most severe duodenal ulcer and may certainly be employed in cases with pyloric stenosis in association with selective vagotomy. The disadvantage of gastrojejunostomy is the tendency for bilious vomiting to occur and iron deficient anaemia has been reported in nearly half the patients in the long term after operation.

1a, b & c

Anatomy

The anterior vagus gives off hepatic branches that supply the liver, gall bladder and first part of the duodenum as well as the anterior aspect of the stomach (*a*). In 20 per cent of patients, the anterior vagus is double (*b*), in which case each nerve provides an hepatic branch.

It is rare (less than 1 per cent) for the posterior vagus to be multiple (*c*). Occasionally, a branch is given off from its left side which passes downwards through or close to the left crus of the diaphragm and thence to the posterior aspect of the fundus of the stomach.

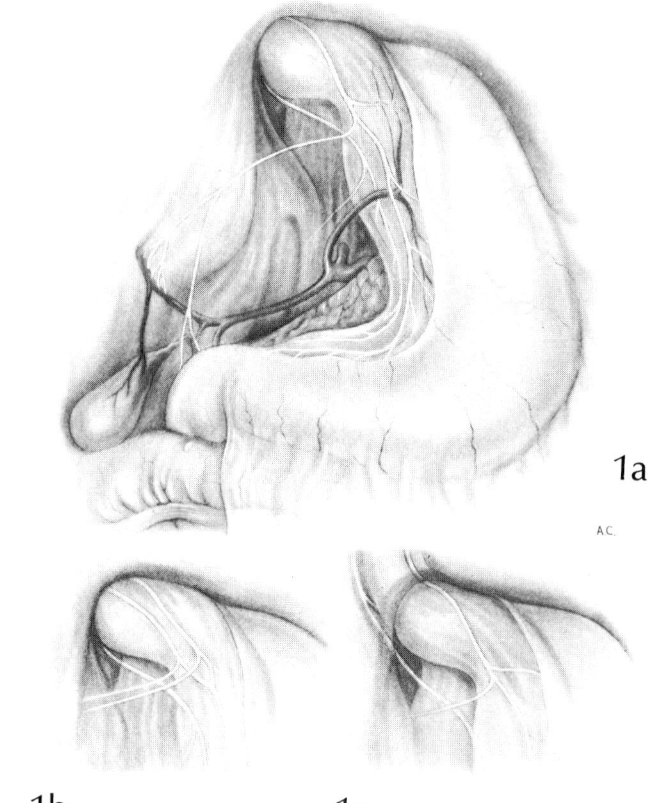

1a

1b 1c

2

Exposure

Nowhere is exposure more important than in the surgery of the hiatal region of the stomach. An upper right paramedian incision with an extension to the xiphisternum is recommended and has the advantage of allowing a two-layer closure. If greater exposure is required the tip of the xiphoid may be excised.

A large, four-bladed retractor is inserted and the superior blade pulled upwards by a rope attached to its handle. This rope passes over a horizontal bar placed between 30 and 45 cm above the patient's face so as to exert both an upward and an anterior lift on the retractor. In order to encourage the abdominal viscera to descend slightly and also to counter the upward pull of the retractor the operating table is tilted head-up by 5°–10°. If the upward pull of the retractor is too strong the venous return to the heart may be interfered with.

It is usually an advantage if the left triangular ligament of the liver is divided and the left lobe retracted to the right by folding it under and holding it in place beneath a pack with a Deever's retractor.

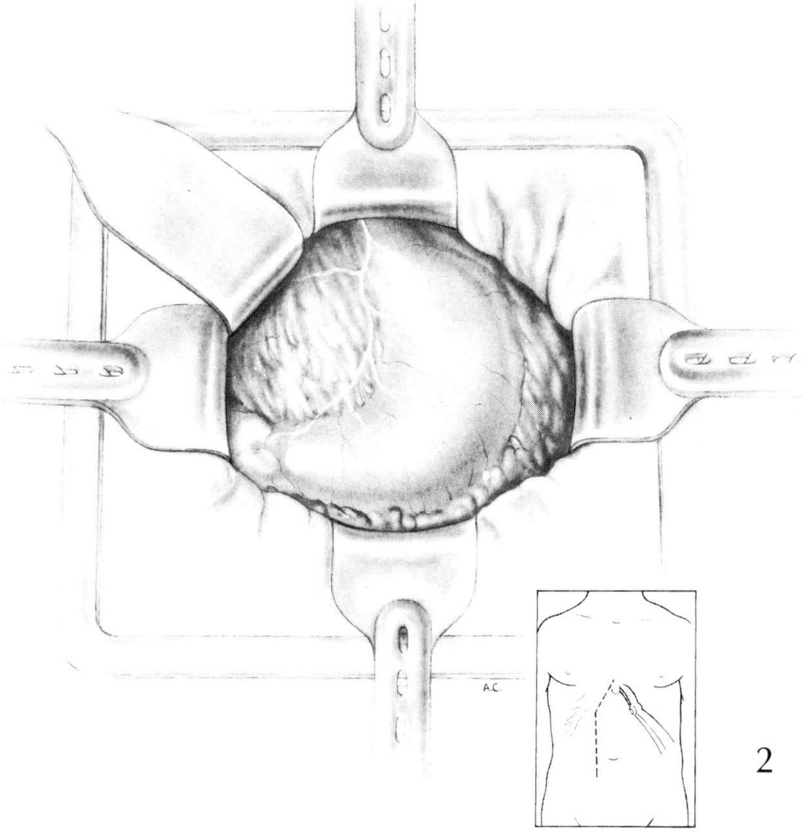

2

The operations

TRUNCAL VAGOTOMY

3

The peritoneum at the junction of the oesophagus with the stomach is incised and, after gentle blunt dissection with a small swab, the anterior vagus nerve can be seen.

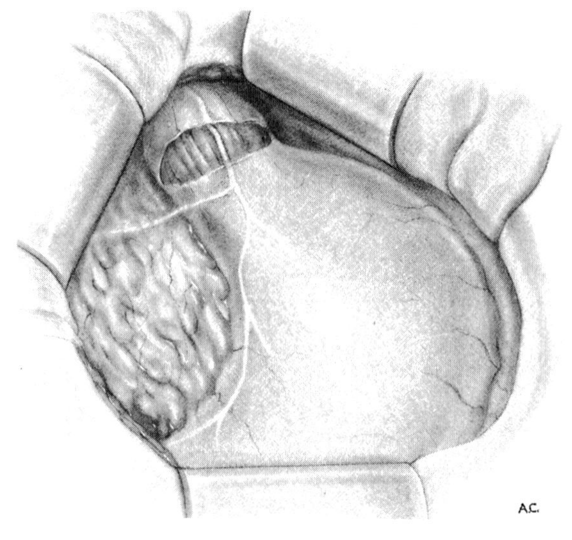

3

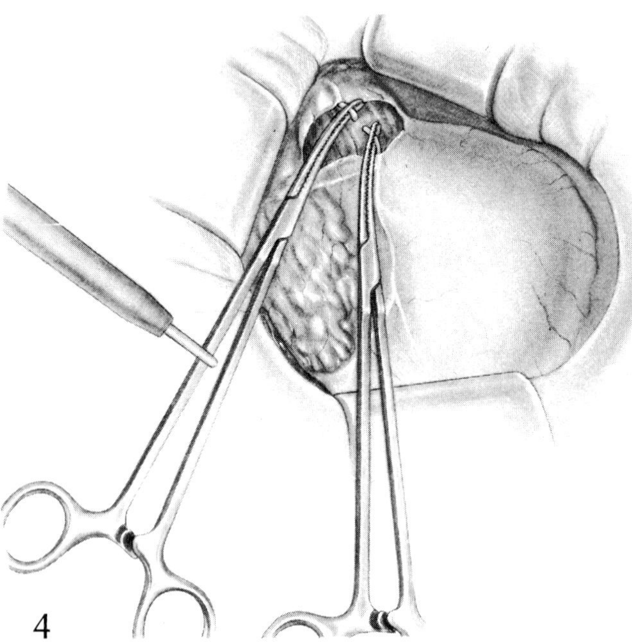

4

4

The anterior vagus is grasped by Lloyd-Davies' artery forceps and approximately 2 cm are excised. The ends of the nerves are then coagulated with the diathermy. This ensures complete destruction of about 5 cm of the nerve. The ends of the nerve may then be tied with thread in order to block the neural tubes and create small granulomas which will have the effect of obstructing regeneration.

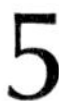

5

The oesophagus is then mobilized by gently passing the right forefinger around it. Care must be exercised not to tear the splenic capsule via its attachment to the left diaphragmatic crus. Some surgeons employ an oesophageal tube but this tends to form a rather rigid structure which can itself damage the oesophagus. It is possible for the oesophagus to be torn from the stomach but this is fortunately rare and occurs in patients with friable organs, for example obese women who have been on steroids.

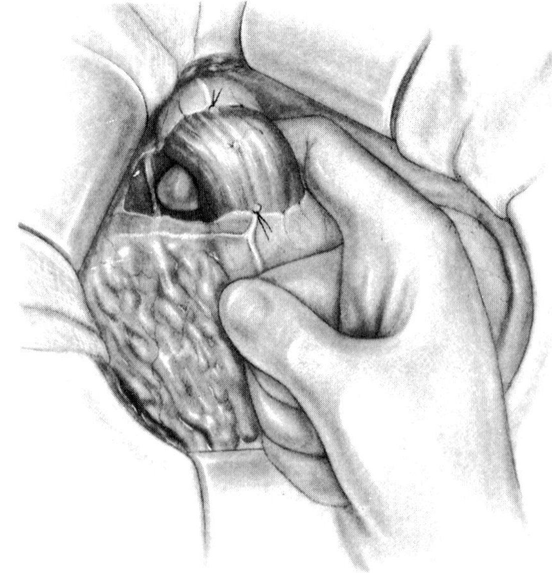

5

6

A rubber tube is passed around the back of the oesophagus; a curved clamp such as a bronchus clamp is ideal for this manoeuvre. The rubber tube can then be used gently to pull the oesophagus away from the underlying aorta. With the tip of the right index finger passed around the left hand side of the oesophagus, the posterior vagus can be palpated lying between the crura and a little to the right of the oesophagus at its junction with the stomach. It cannot be emphasized too strongly that it is a substantial structure and can be felt as a cord passing up into the posterior mediastinum. If a vagus nerve is missed at operation, invariably this is found to have been the posterior one.

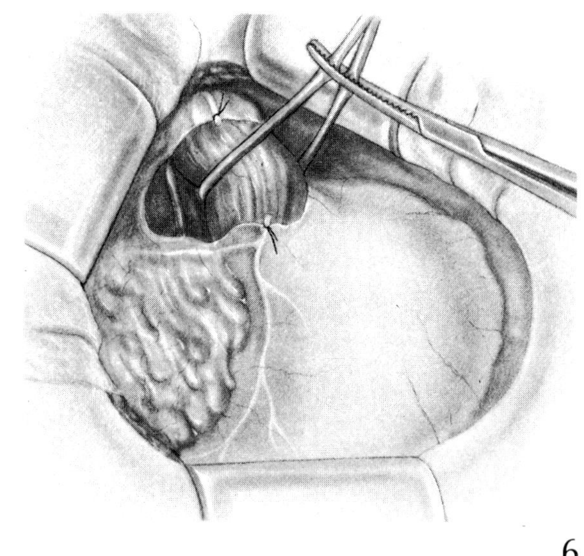

6

7

In the same way as with the anterior nerve the posterior vagus is grasped by two Lloyd-Davies' forceps and 2 cm or so are excised. The ends are diathermied and may then be tied with thread.

There is no need for the hiatus to be repaired; this is, in any case, impossible.

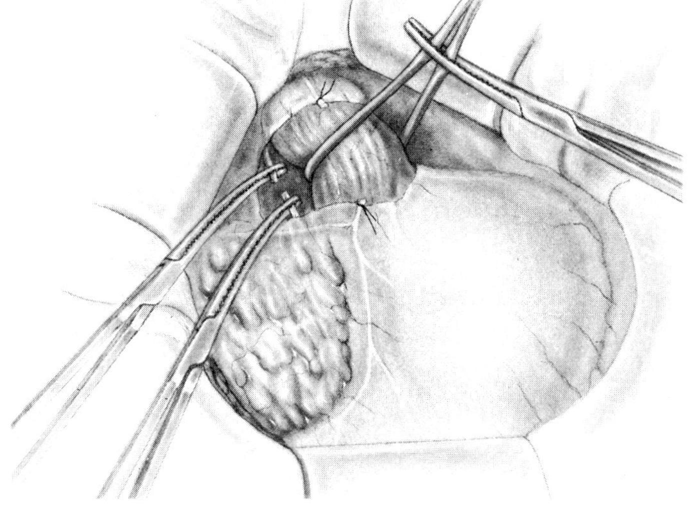

7

SELECTIVE VAGOTOMY

8

This variation of vagotomy was introduced because of the realization that there is no need, on anatomical grounds, to divide any more of the nerve supply to the abdominal viscera than that which passes to the stomach. Thus both afferent and efferent nerves to the abdominal viscera other than the stomach are preserved. The sites of division are shown.

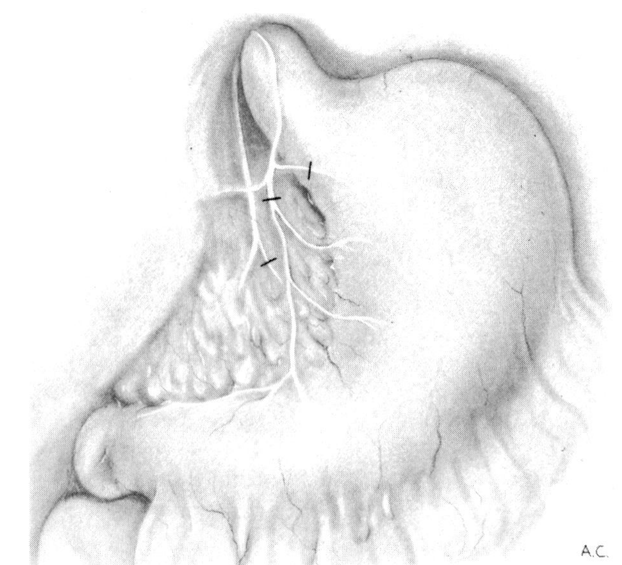

8

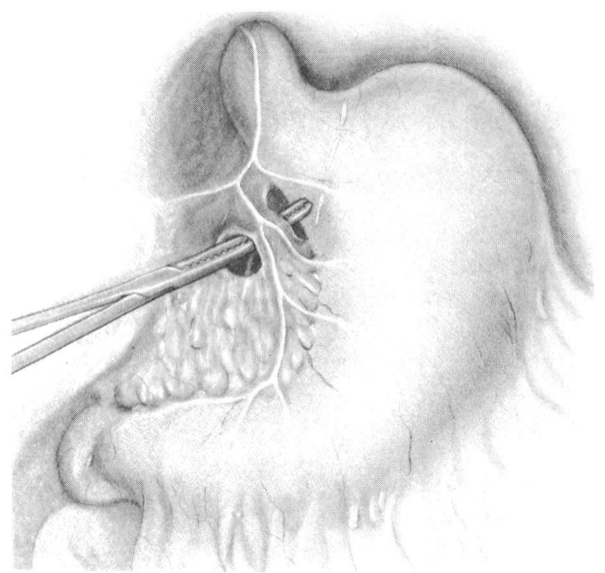

9

9

A hole is made in the lesser omentum and a curved haemostat is passed behind the descending branches of the left gastric artery and vein to emerge precisely at the lesser curve of the stomach. The illustration shows the nerves, which can certainly be seen in life, but in fact the dissection is directed at the vessels. The pedicles are ligated with 2/0 thread and in so doing the nerves are divided as well. The peritoneum is divided across the front of the stomach well below the oesophagogastric boundary (shown on the illustration as a series of white lines). It is helpful at this stage to divide the attachment of the spleen to the left crus and expose the left side of the oesophagus, taking care not to cause annoying bleeding from the left phrenic vessels as they course along the undersurface of the diaphragm. The peritoneal incision across the front of the stomach marks the line of the dissection and if carried out at this point prevents 'straying' into the region of the hepatic branches as they leave the main anterior nerve.

10

The ligation and division of vessels and nerves is now carried across the front of the stomach until the muscle fibres are exposed.

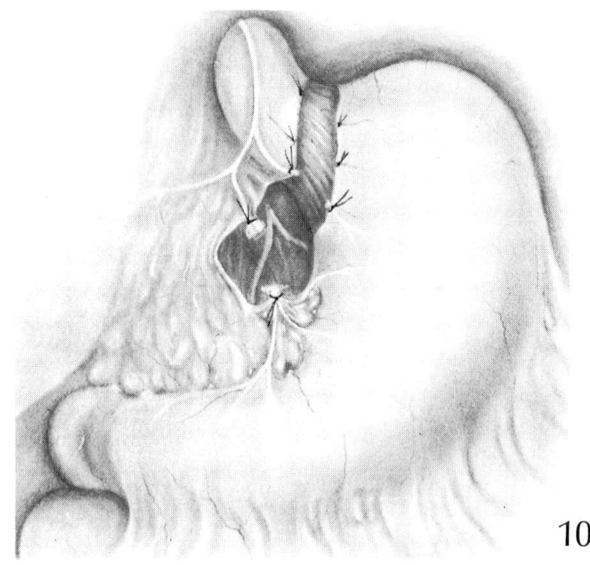

10

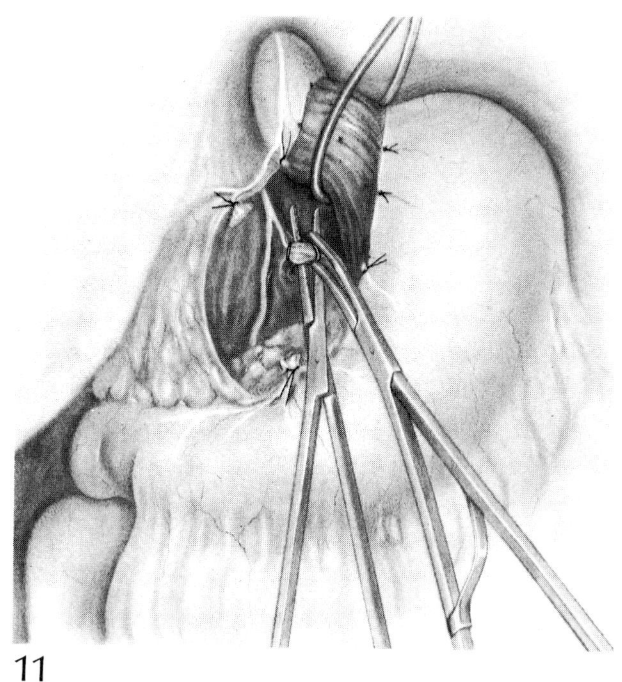

11

11

As with the truncal operation a rubber sling is passed around the oesophagus which is lifted forwards.

The dissection continues along the right side of the oesophagus with ligation and division of reasonably small neurovascular pedicles. Providing proximity to the oesophageal wall is maintained the gastric branch from the posterior nerve will be divided without damage to the main (and larger) posterior trunk which passes along the upper border of the left gastric artery to the coeliac plexus. It is often convenient to use clips to secure these pedicles.

12

The operation is completed by ensuring that no small fibres exist along the wall of the oesophagus which should be clear for at least 5 cm. It is possible to see the main posterior vagus lying between the crura of the diaphragm at this stage and if a small branch leaves its left side above the left crus, then this branch should be divided.

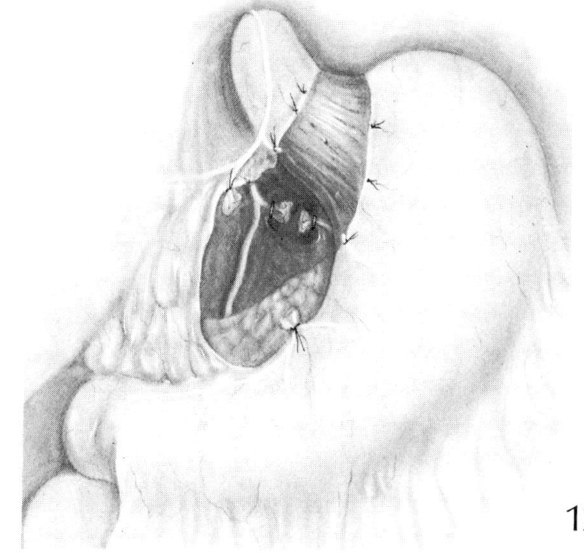

12

PYLOROPLASTY

13

Before this can be carried out properly, adequate mobilization of the first and second part of the duodenum is required. This is performed by dividing the peritoneum along the lateral side of the duodenum, taking care not to damage the common bile duct above or the hepatic flexure of the colon below. The duodenum is then swept towards the midline by means of a swab and mobilization is not complete until the inferior vena cava is exposed.

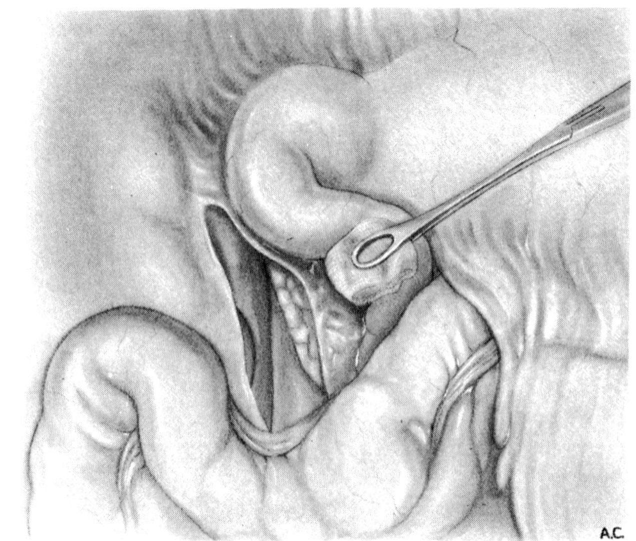

13

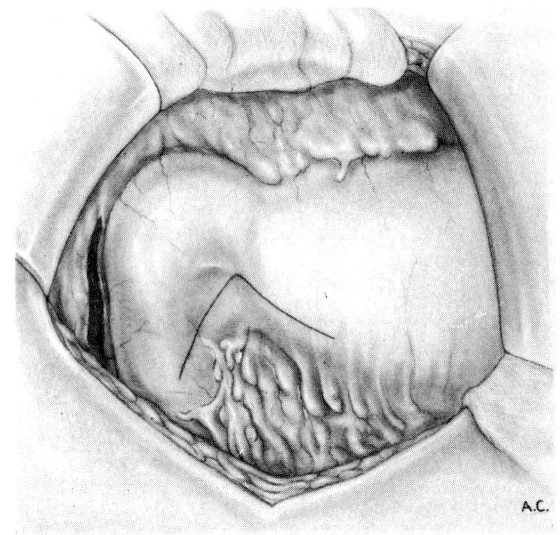

14

14

The gastroduodenal incision is an inverted 'V' with its apex centred on the pyloric ring; each limb is 5 cm long. It has been found to be advantageous to measure the length of each incision with a ruler and a pair of dividers because although it is easy to achieve the correct length on the antrum, there is a tendency to skimp on the duodenal side. The contents of both the stomach and the duodenum are sterile but the rest of the abdominal viscera should be packed off at this stage and suction used to control spillage. The incision may be made with a knife or diathermy current.

15

A pair of Babcock forceps is placed on the divided pyloric ring and two stay sutures of 2/0 chromic catgut are placed at each end of the incision. .

15

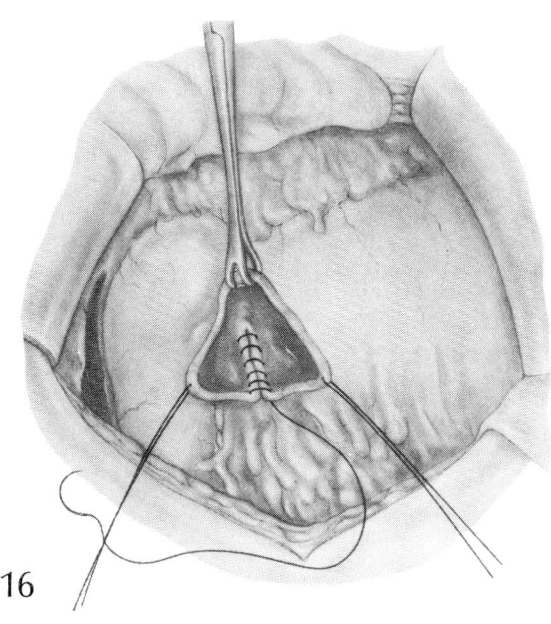

16

16

The pyloroplasty is then closed using a continuous suture of 2/0 chromic catgut starting at the inferior end of the pyloric ring.

17

As the posterior suture line progresses, providing both limbs of the incision are of the same length, the stay sutures come together at the inferior angle of the pyloroplasty.

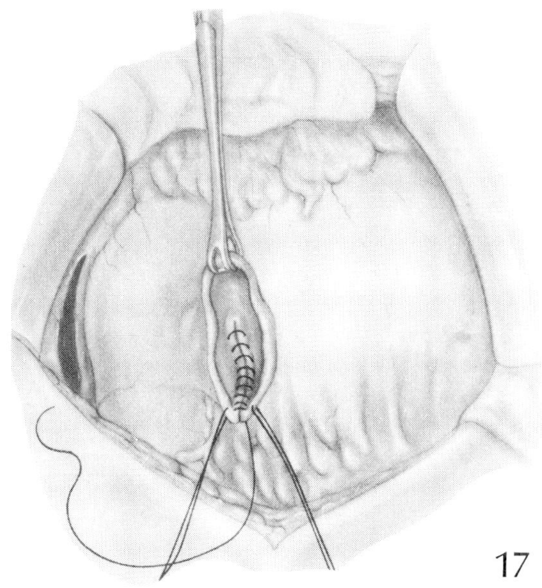

17

18

The single catgut suture is continued along the anterior aspect. A simple through-and-through suture has been found satisfactory, with inversion of the mucosa achieved by taking a larger 'bite' of the seromuscular layer and a smaller 'bite' of the mucosa. The two stay sutures are tied together on completion of the anterior suture line.

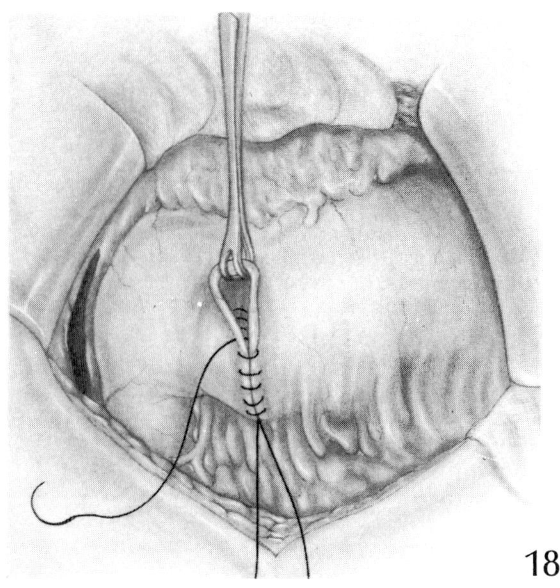

18

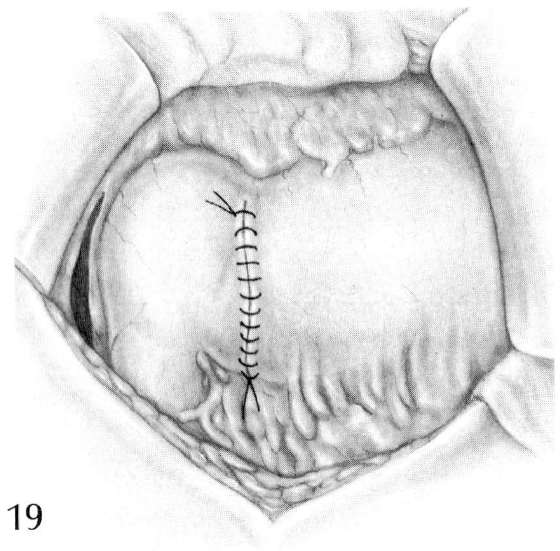

19

19

The completed single-layer closure. If there is anxiety about any part of the suture line, it can be reinforced by several interrupted 2/0 chromic catgut sutures. It is also possible to tack a piece of adjacent omentum over the suture line.

GASTROJEJUNOSTOMY

20

An anterior, juxtapyloric gastrojejunostomy is used. A 5 cm fold of anterior stomach wall is picked up by means of two Babcock forceps.

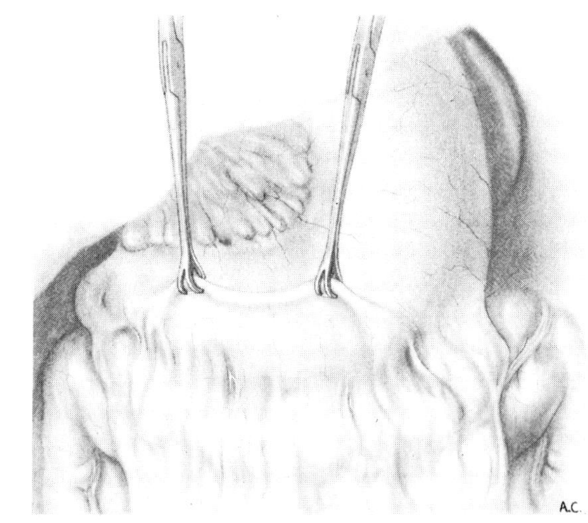

20

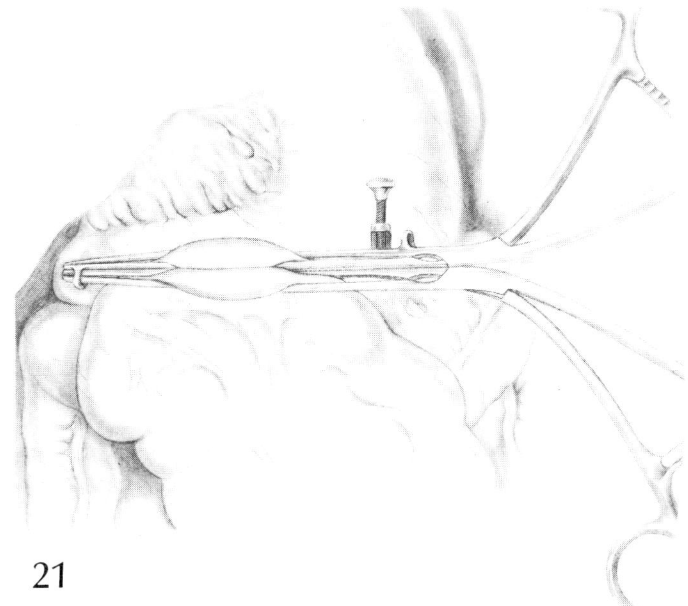

21

21

The first loop of jejunum is then brought over the front of the colon. The afferent loop is made as short as possible but sufficient length is allowed so that the colon will lie snugly beneath the jejunum when the anastomosis is completed.

A pair of Lane's gastrojejunostomy clamps is then applied taking care to pull an adequate fold of both stomach and jejunum through the blades of the clamp. The rest of the abdominal viscera are packed off and a sucker made ready before the bowel is opened.

22

The posterior seromuscular suture (Lembert) of 2/0 chromic catgut is inserted working from right to left. This is locked at the left-hand end of the anastomosis. Before there is any spillage of intestinal contents a red-coloured towel is placed around the Lane's clamp, the handles of which are tucked into a pocket made especially for them. This prevents the sutures from becoming entangled with the instruments and reminds the operators not to allow spillage of any potentially infected material. Both stomach and jejunum are then opened for about 4 cm, each incision being of exactly the same length.

A second 2/0 catgut suture is used for the all-coats stitch. This is started at the right-hand end of the anastomosis by a 'square' stitch.

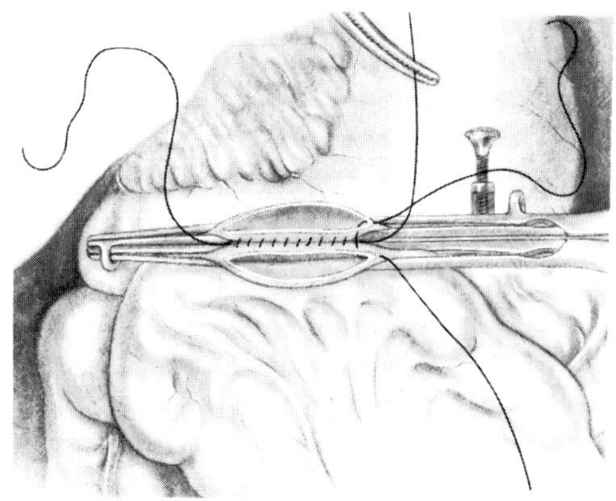

22

23

The end of the all-coats suture is grasped as a loop in order to distinguish it from the seromuscular one. It is then continued as a simple over-and-over stitch, care being taken to pass the needle through both seromuscular and mucosal layers as the mucosa can sometimes slip out of sight and be missed.

A 30 mm round-bodied, half-circle needle can be used but if preferred, a 60 mm round-bodied, half-circle needle can be held in the hand, thus obviating the need for a needle-holder and increasing slightly the speed of performance of the anastomosis.

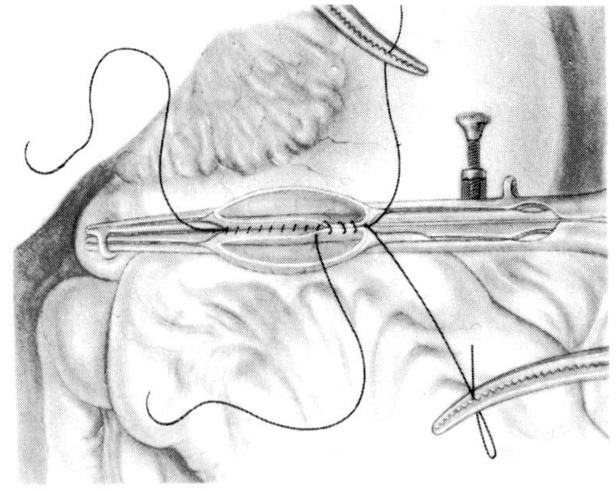

23

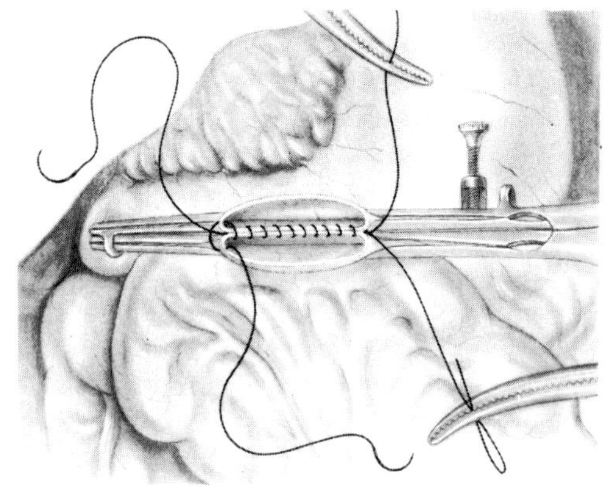

24

24

The left-hand corner is negotiated with the all-coats suture by means of one or two Connell stitches. More than this results in too great an inversion of tissue with compromise of the size of the stoma.

25

After the corner the anterior suture line is completed with a simple over-and-over technique. As with the pyloroplasty the mucosa is inverted by taking a larger 'bite' on the serosa and a smaller one on the mucosa.

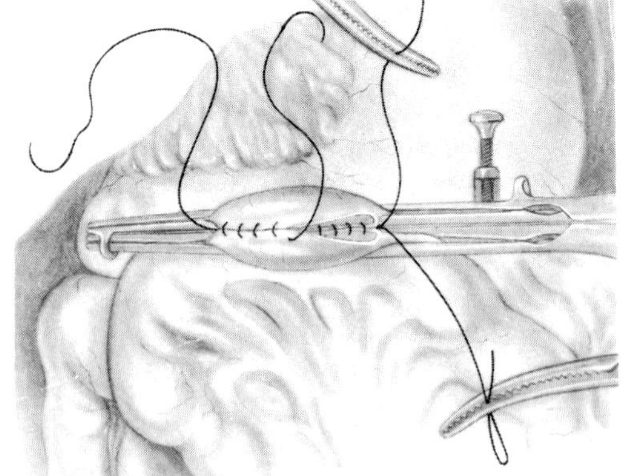

25

26

When the all-coats layer is complete, the suture is tied to its own end. The Lane's clamps are then released and the suture line carefully checked to see if any bleeding is occurring. One of the Lane's clamps is placed behind the anastomosis to hold it up for the completion of the seromuscular suture. This is then carried out without too great inversion of tissue and the suture is tied to its own end. Finally, the anastomosis is checked to make sure that there is at least a two- or three-finger stoma.

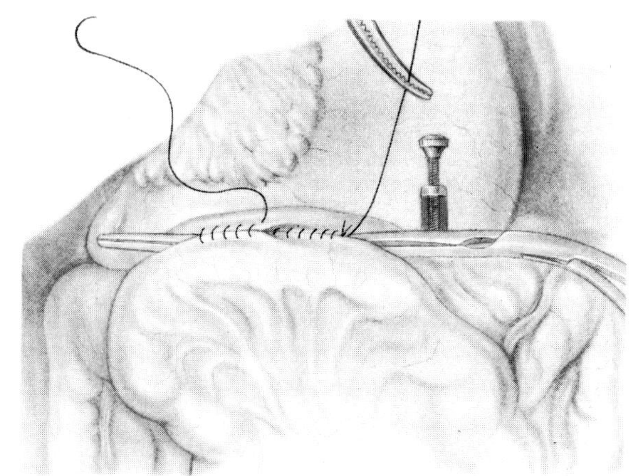

26

Postoperative care

Generally, this is similar for patients who have had either truncal or selective vagotomy with either pyloroplasty or gastrojejunostomy.

Maintenance of fluid and electrolyte balance

By intravenous means

Rigid intravenous regimens are to be avoided because it is self-evident that a large man operated on in warm weather will require more water and sodium than for example a small woman in cooler weather. All patients require more intravenous fluid in the first 24 h than subsequently. Sufficient fluid is given to ensure that the patient is not too thirsty and has a urinary output of at least 1000 ml in the first postoperative 24 h. The amount required ranges from 5 litres to as little as 3 litres with between 150 and 300 mmol of sodium. For the next 2 or 3 days, that is until flatus has been passed and the intravenous fluid can be withdrawn, the volume required is reduced to approximately the urinary output plus 1 litre of water, with 150 mmol of sodium per 24 h.

By oral means

The majority of patients do not require an indwelling gastric tube. In addition, the patient will be more comfortable if allowed sips of water to keep the mucous membrane of the mouth moist. If too much water is given, it will undoubtedly remain in the stomach and cause discomfort. If there is any evidence of a full stomach in the early postoperative phase, a nasogastric tube should be passed and, after all fluid has been withdrawn, left on open drainage. It is then removed when aspiration each 4 h does not produce significant aspirate.

As bowel sounds return, usually after 2–3 days, the oral water is increased stepwise from 50 to 100 ml/h; free fluids are allowed after the first passage of flatus.

From this point mixed fluids including tea and squashes according to the patient's preference are allowed and, if tolerated for 24 h, can be followed by a light diet. This point is usually reached on the fouth or fifth postoperative day.

The chest

As soon as the patient has recovered from the anaesthetic, he is nursed in a sitting-up position. Inhalations of steam with tincture benzoin Co., together with breathing exercises under the direction of a physiotherapist, will prevent mucus retention with pulmonary collapse.

The locomotor system

All patients are encouraged to stand, with help, and to sit out of bed on the first postoperative day. This helps to maintain balancing and righting reflexes which is particularly important in older patients.

The skin

It is of course standard nursing practice to make sure that the patient does not lie for too long in one position. This is particularly important in thin people, for example those patients who have had pyloric stenosis.

Reference

1. Goligher, J. C., Feather, D. B., Hall, R. *et al.* Several standard elective operations for duodenal ulcer. Annals of Surgery 1979; 189: 18–24

2. Finney, J. M. T. A new method of pyloroplasty. Bulletin of Johns Hopkins Hospital 1902; 13: 155–158

Parietal cell (highly selective) vagotomy for duodenal ulcer

E. Amdrup MD, PhD
Professor of Surgery, University of Aarhus;
Chief Surgeon, Surgical Gastroenterological Department L,
Kommunehospitalet, Aarhus, Denmark

Introduction

1

The vagal nerve trunks pass with the oesophagus through the hiatus to the abdomen. The purpose of vagotomy is to denervate the parietal cell area in the corpus of the stomach and thereby obtain a reduction in gastric acid secretion. The section can be performed at three levels: as a truncal (gastric and extragastric) vagotomy (TV), a selective gastric vagotomy (SGV) or a parietal cell vagotomy (PCV). The latter procedure leaves the antral innervation intact and the antral motility virtually unchanged. The main advantage of PCV is that it causes only minimal alterations in gastric emptying of fluids and solids. Thus, a drainage operation is unnecessary and no dumping or diarrhoea follows the operation[1]. The author uses PCV in elective surgery for non-obstructive duodenal ulcer and as an introduction to antireflux cardioplasty. He also uses it, together with suture closure, in cases of perforation in patients with chronic ulcer disease.

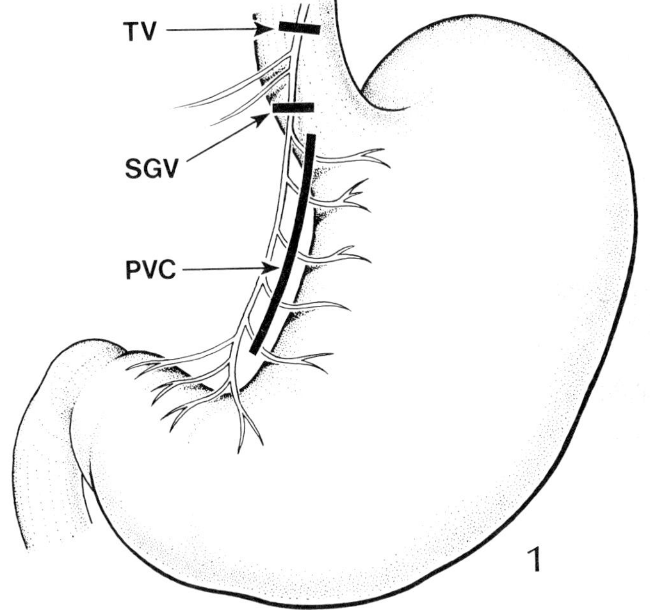

1

The operation

2

Position of patient

Elevation of the patient's upper trunk keeping the xiphoid as the highest point is recommended. This causes the organs to sink caudally and facilitates access to the hiatus region.

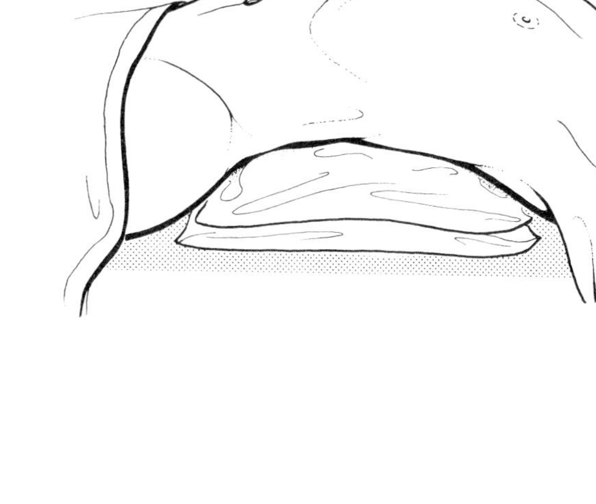

2

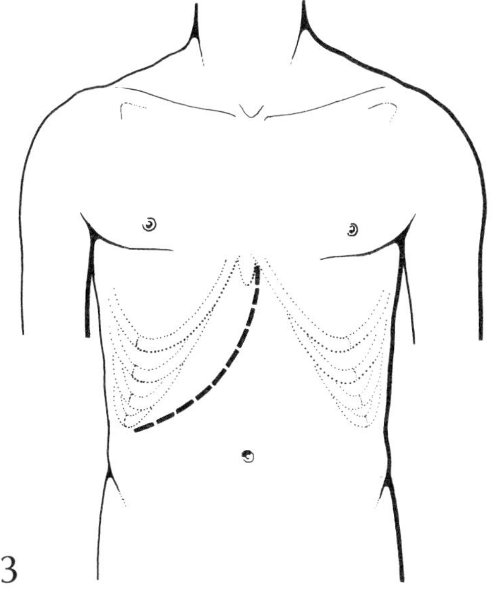

3

3

Incisions

It is possible to perform a PCV through a midline incision but the author strongly recommends a modified Kehr incision, i.e. a short paramedian incision beginning in the angle between the left costal margin and the xiphoid and continued into a right subcostal incision. The xiphoid may be excised if it is large. A rib-lifting retractor (Rochard, Aesculap 1973, 708–711) is extremely helpful and facilitates satisfactory acces even in fat patients. The liver is lifted with a strong retractor, mobilization being unnecessary.

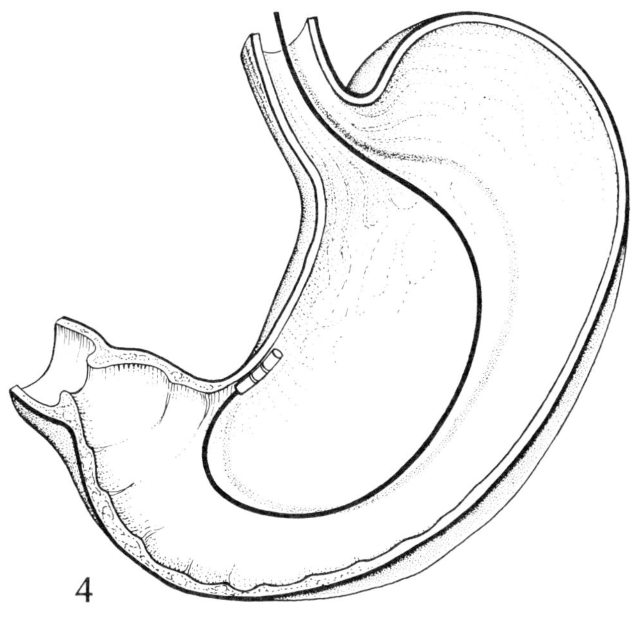

4

4

Mapping the antrum/corpus boundary

The boundary between the antrum and the acid-secreting corpus (the physiological boundary) may be defined by an intragastric pH electrode. Acid secretion is stimulated by pentagastrin given when the skin is incised, in the same dose as used in the preoperative gastric function test. The pH electrode is passed through the oesophagus, and its tip is pulled into the stomach and pressed into the mucous membrane at the lesser curve. At the boundary, movement of the tip of the pH electrode within less than 1 cm effects an abrupt change in pH from acid to neutral and vice versa. Most surgeons omit this part of the procedure, proceeding as described below.

5

Hereafter the assistant pulls the stomach firmly downwards. A thick nasogastric tube along the greater curve facilitates the grip. The non-elastic nerves stand up as tight strings, often visible and easily palpable by the surgeon's fingertip. The anterior gastric nerve of Latarjet is followed down to the point where it enters the stomach. This and the corresponding posterior nerve have to be spared and the point (the anatomical boundary) is marked with a suture stitch.

The anatomical boundary is usually 1–2 cm lower than that estimated by the pH electrode. If they coincide, one may elect also to cut the direct continuations of the nerves of Latarjet and depend on smaller more distal nerve twigs. However, this involves a risk of gastric stasis.

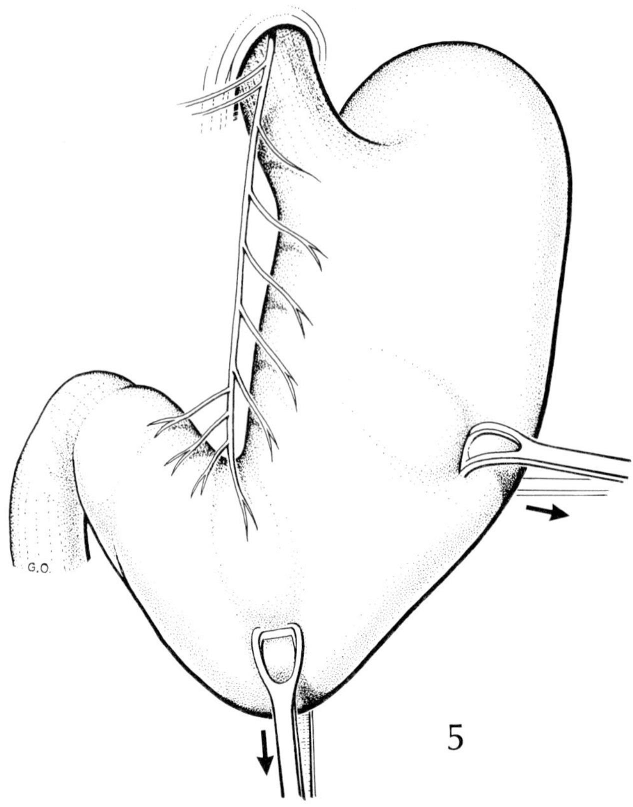

5

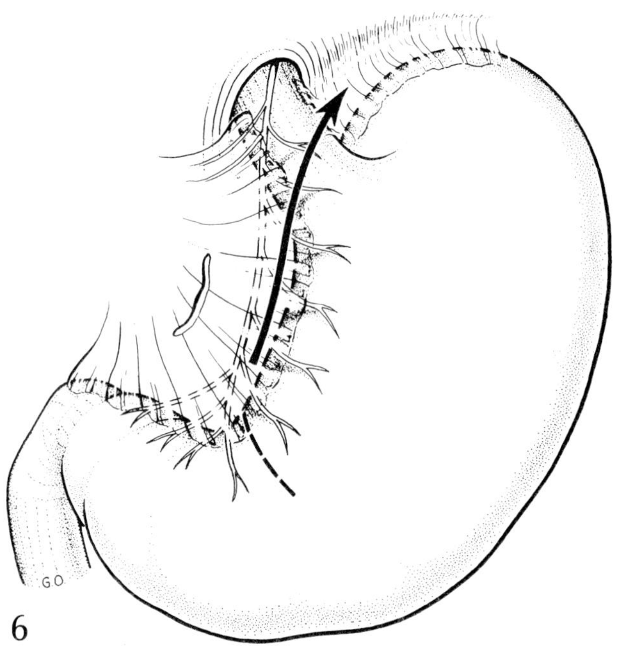

6

Dissection of stomach from omentum

6

This is performed from below upwards starting a few centimetres proximal to the anatomical boundary. An opening is made in the avascular part of the lesser omentum, distal to the hepatic branches of the vagus.

7

The left index finger is passed behind the omentum and stomach, lifting these structure anteriorly.

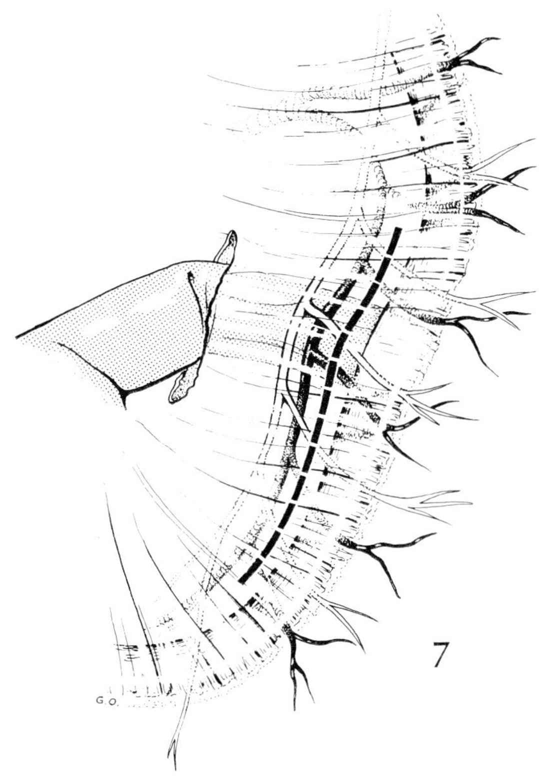

7

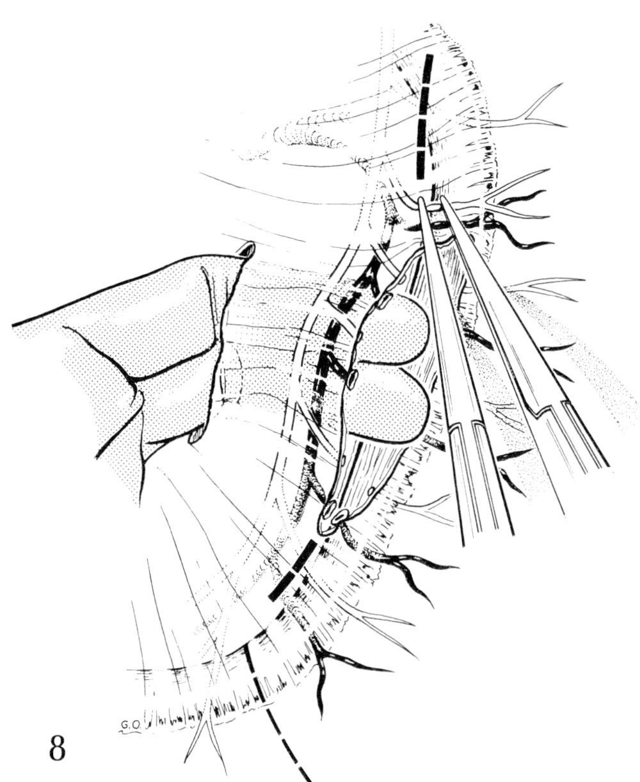

8

8

Adhesions in the lesser sac are cleared by dissection with the finger until the stomach is completely mobile. This should not be forgotten as it facilitates the following steps considerably. The serosa is cut along the lesser curve. Vascular branches from the gastric vessels to the stomach are isolated, clamped, cut and ligated as close to the stomach as possible, one after the other. Long slender artery forceps (Heiss, Martin 1978, 13-423-20) are recommended. The surgeon works along the lesser curve, taking first the anterior and then the posterior vessels. Numerous small nerve branches are seen and cut at the same time, but no special effort is made to locate the gastric nerves or the vagal trunks. The gap between the omentum and the stomach widens. This allows first one, then two fingers to separate the structures from behind.

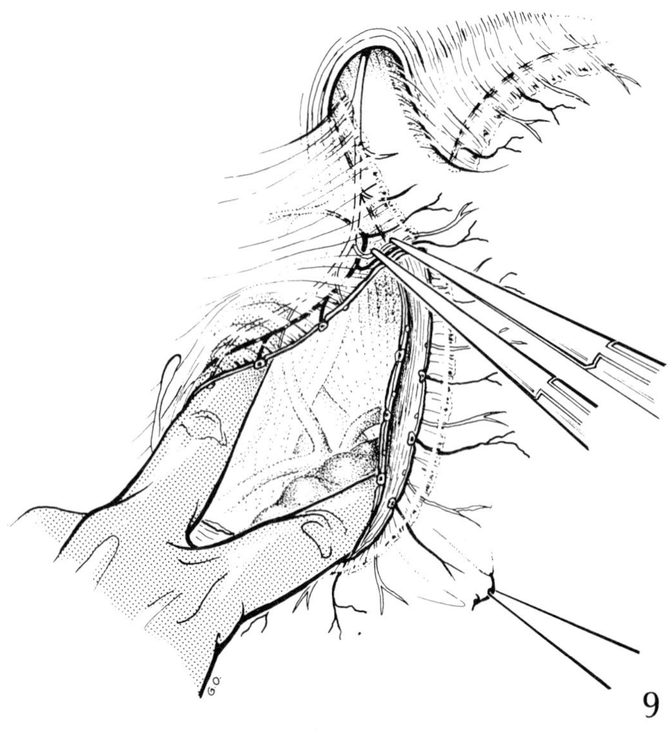

9

9

To help the surgeon to stick to the cleavage the assistant may pull a holding stitch in the lesser curve. The dissection is continued up to the cardia where the presence of longitudinal muscle fibres shows that the oesophagus has been reached. It is now usually easier to separate the stomach and the omentum using the left second and third fingers from in front.

10

10

It is important to continue the ascending dissection carefully past the cardiac region and up on the right side of the oesophagus so that the oesophagus can be encircled with the left index finger. This manoeuvre is dangerous if undertaken before the right side of the oesophagus has been identified. Perforation of the posterior stomach wall has been reported.

11

A rubber tube can now be passed around the oesophagus. By pulling downwards and to the right the tissues to the left of the oesphagus can be searched for nerves to the fundus of the stomach. This is important as large vagal nerve branches ('nervus criminalis') can be pushed to the left during the finger dissection of the oesophagus.

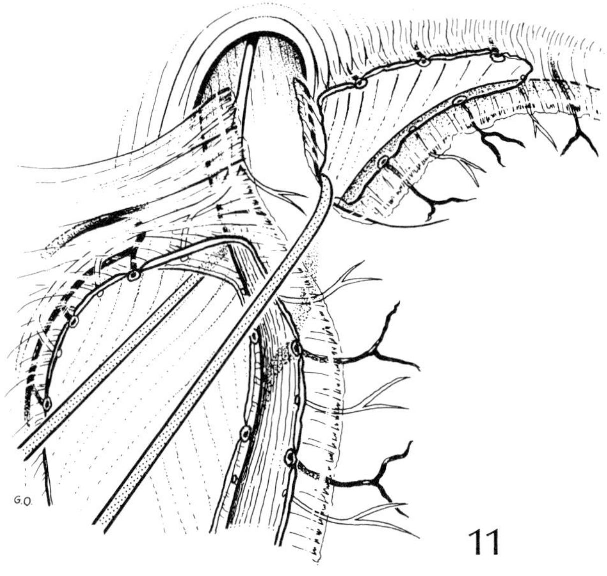

11

12

The oesophagus is now lifted anteriorly and together with the stomach completely separated from the posterior abdominal wall. Nerve fibres from the posterior trunk may pass to the stomach across this gap and have to be divided. When this is complete 5–6 cm of the oesophagus have been isolated. A circumferential search for nerves descending along the oesophagus (just as in a proper truncal and in selective gastric vagotomy) includes this part of the procedure. The oesophagus is then the only structure connecting the corpus of the stomach with mediastinum.

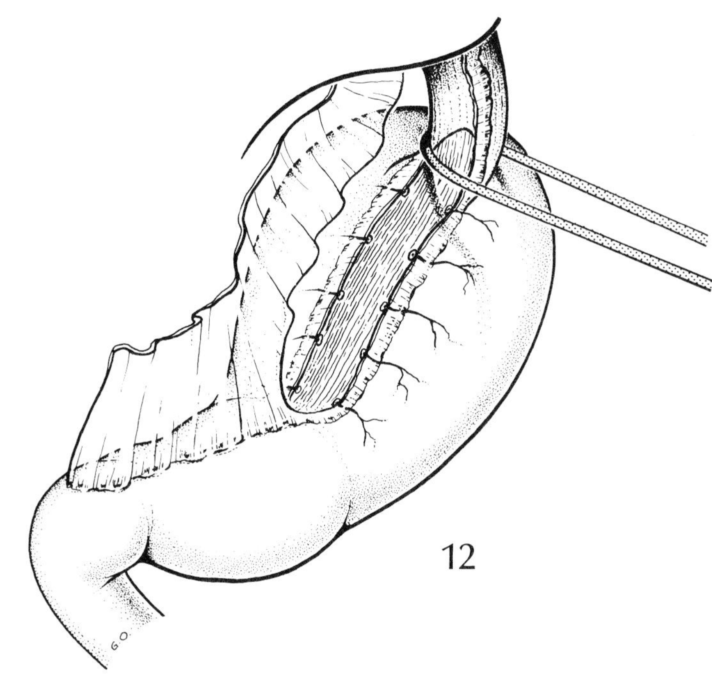

12

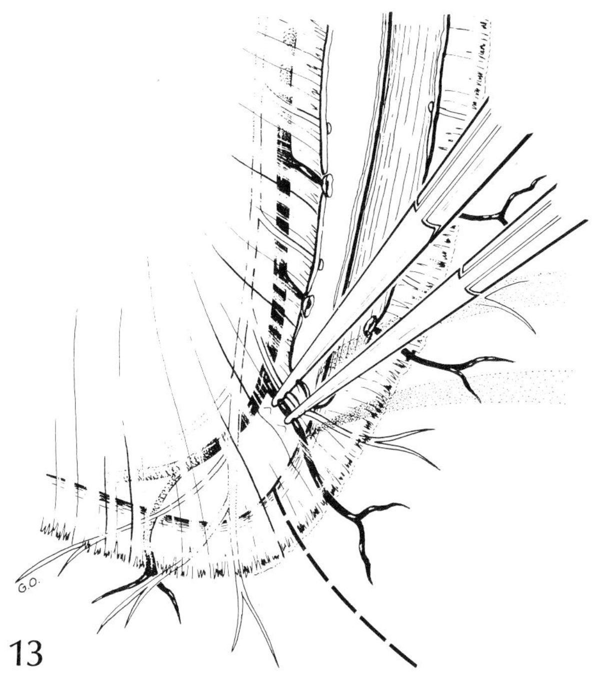

13

13

The final dissection at the boundary is left until last because traction in the omentum during the upper dissection may result in damage to vessels in this area. If no tissue is left to protect the nerves to be preserved they may be crushed during clamping of neighbouring bleeding vessels.

The assistant again pulls the stomach downwards, the main anterior and posterior nerves of Latarjet are located by palpation and the lesser curve of the stomach is dissected free of the omentum down to these nerves. Suture of the serosa on the naked lesser curve is unnecessary. No drains are used.

Postoperative care

A gastric tube is unnecessary. If used it can be removed the day after surgery when the patient can drink freely. A full diet is usually tolerated on the fourth to fifth day and the patient can then leave the hospital.

Comments

Vagotomy of the parietal cell mass is the aim of all types of vagotomy. The selective denervation of that area of the stomach containing these cells requires a careful technique, especially to avoid damage to the gastric nerves and their antral branches. The upper part of the dissection carries the same risk of leaving vagally innervated parietal cell areas as truncal or selective gastric vagotomy, no more and no less. However, PCV involves a further risk of being incomplete if the dissection at the corpus/antrum boundary is not performed extremely carefully.

PCV has only been in clinical use since 1969 and th long-term recurrence rate is still unknown. A 5 yea recurrence rate of about 5–10 per cent may be expecte least in experienced hands and when used for duoden ulcer. However, there is increasing evidence of a signi cantly higher recurrence rate after PCV for prepylor ulcer[2], which emphasizes the importance of careful end scopy before operation.

References

1. Amdrup, E., Andersen, D. Høstrup, H. The Aarhus County vagotomy trial. I. An interim report on primary results and incidence of sequelae following parietal cell vagotomy and selective gastric vagotomy in 748 patients. World Journal of Surgery 1978; 2: 85–90

2. Andersen, D., Høstrup, H. Amdrup, E. The Aarhus County vagotomy trial. II. An interim report on reduction in acid secretion and ulcer recurrence rate following parietal cell vagotomy and selective gastric vagotomy. World Journal of Surgery 1978; 2: 91–100

Partial gastrectomy

Charles G. Clark MD, ChM, FRCS, FRCS (Ed.)
Professor of Surgery and Director of Surgical Unit,
University College Hospital, London

Preoperative

Indications

For the elective treatment of chronic gastric, duodenal or stomal (anastomotic) ulcer; for the treatment of recurrent or persistent ulceration after vagotomy, with or without drainage; for the treatment of complications of peptic ulcer (e.g. haemorrhage).

For the treatment of simple tumours of the stomach that are likely to ulcerate or bleed (e.g. leiomyoma, neurilemmoma) or have a malignant potential (e.g. multiple adenomatous polyps).

Rare indications are the treatment of gastric strangulation, recurrent gastric volvulus, extensive stenosis or infection (e.g. tuberculosis).

The Billroth I gastroduodenal anastomosis is favoured for most patients with gastric ulcer. For duodenal ulcer and for gastric ulcer associated with duodenal ulcer or stenosis, the Polya-type gastrojejunal anastomosis is less likely to lead to recurrence.

Preoperative preparation

General supportive measures to correct anaemia and improve nutrition or correct vitamin deficiency may require several days of intravenous therapy. A decision whether to attempt to reduce the size of the ulcer by carbenoxolone (gastric) or histamine H_2 antagonists such as cimetidine (duodenal) requires judgement in the individual circumstance. Gastric lavage is important in patients with pyloric stenosis. Operation after a period of days or weeks of hospitalization appears to carry an increased risk of thromboembolism.

Anaesthesia and position of patient

General anaesthesia using an endotracheal tube with relaxants is to be preferred but local or epidural anaesthesia can be employed. The patient maintains a dorsal position and one or both arms may be extended and fixed at right angles to facilitate access to veins by the anaesthetist.

The operation

The incision

A midline epigastric or right upper paramedian incision is commonly used, sometimes after infiltrating the line of incision with 1:200 000 adrenaline (conveniently at hand with solutions of 0.5 per cent lignocaine). In obese subjects access to the duodenum may be facilitated by a transverse incision or an oblique 'sabre slash' incision which resembles the Kocher subcostal cholecystectomy incision but is extended over the midline and onto the left costal margin opposite the ninth costal cartilage.

General exposure and exploration

On opening the peritoneal cavity the ligamentum teres may require division close to the liver. The stomach and duodenum are inspected to define the site and extent of ulceration. The hiatus should also be examined for evidence of herniation. A general abdominal exploration to exclude other disease is then carried out.

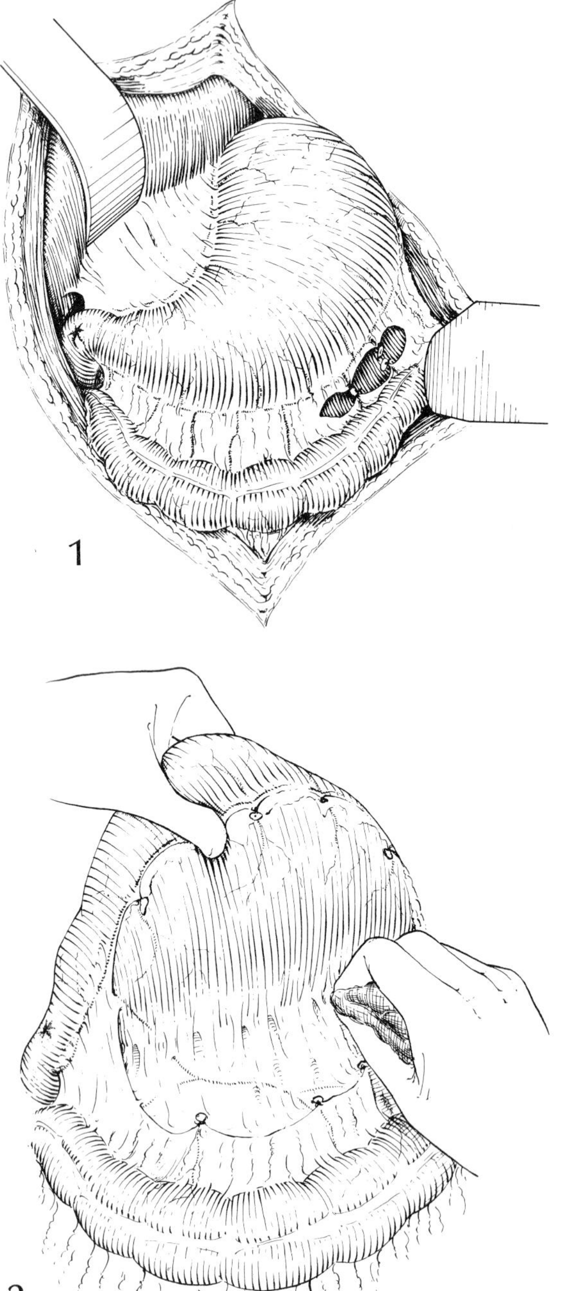

Preliminary mobilization of the stomach

1

Division of the gastrocolic omentum

The division begins in the avascular area to the left, below the short gastric vessels, and outside the gastroepiploic arch. Division of all the epiploic branches of the gastroepiploic is achieved by division between ligatures or between forceps, working from left to right. Division is easiest outside the arcade but in obese patients it may be judicious to remove the whole of the greater omentum from the colon to minimize the risk of postoperative fat necrosis. Alternatively the risk of omental fat necrosis is reduced if the vessels are divided within the arcade. (In the illustration the omentum is shown to be less enveloping than it usually is – when it obscures the transverse colon.)

2

Separation of the mesocolon

The stomach is turned upwards and medially to allow division of adhesions between the posterior wall and the mesocolon, which is swept downwards by gauze dissection, particular care being taken with the middle colic vessels which lie closely applied to the right gastroepiploic vessels. Sharp dissection may occasionally be required as the dissection proceeds to the right to expose the posterior wall of the duodenum. Here fine forceps are required to deal with vessels until the posterior duodenal wall is cleared to expose the gastroduodenal artery.

Mobilization of the duodenum

3

Division of the right gastroepiploic pedicle

Drawing the stomach upwards and to the right exposes the right gastroepiploic vessels which should be divided close to and below the pylorus. The duodenum is then cleared by applying the fine forceps to the small vessels and dividing them to dissect the duodenum free to a point about 1 cm distal to the proposed line of section.

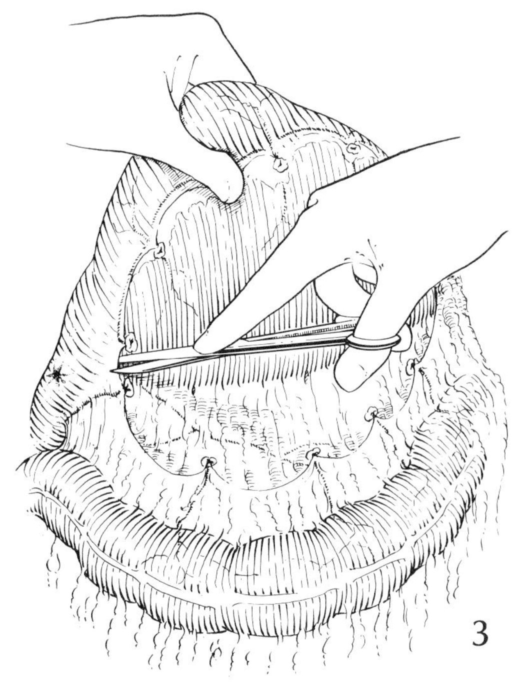

3

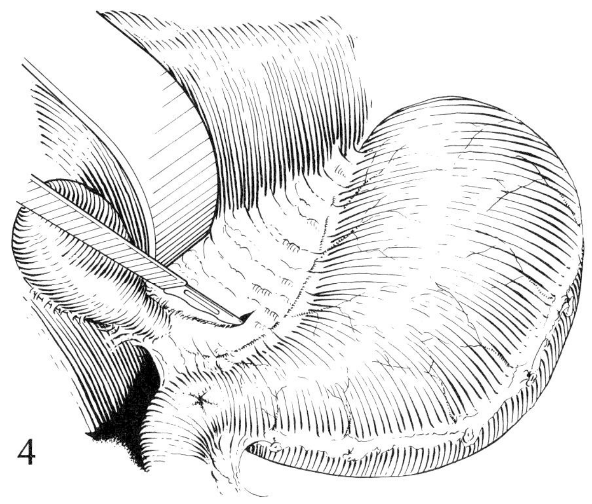

4

4

Exposure of the right gastric pedicle

Drawing the stomach down and to the left exposes the right gastric vessels. Opening through an avascular area of the left omentum these vessels are cleared, though deformity or scarring of the superior part of the duodenum may require sharp dissection to clear the pedicle. The right gastric vessels are now divided between ligatures and the remainder of the duodenum freed by ligating small vessels as described for the inferior part of the duodenum.

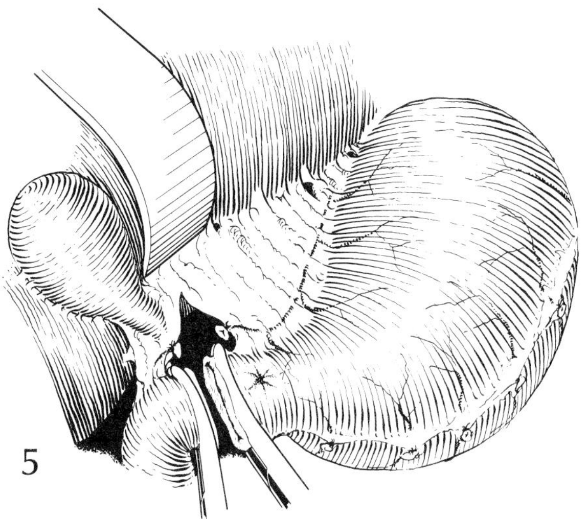

5

5

Transection of the duodenum

The duodenum is divided between crushing clamps, and a gauze swab is used to cover the proximal part. This step may be deferred until all gastric vessels have been divided, but in some cases it is essential for this step to be performed first in order to obtain good access to the left gastric vessels by traction on the stomach. As much healthy duodenum as possible should be preserved to make duodenal closure easy and safe. In postbulbar ulcer it may be difficult or unwise to attempt too liberal a dissection and alternative methods of dealing with the duodenum may be required.

Division of the duodenum between a crushing clamp and a duodenal occlusion clamp is also used, a method of some advantage if the duodenal stump is short.

Closure of the duodenum

Several methods are used depending on circumstances.

6 & 7

If an occlusion clamp has been applied, the duodenum should be closed first by an inverting layer of continuous catgut followed by fine interrupted silk sutures or a single silk purse-string suture.

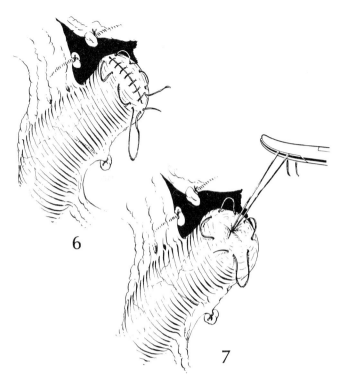

6

7

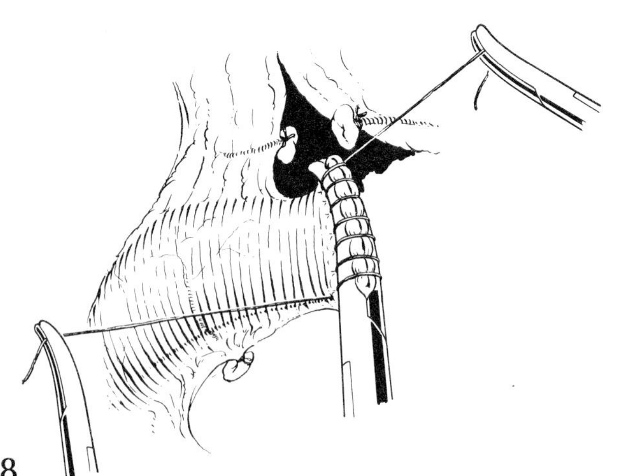
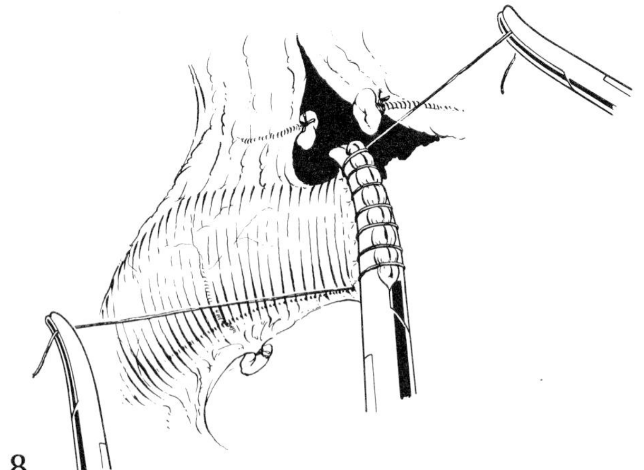
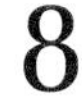

8

8

An alternative method is used where the duodenal stump is short. With the clamp in position a continuous over-and-over suture of catgut is inserted and then drawn tight as the clamp is removed. Thereafter silk sutures are again used.

9

When there is difficulty in closing the duodenum because of scarring and oedema, no attempt should be made to do so. In these circumstances the safest course is to place a wide-bore tube into the duodenum and close the duodenum around it. A foley catheter is sometimes convenient for this purpose. *A controlled fistula is safer than an uncontrolled one,* and the tube may be removed after 10 days.

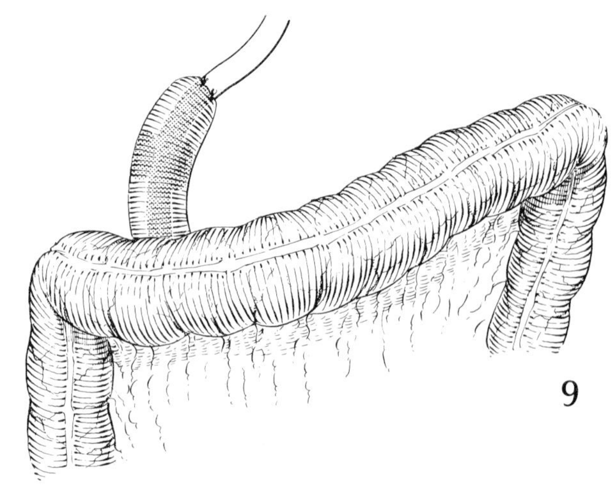

9

Mobilization of the lesser curve of stomach

10

In a thin subject the vessels on the lesser curve of the stomach may be dealt with before division of the duodenum. In obese subjects division of the duodenum facilitates this manoeuvre. The stomach is held forward and the lesser omentum is both examined and palpated for an accessory hepatic artery running from the left gastric artery to the liver. If found it should be preserved, though it is only at risk when the left gastric vessels are divided near their origin in operations for gastric carcinoma. Such division is not necessary for peptic ulcer and the lesser omentum should be divided to expose the left gastric artery at the point where it divides into ascending and descending branches. Posterior adhesions may require division at this point to provide clear exposure of the vessels. With the stomach pulled to the left, the finger and thumb palpate the left gastric vessels. A forceps is thrust through the omentum near the lesser curve and, using this to separate ascending and descending branches, two forceps (such as Maingot's) are applied proximally and one distally and the descending branch of the left gastric is divided between them.

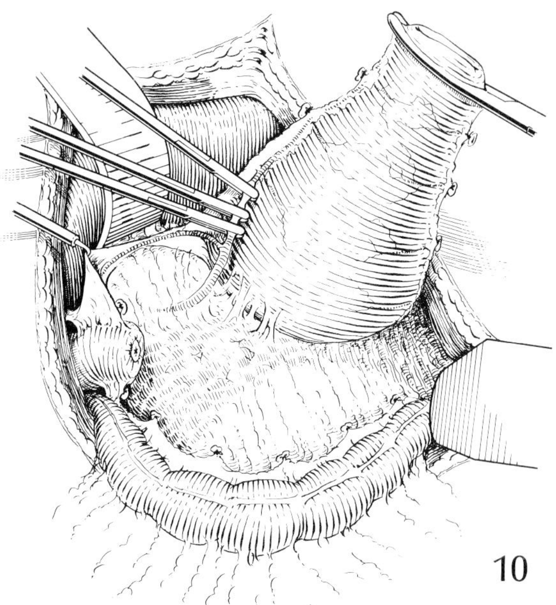

10

11

Division of the left gastric pedicle

Double ligatures of strong silk are applied proximally and one distally. The main branch of the left gastric artery is preserved since its division would entail cutting or ligating the posterior branch of the vagus nerve going to the coeliac axis. The distal ligature on the descending branch of the left gastric may be held by a strong suture or as illustrated by forceps to enable stripping and ligation of vessels on the lesser curve downwards for a distance of 2 or 3 cm to facilitate subsequent anastomosis.

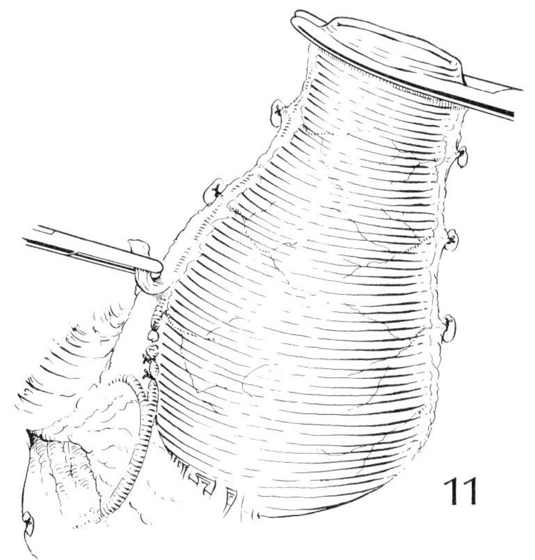

11

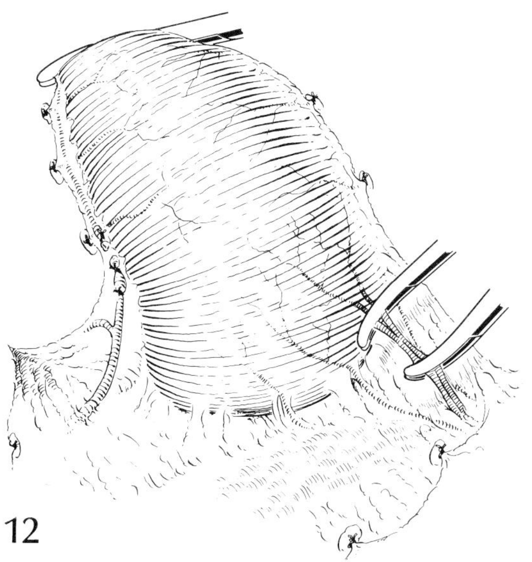

12

12

Mobilization of the greater curve and exposure of short gastric vessels

The colon is pulled downwards by an assistant and the stomach pulled to the right to expose the remainder of the left side of the greater omentum. The gastroepiploic is ligated and the short gastric vessels exposed. The lower two or three are divided between forceps or ligatures. The stomach is now cleared and the site for anastomosis selected. In general a two-thirds gastrectomy is carried out for peptic ulcer but this may be difficult to judge. If the line of section follows the point about 2 cm below the division of the left gastric descending branch on the lesser curve and extends towards the lowest (divided) short gastric vessel, this is a reasonable approximation.

13

The antecolic gastrojejunal anastomosis

This technique should probably only be used when the retrocolic method is inappropriate because of a short transverse mesocolon, dense adhesions, or for expediency during an emergency procedure. Its principal disadvantage is the longer loop of small intestine required for anastomosis. Its only advantage is accessibility should further surgery be required.

The Lane's twin clamp is a simple method of performing anastomosis. The first clamp is placed across the stomach at the level selected. The stomach is then pulled over the left costal margin to expose the posterior wall. The upper jejunum is pulled into the wound and the afferent loop held towards the lesser curve, when the second clamp may be aplied and the two clamps locked together. The afferent loop should be as short as possible and no more than 10–12 cm from the duodenojejunal flexure; the apex of the first jejunal arcade marks an appropriate length. It is preferable if the length of jejunum in the clamp slightly exceeds the length of stomach for easy control of end sutures.

A posterior seromuscular suture is now inserted either of continuous catgut or interrupted fine silk. If catgut, it begins to the left and ends on the lesser curve aspect of the stomach where a hitch-knot temporarily secures it.

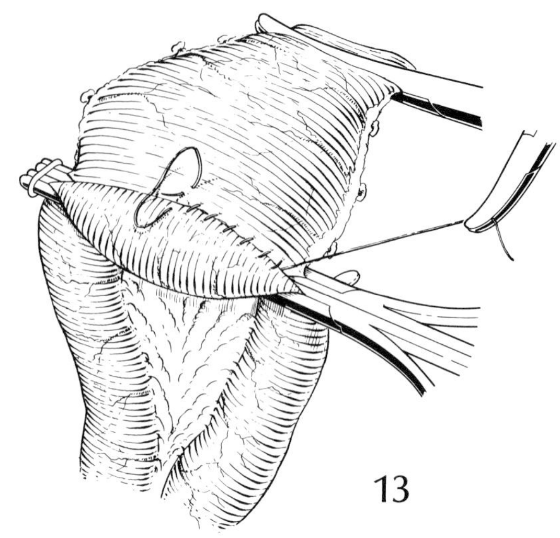

13

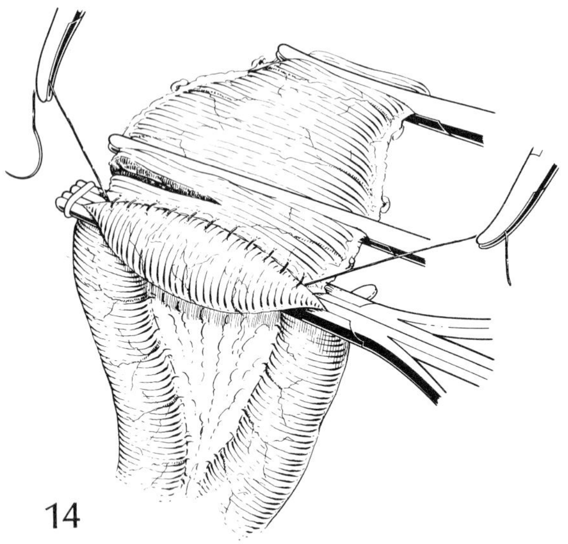

14

14

Formation of a valve

It is doubtful if a valve has any real physiological function but it does offer aded protection to the suture line of the stomach. There appears to be no physiological advantage over whole-width gastrojejunal anastomosis.

A Payr's clamp is applied across the whole stomach about 1 cm above the Lane's clamp. The surgeon should err on the side of more rather than less for the excess can be trimmed. It is expedient to divide the stomach with a swab behind to contain any spillage from the remnant. The specimen is removed and the reconstruction commences. The width of the stoma is first estimated which ideally should equal the width of the small intestine. In general 5–6 cm is adequate.

15

Closure of the valve

The valve is closed by a continuous catgut suture after suitable trimming of the cut edges. If the stomach has been cut too close to the Lane's clamp this may prove difficult and require a subsequent continuous suture for haemostasis and further inversion. The closure of the valve proceeds to a point determined by the width of the anastomosis where a hitch-knot is applied.

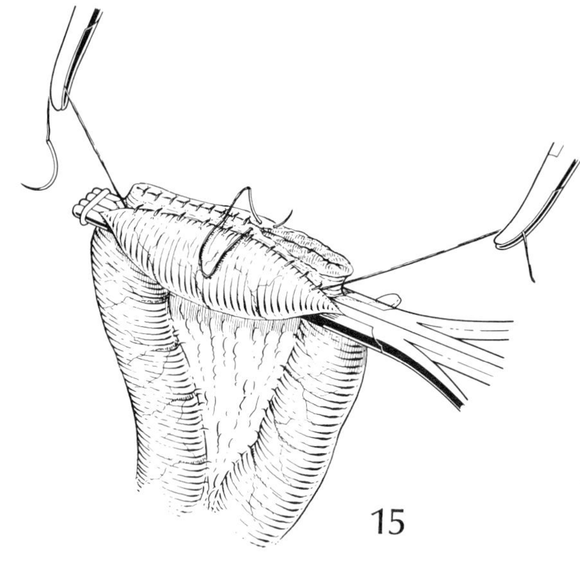

15

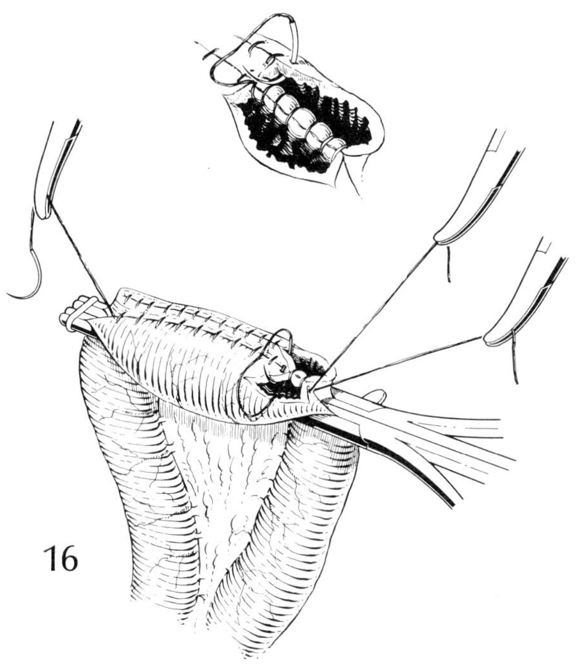

16

The stoma

16

The jejunum is incised opposite the remaining open part of the stomach leaving a seromuscular margin of about 3 mm. Either using a separate suture or continuing with the suture used to close the valve, an all-coats posterior suture is now applied. This through-and-through, over-and-over suture should err on the side of deep bites and the number of sutures per centimetre is irrelevant provided that all the mucosa (particularly jejunal) is enclosed.

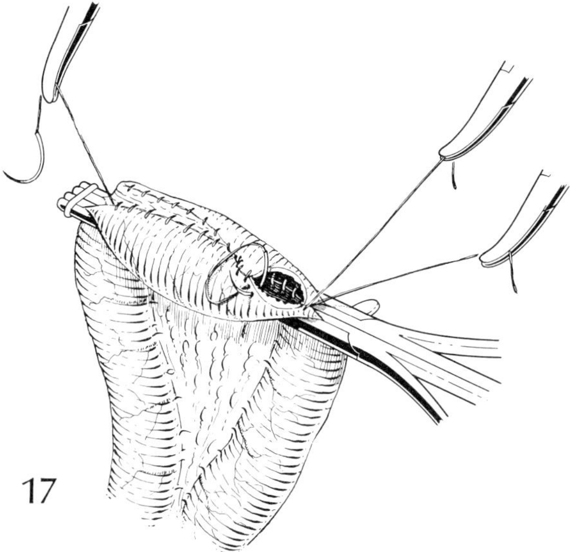

17

17

The anterior all-coats layer

The end of the posterior wall is completed by bringing the suture externally and using a hitch-knot. The anterior layer is begun using a Connell stitch, inverting the mucosa as the suture proceeds from left to right. When the suture reaches the previously constructed valve it can either be tied there if a separate anastomotic catgut suture has been used or, if not, continued along the valve as a supplementary suture for added security. The Lane's clamp may now be removed and the valve and anastomosis inspected for bleeding. If required, interrupted catgut sutures are applied.

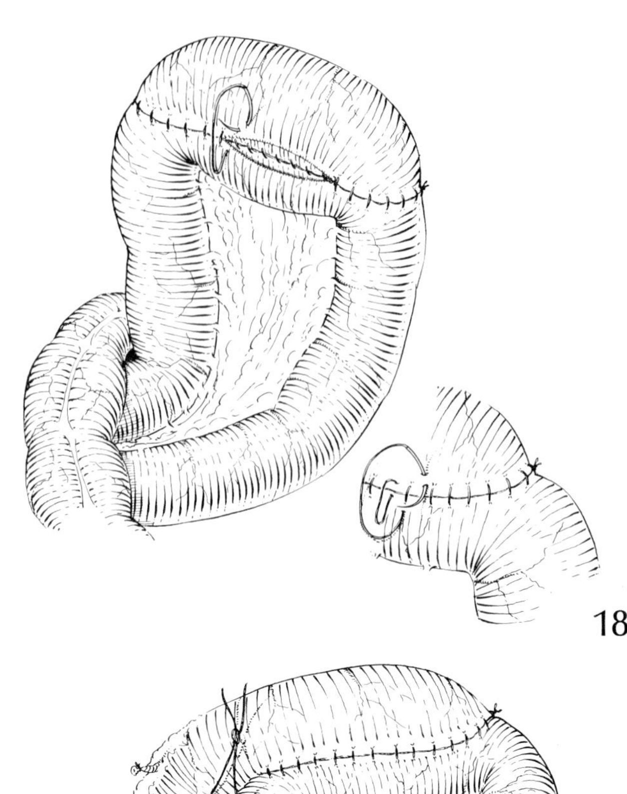
18

18 & 19

The anterior seromuscular layer

If catgut has been used the posterior seromuscular suture is continued along the anterior surface of the valve and anastomosis, eventually joining the initial suture starting the posterior seromuscular stitch.

It is sometimes recommended that a final suture be placed at the junction of afferent loop with lesser curve to support the stomach.

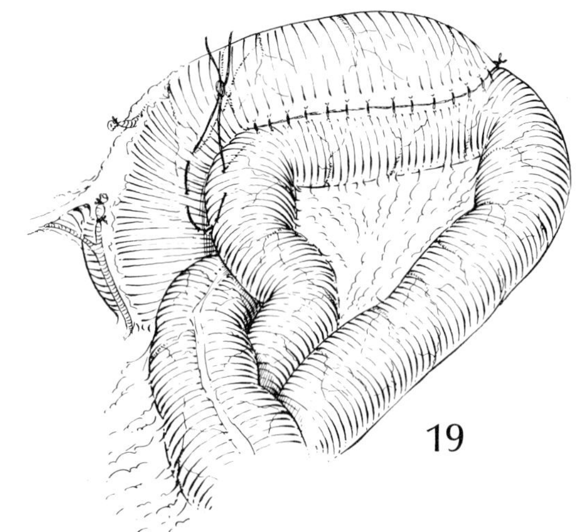
19

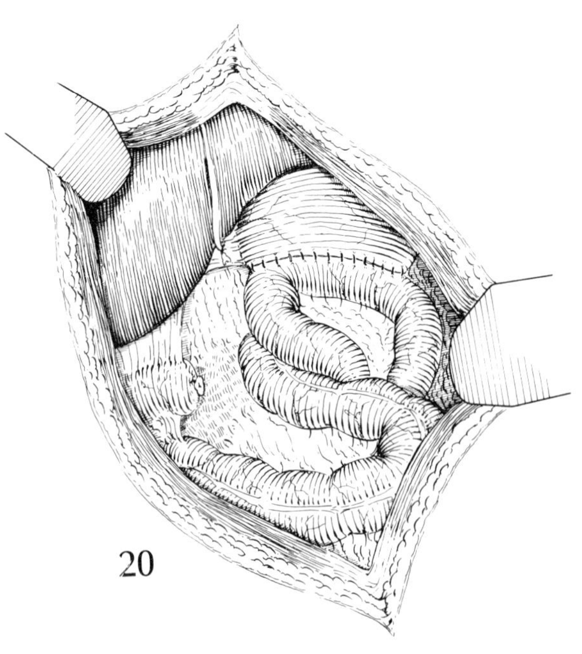
20

20

Final placement and inspection

The colon is now drawn as far to the right as possible to prevent its weight hanging on the afferent jejunal loop. When the stomach and jejunum are returned to the abdomen the anastomosis lies transversely.

Before closing the abdomen a general inspection for bleeding is carried out with particular reference to the spleen, vascular pedicles and omentum. Whether the abdomen is drained or not is a mattter of individual preference but if any difficulty is encountered with duodenal closure drainage is wise.

THE RETROCOLIC GASTROJEJUNAL ANASTOMOSIS

The stomach is mobilized and prepared for transection, as already described.

21

Incision of the mescolon

The transverse colon is lifted up and the mesocolon inspected to define an avascular area usually to the left of the middle colic vessels. It is incised unless the mesocolon is very short, fatty or scarred. Occasionally a transverse incision will be more expedient.

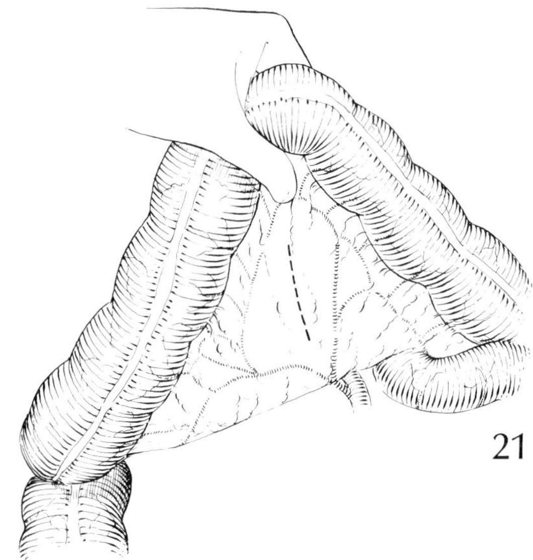
21

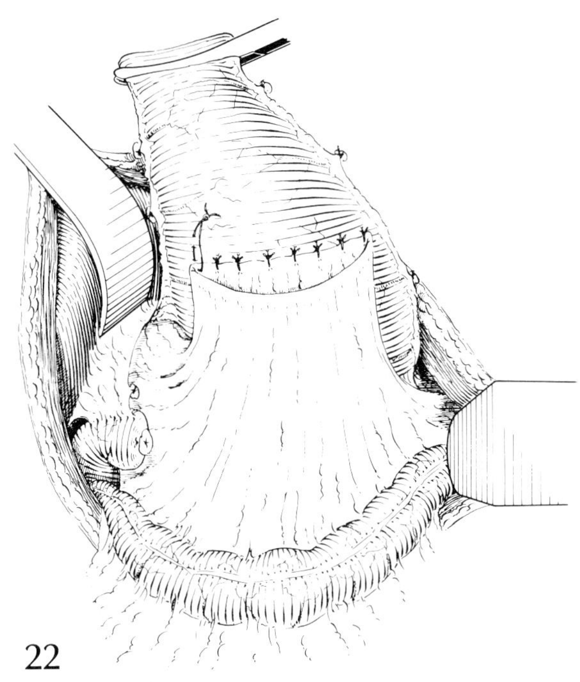
22

Attachment of mesocolon to stomach

22

The stomach is drawn forwards and to the left and the proposed line of transection selected. Below this the inferior part of the mesocolon is attached by interrupted or continuous suture to the posterior wall of the stomach.

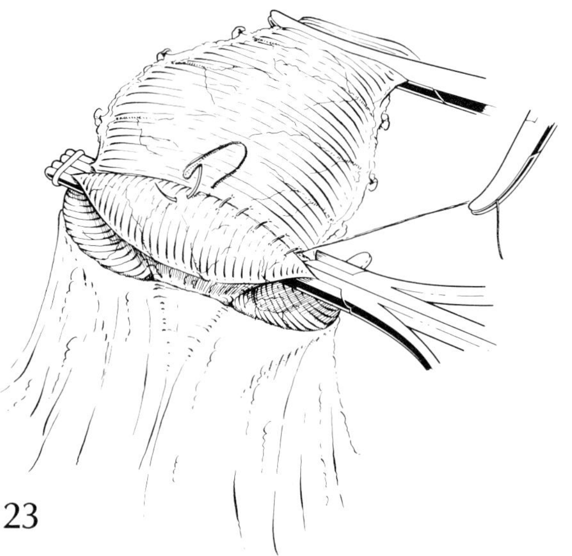
23

Application of clamps and anastomosis

23

The proximal jejunal loop is drawn through the hole in the mesocolon, taking a point approximately 8 cm below the duodenojejunal flexure which will be sutured to the lesser curve aspect of the stomach. The anastomosis proceeds as shown in *Illustrations 13–19*.

The formation of a valve is a matter of choice. It reduces the size of the gastric stoma to some extent and adds protection to the suture line of the closed part of the stomach. It may be necessary to reverse the jejunal loop and bring the proximal jejunum to the greater curvature aspect of the stomach. In such cases it is important not to leave the efferent loop sutured too high on the lesser curve as obstruction to gastric emptying may result.

24

Anterior attachment of mesocolon to stomach

The jejunum and anastomosis is brought through the mesocolon to lie below it. Using interrupted or continuous sutures the anterior part of the mesocolon is sutured to the wall of the stomach above the line of the anastomosis.

The anastomosis should finally lie in the left part of the abdomen. In both antecolic and retrocolic gastrojejunostomy a space is left between the afferent loop in front and the mesocolon or colon behind. This is a potential source of herniation. Some surgeons prefer that these spaces should be closed by interrupted sutures.

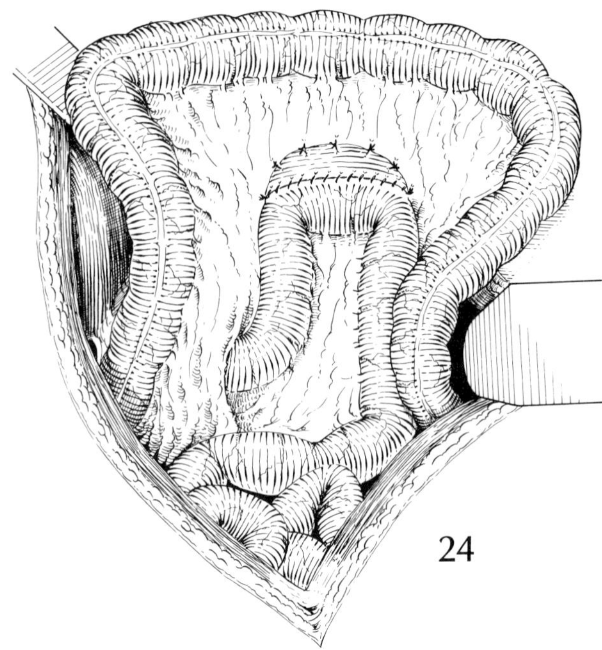

24

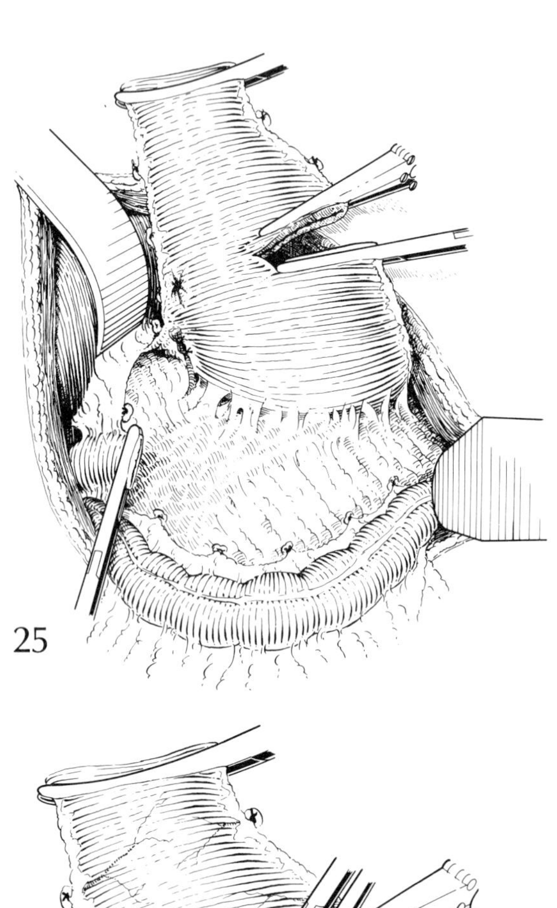

25

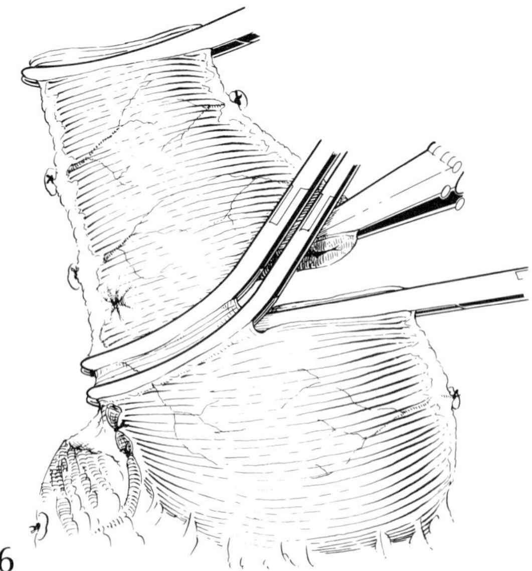

26

THE GASTRODUODENAL OR BILLROTH I (PÉAN) ANASTOMOSIS

Mobilization of the stomach proceeds as shown in *Illustrations 1–5*. The duodenum after division is covered with a small swab to await anastomosis. The stomach is further mobilized for transection as shown in *Illustrations 10–12*.

Transection of the stomach

25

Construction of the gastric stoma

The stomach is lifted forward and a light Lang Stevenson or similar clamp is placed from the greater curvature side across approximately half a stomach to form the stoma. A Payr's crushing clamp is placed distally and the stomach partly divided between the two.

26

The lesser curve

A curved crushing Parker-Kerr clamp is placed from the tip of the light stomach clamp to skirt the margin of the ulcer, and this defines the new lesser curve. A second clamp is applied distally and the stomach is divided between these two clamps and the specimen removed. Alternatively a non-crushing clamp can be used to define the lesser curvature but this has a tendency to slip unless access is good.

Formation of a new lesser curve

27

The all-coats layer

If a suitable clamp such as a Parker-Kerr can be applied, a continuous catgut suture applied over the clamp is inserted and when the clamp is removed the suture is drawn tight, one loop at a time. Sometimes the clamp is difficult to apply in which case suturing is commenced after incising the stomach at the appropriate level and continuing to incise and suture as the resection proceeds.

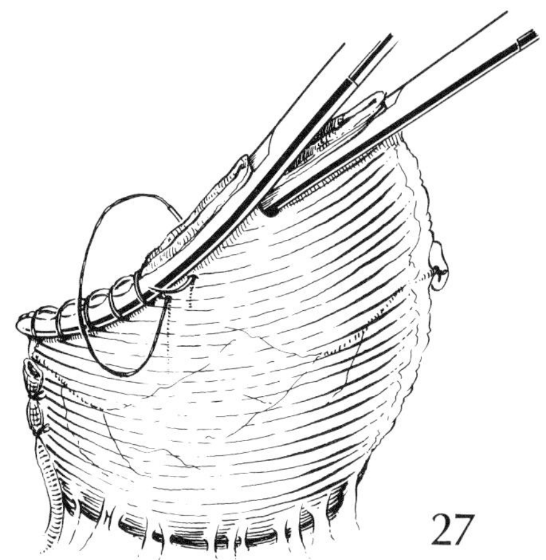

27

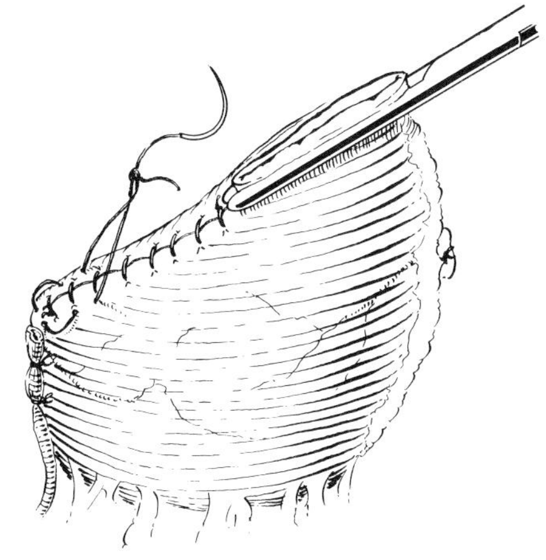

28

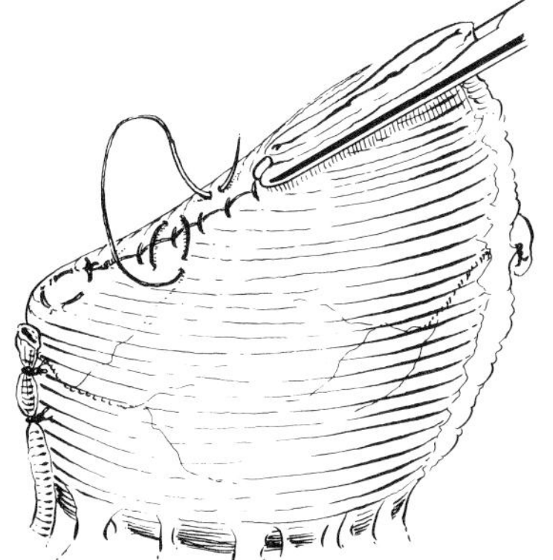

29

28 & 29

The seromuscular layer

The previous suture line is buried either by means of a continuous suture of catgut from the lesser curve downwards or by interrupted silk sutures.

The anastomosis

30

Posterior seromuscular layer

The two light clamps on stomach and duodenum are approximated and the posterior seromuscular suture of catgut is commenced at the greater curve of the stomach. Either a loose spiral ('cork-screw stitch') suture is inserted until the posterior layer has been completed or alternatively the suture may be locked at the greater curve aspect and inserted and drawn tight as it proceeds. The suture passes through the superior duodenal wall and then both posterior and anterior gastric walls above the seromuscular stitch of the lesser curve and is locked with a hitch-knot in preparation for completion later on the anterior aspect of the anastomosis.

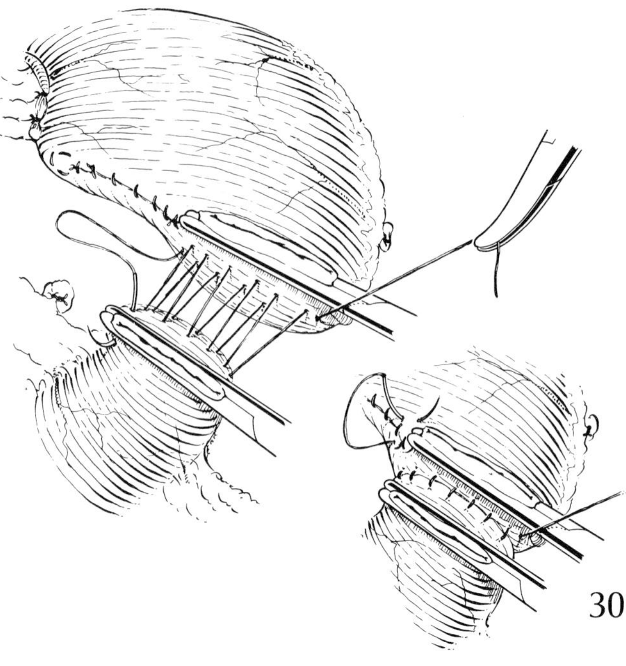

30

31

The posterior all-coats layer

The posterior all-coats layer of continuous catgut, begins at the greater curvature aspect and small close sutures are used to fasten down the redundant folds of mucosa.

32 & 33

The anterior all-coats layer

The corner of the lesser curve is turned and inverted and the anterior suture inserted as shown in *Illustration 17*. Any disparity in size can be overcome by making a small longitudinal incision in the anterior wall of the duodenum.

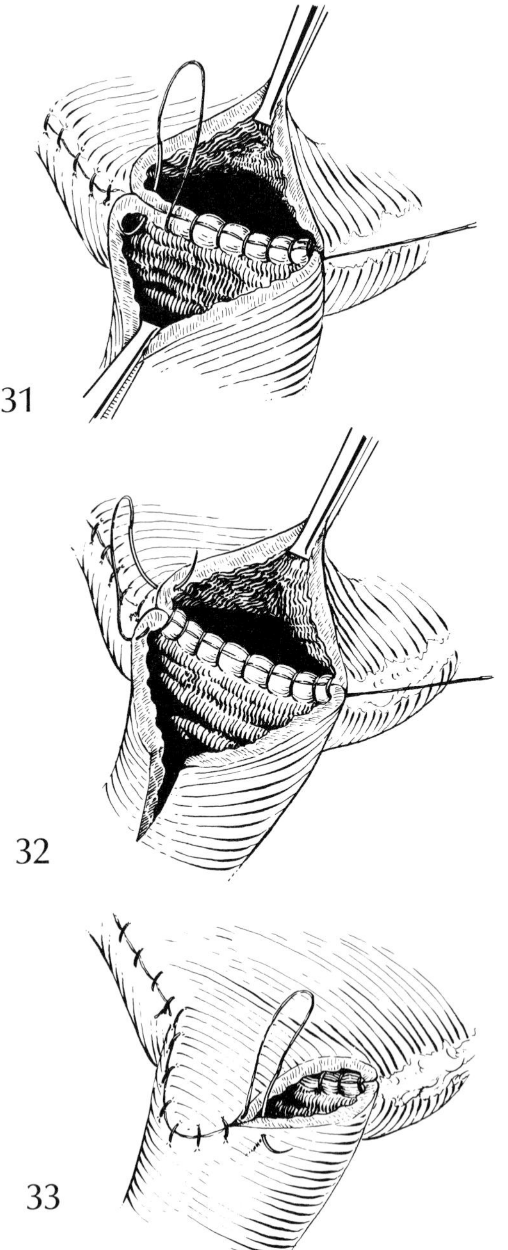

31

32

33

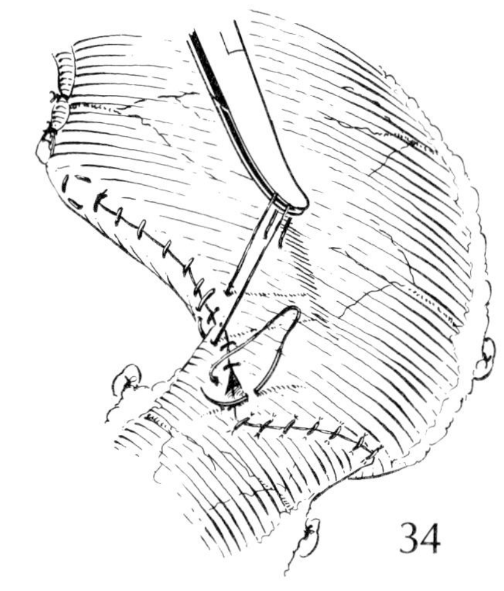

34

34 & 35

The anterior seromuscular layer

The critical angle between the closed lesser curve and the superior border of the duodenum is reinforced by an additional suture which is inserted first through the anterior wall of the stomach, then the posterior wall, then the superior part of the duodenum and tied.

If difficulty is experienced with the duodenum it is sometimes convenient to mobilize it by dividing the peritoneum along its lateral border. On completion of the anastomosis, some surgeons prefer to support the stomach and draw it towards the right by inserting a few sutures between the new lesser curve and either the right gastric pedicle or the remains of the hepatogastric ligament.

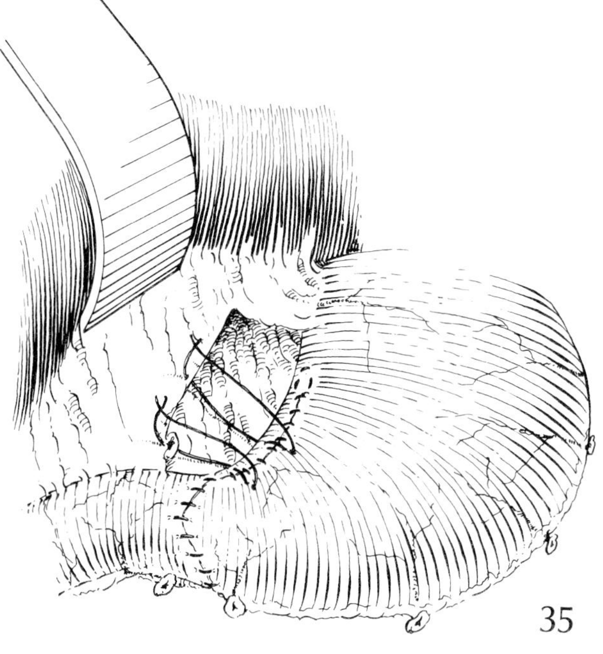

35

The difficult ulcer

THE POSTERIOR PENETRATING DUODENAL ULCER

36

Method 1

For an ulcer situated in the second part of the duodenum with a healthy duodenal bulb (a rare event) the duodenum is dissected in the usual manner. The transection is made as near to the pylorus as possible and the duodenal stump closed by the method shown in *Illustrations 5–8*.

Method 2: Open closure of the duodenum distal to the ulcer

For the posterior penetrating ulcer in the first part of the duodenum, exposure and mobilization proceed in the usual manner until the right gastric pedicle has been divided and the superior border of the duodenum dissected.

The duodenum is entered by blunt dissection and, if the posterior wall is destroyed by ulceration, by far the safest method is to suture the duodenum around a drainage tube, which should be left in position for at least 10 days. This is prefereable to any form of dissection (*see Illustration 9*).

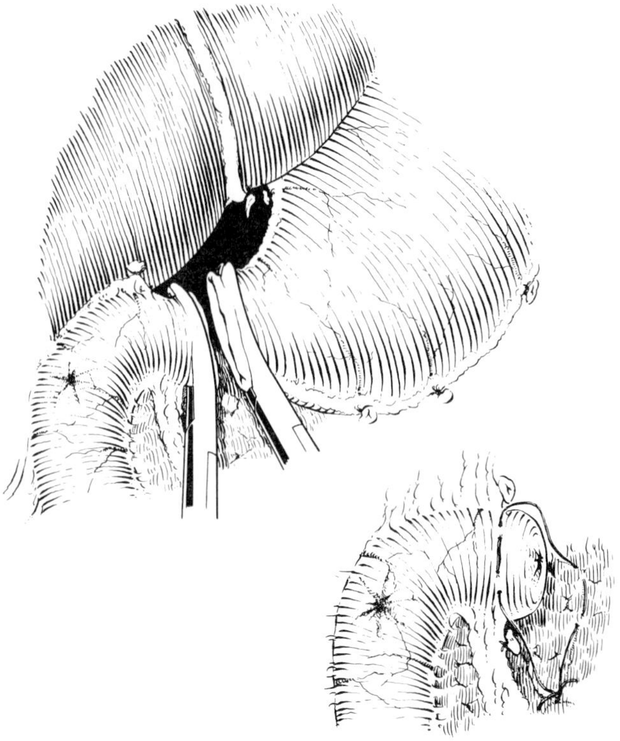

36

37–41

Method 3

In some cases dissection can be carried out by inserting a finger into the lumen of the duodenum and using a knife. The posterior duodenal wall beyond the ulcer is freed from the scarred pancreatic tissue for 1 cm in order to effect a closure. Continuous over-and-over and inverting suture is used to draw the anterior wall well over to the scarred pancreas.

The great danger is disruption of the duodenal closure. Where doubt exists, the method of inserting a tube is by far the safest. Alternative methods of dissecting beyond the ulcer, performing a difficult closure, even with overlaying of omentum, are best avoided.

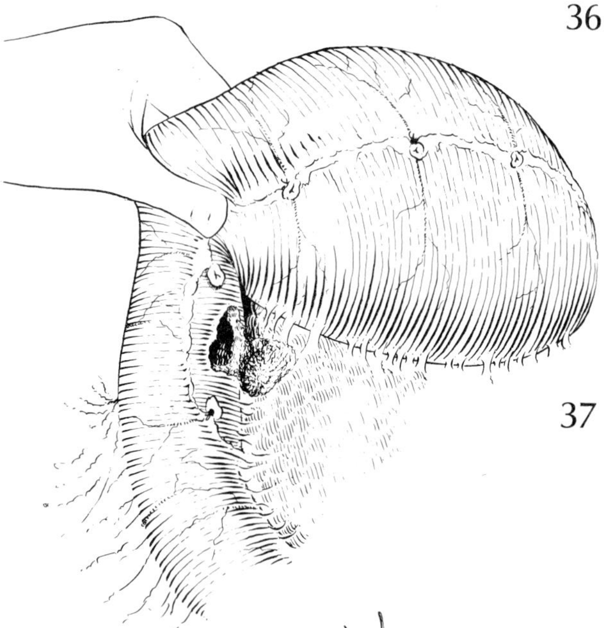

37

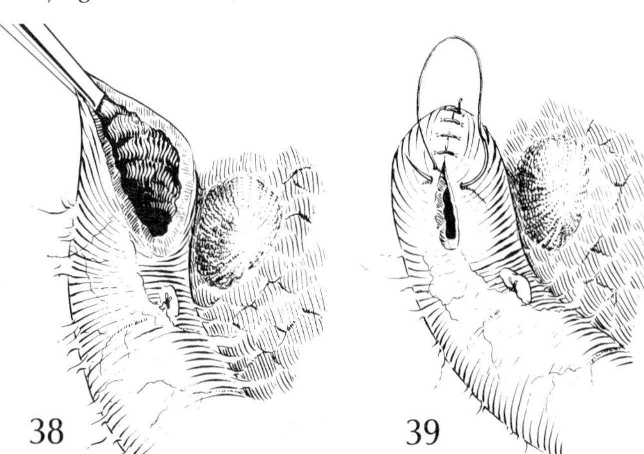

38 39 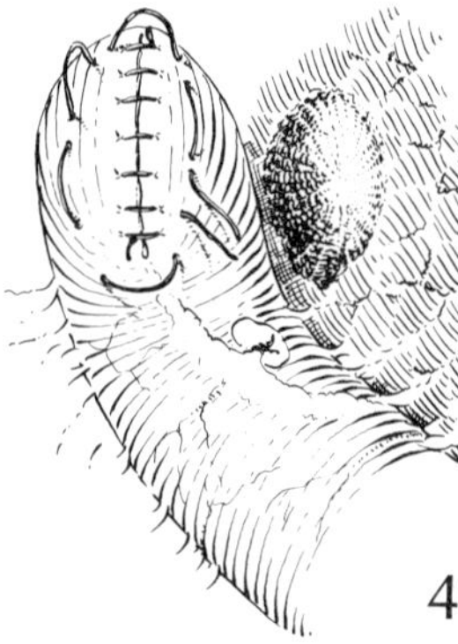 40 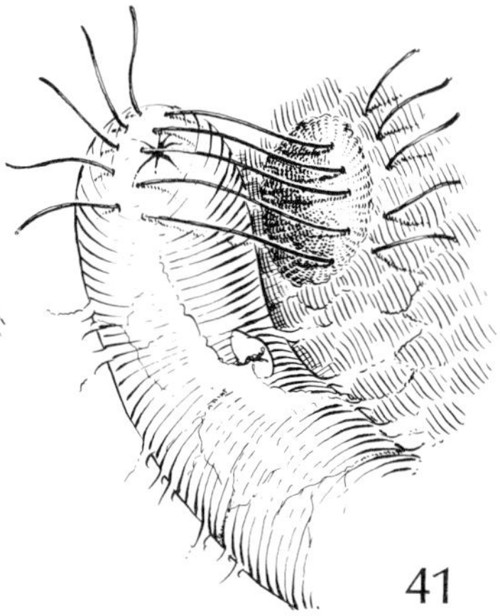 41

Method 4: Prepyloric closure

This method is sometimes adopted in patients with recurrent ulceration after previous surgery.

42

If the duodenal ulcer has caused distortion and great fixation of the duodenum but the pylorus is healthy, the stomach is mobilized as before, two Payr's clamps are applied to the stomach in the region of the antrum about 5 cm proximal to the pyloroduodenal junction.

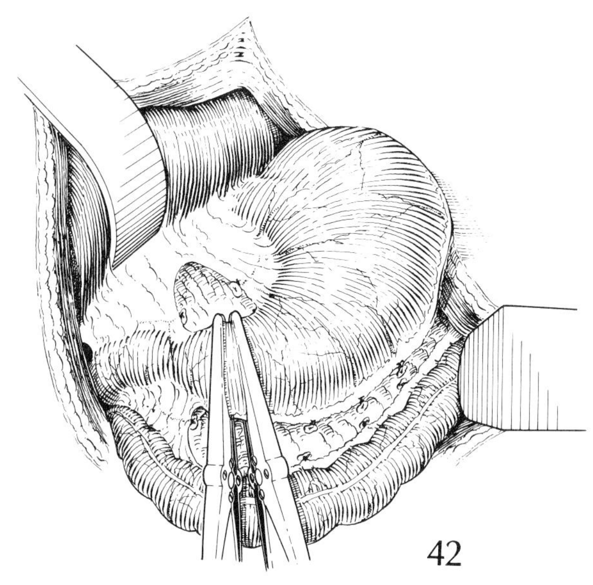

42

43

43

Seromuscular dissection

An incision is made immediately distal to the clamp on the antrum and the seromuscular coats are dissected free from the mucosa down to the pyloric ring, small perforating vessels being ligated as they are encountered. This dissection can sometimes be facilitated by injecting 1:200 000 adrenaline between muscle and mucosa (use 0.5 per cent xylocaine with adrenaline).

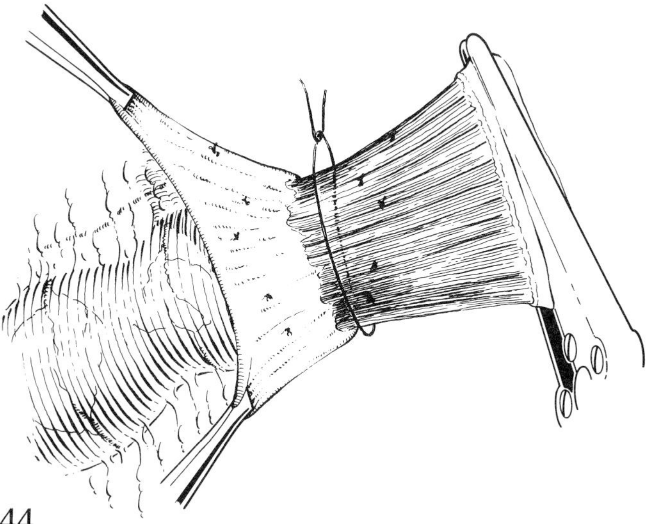

44

44

Closure of the pyloric mucosa

A simple ligature is tied round the pyloric mucosa at this level and the redundant tissue removed.

45 & 46

Closure of the seromuscular layer

The seromuscular stump is now closed by a series of sutures inverting the pyloric muscle, and completing this by a further inverting layer. This method has seldom any application at the present time and carries the danger of leaving some antral mucosa exposed by reflux to duodenal content. This results in the liberation of gastrin and is liable to lead to the early onset of recurrent ulcer. Either the method of inserting a wide-bore tube or an alternative operation such as vagotomy and gastroenterostomy is preferable.

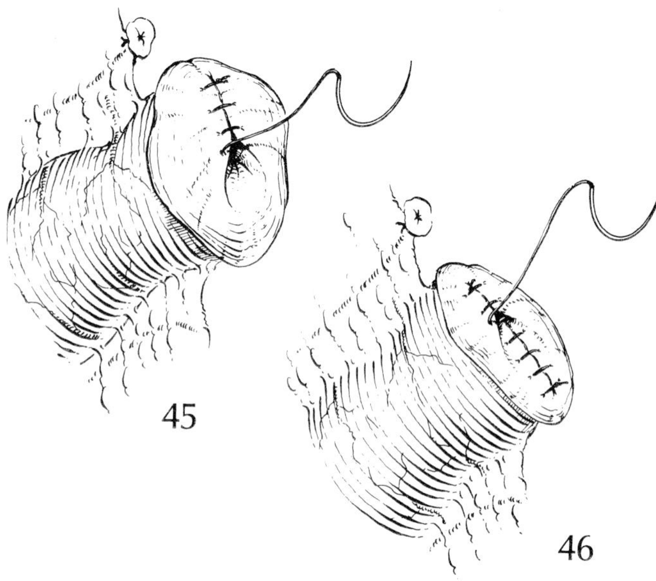

THE HIGH POSTERIOR PENETRATING ULCER

Partial gastrectomy below the ulcer

If resection of a simple gastric ulcer appears to be especially difficult or hazardous, it is quite proper to carry out a limited resection, leaving the ulcer *in situ*. In such cases, preliminary and preferably multiple biopsies of the edge of the ulcer should be obtained and submitted to frozen section to exclude carcinoma. If the ulcer is benign, resection below the ulcer is done and a gastrojejunal reconstruction is performed. This operation is not suitable for a bleeding ulcer.

Partial gastrectomy removing the ulcer

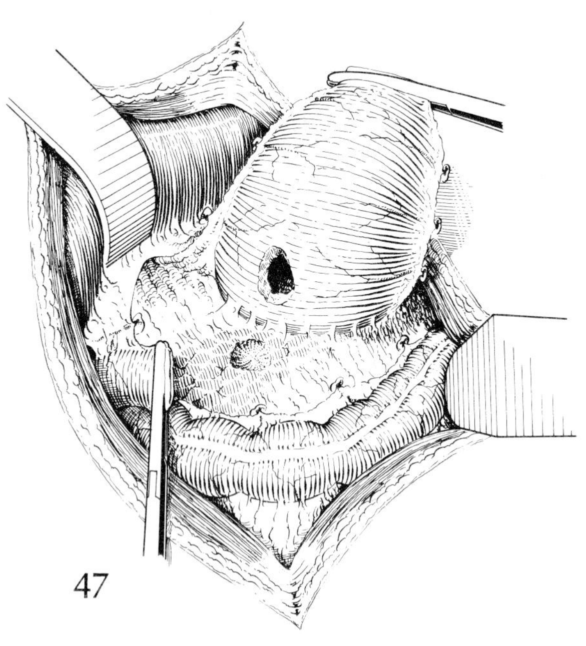

47

Separation of stomach from ulcer bed

After dividing the duodenum the stomach is turned over to the left to expose the adherent area and using the thumb and forefinger the ulcer is 'pinched off' the penetrated structure, usually the pancreas.

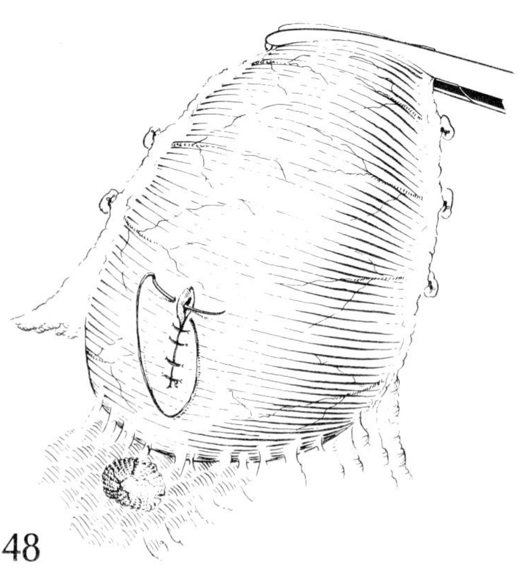

48

Closure of gastric wound

After aspirating the stomach contents through the hole in the posterior wall of the stomach, the hole may be temporarily closed with sutures to prevent spillage. The stomach can now be drawn out of the wound, downwards and to the left to expose the left gastric and the short gastric vessels which are dissected and divided as shown in *Illustrations 10–12*.

The Pauchet procedure and the rotation manoeuvre

The Pauchet procedure taking a tongue of lesser curve containing the ulcer, is used for any high lesser curvature lesion. It may be combined with the rotation manoeuvre if the ulcer is situated on the posterior wall of the stomach.

49

The ulcer is grasped between thumb and forefinger and held as though it were situated on the lesser curve, by pulling the posterior wall forwards. The true lesser curve will not be lying anteriorly and the greater curve posteriorly. Clamps are applied at the selected level across the anterior wall of the stomach, which now forms a new greater curve.

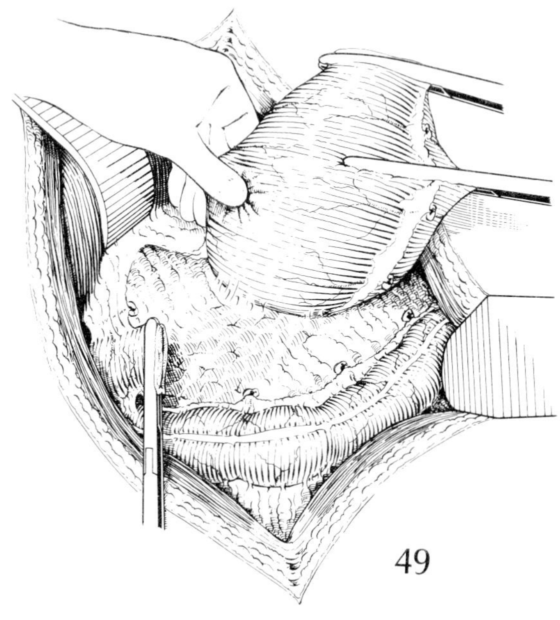

49

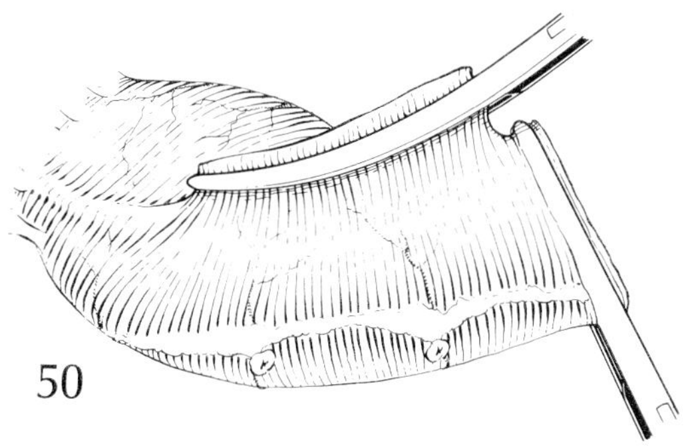

50

50

The gastric transection

Transection is made distal to the clamp and a Parker-Kerr clamp is applied on the posterior wall of the stomach to skirt the ulcer and form a new lesser curve. Transection distal to the Parker-Kerr clamp allows a tongue-shaped segment of posterior wall containing the ulcer to be removed. Closure of the lesser curve proceeds as in the manner depicted in *Illustrations 27–29*.

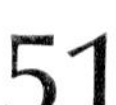

51

Duodenogastric approximation

The gastric remnant and the duodenum are approximated and a Billroth I anastomosis carried out as shown in *Illustrations 30–35*.

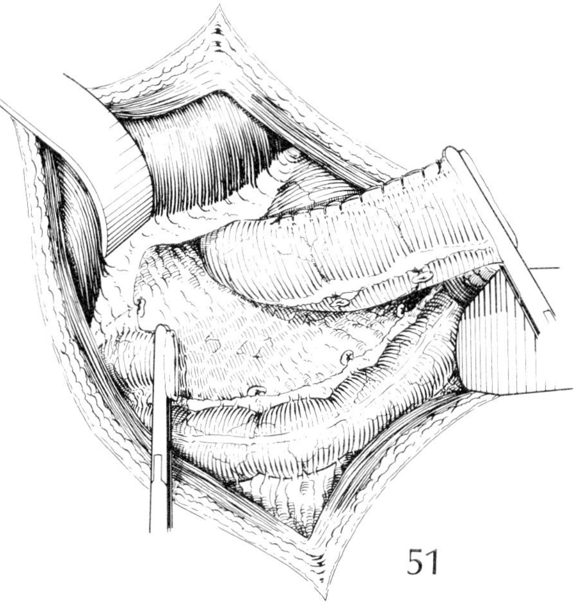

51

52

THE VERY HIGH SUBCARDIAC ULCER

If the ulcer is too high for the Parker-Kerr clamps to be placed above it, the tongue-shaped piece of lesser curve containing the ulcer is excised free-hand, segment by segment, proceeding from below, the cut edges being closed with a continuous all-coats suture as the incision is carried further up towards the cardia.

This suture line is buried with a continuous seromuscular suture as previously described, care being taken to avoid undue narrowing of the oesophagus if the incision encroaches on the cardia.

53

THE HOUR-GLASS STOMACH

The presence of hour-glass contracture may make gastric resection difficult. Nevertheless gastrectomy is preferable to procedures such as gastrogastrostomy or gastrojejunal anastomosis above the narrowed area. As much stomach should be conserved as possible but manoeuvres such as resection below the ulcer and widening the narrowed portion of the stomach by a longitudinal incision and suturing transversely should be avoided. It is usually possible to excise round the ulcer at the expense of the lesser curve by leaving a larger portion of greater curve to give an adequate gastric remnant. Either a gastroduodenal anastomosis or a gastrojejunal anastomosis can be performed as appropriate.

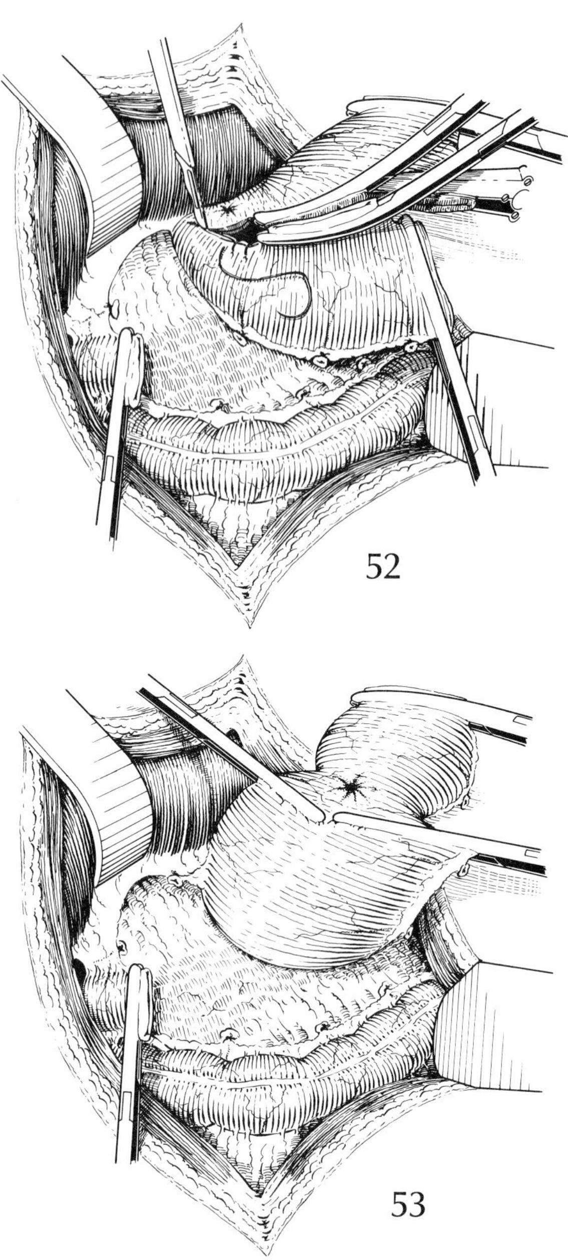

52

53

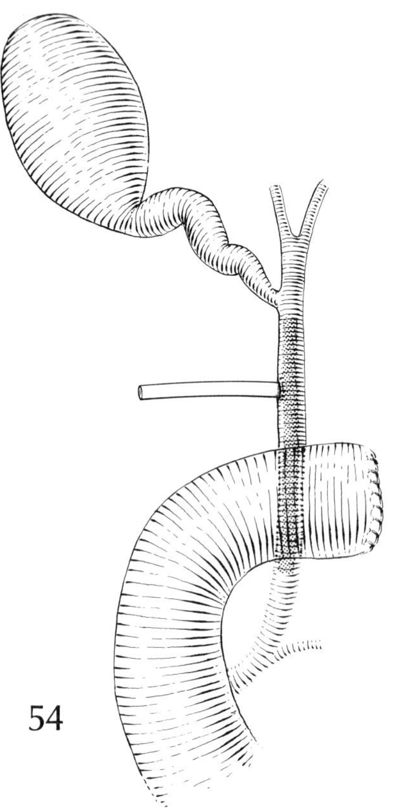

54

54

LAHEY'S PROCEDURE

This uses intubation of the common bile duct to help identify its position where there is intense inflammatory reaction and distortion around the duodenum, particularly the posterosuperior aspects. Even so in very exceptional circumstances the common duct may be cut into. No attempt should be made to repair it in these circumstances, for the tissues are too rigid with inflammation. Instead reliance should be placed on prolonged T-tube drainage, but care must be taken that the T-tube does not pass through the ampulla into the duodenum, for this courts the risk of pancreatitis.

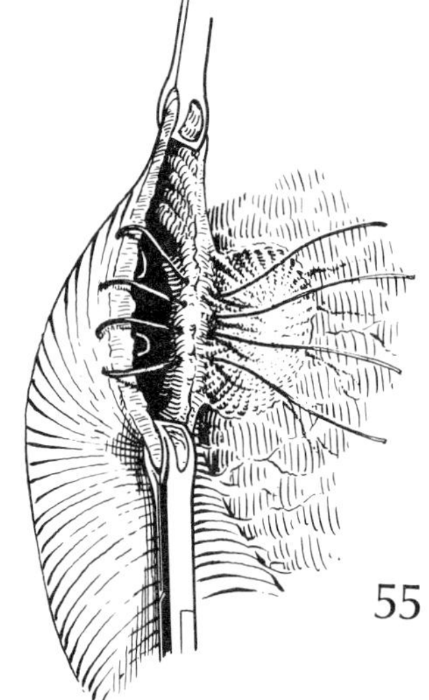

55

55, 56 & 57

NISSEN'S METHOD

Where difficulty is anticipated or experienced in dissecting free the posterior wall of the cut edge of the duodenum from the ulcer, the duodenum can be closed using the technique of suturing the edge of the ulcer to an inverting anterior edge of duodenum, either by a running stitch or interrupted sutures.

Provided the duodenum is sufficiently mobile and pliable, a second layer is inserted to approximate the distal edge of the ulcer crater to the anterior duodenal wall, and this may then be reinforced by omentum. In effect the duodenal stump is buried in the ulcer crater.

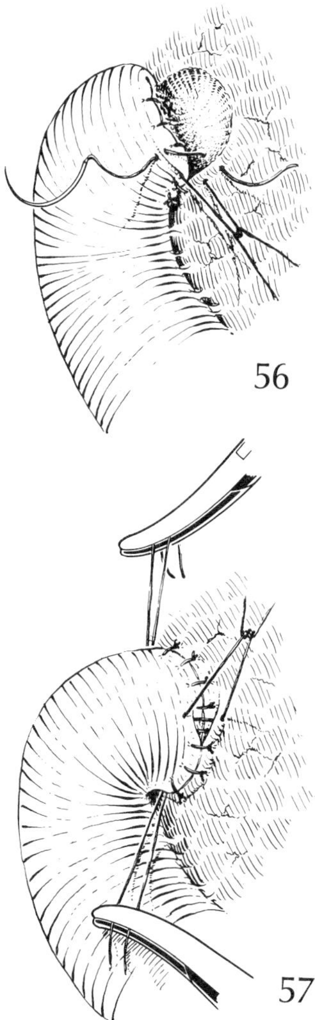

56

57

Special postoperative care and complications

Whether or not a nasogastric tube is used postoperatively is a matter of individual choice. As a means of decompressing the gut it is probably not required, because the gut will be relatively paralysed until challenged. Its sole purpose may be to warn of bleeding from the suture line. Similar reservations pertain to the use of temporary gastrostomy tubes which are difficult to position after gastric resection. There may be a place for gastric decompression after a Billroth I operation particularly if vagotomy has also been used. Gastric retention or delayed emptying is not uncommon.

Intravenous infusion is generally employed in patients after partial gastrectomy though fluids can usually be tolerated after the first 24–48 h. Full fluids should be accepted by the fourth or fifth day, followed by a light diet, preferably of the 'sloppy' type, for a few days. In no circumstances should the patient be advised a special diet after discharge. If the operation does not allow the patient freedom of choice, then it is inadequate. Patients suffering from postgastrectomy problems such as dumping may require dietary advice but for the remainder encouragement to eat a normal varied diet is important to avoid nutritional problems.

Postoperative haemorrhage

Collapse from haemorrhage after gastrectomy has two main causes; bleeding from the suture line or splenic damage. The former will result in haematemesis or melaena and depending on severity may require intervention. Reoperation and gastrotomy to reveal the source of the bleeding will determine the course to be followed. The spleen is vulnerable in gastric surgery and a tear in the capsule may go unnoticed, later resulting in severe haemorrhage requiring reoperation and splenectomy. Current enthusiasm to preserve the torn spleen should be confined to the primary operation. To attempt splenic preservation at reoperation for severe haemorrhage is an unjustifiable risk.

Duodenal stump or suture line leakage

The signs of peritonitis after operation are often less obvious. If leakage occurs within the first 3 days (rare) resuture may be the best treatment. If later, a conservative approach with intravenous hyperalimentation may be required. It is generally unwise to attempt to resuture the duodenum. The insertion of a drainage tube with the duodenum closed round it is far safer.

Rare complications

Fat necrosis of the omentum, gangrene of the gastric remnant and necrotizing enteritis are extremely uncommon but do arise and present with abdominal pain and collapse. Where an intra-abdominal disaster is suspected, a relaparotomy should not be discouraged with one exception: pancreatitis may result from dissection of a posterior ulcer (usually duodenal). It is usually a mild form which responds to symptomatic treatment.

Remedial surgery for postgastric surgery complications

A. Cuschieri MD, ChM, FRCS(Ed.), FRCS
Professor and Head of Department of Surgery,
Ninewells Hospital and Medical School, University of Dundee

Aside from recurrent ulceration, a substantial cohort of patients (30–40 per cent) after gastric surgery for chronic peptic ulcer disease suffer from a variety of symptoms and long-term complications attributed to the altered physiology and anatomy of the upper gastrointestinal tract. In some of these patients the symptoms are severe, intractable and lead to chronic ill health and malnutrition. Disabling symptoms after gastric surgery are more commonly encountered in the younger age group usually in patients after surgical treatment before the age of 35 years, in females and in patients with Polya (Kroenlein) gastric resections. The retrospective experience with highly selective vagotomy to date indicates that the incidence of severe disabling symptoms is reduced but not completely abolished by this procedure although some clinical trials have not shown any significant difference in the short term between this operation and truncal vagotomy with drainage[1,2].

The management of patients with severe disabling symptoms after gastric surgery remains anecdotal and problematic. There have been few clinical trials of remedial surgical operations and indeed these are difficult to set up because of the many variables involved. This chapter is based on a personal experience with 165 patients undergoing remedial surgery for postgastric surgery complications over a period of 16 years.

General principles

1. Despite the well described syndromes and clinical classifications of the various disorders, pure syndromes are rare and a substantial majority of patients present with a mixed clinical picture. However usually they have a dominant symptom which can be elucidated only by a careful and detailed history of the events occurring during bad days. Treatment should be directed towards the abolition or improvement of this symptom first.
2. As a rule, symptoms tend to improve with time and remedial surgery should not be contemplated until 1½–2 years have elapsed and conservative treatment has failed.
3. Expert dietary management is essential and constitutes the mainstay in patients with postgastrectomy hypoglycaemia and in patients with mild to moderate vasomotor dumping. Methoxy pectin which reduces the gastric emptying rate is particularly beneficial in these patients[3].
4. A detailed investigation of the gastrointestinal tract is necessary to outline the pathological anatomy and physiology of these patients.
5. Joint management with a gastroenterologist improves the outcome and is required for the independent assessment of the results of the various remedial surgical procedures.
6. The nature of the remedial surgical procedure for a given complication is influenced by the previous surgery, the nutritional state of the patient and the results of special investigations.
7. Psychiatric/psychological assessment may occasionally be required although this aspect has been overemphasized. More often than not the psychoneurotic manifestations are secondary to the chronic disabling gastrointestinal symptoms and subside with abolition or amelioration of the latter by successful management.

Investigations

Radiology

The key investigation consists of the galactose (200 g)-barium meal and follow-through which enables a crude but visual assessment of the stomach emptying of a hyperosmolar meal and the response of the small intestine to such an osmotic load. This meal should precipitate an attack of vasomotor dumping in all patients who complain of this disorder and it will outline the characteristic small bowel dilatation. In patients with diarrhoea, the galactose-barium meal will demonstrate gross intestinal hurry with the meal reaching the caecum within 10 min of the gastric emptying.

Endoscopy

This is necessary to ascertain the exact anatomy, the size of the gastric reservoir, the extent of duodenogastric reflux of bile and recurrent ulceration, the state of the gastric mucosa and the presence of reflux oesophagitis.

Gastric acid secretory studies

The maximal secretory output in response to pentagastrin and the insulin test are used to establish a baseline and to determine the completeness of previously performed vagotomy. It is essential that all procedures involving jejunal loop transfers, pouch constructions and Roux-en-Y diversions should be accompanied by a complete truncal vagotomy to prevent jejunal ulceration. Revagotomy as part of the remedial surgical procedure was found to be necessary in 11 per cent of patients in this series.

Gastric emptying

Only a crude estimate of the rate and pattern of gastric emptying can be obtained from the barium meal. Gastric emptying is best studied using a radioactively labelled meal of known osmolality with the patient sitting during the upper abdominal scanning with a γ-camera. The pattern of gastric emptying, the 10 min emptying, the $T_{1/2}$ and the per cent retention at 60 min are the most useful indices in the assessment of these patients.

Tests for duodenogastric reflux

A crude indication of the extent of bile reflux and the severity of the associated gastritis is obtained by oesophagogastroscopy. Estimation of bile salt concentration and Na^+ in gastric juice following intubation has been used to quantitate duodenogastric influx, but in general there is little correlation between objective findings and clinical symptoms. More recently the use of biliary excretion scanning before and after intravenous cholecystokinin or milk meal has been adopted to quantitate the extent of duodenogastric reflux[4] although it is too early to assess its value in the management of these patients.

Oesophageal function tests

A significant percentage of patients with bilious vomiting have gross cardio-oesophageal incompetence and in the author's experience the degree of oesophagitis correlates well with the severity of symptoms. Oesophageal manometry and motility studies are necessary in this group of patients as they may indicate the need for an antireflux procedure rather than a major reconstructive or diversional operation.

Medical therapy

There is no indication for surgical intervention in patients with mild to moderate vasomotor dumping and in patients with postgastrectomy reactive hypoglycaemia (late dumping). All patients with diarrhoea should be investigated medically to exclude malabsorption, and the exact mechanism thereof determined. Initially treatment is conservative with intestinal sedatives and bile salt binding agents (cholestyramine or activated charcoal). Surgery is undertaken if the above management fails, if the diarrhoea is intractable or if a surgically correctable lesion is encountered on investigation.

Preoperative care

Severe symptoms are usually attended by a diminished dietary intake and largely because of this, the patients are frequently malnourished. Preoperative parenteral nutrition for a period of 2 weeks should be instituted in patients with significant weight loss and biochemical evidence of malnutrition. The parenteral feeding is continued over the postoperative period until the patient is able to ingest an adequate well balanced diet.

Anaemia is often present. It is usually of the iron-deficient type though a macrocytic picture may be found in patients with previous subtotal/total gastric resections. Further investigation is required with serum B12 and folate levels in addition to a bone marrow biopsy. Correction of the anaemia is desirable before all major surgical reconstructions. A macrocytic anaemia may be the result of bacterial overgrowth when it is usually associated with hypoproteinaemia and steatorrhoea.

Remedial operations

Vasomotor dumping

A useful classification of this syndrome is that of Fenger *et al.*[5] into slight, moderate and severe. Dumping is judged to be slight when attacks are infrequent and the capacity for work is normal. By contrast, in severe dumping the attacks are frequent, severe and accompanied by evidence of malnutrition and a marked reduction of the ability for work. Only patients with severe and persistent dumping symptoms despite adequate dietary management should be considered for remedial surgical treatment. The exact procedure depends on the nature of the previous surgical intervention(s), the objective being to slow down the rapid gastric emptying which underlies the pathophysiology of this condition.

VASOMOTOR DUMPING IN PATIENTS AFTER TRUNCAL VAGOTOMY AND DRAINAGE

The easiest patients to manage are those with a gastroenterostomy where the initial treatment consists of taking down the gastroenterostomy. Excellent results have been obtained in 8 out of 10 patients operated on by the author. Two patients developed evidence of hold up and antral ulceration within 5 years and required further treatment with antrectomy and isoperistaltic jejunal interposition. Although the results of pyloric reconstruction after Heineke-Mikulicz (H-M) pyloroplasty are less certain, the procedure is simple and undoubtedly effective in some patients[6,7]. Good and substantial palliation was obtained by the author in 3 out of 5 patients. The failures were subsequently treated by an antrectomy and isoperistaltic interposition.

Technique of pyloric reconstruction after H-M pyloroplasty

The incision

For remedial gastric surgery, the author's preference is for a midline epigastric incision which skirts the right side of the umbilicus. If the patient has a wide subcostal angle an oblique epigastric approach gives excellent exposure. This incision starts at the upper third of the left costal margin, crosses the epigastrium and runs 2 cm below and parallel to the right costal margin.

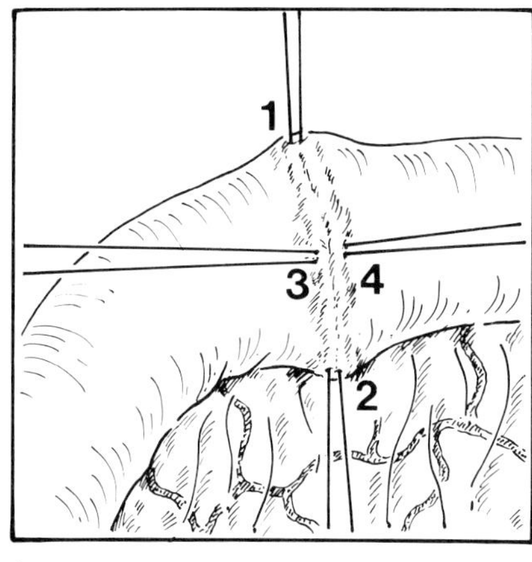

1

1

Exposure of pyloroplasty and insertion of stay sutures

Dense adhesions often bind the pyloroplasty to the undersurface of the right lobe of the liver, gall bladder, greater omentum and hepatic flexure. These have to be carefully divided until the normal anatomy is displayed and the entire extent of the antroduodenal scar is clearly visible. Black silk (3/0) stay sutures are inserted at the proximal (1) and distal end of the scar (2) and at either side of its midpoint (3, 4).

2a & b

Duodenoantrotomy through pyloroplasty scar

The antroduodenal region is opened by scalpel incision of the entire length of the pyloroplasty scar.

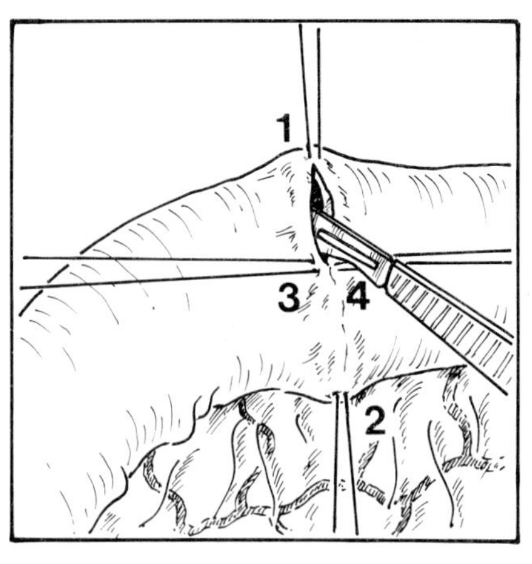

2a

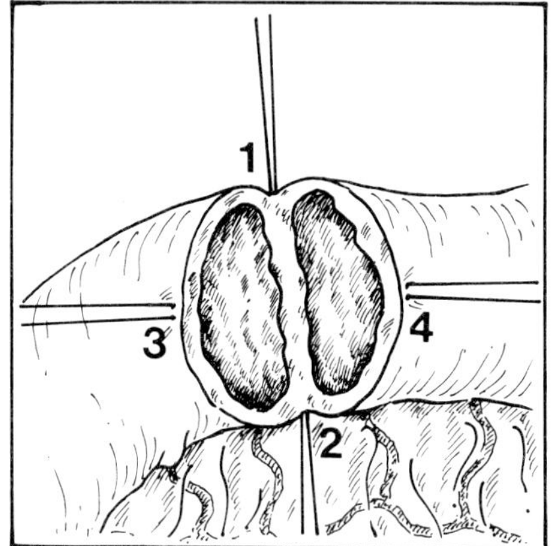

2b

3

The normal alignment of the duodenum and pyloric musculature is achieved by distraction of the midline stay sutures (3, 4) and overlapping and then traction of stay sutures (1, 2).

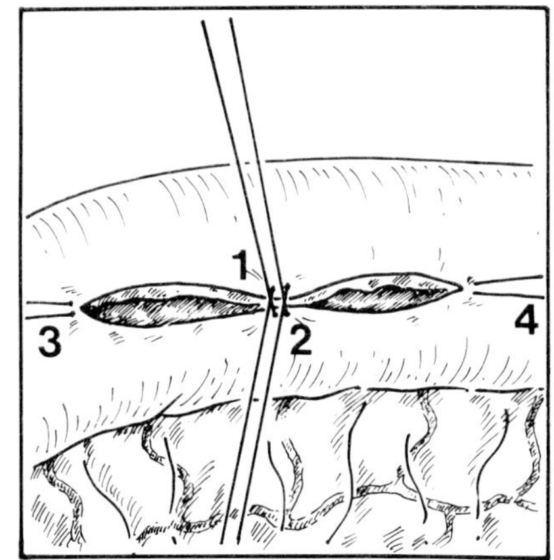

3

4

Suture of incision and closure

The duodenum is closed by carefully placed interrupted 3/0 black silk sutures. A nasogastric tube is inserted before closure of the abdomen and the tip positioned immediately proximal to the suture line. A silicone tube drain is left via a separate stab wound to the antroduodenal suture line.

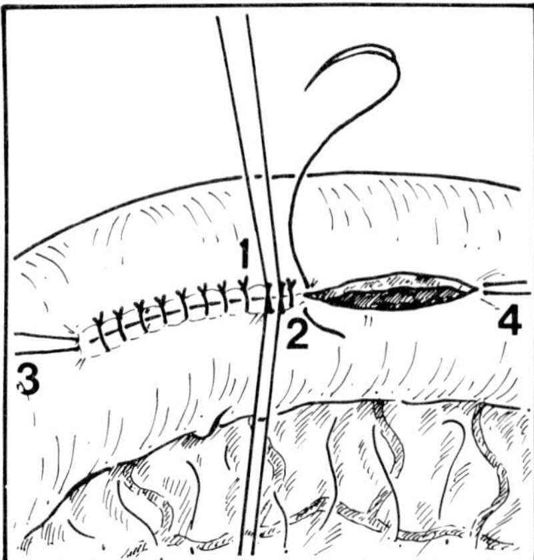

4

VASOMOTOR DUMPING AFTER PARTIAL GASTRECTOMY (POLYA, BILLROTH II)

The most commonly used operation has been the interposition of a jejunal segment between the gastric remnant and the duodenum. Considerable controversy still exists regarding whether the interposed loop should be anti- or isoperistaltic. The antiperistaltic interposition has been generally favoured[8, 9, 10]. However in a controlled clinical trial[11] the author found the two procedures to be equally effective in relieving vasomotor dumping symptoms, but the isoperistaltic interposition was not attended by serious complications such as severe bile reflux gastritis and stenosis of the proximal anastomosis encountered in some patients within the antiperistaltic group.

5

In any event it is important that the anatomy of the small intestinal loops is displayed before a jejunal segment is isolated. Certain loops of jejunum lie normally in an antiperistaltic position with respect to the ligament of Treitz and unless care is taken an unintentional antiperistaltic interposition can be effected or reversal of the loop may paradoxically result in an isoperistaltic interposition.

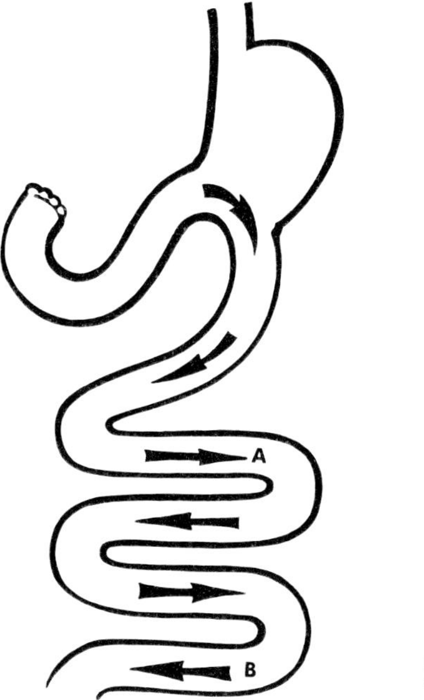

5

Loop A is antiperistaltic and would be changed into an isoperistaltic segment if it were reversed. Loop B is isoperistaltic and would need reversal if an antiperistaltic interposition between stomach remnant and duodenum is contemplated

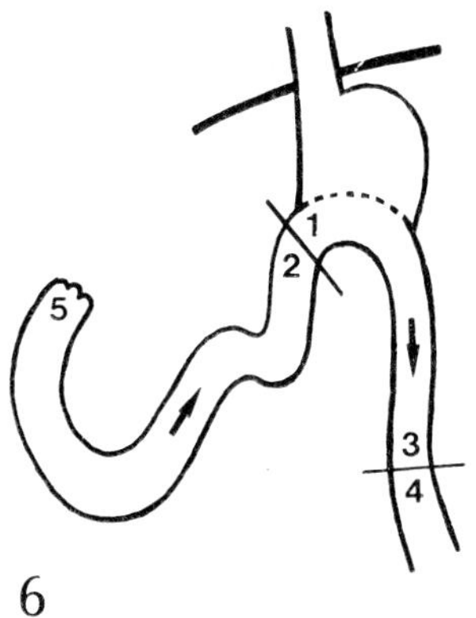

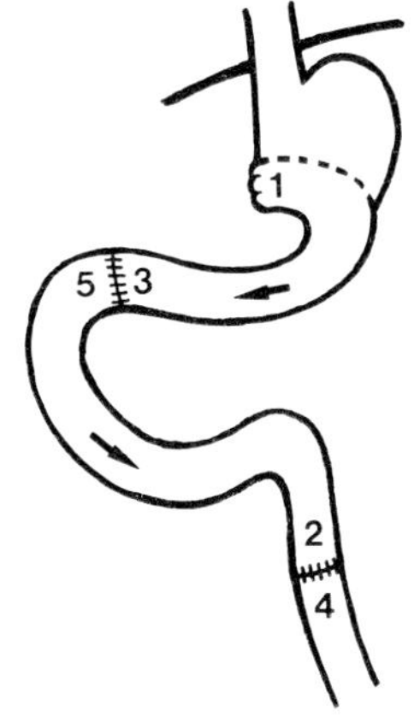

6

6

Soupault Bucaille procedure

In patients with Polya gastrectomy an isoperistaltic interposition may be performed by the Soupault Bucaille procedure when the efferent loop is transected some 12–15 cm from the stomach remnant and the proximal cut end anastomosed to the duodenal stump. The distal cut end of the efferent loop is then anastomosed to the afferent loop after the latter has been taken down from its junction with the stomach remnant.

7

Exposure and vagotomy

Through a midline incision the anatomy is displayed by division of the relevant adhesions. The entire stomach remnant requires mobilization usually from the undersurface of the liver and diaphragm. In addition the gastrojejunostomy or gastroduodenostomy should be displayed. Often adhesions involving the liver, gall bladder and hepatic flexure of the colon require division. An adequate mobilization of the second part of the duodenum by division of the peritoneum of the subhepatic pouch is essential for a safe anastomosis with the transposed jejunal loop. It is good policy to identify the bile duct at this stage. A truncal vagotomy is performed after division of the left triangular ligament of the liver and mobilization of the gastro-oesophageal junction. In previously vagotomized patients with a positive insulin test, exploration for the intact vagal trunk(s) and revagotomy must be done.

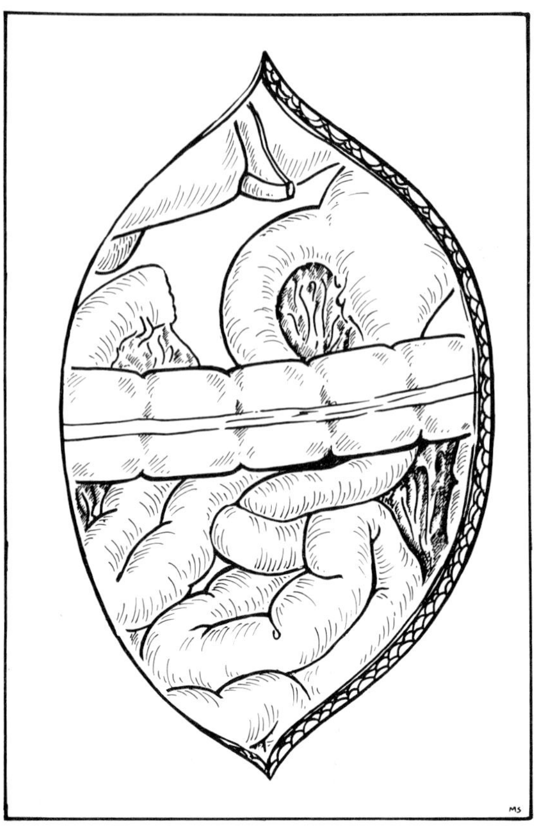

7

8

Two curved non-crushing clamps are applied on either side of the mobilized gastrojejunal anastomosis which is then disconnected along the junction of the jejunal loop to the stomach remnant preferably by scalpel incision. In patients with Billroth I gastrectomy, separation of the stomach from the duodenum should be delayed until after the construction of the jejunal loop to avoid contamination and prolonged clamping of the duodenum and stomach remnant.

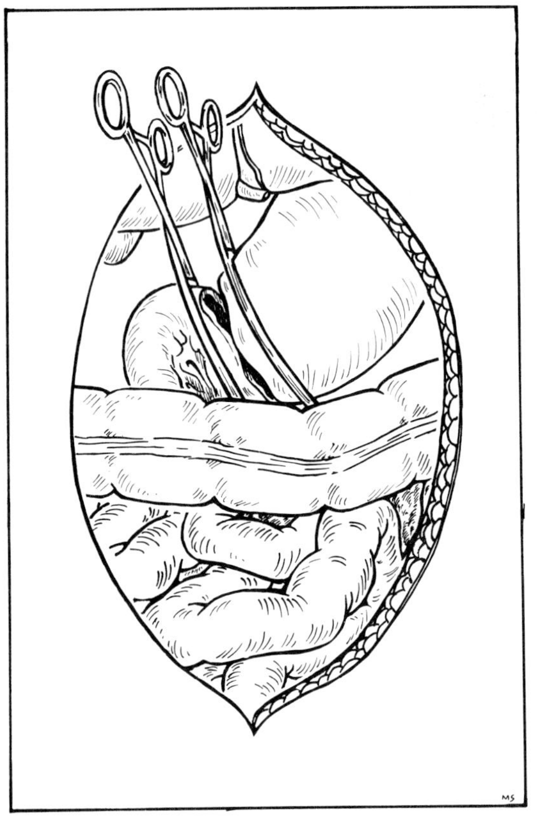

8

9

The detached jejunum is closed transversely with a single layer of 3/0 black silk interrupted seromuscular sutures. It is then replaced below the transverse mesocolon.

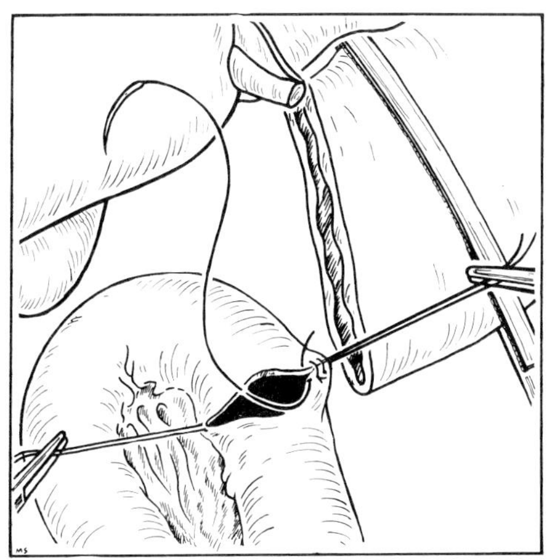

9

10

10

Choice of jejunal segment

A suitable segment of upper jejunum is selected and its lie in relation to the ligament of Treitz determined. Important factors which determine the choice of a particular segment of jejunum include freedom from adhesions of the bowel segment concerned and its mesentery, and the anatomy of the mesenteric arcades. The loop is measured along its antimesenteric border in the unstretched state. For antiperistaltic interpositions a length of 10–12.5 cm is marked by means of stay seromuscular sutures on the antimesenteric border of the gut. Isoperistaltic loops can be made longer without any risk of gastric retention and their recommended length varies from 12.5 to 20 cm, although the author's preference is for a 15 cm loop as this has been shown to result in a gastric emptying pattern that approximates to the normal[12].

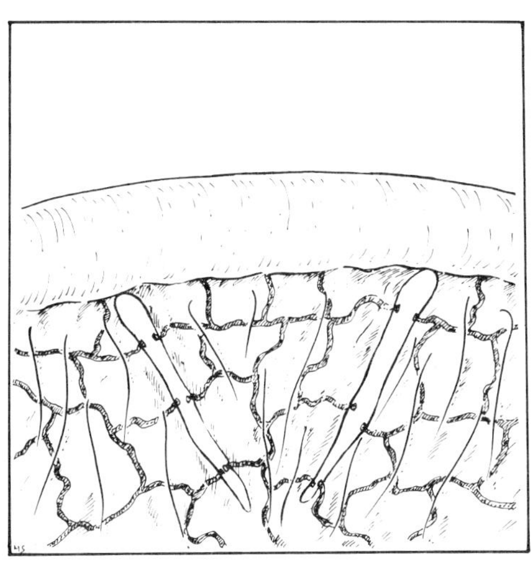

11

11

Construction of mesenteric vascular pedicle

The main vessels to the jejunal segment are identified and the vessels crossing the proposed line of division of the mesentery are individually ligated. The mesentery is then divided as far as the bowel edges on either side of the vascular pedicle.

12

Separation of jejunal segment

Non-crushing clamps are applied to the jejunum on either side of the demarcated segment and the small bowel transected at either end.

12

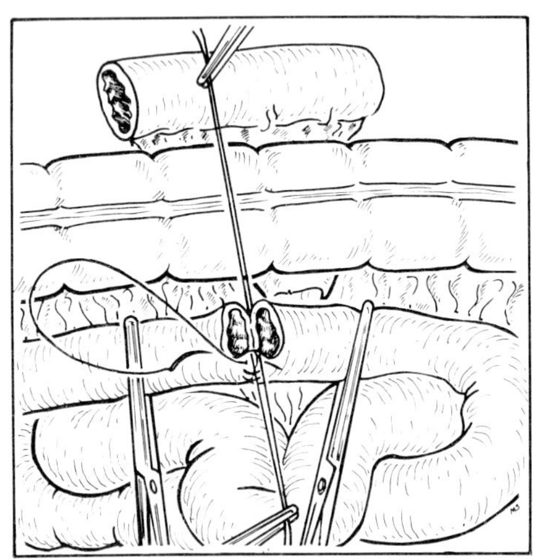

13

13

Transposition of jejunal loop to supracolic compartment and restoration of continuity of jejunum

The isolated loop is transferred to the supracolic compartment through the gap in the transverse mesocolon left after the posterior gastrojejunostomy was taken down. It is kept in between two moist gauze swabs in this compartment. The mesenteric pedicle of the transposed jejunal segment is sutured to the edges of the defect in the mesocolon which is then closed. The continuity of the jejunum is restored by means of an end-to-end anastomosis which is carried out in a single-layer technique with interrupted 3/0 black silk sutures.

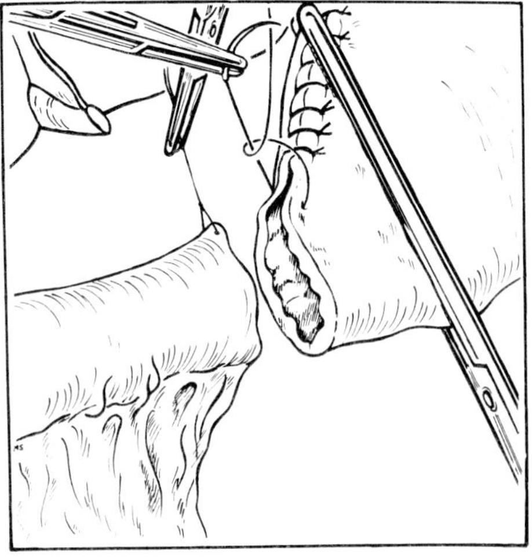

14

14

Preparation of gastric remnant

The gastric remnant is trimmed and its distal open end is partially closed with interrupted 3/0 black silk sutures to approximate its circumference to that of the jejunal loop. In patients with Billroth I anastomosis the stomach remnant is disconnected from the duodenum at this stage.

15

Jejunogastric anastomosis

This end-to-end anastomosis is carried out using a single-layer technique with 3/0 black silk interrupted seromuscular sutures. Two stay sutures are inserted at each end, and the posterior part of the anastomosis is sutured first.

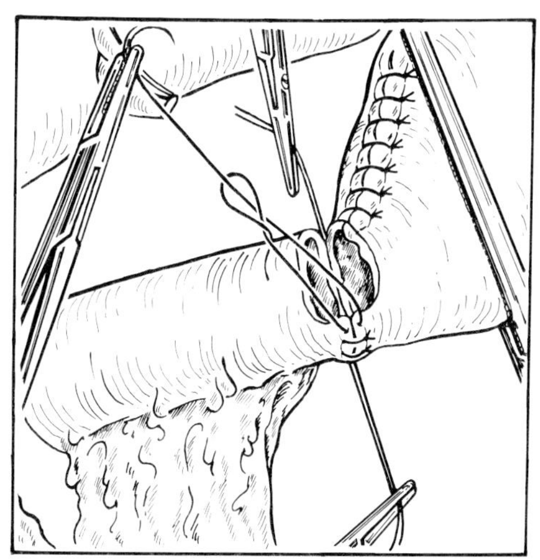

15

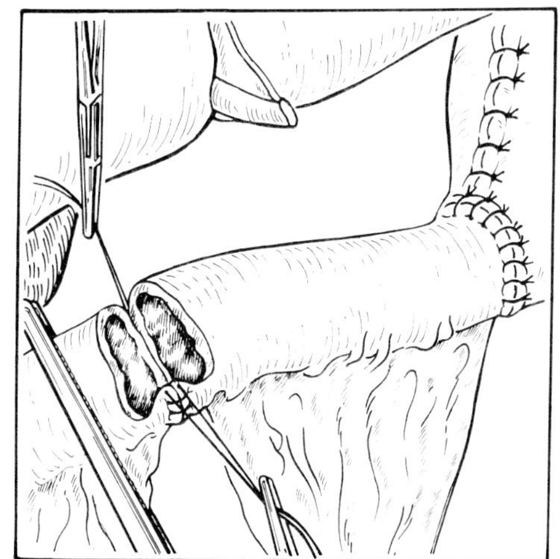

16a

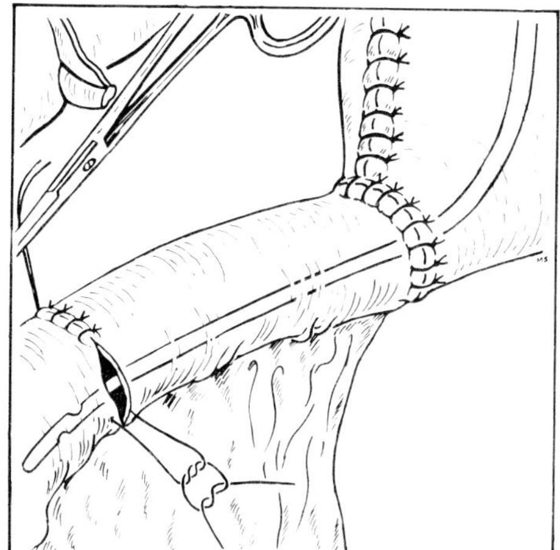

16b

Duodenojejunal anastomosis

16a & b

Whenever technically possible this anastomosis is carried out in an end-to-end fashion using a single-layer technique with interrupted 3/0 black silk seromuscular sutures. Before completion of the duodenojejunal anastomosis, the nasogastric tube is passed through the jejunal loop into the duodenum beyond the anastomosis.

If the duodenal stump is short, fibrosed and densely adherent to the head of the pancreas, the distal end of the jejunal loop can be anastomosed to the second part of the duodenum in an end-to-side fashion. This procedure is technically easy if adequate mobilization of the duodenum and head of the pancreas is performed initially.

17

Drainage and closure

Side holes are cut out in a silicone tube drain and this is then introduced through a separate stab wound. The drain is made to lie alongside the interposed jejunal loop. The abdominal wound is then closed with 2/0 black silk.

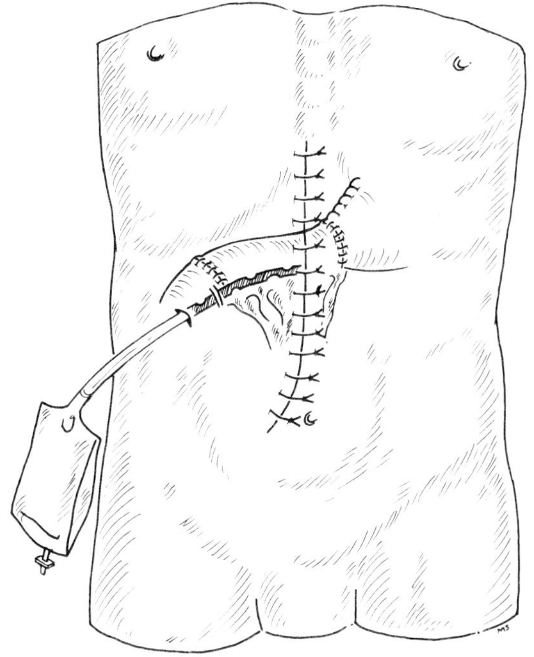

17

VASOMOTOR DUMPING AND SMALL STOMACH SYNDROME AFTER TOTAL/SUBTOTAL GASTRECTOMY

Although these patients experience vasomotor dumping as their dominant symptom, they also suffer from postcibal epigastric discomfort and fullness with early satiety. The entire symptom complex is often referred to as the small gastric remnant syndrome.

These patients, who are usually malnourished and anaemic, are the most difficult to manage. In the author's experience medical therapy is seldom successful and remedial surgery should be undertaken before the development of gross malnutrition and long-term postgastrectomy complications. Surgical treatment is designed to restore a reservoir between the oesophagogastric junction and the upper small bowel. Several procedures have been used but none have been adequately evaluated in the long term.

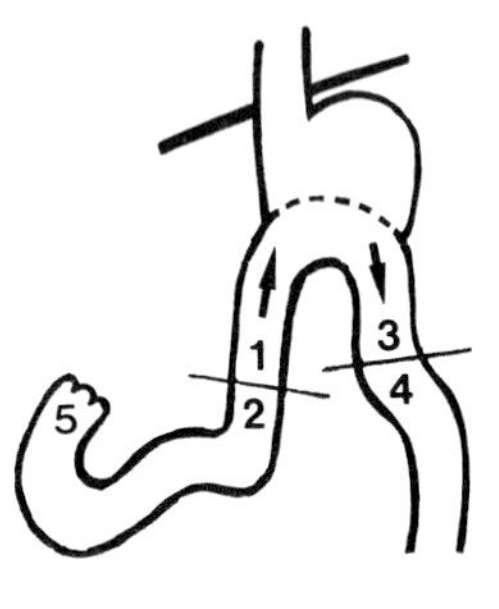

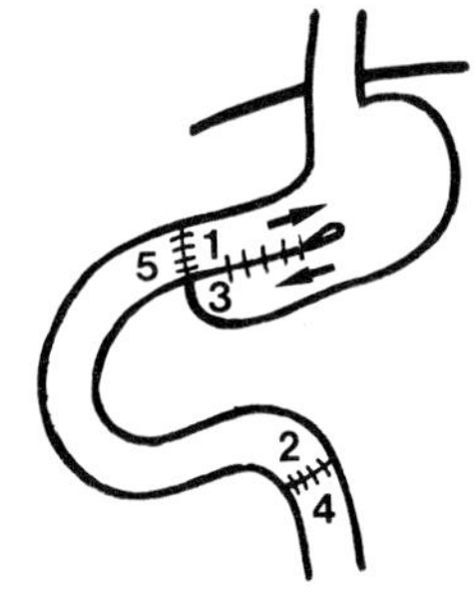

18

18

Poth pouch

In this procedure described by Poth[13], the gastroenterostomy is retained but both afferent and efferent limbs are divided 10–12 cm from the gastric remnant. The proximal cut end of the efferent (isoperistaltic) limb is closed and the distal end of the afferent limb (antiperistaltic) is anastomosed to the duodenal stump. The proximal end of the afferent limb is then joined to the distal end of the efferent limb. A long enteroenteric anastomosis is then performed between the two jejunal segments. The resulting reservoir receives an isoperistaltic inflow from the gastric remnant and has an antiperistaltic conduit to the duodenum.

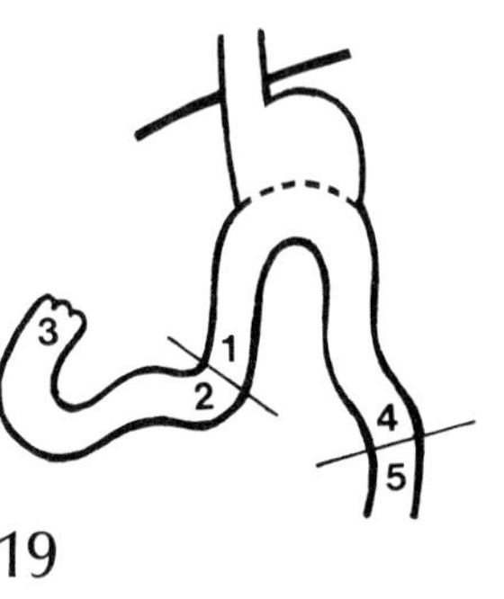

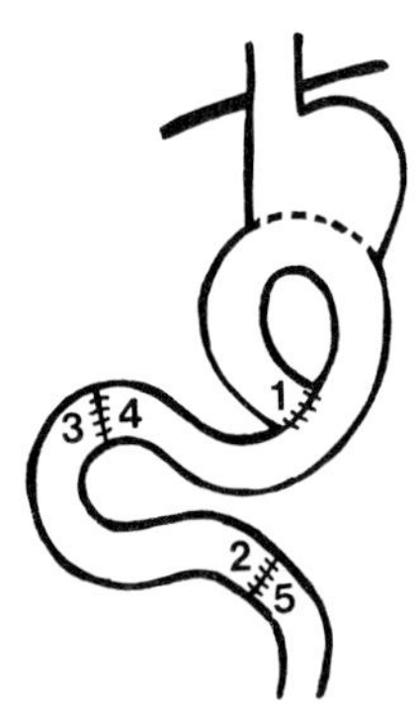

19

19

Circular loops

Both isoperistaltic and antiperistaltic circular loops are constructed distal to the gastroenterostomy after transection of both limbs 10–12 cm from the junction with the stomach remnant. The author has no personal experience with circular loops except for their removal in 3 patients because of the development of severe bacterial overgrowth and malabsorption.

20

Hunt-Lawrence pouch

This was first described by Hunt[14] and subsequently modified by Lawrence[15]. The afferent jejunal limb is divided 10–12 cm from the gastroenterostomy and its distal end closed. A long enteroenteric anastomosis is then performed between the closed afferent limb and the adjacent efferent limb. The proximal end of the afferent limb is then anastomosed end-to-side to the efferent limb (Roux-en-Y) some 40–60 cm distal to the gastrojejunostomy. The Hunt-Lawrence pouch has been most commonly used as a primary reconstructive procedure at the time of total/subtotal gastrectomy. A modification of the Hunt-Lawrence pouch is advocated by Lygidakis with two enteroenteric anastomoses between the closed afferent limb and the efferent limb.

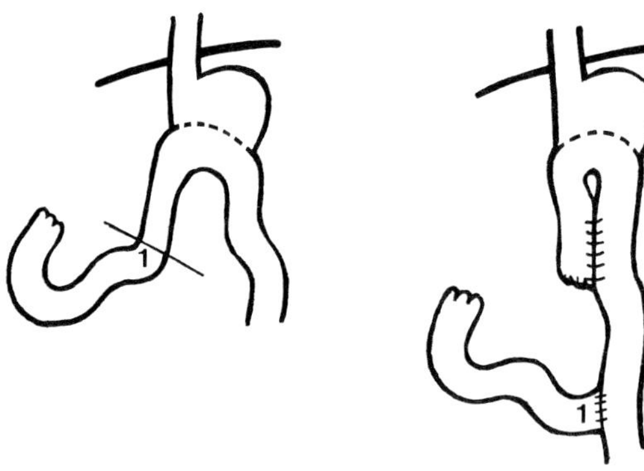

20

21

Tanner Roux-19 procedure

The author has no experience of this procedure, first reported in 1954[16], except to take one down because of severe malabsorption due to bacterial overgrowth. The operation entails the division of the afferent limb at an appropriate distance from the stomach remnant and its anastomosis in an end-to-side fashion to the efferent limb 10–15 cm distal to the gastrojejunostomy. The proximal divided end of the afferent limb is then anastomosed to the efferent limb as a Roux-en-Y 60 cm distal to the gastroenterostomy.

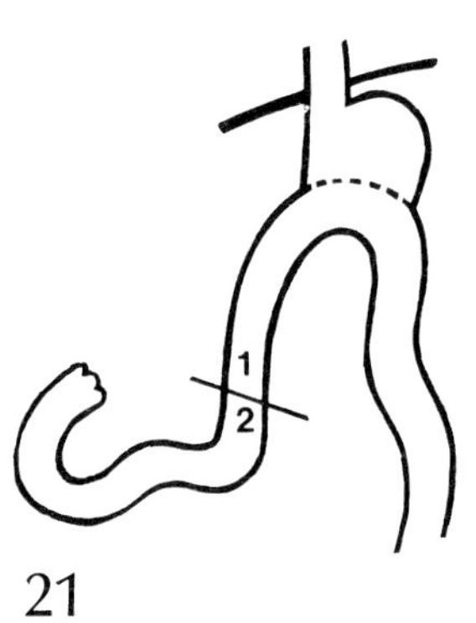

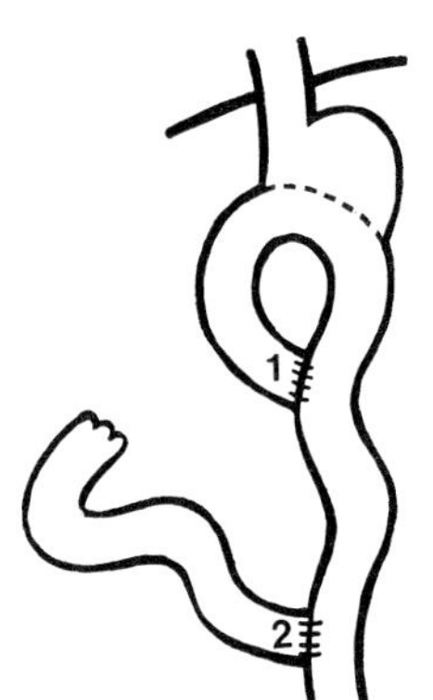

21

22

Hays pouch

This consists of a triple limb pouch between the stomach remnant and the duodenal stump[17]. The long-term results have been poor because of dilatation and stasis within the pouch[18, 19].

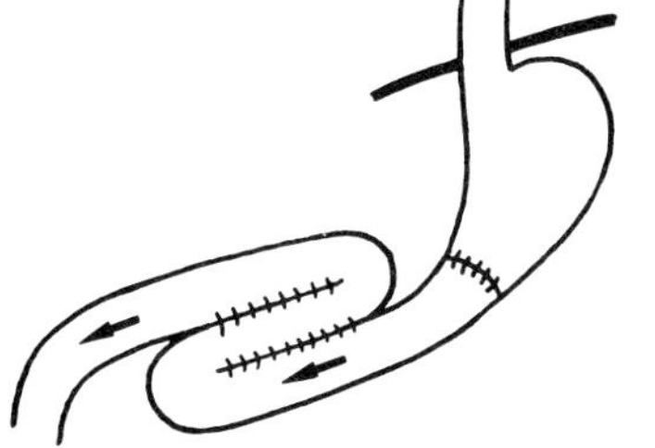

22

The author's procedure

The following operation has been performed in 8 subjects with severe malnutrition and disabling symptoms after high subtotal Polya gastrectomy. In addition the operation was undertaken in 10 subjects as a primary reconstructive procedure at the time of subtotal gastrectomy. The results over a period of 10 years have been good in 13 patients with a reasonable weight gain and absence of severe disabling symptoms. No long-term bacterial overgrowth problems have been encountered. Early satiety, post-prandial fullness and heartburn have been the residual complaints in 5 patients but these symptoms have improved with medical therapy.

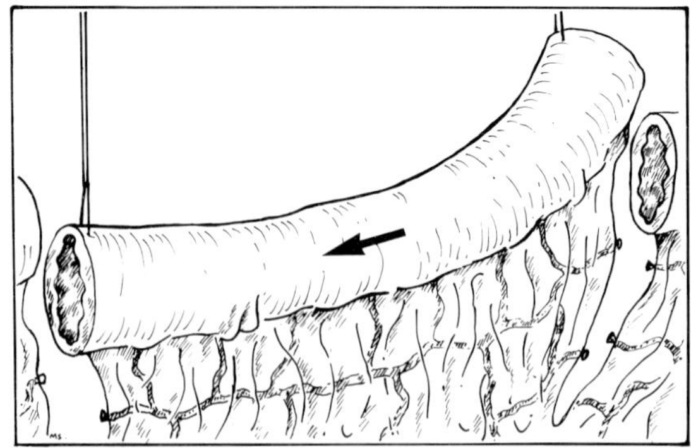

23

23

The procedure consists of isolating a 30 cm isoperistaltic jejunal segment.

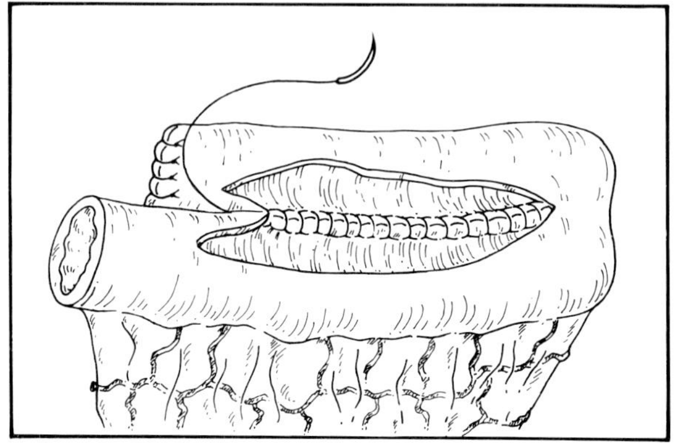

24

24

This is then folded on itself such that the lower limb is longer by 5 cm. The proximal end of the loop is closed with a single layer of interrupted 3/0 black silk sutures.

A long enteroenteric anastomosis is then performed between the two limbs using a two-layer technique with interrupted 3/0 black silk sutures and 2/0 chromic catgut.

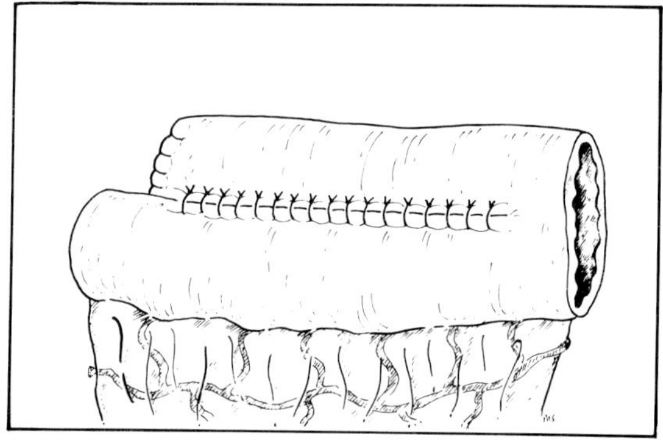

25

25

A 2 cm ellipse is cut out at the apex of the loop which is then anastomosed to the gastric remnant using a single-layer technique with non-absorbable sutures. Two stay sutures are inserted, one at either end, and the posterior part of the anastomosis is completed first.

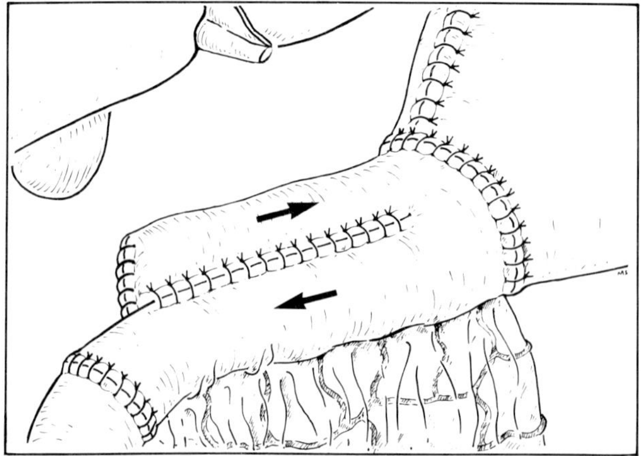

26

26

The distal end of the loop is then anastomosed to the duodenal stump using a similar one-layer technique with interrupted non-absorbable seromuscular sutures.

Reflux gastritis and bilious vomiting

Patients who complain of bile vomiting and abdominal pain after gastric surgery comprise a heterogenous group. They require full investigation to establish the exact pathology.

The most common are patients with *reflux gastritis* who complain of epigastric pain, nausea and vomiting in the early postprandial period. The pain is commonly burning and is not relieved by antacids. The vomit is either liquid bile or consists of food mixed with bile. The endoscopic findings include bile reflux, gastritis with an oedematous friable mucosa and superficial erosions. Often these patients are malnourished and anaemic.

Bile vomiting may be due to *intermittent obstruction* of either the afferent or efferent limb of a gastrojejunal anastomosis. In the afferent loop syndrome the pain is relieved by the vomiting which is often projectile and consists of fluid bilious material. Chronic efferent loop obstruction from adhesions, internal herniation or intussusception is best diagnosed by a barium meal.

Bilious vomiting may also be a dominant symptom in patients with *recurrent ulceration* and subsides with effective therapy for the underlying ulcer.

An important group consists of patients with gross *cardio-oesophageal incompetence* with or without a demonstrable hiatus hernia. These patients experience severe heartburn in addition to the bilious vomiting and have an associated oesophagitis; untreated, they may develop benign oesophageal stricture. It has been the author's practice to treat this group with antireflux operation.

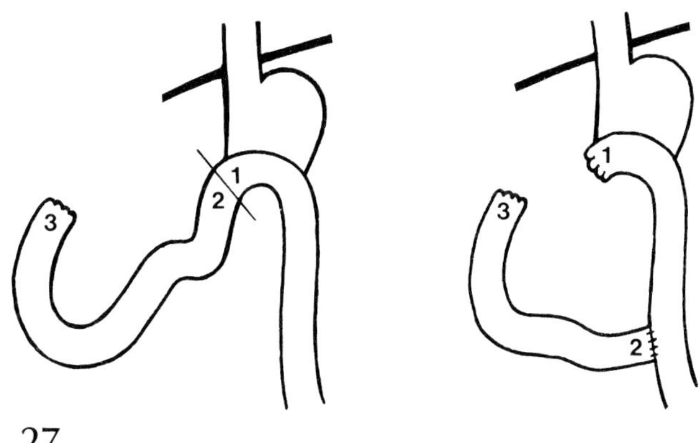

27

Not infrequently symptomatic reflux gastritis will improve with time. Initially therefore treatment is medical, with metoclopramide which is effective in promoting emptying in patients after partial gastrectomy and truncal vagotomy, and bile salt binding agents which are at times effective in this condition. Surgical treatment is considered only if symptoms persist despite medical therapy.

REFLUX GASTRITIS AFTER VAGOTOMY AND DRAINAGE

The author has obtained excellent results in patients with reflux gastritis following vagotomy and gastrojejunostomy by taking down the anastomosis between the stomach and small intestine. Gastric hold-up has occurred in 2 out of 11 patients, both of whom developed antral ulceration and required antrectomy and isoperistaltic interposition.

The results of 3 patients with pyloric reconstruction for reflux gastritis following vagotomy and H-M pyloroplasty performed by the author have been poor, and these patients are best treated by antrectomy and an isoperistaltic (15 cm) jejunal interposition.

REFLUX GASTRITIS AFTER POLYA GASTRECTOMY

Surgical treatment consists of either a Roux-en-Y diversion or an isoperistaltic jejunal interposition. Most experts favour the former procedure because of its technical simplicity and overall better reported results[20, 21] although there has not been a clinical trial of these two operations. Irrespective of which procedure is used, a truncal vagotomy is performed to prevent recurrent ulceration.

Roux-en-Y diversion

27

The afferent loop of the gastroenterostomy is divided near the stomach remnant and the distal end closed. The proximal end of the afferent loop is then anastomosed end-to-side to the efferent loop at least 40 cm and preferably 60 cm distal to the stomach remnant. Roux loops shorter than 40 cm are usually ineffective in eliminating reflux.

Roux-en-Y diversion after a Billroth I gastrectomy consists of mobilization with subsequent division of the gastroduodenal anastomosis and closure of the duodenal stump. Some trimming of the gastric remnant is advisable before anastomosis to the long limb of the Roux-en-Y loop.

Isoperistaltic jejunal interposition

The author favours this procedure for reflux gastritis after partial gastrectomy. The isoperistaltic interposition can be effected by the Soupault Bucaille procedure. If not, an isolated jejunal loop is transferred to the supracolic compartment. The optimal length of the loop in the author's experience has been 16–20 cm. Longer loops tend to kink and cause gastric outlet obstruction. The author has obtained a satisfactory result in 38 patients out of 45 treated with isoperistaltic interposition for reflux gastritis.

Diarrhoea and malabsorption

The reported incidence of diarrhoea after gastric surgery varies considerably. This is in part due to the lack of an agreed definition of diarrhoea. Although most commonly reported after truncal vagotomy and drainage, diarrhoea may follow partial gastrectomy or Roux-en-Y procedures to divert bile from the gastric remnant where this is usually associated with bacterial overgrowth and malabsorption.

Three patterns of diarrhoea are encountered after vagotomy[22]. The first consists of frequent loose motions often considered beneficial by previously constipated patients. The second variety consists of intermittent episodes of short-lived diarrhoea with normal bowel habits in between attacks. The third pattern consists of severe episodic explosive watery diarrhoea which is often associated with incontinence and malnutrition. Both the intermittent and the severe episodic diarrhoea may occur alone or in conjunction with other symptoms, most commonly vasomotor dumping. Despite the high figures reported in the literature on the incidence of postvagotomy diarrhoea, the severe and intractable disorder is encountered in less than 2 per cent of patients.

All patients with diarrhoea as a persistent dominant symptom should have faecal fat estimation. If steatorrhoea is established in this way then a complete malabsorption survey, including tests of small bowel function, jejunal mucosal biopsy and the ^{14}C cholate breath test for bacterial overgrowth, should be done. Out of a series of 21 patients with severe postvagotomy diarrhoea referred to the author the 3 patients with steatorrhoea were found to have significant but correctable pathology: adult coeliac disease, gastroileostomy and bacterial overgrowth due to a long and distended afferent loop.

The author has had to take down circular loops, Roux-19 procedures and some long Roux-en-Y diversions because of diarrhoea and malabsorption 5–10 years later. All patients improved with restoration of gastroduodenal continuity via an interposed jejunal loop.

The treatment of diarrhoea in the absence of a correctable cause remains problematic. Patients with mild or intermittent diarrhoea should be treated medically. Both intestinal sedatives and dietary manipulations are ineffective in the long term but substantial improvement is often obtained with bile salt binding agents as these patients excrete abnormal amounts of chenodeoxycholate in the faeces. However in the author's experience no patient with severe and intractable diarrhoea has obtained sustained palliation with either cholestyramine or activated charcoal.

SURGICAL PROCEDURES FOR INTRACTABLE DIARRHOEA

Reversed jejunal segment

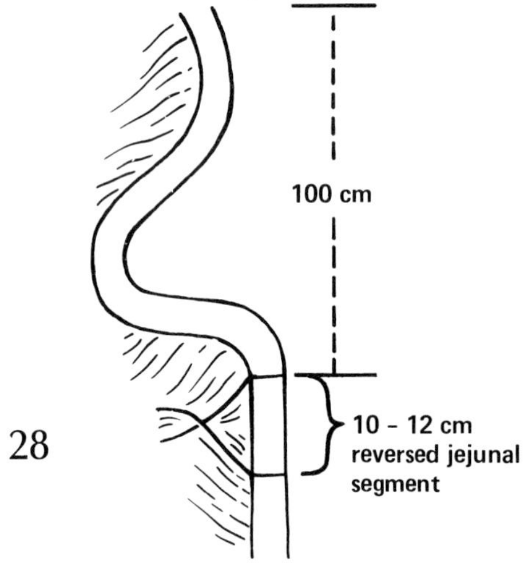

28

28

Herrington-Sawyers' procedure[23] consists of the reversal of a 10–12 cm jejunal segment some 100 cm distal to the ligament of Treitz. The jejunal segment is first isolated, rotated 180° and then reanastomosed at either end to the proximal and distal small bowel. This procedure is based on the experimental work of Hammer *et al.*[24] who reported a beneficial effect on survival by a reversed segment after massive small bowel resection. The author has performed this operation on 6 patients with one long-term beneficial effect. Complications which necessitated removal of the reversed jejunal segment in 3 patients were severe attacks of postprandial colic and distention, severe eructations of foul air and recurrent ulceration associated with hypersecretion of acid.

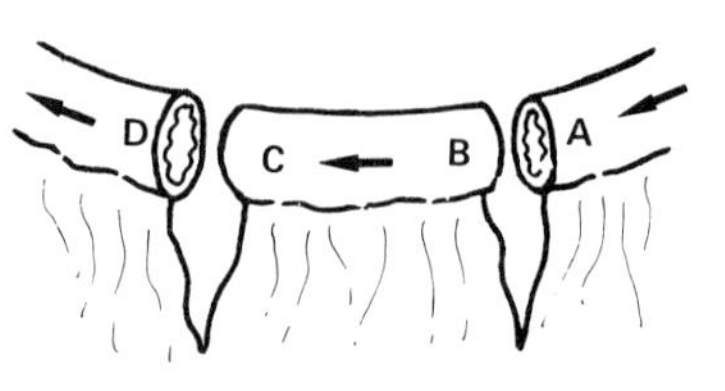

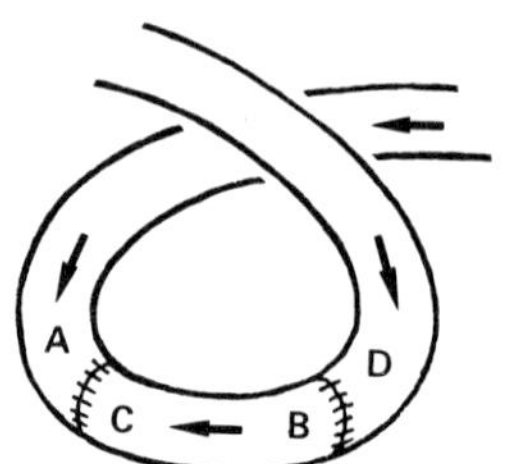

29

29

The Poth procedure[25] is essentially a jejunal antiperistaltic segment created by isolating a 20 cm loop and then transposing the proximal and distal small bowel to the opposite ends of the isolated loop, thereby creating an antiperistaltic segment without reversal. The author has no experience of this procedure and is unaware of any large reported series.

Antiperistaltic ileal segments

The author has found that procedures involving the creation of a distal antiperistaltic segment some 40 cm from the ileocaecal valve to be the most beneficial procedure for severe and disabling diarrhoea after gastric surgery. An ileal loop some 8 cm long is isolated. It is then rotated 180° about its pedicle before reanastomosis in continuity with the small bowel. Alternatively the antiperistaltic effect can be achieved by the Poth manoeuvre or a modification of it described by Rygick[26]. Relief from the diarrhoea in 7 out of 8 patients has been obtained by the author using a distal ileal antiperistaltic segment without any severe complications. As one patient subsequently developed appendicitis which caused diagnostic difficulties and technical problems during the appendicectomy because of involvement of the antiperistaltic segment in the appendix mass, the author now routinely includes an appendicectomy as part of the procedure. The Poth and the Rygick methods of creating an antiperistaltic segment without reversal are equally safe but patients are prone to attacks of postprandial colicky abdominal pain, which however tend to subside after several months.

The Rygick procedure

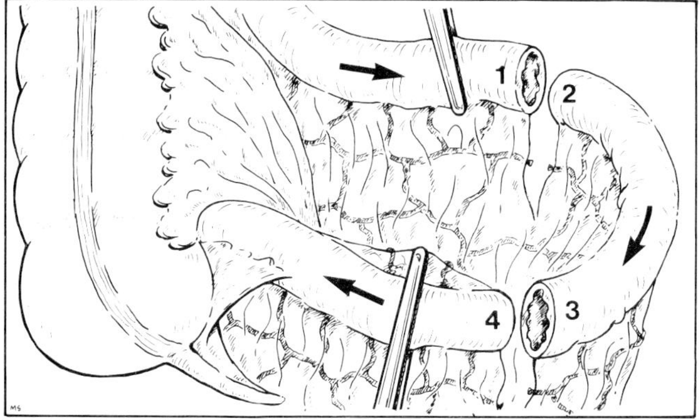

30

30

A 12 cm segment of ileum is isolated some 40 cm from the ileocaecal valve.

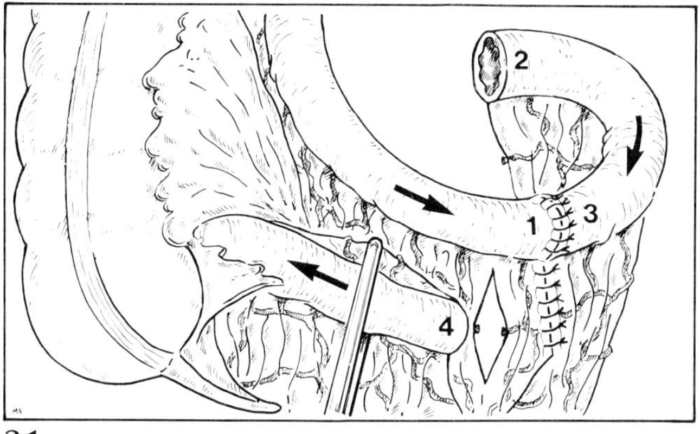

31

31

The proximal small bowel is anastomosed to the distal end of the isolated loop.

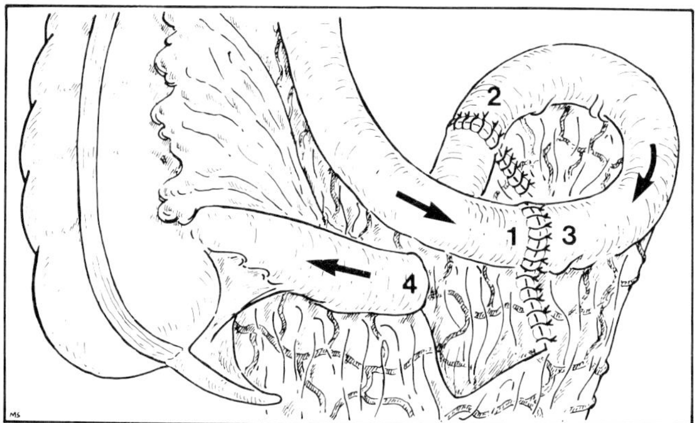

32

32

A small window is created in the mesentery through which the distal small bowel is passed before its anastomosis to the proximal end of the isolated segment. Both anastomoses are carried out in a single-layer technique with 3/0 non-absorbable interrupted seromuscular sutures. The mesenteric gaps are then closed with interrupted sutures.

References

1. Koffman, C. G., Elder, J. B., Gillespie, I. E. *et al.* A prospective randomized trial of vagotomy in chronic duodenal ulceration. British Journal of Surgery 1979; 66: 145–148

2. Christiansen, J., Jensen, H. E., Elby-Poulsen, P., Bardram, L., Henriksen, F. W. Prospective controlled vagotomy trial for duodenal ulcer. Annals of Surgery 1981; 193: 49–55

3. Leeds, A. R., Ralphs, D. N. L., Ebied, F., Metz, G., Dilawari, J. B. Pectin in the dumping syndrome: reduction of symptoms and plasma volume changes. Lancet 1981; 1: 1075–1078

4. Mackie, C. R., Wisbey, M., Cuschieri, A. Milk-^{99}Tc^{m} EHIDA test for enterogastric bile reflux. British Journal of Surgery 1981; 68: 351

5. Fenger, H. J., Gudmand-Hoyer, E., Kallenhauge, H. E., Andreassen, M. Clinical experience with isoperistaltic interposition of a jejunal segment for the incapacitating dumping syndrome. Annals of Surgery 1971; 175: 274–278

6. Regan, J. F., Schmutzer, K. J., Stemmer, E. A. Procedures of value for the prevention and cure of dumping after vagotomy and pyloroplasty. American Journal of Surgery 1972; 124: 279–286

7. Christiansen, P. M., Hart-Hansen, O., Pedersen, T. Reconstruction of the pylorus for postvagotomy diarrhoea and dumping. British Journal of Surgery 1974; 61: 519–520

8. Sawyers, J. L., Herrington, J. L., Jr. Superiority of antiperistaltic jejunal segments in management of severe dumping symptoms. Annals of Surgery 1973; 178: 311–321

9. Herrington, J. L., Jr. Reversed jejunal segment one year after operation. American Journal of Surgery 1970; 119: 340–342

10. Alexander-Williams, J. Gastric reconstructive surgery. Annals of the Royal College of Surgeons of England 1973; 52: 1–17

11. Cuschieri, A. Isoperistaltic and antiperistaltic jejunal interposition for the dumping syndrome. A comparative study. Journal of the Royal College of Surgeons of Edinburgh 1977; 22: 319–324

12. Mackie, C. R., Hall, A. W., Clark, J., Wisbey, M., Baker, P. R., Cuschieri, A. The effect of isoperistaltic jejunal interposition upon gastric emptying. Surgery, Gynecology and Obstetrics 1981; 153: 813–819

13. Poth, E. J. The dumping syndrome and its surgical treatment. American Surgeon 1957; 23: 1097–2013

14. Hunt, C. J. Construction of a food pouch from segment of jejunum as a substitute for stomach in total gastrectomy. Archives of Surgery 1952; 64: 601–608

15. Lawrence, W. J., Jr. Reservoir construction after total gastrectomy. Annals of Surgery 1962; 155: 191–198

16. Tanner, N. C. Surgery of peptic ulceration and its complications. Postgraduate Medical Journal 1954; 30: 448–465

17. Hays, R. P. Anatomic and physiologic reconstruction following total gastrectomy by the use of a jejunal food pouch. Surgical Forum 1953; 4: 291–295

18. Woodward, E. R., Hastings, N. Surgical treatment of the postgastrectomy dumping syndrome. Surgery, Gynecology and Obstetrics 1960; 111: 429–437

19. Nelson, A. R. Simpler surgery in the treatment of postgastrectomy malnutrition. American Journal of Surgery 1972; 124: 750–753

20. Drapanas, T., Bethea, M. Reflux gastritis following gastric surgery. Annals of Surgery 1974; 179: 618–627

21. Herrington, J. L., Jr, Sawyers, J. L., Whitehead, W. A. Surgical management of reflux gastritis. Annals of Surgery 1974; 180: 526–537

22. Logan, H. Steatorrhoea and diarrhoea after vagotomy: A comparison of drainage procedures. Gut 1964; 5: 188–191

23. Herrington, J. L., Jr, Edwards, W. H., Carter, J. H., Sawyers, J. L. Treatment of severe postvagotomy diarrhoea by reversed jejunal segment. Annals of Surgery 1968; 168: 522–541

24. Hammer, J. M., Seay, T. H., Johnston, R. L., Hill, E. J., Prust, F. H., Campbell, R. J. The effect of antiperistaltic bowel segments on intestinal emptying time. Archives of Surgery 1959; 79: 537–541

25. Poth, E. J. The use of gastrointestinal reversal in surgical procedures. American Journal of Surgery 1969; 118: 893–899

26. Rygick, A. V., Nasarov, L. V. Antiperistaltic displacement of an ileo loop without twisting its mesentery. Diseases of the Colon and Rectum 1969; 12: 409–502

Perforated peptic ulcer

N. A. Matheson ChM, FRCS, FRCS(Ed.)
Consultant Surgeon, Aberdeen General Hospitals

Preoperative

Indications

Most patients with perforated peptic ulcer should be treated by operation, but there is a small place for conservative management. Those who have typical symptoms but of short duration with improvement by the time of hospital admission and in whom the signs of peritoneal irritation are localized may, particularly when free gas is absent or minimal, have a small perforation which has already been sealed off with fibrin, omentum or an adjacent viscus. Therefore, operation is avoidable and treatment is by withholding oral fluids and the institution of continuous gastric decompression using a vented naso-gastric tube. Recovery is usually dramatically rapid but a state of preparedness should be kept lest there be evidence of renewed peritoneal contamination. Such a policy is particularly appropriate if, in addition to the above criteria, there is no antecedent dyspeptic history – a circumstance which is in favour of an acute rather than a chronic duodenal ulcer. Non-operative management is less attractive in women than in men because women who perforate are more likely to have a gastric than a duodenal ulcer.

In elderly patients with advanced cardiac or respiratory disease the benefit of operation must be weighed against its hazards. In some of these patients, and in those who refuse operation, non-operative management may be the best treatment whatever the severity of clinical signs and should be pursued with vigour and enthusiasm rather than in a spirit of hopelessness.

Preoperative treatment

The first essential of preoperative treatment is pain relief. Whoever is responsible for management decisions must lose no time in arranging effective analgesia usually with an adequate dose of morphine given slowly intravenously. Once this has been done a vented nasogastric tube is passed for continuous gastric decompression and arrangements are made for operation without delay. To avoid unnecessary discomfort, the abdominal skin should not be shaved until the patient is anaesthetized. An intravenous infusion is established but it is not usual for those who now arrive in hospital soon after perforation to show deficits in extracellular fluid of an extent that require the operation to be delayed for their correction.

Choice of procedure

Before opening the abdomen it is usually possible to make a provisional decision on what operation is to be done. Simple closure of a duodenal perforation fulfils the principles of emergency surgery, gives excellent immediate results and is safe in inexperienced hands. Unfortunately, two-thirds of patients who have had a perforated duodenal ulcer simply closed have recurrence of troublesome dyspeptic symptoms. Therefore, there is an increasing tendency to use a definitive procedure, usually vagotomy but occasionally partial gastrectomy, in patients who merit it on the basis of the severity and length of their antecedent history taken in conjunction with their present perforation. Earlier fears that vagotomy in the presence of peritoneal contamination would lead to mediastinitis appear groundless, though it is for this reason that some apply a deadline of 8 h from the time of perforation after which vagotomy is held to be unsafe. With experience the use of a definitive procedure in selected patients is not associated with increased mortality. However, the outcome of widespread adoption of such a practice in perforated duodenal ulcer, with resulting relaxation in the criteria of selection and with the inexperienced tempted to 'try their hands', is at best uncertain. Therefore, in general, simple closure remains the procedure of choice except in well chosen circumstances.

When perforation of a duodenal ulcer is associated with haemorrhage, a definitive procedure with control of the site of bleeding is mandatory.

In perforated gastric ulcer the choice of procedure is influenced by the fact that one-third of perforated gastric ulcers prove to be malignant. Biopsy is unreliable in establishing the nature of the perforated ulcer. In addition, a perforated gastric ulcer, which is often larger and whose edges are more friable than a perforated duodenal ulcer, is liable to break down or bleed after simple closure. Therefore, with few exceptions, perforated gastric ulcer is best treated by partial gastrectomy.

If a patient who has previously had a gastrojejunal anastomosis with or without gastric resection presents with the features of perforated ulcer, a diagnosis of perforated stomal ulcer may be made with confidence. After vagotomy such an occurrence is rare. The perforation, which is jejunal and close to the stoma, may be treated with good immediate results by simple closure but recurrence is inevitable. Therefore, if the experience of the operator and the patient's condition are such that it may be undertaken without additional hazard to survival, a procedure to diminish acid secretion further is appropriate and will vary according to the original operation.

The operations

Choice of incision

The best incision for emergency abdominal surgery is through the midline. An upper midline incision is attractively simple, rapidly made and involves less tissue trauma than incisions across muscle planes. Such an incision may be freely extended and gives excellent access either for simple closure or for a definitive operation. Reoperation, if necessary later, is straightforward through a midline scar. The possible criticism that midline incisions are prone to dehiscence and herniation is answered by the use of a mass closure technique.

Though it is possible to close a perforated duodenal ulcer through a small incision, efficient management of gross peritoneal contamination requires that the incision be large enough for the hand to be inserted through it – smallness of the incision is an undesirable aim.

If a definitive procedure is decided upon, the midline incision is made from xiphoid to umbilicus. Though easily done it is seldom necessary to extend it beyond the umbilicus. The skin incision need not extend cephalad beyond the tip of the xiphoid, but exposure to the oesophageal hiatus may be improved by dividing the fibromuscular attachments and the underlying peritoneum to the left of the xiphoid to enter the apex of the angle between the xiphoid and the left costal margin. The margins of the resulting space are rigid but a Deaver retractor can be accommodated to facilitate exposure of the hiatus during vagotomy. Even better exposure is given by the use of a sternal lifting retractor connected by chain to a rigid overbar fixed to the operating table. If this is available the costoxiphoid angle need not be entered.

PERFORATED DUODENAL ULCER – SIMPLE CLOSURE

Once the peritoneum has been opened and the diagnosis confirmed, gastrointestinal contents are removed from the peritoneal cavity by suction. This is facilitated by insinuating a hand between viscera and abdominal wall to make a space into which the sucker may be inserted. Both subphrenic spaces, the paracolic gutters and the pelvis are dealt with in turn. It is rational then, or after the perforation is closed, to wash out the peritoneal cavity with 2–3 litres of saline with or without an antibiotic.

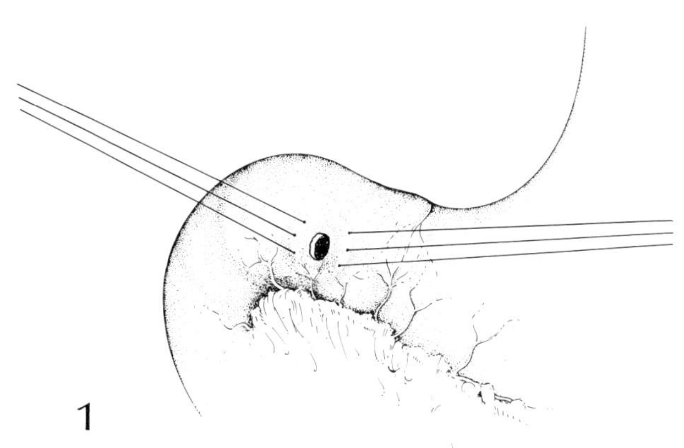

1

1

The right margin of the incision is retracted and the assistant draws the stomach and pylorus to the left by traction on a gauze swab thereby improving access to the site of perforation. Most duodenal perforations are small and easily closed. The simplest method which has amply stood the test of time is to plug the defect with a convenient frond of omentum. Sutures of 0/0 or 2/0 chromic catgut on an atraumatic 30 mm needle are passed through all layers of the duodenal wall sufficiently far from the margin of the perforation that they are unlikely to tear out because of friability. More than three such stitches are seldom necessary and in a small perforation, two may suffice. After placement, the sutures are left long and may be held in the tip of an artery forceps.

2 & 3

A convenient frond of omentum with enough bulk to plug the defect is grasped in the tip of an artery forceps and drawn over the perforation to be held in place by the assistant. The stitches are then tied over the omental plug, top and bottom stitches being tied first so that tension on the middle stitch, which is the most likely to cut out, is reduced. However, cutting out should be avoided by tying each stitch with just sufficient tension to retain the omental plug snugly in position.

Drainage of the peritoneal cavity is unnecessary.

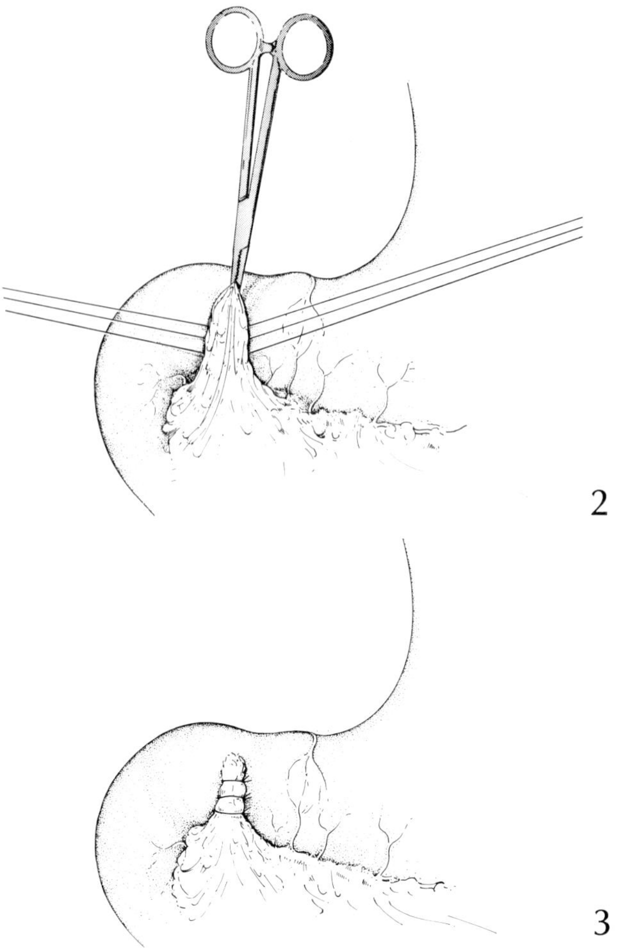

PERFORATION WITH OBSTRUCTION

At times a perforated duodenal ulcer may be associated with so much surrounding oedema that duodenal obstruction may appear to be a hazard after operation, leading the inexperienced to take refuge by making a gastrojejunostomy. Duodenal obstruction associated with perforation is not often of lasting significance and almost never cicatricial. Therefore, an additional procedure to relieve such obstruction is seldom necessary. However, in the infrequent circumstance in which obstruction appears inevitable were the perforation closed, a definitive operation is indicated and a gastroenterostomy alone should definitely be avoided.

PERFORATION WITH HAEMORRHAGE

Although posterior ulcers are more likely to bleed, anterior ulcers are not free from similar risk. Infrequently, perforation and haemorrhage from an anterior ulcer may coexist.

Simple closure of a perforated duodenal ulcer which is associated with clinically apparent bleeding is unreliable and exposes the patient to the risk of a second procedure for its arrest. Therefore, a definitive procedure which will effect immediate and, as far as possible, lasting control of the bleeding site is the aim. Though the source of bleeding is related to the perforated ulcer rather than to the unlikely coexistence of a posterior ulcer which has bled simultaneously, it may not be from the edge of the perforation, which is but the deepest part of the ulcer crater and does not always coincide with the whole extent of underlying mucosal denudation. In such patients permanent control of the source of bleeding through a pylorotomy incision is less certainly achieved than in patients with bleeding alone. Thus, truncal vagotomy and pyloroplasty, though a possible approach, is not ideal. Similarly, simple closure combined with truncal vagotomy and gastroenterostomy cannot be relied on to control the bleeding. Therefore, when perforation and bleeding occur simultaneously, partial gastrectomy of the Billroth II (Kronlein-Polya) type is advisable.

DEFINITIVE OPERATION FOR PERFORATED DUODENAL ULCER

Indications

Apart from the special circumstances of perforated duodenal ulcer associated with bleeding, the propriety of treating a patient definitively at the time of otherwise uncomplicated perforation should always be considered. If perforation or bleeding has occurred on a previous occasion or if the patient's previous dyspeptic symptoms would justify elective operation in the absence of perforation then clear-cut indications for definitive treatment exist. Such treatment should also be considered in any patient with perforation whose past symptoms clearly indicate chronic duodenal ulcer inasmuch as a definitive procedure will very likely be necessary in the future. However, the frequency with which a definitive operation is done for perforated duodenal ulcer will rightly depend on the skill of the operator. Should he lack experience of operating electively for duodenal ulcer, simple closure remains a safe and straightforward procedure which gives excellent immediate results.

Because bacterial contamination of the peritoneal fluid increases with time it has been customary to impose a time limit beyond which a definitive procedure is considered inadvisable. Though a risk of mediastinal infection introduced at vagotomy has been over-emphasized it is nevertheless a sound principle to limit surgical procedures to a minimum in the presence of peritoneal sepsis. Therefore if 12 h or more have passed since the time of perforation, intent should be concentrated on saving life; definitive treatment should probably be avoided in favour of simple closure with peritoneal lavage.

Choice of operations

The choice of operation is influenced by the procedure with which the operator is accustomed to treat duodenal ulcer electively. Occasionally, however, it may be necessary to depart from habit and the case for partial gastrectomy as the most reliable operation for perforated duodenal ulcer complicated by bleeding has already been considered. There are also infrequent circumstances where the size of the perforation, particularly in awkwardly situated superior ulcers, and the friability of the adjacent duodenal wall is such that partial gastrectomy is the safest operation. Such conditions apply in particular to recurrent perforation some days after simple closure.

Except in these difficult situations vagotomy is as appropriate in the presence of perforation as it is electively. Highly selective vagotomy (proximal gastric vagotomy, parietal cell vagotomy) properly done gives better results electively than truncal vagotomy and drainage and is currently the procedure of choice in elective duodenal ulcer surgery. The operation, however, is both technically demanding and time-consuming and without special experience and a slim patient can seldom be appropriate as an emergency procedure. Therefore, for most perforated duodenal ulcers a decision in favour of definitive operation will mean truncal vagotomy with a drainage procedure together with acceptance that the long-term results of such a combination will be inferior to those of highly selective vagotomy.

Previously we have advocated truncal vagotomy and pyloroplasty in perforated duodenal ulcer but there is increasing awareness of the imperfect results of operations that destroy normal gastric emptying. In addition, symptomatic disturbances of gastric emptying secondary to gastric drainage are more amenable to later surgical correction after gastroenterostomy in which dismantling the anastomosis is much easier than attempting to reconstruct the pylorus after pyloroplasty. Accordingly, the pylorus should usually be preserved and most definitive operations for perforated duodenal ulcer will therefore comprise closure of the perforation, truncal vagotomy and gastroenterostomy. In practice the combination is unfortunate in that first, gastroenterostomy is not so simple for the inexperienced as pyloroplasty; second, the postoperative course may not be so smooth; and third, the long-term results are inferior to highly selective vagotomy. In effect a decision in favour of definitive treatment for perforated duodenal ulcer has to be carefully weighed against these disadvantages and simple closure will often be a sound decision.

PERFORATED GASTRIC ULCER

Most patients found to have a perforated gastric ulcer are best treated by partial gastrectomy with gastroduodenal anastomosis (Billroth I). Such a choice is based first, on the high incidence of malignancy in perforated gastric ulcer, a situation which does not lend itself to diagnosis by peroperative biopsy with frozen section, and second, on the fact that gastric perforations are often large and difficult to close. In addition, the likelihood of a need for definitive treatment in the future after perforation is high. Therefore, partial gastrectomy is the treatment of choice other than in exceptional circumstances. Techniques of partial gastrectomy are described on pp. 219–238 in this volume.

Simple closure of a perforated gastric ulcer is appropriate when the ulcer is pyloric or immediately prepyloric in that such ulcers are akin to duodenal ulcers. It may also be appropriate in the unusual patient who presents with perforation of a small acute ulcer as a complication of steroid administration or of stress. In addition, closure may be the best course in a desperately ill patient in whom speed and minimal tissue trauma may be of over-riding importance.

Simple closure of a perforated gastric ulcer may be carried out in the same way as for a duodenal ulcer.

PERFORATED STOMAL ULCER

Perforated stomal ulcer may be treated by simple closure with good immediate results. Such a policy has the advantage of being within the capabilities of the inexperienced and of providing for further investigation with regard to acid secretory status before a later planned procedure. Nevertheless, assuming the experience and competence of the surgeon and the fitness of the patient, it is better to undertake a procedure to reduce further acid secretion at the time of perforation. Such a procedure will depend on the original operation. If this were simple gastroenterostomy truncal vagotomy should be added to closure of the perforation. Conversion to partial gastrectomy (Billroth II, Kronlein-Polya) may give marginally better results in theory but vagotomy is a much simpler procedure and therefore more appropriate in the presence of perforation. Should the original operation have been partial gastrectomy, truncal vagotomy is also appropriate. Perforation of a stomal ulcer is a rarity after vagotomy and gastroenterostomy. Should it be encountered, revagotomy with antrectomy or conversion to partial gastrectomy (Billroth II, Kronlein-Polya) are suitable alternatives but require that the operator be thoroughly experienced in gastric surgery. Failing such experience, the safe course is to rely on simple closure.

Operative treatment for bleeding ulcer

P. S. Hunt MS, FRACS
Surgeon, Prince Henry's Hospital, Melbourne;
Associate Professor, Monash University, Melbourne

Introduction

The essence of good treatment of bleeding peptic ulcer is early diagnosis and timely surgery when appropriate. The management of these patients should be centralized in a special unit under the care of both an endoscopist and a surgeon. The endoscopist is responsible for early diagnosis and resuscitation; the surgeon takes over the management when the criteria for surgery are met. The usual mortality rates of 10–12 per cent with bleeding ulcer can be reduced to the region of 3–5 per cent in such a unit.

Endoscopy should be performed within 12 h of admission. This can produce a diagnostic rate of 95 per cent making unnecessary other methods of diagnosis such as barium meal and angiography. In most patients endoscopy identifies a single major cause of bleeding for which a specific surgical procedure is appropriate. Early diagnosis is the basis of planned management and rarely should surgeons have to operate on an undiagnosed patient or have to perform gastrotomy to look for a lesion. The 24 h after operation are critical and cardiorespiratory problems can cause death during this period. Most patients should be ventilated postoperatively in an intensive care unit until circulation is stable.

Unless indicated otherwise the cross-references in this chapter refer to *Operative Surgery: Alimentary Tract and Abdominal Wall, Volume 1, 4th Edition*

Indications for surgery in bleeding peptic ulcer

The three major prognostic factors are an age of over 50 years, shock on admission, and continued or recurrent bleeding in hospital. Patients who are shocked on admission are generally those who rebleed from a large vessel. Thus the two indications for surgery *after optimal resuscitation are*:

1. shock and an age greater than 50 years on admission;
2. continued or recurrent bleeding requiring 5 or more units of blood transfusion.

In the occasional patient who has terminal disease in other systems or is very old, consideration should be given to non-operative management.

These rules should apply to chronic gastric and duodenal ulcer and to erosive gastritis. Recently, erosive gastritis is a less frequent cause of upper gastrointestinal haemorrhage and bleeding from the entire stomach mucosa is now unusual. In the small group of patients who continue to bleed slowly from erosive gastritis, cimetidine will control bleeding in most cases. It is important to emphasize that cimetidine does not influence the early course of bleeding chronic peptic ulcer. The majority of patients with haematemesis and melaena caused by stress are in intensive care units or on steroids and immunosuppressive drugs. In the majority of such cases bleeding is from a large penetrating duodenal ulcer. Early endoscopy is essential and the indications for surgery must be strictly applied. The presence of active bleeding, visible vessel or clot, in the base of a chronic peptic ulcer are endoscopic findings which strengthen the indication for urgent surgery in these patients.

Application of this policy leads to an operative rate of about 35 per cent, with 25 per cent for shock in patients aged over 50 years and 5–10 per cent for continued or recurrent bleeding. In a special unit, operative mortality can be reduced to the region of 3–4 per cent for chronic peptic ulcer[1, 2].

Recognition of shock

The protocol should define clearly the criteria for the presence of shock. Optimal resuscitation should also be defined, especially in relation to the timing of surgery, and depends upon the rate of bleeding. Immediate blood transfusion is indicated if shock is present and should begin before endoscopy. The criteria for the diagnosis of shock are as follows.

1. Peripheral circulatory failure.
2. A pulse rate higher than 100/min.
3. Postural hypotension with a fall in blood pressure below 100 mmHg or more than 20 mmHg on sitting upright, associated with peripheral circulatory failure. This state of 'compensated shock' can be seen after significant blod loss in aged hypertensive and in younger patients. A central venous line is a most valuable method of monitoring when there is massive bleeding in the presence of heart failure. Swan-Ganz catheters in the pulmonary artery give more information but require expertise which is not always available.

Some patients, especially alcoholics with minimal blood loss, have hypovolaemia caused by vomiting. They have either tachycardia or brachycardia, pallor and postural hypotension. The haemoglobin is usually near normal and urgent surgery for chronic peptic ulcer is not indicated in this group unless there is continued bleeding.

Clinical observation

The other indication for surgery is the presence of continued or recurrent bleeding. There is an increased risk of rebleeding in aged patients with chronic peptic ulceration. When transfusion of 5 or more units of blood is necessary, surgery is indicated. An observation chart which records vital signs is useful but is no substitute for frequent clinical observation and experienced nursing care. Rebleeding is usually revealed by melaena. However, massive haemorrhage may occur without melaena and the patient can die suddenly after appearing to be in a satisfactory condition – a situation usually seen in the old with gastric ulcer. Such patients should therefore be subjected to urgent surgery when there is shock on admission. The use of a nasogastric tube is essential in mentally confused patients who may aspirate (and need surgery) but it should be removed as soon as possible after the bleeding has stopped and early feeding should then be started. Occasionally nasogastric aspiration is necessary to verify that there is blood in the stomach and thus exclude a lower gastrointestinal cause of haemorrhage. Endotracheal intubation may be indicated in some mentally confused and massively bleeding patients before endoscopy to minimize the chance of aspiration.

General technical points

Meticulous haemostasis is particularly important in these patients to reduce the incidence of both intraperitoneal and anastomotic haemorrhage. Tissue oedema also poses problems as there is a tendency for stitches to cut through, and it is desirable to use 2/0 rather than 3/0 calibre suture materials. Two-layer anastomoses are preferable but the presence of oedema makes infolding a possible cause of postoperative obstruction. The haemostatic inner all-coats layer is best performed by the Schmeiden method. Here tension is applied from the mucosal side of the anastomosis so that the cut edges of bowel are better apposed and less bulky when infolded with interrupted serosal sutures. Patients with bleeding gastric ulcers have hypochlorhydria and microfloral overgrowth in their stomachs, and are to be treated similarly to those having large bowel surgery in order to reduce infection. Extra care must be taken to avoid damage to the spleen. This can easily happen in this form of upper gastrointestinal surgery and may go unrecognized. Furthermore, there is an increased incidence of sepsis in patients after splenectomy, making removal of the spleen undesirable. The use of a continuous 2/0 synthetic monofilament posterior layer for anastomosis is useful. This suture gives a more watertight closure posteriorly and is easier to insert because tension is applied after it has been passed through the serosa, allowing for adjustment of disparate lumina. Also, because these sutures are elastic there is less tension and tendency to cut through oedematous tissue.

Special causes

Bleeding in the 'Mallory-Weiss syndrome' is caused by a gastro-oesophageal tear and usually stops without operation. Surgery is necessary in only about 1–2 per cent of patients. Bleeding from a submucosal artery in a localized area of erosive gastritis can be a worrying diagnostic problem. Generally this lesion is confused with the Mallory-Weiss syndrome and occasionally with bleeding oesophageal varices, as these small ulcers are often high in the posterior wall of the stomach. It may be necessary to perform a gastrotomy to define the lesion, when the bleeding vessel can usually be felt rather than seen.

There is a tendency for rebleeding to occur and gastrectomy is usually necessary although vagotomy, pyloroplasty and ligation of the left gastric pedicle is usually a satisfactory way to control bleeding from a fundal vessel. If oesophageal varices are found to be the cause of bleeding, the abdomen should be closed and balloon tamponade instituted or EEA stapling of the distal oesophagus performed (see p. 403 in this volume). Occasionally, lesions seen endoscopically cannot be identified at operation and in such cases gastrectomy can be done relying on previous endoscopic localization. During resection the ulcer can usually be felt by palpation of the mucosa before completing the anastomosis. With stomal ulcers, vagotomy is essential for the control of bleeding and the prevention of further recurrence, whether due to chronic stomal ulceration or to alkaline reflux gastritis.

Duodenal ulcer

Vagotomy, pyloroplasty and oversewing of the bleeding site is the most satisfactory emergency procedure for all age groups. There are two essential technical points. First, vagotomy must be complete. Second, ligation of the bleeding point must not be hurried or inadequate, leading to early postoperative bleeding. While vagotomy and pyloroplasty is the preferred procedure, once in every 4 or 5 cases it is best to change the operative plan and perform an antecolic Schoemaker Billroth II (Polya) gastrectomy. If possible the decision to perform gastrectomy should be made before pylorotomy because this makes duodenal closure more difficult. If the vagus nerves seem likely to be inaccessible, or if the ulcer is large so that pyloroplasty and control of bleeding will be difficult, gastrectomy should be done. Perforation with haemorrhage is an absolute indication for partial gastrectomy. There are other relative indications. A patient who is obese, has a deep chest, a fatty infiltrated liver with an enlarged left lobe, some degree of portal hypertension with para-oesophageal collateral vein development and retroperitoneal oedema is best treated by partial gastrectomy. In such patients access and exposure may be poor with increased danger of local haemorrhage, splenic damage or perforation of the oesophagus. The presence of oesophagitis may also influence the decision, though in such cases fundoplication can usually be added to vagotomy and pyloroplasty. With very large ulcers associated with marked oedema, pyloric stenosis and extension of the ulcer to the superior duodenal border, there is a tendency for the duodenum to fall apart and a change in plan may be indicated. Large ulcers also pose problems with control of the bleeding point, especially when bleeding is from the periphery of the ulcer rather than a central vessel. In these circumstances, by the time bleeding has been controlled, it is not possible to perform a satisfactory pyloroplasty.

The main advantage of an antecolic Schoemaker Billroth II procedure is that an adequate two-thirds or more gastric resection can be combined with a short non-angulated afferent loop. Antral resection and the creation of a new lesser curve produces a tubular gastric remnant. The short afferent loop reduces the incidence of both afferent loop obstruction and duodenal stump leakage.

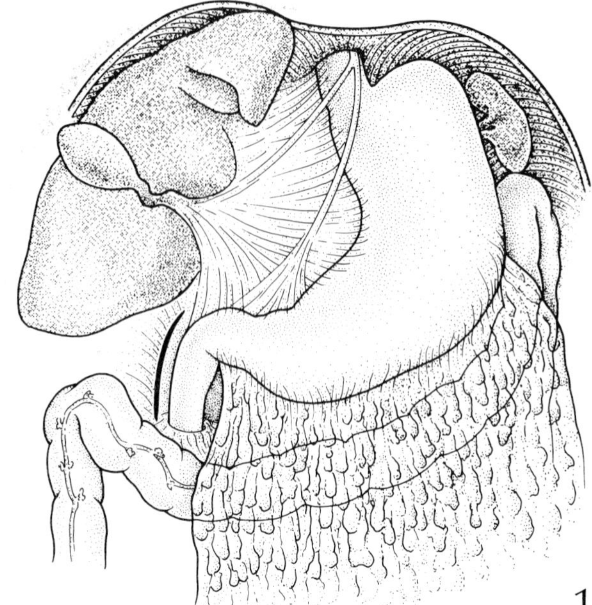

1

The operation

PYLOROPLASTY

1 & 2

An upper midline incision is most suitable for the exposure of a bleeding ulcer. Such placement is also best for vagotomy as well as giving a satisfactory duodenal exposure although in some obese individuals it may be necessary to extend the incision up to 5 cm below and to the right of the umbilicus. Pylorotomy is performed before vagotomy in the bleeding patient. Adhesions between the liver, gall bladder and duodenum are divided. The duodenum is mobilized by a Kocher manoeuvre. Adhesions and oedema may make it difficult to find the retropancreatic plane and care is necessary. However duodenal mobilization is necessary in order to gain a satisfactory two-layer closure of a pyloroplasty.

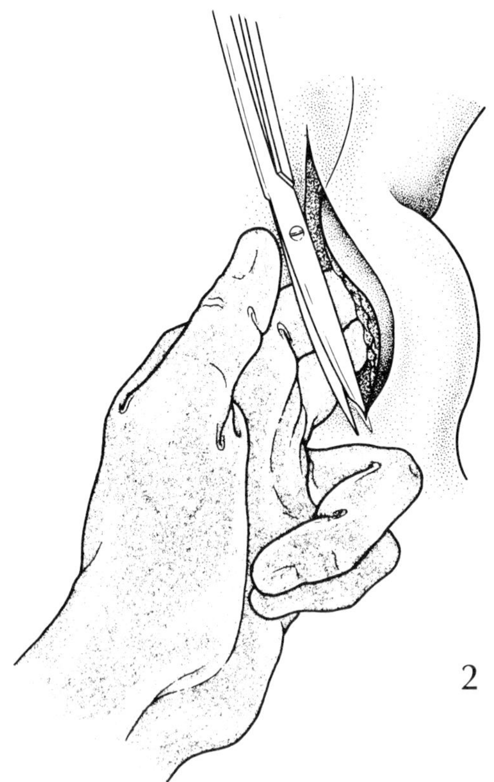

2

3

Pylorotomy can be performed using cutting diathermy. The incision is extended 3–4 cm into both the stomach and duodenum. This is a little longer than is necessary in the elective situation in order to get better access to the bleeding point. A pair of Babcock forceps is placed on the divided pyloric ring.

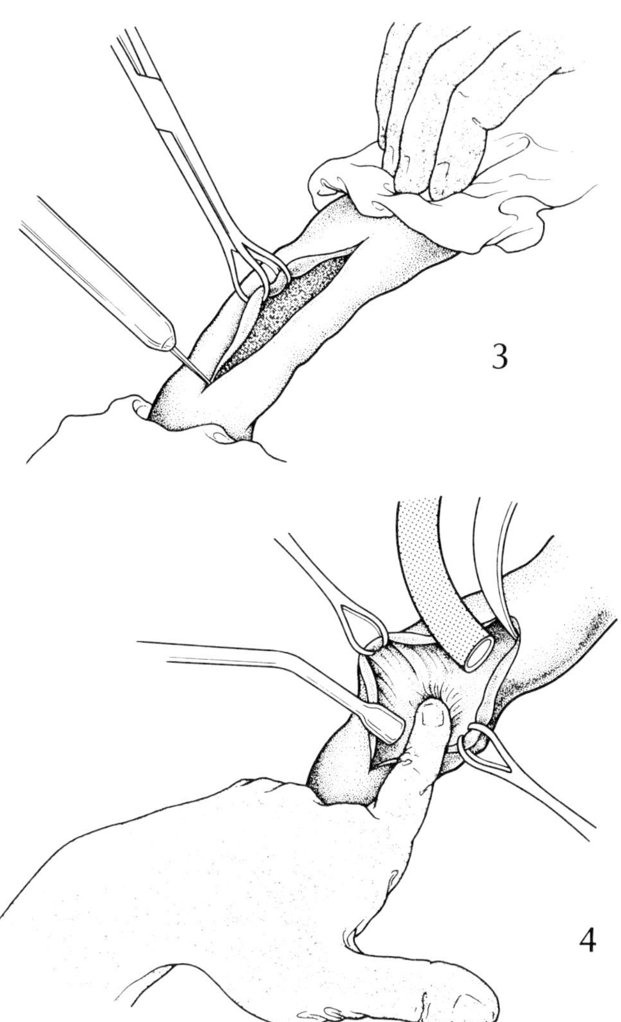

4

It is common to find at operation that bleeding from duodenal ulcer seems to have stopped. The stomach usually contains little blood, but further down the alimentary tract blood can be seen as a bluish discoloration of the small and large bowel. The duodenal ulcer is usually posterior and can readily be felt tethered to the pancreas. With severe bleeding the stomach may be full of blood which must be sucked out after pylorotomy, while finger pressure is applied to the bleeding point. Two suckers are useful at this point, one with a metal nozzle for blood and bile and the other with the tubing alone to pick up clot. With the index finger on the bleeding vessel a narrow Deaver retractor is inserted into the stomach, the stomach emptied of blood clot and blood and bile sucked away. After about 5 min of finger pressure, the bleeding can be controlled for a time, which also allows for further resuscitation.

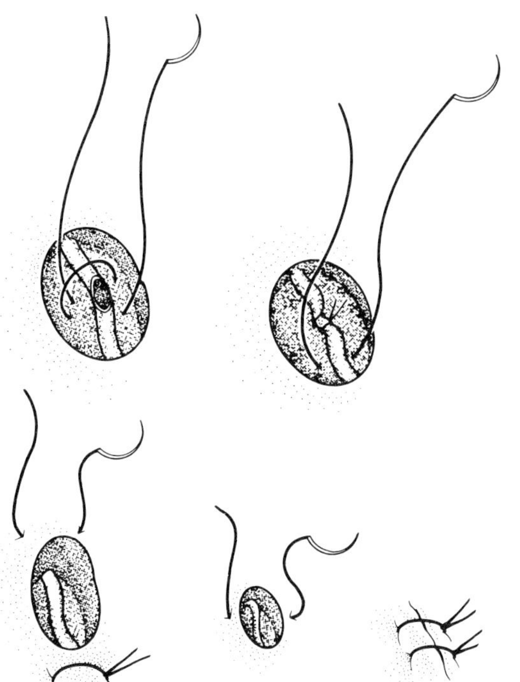

5

5

The bleeding point, which is usually in the side of the gastroduodenal artery, is oversewn with an atraumatic 2/0 silk suture and the bleeding vessel is then ligated above and below. Smaller ulcers and those of intermediate size in which it is difficult to close the ulcer or gain access to the vessel can be closed *in toto*. The vessel is ligated above and below the bleeding point at the mucosal ulcer edge. The common bile duct is 1–1.5 cm to the right of the gastroduodenal artery so damage to the duct is avoidable with first part duodenal ulcers. On occasions there may be more than one bleeding point as there are as many as four arterial tributaries in the base of the ulcer which may need separate ligation. Control of bleeding must be entirely satisfactory before proceeding to pyloroplasty.

6 & 7

Two-layer transverse Heineke-Mikulicz closure of a pyloroplasty is satisfactory in most cases. Care must be taken to avoid excess infolding of the oedematous mucosa which may later cause obstruction. This is best done by using a Schmeiden stitch.

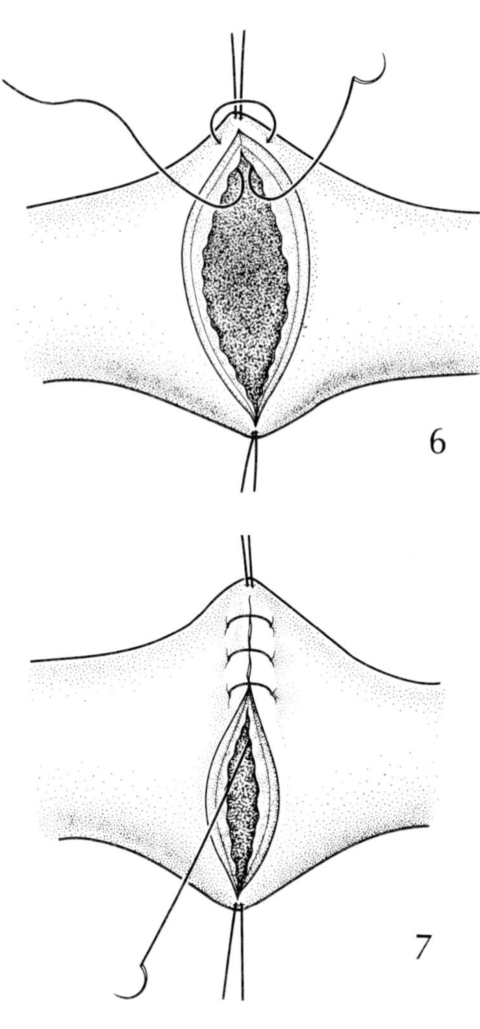

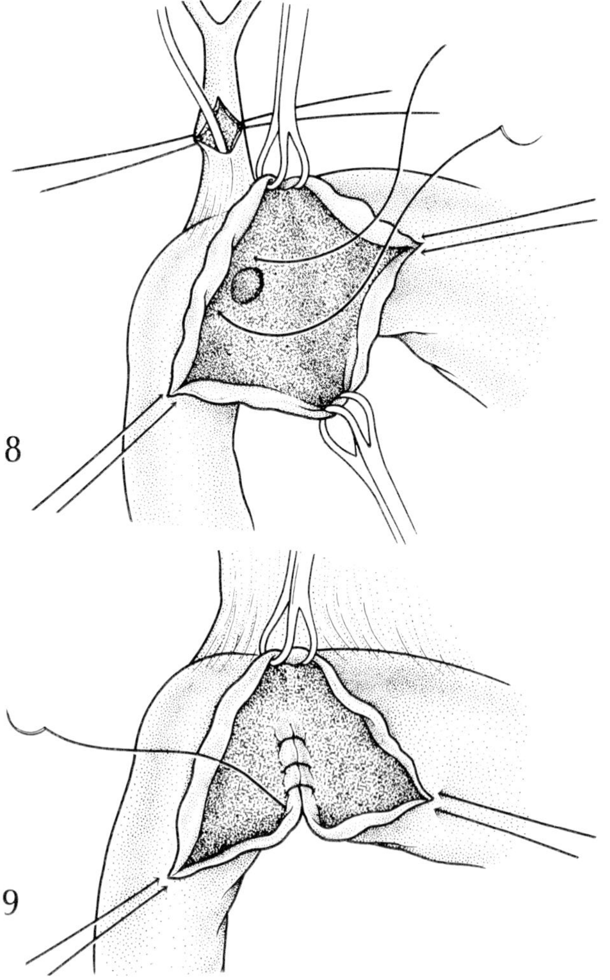

8 & 9

With a long pylorotomy for more distal ulcers it may be better to create a Finney pyloroplasty. Mobilization of the second and third parts of the duodenum is essential and the lower half of the pylorotomy is closed in the same way as a posterior layer of a gastroduodenal anastomosis. With these more distal ulcers it is wise to open the bile duct and insert a Bakes' dilator before control of bleeding to identify the duct and ampulla of Vater.

VAGOTOMY

To ensure that complete vagotomy is performed the procedure should be carried out at the site of the most constant vagal anatomy. This is at the cardio-oesophageal angle rather than the oesophageal hiatus where the vagal plexus may still persist. At the distal oesophagus the most expeditious procedure is an anterior selective and posterior truncal vagotomy. Attention must be paid to three landmarks to be sure of complete isolation of vagal fibres. These are: on the right, the lesser omentum below the hepatic branches of the anterior vagus; on the left, the cardio-oesophageal angle of His; and posteriorly, the posterior vagal trunk just proximal to its coeliac branch. A nasogastric tube should be present as a guide for dissection of the oesophagus. Highly selective vagotomy is the procedure of choice for the elective treatment of duodenal ulcer (see pp. 223–231), but is an inappropriate method in patients with bleeding.

10

With vagotomy at the level of the cardio-oesophageal junction, dissection can often proceed below the left lobe of the liver or if necessary the left triangular ligament can be divided and the left lobe turned to the right. Scissor dissection starts to the left of the distal oesophagus at the angle of His, opening a path posterior to the oesphagus. Short free adhesions to the anterior spleen are divided and the superior border of the gastric fundus is dissected away from the retroperitoneum for about 2–3 cm to the uppermost short gastric artery. Occasionally, when access is difficult, it helps to mobilize the oesphagus by division of the anterior vagus first at the level of the cardio-oesophageal angle.

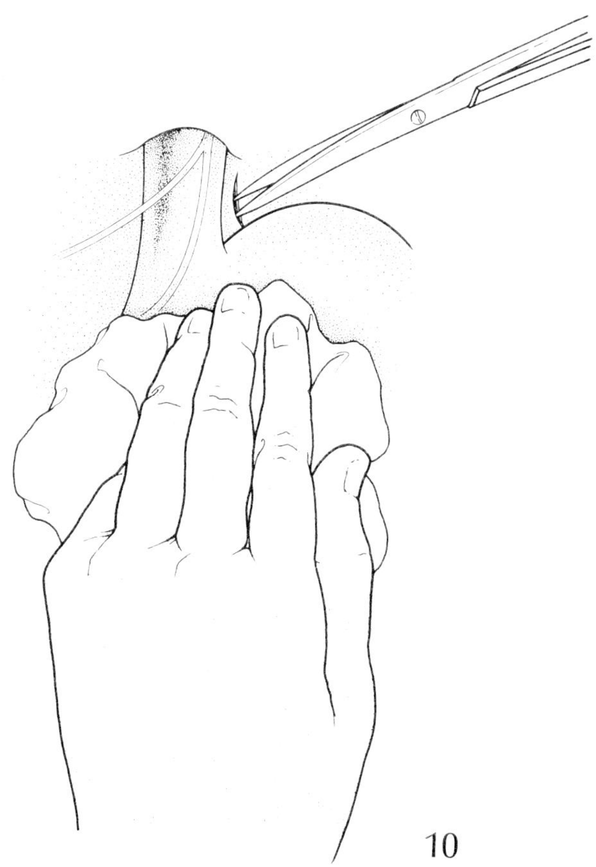

10

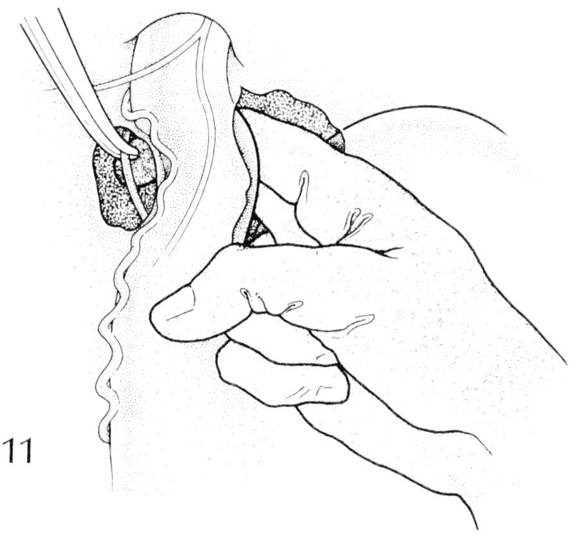

11

11

Finger dissection is continued posterior to the distal oesophagus with the aim of identifying the posterior vagal trunk–coeliac division in the areolar tissue of the gastropancreatic fold. Dissection is continued behind the posterior trunk just above this branch until the peritoneum of the right surface of the gastropancreatic fold is encountered. The fingertip is then pushed gently through this surface and through the lesser omentum below the hepatic branches of the anterior vagus. If the posterior trunk is readily palpable it can be divided at this point of the procedure. It is pushed to the right on the tip of the index finger, clamped above and below with metallic clips and a 1 cm segment removed.

12

Two fingers or a Lahey clamp are then passed along the path of finger dissection to grasp and pull back a 12–14 Fr red rubber catheter for distal oesophageal traction.

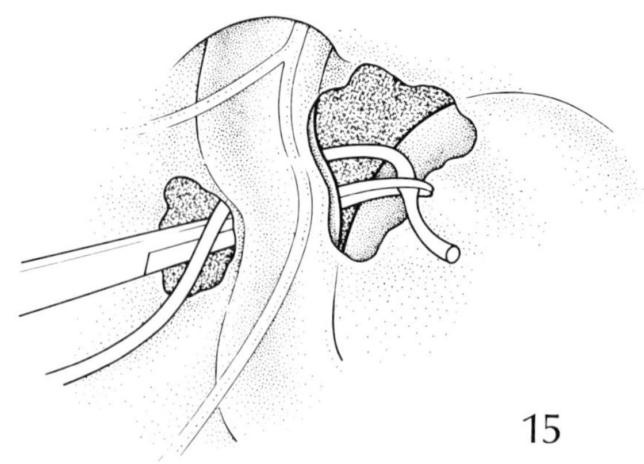

15

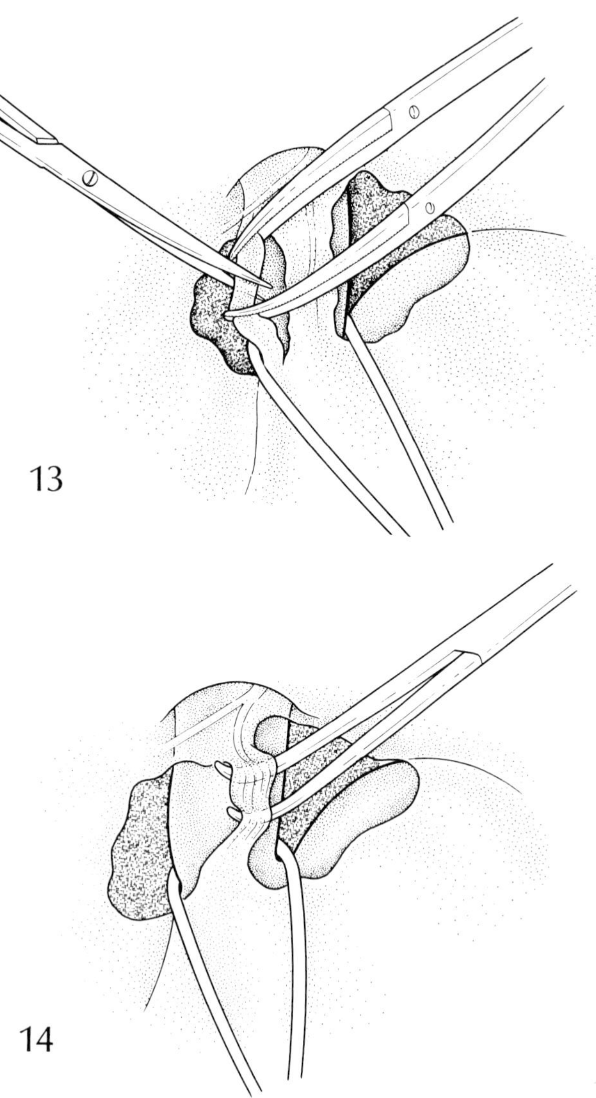

13

14

13 & 14

The anterior vagus is divided in two steps. First the areolar tissue containing branches of the anterior vagus and ascending branches of the left gastric artery is dissected free from the right anterior oesophagus using a Lahey clamp, and is clamped and divided. A plane is then found either with finger dissection or a Lahey right-angled clamp on the anterior surface of the distal oesophagus. The tissue superficial to this is lifted free from the distal oesophagus, clamped and divided. This layer includes all the anterior vagal fibres.

Using the red rubber sling to produce traction on the distal oesophagus, any residual fibres can be felt as fine tense strands and divided. Some intramuscular nerve fibres may occasionally need to be divided. After lifting the oesophagus forward, the distal oesophagus is cleared posteriorly off areolar tissue for approximately 5–7 cm up to the hiatus. This ensures that any higher branches of the posterior vagus (usually passing to the left – the 'criminal' nerves of Grassi) can be divided. Haemostasis is checked before and after removal of the red rubber traction tube, and the spleen is inspected for damage.

PARTIAL GASTRECTOMY

15

The antecolic Schoemaker Billroth II procedure is started by mobilizing the greater curve of the stomach, dividing the short branches from the left gastroepiploic vessels to the stomach, down to the pylorus. It is desirable to keep inside the gastroepiploic vessels to preserve the omental blood supply. To avoid damaging the middle colic artery, it is necessary to sweep the transverse mesocolon away from the posterior surface of the pyloric antrum. The lesser sac is almost always obliterated at this point.

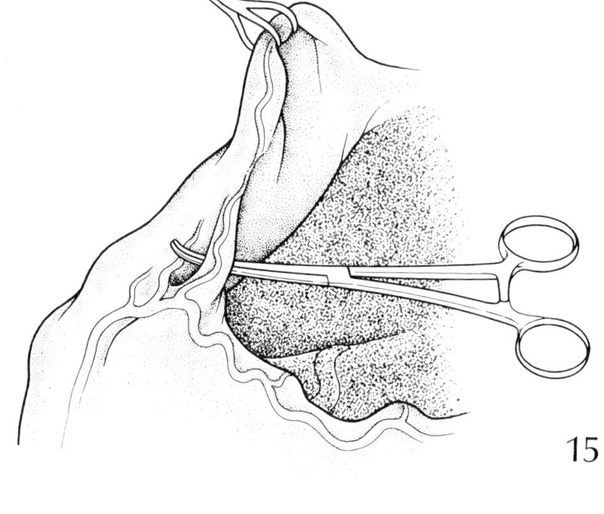

15

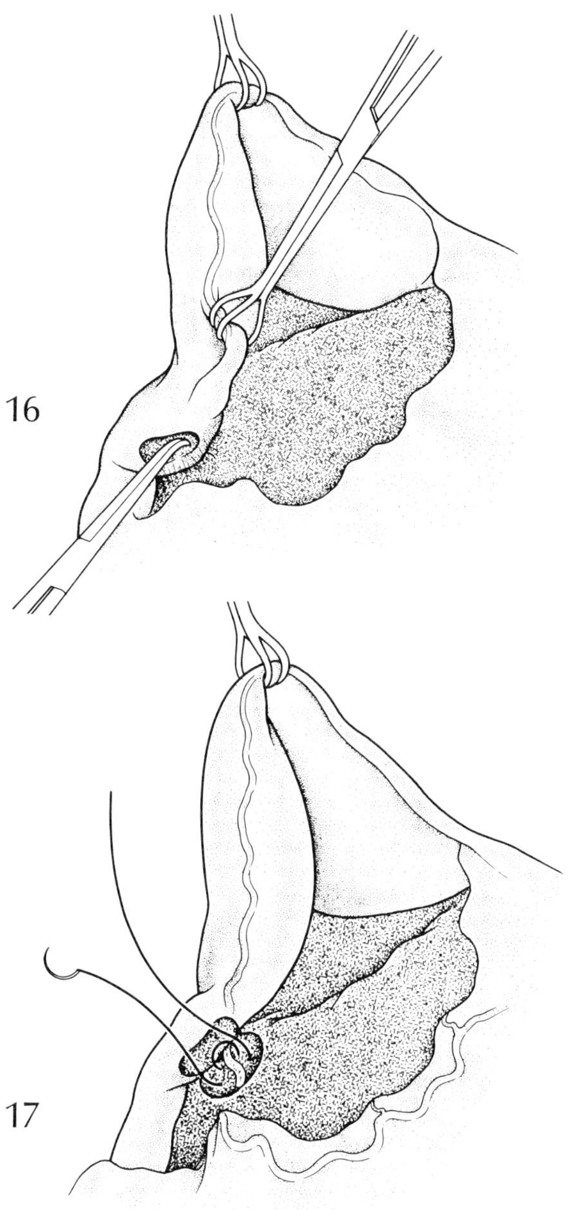

16

17

16 & 17

The greater curve is held up and to the right with Babcock forceps and adhesions between the antrum and the pancreas are divided as far as the edge of the posterior duodenal ulcer. By using the finger or artery forceps for blunt dissection the ulcer crater can be broken into, exposing the gastroduodenal artery in its base. Clots can then be sucked away and finger pressure applied to the bleeding point if necessary. The vessel is then oversewn.

18

The right gastric artery can then be divided. The index finger of the left hand is inserted through the filmy portion of the lesser omentum and behind the right gastric vessels just distal to the pylorus. The vessels are dissected from the wall of the duodenum using Lahey forceps, then clamped and divided.

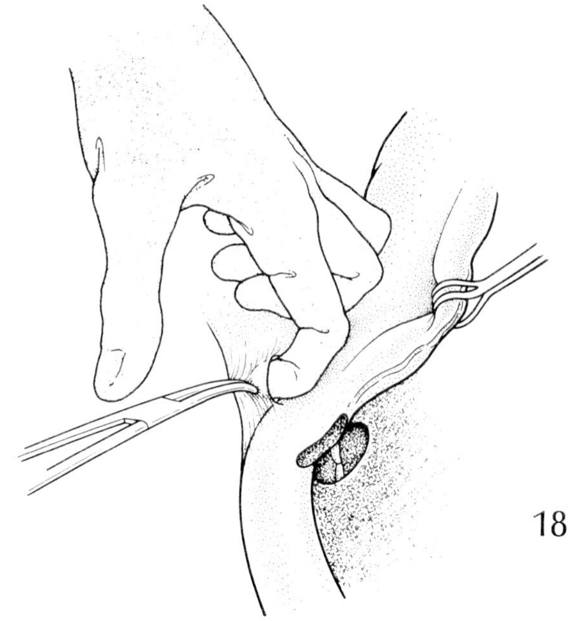

18

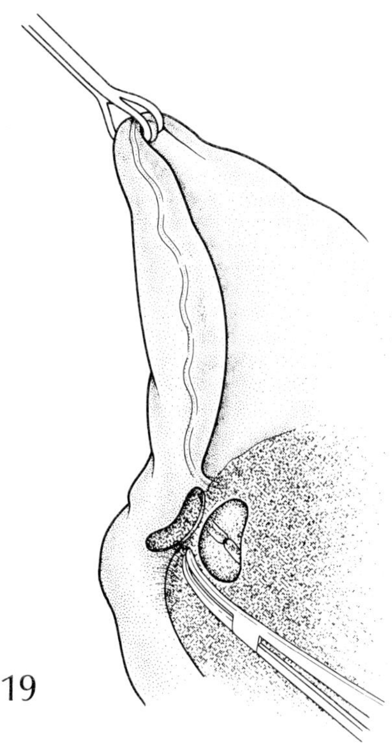

19

19

The crucial point of the dissection comes at the distal edge of the ulcer. Keeping close to the wall of the duodenum the medial wall is mobilized from the fibrotic distal edge of the ulcer for about 1 cm. This is best done by spreading artery forceps and starting a plane above and below on the duodenal wall about 1 cm distal to the ulcer. It helps to maintain traction on the stomach but with large ulcers the duodenum can come apart unless traction is gentle. The anterior wall of the duodenum is divided just distal to the duodenal bulb after completion of the medial dissection. Cetrimide-soaked gauze is tied over a Kocher clamp applied to the divided end of the stomach.

20

Occasionally, adequate mobilization of the duodenum beyond the ulcer is not possible and it is then wise to use catheter drainage of the duodenum to establish a controlled duodenal fistula should a Nissen closure of the anterior wall to the ulcer edge be necessary. It may be useful to insert a Bakes' dilator into the bile duct during dissection if the ulcer involves the second part of the duodenum, to identify the duct and ampulla of Vater.

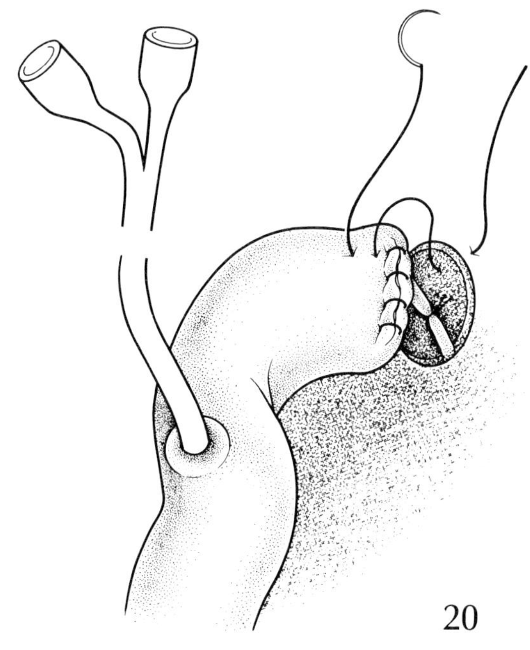

20

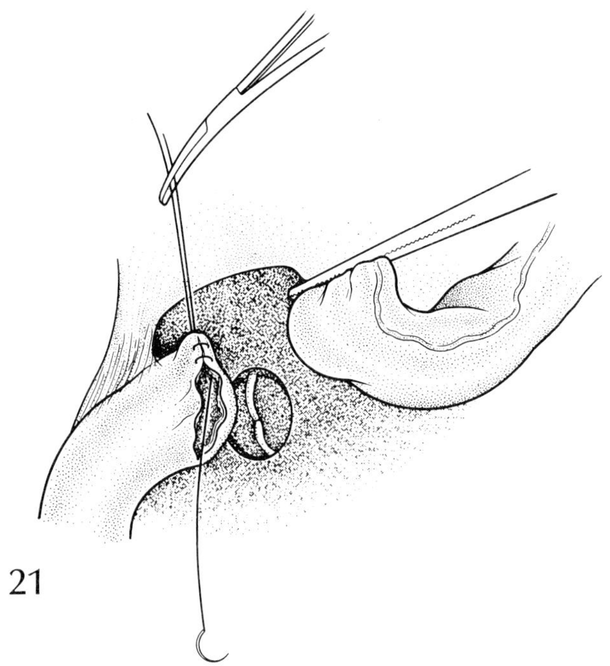

21

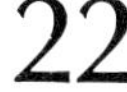

21

In normal circumstances, a two-layer closure of the duodenum is performed. The intial layer is a continuous all-coats 2/0 polyglycolic acid Schmeiden stitch, followed by interrupted serosal 2/0 silk stitches plus an omental patch.

22

The stomach is pulled down and to the left. The index finger of the left hand is then inserted behind areolar tissue on the lesser curve distal to the left gastric artery. A plane is opened between the lesser curve and the descending left gastric vessels which are clamped and divided.

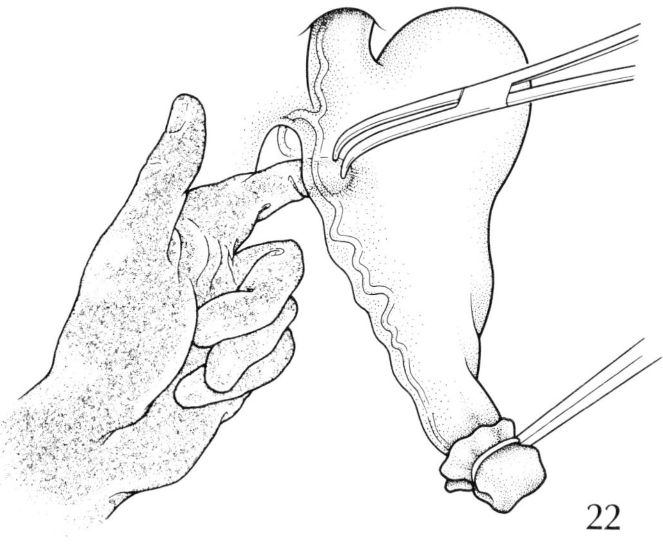

22

23 & 24

Traction is maintained on the stomach downwards and towards the left and the Lang-Stevenson clamp applied across the stomach about 5–6 cm from the greater curve at or above the lowest short gastric vessel. At this point one should define the duodenojejunal flexure and select a loop of proximal jejunum for anastomosis. A straight Kocher clamp is then applied parallel and distal to the first clamp and the stomach is divided between these two clamps. To prevent the clamp slipping, a cuff of stomach is left distal to the proximal clamp. A Parker-Kerr clamp is then applied from the end of this division to high on the lesser curve in the area previously cleared. A marking all-coats stitch of 2/0 polyglycolic acid is inserted high on the lesser curve, obliterating exposed muscle in this area and reproducing serosal apposition. If this suture is not used, the divided lesser curve may slip out of the tip of the clamp.

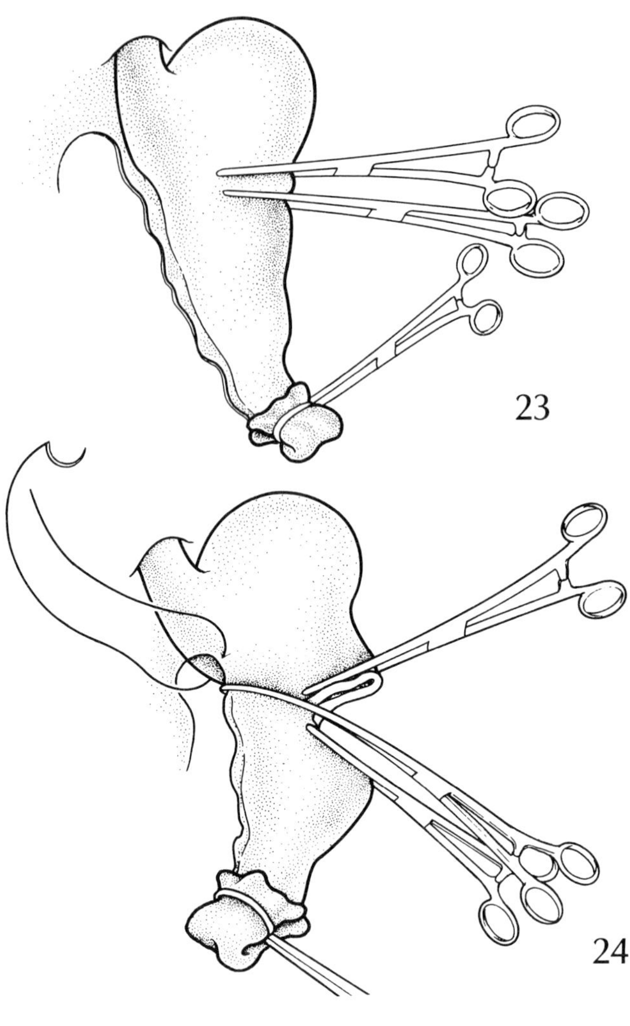

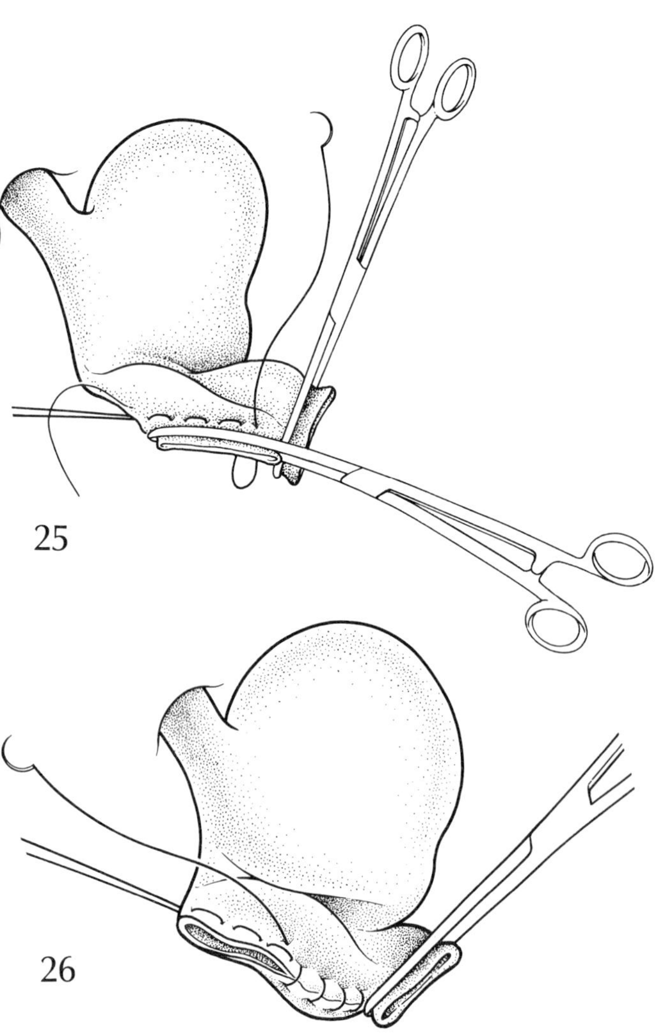

25 & 26

The distal stomach is then removed by cutting along the inferior border of the Parker-Kerr clamp with a scalpel. The new lesser curve is sealed with a to-and-fro or sewing-machine stitch proximal to the Parker-Kerr clamp. The same suture returns as a continuous all-coats layer from distally to the proximal lesser curve. The closure of the new lesser curve is completed with interrupted serosal sutures of 2/0 silk. Particular care should be taken with haemostasis and small bleeding vessels are ligated individually. This completes the Schoemaker closure and the formation of a new lesser curve.

27

The jejunum is brought up and a posterior serosal continuous layer of monofilament 2/0 Prolene is started from the left side. At this point the redundant portion of gastric mucosa is excised with a scalpel from the Lang-Stevenson clamp. The posterior layer should be on the superior surface and parallel to the mesenteric border of the jejunum to avoid torsion.

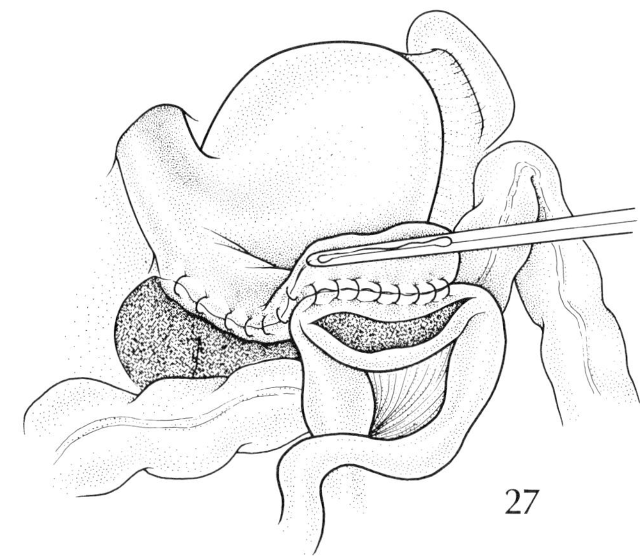

27

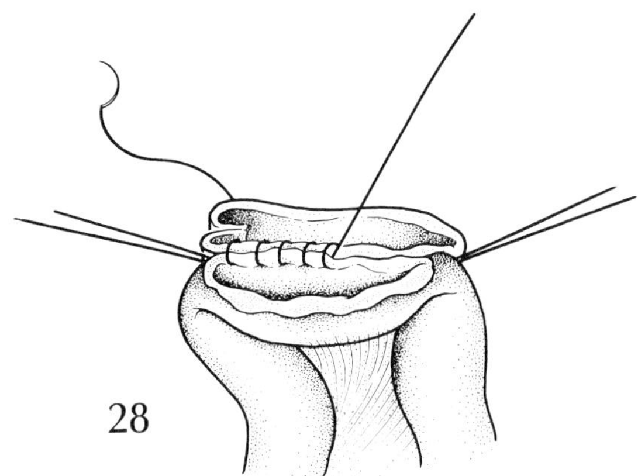

28

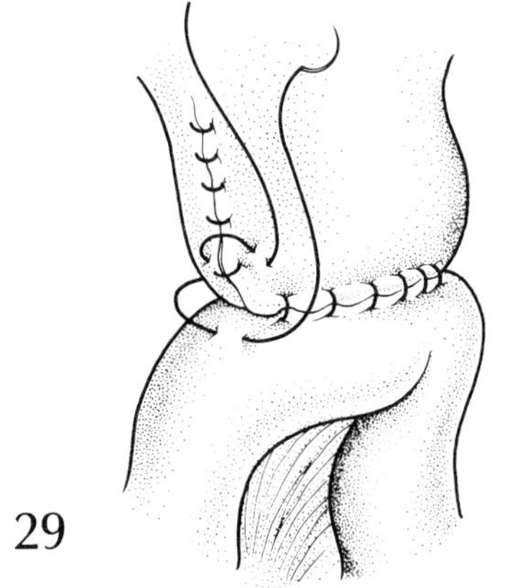

29

28 & 29

An opening is made on the superior surface of the jejunum with a scalpel. The all-coats layer of continuous 2/0 polyglycolic acid is then started at the midpoint of the posterior wall and continued around in both directions with two separate sutures to meet in the anterior midline. This brings a continuous invaginating Connell suture through the critical angle at the right jejunogastric junction. For better apposition the suture is carried onto the anterior wall as a Schmeiden stitch, applying tension to the suture by pulling through from the mucosal side.

Finally the anterior layer is completed with interrupted 2/0 silk producing a stoma of approximately 5 cm. A purse-string serosal suture is inserted at the critical angle between the new lesser curve and the jejunogastric anastomosis. The transverse colon is pulled well to the right leaving a short direct afferent limb of jejunum to the gastric remnant which lies high and to the left.

GASTRIC ULCER

Billroth I gastrectomy is preferable to vagotomy and pyloroplasty for bleeding gastric ulcer. This is because of a lower rebleeding rate and the possibility of cancer being present: at endoscopy in these cases it is difficult to be sure whether an ulcer is malignant or benign. The incidence of carcinoma in ulcers coming to urgent operation is approximately 10 per cent. In about 20 per cent of operations for bleeding gastric ulcer a Billroth II anastomosis is desirable. This is the case when there is duodenal scarring, high gastric ulcer with a small stomach or the possibility of cancer. In general, any anastomosis of the Billroth I type which is under tension is inappropriate. With prepyloric ulcers, vagotomy should be added to Billroth I antrectomy.

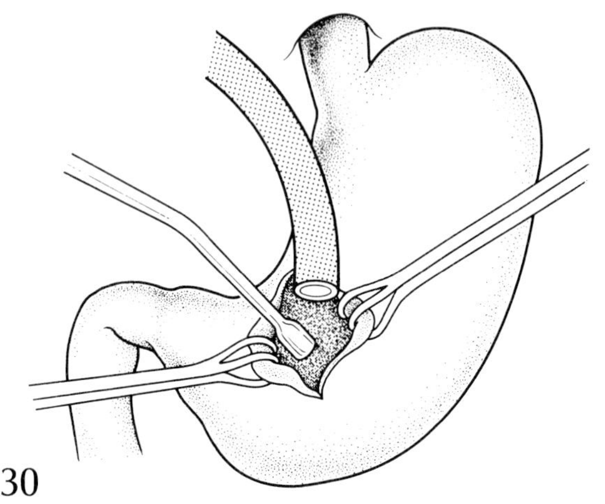

30

30

Occasionally, the stomach with a bleeding gastric ulcer is grossly distended with blood and clot. In this situation a gastrotomy may first be necessary to evacuate clot. An incision is made vertically on the anterior wall of the stomach close to the lesser curve. Generally there is an air pocket above the clot and Babcock clamps can be applied to either side of the gastrostomy to minimize spillage. Two suckers are useful, one with a metal nozzle for bile and one without, to remove clot. It is important to avoid contamination of the peritoneal cavity and the area should be packed off. Bleeding often stops spontaneously once the stomach has been emptied, or if not, it can be controlled by finger or sponge pressure for 5 min before proceeding with resection.

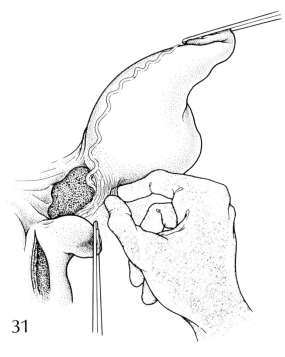

31

31

After mobilization of the greater curve the duodenum is clamped just distal to the pylorus with a Lang-Stevenson clamp. It is often necessary to perform an adequate Kocher manoeuvre before anastomosis. The stomach is then divided and turned upward and to the left to expose the left gastric pedicle. The ulcer can be seen at this point and is pinched off the pancreas, often breaking into the gastric lumen. The bleeding vessel on the ulcer base left in the posterior abdominal wall should then be ligated and the ulcer opening in the stomach closed with a continuous suture. It is generally possible to place a curved Parker-Kerr clamp above the ulcer to the lesser curve and the distal part of the stomach, including the ulcer, is removed.

32

With high gastric ulcers it may be necessary to do a Pauchet manoeuvre. A stay suture is placed high on the lesser curve just distal to the cardio-oesophageal junction and a nasogastric tube or a large bougie should be passed down the oesophagus to make sure that the lumen of the oesophagogastric junction is not compromised. The lesser curve is then opened just distal to the marking stay suture with cutting diathermy and the ulcer identified. Incision of the stomach is carried down anteriorly and posteriorly to include a tongue of stomach containing the ulcer. It may be necessary to turn the Lang-Stevenson clamp onto the anterior wall of the stomach creating a new greater curve, shifting the new sutured lesser curve from posterior to the right.

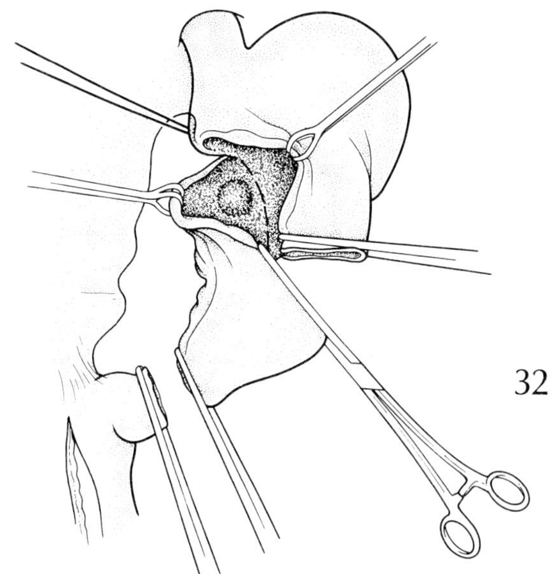

32

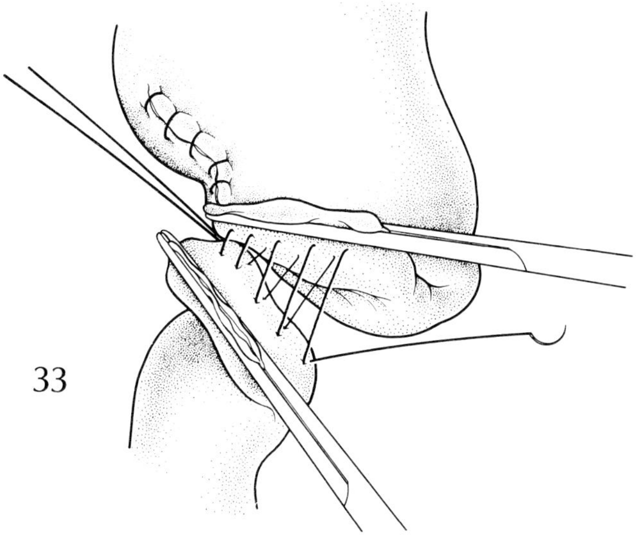

33

33

A continuous monofilament posterior layer of 2/0 Prolene is used to start the gastroduodenal anastomosis. The suture can be used to adjust the lumen but should not narrow it. Occasionally if there is a disparity of the lumen a Horsely slit can be useful. This is performed at the anterior midpoint of the duodenum to widen the duodenal lumen. If the anastomosis seems narrow a nasogastric tube can be passed through it into the distal duodenum.

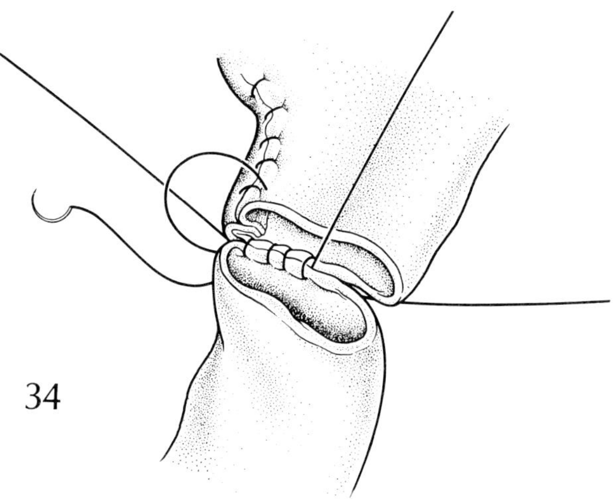

34

34

The all-coats layer is then started from the midline posteriorly using 2/0 polyglycolic acid and continued to the midline anteriorly. The anterior layer is completed with interrupted 2/0 silk and a purse-string suture is placed on the medial side at the junction of the new lesser curve and the gastroduodenal anastomosis.

EROSIVE GASTRITIS

Erosive gastritis is best treated by high Billroth I gastrectomy. With adequate mobilization of the duodenum and division of three or four short gastric vessels it is usually possible to do an 85 per cent subtotal gastrectomy and still achieve a Billroth I anastomosis without tension. Residual ulcers in the fundus seen during this anastomosis can be underrun. It is rarely necessary to perform a total gastrectomy.

WOUND CLOSURE AND DRAINAGE

Many patients treated surgically for bleeding ulcer are poorly nourished and elderly, and the upper midline incision is likely to heal poorly. Mass closure with continuous monofilament nylon (*see* p. 129 in this volume) is safer than absorbable sutures and through-and-through 'tension sutures', using Emasy buttons, are an excellent safeguard against burst abdomen. Drainage of the subcutaneous space with Penrose drains can reduce infection of haematoma. Despite the greatest care with haemostasis, there are two areas which may continue to ooze – under the cupola of the left diaphragm and the region of the isolated ulcer base after gastrostomy. It is wise to insert an intraperitoneal drain for at least 48 h.

Postoperative care

Early postoperative complications in these patients include intraperitoneal haemorrhage, myocardial failure and infarction, deteriorating respiratory function and aspiration accidents. Vital organ function, especially myocardial, must be preserved by maintenance of an adequate circulating volume. This is achieved by reference to heart rate, blood pressure, pulse pressure, the jugular or central venous pressure, peripheral perfusion and urine output. It is important not to fix on one variable. If the patient is thought to be plasma-volume depleted, intraperitoneal haemorrhage should be considered as a cause. The *rate* of infusion of blood, plasma or saline should be determined by the venous pressure response. The choice between these isotonic sodium fluids will be based on a need to maintain an adequate haemoglobin and plasma oncotic pressure.

Respiratory problems may develop insidiously and should be anticipated, especially in those with chronic airway disease. Respiratory infection can occur early, and lead to the need for prolonged intensive care. The prevention of this complication is interrelated with the maintenance of cardiac funtion. Whilst particular care must be taken to prevent hypovolaemia, volume loading to correct this should be done cautiously. Sudden increases in venous return may promote an increase in sodium and water in the lung, with consequent deterioration in pulmonary gas transfer. Thus in patients with evidence of lung disease, consideration should be given to measuring the left atrial pressure to optimize fluid therapy. Ideal ventilating patterns should combine an adequate tidal and minute volume with relatively low inspiratory flow rates. Sodium balance is vital because of the tendency of these patients to retain sodium and water in the lung. This will require frequent measurements of urine sodium levels.

References

1. Hunt, P. S., Hansky, J., Korman, M. G. Mortality in haematemesis and melaena: a prospective study. British Medical Journal 1979; 1: 1238–1240

2. Hunt, P. S., Korman, M. G., Hansky, J., Marshall, R. D., Peck, G. S., McCann, W. J. Bleeding duodenal ulcer: reduction in mortality with a planned approach. British Journal of Surgery 1979; 66: 633–635

Total gastrectomy for cancer

Hugh Dudley ChM, FRCS (Ed.), FRACS, FRCS
Professor of Surgery, St Mary's Hospital, London

Introduction

Surgeons cannot claim to make a large contribution to long survival in gastric cancer. The best results are in node-negative, non-penetrating lesions where even then survival rates of 40 per cent at 5 years are the exception rather than the rule. Even more favourable factors are mucosal involvement only[1], follicular hyperplasia in the regional nodes[2] and a well differentiated histological pattern[3].

However, though the outlook for survival is mediocre, the surgical role extends to proper palliation by restoring reasonably normal swallowing and digestion and removing tumour bulk. The latter may well be of greater importance in the future as chemotherapeutic and immunotherapeutic techniques become more tumour specific. In the meantime, the surgeon must, in gastric cancer as in other malignancies, accept that most of his patients will not long survive but that he must do his best for his individual patient. The author believes that, provided the mortality can be kept to a reasonable level (less than 10 per cent), a total gastrectomy is still the best method of palliation and, where the factors favour the patient, provides best chance of cure.

Total gastrectomy cannot be undertaken with minimal mortality and morbidity unless considerable attention is paid to preoperative and postoperative management. Preoperatively, most of these patients are malnourished. Within the time available before surgery (usually no more than 2 weeks), the patient cannot gain much weight, but he can be put into positive nitrogen balance by intensive parenteral nutrition. A patient who is gaining weight will also be less likely to have inadequate responses in immunological terms. We have to admit that, at the time of writing, we are still far from understanding all the details of specific deficiencies in macro- and micronutrients which affect convalescence after injury. However, whether nutritional repletion is by tube passed through the lesion or preferably by total parenteral nutrition using a central venous catheter, we must now concede that it is not worth operating on patients whose nutritional decline is unarrested and who are not provided with a balanced regimen.

The other major factor in postoperative mortality is respiratory failure. In part, this can be attributed to the weakness of respiratory effort which is in turn the consequence of poor nutrition; in part, it is the inevitability of the association of respiratory disease with an aging urban population; finally, patients with vomiting and/or dysphagia may well have laryngeal spill, particularly if their cough reflex is weak. Thus, intensive physiotherapy should be used wherever possible. In addition, a short (not more than 24 h) course of parenteral antibiotics which spans the period of operation should be used to minimize the effects of colonization of the lungs by intestinal organisms. As with other upper gastrointestinal procedures, we use a cephalosporin given with the premedication, at 6 h and at 12 h.

Specific instructions to the patient about the nature of the incision and its effects in causing pain are useful. In addition, it is wise to warn the patient that a period of artificial ventilation by transoral or transnasal tracheal tube may be necessary and that where such facilities exist, he or she may wake in the intensive care unit. Whenever possible it is desirable to have the staff of that unit visit the patient preoperatively.

General measures of preparation are pursued as for any major surgical procedure. Oral hygiene is attended to and a loaded colon is emptied. In obstructed patients, a nasogastric tube is placed 3 days before surgery and twice daily lavage carried out with copious amounts of water. When a nasogastric tube is in position it is futile to give the patient oral food or fluids. Rather, continuous suction should be instituted which will rapidly lead to a decline in the volume of aspirate to less than half a litre daily and to a contracted and manageable stomach at operation.

The operation

The objective of the radical operation for cancer of the stomach is the removal of that organ, the spleen (hilar nodes), greater omentum (diffuse and subpyloric nodes), body and tail of the pancreas (supra- and infrapancreatic nodes) *en bloc*. In addition, the clusters in the porta hepatis (right gastric nodes) and around the coeliac axis (left gastric nodes) can be dissected by working in the adventitial plane of these vessels. The operation can be done through the abdomen or the chest: in a thin individual with a distal carcinoma the former is entirely adequate provided a very long incision is made so as to permit retraction of the wound edge well out to the left paracolic gutter.

A useful adjunct is to split the sternum as high as the fourth interspace (see chapter on 'Access to the abdomen and lower chest', pp. 126–145 in this volume). However, in a heavily built patient with a body or fundal tumour, a transthoracic exposure is greatly to be preferred. In such circumstances, the coeliac axis is approached from the side, so permitting an accurate dissection and a clean sweep of all the retroperitoneal tissues away from the front of the aorta and the crus. Either a standard thoracotomy through the bed of the eighth rib or a thoracoabdominal incision in the same line may be used (see p. 142 in this volume). The latter is to be preferred and if carried well across the midline permits very easy closure of the duodenal stump.

Resectability (as distinct from curability) is established by ascertaining that infiltration of the posterior abdominal wall, superior mesenteric vein or liver is not such as to pose technical problems. The surgeon may yet elect to retreat if there are multiple liver metastases or peritoneal seedlings because palliation by resection is unlikely to give the patient a qualitative gain in survival.

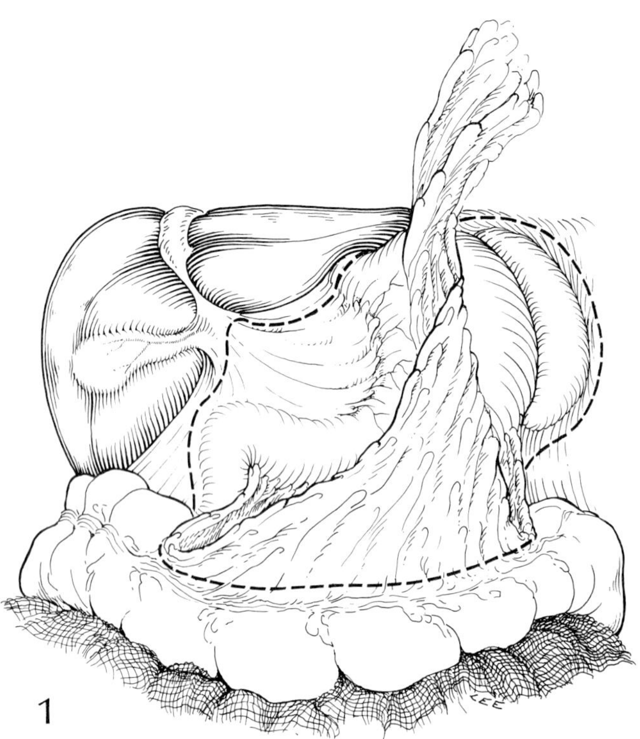

1

1

The resection is undertaken *away* from the tumour on the line of the peritoneal incision shown. It may begin anywhere on this line but the author's preference is to start either at the left lateral end of the bloodless attachment of the greater omentum to the transverse colon, or at the oesophageal hiatus.

2

If the first course is chosen the peritoneal incision passes downwards and medially into the wedge of posterior parietal peritoneum which is interposed between the left edge of the transverse mesocolon and the lower border of the body and tail of the pancreas. Here, on a slightly anterior plane, the greater omentum is draped over and attached to the front of the splenic flexure. The omentum's attachment is normally bloodless from this point to the hepatic flexure.

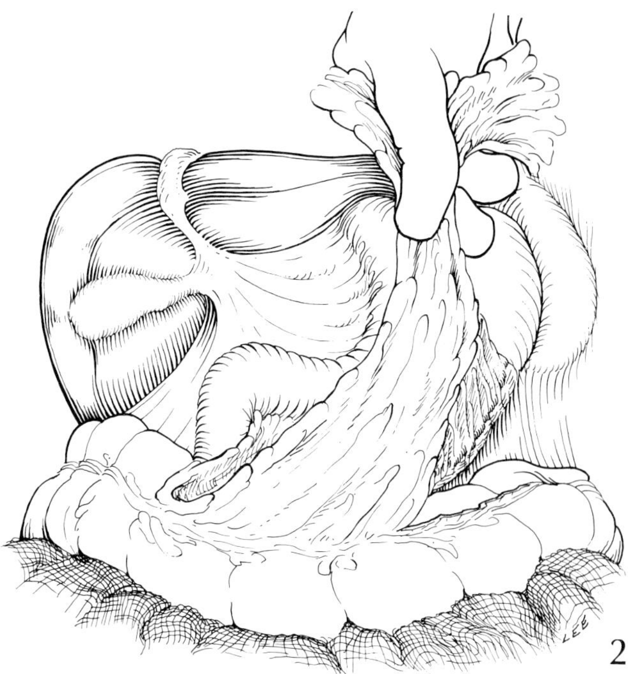

2

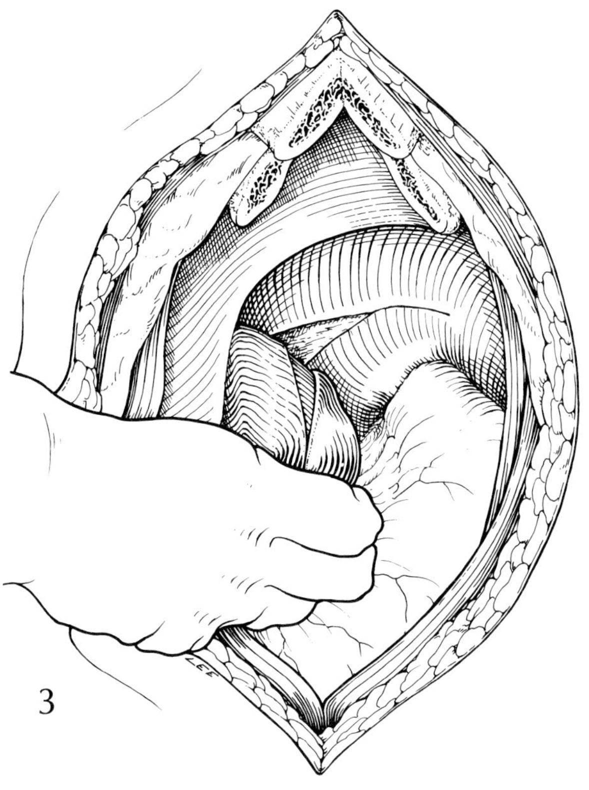

3

3

The alternative starting point is at the oesophageal hiatus where it is first necessary to divide the left triangular ligament of the liver and turn the left lobe downwards and to the right. This exposes the parietal peritoneum flowing over the diaphragm on to the oesophagus and thus permits entry into the cirumferential peritoneal dissection described above. From here it is possible to take the dissection either to the left or the right, stripping the peritoneum downwards into the hiatus.

4

Dissection of the greater omentum proceeds to the right and separates this structure from the transverse colon in the bloodless line of Pauchet. Often in the elderly the omentum is plastered against the anterior aspect of the transverse mesocolon. Sometimes it is possible to strike the plane by blunt dissection but a piecemeal approach may be required. The objective is to lift the whole omentum up and so expose the transverse mesocolon. Occasionally the tumour may involve this structure in which case the middle colic artery is divided at its root. The colon's vascularity is then observed throughout the rest of the procedure and a transverse colectomy done if there is any doubt about viability.

Lifting the omentum up exposes the right gastroepiploic artery at its origin, though in order to do so a few filmy attachments of the right border of the greater omentum to the lower aspect of the first part of the duodenum may need to be divided. The dissection here is lateromedial to ensure that the subpyloric glands are included.

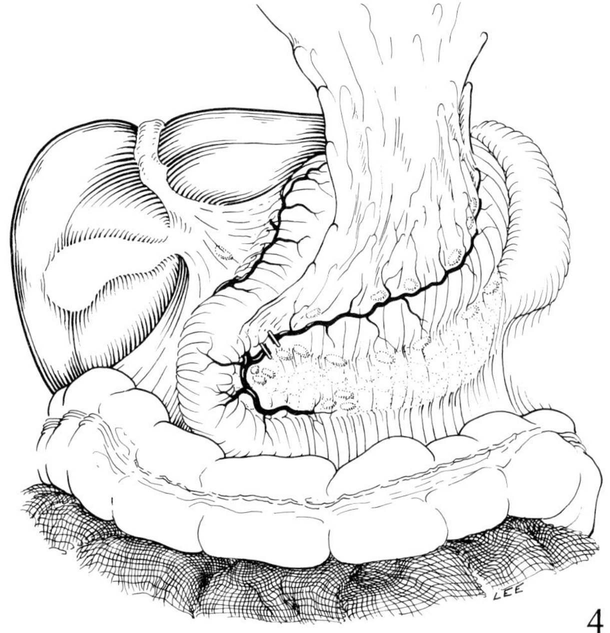

4

5

It is next convenient to mobilize the duodenum because the line of peritoneal dissection required takes the operator up across the porta hepatis to expose the common bile duct and hepatic vessels, thus allowing nodes that lie on their anterior aspect to be swept to the left.

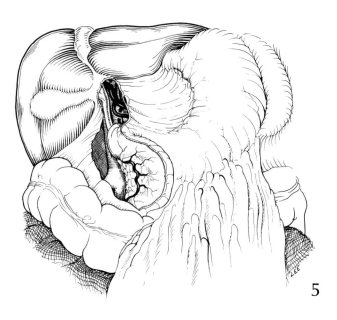

5

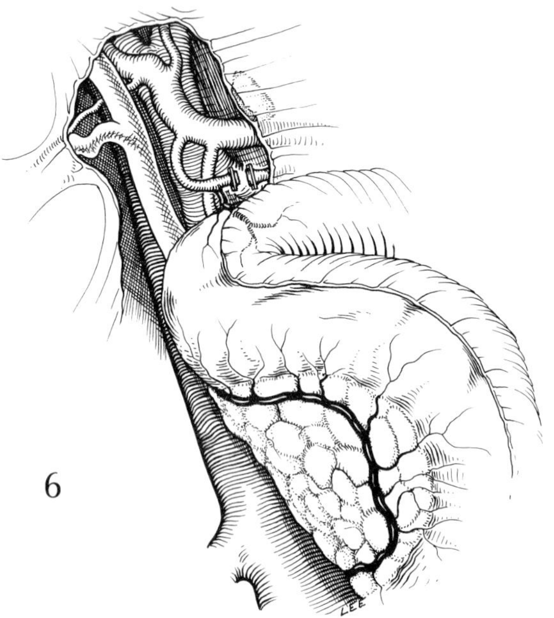

6

6

The anatomy is variable but the right gastric artery should be ligated or clipped as convenient and the main trunks of the hepatic and gastroduodenal vessels cleared by displacing all tissue to the left.

7

The duodenum is now virtually completely free though the right reflexion of the lesser sac (not shown) may need to be divided posteriorly.

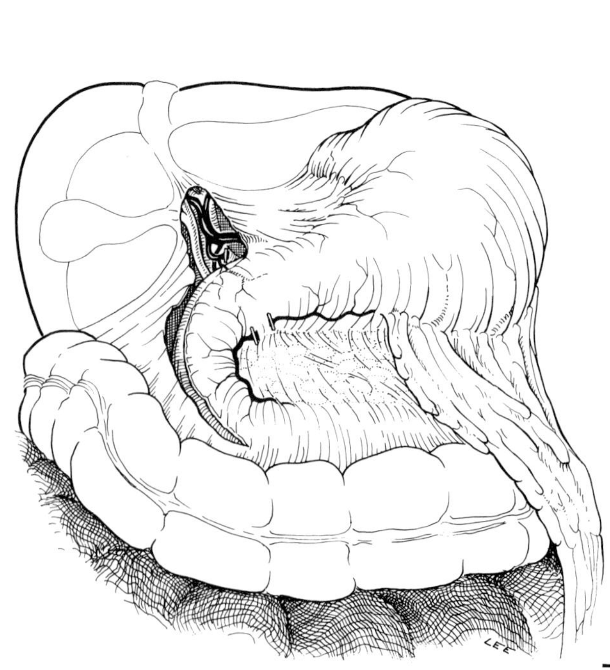

7

8

It is then possible to insinuate a clamp behind the duodenum and transect it. Turning the stomach to the left will begin to expose the upper border of the pancreas and the coeliac axis.

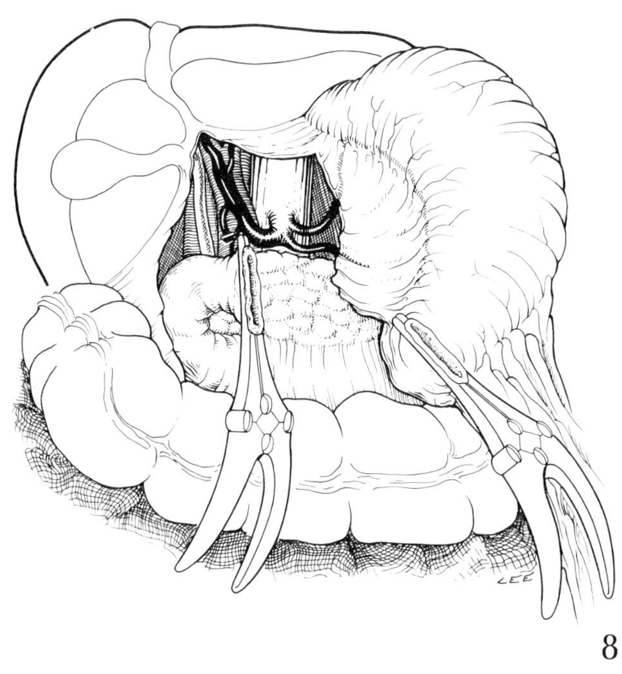

8

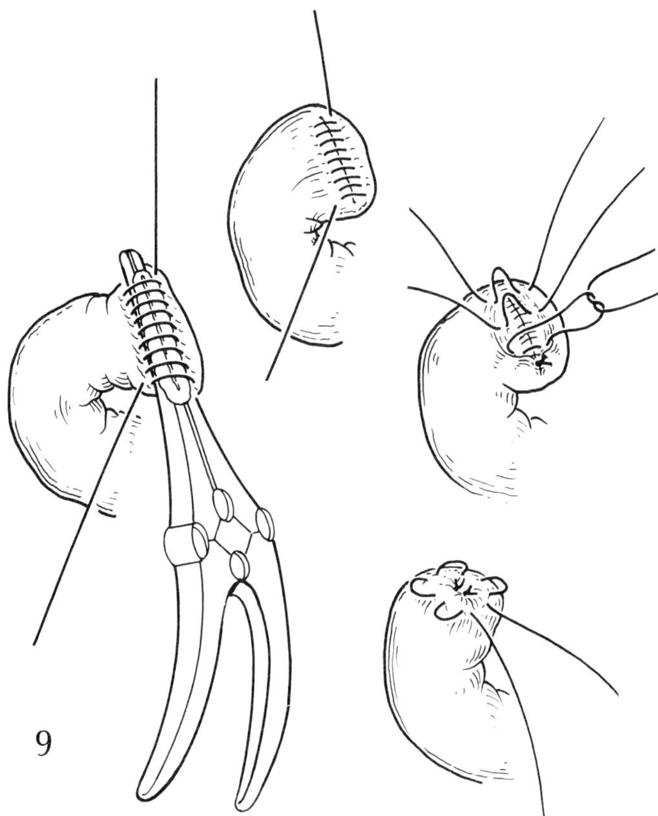

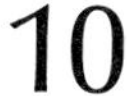

9

9

Duodenal stump closure can by any number of different tecniques (see p. 222 in this volume). That used by author is shown. The inner continuous layer is in polydioxanone, the outer layer and the purse-string with braided polyamide (nylon) or polypropylene.

10

The dissection then proceeds to mobilize the free edge of the lesser omentum around to the left across the anterior face of the oesophagus and down around the lienorenal ligament lateral to the spleen.

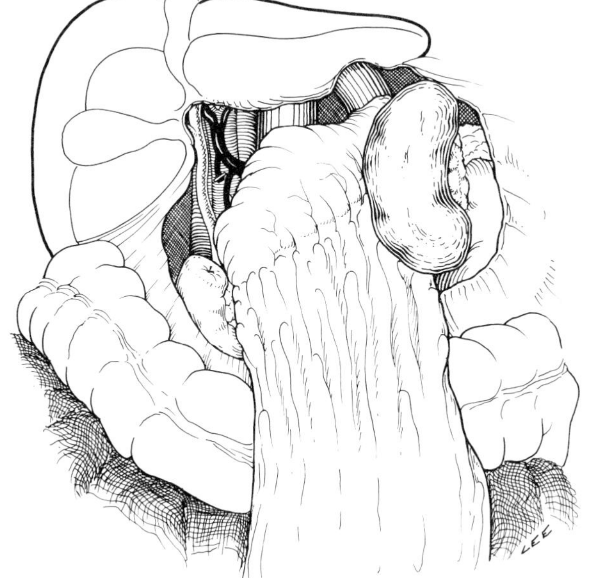

10

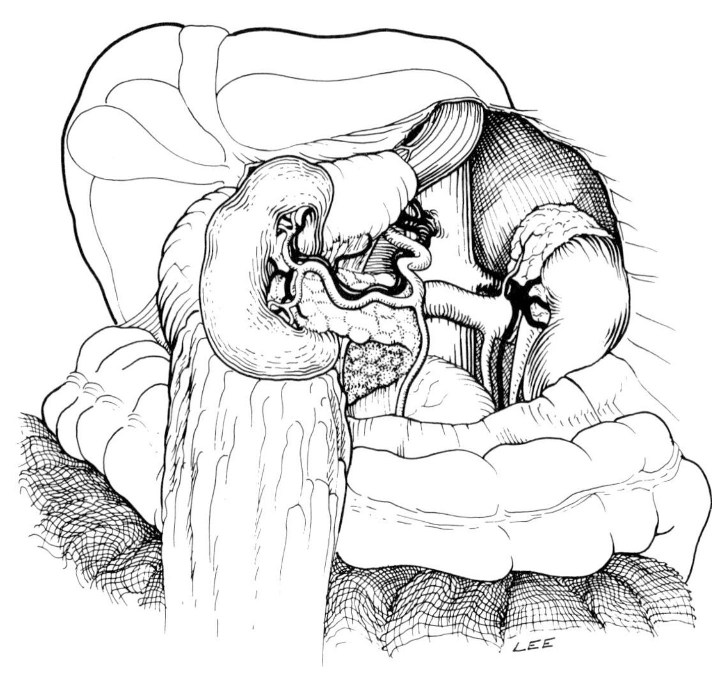

11a

11a & b

It is now possible to dissect in the areolar tissue behind the splenic pedicle and anterior to kidney and adrenal. As the stomach and spleen are reflected medially it is possible to see the coeliac axis from this aspect and:

(*a*) make a precise dissection of the lymph nodes;
(*b*) divide the splenic artery close to its origin and the splenic vein close to the confluence of it and the inferior mesenteric veins.

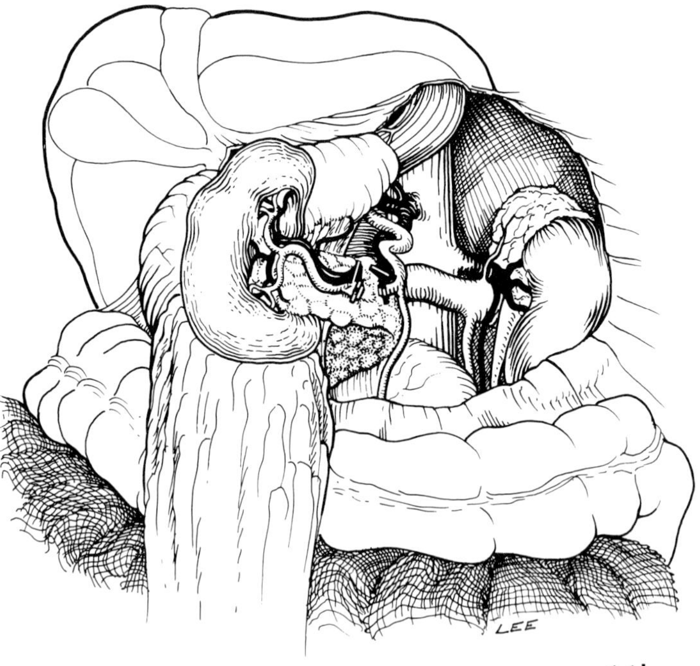

11b

12

The next step is to transect the pancreas. A soft right-angled clamp is applied to the gland and a knife used to make a precise division. As this is done the duct comes into view and is precisely identified, transfixed and clipped or ligated. A mesh work of vessels behind may require attention but the next objective is to divide the left gastric artery.

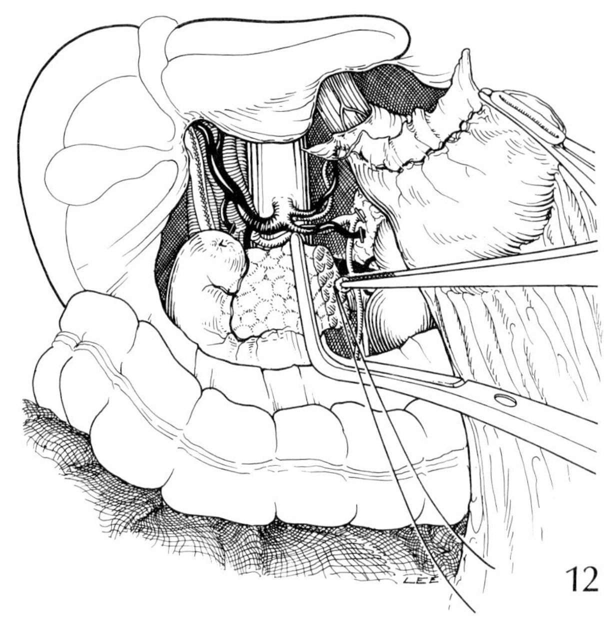

12

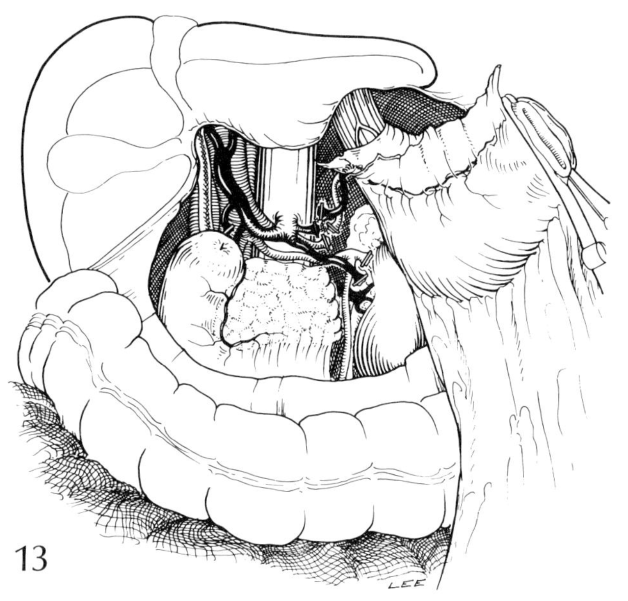

13

13

Traction on the mass of tissue – stomach, spleen, omentum and body and tail of the pancreas – now exposes the last major branch of the coeliac axis – the left gastric. This is divided so freeing the block dissection.

14

Additional oesophageal length is desirable at all times but essential if the aproach has been via the abdomen. Division of the vagal trunks – here shown anteriorly – permits delivery of 6–8 cm of oesophagus into the abdomen.

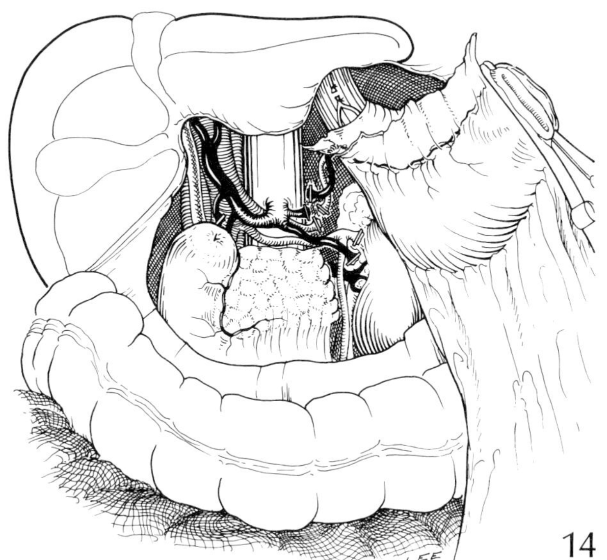

14

Oesophagojejunostomy

The simplest reconstruction is by end-to-end or end-to-side oesophagojejunostomy. There is little evidence to support any more complex approach. Great care must be taken in fashioning a Roux loop – one of the most useful techniques available to the gastrointestinal surgeon.

15

A loop is identified as close to the duodenojejunal flexure as possible which has the appropriate pattern of vascular arcade.

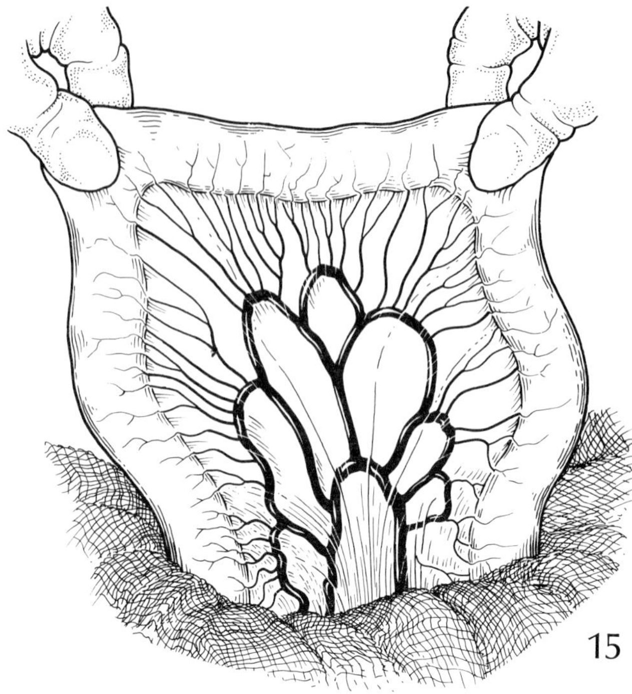

15

16

A line of dissection is next chosen to give the appropriate length of loop which will bridge the gap.

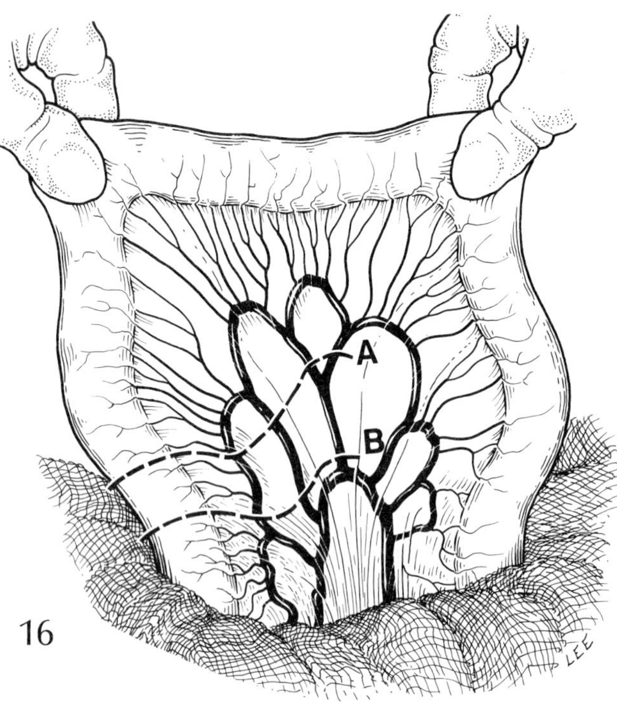

16

17

Careful incisions are then made in the mesentery with a knife and the individual vessels clipped or ligatured. Mass ligature should not be done as intramesenteric haematoma is almost inevitable.

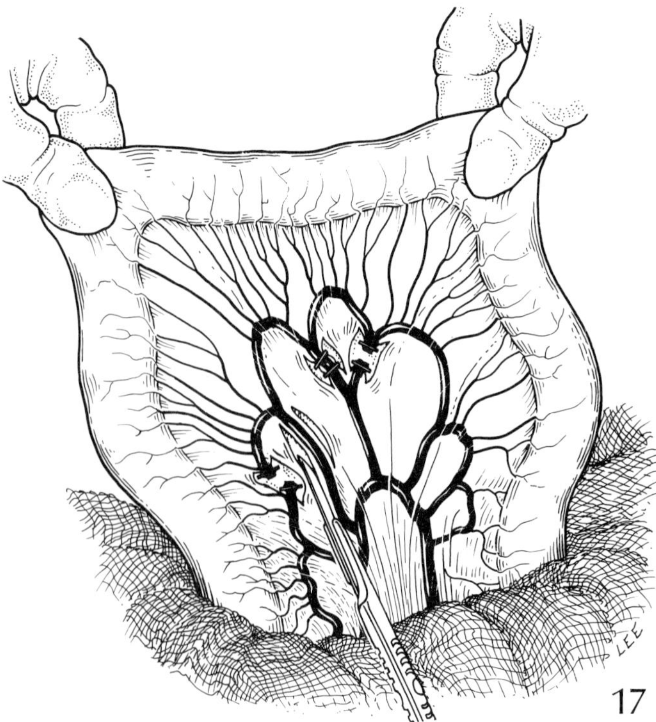

17

18

The ultimate line of dissection now isolates a loop which is dependent on one, two or three arcades. In this illustration the vascular division has been moved back on the loop side to provide alternative venous drainage pathways. This is desirable but not essential.

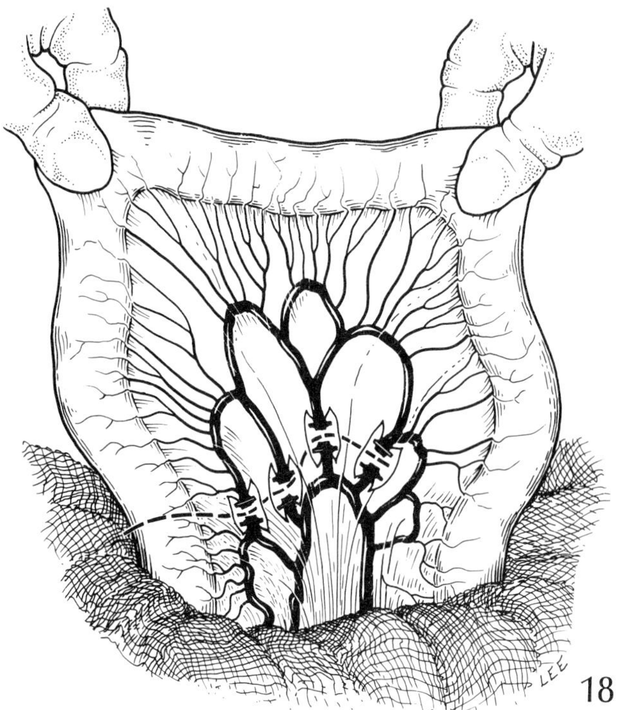

18

19

The loop is then transected between soft clamps.

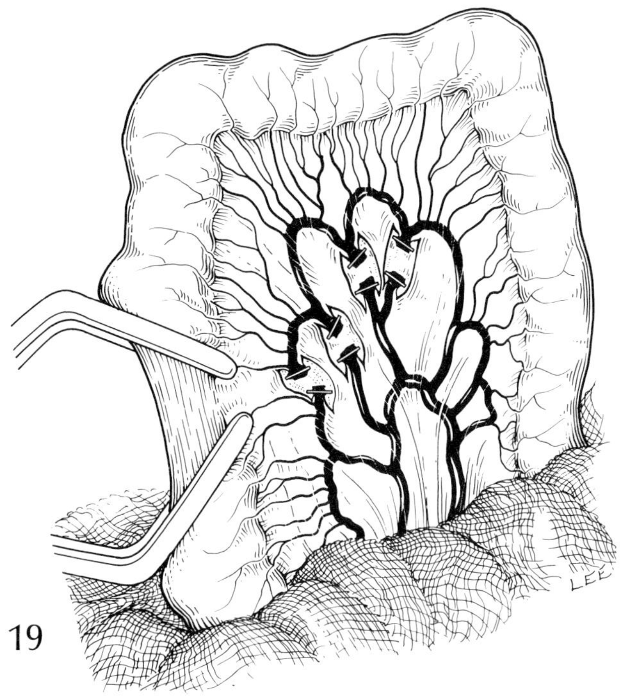

19

20

The preferred route for reconstruction after total gastrectomy is retrocolic. An avascular area is found in the transverse mesocolon and the mobilized loop brought up to be in relation to the divided oesophagus. It is convenient to apply the soft clamp from above and so draw the loop up.

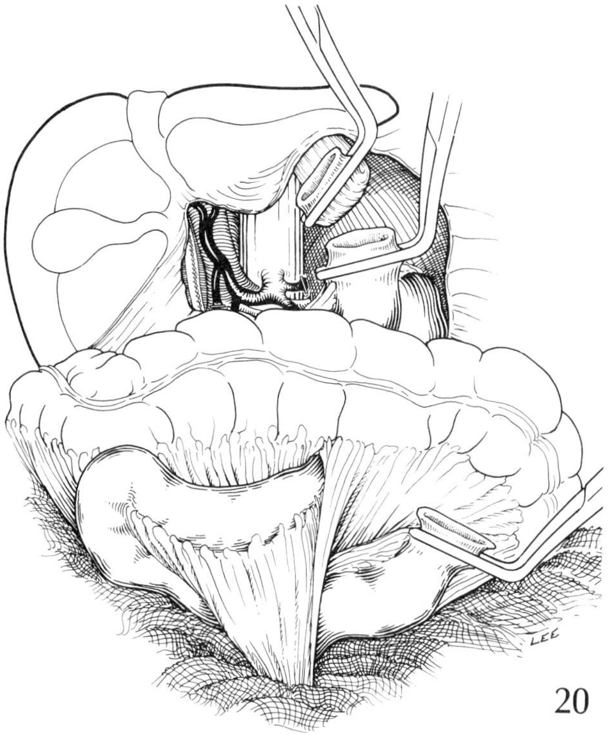

20

Jejunojejunostomy

21a & b

The restoration of intestinal continuity is achieved by end-to-side jejunojejunostomy. The lie of the loop determines whether the jejunojejunal anastomosis is done laterally (*a*) or medially (*b*) but in either case the cut edge of mesentery is joined to the surface of the mesentery of the afferent loop so as to eliminate a potential aperture through which a hernia could take place.

Either a conventional sutured anastomosis or a stapling technique may be used.

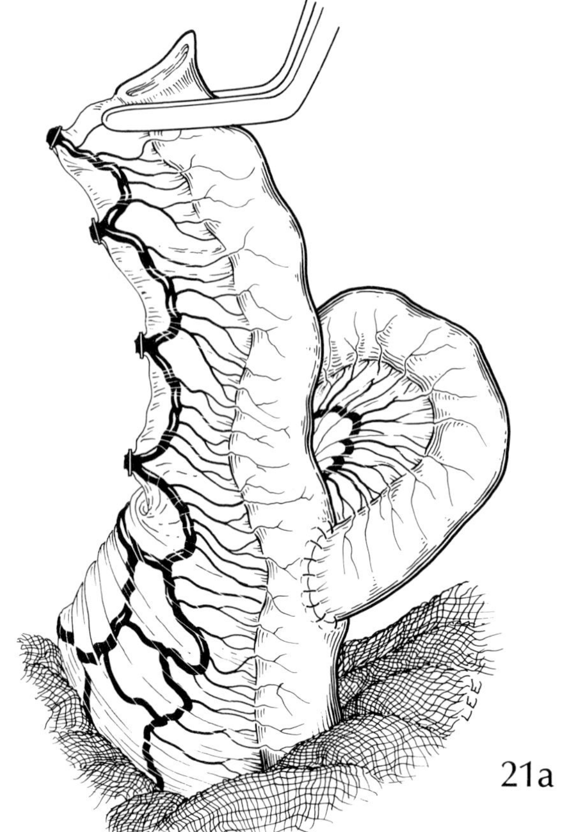

21a

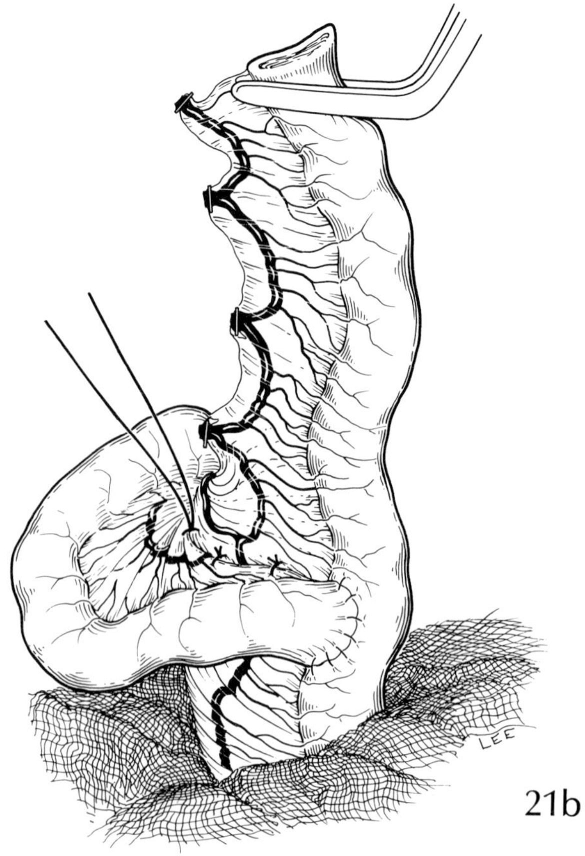

21b

Suture technique

22 & 23

For many years the author has used, without clinical leakage, a single layer of interrupted non-absorbable sutures (braided polyamide) inserted as shown. Others have employed different materials, e.g. stainless steel, with similar results. Meticulous placement and sympathetic tying of the knots so as to avoid strangulation are more important than the suture material used.

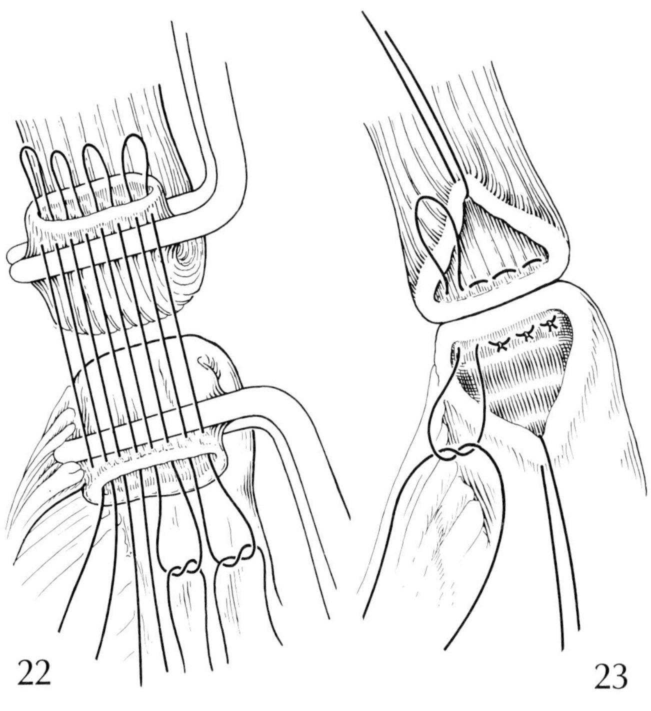

22 23

24

The anastomosis is reperitonealized by tacking the serosal surface of the jejunum to the cut edge of diaphragmatic peritoneum.

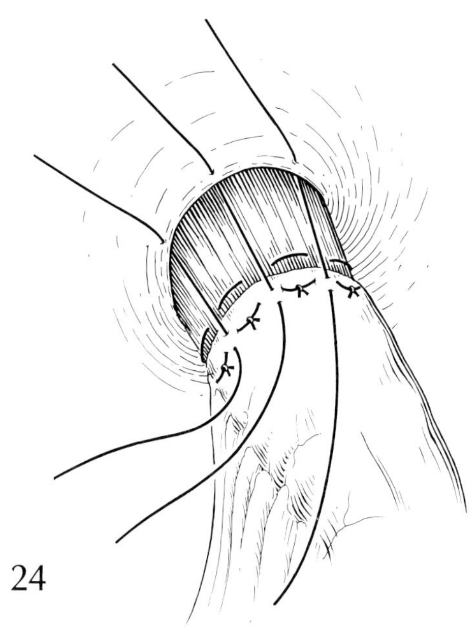

24

25

The completed procedure is shown. A supplementary jejunostomy into the efferent loop allows early resumption of enteral feeding.

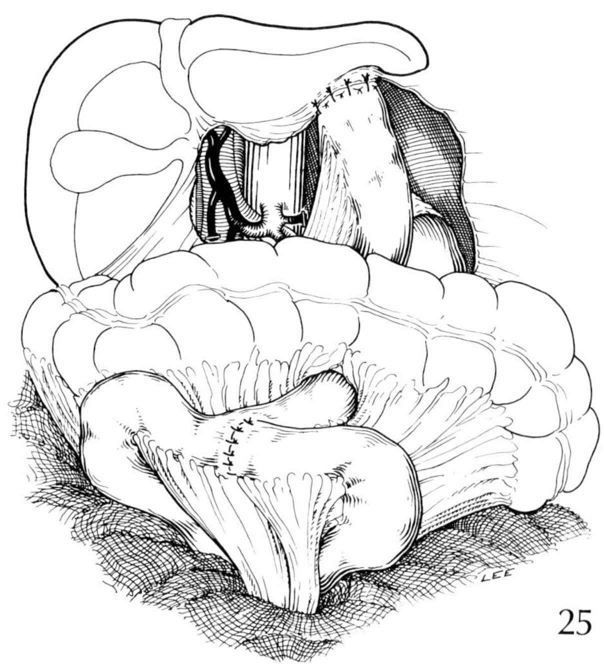

25

Stapling technique

26

The staples can be introduced conventionally through a small enterostomy in the jejunal loop.

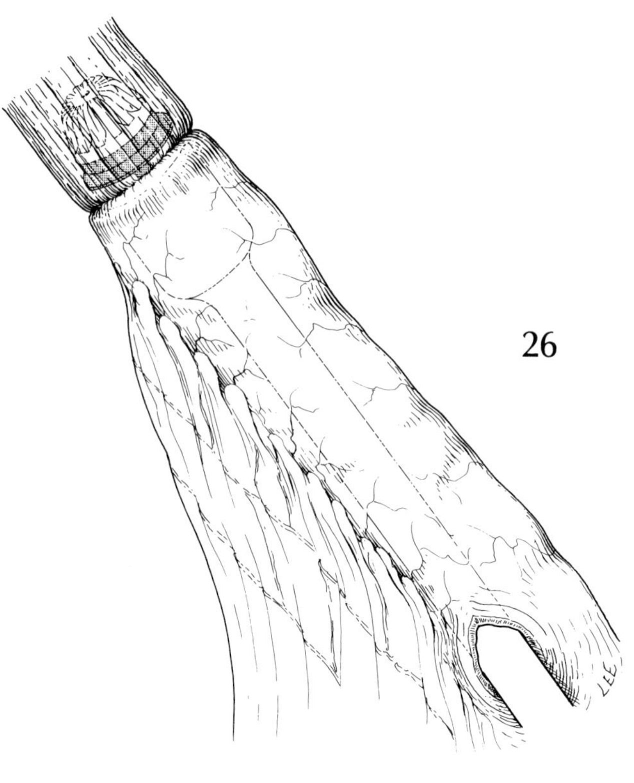

26

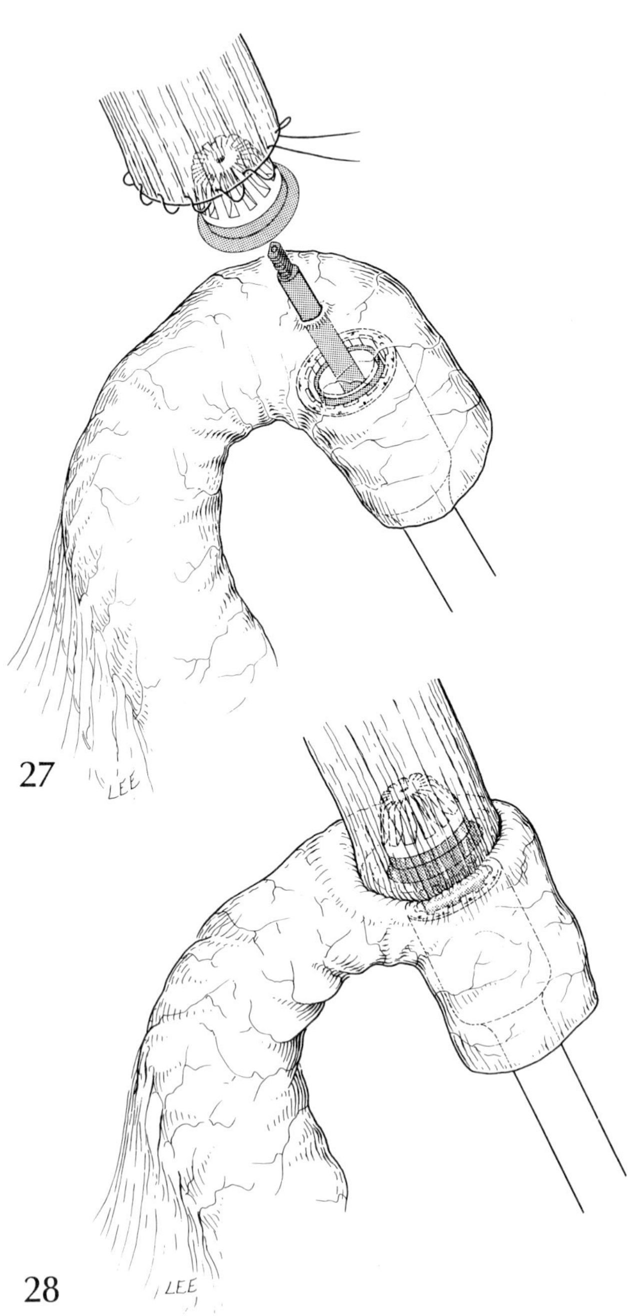

27

28

27 & 28

Alternatively, if the loop is turned over it is possible and desirable to insert the stapler without its head through the open jejunal mouth and on through the wall of jejunum to present an end-to-side oesophagojejunostomy.

29

The open wall of the jejunum is closed by conventional techniques or by linear stapling.

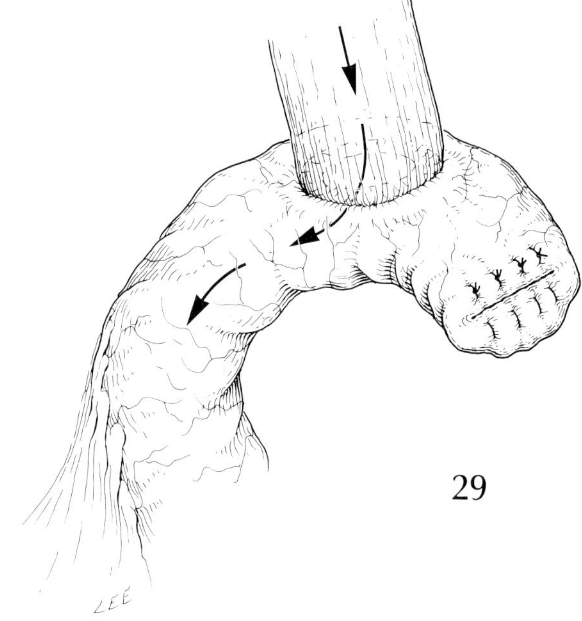

29

Postoperative care

Postoperative management is dictated by the physical circumstances of the case. An abdominal total gastrectomy in a relatively healthy middle-aged patient will occasion no more disturbance than, say, a cholecystectomy. Oral fluids are withheld for 48 h and then, in the presence of normal small bowel activity on auscultation, instituted rapidly and increased so that a full intake is achieved over the ensuing 36 h. Thereafter, provided the patient is prepared to chew adequately, any solid food can be taken, but it will be 7–10 days before a full energy intake is achieved. The author believes it is important to encourage the patient to regard himself as dietetically normal until proved otherwise and the surgeon has an important task to convince the patient that, though he now lacks a stomach,he is able to eat virtually normally.

On occasion, the surgeon may doubt the integrity of the anastomosis. A useful check is to administer 40 ml of water-soluble contrast medium on or about the fifth day and to expose a chest film at 5 min and an abdominal film at 40 min. The first establishes whether or not there is a hold up (rare) or radiological leakage (about 8–10 per cent), the second if small bowel propulsion is adequate beyond the anastomosis. Any abnormality at the suture line is an indication for caution in the administration of oral fluids. Most radiologically demonstrated leaks are asymptomatic and restriction of fluids for a week is all that is necessary. If total parenteral nutrition is not available for postoperative support, thought should be given to the establishment of a jejunostomy distal to the enteroenterostomy at the time of surgery. Though jejunostomy feeding can be difficult to establish and sustain, careful drip feeding of low residue, iso-osmolal feeds can do almost as much as parenteral nutrition until oral intake is re-established.

References

1. Fielding, W. L., Ellis, D. J., Jones, B. G. *et al.* Natural history of 'early' gastric cancer: results of a 10-year regional survey. British Medical Journal 1980; 281: 965–967

2. Black, M. M., Opler, S. R., Speer, F. D. Microscopic structure of gastric carcinomas and their regional lymph nodes in relation to survival. Surgery, Gynecology and Obstetrics 1954; 98: 725–734

3. Ishii, T., Ikegami, N., Hosoda, Y., Koide, O., Kaneko, M. The biological behaviour of gastric cancer. Journal of Pathology 1981; 134: 97–115

Appendicectomy

P. E. A. Savage MS, FRCS
Consultant Surgeon, Queen Mary's Hospital, Sidcup, Kent

Preoperative

Principles and justification

Appendicectomy is indicated whenever a diagnosis of acute appendicitis is made within 4–5 days of the onset of symptoms. During this period, any palpable swelling in the right iliac fossa is almost certainly an *appendix mass*, the structures involved in which may be separated safely be gentle dissection. The operation should be performed at the earliest opportunity compatible with the safe administration of a general anaesthetic. This is particularly important in children, in whom the rapid progression of the disease to peritonitis is a constant hazard.

A clinical diagnosis of non-specific mesenteric lymphadenitis in a child who has not had an appendicectomy should be confirmed at operation and the appendix removed. The appendix should also be removed if, at operation for acute appendicitis, the clinical features are found to be due to 'terminal ileitis' provided that there is no macroscopic evidence of involvement of the caecum or the appendix.

Appendicectomy is also indicated in patients with recurrent bouts of right iliac fossa pain in whom a diagnosis of chronic or recurrent subacute appendicitis has been made. Although macroscopically the appendix appears normal and the microscopic findings are unremarkable, examination of the lumen usually reveals a faecolith or other debris. The appendix may be removed during some other intra-abdominal procedure if access is easy, the appendix obviously abnormal and the risk of contaminating the primary operative site minimal.

Appendicectomy is contraindicated when a patient presents with a history of more than 5 days' duration and a right iliac fossa swelling that is almost certainly an *appendix abscess*.

Special preoperative preparation

If there are signs of peritonitis or if vomiting has been a marked feature of the illness, the stomach should be emptied by a nasogastric tube and an intravenous infusion set up. All patients should be given an anti-anaerobic agent such as metronidazole suppository with their premedication (adults 1 g; children 500 mg).

Anaesthesia

Four hours should have elapsed since the patient last ate or drank. After suitable premedication, general anaesthesia is induced and anaesthesia maintained with endotracheal intubation.

The operation

Position of patient

The patient is placed supine on the operating table and the diathermy pad positioned. Tilting the table may be helpful during the operation.

Preparation and towelling of the skin

The skin should be prepared as for a laparotomy, the antiseptic solution reaching from the nipples to the upper thigh. Four sheets are arranged to leave exposed the midline, the umbilicus, the anterosuperior iliac spine and the right flank.

1

Choice of incision

A transverse incision centred over the area of maximum tenderness gives the best approach to the inflamed appendix and the most satisfactory cosmetic result. An incision no more than 5cm long is adequate in the first instance but should be extended without hesitation if difficulties are encountered. Should the diagnosis prove to be incorrect, either the incision may be closed and a more appropriate one made, or the existing incision may be converted to a Pfannenstiel approach (see p. 43) if this will give adequate access.

In the presence of peritonitis a right paramedian incision allows a more adequate exploration and peritoneal toilet to be performed.

A long oblique muscle-cutting incision may be necessary in a fat patient in order to achieve a safe and adequate exposure.

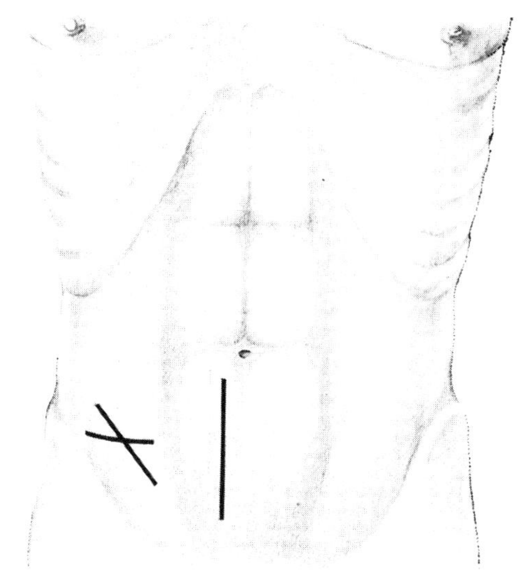

1

2

Incising the external oblique aponeurosis

After the skin, subcutaneous fat and membranous layer of the superficial fascia have been incised the external oblique aponeurosis is nicked with a scalpel and divided in the line of its fibres with scissors.

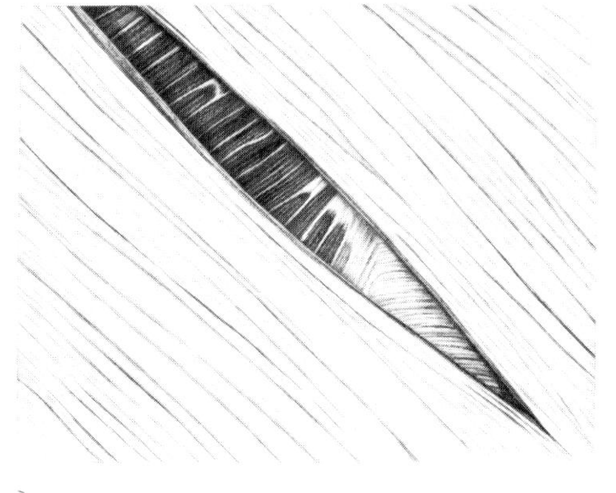

2

3

Incising the internal oblique insertion

Splitting the internal oblique and transversus abdominis muscles is most easily achieved by grasping the edge of the rectus sheath with two tissue forceps and dividing the insertion of the internal oblique transversely with a scalpel.

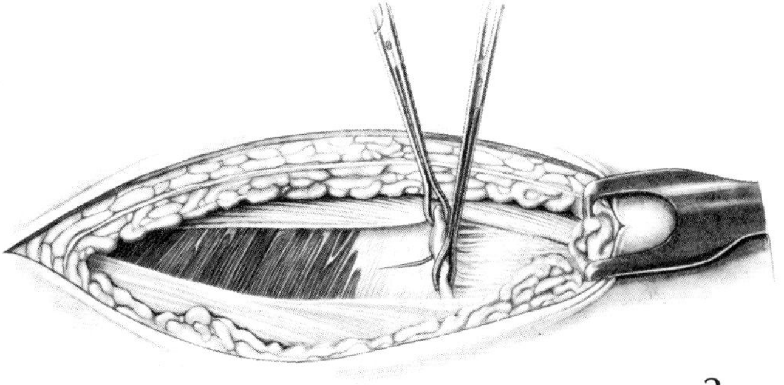

3

4

Splitting the internal oblique and transversus abdominis

The jaws of a large artery forceps are carefully inserted in a medial direction and opened to split the fibres of the internal oblique and transversus abdominis muscle fibres further and allow the insertion of retractors to provide adequate exposure.

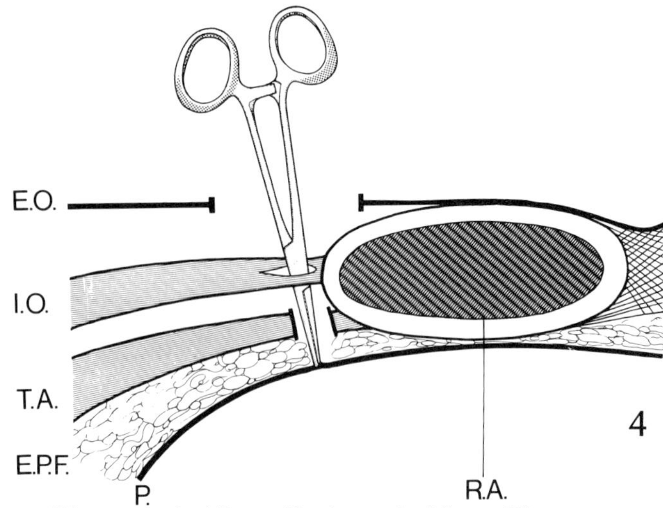

EO = external oblique; IO = internal oblique; TA = transversus abdominis; EPF = extraperitoneal fat; P = peritoneum; RA = rectus abdominis

5

Incising the peritoneum

Any extraperitoneal fat is cleared by blunt dissection from the peritoneum which is picked up between two artery forceps. After making sure that no bowel has been inadvertently trapped by feeling the layers of the peritoneum between thumb and index finger, the peritoneum is carefully incised with a scalpel. Once the peritoneum has been opened the incision is extended in a transverse direction using scissors and the retractors are reinserted and lifted to allow air to enter the peritoneal cavity. Any peritoneal fluid is aspirated, a sample being saved for bacteriological examination.

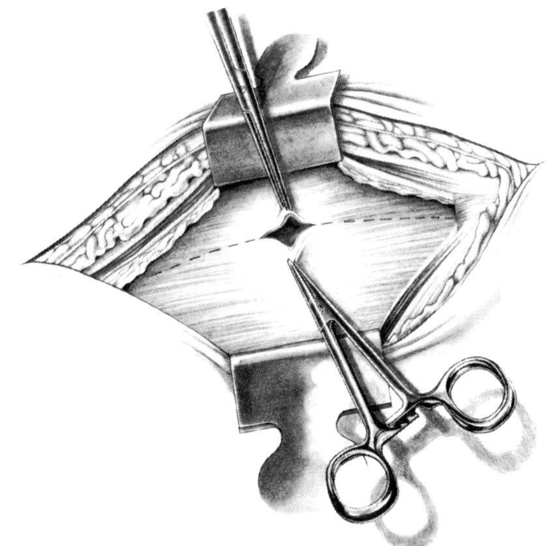

6

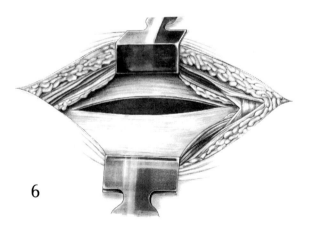

6

Extension of incision medially

Additional exposure medially may be obtained by dividing the anterior and posterior layers of the rectus sheath and retracting the rectus abdominis muscle medially. Too vigorous retraction may tear the inferior epigastric vessels necessitating a further extension of the incision to control the bleeding.

7 & 8

Extension of incision laterally

Safe extraction of a retrocaecal appendix may require additional exposure laterally by incising the abdominal wall muscles obliquely and, if necessary, extending the skin incision in the same direction.

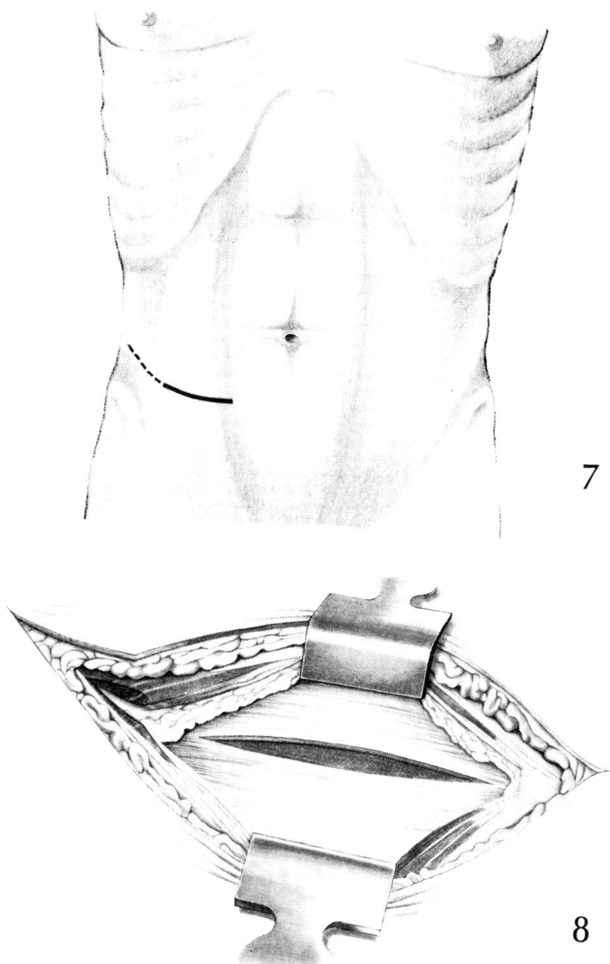

7

8

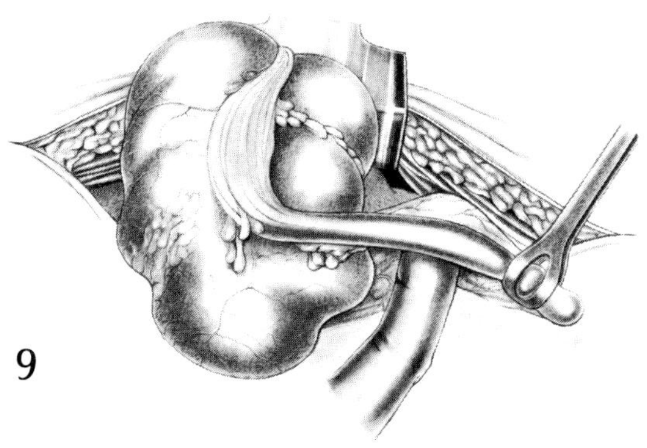

9

9

Delivering the appendix

The caecum is identified by the presence of taeniae coli on its surface, and an index finger is passed down the paracolic gutter and below the caecum to locate the appendix. Any inflammatory adhesions on the *lateral* side of the appendix can be freed safely with the finger and the organ delivered to the surface of the wound. If difficulty is encountered, in either locating or delivering the appendix, the caecum is first grasped with non-toothed forceps and delivered to the surface; then the bowel is held firmly with a swab and gently rocked to and fro while the caecum is progressively delivered until the taeniae coli can be followed down to the appendix. At the earliest opportunity a Babcock's tissue forceps is placed around the appendix. Attempts to push or pull the appendix out forcibly should be resisted, particularly if it is gangrenous and likely to burst.

10 & 11

Securing the appendicular vessels

Once the appendix has been delivered, the appendicular vessels are clipped, divided and ligated. When the mesentery is oedematous, the artery forceps are placed close to the appendix and small bites taken. For added security a transfixion stitch is passed through each side of the mesentery.

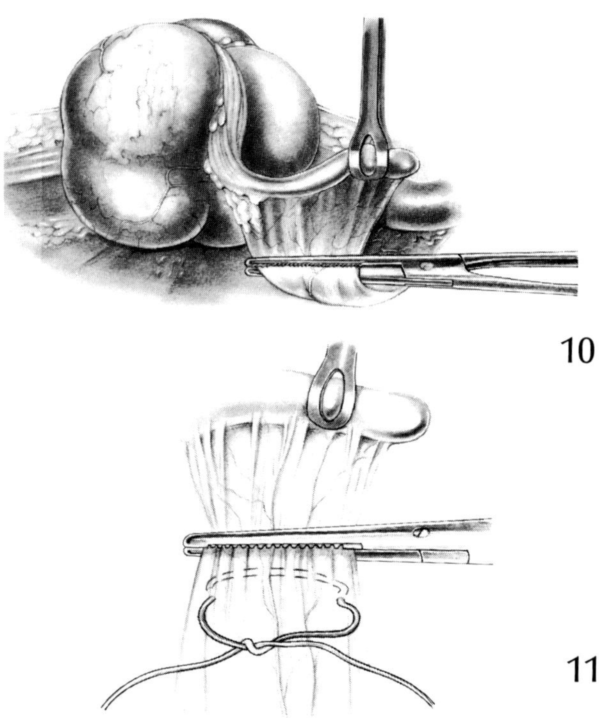

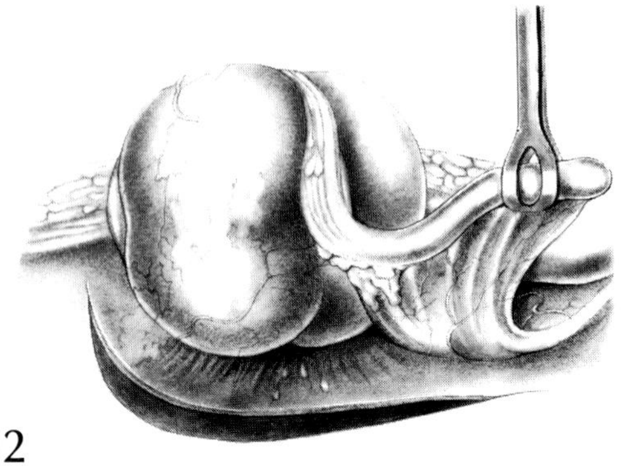

10

11

12

Retrieving a lost appendicular artery

If the appendicular artery is lost it retracts behind the terminal ileum. Gentle traction on the caecum may bring the vessel into view, but if it cannot be retrieved easily without risk of damaging the ileum or mesenteric vessels, the incision is extended and the caecum mobilized by dividing the parietal peritoneum. The artery may then be safely secured.

12

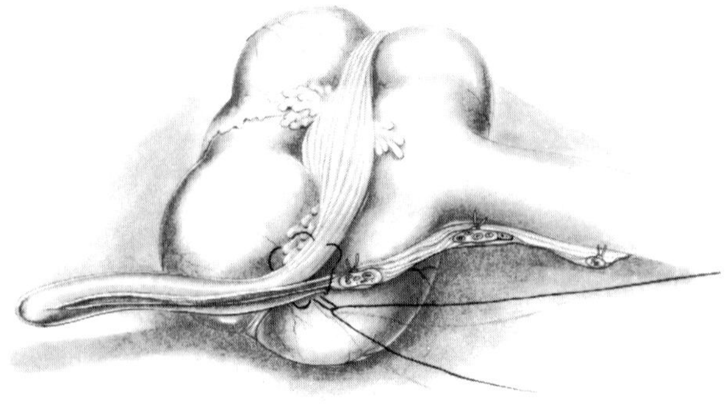

13

13

Insertion of purse-string suture

With the appendix held vertically, a purse-string seromuscular suture of 2/0 chromic catgut is inserted 1 cm from the base of the appendix.

14, 15 & 16

Ligation and invagination of appendix stump

The appendix is crushed at its base with an artery forceps and the crushed area ligated with 2/0 chromic catgut. The appendix is then divided with a scalpel and the stump invaginated into the caecum where it is retained by tightening and tying the purse-string suture.

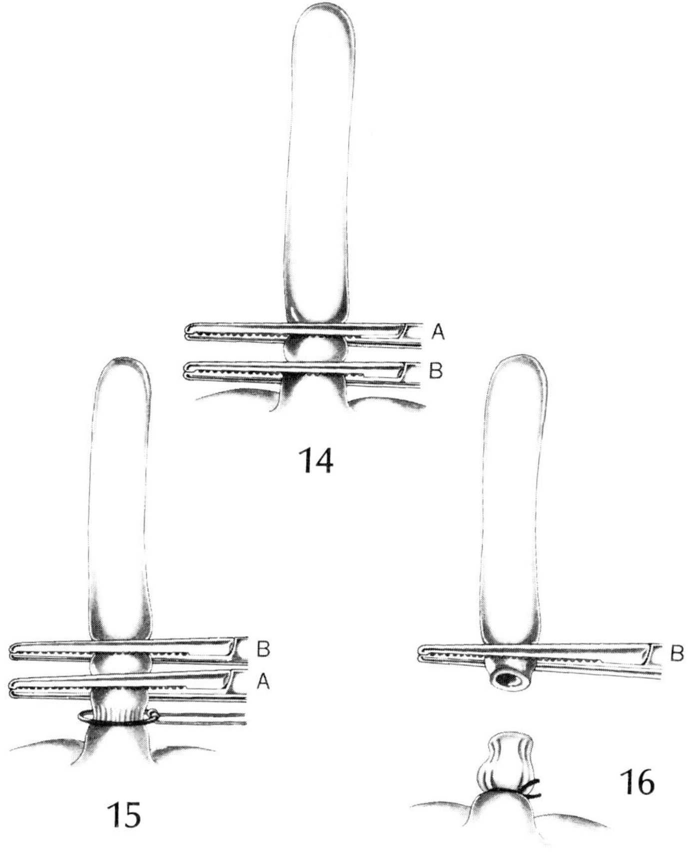

Local exploration

The site of invagination is examined together with the appendicular mesentery to make sure that haemostasis is secure. In the absence of peritonitis the existence of a Meckel's diverticulum should be excluded by examining the last 1 m of the ileum. Once the terminal ileum has been picked up at its junction with the caecum subsequent manipulations are easier if the caecum itself is returned to the peritoneal cavity. The uterus and right ovary are usually within reach of the examining finger. The presence of abnormal mesenteric lymph nodes is noted.

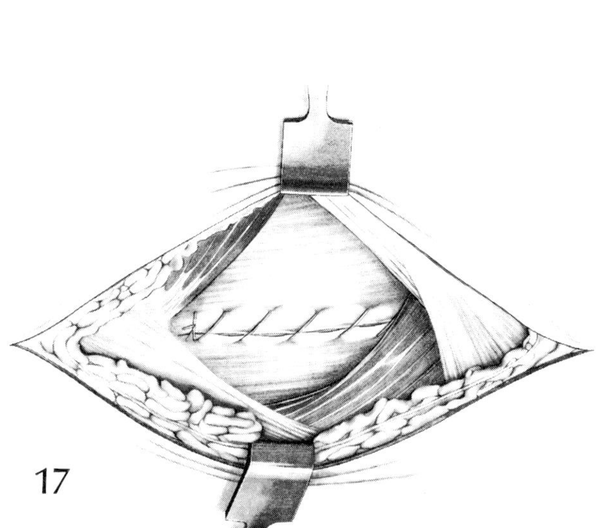
17

17

Closure of peritoneum

To close the incision four artery forceps are placed on the peritoneum, which is sutured with a continuous absorbable suture, care being taken not to pick up a piece of bowel with the needle.

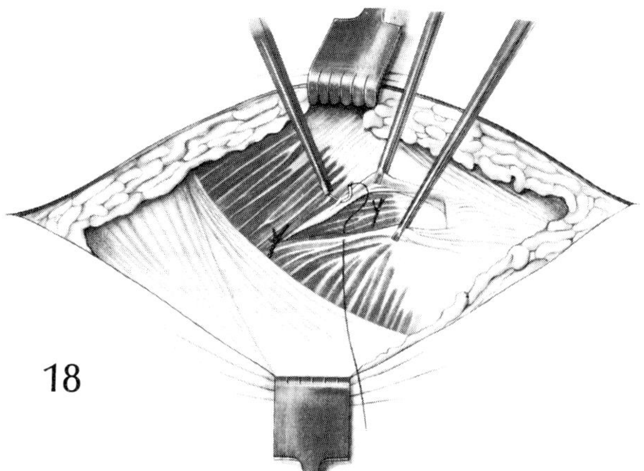
18

18

Closure of muscles

The muscles of the abdominal wall are closed in layers, the transversus abdominis and the epimysium of the internal oblique muscle being approximated with interrupted absorbable sutures.

19

Closure of external oblique, fat and skin

The external oblique muscle and aponeurosis is closed with a continuous suture of absorbable material, the dead space is obliterated with a fat stitch and the skin closed with interrupted or subcuticular sutures. If the wound has been contaminated, antibiotic or antiseptic powder may be applied to the layers of the wound. In particularly obese patients it is generally wise to drain the subcutaneous tissue with a corrugated drain placed via a separate stab incision.

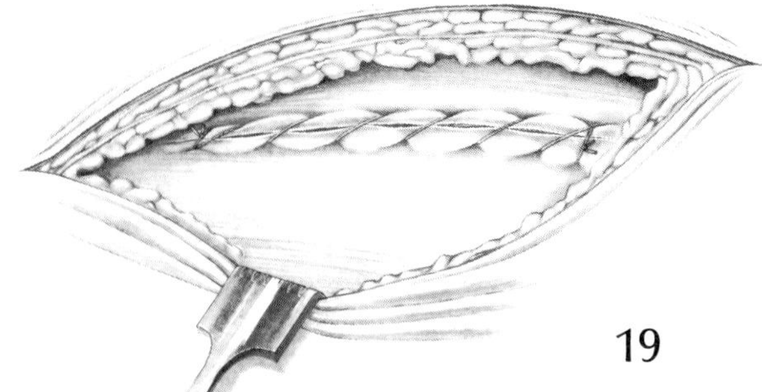
19

20

Retrograde appendicectomy

An adherent inflamed retrocaecal appendix is best removed by the technique of retrograde appendicectomy. Having identified and delivered the caecum, the appendix is clamped, divided and ligated at its base, the stump being invaginated with a purse-string suture. *The caecum is replaced in the peritoneal cavity.* The mesoappendix close to the appendix is clamped and divided, taking small bites until the the whole organ can be removed, after which the vessels may be ligated. If the appendix bed is oozing, a *soft* drain is inserted down to the area via a separate stab incision in the flank. The drain is sutured to the skin and for added security is transfixed with a safety pin.

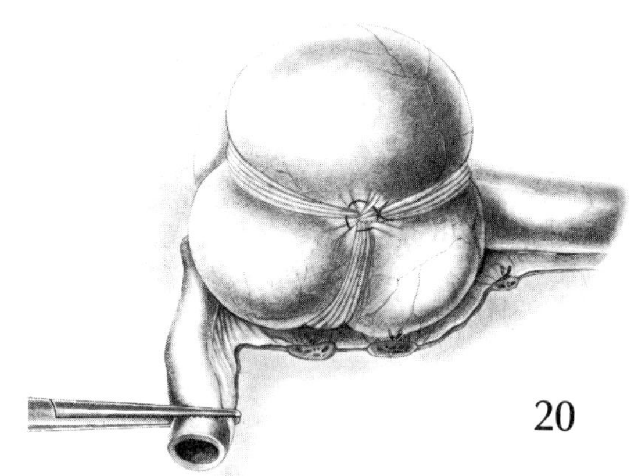
20

Postoperative care

Postoperatively the patient is kept under observation and adequate analgesics and antinauseants given as required. A 5 day course of metronidazole is prescribed, a 1 g metronidazole suppository being inserted rectally every 8 h until the patient is able to take the drug orally, when the prescription is changed to 200 mg 8 hourly.

Complications

Wound infection

The development of pain in the wound associated with a fever and local signs of inflammation indicate a wound infection. A mild cellulitis may respond to a course of broad-spectrum antibiotics or an increased dose of metronidazole, but it will often be necessary to drain the wound by inserting a pair of sinus forceps into the most inflamed and indurated area.

Intestinal fistula

The development of a faecal fistula suggests damage to the caecum or terminal ileum. A retained swab, Crohn's disease or actinomycosis must be excluded. Initial treatment should be conservative, with an elemental diet, but subsequent re-exploration may be advisable.

Pylephlebitis

The development of a fever, rigors and jaundice suggests the rare complication of pylephlebitis. After blood cultures have been taken, active treatment with intravenous antibiotics and other supportive measures should be instituted.

Splenectomy, partial splenectomy, staging laparotomy

Miles Irving MD, ChM, FRCS
Professor of Surgery and Consultant Surgeon, Hope Hospital, Salford

David Gough FRCS, FRCS(Ed.), FRACS, DCH
Consultant Paediatric Surgeon, Royal Manchester Children's Hospital, Pendlebury, Manchester

Introduction

The traditional indications for splenectomy, i.e. trauma, hereditary spherocytosis, idiopathic thrombocytopaenic purpura, cysts and tumours and as part of radical upper abdominal surgery such as total gastrectomy, remain the principal reasons for this operation. However, splenectomy is now being increasingly used in the management of conditions where it was once thought to be contraindicated. Thus, it is now requested for patients with chronic lymphocytic leukaemia, chronic granulocytic (myeloid) leukaemia, the lymphomas and hypersplenism from a variety of causes.

Parallel with the recognition of the benefits of splenectomy has come a realization of the danger from serious infection (particularly pneumococcal) that may follow, even years later, in children and adults[1,2].

As a consequence it is now suggested that in those cases where splenectomy is not an essential part of treatment every effort should be made to conserve part or all of the spleen. Whether this advice is sensible in the adult remains to be seen. It may well be that prevention of death from overwhelming septicaemia may be counterbalanced by the postoperative mortality and morbidity of attempts at splenic preservation. If total removal is necessary it seems reasonable on present evidence to give prophylactic antimicrobial treatment for at least 2 years afterwards. Alternatively, an attempt should be made to vaccinate the patient against pneumococcal sepsis.

Preoperative

Indications

Trauma

Where the spleen is avulsed or fragmented splenectomy is the only feasible treatment. However, where it is lacerated, or only a segment is avulsed, conservative treatment or partial splenectomy should be attempted even if in the end splenectomy has to be resorted to. Unrecognized traumatic splenic injury of mild degree has probably gone untreated for years without harm. Recent diagnostic methods have established that a planned non-operative approach for selected cases of traumatic rupture of the spleen is both safe and effective[3].

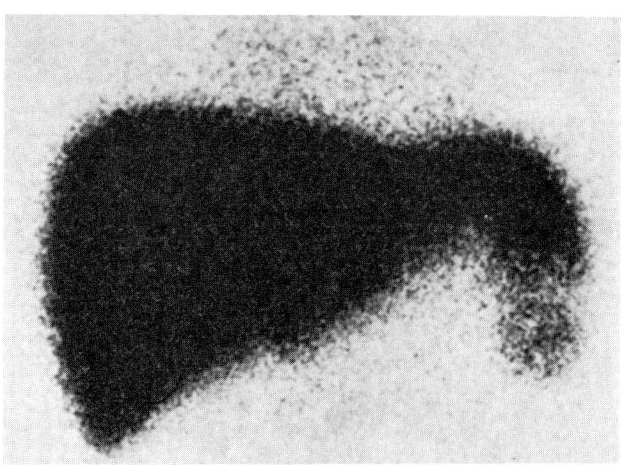

1

The relatively non-invasive investigation of radionuclide imaging using technetium is able to show evidence of splenic injury in a large proportion of cases. The illustration shows a lower pole splenic injury which was managed without surgery. Because delayed splenic rupture is almost unknown in children, and in this age group the spleen is often the only organ injured, this policy has gained most support amongst the ranks of paediatric surgeons. Autotransplantation of splenic fragments as free grafts can occur naturally after injury but is of no proven benefit as a planned surgical procedure.

Hypersplenism

In this state the spleen, which is usually enlarged, is destroying one or more components of the blood, e.g. erythrocytes, leucocytes and platelets, at a rate in excess of the ability of the marrow to produce them. This may be the result of abnormalities of the cells, which are more easily destroyed than normally, or enlargement of the spleen resulting in stagnation of the blood cells with their consequent destruction. Hereditary spherocytosis, sickle cell anaemia, idiopathic thrombocytopaenia and splenic anaemia due to portal hypertension and lymphomatous infiltration of the spleen can be classified under this heading.

Leukaemias

Haematologists now consider that chronic lymphocytic leukaemias, chronic granulocytic leukaemia and variants such as hairy cell leukaemia can be treated more effectively if the spleen is removed. The operation has to be done when the patient is in good condition and free from infection. It is contraindicated in acute leukaemias, blast crises, and when the patient is deteriorating and/or infected.

Incidental

Splenectomy is often necessary during the course of major upper abdominal surgery such as total gastrectomy or pancreatectomy. However, every effort should be made to preserve the spleen in these operations as long as conservation does not compromise the clearance of malignant disease.

Giant splenomegaly

In some diseases, such as myelofibrosis, the spleen grows to such a huge size that the weight becomes unbearable for the patient and in addition is prone to repeated painful infarction. In these circumstances splenectomy is worthwhile.

Cysts, tumours, abscess, torsion, splenic artery aneurysm

In these rare conditions splenectomy is necessary to establish the diagnosis as well as to treat the disease.

Staging laparotomy

Splenectomy is still considered by most of those who treat Hodgkin's disease to be an integral part of the staging of Clinical Stages I and II of the disease. In many instances Stage III disease is also included. However, its value is being increasingly challenged, especially by paediatric oncologists, as the mortality rates from late systemic infection have approached 10 per cent in patients subjected to staging laparotomy and splenectomy for Hodgkin's disease. Indeed, some paediatric oncologists now regard splenectomy or even partial splenectomy as unnecessary in the management of Hodgkin's disease in children. When evidence of splenic involvement is requested by the medical oncologists partial splenectomy has a place although it carries a risk of missing splenic disease in 10 per cent of patients[4].

Preoperative preparation

Close consultation with the haematologist and medical oncologist is essential in patients undergoing splenectomy for lymphoma or a haematological disorder. The surgeon should ensure that the haemoglobin and white cell count have been recently measured and the bone marrow assessed. Anaemia, leucopaenia and thrombocytopaenia are not in themselves contraindications to operation as long as the bone marrow shows evidence of ability to produce these cells. There is rarely any benefit to be obtained from splenectomy for hypersplenism if the marrow is aplastic or totally replaced by tumour. If there is doubt about the role of the spleen in red cell or platelet destruction survival studies with ^{51}Cr-labelled cells can be informative. In cases of haemolytic anaemia the gall bladder should be investigated to see if it contains stones.

The surgeon should encourage his colleagues to refer patients for splenectomy before the underlying disease has progressed to the point where the patient is subject to serious infections. Splenectomy in infected hypersplenic patients almost never succeeds in improving their condition.

Before operation for uncomplicated splenectomy 2 units of blood should be cross-matched. For large spleens, where there is a possibility of multiple vascular adhesions, up to 6 units of blood should be prepared. Platelet infusions should be ordered for severely thrombocytopaenic patients but should not be given until the splenic artery has been tied. In cases of traumatic rupture of the spleen preoperative colloid and blood transfusion to resuscitate the patient is mandatory.

The patient should be shaved from nipples to midthigh. A nasogastric tube is passed.

The operations

Anaesthesia

An endotracheal tube and muscle relaxation are essential. The anaesthetist should be warned that in difficult cases it may be necessary to divide the left costal margin and open the thorax. Prophylaxis against venous thrombosis should be commenced using intermittent calf compression with pneumatic leg cuffs, supplemented by intravenous dextran when induction of anaesthesia begins.

ELECTIVE SPLENECTOMY FOR NORMAL-SIZED OR SLIGHTLY ENLARGED SPLEEN

Position of patient

Supine with a sandbag under the left lower ribs.

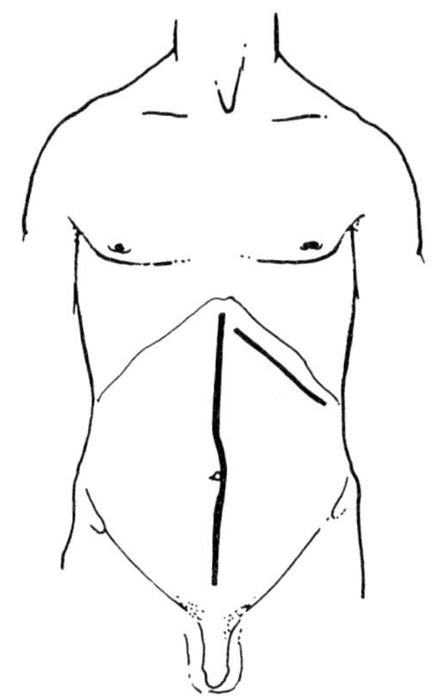

2

2

The incision

Long midline or left subcostal muscle cutting.

Exploration

General exploration should commence with examination of the spleen, taking care not to tear any adhesions. The splenic hilum should be palpated for lymph node enlargement. The liver should be examined for the presence of cirrhosis and tumour infiltration. The gall bladder should be palpated as, in cases of haemolytic anaemia, it frequently contains stones. In this event it should be removed.

A careful examination for the presence of accessory spleens is carried out paying particular attention to the gastrosplenic ligament, the mesocolon and the upper border of the pancreas.

Splenectomy

The operator's right hand should be slid gently over the convex diaphragmatic surface of the spleen. In most cases it will do so without obstruction down to the lienorenal ligament. If adhesions are encountered they should not be broken down but dealt with in the manner described later.

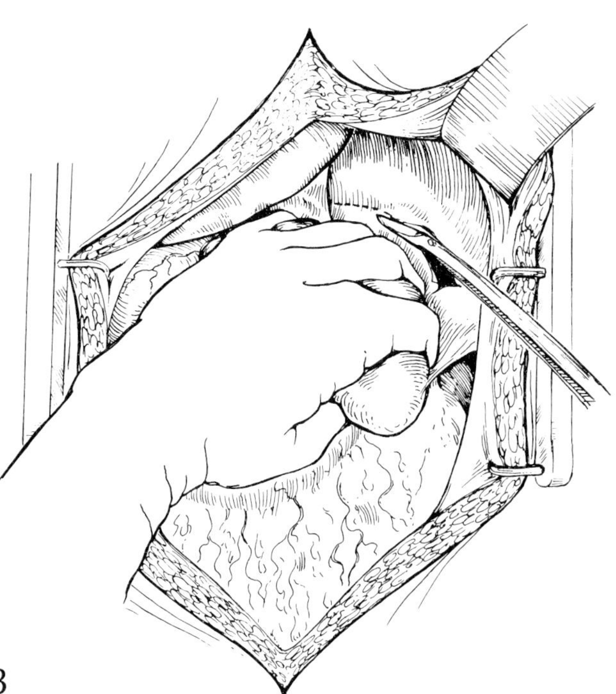

3

3

Mobilization of the spleen

The operator now substitutes his left hand for his right and gently pulls the spleen up towards the abdominal incision to that the taut posterior leaf of the lienorenal ligament is clearly demonstrated. This is then incised with scissors along its full length allowing the posterior surface of the spleen and the contents of the hilum to be drawn up into the wound.

Division of vessels

4

At this stage a band of short gastric vessels passing to the upper pole of the spleen in the top of the gastrosplenic ligament may limit mobilization. They should be divided between artery forceps and ligated with 0 silk. Care must be taken not to include any of the stomach wall in the ligatures as this can lead to a gastric fistula.

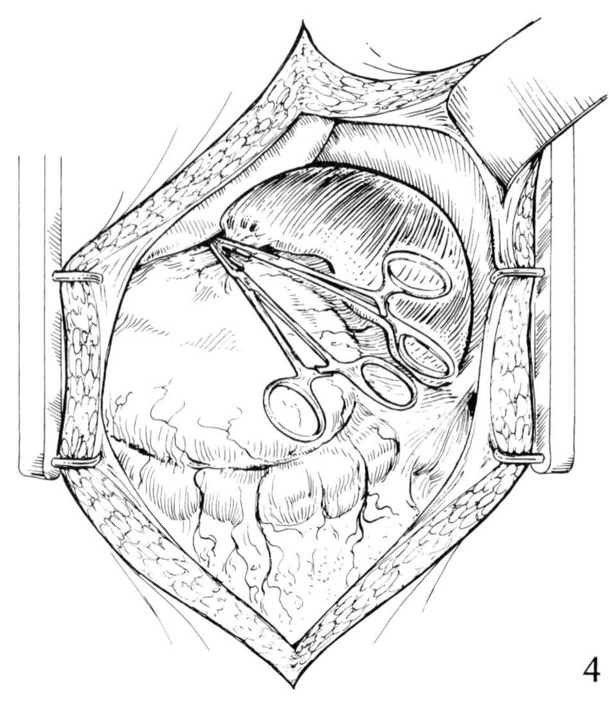

4

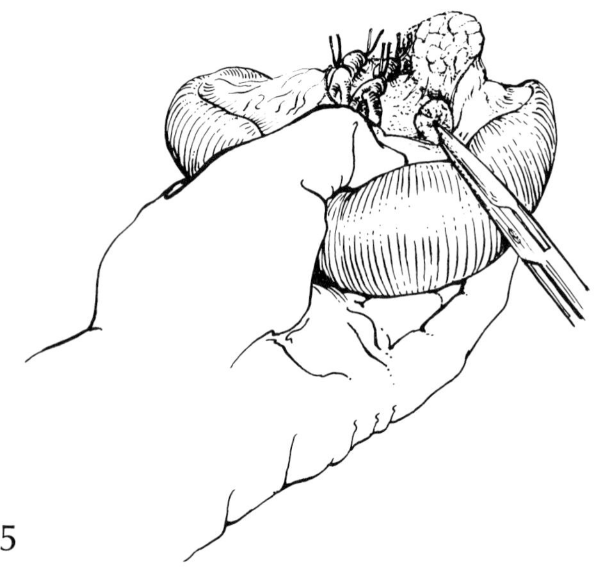

5

5

Attention is then turned to the posterior aspect of the splenic hilum. The tail of the pancreas is identified and carefully dissected from the hilum using scissors and gauze pledgets. Bleeding from small vessels can be arrested by diathermy coagulation. The splenic artery and vein are dissected out and ligated in continuity with strong linen thread. The artery should be ligated before the vein. The vessels are then divided between the ligatures. In thrombocytopaenic patients platelet infusions should be given at this stage.

Division of the gastrosplenic ligament

6

The spleen is then turned over to demonstrate the gastrosplenic ligament which is divided piecemeal between ligatures. This exposes the anterior leaf of the lienorenal ligament which, apart from a few small vessels, should be avascular. It is divided by dissection with the scissors, continued care being taken not to damage the pancreas. The spleen can now be removed. Haemostasis is secured by diathermy or suture ligation of any bleeding vessels in the residual splenic pedicle. If there has been extensive dissection in the left hypochondrium a low pressure suction drainage catheter should be placed in the subdiaphragmatic space.

The abdominal wound is then closed in layers.

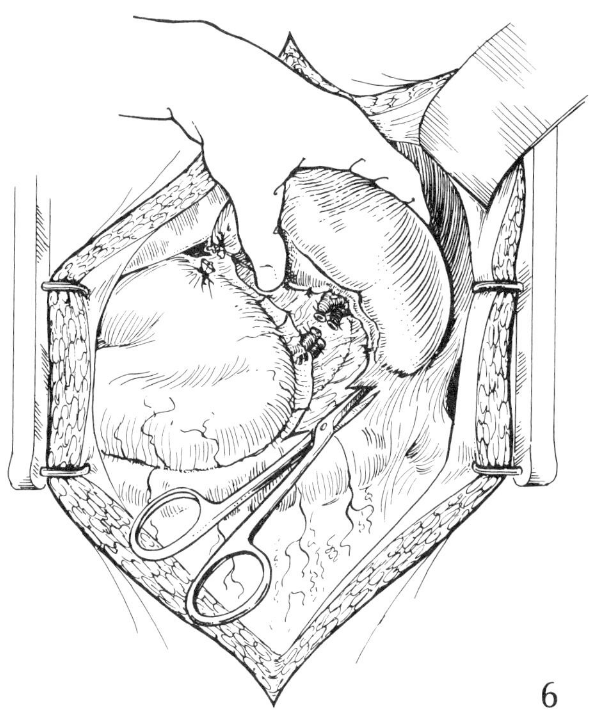

6

MODIFICATION OF TECHNIQUE FOR RUPTURED SPLEEN

The principles of the operation are the same. The additional problems are the initial control of haemorrhage, the detection of associated injuries and the desirability of conserving the spleen where possible.

The incision

This should always be a long midline incision which allows free and rapid access to other viscera that may also be damaged.

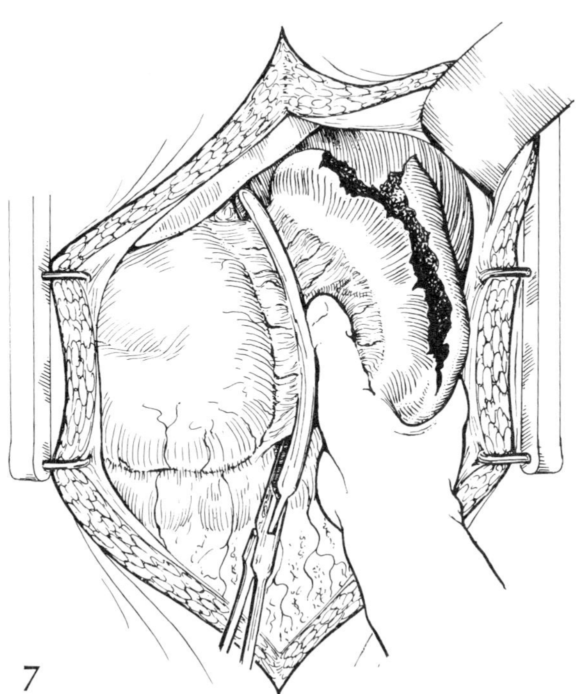

7

Control of bleeding

7

It is first necessary to remove the blood and clot in the left hypochondrium by scooping, mopping and suction. An assistant strongly lifts the left costal margin with a retractor and the surgeon's right hand is thrust down to the splenic hilum where, in cases of continuing vigorous bleeding, the vessels are grasped between finger and thumb.

If at this stage the patient is grossly shocked squeezing should be maintained until the anaethetist has corrected the hypovolaemia. Where prolonged compression is necessary it may be made easier by occluding all the hilar structures with a non-crushing intestinal clamp.

Once the situation has stabilized and it is ascertained that the spleen is so badly damaged that no form of conservation or repair is possible, splenectomy should be carried out in a manner as near as possible to that described for elective splenectomy. The surgeon should avoid the temptation to apply forceps in a blind fashion and to mass-ligature structures in the splenic hilum as it is in this way that the gastric wall and pancreatic tail are damaged. However, in certain cases it can be very difficult to isolate and ligate the major vessels, and in this situation the clamped tissues can be transfixed and ligated with strong thread sutures.

CONSERVATION, REPAIR AND PARTIAL SPLENECTOMY FOR RUPTURED SPLEEN

Conservative treatment

Although non-operative treatment is well established, and it is now evident that with careful observation and circulatory support from transfusion certain ruptured spleens can be left *in situ* to heal, it remains a difficult policy to adopt in the treatment of patients with abdominal injuries. The hazards are obvious, other injuries can be missed, bleeding can recur and delayed rupture is a risk. It does not simplify the treatment of injured patients but makes it more complex. It is a policy which must be abandoned where continuous bleeding is evident and where other injuries are suspected.

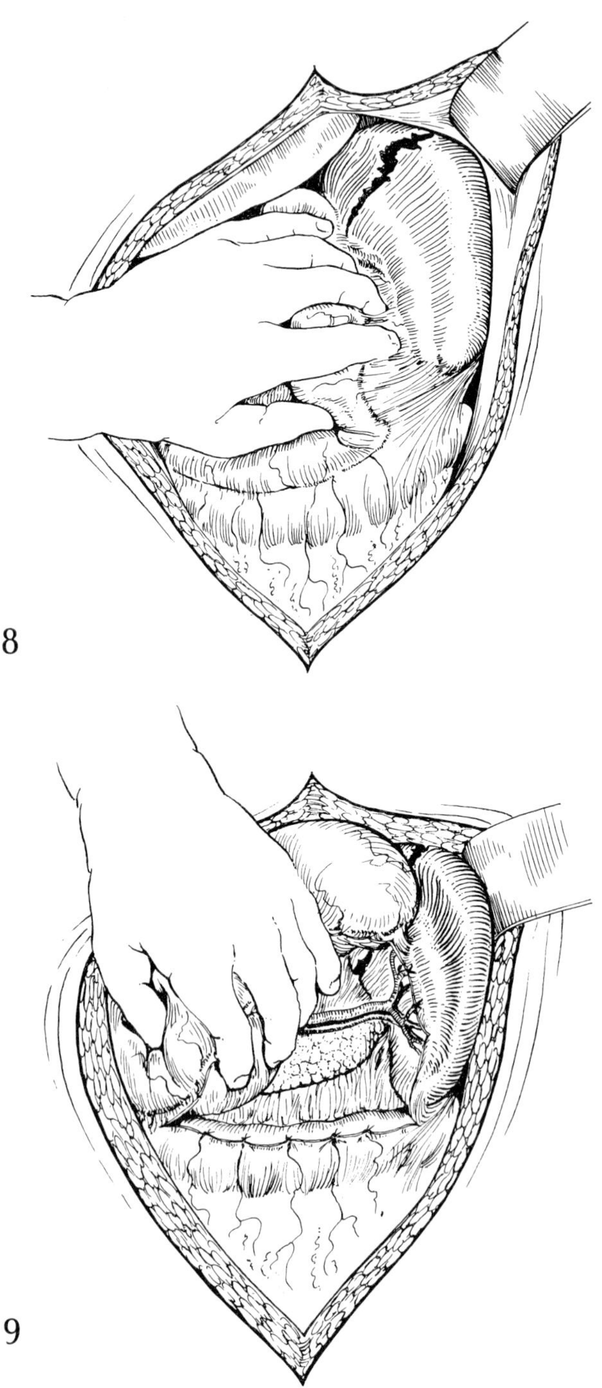

8

9

8 & 9

The decision to leave a spleen to heal spontaneously can also be taken at operation. Where a minor splenic injury is seen and bleeding has ceased, inspection of the area can be made by retraction and without dividing the lienorenal ligament. Entry to the lesser sac is gained for examination of the splenic hilum, pancreas and retroperitoneal tissues. If these areas are free from damage and haematoma the spleen can be left *in situ* and the abdomen closed with suction drainage to the area of the spleen. This represents simply a return to the proven safety of non-operative treatment. In some cases persistent oozing of blood from the torn splenic substance may be controlled by the local application of dry microfibrillar collagen (Avitene).

10

Splenorraphy

Suture of splenic lacerations is advocated by some authorities, but where haemorrhage has ceased it is probably unnecessary and may even cause bleeding to recommence. However, where bleeding is still continuing from an easily accessible laceration in the lower pole of the spleen the insertion of 0 polyglycolic acid sutures, combined with ligation in continuity of the relevant polar artery, may achieve control. However, if active bleeding continues then our advice is not to persist with suturing but to perform total or partial splenectomy.

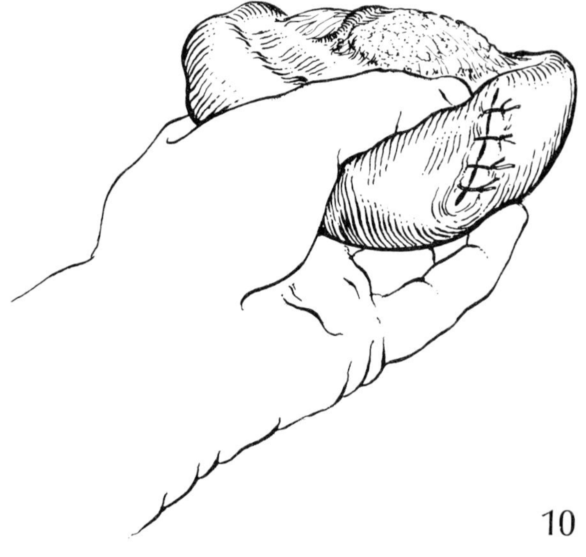

10

Partial splenectomy

Should a fragment of spleen be completely or partially avulsed, usually at the upper or lower poles, then a different policy can be adopted.

11

The spleen is fully mobilized as previously described by dividing the lienorenal and gastrosplenic attachments. The splenic pedicle is grasped by the assistant and compressed while the tail of the pancreas is dissected bluntly from the hilum and the vessels are exposed. Dissection close to the capsule exposes the relevant polar artery which is encircled and doubly ligated with thread or occluded with metal clips.

12

Wedge resection is accomplished using cutting diathermy and mattress sutures of '0' polyglycolic acid are used to control oozing from the open edge. After satisfactory haemostasis is obtained the abdomen is closed with suction drainage to the splenic area. This procedure is probably only of value if more than half the spleen is preserved.

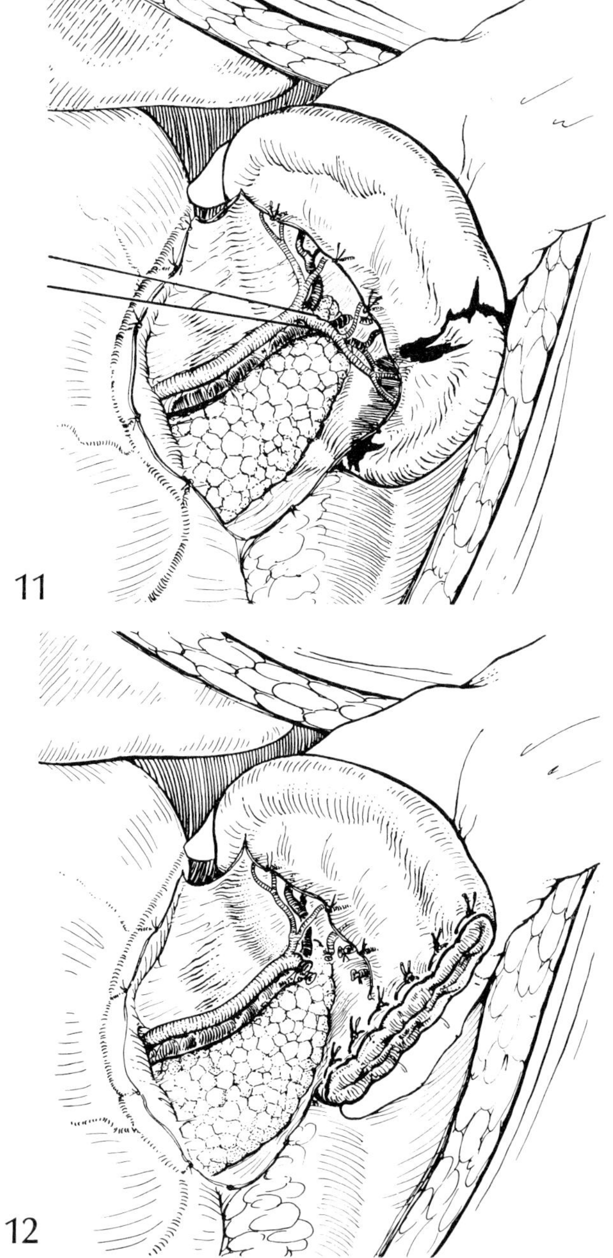

11

12

MODIFICATION OF TECHNIQUE FOR GIANT SPLEEN AND THE MANAGEMENT OF SPLENIC ADHESIONS

Providing they are mobile, huge spleens such as occur in myelofibrosis, chronic granulocytic leukaemia and the tropical splenomegalies are often easier to remove than small ones.

13

The incision

An oblique incision in the line of the ninth rib from the costal margin to the right iliac fossa. The incision may have to be very long to permit mobilization and delivery of the spleen.

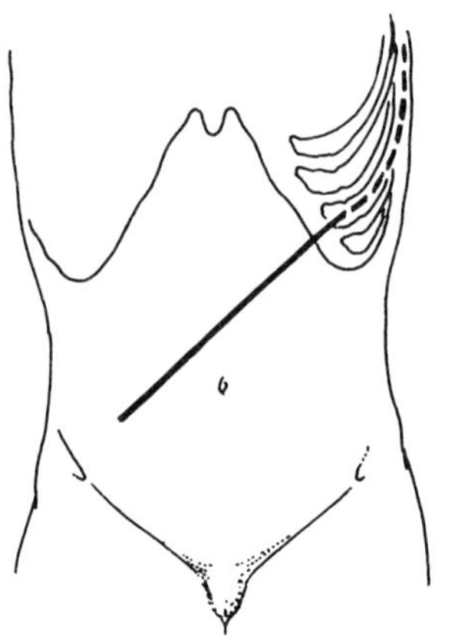

13

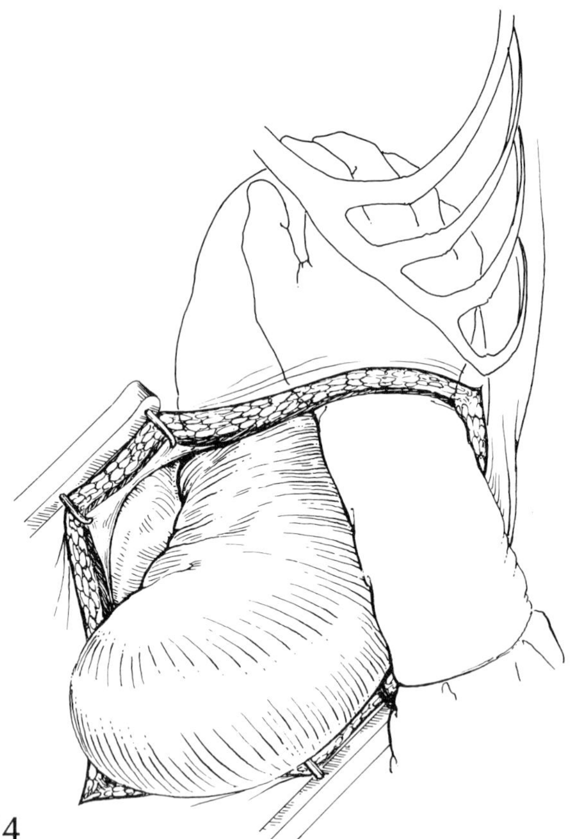

14

14

Mobilization

The abdominal section of the incision is opened and the surface of the spleen exposed. If the spleen is mobile and there are no adhesions the organ can usually be easily delivered from the abdomen because all the ligaments have been stretched. The technique of removal is then essentially the same as that already described for elective removal of a normally sized spleen.

The management of splenic adhesions

Problems arise when the spleen is covered with vascular adhesions connecting it to the diaphragm and parietal peritoneum. In such circumstances the surgeon should not try and deliver the organ from the abdomen nor break down the adhesions by blunt dissection.

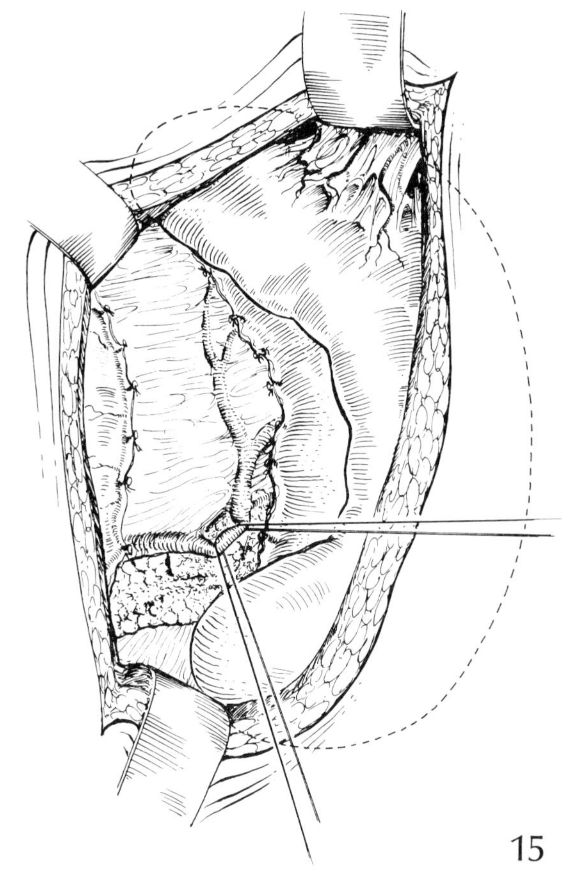

15

15

The first step is to divide the gastrosplenic ligament, enter the lesser sac and expose the splenic artery at the upper border of the pancreas. The artery should be tied in continuity at the apex of one of its convolutions with strong linen thread ligatures (2 gauge) passed round it on an aneurysm needle.

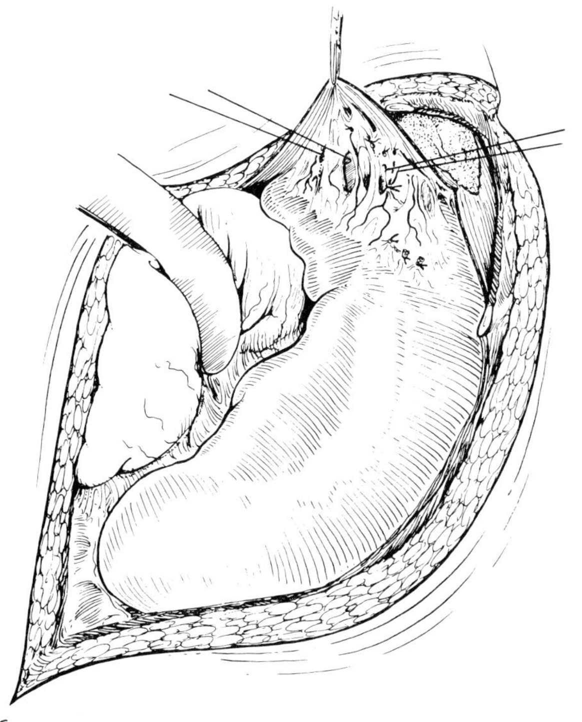

16

16

The adhesions should then be carefully assessed. If they are few and can be easily divided between clamps under direct vision without opening the chest it is permissible to proceed in this manner.

If however there are many and they are thick and vascular the incision should be extended, the costal margin divided and the thorax opened through the bed of the ninth rib. The diaphragm should be divided as far as necessary to allow good access to the adhesions. The adhesions should be divided and ligated individually until the lienorenal ligament is reached. Thereafter the operation can proceed as described above for elective splenectomy.

Management of the diaphragm after removal of a spleen covered with adhesions

17

When a giant spleen with multiple adhesions is removed the surgeon may occasionally be left with a huge bed consisting of a large floppy diaphragm covered with raw oozing areas. This situation can be difficult to deal with and is virtually never completely controllable by diathermy coagulation, suction drains or haemostatic gauze. The most effective technique to control oozing is plication of the diaphragm with a series of firmly tied parallel 0 polyglycolic (Dexon) sutures inserted at 5 cm intervals, until bleeding is controlled.

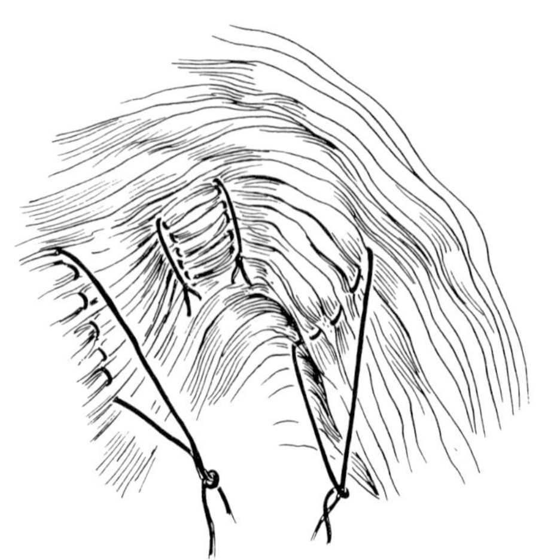

17

MODIFICATION OF TECHNIQUE IN STAGING LAPAROTOMY FOR HODGKIN'S DISEASE

The incision

Long midline to allow access to the liver and the coeliac, mesenteric, para-aortic and iliac nodes in addition to the spleen.

Procedure

The operation to remove the spleen is essentially the same as that described for elective splenectomy, with one modification. When the vessels have been isolated and divided the proximal ends should be marked with 3 or 4 medium metal clips.

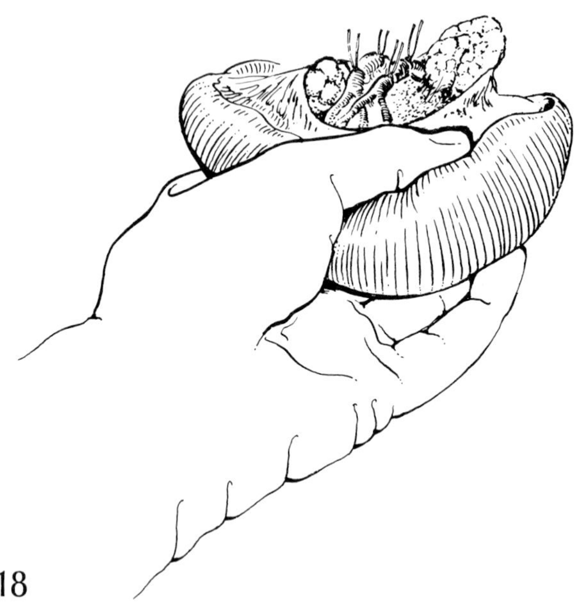

18

18

Whilst the spleen is being removed it is examined to ensure that it contains lymph nodes in the hilum. If not, the area of the remaining pedicle must be examined for suitable nodes and one removed.

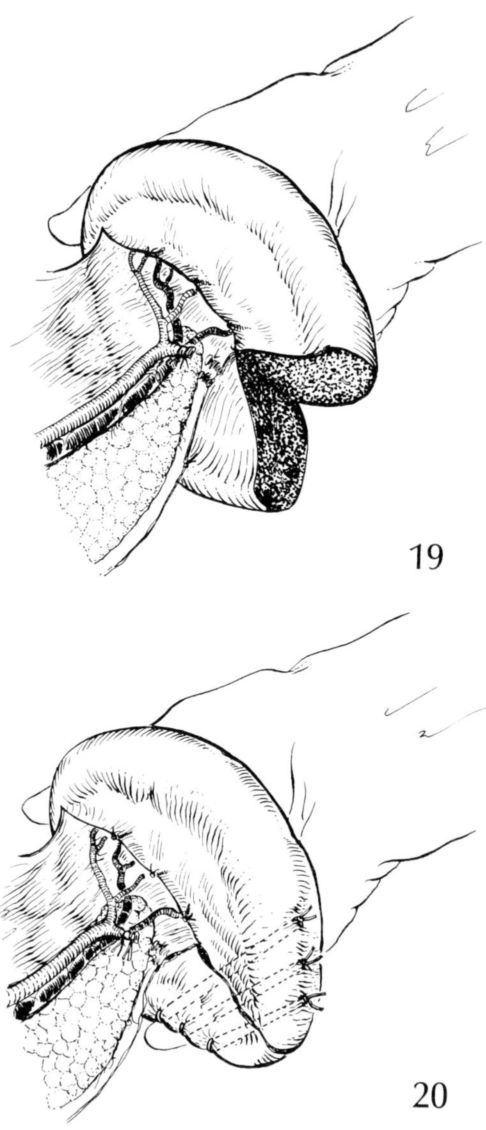

19

20

19 & 20

Where it is decided that only partial splenectomy should be undertaken the spleen is fully mobilized, as previously described. The tail of the pancreas is dissected from the hilum and a hilar lymph node identified and removed. The lower polar artery is dissected and doubly ligated in continuity with 00 silk thread. A wedge of the lower pole of the spleen is then resected with the cutting diathermy and the resulting 'fish mouth' defect closed with interrupted mattress sutures of 0 polyglycolic acid.

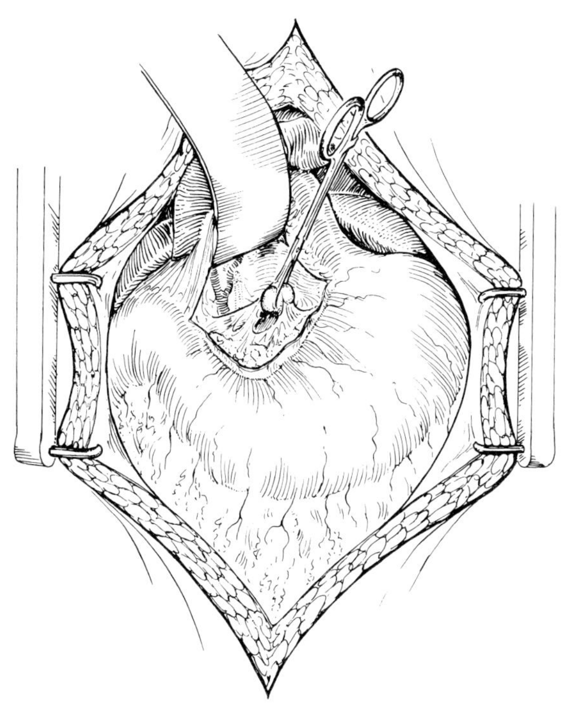

21

21

Following splenectomy the main abdominal lymph node groups are palpated and representative nodes taken from each. Some guidance as to the existence and site of enlarged nodes may have been obtained before operation from lymphangiography or CAT scanning. The nodes in the distribution of the coeliac axis are examined, particular attention being paid to the porta hepatis. Any obviously enlarged node is removed and the site marked by clips. In the absence of enlarged nodes the gastrohepatic omentum is divided to expose the upper border of the pancreas along which two or three nodes can usually be seen. One of these is dissected free and grasped with Babcock forceps following which it can be easily removed.

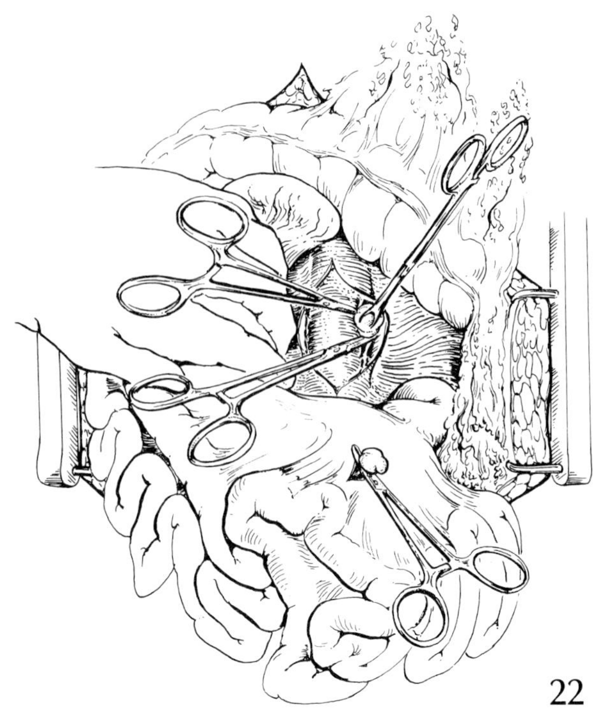

22

22 & 23

Attention is then paid to the para-aortic nodes. The transverse colon is lifted up and the small bowel mesentery displaced upwards and to the patient's right. This reveals the abdominal aorta and vena cava. The peritoneum over the vessels is divided and the lymph nodes on both sides of the aorta palpated from beneath the third part of the duodenum superiorly to the level of the bifurcation inferiorly. Any obviously enlarged node is removed. In the absence of enlarged nodes a normal-sized node is dissected from either side of the aorta.

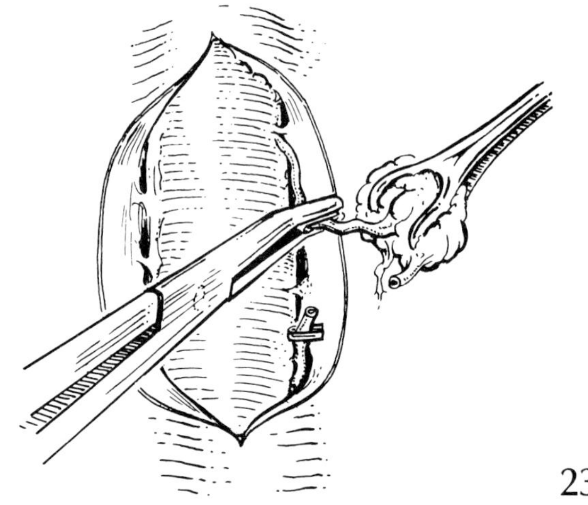

23

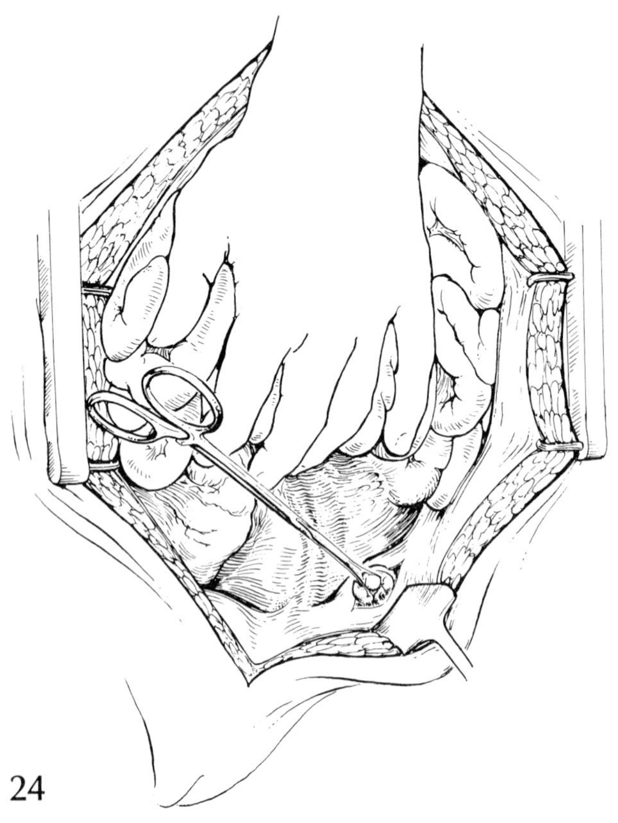

24

24

The nodes along the iliac vessels are palpated. In the absence of obvious abnormality, representative nodes are removed from alongside the external iliac artery on each side at the point where the artery passes under the inguinal ligament. The small bowel mesentery is displayed and any enlarged node is sampled taking care not to damage the mesenteric vasculature. Biopsy sites, other than in the mesentery are marked with clips.

It is usual to remove the vermiform appendix at this stage of the operation.

Postoperative management following splenectomy or partial splenectomy

Most patients have an uncomplicated postoperative course. Suction drainage from the splenic bed usually diminishes to the point where the drains can be removed on the second postoperative day.

Intravenous infusion of crystalloids to maintain hydration is usually necessary for about 48 h and nasogastric suction can be discontinued after 24 h unless aspirates remain high. Skin sutures can be removed on the seventh day. In thrombocytopaenic patients considerable bruising of the skin around the wound may occur but this is usually of little consequence and resolves spontaneously.

Many patients develop some effusion and collapse of the left lower lobe of the lung which usually responds to physiotherapy. The thrombocytosis that follows splenectomy is no cause for alarm although if the count goes above 1 million it is reasonable to give aspirin by mouth until the count falls.

It is now recognized that, even in adults, there is an increased risk of late systemic infection following splenectomy. Prophylaxis against this should be by the use of either an antipneumococcal vaccine or regular therapy with oral penicillin for at least 2 years after operation.

References

1. Singer, D. B. Post splenectomy sepsis. In: Rosenberg, H. S., Bolande, R. P. eds. Perspectives in paediatric pathology. Chicago: Year Book Medical Publishers, 1973: 285–311

2. Robinette, C. D., Fraumeni, J. F. Splenectomy and subsequent mortality in veterans of the 1939–45 war. Lancet 1977; 2: 127–129

3. Shandling, B. Splenectomy for trauma, a second look. Archives of Surgery 1976; 3: 1325–1326

4. Dearth, J. C., Gilchrist, G. S., Telander, R. L., O'Connell, M. J., Weiland, L. H. Partial splenectomy for staging Hodgkin's disease. Risk of false negative results. New England Journal of Medicine 1978; 299: 345–346

Cholecystectomy, cholecystostomy and exploration of the common duct

A. A. Gunn ChM, FRCS (Ed.)
Consultant Surgeon, Bangour Hospital, Broxburn, West Lothian, Scotland

Primary operation for benign disease of the biliary tract has become the commonest general surgical operation in the last 5 years, exceeding appendicectomy and herniorrhaphy[1]. Many factors may be involved, including change in the use of hospital beds, the management of patients, the indications for operation and the incidence of the disease. In particular, there has been an increase in the frequency and severity of cholecystitis in women under the age of 40 years. One associated feature is the prevalence of the use of the contraceptive pill.

The operations can be done with a mortality of less than 1 per cent[2] but disregard for careful preparation, surgical anatomy, surgical technique and postoperative management can lead to disaster. This in part explains why the UK national mortality rate for biliary surgery is nearly five times greater[3].

Preoperative preparation

Many of the patients are elderly and have other diseases that require assessment before operative treatment. The majority are obese which increases the technical difficulties for the surgeon and makes postoperative complications more likely. Weight reduction under the control of the dietitian is possible but is achieved more easily if a target weight is selected with a provisional date for admission. The common use of the contraceptive pill adds a further, though small, risk of venous thrombosis and it is advisable that administration should be stopped at least 6 weeks before surgery. If this is not possible then full prophylactic measures must be instituted.

Assessment includes history of disease in the patient and his family, urine and blood tests and a chest X-ray. The blood urea level must be measured because many of the patients are not only obese but also multiparous with a history of recurrent urinary tract infection. Renal failure is an uncommon but serious complication of biliary surgery. Postoperative atelectasis occurs in more than half the patients and preoperative physiotherapy, cessation of smoking and, in some patients, antibiotic cover are required. Myocardial infarction is a cause of death and a baseline ECG is justified in those at risk.

Liver function tests may suggest obstruction or hepatic insufficiency which sets a limit on the value of oral or intravenous cholecystography. Such abnormal findings are frequently, though not always, associated with a stone or stricture in the common bile duct. Ultrasound is becoming increasingly valuable in the diagnostic pathway. An abnormal prothrombin activity necessitates preoperative treatment with Vitamin K to reduce the risk of haemorrhage.

Jaundiced patients have a high risk of postoperative renal failure which can be reduced by operating during diuresis produced by a fluid load aided by mannitol infusion[4].

Postoperative morbidity studies reveal that infection is the major problem and is more common in the 25–30 per cent of patients who have infected bile[5]. This is more frequent with age over 50 years, a history of jaundice, a tender palpable gall bladder with a pyrexia or leucocytosis, a non-functioning gall bladder, abnormal liver function tests and abnormalities in the common duct. Where three or more of these are present, there is evidence that pre- and postoperative antibiotics can reduce the morbidity. The antibiotic selected should be known to be effective against the organisms as judged by previous experience. The common organisms are *Escherichia coli* and *Streptococcus faecalis*. It is important to appreciate that the aim is to produce adequate blood and tissue levels rather than to select an antibiotic that is secreted in high concentration in the bile. Studies show that this reduces the expected rate of positive culture on drainage fluid and, to a certain extent, the incidence of positive culture within the gall bladder.

The patient's blood should be grouped in case transfusion is necessary and the patient kept as mobile as possible to reduce the incidence of deep vein thrombosis. An intravenous infusion and an intragastric tube should be in place before anaesthesia. A catheter is also required in the jaundiced patient to monitor urinary output.

The cross-references in this chapter refer to *Operative Surgery: Alimentary Tract and Abdominal Wall, Volume 2, 4th Edition*

Anaesthesia

General anaesthesia for gall bladder surgery is essentially no different from that of any intra-abdominal operation. However, there are a few points of particular interest to the anaesthetist. The presence of abnormal liver function tests requires caution to be taken according to the degree of abnormality with the dosage of all drugs used, as almost all depend on the liver for their detoxication. In particular, the use of halothane is contraindicated in the presence of abnormal liver function in view of the remote possibility that it may be a cause of postoperative jaundice.

General anaesthesia must produce an asleep, analgesic patient with good muscle relaxation and a stable blood pressure. Premedication with papaveretum (Omnopon) 10–20 mg according to age and physical state plus atropine 0.6 mg produces a calm, drowsy patient before anaesthesia. Induction of anaesthesia is produced by a 'sleep dose' of methohexitone, 60–80 mg usually, and relaxation by using long-acting competitive neuromuscular blocking agents such as alcuronium 15 mg or pancuronium 4–6 mg. Nitrous oxide and oxygen in a 70:30 ratio will keep the patient asleep and analgesia is produced by the intravenous injection of fentanyl 0.1 mg. Fentanyl is a very powerful analgesic whose actions lasts 25–30 min and further incremental doses of 0.05–0.1 mg can be given during the operation. The muscle relaxation must be reversed at the end of the operation by giving atropine 1.2 mg and neostigmine 2.5 mg.

Care must also be taken during the operation with the placing of the deep retractors to avoid kinking of the inferior vena cava with the resulting drop in venous return to the heart and consequent diminished cardiac output. Intravenous atropine 0.6 mg given just before the operative cholangiogram helps to diminish any spasm of the sphincter of Oddi and, because most nasogastric tubes have a metal tip incorporated in their manufacture, the nasogastric tube must be withdrawn well into the stomach. It has been shown that this metal tip can overlie the lower end of the bile duct system on X-ray with the possibility of masking the presence of a retained gallstone within the duct system.

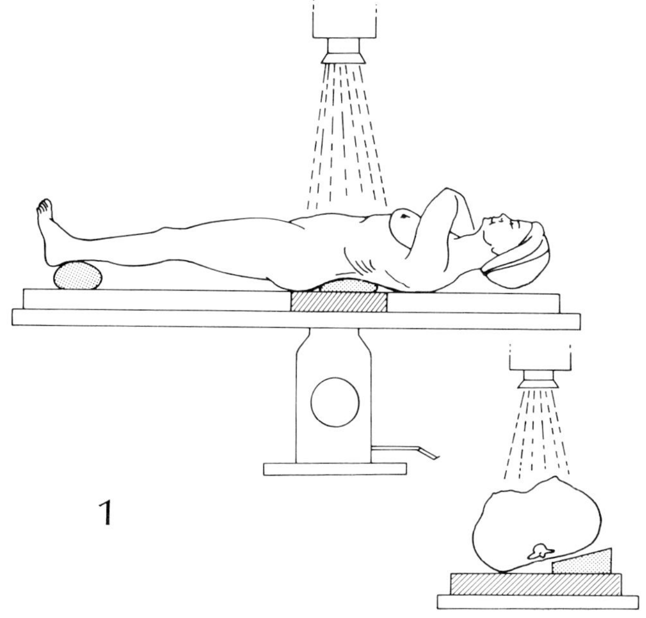

1

1

Position of patient

The patient is placed on the cassette changer table top so that the tip of the ninth costal cartilage is opposite the centre of the grid. Foam wedges are placed under the lower left ribs and the left buttock so that the common bile duct will not be superimposed on the lumbar spine on the cholangiogram. The plane of the grid remains at right angles to the X-ray beam in order to give clear definition. A foam pillow is inserted under the ankles to raise the calves off the table.

The incisions

2

The incisions most commonly advocated are the right upper paramedian (*1*), a Kocher's right subcostal (*2*) or a midline incision (*3*). The surgeon stands on the right side of the table for the paramedian and Kocher's but on the left for the midline. Personal preference is the main reason for selection but in the obese patient or where there is a wide costal angle a Kocher's incision is preferred. Each incision gives good exposure and can be extended if required. The Kocher's incision can be turned superiorly to the xiphoid process or continued into the left subcostal region.

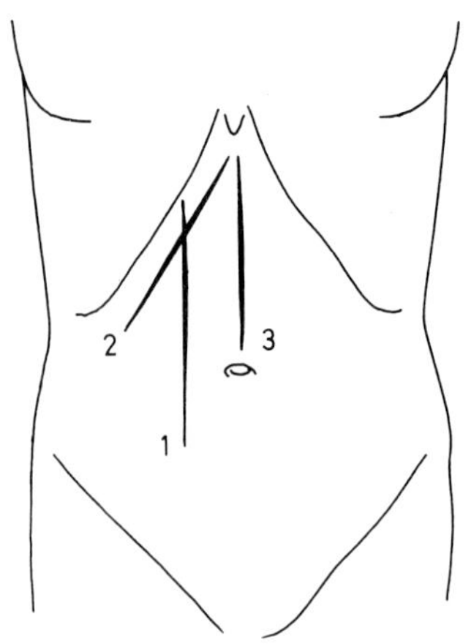

2

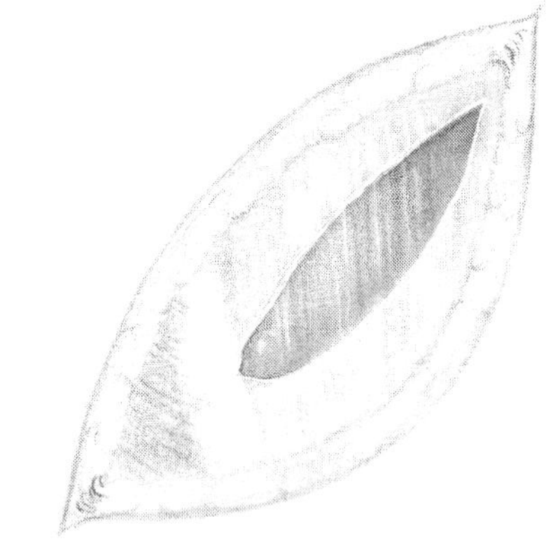
3

3, 4 & 5

Right Kocher's incision

The incision is placed 4 cm below and parallel to the costal margin and extends from the epigastrium in the midline to the eighth or ninth costal cartilage. The anterior sheath is opened in the line of the incision until both edges of the muscle which can then be stretched over two fingers and gradually divided; before division, any vessels are caught with some muscle as they tend to retract deep to the muscle. The peritoneum is opened between forceps and if this fails to give adequate exposure, the muscle layers are divided laterally, taking care to avoid damaging the ninth intercostal nerve.

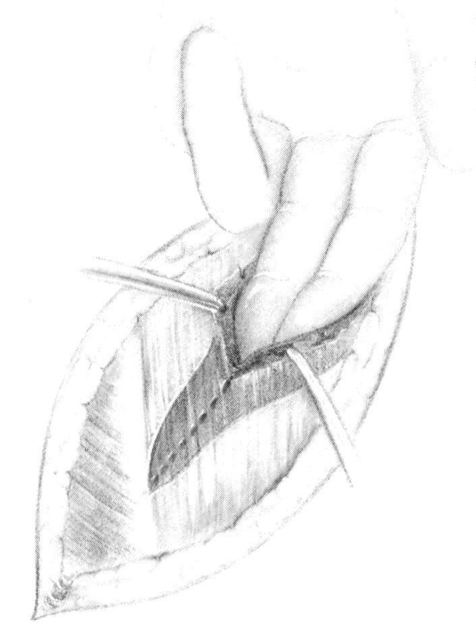
4

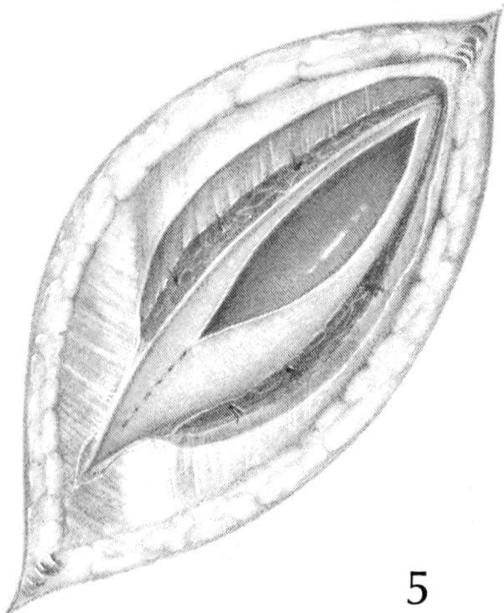
5

Abdominal drainage

6 & 7

Drains are extremely valuable if correctly selected and placed and used intelligently. Experience has shown that Redivac or other closed suction drains are effective. Two should be used: the first lies vertically, posterior to the right lobe of the liver; the second arches across the front of the oesophagus, under the left lobe of the liver, with its tip on the lesser omentum. The drains should be checked daily to see that they have not become blocked.

Drains were initially successfully used to remove air from under the diaphragm and thereby reduce basal atelectasis[6]. The studies showed that the mean volume of blood and bile was in excess of 200 ml. Any large collections lead to complications which carry a high morbidity. Care must therefore be taken to prevent them and, should they occur, to ensure that treatment can be speedily instituted. Bile comes from leakage from the gall bladder bed or, more rarely, when a ligature comes off. Subphrenic collections are not uncommon and, if the bile is infected, may result in an abscess or peritonitis. The drain not only removes these potentially dangerous collections but also reveals the nature and volume of drainage. Haemorrhage is easily diagnosed, but biliary peritonitis is much more insidious in clinical presentation and drains are invaluable in early detection. Rarely, large collections of bile occur in the subphrenic and subhepatic positions and, by displacing the liver and obstructing the cava, cause sudden collapse of the patient (Waltman Walters syndrome); with proper techniques and drainage this should not occur.

Wound closure

Personal preference varies but the author uses continuous polyglycolic acid in two layers – peritoneum and posterior rectus sheath, anterior rectus sheath – with interrupted sutures of similar material to re-appose the subcutaneous tissues and subcuticular polyglycolic acid for the skin.

Postoperative care

Analgesia Papaveretum (Omnopon) 10–20 mg hourly as required. Morphine preparations tend to produce spasm of the sphincter of Oddi and if repeated doses are necessary, the addition of an antispasmodic drug such as atropine 0.6 mg or buscopan 15 mg should be considered.

Antibiotics Preoperatively antibiotics may have been prescribed because it was thought that the bile was likely to be infected. Postoperatively treatment can be stopped if the bile is shown to be sterile but the author continues antibiotic therapy if the drainage material from T-tube or drains remains positive.

Intravenous fluids Five per cent dextrose and 0.9 per cent saline are given as indicated by routine assessment of fluid and electrolyte balance. Urinary output should be monitored closely to ensure adequate diuresis.

Intragastric drainage This is not required as a routine unless indicated for signs of gastric hold-up – nausea, vomiting, hiccups, distension or shoulder-tip pain – occurring in about 10 per cent of patients. Exceptions to

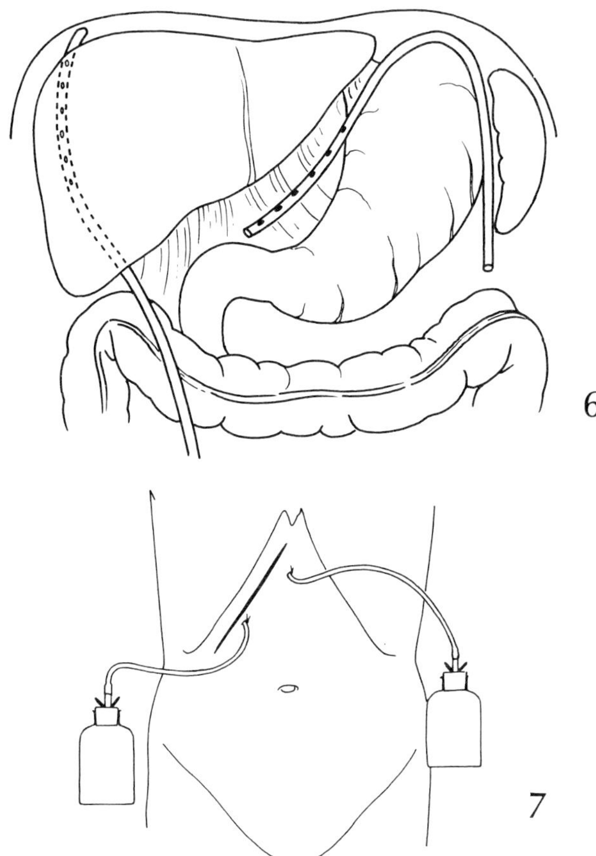

this rule include patients who have required duodenotomy or additional gastric surgery.

Physiotherapy Essential to encourage respiration and to keep the limbs mobile.

Subsequent management depends on the progress of the patient but normally oral fluids can be introduced after 24–48 h and the intravenous fluids withdrawn. The patient should be encouraged to walk within the first 24 h and, provided home support is available, can be discharged in 7–10 days.

Postoperative complications

The incidence of complications varies with many factors including the patient, the stage of the disease, the skill of the surgical team and the postoperative care. Every endeavour must be made to prevent, diagnose and treat each complication if morbidity and mortality are to approach an acceptable level.

The commonest complications, as in every major abdominal operation, are pulmonary atelectasis (50 per cent), deep vein thrombosis (25 per cent, if looked for) and wound infection (4 per cent). Major pulmonary embolus is less common though the true incidence of minor episodes is difficult to establish. The other general complications – wound disruption, ileus, haemorrhage and subphrenic abscess – should occur in less than 1 per cent of patients.

The specific complications which occur in less than 1 per cent of patients include biliary fistula, septicaemia, biliary peritonitis, bacteriogenic shock and Waltman Walters syndrome.

CHOLECYSTECTOMY

Cholecystectomy is the primary operation for cholecystitis and can be associated with a mortality of less than 0.2 per cent. The fact that this figure is not repeated in national statistics is the result of failure to recognize technical problems and to display the anatomy in each patient. Congenital abnormalities are frequent in the origin, course and number of the cystic arteries, in the termination of the cystic duct (the level, the side of the common hepatic duct), and the site of entry of the common bile duct into the duodenum (about 20 per cent end at a lower level than described in the anatomy textbooks). However, despite these anatomical problems, the surgeon is advised to follow the cystic artery to the gall bladder and the cystic duct to the common duct as well as to the gall bladder before any ligatures are tied. In this way, the worry about possible anatomical variations is reduced.

Cholecystectomy is the basic operation for chronic cholecystitis and, many surgeons believe, for patients with acute cholecystitis with acute symptoms of less than 7 days, provided the surgeon has the necessary experience. Ideally cholecystectomy for acute cholecystitis should be done on the next convenient operation list with full assistance after appropriate investigation and preoperative treatment. The oedema present at this stage aids the surgeon, whereas with a longer history, granulation tissue and adhesions make operation more hazardous. Such patients are less likely to perforate (never, in the author's experience) and are best treated conservatively with elective cholecystectomy later. Retrograde mobilization of the gall bladder may be extremely helpful in a difficult situation, allowing the 'pedicle' of neck of gall bladder and artery to be identified.

Contraindications

Poor risk, aged or feeble patients may require cholecystectomy but an effort must be made to reach the optimal state before the operation. In some of these patients the symptoms can be adequately controlled by a low fat diet and antispasmodic drugs. The author has used chenodeoxycholic acid in this situation and, although the stones have not changed, the symptoms have been reduced. Obesity is not a contraindication but can be reduced by dietary advice and supervision.

Preoperative preparation

Preoperative preparation, anaesthesia and position on the operating table have been described. The incision is a Kocher's, right paramedian or midline. Exploration proceeds in a systematic way and particular note should be made of the hiatus, stomach, duodenum, liver, pancreas and colon.

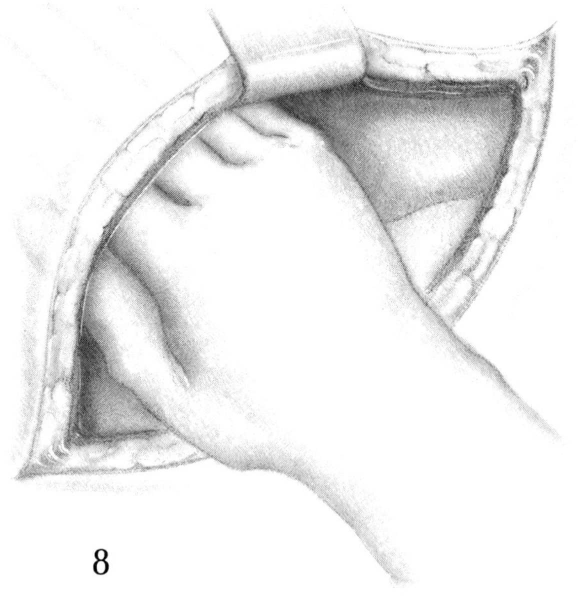

8

The operation

8

Exposure

The right hand can be introduced over the right lobe of the liver to allow entry of air into the subdiaphragmatic area, thereby permitting the liver to descend and making visualization easier.

9

Packing

The gall bladder is grasped with Mayo's forceps, one near the fundus and the second on Hartmann's pouch. With both forceps held in one hand the gall bladder is lifted towards the edge of the wound. Any adhesions to the omentum, colon or duodenum are divided and a pack is placed over these structures, allowing retraction inferiorly with a broad-bladed Deever's retractor or by the assistant's hand. A second narrow-bladed Deever's retractor is inserted over the lesser omentum near the free border with traction to the left – a pack may be required in some patients to aid this manoeuvre. If a second assistant is available, a short-bladed retractor placed under the costal margin is helpful in getting the maximum exposure.

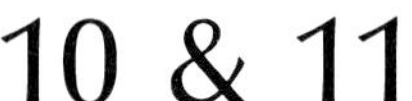

10 & 11

Inspection

The anatomy of the biliary tree is assessed by carefully dividing the peritoneum on the anterior aspect of the cystic duct and continuing into the anterior layer of the lesser omentum overlying the common bile duct. The diameter of the cystic duct and the common bile duct are noted and, by blunt dissection with a pledget, a triangle bounded by the cystic duct, common bile duct and the porta hepatis is exposed. The cystic artery is seen in this triangle in most patients. Before the surgeon proceeds he must have a clear picture of the arrangement of the duct system and the arterial supply. Failure to appreciate variation may result in division of the common bile duct, hepatic artery or right hepatic artery.

Operative cholangiogram

This examination is essential at this stage, not only to detect stones or stricture, but also to confirm the anatomy of the duct system before palpation of the lower end of the common duct. The surgeon usually prefers one method but must be prepared to use one of the alternatives if the method of choice is difficult.

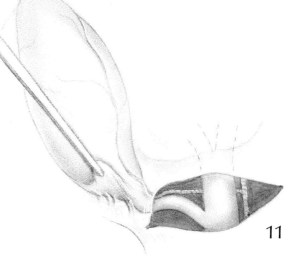

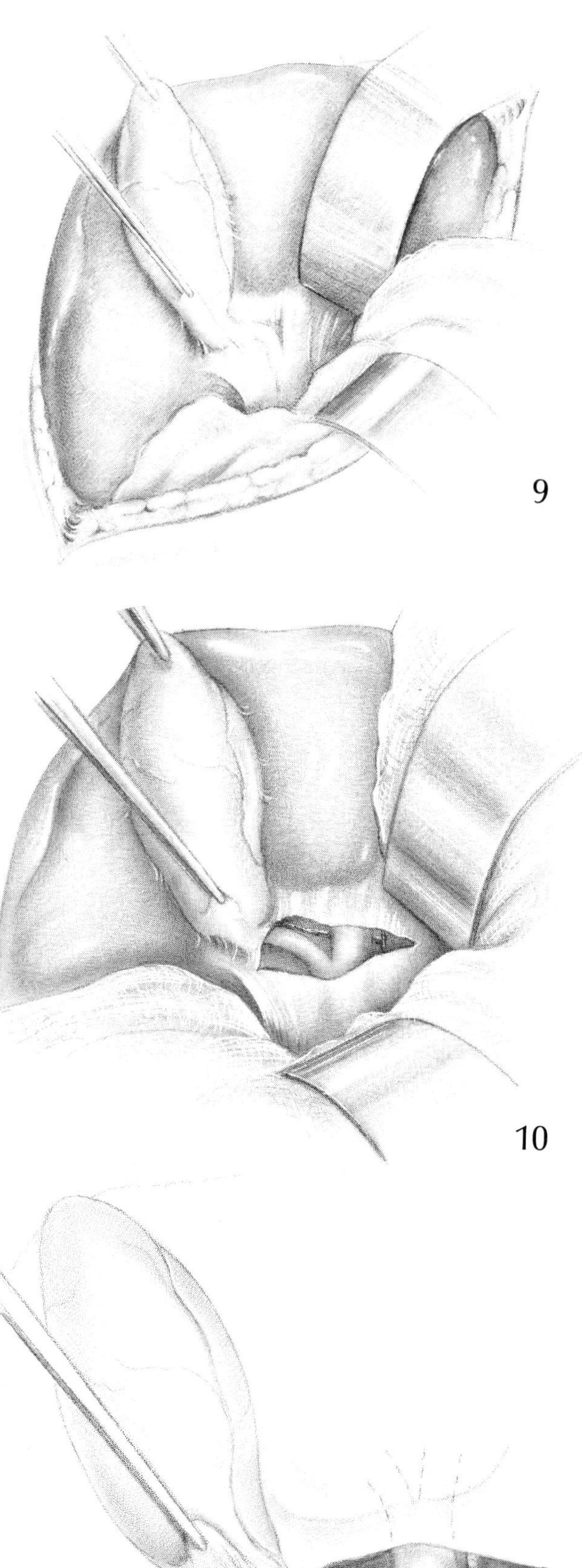

9

10

11

12

Palpation of lower end of common bile duct and pancreas

The index finger of the left hand is inserted into the foramen of Winslow, with the thumb lying anterior to the lesser omentum. The peritoneal reflection between the duodenum, pancreas and inferior vena cava is broken by a downward movement, allowing the index finger to lie posterior to the second part of the duodenum and the head of the pancreas; the thumb slides down anterior to the pancreas, allowing bidigital examination. The pancreas is normally lobular and firm in texture but may be thickened by inflammation or stony hard because of tumour. The anatomical site of tumour of the ampulla will have been demonstrated by the cholangiogram and palpation may reveal a stone or a mass suggestive of a tumour in the pancreas, ampulla or duodenum.

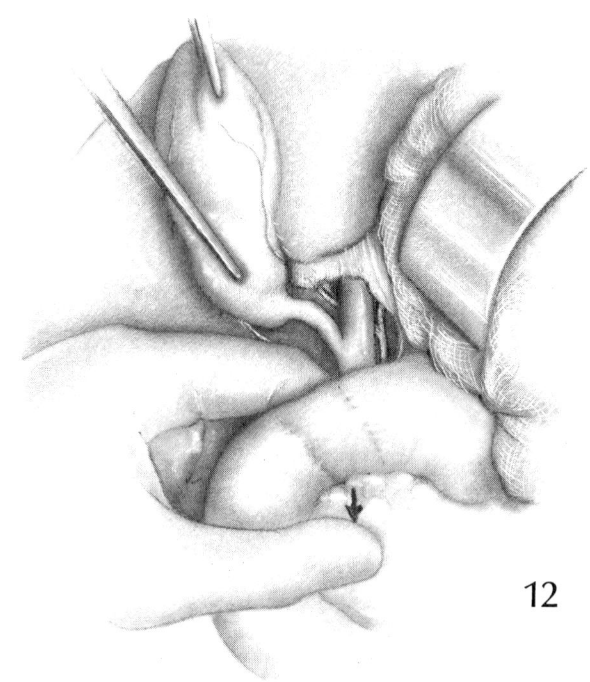

12

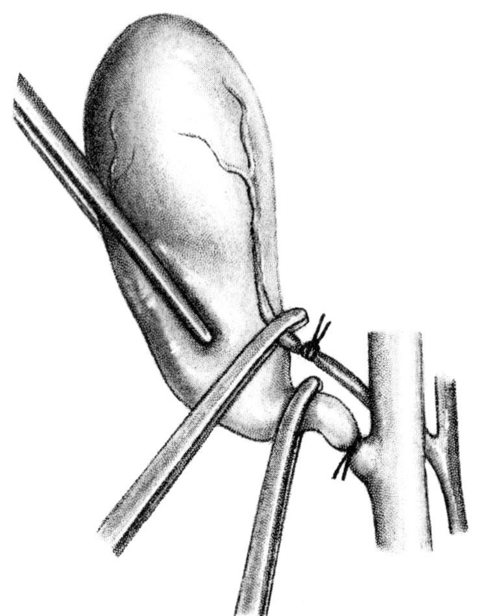

13

Ligation of cystic duct and artery

The artery should be ligated and divided first because division of the duct before the artery can result in excessive tension on the latter which can then tear and retract into the porta hepatis. However, this is a rule which at times has to be broken, but the danger must be recognized.

The forceps on the gall bladder are held in the left hand to produce tension and the cystic artery is cleared of soft tissue with a pledget held in cholecystectomy forceps. The artery is followed to the gall bladder and ligated close to the edge of the gall bladder wall. A cholecystectomy forceps is placed on the artery at least 2 mm away from the ligature and the vessel divided. Silk or polyglycolic acid suture with at least three throws should be used to achieve a firm holding knot.

The cystic duct is cleared in a similar manner to expose the junction with the common bile duct. A polyglycolic acid ligature is used to tie the duct close to the wall of the common duct and a cholecystectomy forceps is placed on the duct nearer to the gall bladder. The duct is divided, leaving a stump of at least 2 mm to ensure a safe ligature. A silk or other non-absorbable ligature should not be used because this can erode into the lumen and form the nidus for a stone.

14

Removal of the gall bladder

The two cholecystectomy forceps are held in the palm of the left hand to put tension on the tissues between the gall bladder and the liver. The index finger of the right hand is inserted between the neck of the gall bladder and the gall bladder bed and used to separate them with gentle blunt dissection. This method reveals tight strands which should be caught in forceps before division because they usually contain additional vessels. The edges of the mesentery will become apparent and are cut with scissors or a knife; extra tension without such division may cause stripping of the capsule of the liver.

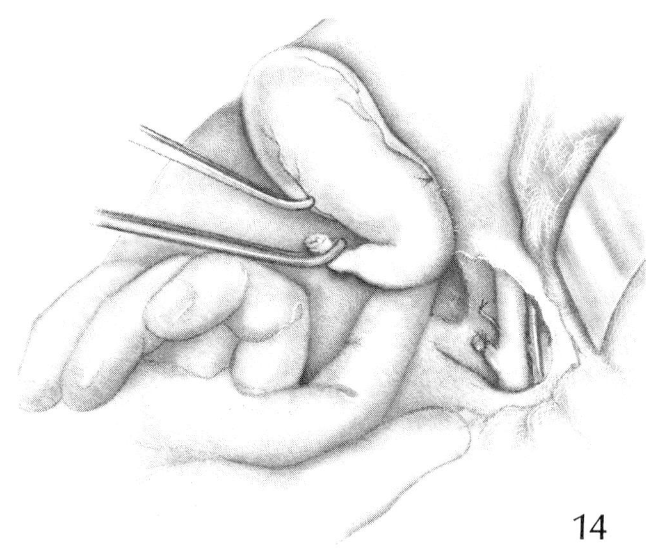

14

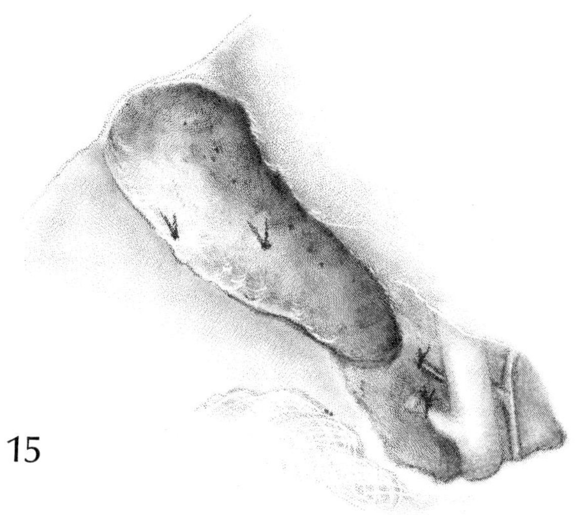

15

15

The gall bladder bed

After removal of the gall bladder, the bed is inspected for any bleeding points which are caught and ligated; these are usually in the edges of the mesentery. When the edges of the mesentery are well formed they may be sutured but stitches should not be inserted in the liver because bleeding occurs from the stitch holes. Any persistent oozing from the bed can be controlled by a small pack of haemostatic gauze.

Final assessment and closure

The operative field is inspected with particular reference to the ligatures on the arteries and the cystic duct. The wound is closed in layers as described, with drains in the right subdiaphragmatic area and the left subhepatic position anterior to the lesser omentum.

CHOLECYSTOSTOMY

Cholecystostomy used to be considered as the operation of choice for patients who required surgical treatment for acute cholecystitis. To a degree this view may have originated before supportive treatment (intravenous therapy and antibiotics in particular), which could carry the patient through the definitive procedure of cholecystectomy, had been developed. As a consequence, treatment of an acute attack was initially conservative, so that if surgery was called for because the patient's general or local condition deteriorated, technical difficulties such as adhesions, vascularity and necrosis of the gall bladder wall were found. Even cholecystostomy was then associated with a high mortality. Cholecystostomy also has several inherent difficulties.

1. It can be difficult to remove the obstructing stone.
2. The procedure can result in contamination of the wound and peritoneum by the bile from the gall bladder which is infected in over 30 per cent of patients with acute cholecystitis.
3. A mucous fistula persists if the obstruction is not removed, making the second operation difficult.
4. It is likely that the sutures anchoring the drainage tube will cut out if the gall bladder wall is ischaemic and this can result in biliary peritonitis.

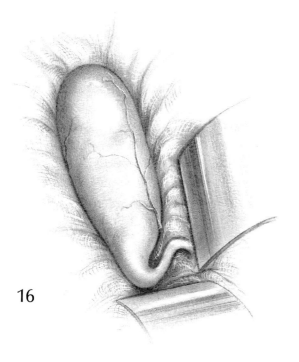

Cholecystostomy should be avoided except, possibly, in the following situations.

Acute cholecystitis

1. When cholecystectomy would present technical difficulties, as with dense or vascular adhesions, inflammation or abscess obscuring the anatomy.
2. When an inexperienced surgeon has no alternative but to operate on advanced acute cholecystitis and has no experienced colleague available.
3. When the condition of the patient is grave from toxaemia, jaundice or other disease.
4. When decompression of the biliary tract is necessary in suppurative cholangitis and inflammation around the common duct makes choledochotomy impossible.

Acute pancreatitis

Operation is necessary for some patients with pancreatitis in whom drainage of the common bile duct may not be possible. In this situation, cholecystostomy allows decompression of the biliary system.

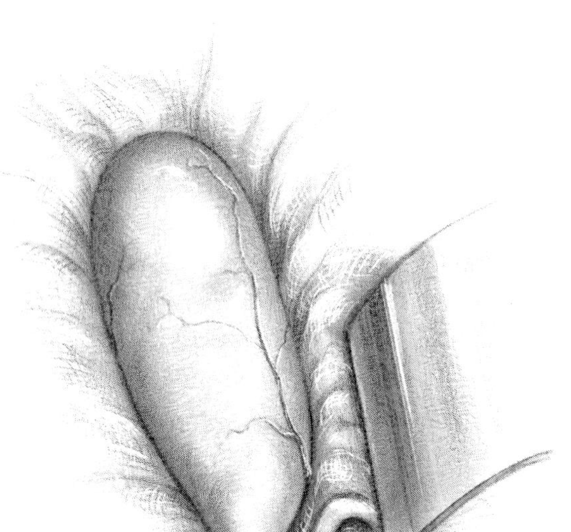

16

The operation

Preoperative preparation, position of patient on table and incisions are as for cholecystectomy.

16

Exposure

The gall bladder is exposed in the standard manner, any adhesions are divided and packs are inserted to protect not only the surrounding tissues but also the wound edges.

17

Decompression of the gall bladder

Forceps are not put on to the gall bladder until it has been decompressed. To do this the organ is held with the right hand and a trocar (Mayo Ochsner) inserted into the fundus. The trocar point is withdrawn leaving the cannula in place, so permitting emptying of the gall bladder.

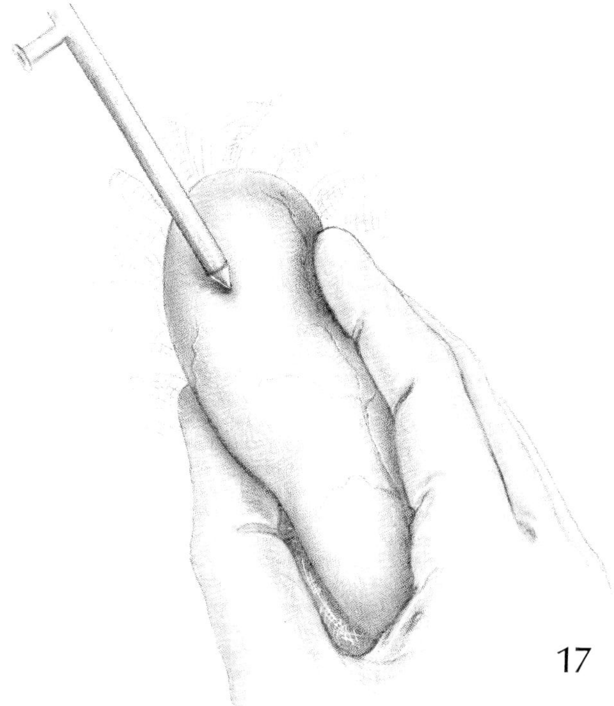

17

18

Opening the gall bladder

The cannula is gradually withdrawn and a light occlusion clamp placed across the fundus to prevent leakage. The edges of the opening are gently grasped in Babcock's tissue forceps and the opening enlarged with scissors to about 3 cm.

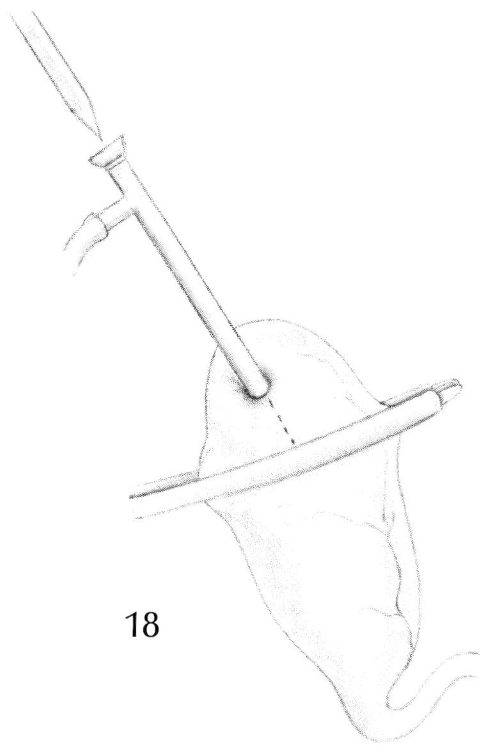

18

19

Removal of obstruction

The clamp is removed and the contents aspirated with a sucker. A dry swab is inserted with the finger so that small stones can be picked up. Palpation will reveal most stones at the neck of the gall bladder and many of these can be milked up and removed.

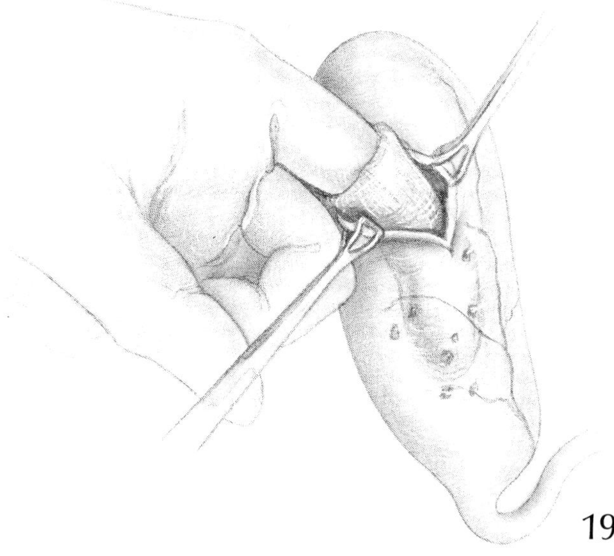

19

20

Insertion of drain

A purse-string suture of 2/0 catgut is inserted around the healthy margin of the opening into the gall bladder. A Foley catheter is introduced through a stab incision in the abdominal wall and led into the gall bladder where the balloon is inflated to about 5 ml. The suture is drawn tight and tied. A second purse-string suture is used to produce an inkwell effect. The ends of the suture are left long so that they can be brought through the stab incision alongside the Foley catheter, thereby anchoring the gall bladder to the deep surface of the wound.

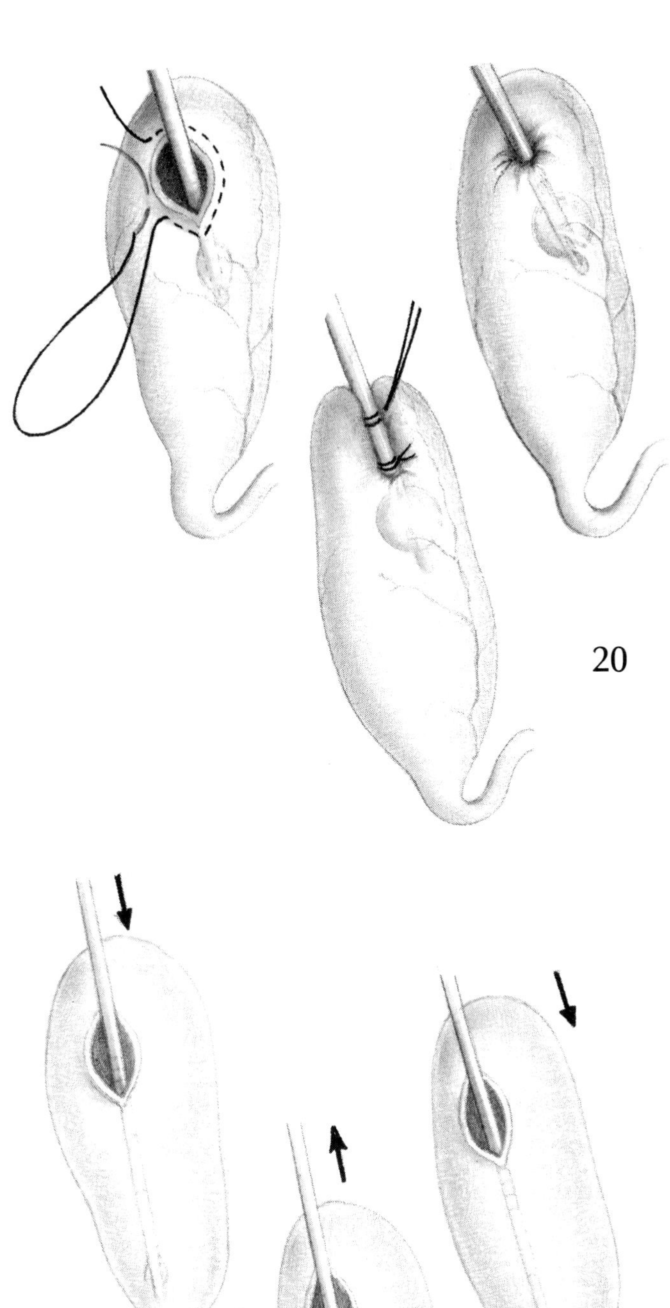

20

Radiological assessment

The radiographer is called, the X-ray head accurately placed and 10–20 ml of Hypaque are injected down the Foley catheter to assess the clearance of the gall bladder and cystic duct and to delineate any abnormalities in the common bile duct.

21

If the gall bladder is still obstructed, the cholecystostomy should be reopened and a further attempt made to clear the obstruction. A Fogarty bile duct catheter can often be passed beyond the stone, and the balloon inflated and withdrawn, bringing the stone with it.

21

Wound closure

The suction (Redivac) drains are inserted and the wound closed. The Foley catheter is anchored with a stitch which is also tied to the ends of the second purse-string suture.

Postoperative management

1. Intravenous fluids.
2. Intragastric drainage with continuous syphon drainage and hourly check aspiration.
3. Antibiotics if indicated by the preoperative assessment and by operative findings.
4. The Foley catheter should be left unclamped and the daily loss noted. On occasions, the loss is considerable and an aliquot should be sent for electrolyte assessment to permit accurate replacement. Further X-rays should be taken between 5 and 10 days after the operation by injecting contrast medium into the Foley catheter. If a patent cystic duct is shown, the Foley catheter can be clamped and if there are no side-effects (pain in the abdomen or shoulder tip, nausea, vomiting or leakage around the Foley catheter) the Foley balloon can be deflated and removed at 10 days. Alternatively, if the gall bladder is still obstructed, it is wise to leave the Foley catheter in place until elective operation is possible, usually about 6 weeks later.

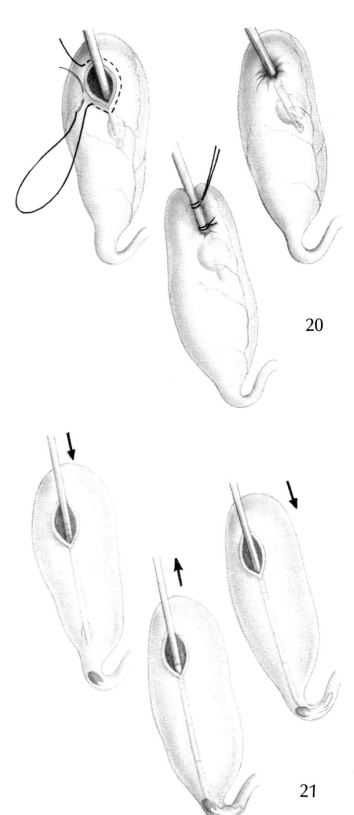

EXPLORATION OF THE COMMON BILE DUCT

The operation of choledochotomy carries a mortality of at least four times greater than cholecystectomy alone. This is partly accounted for by the older age group, the longer operation and the technical difficulties in more advanced disease[7]. The complications that are more frequent are those associated with infection which is in parallel with the increased incidence of positive bile culture in patients who require this operation. Evidence is accumulating that the presence of a T-tube may be responsible for some increase in morbidity as it can be shown that in about 20 per cent of patients there is some leakage of bile around the T-tube in the early postoperative period; this would suggest that the T-tube should be used with discretion. However, discretion is only gained with experience and by careful assessment by radiography or choledochoscopy during the operation. It is possible that ERCP techniques may replace difficult exploration of the common duct, thereby reducing morbidity[8].

Indications

Classically, the indications are recorded as: (*1*) a history of jaundice; (*2*) multiple small stones in the gall bladder; (*3*) a dilated cystic duct; (*4*) induration of the head of the pancreas; (*5*) a dilated common duct; (*6*) a palpable stone in the common duct.

However, analysis of the author's experience and that of others shows that none of the first five are likely to yield more than one in three patients with stones in the duct. Furthermore, 80 per cent of patients admitted for cholecystectomy have at least one of these classical indications. Unfortunately, the lower end of the common duct is difficult to palpate and 30 per cent of patients with stones would be missed if reliance had been placed on this method of assessment. The most accurate method of diagnosis is an operative choledochogram obtained before palpating the duct (*see* pp. 637–643).

Residual disease

It is essential to establish that no stone or stricture remains in the ducts after exploration because it will probably require removal either by dissolution, radiographically controlled techniques, endoscopic withdrawal or a difficult second operation. Some small stones will pass spontaneously. It is reported that 10–20 per cent of explorations of the common duct are incomplete. Cholangiography through the T-tube at operation is disappointing because the contrast medium fails to pass through the sphincter of Oddi in about half of the patients unless a number of successive films are exposed. The fibreoptic choledochoscope can achieve satisfactory visualization provided the ducts are dilated. This instrument is still not widely available. The author finds that postexploration cholangiography with the use of a Foley catheter gives satisfactory films of the duct system (*see* 'Results' section).

Assessment

Preparation, positioning, incision and exposure are the same as for cholecystectomy. The state of the gall bladder, and the diameter of the cystic and common ducts are assessed. An operative choledochogram is obtained (*see* pp. 637–643) and then the common duct and pancreas are palpated while the films are being developed. The gall bladder may be removed during this interval but on occasions is kept as a useful means of traction on the cystic duct. The presence of a stone or stricture is established. The cystic duct and cystic artery are ligated and a third retractor can be placed to retract the liver in a superior direction.

The operation

22

Opening the duct

Stay sutures of 000 catgut are inserted into the common duct near either edge of the anterior aspect about 2 cm above the first part of the duodenum and a longitudinal incision is made with a fine knife. A specimen of bile is taken for culture and the opening into the duct is enlarged inferiorly towards the duodenum.

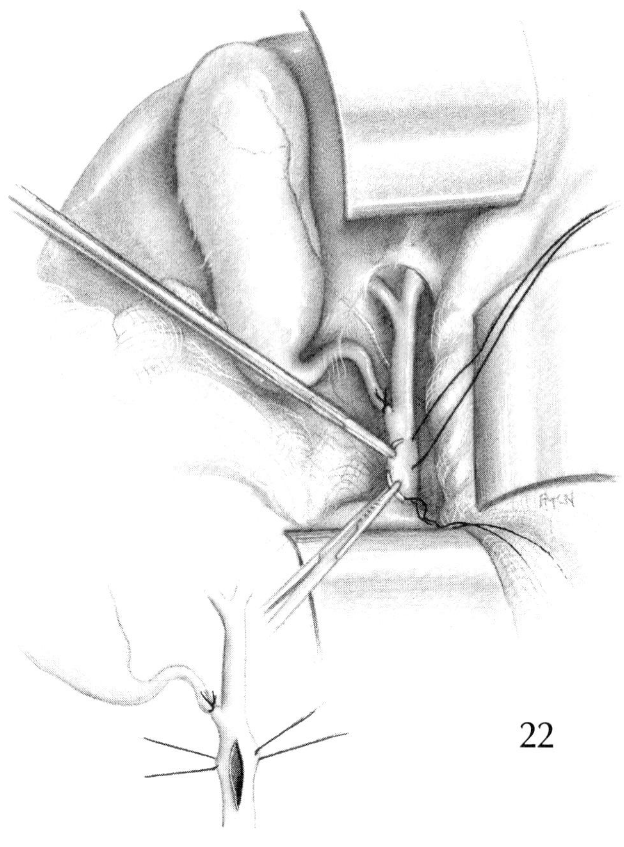

22

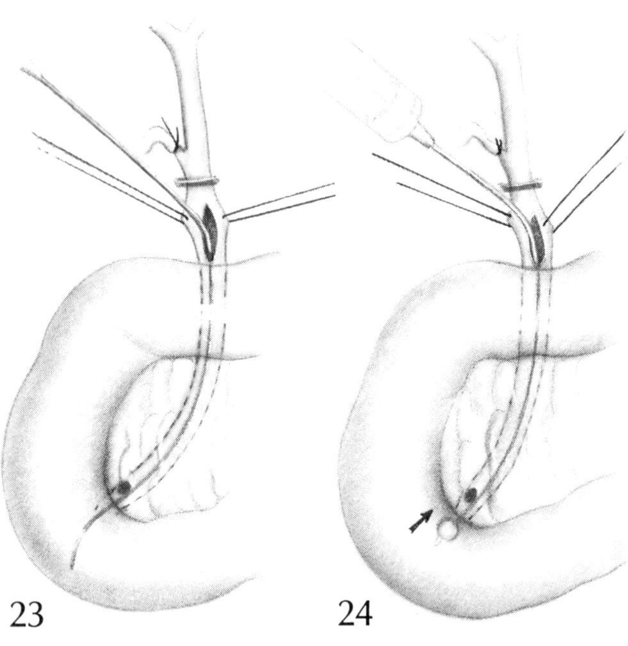

23 24

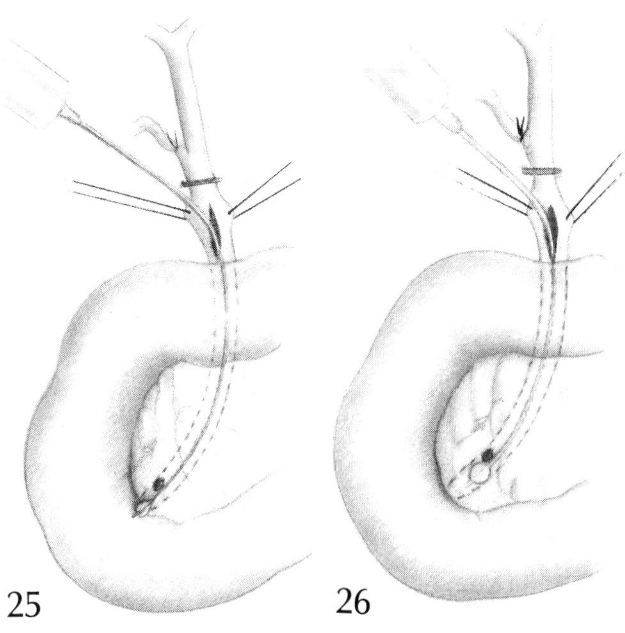

25 26

23–26

Exploration (distal)

A Fogarty catheter[9] is inserted down the common bile duct into the duodenum and the balloon inflated. It may be necessary to release the tension on the inferior retractor because this can obstruct the passage of the catheter. The catheter is gently withdrawn until it is halted by the sphincter of Oddi – usually about 7 cm from the opening of the common duct.

This establishes the position of the sphincter which may not have been visualized on the cholangiogram because of the failure of the contrast medium to pass beyond an obstruction. The lower end of the duct is palpated and a stone may be felt against the catheter above the balloon. A bulldog or similar clamp is placed across the common duct above the opening to prevent any stones escaping into the proximal ducts. The balloon is deflated and the catheter gently brought through the sphincter – this can be traced by the palpating fingers and is recognized by a sudden jerk on the catheter. The balloon is reinflated and is steadily withdrawn, bringing the stone with it. This procedure is repeated until no more stones are withdrawn.

27 & 28

Exploration (proximal)

The catheter is reinserted into the proximal segment and the procedure repeated in the left and right hepatic ducts. The bulldog clip is placed on the common duct below the opening to prevent stones falling into the distal duct. The balloon is inflated until some resistance is felt and withdrawn with the pressure maintained by pressure on the syringe. This is necessary because the lumen of the duct increases in diameter and unless the balloon continues to fill the lumen, a stone may slip past. The bulldog clip is then removed.

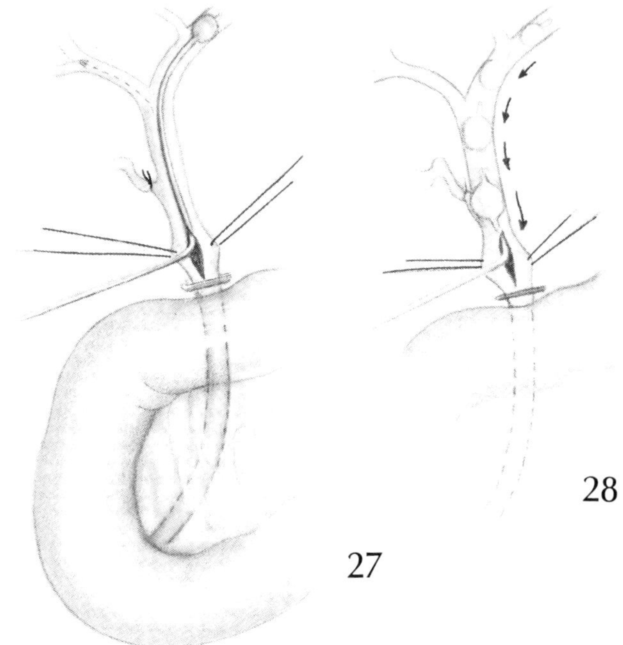

27

28

Reassessment by palpation

The common bile duct above and below is carefully palpated with and without a Fogarty catheter in place.

29

Reassessment by X-ray

The author finds that satisfactory films are obtained by using a modified Foley catheter. The distal end of the catheter is removed beyond the balloon as the terminal portion can look like a stone on subsequent films. The balloon should be inflated to ensure that it has not been damaged. The proximal end is trimmed until it will accept a Luer-Lock syringe.

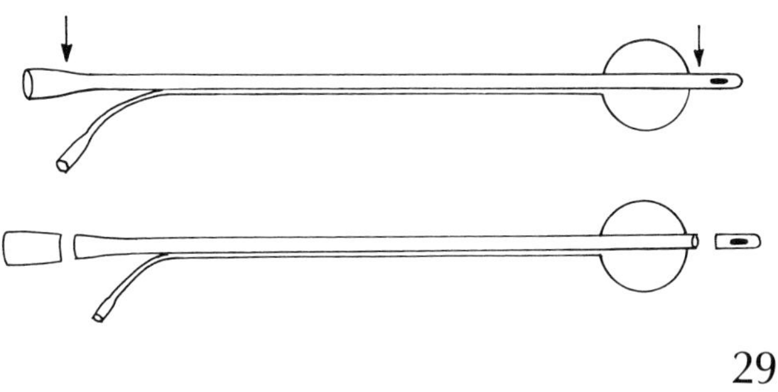

29

30 & 31

The catheter is inserted into the common duct so that the balloon lies just distal to the opening where it is inflated to occlude the duct. This is tested by injecting 5 ml of sterile saline and observing for any reflux around the catheter. After checking the position of the X-ray machine, about 10 ml of Hypaque are injected and a film taken. The balloon is deflated and the procedure repeated with the catheter in the common hepatic duct.

Some surgeons believe that it is important to know the pressure that is required to open the sphincter of Oddi. This can be assessed by attaching a manometer to the Foley catheter into the common bile duct. Alternatively, a choledochoscope can be used to determine the normality of the larger ducts.

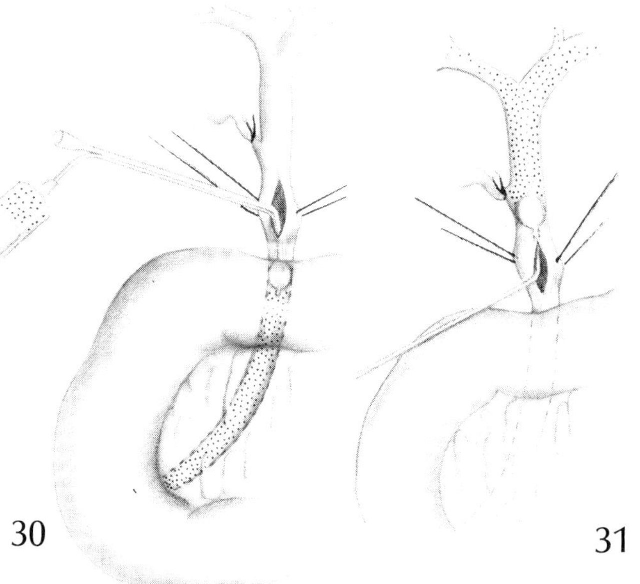

30

31

The fixed stone

32

On occasion a stone remains fixed at the lower end of the common bile duct and cannot be removed by the standard method. A bougie can be gently passed down the duct and an attempt made to dislodge the stone with the aid of the fingers of the left hand gripping the second part of the duodenum.

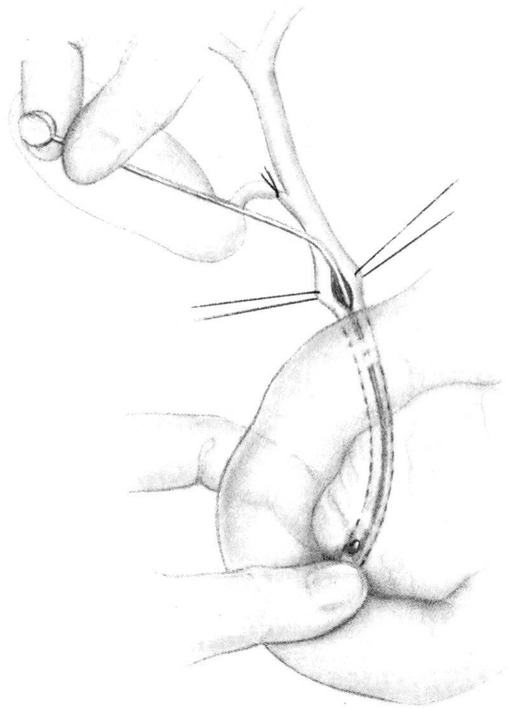

32

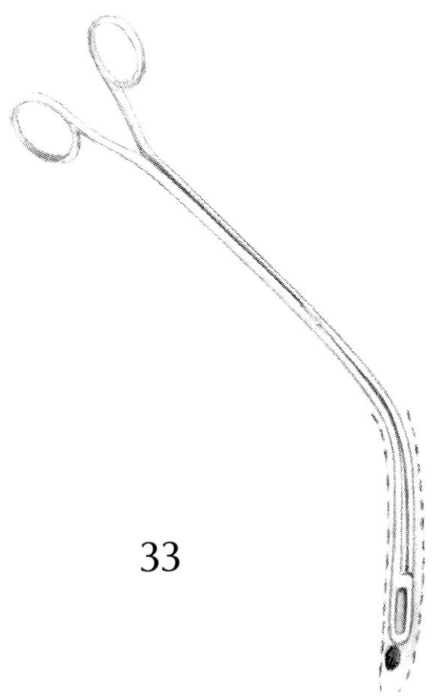

33

33

Alternatively, a Desjardin's forceps can be introduced and carefully positioned around the stone by palpation and then withdrawn. Force must not be used because the duct may be caught between the forceps and damaged.

If these manoeuvres fail to move the stone a duodenotomy is required. Postoperative ERCP has been suggested as an alternative.

34

Closure of the duct (without a T-tube)

A suture of atraumatic 000 catgut is begun just above the opening in the duct and firmly tied with the end held by a small artery forceps which can be used as a fine retractor to elevate the duct. A continuous suture is placed with the bites about 2 mm apart, through each edge of the choledochotomy, care being taken to avoid inclusion of the posterior wall of the duct. The repair is continued just beyond the lower end of the opening and tied firmly.

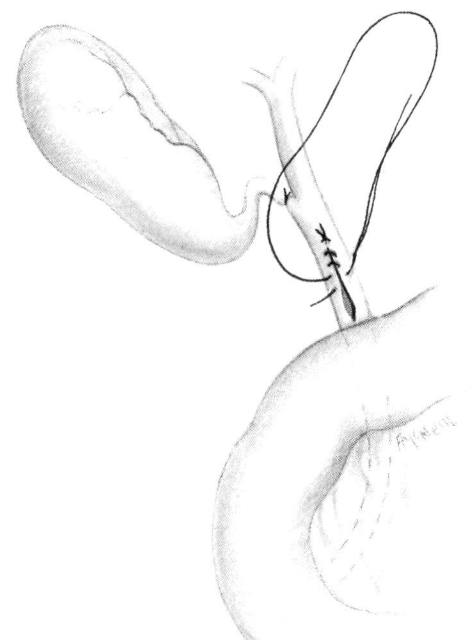

34

Closure of the duct (with a T-tube)

35

Modification of the T-tube

The T-tube is selected according to the size of the common bile duct and should be smaller in diameter to permit passage of bile. The size varies from 8 to 14 Fr. The limbs of the T-tube are shortened to 2–3 cm each to ensure that the upper end does not lie in one hepatic duct and that the lower end does not pass into the duodenum, so blocking the papilla. Half of the diameter of the short limb is filletted off with scissors. The lumen of that part of the tube in the duct is now U-shaped on cross-section, so that blockage of the tube cannot occur. Withdrawal of the tube is also easier.

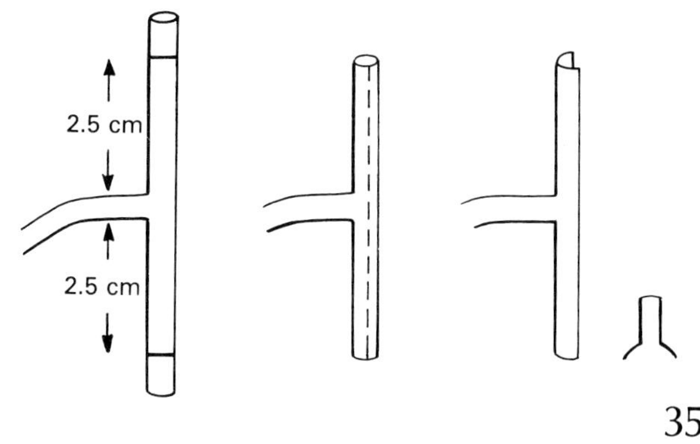

35

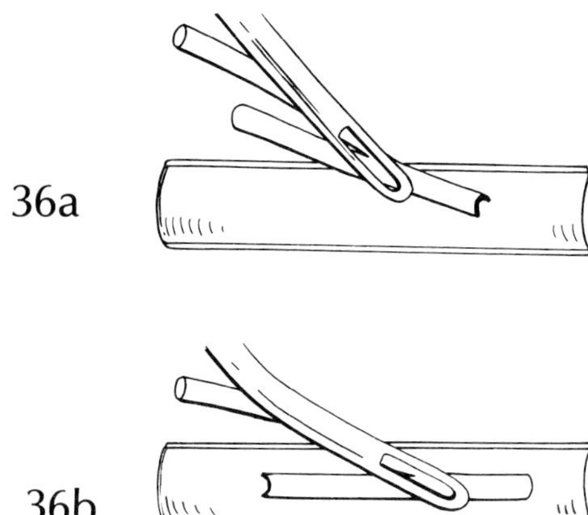
36a
36b

36a & b

Insertion of the T-tube

The T-tube is grasped in a Desjardin's forceps so that the shaft and the distal limb are in line (*a*) and introduced into the common bile duct until the proximal limb slips into the proximal duct (*b*).

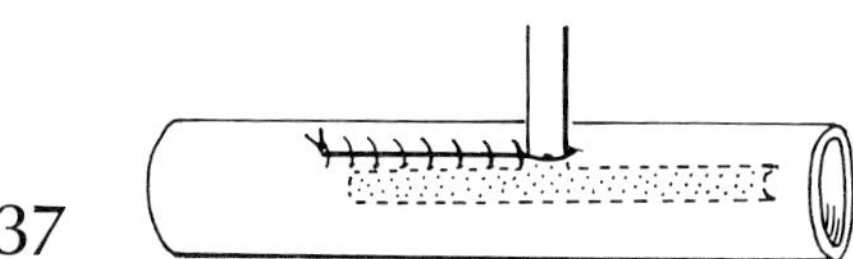
37

37

Closure of the duct

The common bile duct is repaired with 000 atraumatic continuous catgut which begins proximal to the upper end of the opening and is continued inferiorly so that the T-tube is at the lower end of the repair. The T-tube must not be caught in the suture because the duct will then be torn when the tube is removed.

38

Removal of gall bladder and wound closure

The gall bladder is removed as previously described and the ligatures on the cystic duct and artery inspected. The closure of the common bile duct is checked for leakage and, if present, an additional suture can be used. Care must be taken to avoid cutting the previously inserted continuous suture.

A small incision is made in the abdominal wall inferior to the midpoint of the incision and a fine forceps inserted to catch the end of the T-tube which can be brought out and anchored to the skin with a silk suture.* The end of the tube is attached to a bile bag, the suction drains inserted and the wound closed in layers.

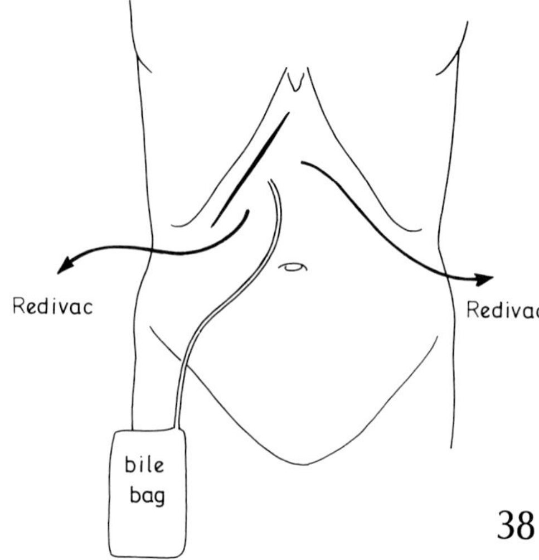

38

Postoperative care

1. Intravenous fluids are continued until the patient can take oral fluids.
2. Oral fluids are usually commenced the following day, 30 ml hourly, unless the patient requires an intragastric tube for nausea, vomiting, shoulder pain, tachycardia, hypotension or hiccups.
3. Analgesia such as phenazocine hydrobromide (Narphen) 4 mg or papaveretum (Omnopon) 10 mg may be required.
4. Fluid and electrolyte balance should be monitored with particular note taken of the urinary output.
5. If antibiotics have been given preoperatively they should be continued until negative culture reports are received from the specimen of gall bladder, the T-tube and drainage fluid.
6. Routine postoperative assessment is maintained.
7. The T-tube is allowed to drain freely into a bile bag for 5 days when it is clipped for 1 h after meals. This is increased by 1 h each day so that by the tenth day the tube is clipped all day. A T-tube cholangiogram is obtained as a final check that the duct system is normal and, if so, the skin suture is withdrawn and the tube removed.

The following problems may arise.

1. Nausea and vomiting due to duct obstruction or irritation of the duodenum by bile leakage; shoulder tip pain due to diaphragmatic irritation by bile; leakage of bile around the T-tube while it is clipped. The T-tube should be allowed to drain freely for 24 h and the trial of clipping repeated. A recurrence of the symptoms requires investigation by a cholangiogram through the T-tube which may reveal profuse leakage from the choledochotomy, a missed stone or stricture, or that the T-tube has partly or completely come out of the duct. The first two findings require operation and the third removal of the T-tube in the first instance and close observation.
2. The final cholangiogram may reveal residual stones or a stricture. If the stone is small the T-tube can be left in place and the patient discharged with arrangements to return for repeat films. A considerable proportion of these will pass spontaneously. Larger stones are less likely to pass and several alternatives should be considered: perfusion with cholic acid; later radiographically controlled removal with instruments such as a Dormia stone-catcher; or endoscopic cannulization of the papilla and removal.
3. Occasionally the T-tube will not come out. Traction from a 0.5 kg weight on the end of the tube is usually sufficient to solve the problem, which is, however, very unlikely to arise if the T-tube has been modified as recommended.
4. A biliary leak may persist after removal of the T-tube but usually stops after 24–48 h. If it does not, a sinogram through the track will reveal the cause.

* It is now believed that the T-tube should be brought out *superior* to the wound to permit removal of residual stones by radiographically controlled techniques.

SPHINCTEROTOMY AND CHOLEDOCHODUODENOSTOMY

Preoperative intravenous cholangiogram, operative cholangiogram or operative exploration may reveal a stone or a stricture at the lower end of the common bile duct. Not uncommonly, X-rays after exploration of the duct show a residual stone or a stricture. Repeat supraduodenal exploration may remove the stone, but it may fail in which case, or with a stricture, a further procedure is necessary: the choice lies between a sphincterotomy and a choledochoduodenostomy (or later ERCP).

Sphincterotomy requires a duodenotomy placed at the level of the sphincter of Oddi, division of the sphincter and suture of the wall of the common bile duct to the duodenum. Care must be taken to avoid damaging the opening of the pancreatic duct and the duodenal closure must be meticulous to prevent leakage or narrowing of the duodenum. Most surgeons leave a T-tube in the common duct as a decompression to permit healing of the suture line. For these various reasons, this operation adds to cholecystectomy and choledochotomy the complications specific to a duodenotomy. These are:

1. a false opening into the duodenum;
2. leakage from the suture line;
3. damage to the pancreatic duct;
4. leakage from the duodenotomy;
5. obstruction of the duodenum.

Morbidity is increased by this procedure, but it has the advantages of facilitating inspection of the papilla, biopsy and pancreatic sialography if required.

Choledochoduodenostomy is the easier of two difficult procedures in that the opening into the common bile duct is used for the anastomosis to the adjacent duodenum. Two channels are available for the passage of bile, a T-tube is unnecessary and there is no large repair of the duodenum. The disadvantages are the absence of confirmation of the nature of the lesion at the papilla and the possibility of reflux from the duodenum into the common bile duct. In the author's experience, symptoms from reflux cholangitis are rare. The majority of patients are elderly and the lesser procedure is advisable but in younger patients or where a tumour is suspected the direct approach is recommended.

The majority of these patients have infected bile and the appropriate antibiotics should be begun preoperatively and continued postoperatively to reduce morbidity.

Sphincterotomy

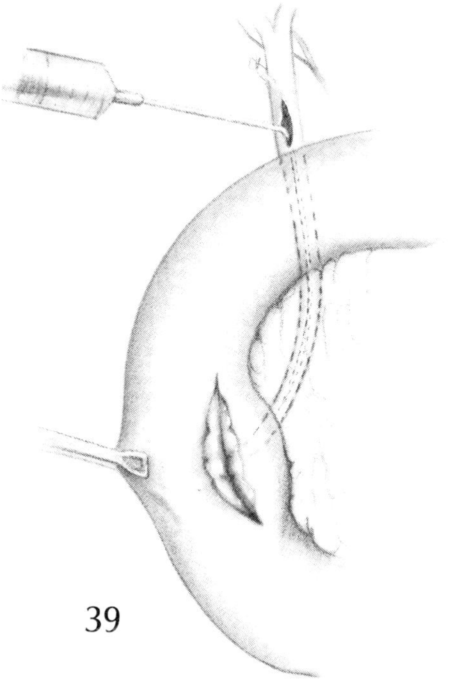

39

39

Identification of the ampulla

The second part of the duodenum is mobilized by dividing the peritoneum lateral to the second part of the duodenum (Kocher's manoeuvre). The Fogarty catheter is passed down the common bile duct into the duodenum, the balloon inflated and the catheter withdrawn until it impacts onto the sphincter. The balloon can be palpated, thereby identifying the ampulla and the level at which the duodenum has to be opened. If the Fogarty catheter cannot be passed into the duodenum, the cholangiogram is reviewed so that an estimate can be made of the site of the sphincter. Instruments should not be passed blindly as they may traumatize the duodenum and a false passage can be created.

A narrow duodenum should be opened longitudinally, whereas a wide duodenum can be opened and closed obliquely. Babcock's forceps are placed on the medial and lateral edge of the anterior surface of the second part of the duodenum at the level of the sphincter. The duodenum is opened with a small knife and the split enlarged to about 4 cm.

40

Sphincter identification

The Babcock's forceps are repositioned on the edges of the opening into the duodenum and the Fogarty catheter will be seen emerging from the opening of the common bile duct. If the catheter could not be passed, a Lister's bougie is passed down the common bile duct and gently pushed against the lower end of the duct; bile will be seen escaping. The bougie can then be made to pass through the sphincter to enter the duodenum.

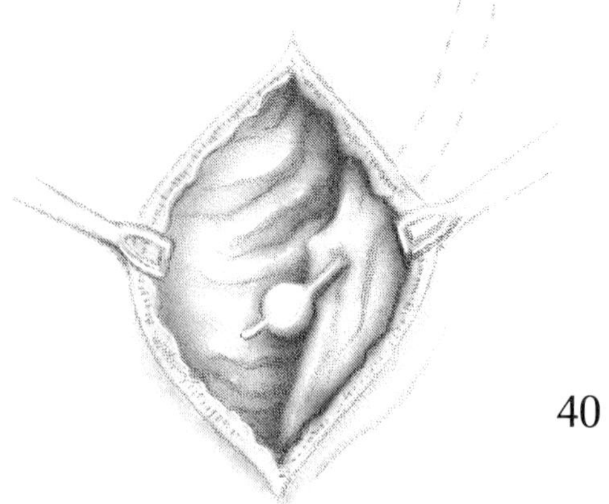

40

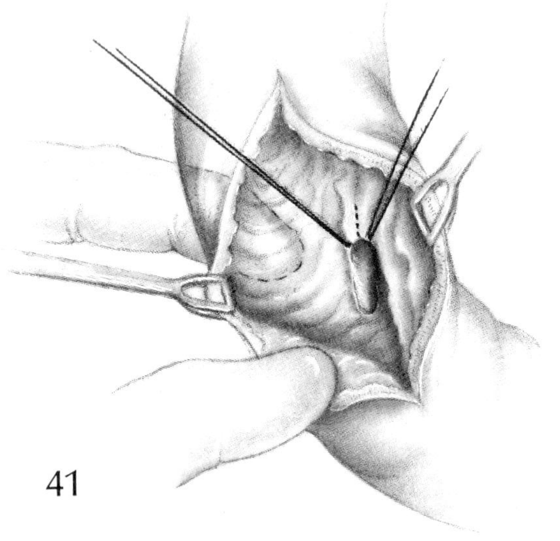

41

Sphincteroplasty

41

The Fogarty catheter or bougie is withdrawn and replaced by an instrument such as a grooved hernia director, suitably bent to allow ease of passage and subsequent manipulation. The groove is of assistance in placing the sutures.

Two 3/0 catgut sutures are placed through the opening of the duct, superolaterally and superomedially (10 and 2 o'clock), tied and held. A fine knife is used to cut the duodenal wall between the sutures.

42

A series of similar sutures is inserted in pairs and the walls of the duodenum and duct further divided, to enlarge the opening gradually until it measures more than 1 cm.

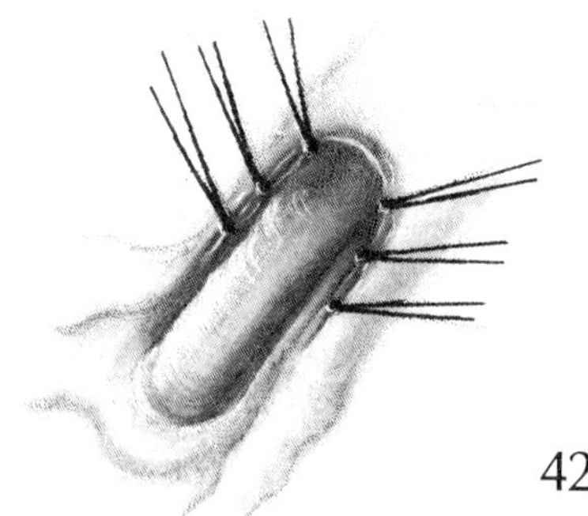

42

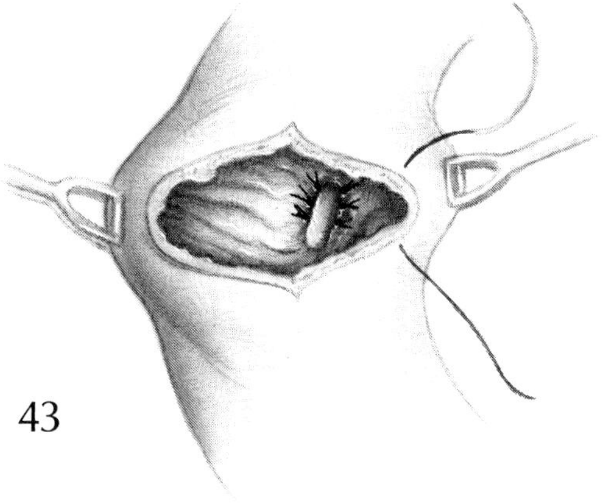
43

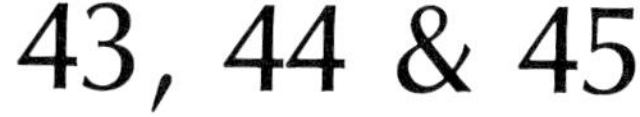

43, 44 & 45

Duodenal closure

The longitudinal opening is made transverse by removing the Babcock's forceps and replacing them on the duodenal wall at the midpoint of the opening. Closure is completed with through-and-through 2/0 catgut sutures followed by interrupted silk.

The operation is completed by T-tube insertion, wound drainage and closure.

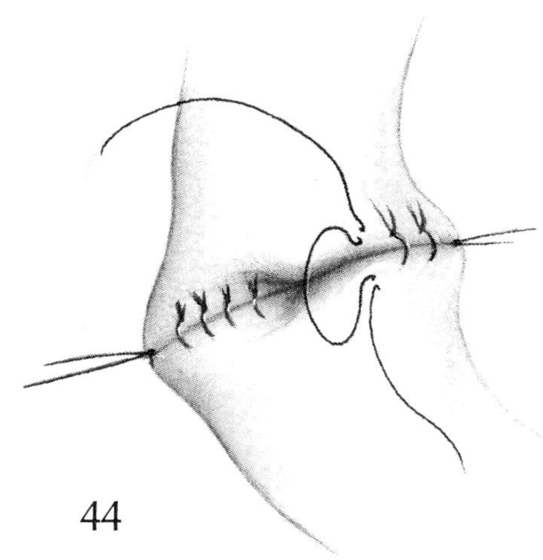
44

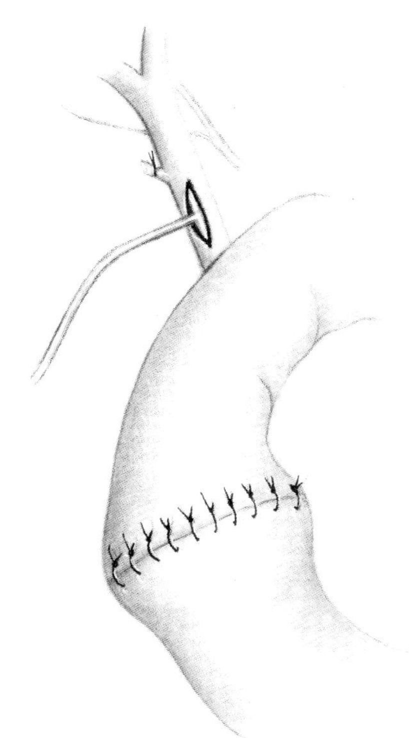
45

PERSONAL RESULTS

Table 1 Personal results (1069 consecutive patients) obtained by prospective recording and analysis by the author on punch cards.

	Cholecystectomy (n = 863)	*Choledochotomy (n = 206)*
Atelectasis*	318	76
Pulmonary embolus†	6	3
Wound infection§	14	14
Wound disruption	8	2
Deep vein thrombosis**	5	2
Wound haematoma	14	2
Biliary fistula	4	5
Biliary peritonitis	4	2
Renal failure	1	1
Bacteriogenic shock	7	2
Subphrenic abscess	13	4
Walter Waltman syndrome	1	0
Other minor	35	8
Death	3	5
No complications	504	99

*Crepitations or positive X-ray. Not all patients had an X-ray so that the incidence is probably higher
†Clinical diagnosis confirmed by X-ray alone. The true incidence will be higher
§A wound discharging fluid with a positive culture
**Clinical or ultrasound signs confirmed by venography but isotope scanning was not done

Table 2 'Foley' intraoperative postcholedochotomy cholangiogram (173 consecutive patients)*

Normal	123
Stone	25
? Stone – repeated – Normal	10
Stricture	7
Unsatisfactory	2
Not done	6

*The author believes that this is a valuable technique. In this series 32 patients had residual disease.

Table 3 Frequency of primary biliary operations (1193 consecutive patients)

Cholecystectomy	915
Choledochotomy	209
Sphincteroplasty	34*
Choledochoduodenostomy	35*

*It is the author's view that choledochoduodenostomy is the easier operation and is now preferred unless sphincteroplasty is essential to remove a fixed stone, to acquire histological material or to carry out pancreatography. Even in this personal series the number of patients requiring an additional procedure is small; nevertheless follow-up reveals no difference in the results of the two groups. Recurrent cholangitis has not been a problem after choledochoduodenostomy.

References

1. Editorial. Scottish Hospital in-patient statistics. London : HMSO (annual)
2. McSherry, C. K., Glenn, F. The instance and cause of death following surgery for non-malignant biliary tract disease. Annals of Surgery 1980; 191: 271–275
3. Editorial. Scottish Hospital in-patient statistics. London: HMSO, 1978
4. Dawson, J. L. Jaundice and anoxic renal damage. Protective effect of mannitol. British Medical Journal 1964; 1: 810–811
5. Haw, C. S., Gunn, A. A. The significance of infection in biliary surgery. Journal of the Royal College of Surgeons of Edinburgh 1973; 18: 209–212
6. Gunn, A. A. Abdominal drainage. British Journal of Surgery 1969; 56: 274–276
7. Orloff, M. J. Importance of surgical technique in prevention of retained and recurrent bile duct stones. World Journal of Surgery 1978; 2: 403–410
8. Cotton, P. B., Vallon, A. G. British experience with duodenoscopic sphincterotomy for removal of bile duct stones. British Journal of Surgery 1981; 68: 373–375
9. Fogarty, T. J., Krippaehne, W. M., Dennis, D. L., Fletcher, W. S. Evaluation of an improved operative technic in common duct surgery. American Journal of Surgery 1968; 116: 177–183

Transduodenal exploration of the bile duct (biliary sphincterotomy)

A. L. G. Peel MA, MChir, FRCS
Consultant Surgeon, North Tees General Hospital, Stockton on Tees, Cleveland

Historical

In 1895 Kocher described an operation in which he had removed a stone impacted in the lower common bile duct transduodenally – creating an internal choledocho-duodenostomy. Three years later McBurney from New York reported a small series of patients undergoing trans-duodenal exploration of the bile duct but he, unlike Kocher, had incised part of Oddi's sphincter, removing the stones through the divided papilla (a sphincterotomy). This approach to the common bile duct is favoured by surgeons in many countries in Europe and North and South America but although there is general agreement on the anatomy of the choledochoduodenal junction much confusion still remains with regard to operative terminology.

Anatomy

1

Oddi's sphincter comprises the main biliary sphincter (sphincter choledochus), which is well developed and constant, and two variable sphincters (sphincter papillae and sphincter pancreaticus), which may be rudimentary or absent. It is important to note that the sphincter choledochus extends beyond the duodenal wall.

A papillotomy divides the mucosa at the tip of the papilla and the fibres of the sphincter papillae when present; a sphincterotomy divides, in addition, the intraduodenal part of the sphincter choledochus. When the cut mucosal edges are sutured it is frequently termed a papillostomy or sphincteroplasty. A total sphincteroplasty however divides all the sphincter fibres surrounding the terminal bile duct and as the incision necessarily extends outside the duodenal wall the cut edges must be sutured to prevent retroperitoneal leakage of duodenal contents.

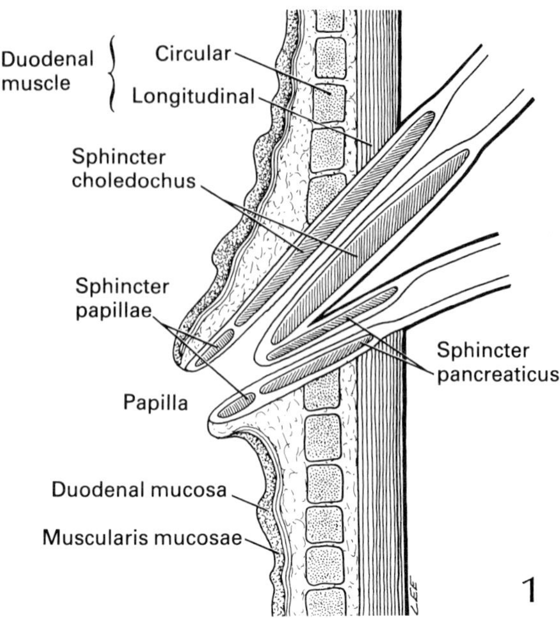

Preoperative

Indications for transduodenal sphincterotomy in biliary tract disease.

Absolute

Impacted stone at the lower end of the common bile duct.
Stenosis of the papilla and sphincter.
Re-exploration (endoscopic sphincterotomy may be preferred when the patient is elderly and frail).

Relative

As the method of choice for patients with multiple common bile duct stones and sludge.

Contraindications

A single large stone in the supraduodenal portion of the common bile duct that does not descend to the sphincteric region.
Multiple facetted stones locked in the bile duct.
Long stricture of terminal common bile duct (chronic pancreatitis).
The presence of acute pancreatitis.

Special precautions

These are necessary if there is a previous history of acute or chronic pancreatitis.

Preoperative preparation

Standard liver function tests should be carried out and any prolongation of the prothrombin time corrected with intramuscular injections of Vitamin K. The bile ducts should then be examined by the appropriate imaging techniques; ultrasonography when available, intravenous cholangiography in the anicteric patient and either percutaneous transhepatic or endoscopic retrograde cholangiography in the jaundiced patient. In the presence of jaundice it is important to ensure adequate hydration. An intravenous infusion of crystalloids is started at least 12 h preoperatively, 200 ml 10 per cent mannitol is given at the induction of anaesthesia and the patient is catheterized in order to monitor the intra and postoperative urinary output. Appropriate antibiotics in a dosage calculated according to the patient's body weight, plasma creatinine concentration and age are administered intravenously at the time of premedication. The author uses cephamandole supplemented by gentamicin unless renal function is compromised.

The operation

Either a right paramedian or Kocher's subcostal incision provides good access to the biliary tree. A full laparotomy, particularly noting the state of the biliary tree, liver, pancreas and duodenum, is carried out. Whenever possible the cystic duct is cannulated using an olivary tipped ureteric catheter (No. 4 Fr). If cannulation fails cholangiography can be carried out by direct puncture of the bile duct using a fine butterfly needle.

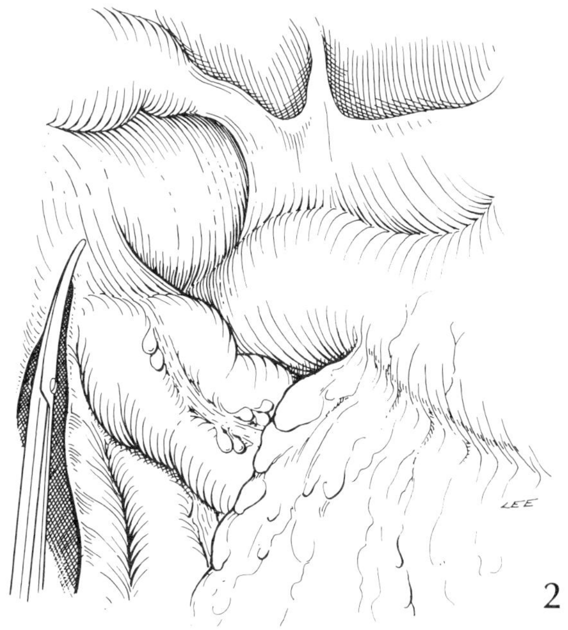

2

2

The hepatic flexure of the colon and proximal transverse colon are mobilized and reflected caudally, exposing the head of the pancreas and the duodenal 'C'.

3

The posterior peritoneum is now incised along the right lateral margin of the second and third parts of the duodenum.

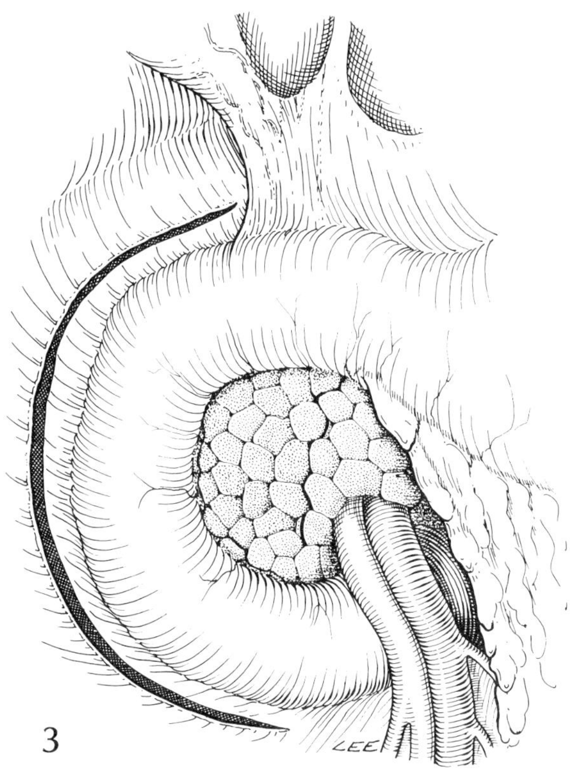

3

4

With a combination of sharp and blunt dissection the duodenum and pancreatic head are mobilized forwards and medially, exposing the gonadal vessels and inferior vena cava. Dissection continues until the aorta is visualized and the third part of the duodenum, proximal to the point where it is crossed by the superior mesenteric vessels, is free.

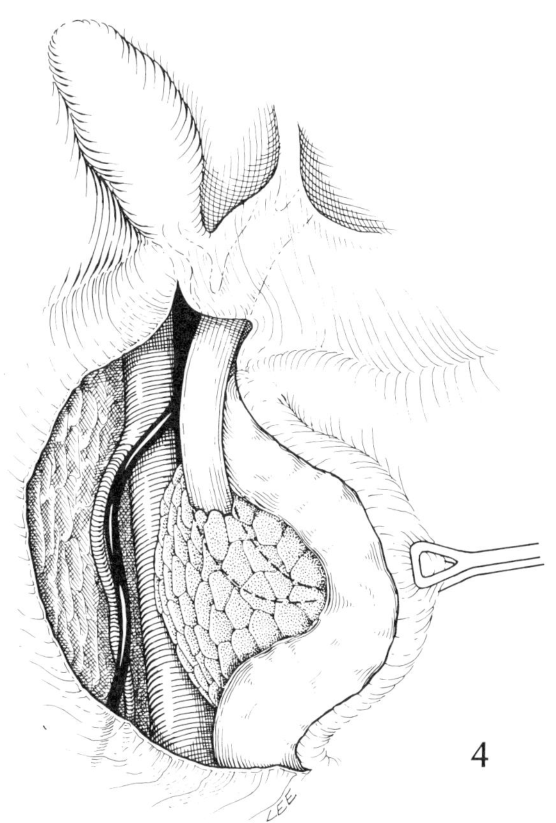

4

5

With the fingers of the left hand behind the duodenum and pancreatic head, the papilla is located on the medial wall of the duodenum with the left thumb. It is often situated more distally in the second or third parts of the duodenum than is commonly appreciated. If difficulty in the identification of the papilla is encountered the ureteric catheter may be advanced down the common bile duct toward the papilla.

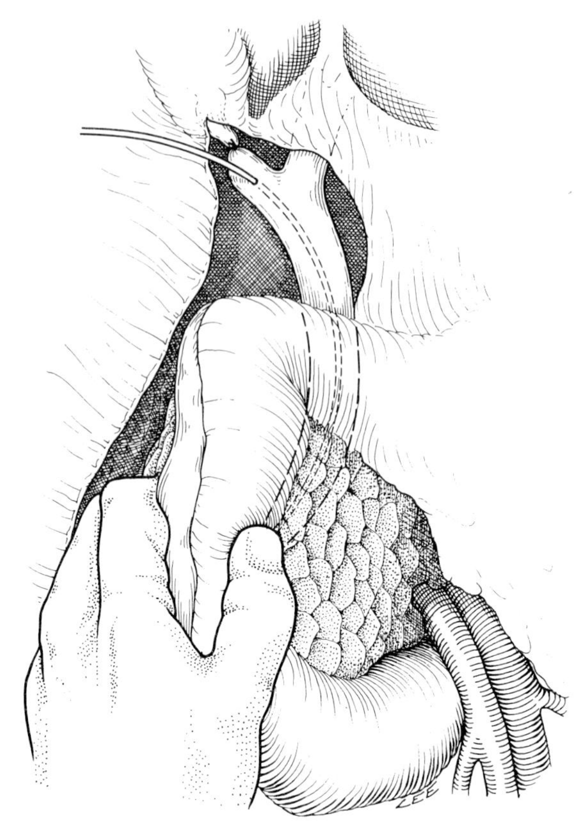

5

6

A small bulldog clip is then placed across the supraduodenal part of the common bile duct in order to prevent calculi slipping back into the common hepatic duct and its tributaries.

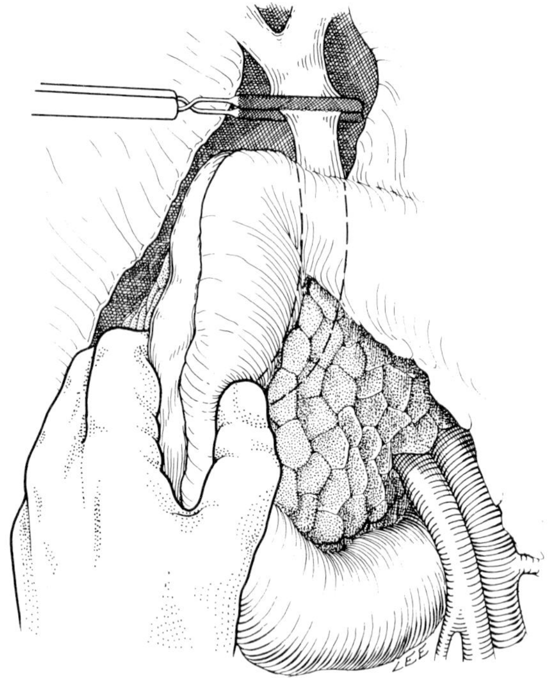

6

7

Stay sutures are inserted into the anterior and posterior duodenal wall at the level of the papilla and the duodenal wall is incised longitudinally or transversely – the author prefers the former since this allows the surgeon greater freedom of access.

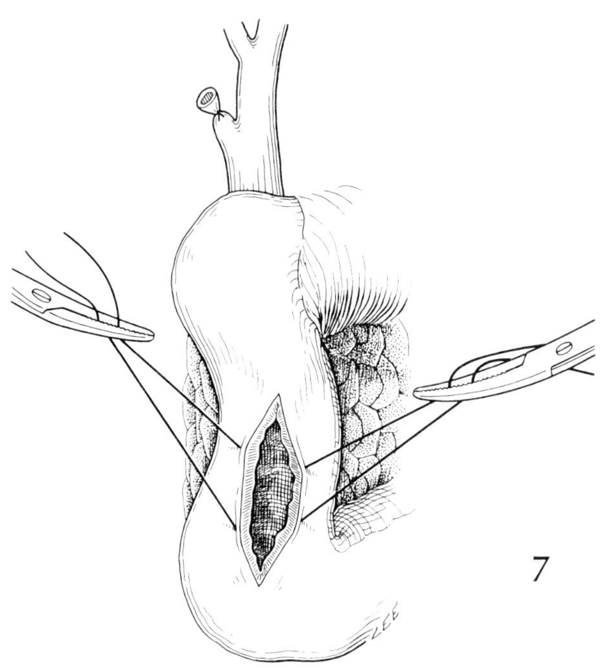

7

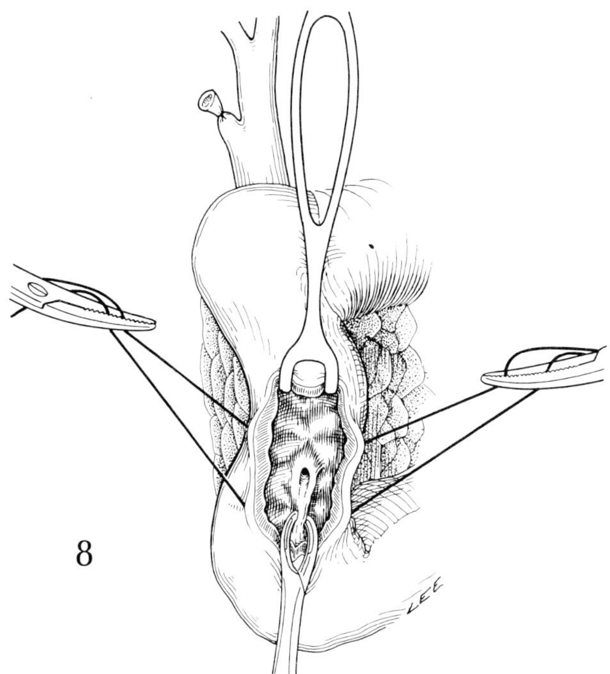

8

8

Babcock tissue forceps are applied to the longitudinal fold distal to the papilla and the latter is drawn into the duodenotomy incision. The first assistant holds the Babcock in his left hand. The exposure may be improved by gently retracting the anterior wall of the proximal duodenum with a Czerny retractor.

9

A grooved director or lacrimal probe is passed into the papillary orifice and thence into the common bile duct. Before starting the sphincterotomy it is essential to ensure that the director has entered the biliary and not the pancreatic tree. This can be confirmed by seeing movement of the tip of the director within the lumen and against the wall of the supraduodenal part of the common bile duct. Entry into the pancreatic duct is most easily avoided by keeping the handle of the grooved director or probe horizontal, thus running the tip of the instrument along the anterior aspect or roof of the common bile duct.

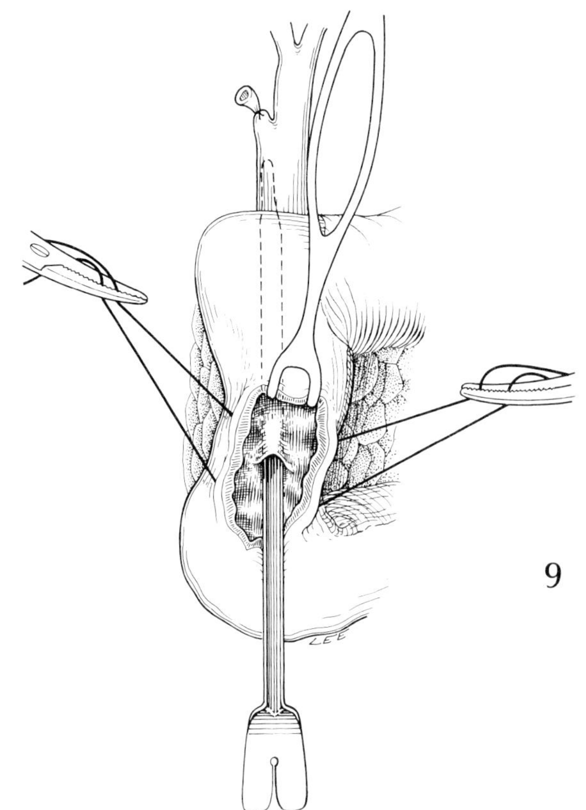

9

10

After insertion of the director into the bile duct the papilla and sphincter are divided in their longitudinal axis at 10 o'clock. The author initiates the sphincterotomy with a scalpel.

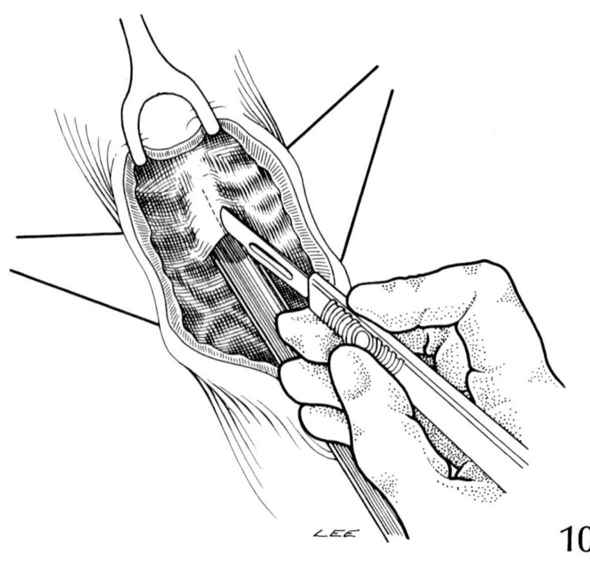

10

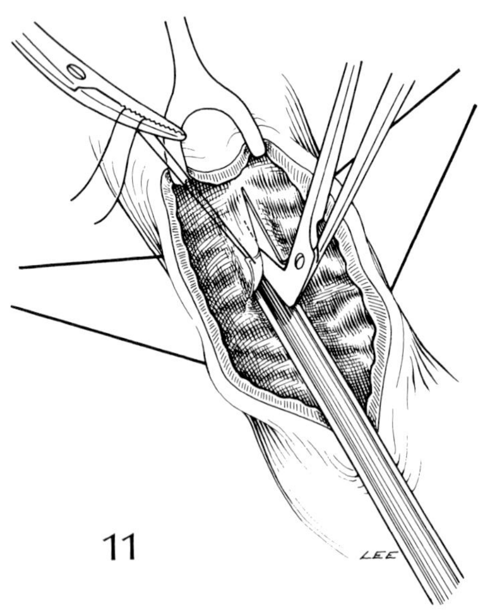

11

11

The incision is completed with Pott's angled scissors and fine catgut sutures may be inserted to keep the cut edges apart, facilitating the exposure of the distal bile duct. The length of the incision is sufficient to permit the easy passage of Desjardin's stone-retrieving forceps into the common bile duct. Complete division of the sphincter with extension of the incision outside the duodenum is not considered essential but if carried out invariably requires the insertion of sutures between duodenal and bile duct mucosa in order to prevent both leakage into the retroduodenal space and bleeding from the circumferential duodenal vessels.

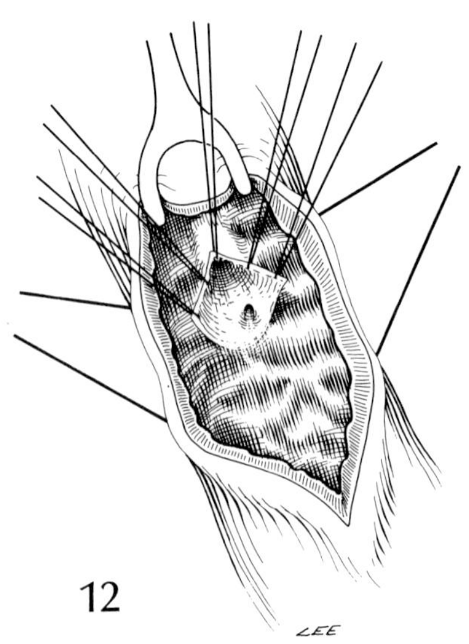

12

12

The pancreatic duct orifice may be identified in the floor of the sphincterotomy by observing the periodic flow of pancreatic juice. Probing the pancreatic duct should be avoided whenever possible.

13

Stones are extracted with Desjardin's forceps and Fogarty balloon catheters.

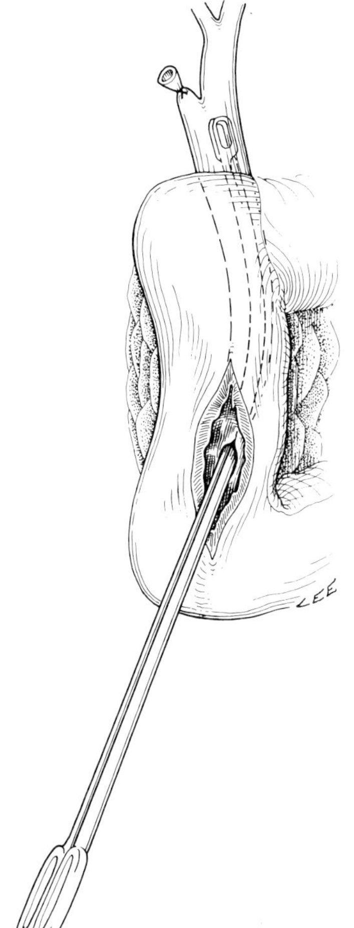

13

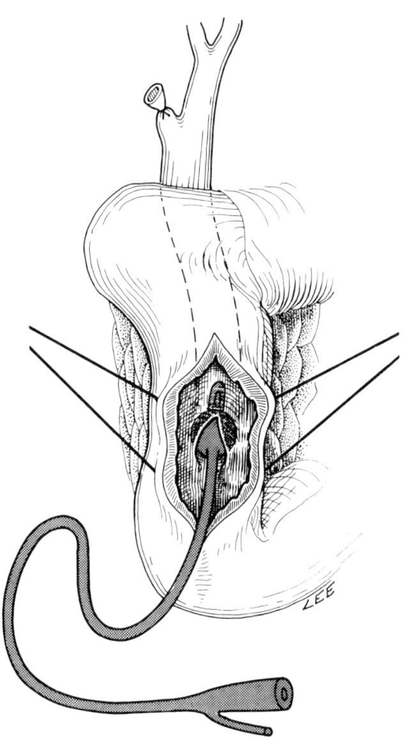

14

14

Clearance of the duct is confirmed by intraoperative postexploratory cholangiography via the sphincterotomy using a Foley balloon catheter.

15

Alternatively, choledochoscopy may be used. For this the author uses the rigid Storz instrument which, when inserted via the sphincterotomy, allows inspection of the right and left hepatic duct and their primary branches. The stay sutures may now be tied or removed – if the former it is important to make certain that those on the superomedial edge of the sphincterotomy have not encircled the pancreatic duct or its orifice.

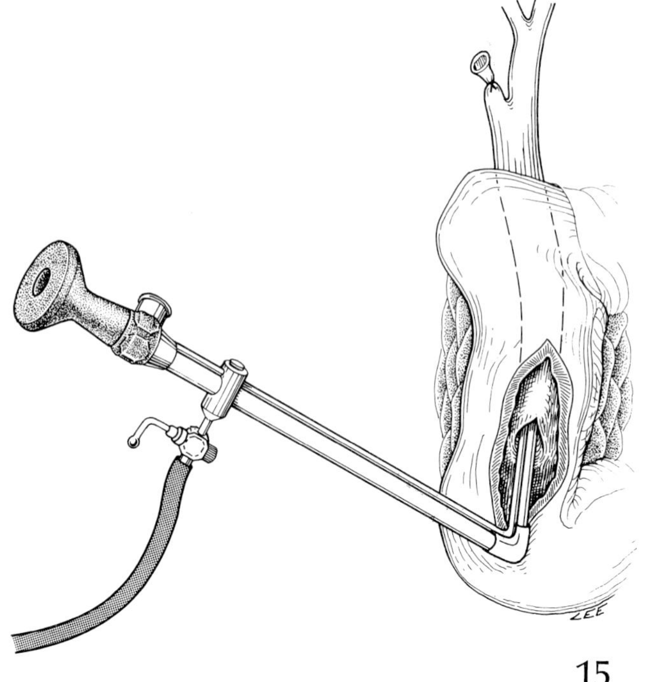

15

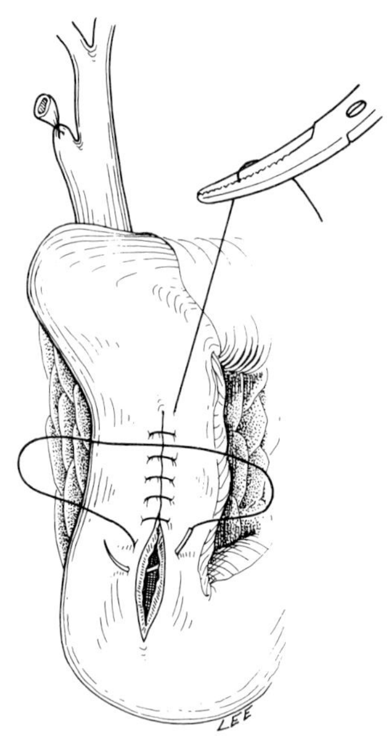

16

16

The duodenotomy is closed in its original axis using a continuous haemostatic suture (catgut) through all layers and fine non-absorbable Lembert sutures. Closure of a longitudinal duodenotomy in a transverse axis is not recommended because the splinting effect of the pancreas along the medial wall of the duodenum will lead to tension on the suture line.

After removal of the gall bladder the cystic duct stump is secured with an absorbable transfixion ligature and the abdomen closed with drainage to the subhepatic pouch (the author prefers the Anderson sump suction system). A T-tube is not usually required in the absence of a supraduodenal choledochotomy.

Postoperative care

Hydration is initially maintained by intravenous fluids and the stomach kept decompressed by nasogastric aspiration. Oral fluids are gradually introduced and intravenous therapy can usually be discontinued on the fourth day. Antibiotics are continued for 72 h. The drain is removed on the third to fourth day according to the volume obtained.

A transient rise in the plasma amylase level may be expected in up to a third of patients in the first 24 h postoperatively but clinical acute pancreatitis is rare.

Complications

The operation requires precision and the avoidance of unnecessary probing and manipulation which may produce oedema and will prolong the operation. Certain authors have reported problems with postoperative bleeding, cholangitis and pancreatitis and measures important in their prevention may be summarised as follows.

Bleeding

Persistent bleeding of the sphincterotomy incision usually arises from a divided circumferential duodenal artery and is best secured by suture.

Cholangitis

It is important to remove all calculi and provide an adequate sphincterotomy with free drainage. Peroperative antibiotics have been shown to reduce the incidence of septic complications.

Acute pancreatitis

The orifice of the pancreatic duct should be identified. Probing is best avoided. It is essential to ensure that no suture encircles the pancreatic duct.

Further reading

Peel, A. L. G., Hermon-Taylor, J., Ritchie, H. D. Technique of transduodenal exploration of the common bile duct. Annals of the Royal College of Surgeons of England 1974; 55: 236–244

Peel, A. L. G., Bourke, J. B., Hermon-Taylor, J., MacLean, A. D. W., Mann, C. V., Ritchie, H. D. How should the common bile duct be explored? Annals of the Royal College of Surgeons of England 1975; 56: 124–134

Choledochoduodenostomy

J. L. Dawson MS, FRCS
Consultant Surgeon, King's College Hospital, London

Preoperative

Indications

Choledochoduodenostomy should be considered in patients who are found to have a dilated common bile duct containing infected bile and biliary mud. Choledochotomy and duct lavage alone are associated with recurrent symptoms in a significant proportion of such patients.

Choledochoduodenostomy is especially suitable for those patients in whom the supraduodenal bile duct is grossly dilated or if there are multiple intrahepatic stones. It may also be used occasionally in patients with oriental suppurative cholangiohepatitis (see p. 724). It may be performed either at the same time as cholecystectomy if appropriate or at re-exploration in a patient with recurrent symptoms.

Contraindications

Choledochoduodenostomy should not be attempted in a patient with a bile duct of normal dimensions. It is best avoided in patients with malignant obstruction of the distal duct as extension of the tumour may well involve the stoma and produce recurrent symptoms.

Preoperative preparation

If the patient has or has had cholangitis, special care is necessary. The patient should have preoperative intravenous fluids. Vitamin K is given by injection if the patient is jaundiced and antibiotics are used prophylactically to minimize the possibility of Gram-negative septicaemia which frequently follows manipulation of the bile duct in patients with cholangitis. Because of the risk of renal failure the urine output should be maintained both during the operation and in the postoperative period by an osmotic diuretic such as mannitol.

The cross-reference in this chapter refers to *Operative Surgery: Alimentary Tract and Abdominal Wall, Volume 2, 4th Edition*

The operation

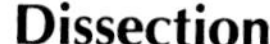

The incision

A Mayo-Robson, Kocher or paramedian incision may be used. It must be of sufficient length to allow good exposure. If the patient is being reoperated on it is far better to reopen the same incision.

Exposure

The right upper quadrant must be adequately dissected to expose the first and second parts of the duodenum, the aditus to the lesser sac and the free edge of the lesser omentum and the liver. It may be necessary to reflect the hepatic flexure of the colon downwards to achieve adequate exposure.

Dissection

If the patient is being re-explored after a previous cholecystectomy the duodenum (or colon) is frequently found adherent to the gall bladder fossa. Careful dissection is required and the pulse of the hepatic artery is an invaluable guide to the position of the bile duct. The bile duct is defined and the contiguous surface of the duodenum is dissected away by dividing the overlying peritoneum. The common bile duct is then opened and a specimen of bile sent for culture. Stones are removed and the duct is cleared of debris by copious lavage with saline. The duodenum is freely mobilized by Kocher's manoeuvre in order to allow it to roll upwards over the anterior surface of the bile duct without tension.

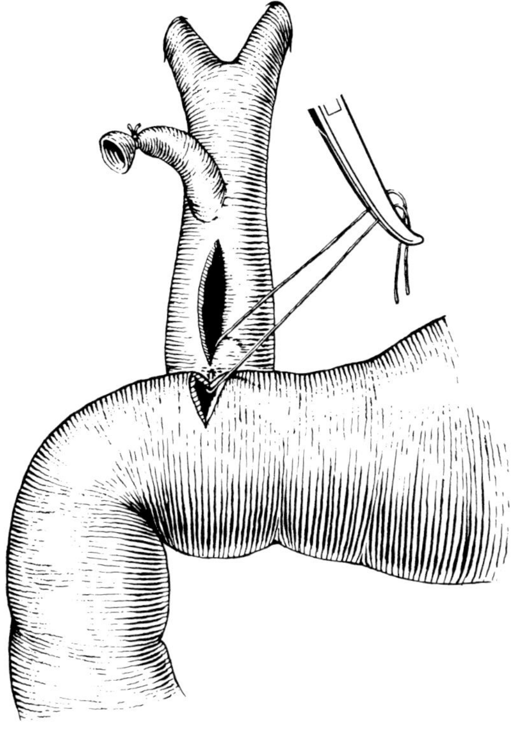

1

The stoma

There is general agreement from the literature that, provided the stoma is made 2.5 cm or more, recurrent symptoms are rare. Occasionally the duct is wide enough to allow the stoma to be placed horizontally but an oblique or vertical stoma is usually necessary.

1

After the duct has been dissected a vertical incision 2.5 cm long is made in its supraduodenal portion and the duodenum is opened in such a way to allow the stoma to be made without tension. The opening in the muscular layer is made with a fine knife. Care is taken to make this opening somewhat smaller than the choledochotomy as it tends to enlarge as suturing proceeds.

The anastomosis is done with interrupted 3/0 chromic catgut sutures beginning in the midline posteriorly. Each interrupted suture is held until the next one is placed gradually working round until the corners of the anastomosis are reached. The knots on the posterior wall are placed in the lumen.

2

Once the corners are reached the sutures are inserted from outside and held.

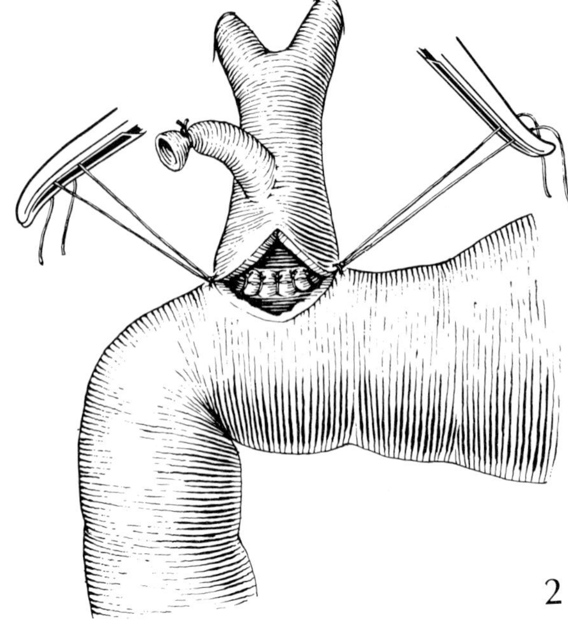

2

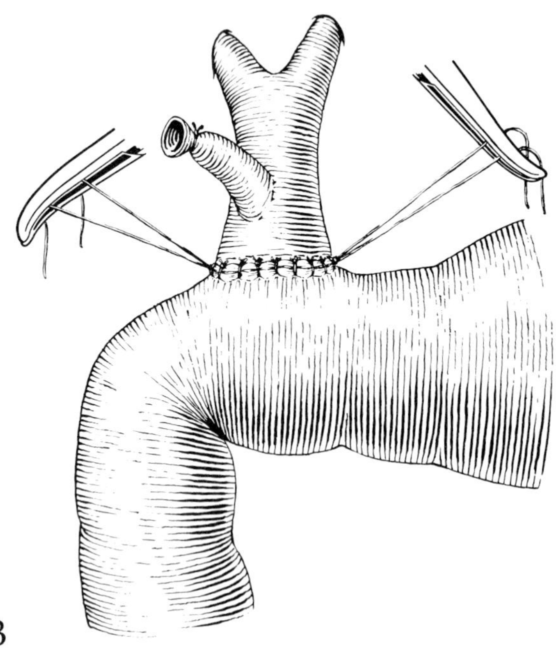

3

3

The anterior wall is then completed.

4

If the common bile duct is thickened then a seromuscular layer may be inserted to cover the anterior layer of the anastomosis but this layer is probably not essential.

No internal splinting is used. Non-absorbable sutures are not necessary and may cause visible redness of the stoma at subsequent endoscopy even if used on the seromuscular layer.

A corrugated drain is placed to the Pouch of Morison and the abdomen closed.

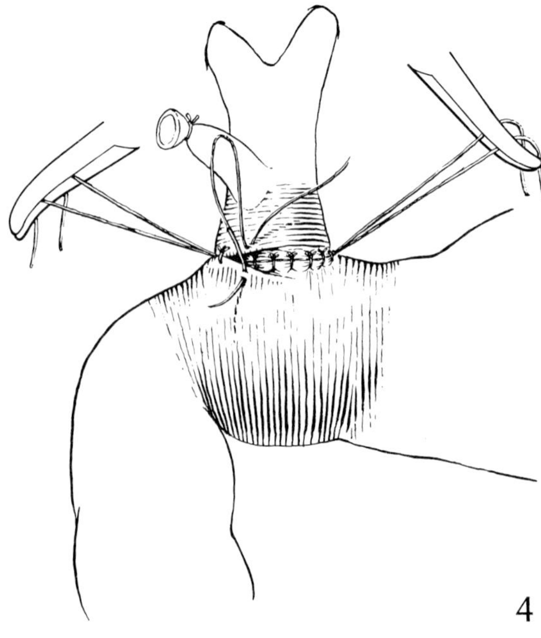

4

Postoperative care

In patients who have or have had ascending cholangitis a careful watch must be kept for evidence of septicaemia in the early postoperative period. The urine output is carefully recorded, especially in jaundiced patients. Nasogastric suction is used and the patient maintained on intravenous fluids until evidence of propulsive peristalsis returns which is usually about the third day.

An adequate stoma size may be confirmed by the presence of gas in the biliary tree on a straight abdominal X-ray (especially if a carbonated drink is given beforehand). Barium studies should show free reflux of barium into and out of the biliary system. The stoma may also be examined directly by fibre-endoscopy.

Results

In most published series the mortality and morbidity rates are low. A small percentage of patients may have a slight biliary leak but this dries up within a few days.

The long-term results of choledochoduodenostomy are uniformly good providing the stoma is made at least 2–2.5 cm in diameter. There is some evidence to show that shrinkage of the stoma may later take place even in symptomless patients.

The incidence of recurrent symptoms is less than 5 per cent in most series.

Further reading

Akiyama, H., Ikezawa, H., Kameya, S., Iwasaki, M., Kuroda, Y., Takeshita, T. Unexpected problems of external choledochoduodenostomy. American Journal of Surgery 1980; 140: 660–665

Dawson, J. L. Renal failure in obstructive jaundice – clinical aspects. Post-Graduate Medical Journal 1975; 51: 510–511

Ham, J. M., Sorby, W. Measurement of stoma size following choledochoduodenostomy by transduodenal cholangiography. British Journal of Surgery 1973; 60: 940–943

Johnson, A. G., Stevens, A. E. Importance of the size of the stoma in choledochoduodenostomy. Gut 1969; 10: 68–70

Madden, J. L., Chun, J. Y., Kandalaft, S., Parekh, M. Choledochoduodenostomy. An unjustly maligned surgical procedure? American Journal of Surgery 1970; 119: 45–54

Thomas, C. G., Nicholson, C. P., Owen, J. Effectiveness of choledochoduodenostomy and transduodenal sphincterotomy in the treatment of benign obstruction of the common duct. Annals of Surgery 1971; 173: 845–856

Pancreaticojejunostomy

Thomas Taylor White MD
Clinical Professor, Department of Surgery,
University of Washington School of Medicine, Seattle, Washington

Introduction

The author used pancreaticojejunostomy as the principal treatment in about 35 per cent of his 227 patients with painful chronic pancreatitis who had dilated pancreatic ducts; another 10 per cent, principally those with small, shrunken pancreases, were treated by a 95 per cent pancreatectomy (Childs). Pain-free patients are treated for steatorrhoea with pancreatin, are advised to abstain from alcohol, receive oral or injected agents to control their diabetes, and undergo choledochoduodenostomy to decompress the biliary tree when the distal end of the bile duct is compressed by pancreatic swelling and/or fibrosis. With this procedure, 82 per cent of the patients can expect relief from pain. Our 22-year follow-up studies show that patients with alcoholism gradually succumb to the disease in spite of this operation, even though they are relieved of pain, and that non-alcoholics lead relatively normal lives.

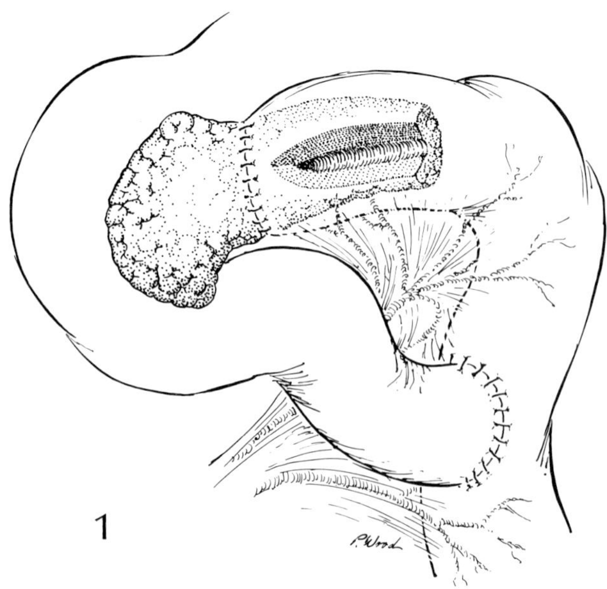

1

1

The original Gillesby-Puestow operation consisted of mobilization of the spleen and tail of the pancreas, followed by resection of the spleen with a small piece of the tip of the pancreatic duct, filleting of the left two-thirds of the pancreatic duct to in front of the portal vein, then invagination of the tail into a Roux-en-Y loop of jejunum. This is now only of historical interest. Experience showed both that extremely heavy bleeding occurred when this technique was used, because of mobilization of the tail of the pancreas, and also that the ductal incision has to be extended further to the right than was originally planned in order to obtain appropriate long-term drainage of the pancreas without persistent pain.

Indications for anterior pancreaticojejunostomy

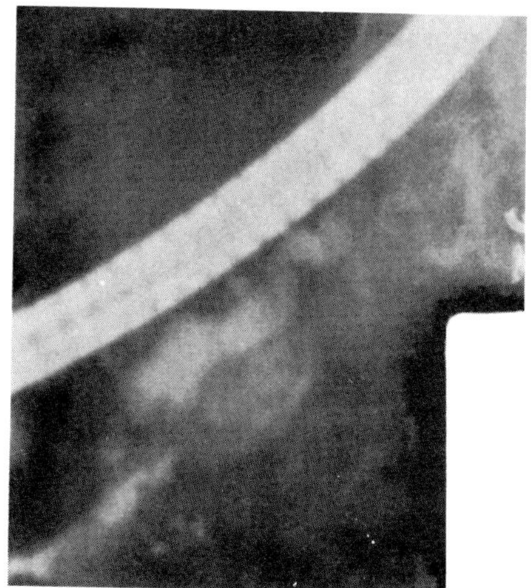

2

2

There has been preoperative endoscopic cannulation of the duodenal papilla with X-rays which demonstrate dilatation of the duct system with or without cyst formation.

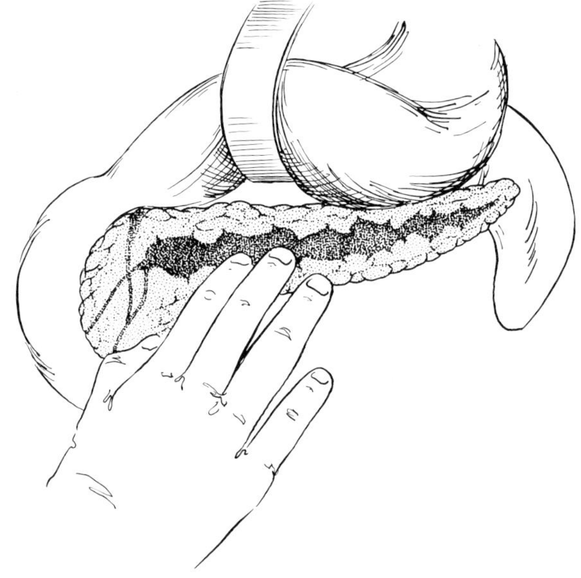

3

3

The duct is dilated on palpation of the anterior surface of the gland.

4

If a pancreatogram has not been obtained prior to operation, a direct pancreatogram is taken at the time of surgery and will demonstrate a dilated duct system.

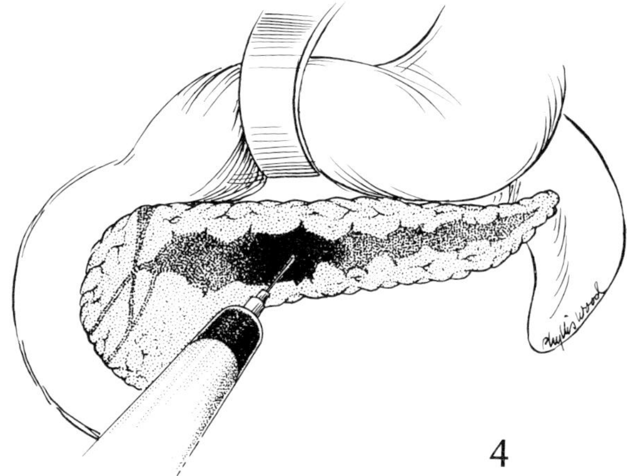

4

The operation

5

The pancreas is exposed by first opening the lesser peritoneal sac by dividing the gastrocolic ligament. The duct has been palpated and a surgical pancreatogram carried out if endoscopic cannulation has not been done preoperatively.

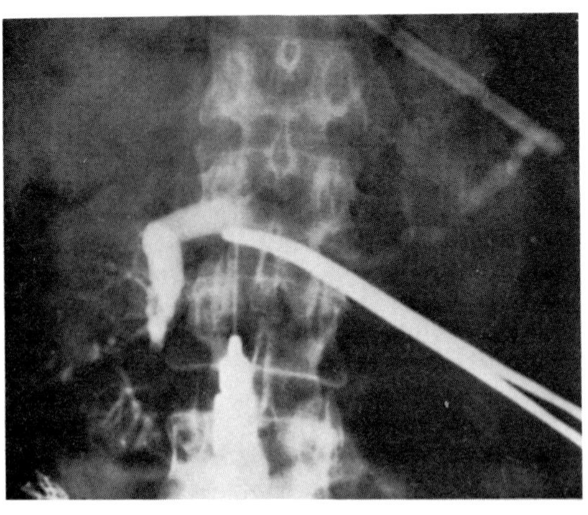

5

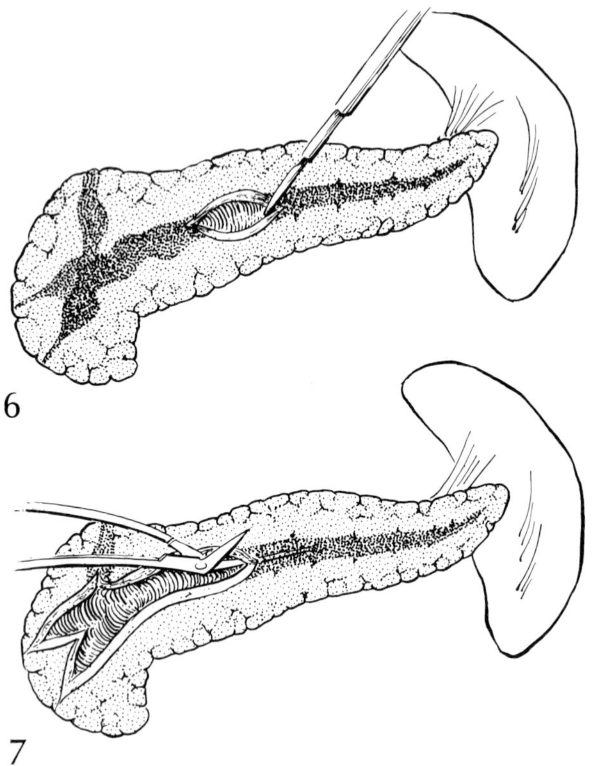

6

7

6 & 7

The pancreatic duct is then opened longitudinally, using a cautery or dura scissors.

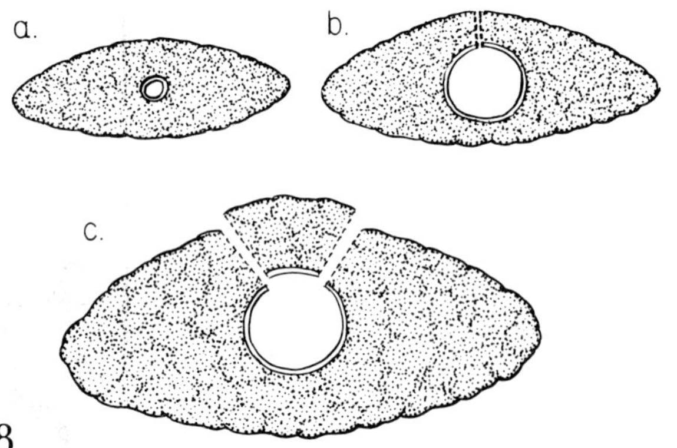

8

8

The relative cross-sectional diameters of the duct and pancreas are shown: the normal pancreatic duct is relatively small (*a*) but is a major proportion of the cross-section in the majority of patients in whom pancreaticojejunostomy is indicated (*b*); finally the duct and gland are both enlarged and boggy (*c*). In the situation shown in (*b*) a single anterior cut will cause the edges of the duct to spring apart. However, in (*c*) a wedge of tissue must be removed from the anterior surface of the pancreas to prevent margins of the duct from falling together.

9

The arterial circulation of the pancreas is shown. There are no major vessels near the anterior surface of the organ until a line about 1 cm to the left of the duodenum, where the anterosuperior and inferior pancreaticoduodenal arteries are to be found.

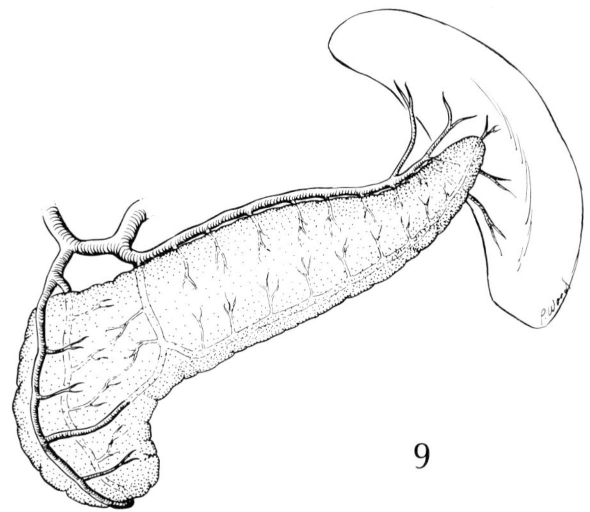

9

10

The Roux loop is next fashioned just beyond the ligament of Treitz after selecting the primary, secondary and tertiary arcades in such a way that they can be divided without loss of blood supply to the loop after it has been transplanted to the front of the pancreas through the opening indicated by the arrow.

10

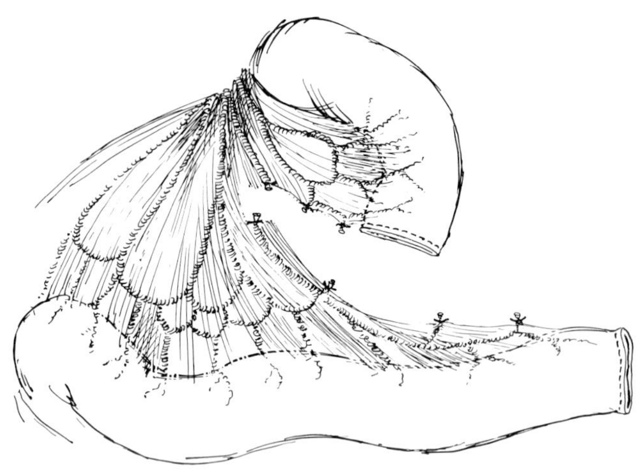

11

11, 12 & 13

The vessels are divided and the gut transected. Though clamps may be usd they are clumsy and in the operator's way. Two rows of staples permit the jejunum to be divided and easily manipulated through the gap in the mesocolon above Treitz's ligament where it lies adjacent to the anterior aspect of the pancreas. The proximal loop lies snugly below the mesocolon while the pancreaticojejunostomy is being done.

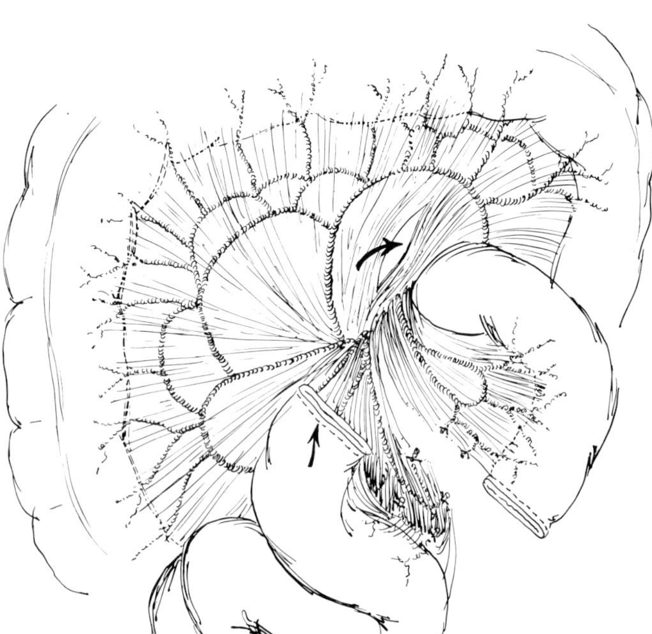

12

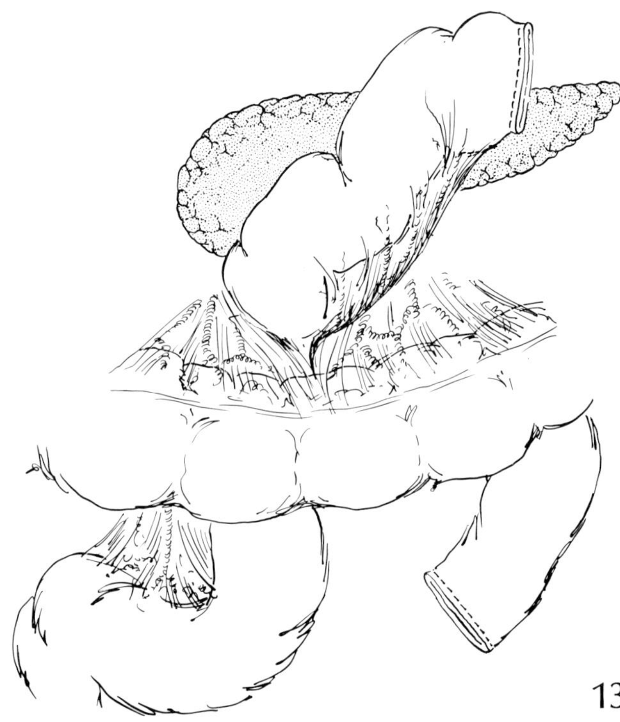

13

14

The jejunum is fixed to the lower edge of the pancreas with interrupted 2/0 sutures.

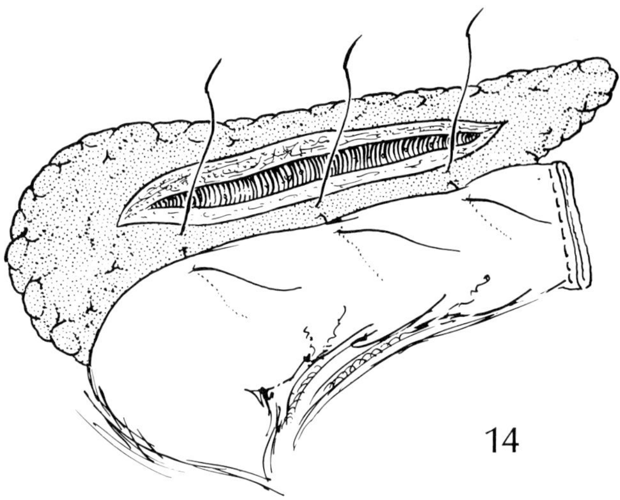

14

15

15

The jejunum is incised as indicated by the dotted line.

16

A running 0 or 2/0 catgut suture attaches the cut edges of the pancreas and jejunum.

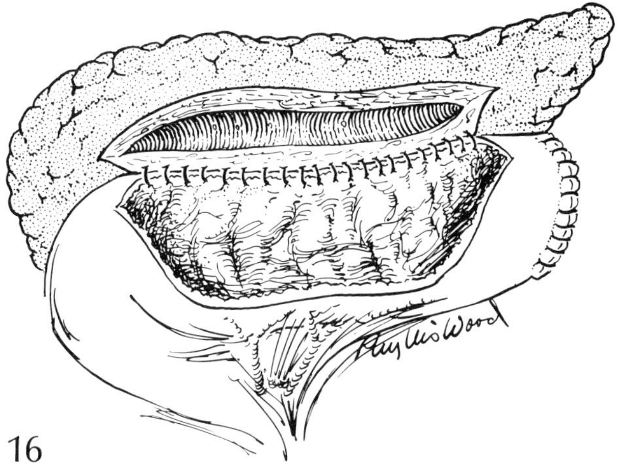

16

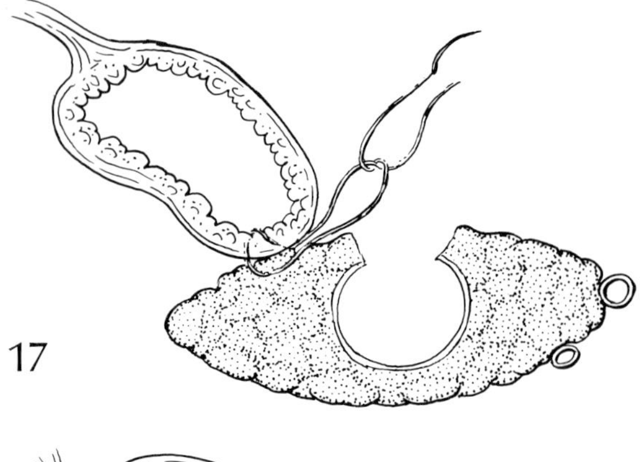

17

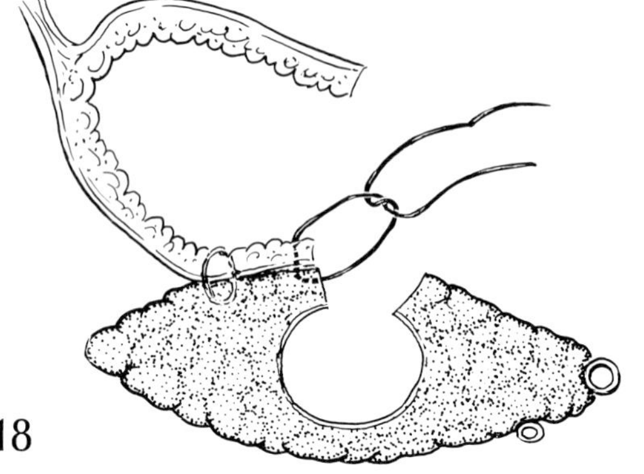

18

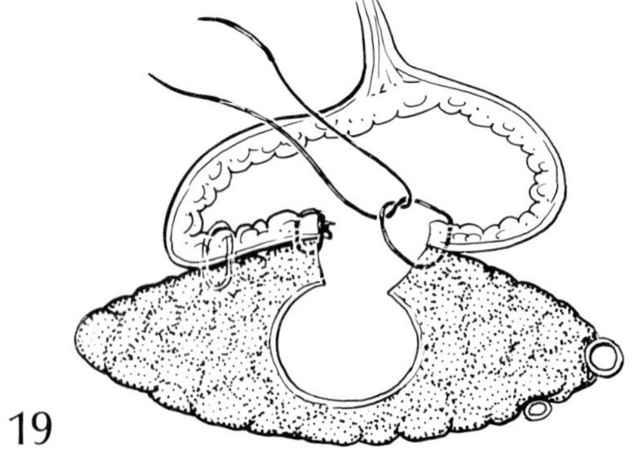

19

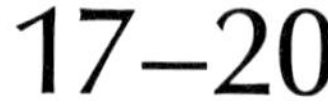

17–20

The whole of the anastomosis is shown in cross-section, completion of the upper suture line being performed by the same technique as the lower.

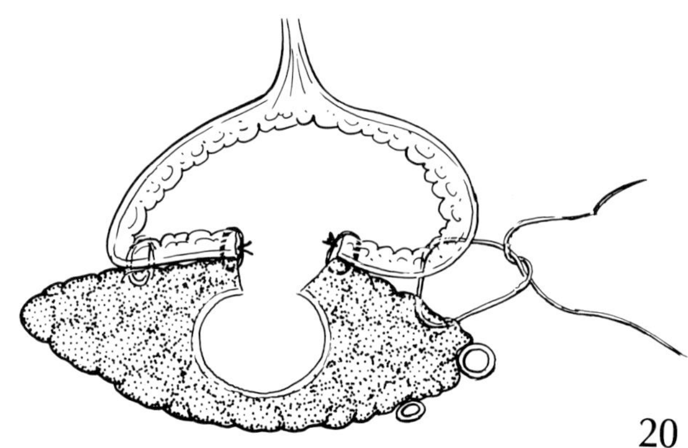

20

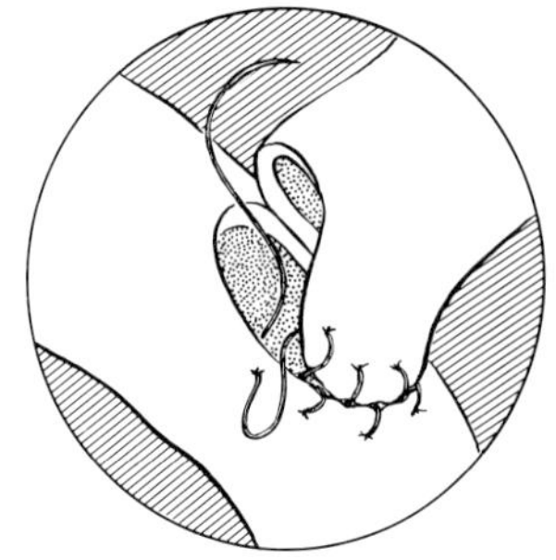

21

21

Anatomical continuity is restored by jejunojejunostomy below the colon, with a single layer of through-and-through sutures.

22

If necessary a choledochojejunostomy can be made to the Roux loop to bypass obstruction of the lower end of the duct. The flow of pancreatic juice (and bile) is shown by the arrows.

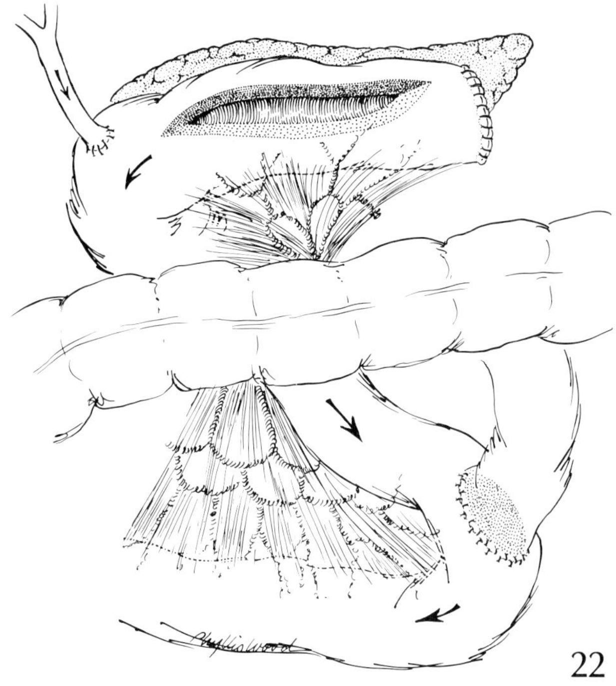

22

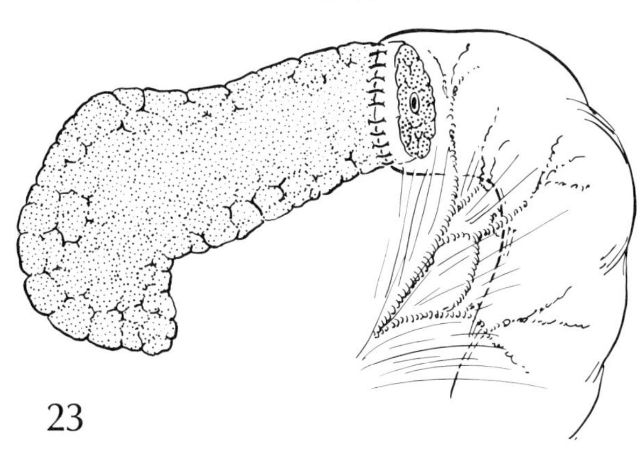

23

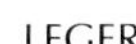

Other operations

23, 24 & 25

The drainage procedures of Du Val, Leger or Mercadier as well as others have not been successful because the small anastomosis used in these procedures soon tends to occlude.

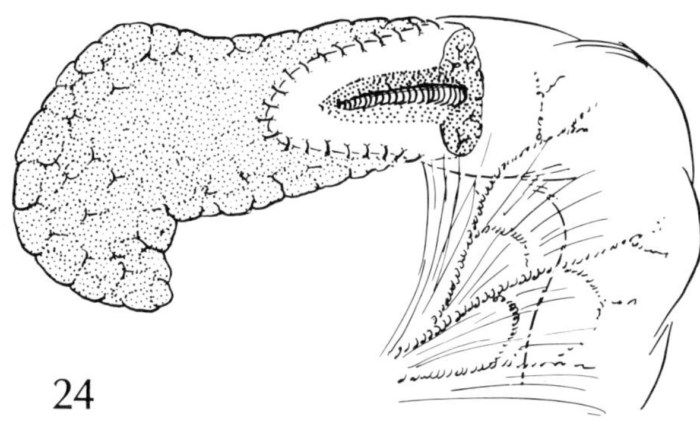

24

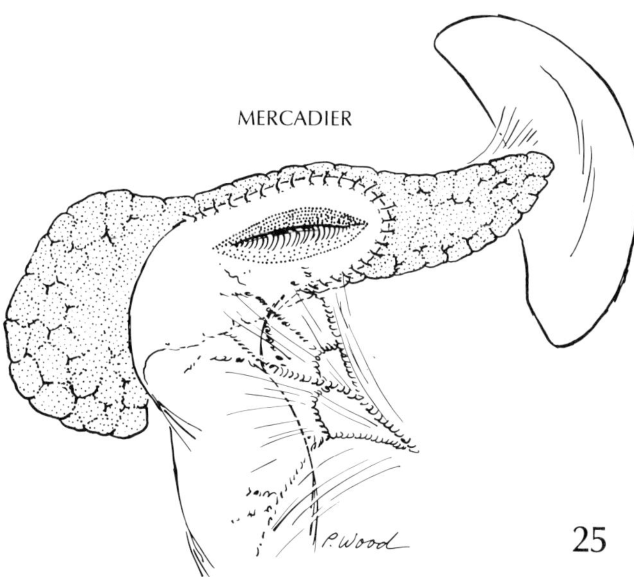

25

26

When a large pancreatic cyst occurs in chronic pancreatitis, the situation is as shown. Simple drainage of the cyst into a Roux-en-Y loop will not relieve the underlying pancreatic duct obstruction and a pancreaticojejunostomy as already described is required.

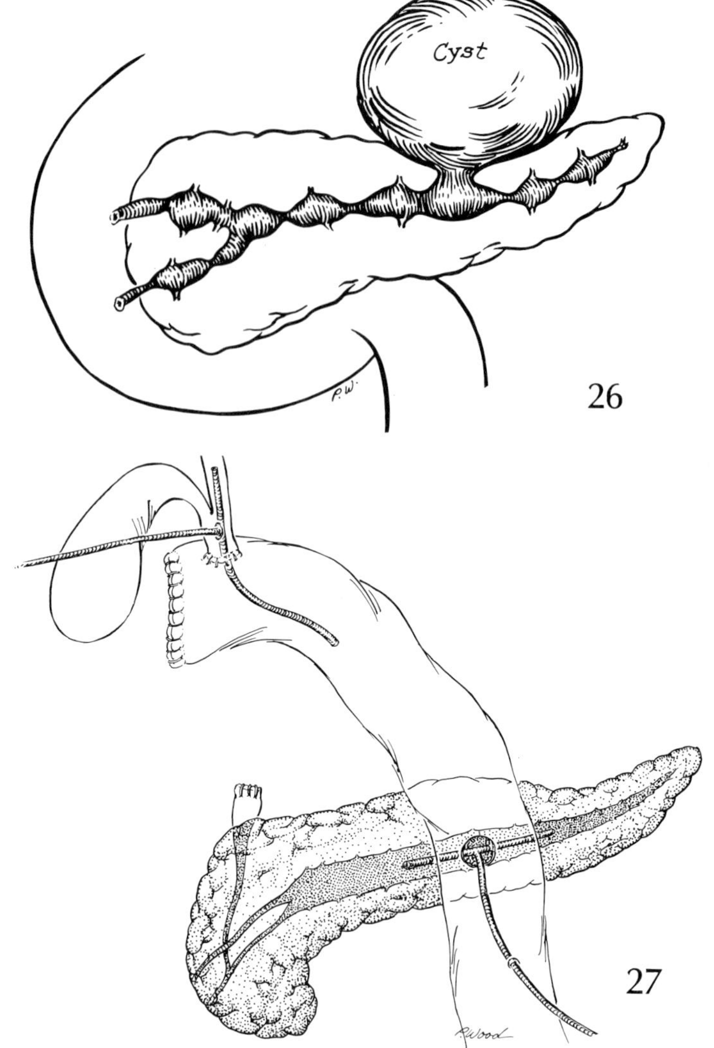

27

Pain caused by obstruction of a normal duct responds well to the procedure described by Cattell in which the Roux loop is brought up to drain the duct side-to-side and decompress the biliary tree if necessary.

Further reading

Gillesby, W. J., Puestow, C. B. Pancreaticojejunostomy for chronic relapsing pancreatitis: an evaluation. Surgery 1961; 50: 859–862

Jordan, G. L., Jr, Howard, J. M. Caudal pancreaticojejunostomy in the management of chronic relapsing pancreatitis. Surgery 1958; 44: 303–311

Leger, L., Lenriot, J. P., Lemaigre, G. Five to twenty year follow-up after surgery for chronic pancreatitis in 148 patients. Annals of Surgery 1974; 180: 185–191

Sato, T., Saitoh Y., Noto, N., Matsuno, K. Appraisal of operative treatment for chronic pancreatitis, with special reference to side-to-side pancreaticojejunostomy. American Journal of Surgery 1975; 129: 621–628

Traverso, L. W., Tompkins, Urrea, P. T., Williams, B. A., Longmire, P. Surgical treatment of chronic pancreatitis. Annals of Surgery 1979; 190: 312–319

Way, L. W., Gadacz, T., Goldman, L. Surgical treatment of chronic pancreatitis. American Journal of Surgery 1974; 127: 202–209

White, T. T. Pancreatitis. Baltimore: Williams and Wilkins, 1966

White, T. T. Surgical treatment of chronic pancreatitis – report of 227 cases. Japanese Journal of Surgery 1981; 11: 1–7

White, T. T., Harrison, R. C. Reoperative gastrointestinal surgery, 2nd ed. Boston: Little, Brown & Co., 1979

White, T. T., Hart, M. J. Pancreaticojejunostomy versus resection in the treatment of chronic pancreatitis. American Journal of Surgery 1979; 138: 129–135

White, T. T., Slavotinek, A. H. Results of surgical treatment of chronic pancreatitis. Annals of Surgery 1979; 189: 217–224

Pancreatoduodenectomy

Michael Knight MS, FRCS
Consultant Surgeon, St George's Hospital
and St James' Hospital, London

Historical aspects

In 1899 Halsted[1] published his account of a limited resection of the periampullary region with reimplantation of the bile duct and pancreatic duct into the duodenal suture line. In was not until 1912, however, that the first serious attempt was made to resect the whole head of the gland. In that year, Kausch[2], in a two-stage procedure, successfully removed the duodenum and head of the pancreas for ampullary carcinoma and restored pancreatointestinal continuity with a formal anastomosis of the pancreatic remnant to the jejunum. The results of this operation in other hands, however, were less successful because of complications relating to the pancreatic anastomosis and the procedure fell into disrepute. At that time it was generally believed that flow of pancreatic juice into the intestine was essential for life but this was questioned in 1935 by Whipple, Parsons and Mullins[3] who proceeded to carry out a radical excision of the head of the pancreas with ligation of the main duct in the residual gland. The resection was preceded, a month earlier, by a gastroenterostomy, ligation and division of the common bile duct and a cholecystogastrostomy, the latter to relieve jaundice which Whipple knew to be associated with a bleeding tendency at operation. The patient lived for over 2 years before dying of metastases. Encouraged by Whipple's success, several other surgeons published their results of the procedure in patients with ampullary carcinoma and in 1937, Brunschwig[4] carried out the operation successfully for carcinoma of the head of pancreas. By the end of the decade, Dam's[5] work on vitamin K was gaining recognition and Whipple in 1940[6] was able, for the first time, to dispense with preliminary bile drainage and proceed to a one-stage pancreatoduodenectomy. Since that time, many modifications to the original technique have been suggested and in particular, because of the crippling effects of pancreatic steatorrhoea in some patients, the formal pancreatojejunal anastomosis was reintroduced.

The cross-reference in this chapter refers to *Operative Surgery: Alimentary Tract and Abdominal Wall, Volume 2, 4th Edition*

Preoperative

Principles and indications

The purpose of the operation of pancreatoduodenectomy is to remove, *en bloc* with adjacent lymph nodes, the head of the pancreas, the duodenum, the pylorus and distal half of the stomach, the gall bladder and the lower end of the common duct; and to restore biliary-pancreatic and gastrointestinal continuity.

Pancreatoduodenectomy is the treatment of choice for operable malignant tumours of the ampulla of Vater, the lower end of the common bile duct, the duodenum and the periampullary region of the head of the pancreas. For this group of patients the operation carries an acceptable mortality and a good chance of long-term survival. Less favourable results, however, have been reported in patients with more extensive carcinomas of the head of the pancreas and this raises the question of whether such a formidable procedure is justifiable in these patients. In trying to answer this question, one must first consider the alternatives such as the palliative bypass operations, chemotherapy and radiotherapy. None of these offers a prospect of cure. Furthermore, what may appear to be a large bulky tumour of the head of the pancreas at laparotomy, may, in fact, be an area of chronic pancreatitis around a small obstructing but potentially curable ampullary carcinoma. A reasonable policy then would be to reserve pancreatoduodenectomy for periampullary tumours including those small tumours of the head of the pancreas originating in the terminal pancreatic duct. For larger tumours, particularly in the younger age group, the operation would be justifiable if the disease process is macroscopically limited to the head of the gland well to the right of the portal vein. Although the 'cure' rate will be low, this approach would seem to provide the best palliation for this group of patients with carcinoma of the head of the pancreas.

Pancreatoduodenectomy for cancer is performed only after careful preliminary dissection has failed to demonstrate any local or metastatic spread of the tumour and in particular any extension into the vena cava, portal vein, superior mesenteric vein and root of the transverse mesocolon. The sequence of the preliminary dissection and mobilization is, therefore, important to avoid any irrevocable step being taken before it is certain that resection can be performed.

The operation of pancreatoduodenectomy may also be indicated for traumatic disruption of the head of the pancreas (*see* volume on *Accident Surgery*, 3rd edition, pp. 296–304), in some patients with chronic pancreatitis limited to the head of the gland and in rare cases of benign tumour such as cystadenoma and islet cell tumour which cannot be removed by more limited resections.

Preoperative preparation

As much information as possible should be obtained about the nature, site, extent and effects of the lesion to be resected and, in particular, evidence should be sought of metastatic spread in patients suspected to have malignant disease. An accurate preoperative diagnosis is nearly always possible using one or more of the following investigations: gastroduodenoscopy and biopsy, upper abdominal ultrasound and computerized axial tomography, percutaneous pancreatic biopsy under imaging control, endoscopic retrograde cholangiopancreatography and brush cytology. Arteriography is occasionally helpful in diagnosis and also provides information about vascular anomalies that might be encountered during the operation.

In jaundiced patients, a complete assessment of hepatic and renal function is essential and the blood is screened for anaemia and coagulation defects. Intramuscular vitamin K is given to correct an abnormal prothrombin time and blood transfusion is occasionally necessary for anaemia caused by chronic blood loss from an ulcerated duodenal or ampullary carcinoma. A significant number of patients with pancreatic malignancy and chronic pancreatitis will be diabetic and in the preoperative period stabilization with soluble insulin will be required.

Prophylactic antibiotics are started just before operation, and to reduce the risk of postoperative renal failure, a 10 per cent solution of mannitol is infused intravenously before induction of anaesthesia. Recently we have studied the effect of oral bile salts (sodium taurocholate 1 g three times a day) given for 2 days before operation and our preliminary findings indicate a beneficial effect on renal function and a reduction in the incidence of postoperative renal failure[7].

Anaesthesia

A combination of light general anaesthesia and a high epidural anaesthetic provides ideal operating conditions with profound muscular relaxation and minimal blood loss[8]. The patient is placed in the supine position on the table equipped for operative radiology.

The operation

1

Incision and preliminary inspection

The abdomen is opened through a right Mayo-Robson or continuous bilateral subcostal (Chevron) incision depending upon the width of the costal angle. In cases of malignant biliary obstruction, the surgeon is usually met by a distended gall bladder and dilated common bile duct, both of which are thin-walled and transparent. In comparison, a common duct dilated because of chronic pancreatitis is usually thick-walled and opaque. The head of the pancreas is now palpated and the body of the gland felt through the lesser omentum. This will give the surgeon some idea whether he is dealing with a tumour localized to the head of the gland or whether there are signs of extensive infiltration. Evidence of metastases is sought in the liver, lymph nodes and peritoneum, not omitting to lift the transverse mesocolon to inspect and palpate the head and uncinate process from below. On many occasions, infiltration at this point has been the only sign that the tumour is unresectable and that palliative bypass surgery should be carried out.

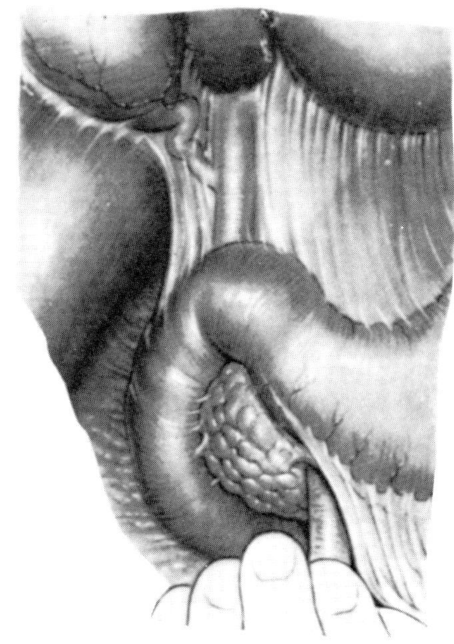

1

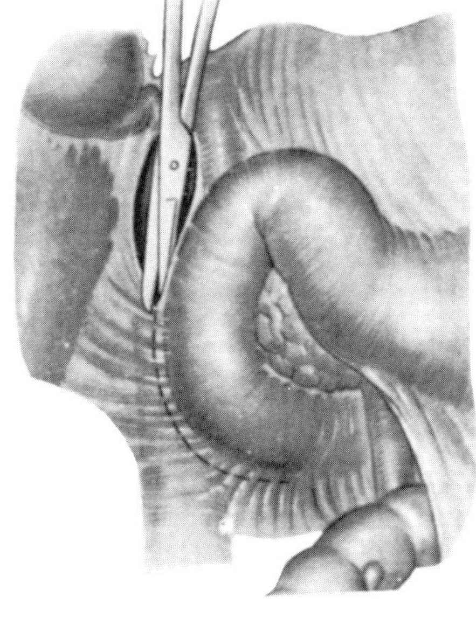

2

Exposure of head of pancreas

2

In the absence of signs of distant or local spread, the surgeon now proceeds to mobilize the hepatic flexure and right transverse colon in a medial and downward direction to expose the duodenum and head of the pancreas. The peritoneum and loose areolar tissue lateral to the second part of the duodenum are then divided to allow the duodenum and head of the pancreas to be lifted forward off the inferior vena cava.

3

The head of the pancreas and ampullary region can now be palpated between fingers and thumb to assess the nature, size and extent of the tumour.

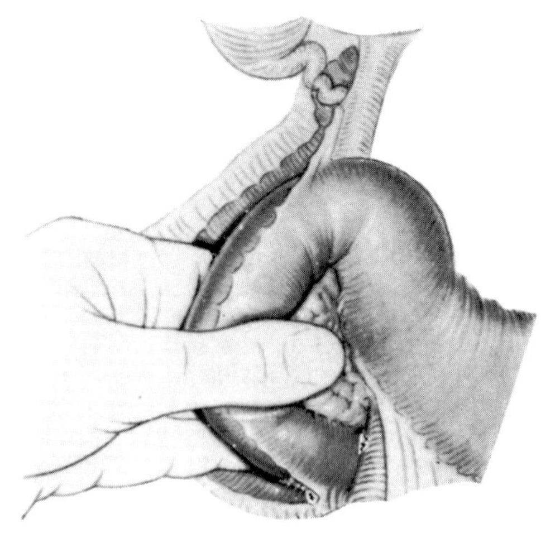
3

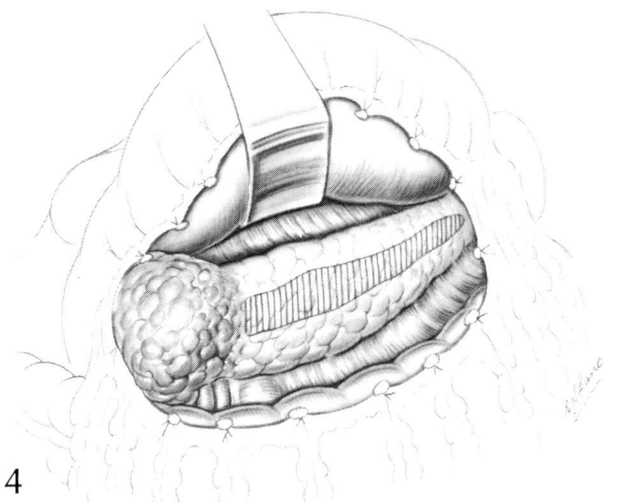
4

4

Examination of body of pancreas

The body of the pancreas is now approached through the gastrocolic omentum and any extension of the malignant process around or to the left of the portal vein noted. The body of the pancreas is usually firm because of chronic obstructive pancreatitis and a dilated pancreatic duct may be palpable through the substance of the gland.

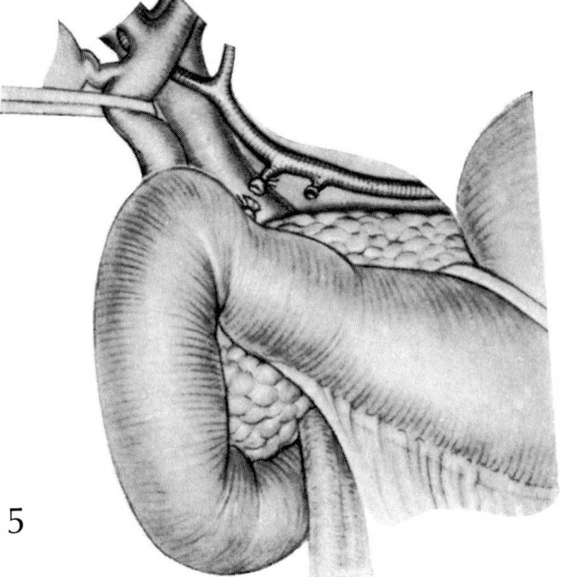
5

5

Retraction of common bile duct; exposure and ligation of right gastric and gastroduodenal arteries

A tape passed round the common bile duct is retracted to the right. The right gastric and gastroduodenal arteries are both identified and divided between ligatures. The portal vein now comes into view, lying deeply behind and medial to the common bile duct, its lower end disappearing behind the pancreas.

6

Finger dissection between pancreas and portal vein

In practice resectability depends mainly upon the freedom of the portal vein and its tributaries from malignant invasion so it is important at this stage, providing no other evidence of inoperability has been encountered, to establish the relationship of the tumour to these vessels.

From above, the index finger of the left hand gently opens up the plane between the pancreas and the anterior surface of the portal vein. The index finger of the right hand similarly opens up from below the space between the pancreas and the front of the superior mesenteric vein. If those fingers meet, lifting the pancreas forwards off the uninvolved vessels, resection can be carried out. If an area of fixity is encountered, force must not be used or disastrous haemorrhage may follow. During this manoeuvre, neither finger should be allowed to stray into the groove between the right lateral aspect of these vessels and the head of the pancreas as this is crossed by several pancreatic veins which may be sheared off.

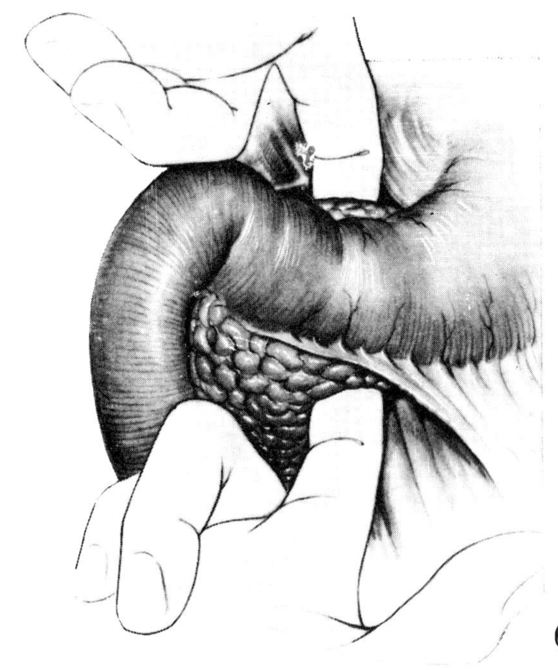

6

7

Division of stomach

Assuming that it has now been decided to proceed with radical resection, the stomach is divided between clamps at a level similar to that of a Polya gastrectomy. A more limited resection would carry the risk of late stomal ulceration after gastrojejunal continuity has been restored.

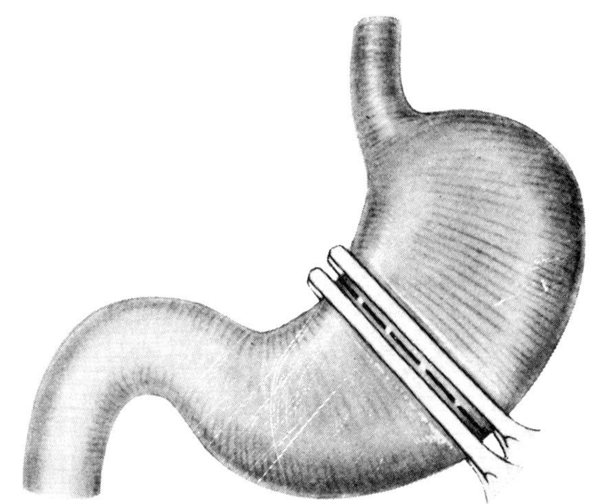

7

8

Division of common bile duct

The bile duct is first incised with a knife at the selected point of division and the escaping bile removed with the sucker. The emptied and collapsed gall bladder and bile duct occupy much less space in the upper abdomen and this makes the rest of the operation a little easier. After division of the bile duct, a bulldog clip is placed on the proximal end. Retraction of the stomach to the right completes the exposure of the head and neck of the pancreas.

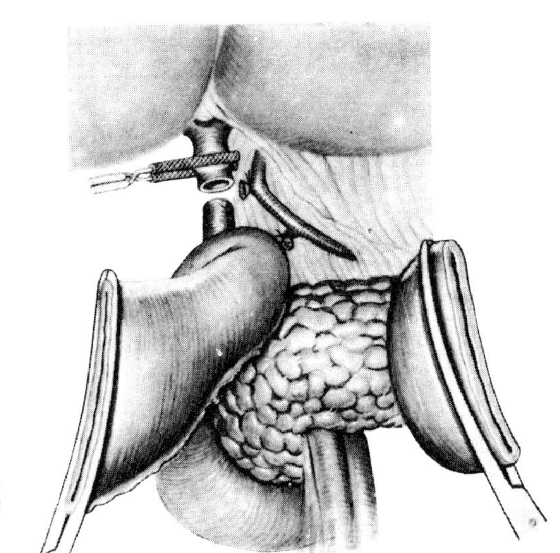

8

9 & 10

Division of pancreas

The body of the pancreas to the left of the portal vein and superior mesenteric artery is mobilized without difficulty from the retroperitoneal tissues. A Kocher dissector is positioned behind the neck of the pancreas and the gland divided between haemostatic stay sutures as shown. A dilated pancreatic duct is usually encountered and after transection retained juice is removed by suction.

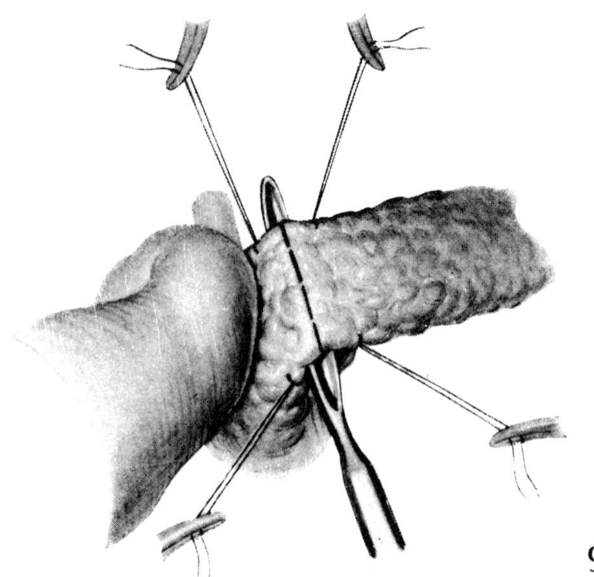

9

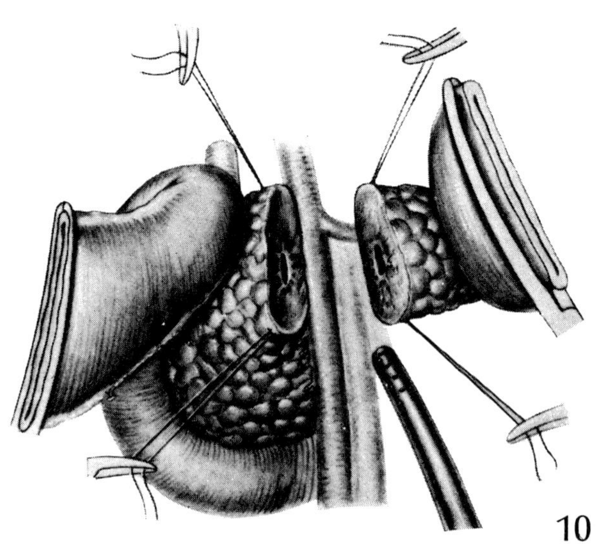

10

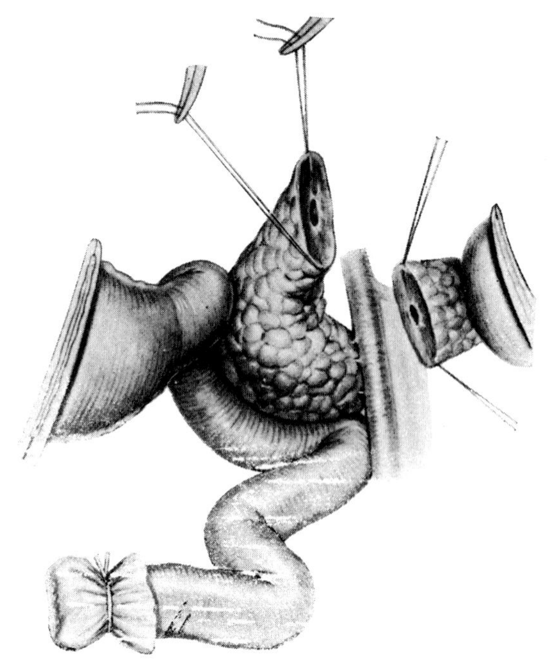

11

Division and mobilization of jejunum

The distal line of section of the alimentary tract may be through the third part of the duodenum, the distal end being closed as a blind stump, or the whole of the duodenum and upper few inches of the jejunum may be removed. This is the better procedure. The next stage of the operation is therefore directed towards the duodenojejunal flexure. The transverse colon is lifted up, the flexure identified and the upper jejunum divided. The proximal end is capped with gauze, the ligament of Treitz incised and the mobilized jejunum brought through to the right of the superior mesenteric vessels.

12

Detachment of duodenum and uncinate process of pancreas from superior mesenteric vessels; preparation for reconstruction

The mass to be removed is now attached only by the small vessels which pass between the duodenum and uncinate process and the superior mesenteric vessels. The largest of these is the inferior pancreatoduodenal artery running from the superior mesenteric artery into the groove between the head of the pancreas and the duodenum. This is carefully secured and divided after which the groove between the superior mesenteric vein and the uncinate process of the pancreas is dissected. If the whole of the uncinate process is stripped off the superior mesenteric vein it is often difficult to secure all the short stout venous channels running from the process into the vein. It is much safer to leave a thin slice of the uncinate process alongside and protecting the vein. The final detachment is, therefore, effected by picking up this thin slice of pancreas with a row of fine artery forceps, clipping and cutting as each is applied and then tying off with fine silk ligatures. The tumour may now be removed and reconstruction begun.

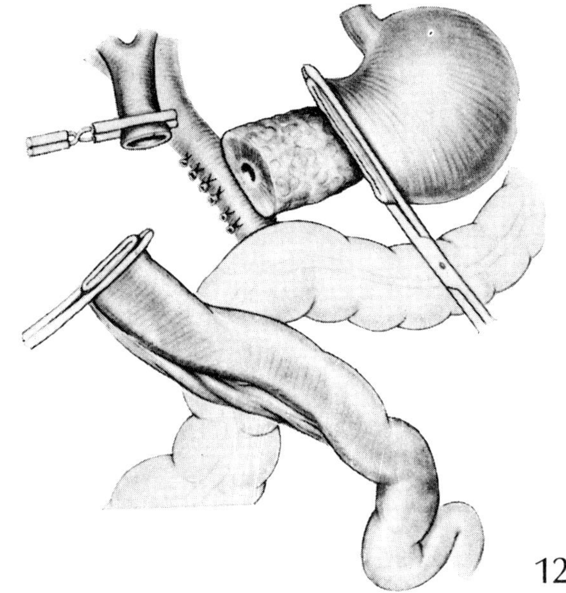

12

13

Anastomosis of bile duct to jejunum

The divided jejunum is now brought up in front of the colon and anastomosed directly to the residual bile duct. An end-to-side anastomosis is quite commonly employed, the open end of the jejunum being closed first; but the bile duct may, if the surgeon wishes, be anastomosed end-to-end to part of the open end of jejunum, the rest of it being closed as shown. Some surgeons employ temporary T-tube drainage of the bile duct with the lower limb of the T-tube extending through the anastomosis into the jejunum. This is a useful step and allows a final cholangiogram to be performed before removal of the tube on the tenth postoperative day.

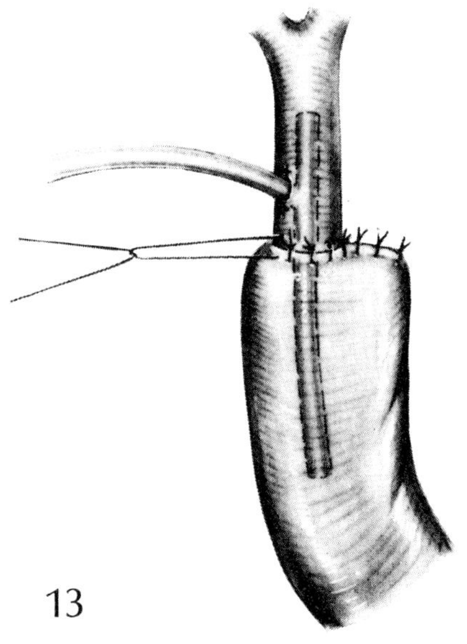

13

14

Anastomosis of pancreas to jejunum

Below the biliary-intestinal anastomosis an oval strip of seromuscular layer is removed to expose the jejunal mucosa. The divided pancreatic substance is now sutured to the seromuscular layer of the jejunum using continous silk, as shown. When the posterior part of this suture line has been completed, a stab incision through the jejunal mucosa opposite the pancreatic duct allows a length of fine Silastic tubing to be threaded up the pancreatic duct in one direction and through into the jejunum in the other. The tubing is then brought out through the jejunal wall at a lower level to pass through the abdominal wall to a collecting apparatus. Occasionally, if the lining of the dilated pancreatic duct is well developed it may be possible to insert three or four fine catgut sutures to approximate the duct to the jejunal mucosa around the tube. The anterior layer of the pancreatointestinal anastomosis is now completed with the continuous silk suture.

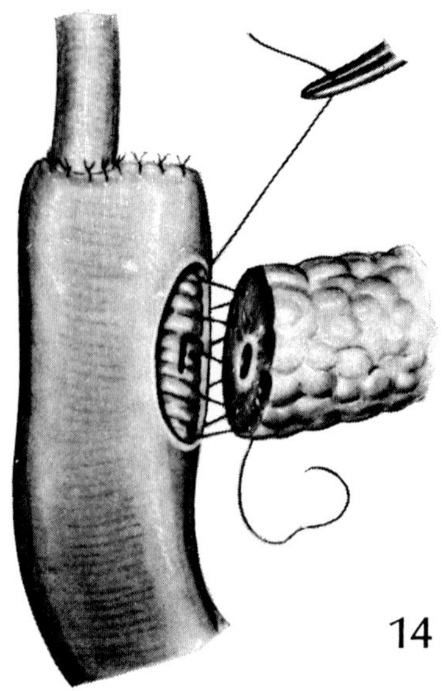

14

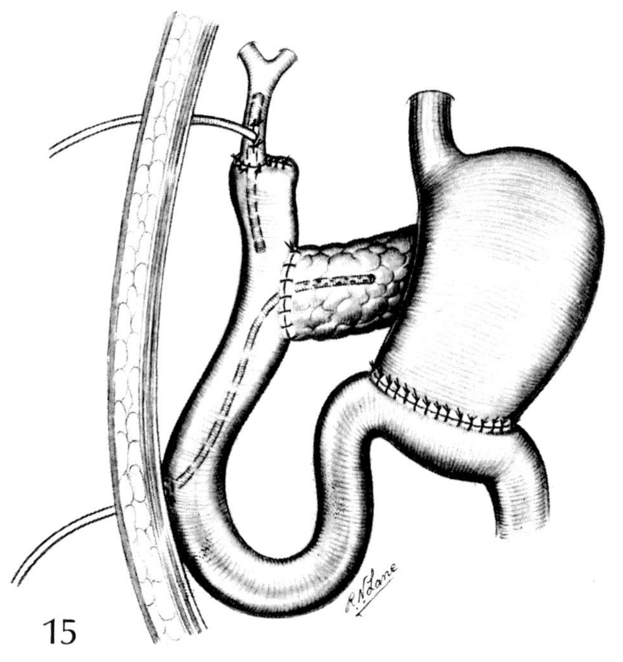

15

15

Gastrojejunostomy; closure of abdomen

Finally, the divided stomach is anastomosed to the side of the jejunum in two layers. Vacuum drains are positioned close to the biliary and pancreatic anastomoses and the abdomen closed in layers.

Alternative methods of dealing with the pancreatic remnant

Ligation of pancreatic duct

Ligation of the main pancreatic duct and oversewing the cut end of the pancreas is a reasonable alternative to a formal anastomosis in those patients with a soft pancreas and small calibre pancreatic duct. Such a gland does not take sutures well and even if an anastomosis is achieved the postoperative fistula rate is high. Ligation of the duct, therefore, avoids a potentially dangerous anastomosis but even so there is no guarantee that a pure pancreatic fistula will not develop. Indeed, in some published series the incidence of fistula is about 50 per cent but these are usually temporary, and the pure pancreatic juice that does leak is said to be less corrosive than that from a disrupted pancreatojejunal anastomosis from which biliary and intestinal secretions also escape.

Invagination of cut end of pancreas into jejunal lumen

Technically it may seem easier to achieve pancreatic-intestinal continuity by invaginating the cut end of the pancreas into the open end of the jejunum, suturing the pancreatic capsule to the jejunal wall. The method, however, has little to recommend it. In particular, the postoperative fistula rate is high even when an indwelling catheter is left inside the duct and there is also considerable doubt whether the pancreatic duct remains open for any length of time in the absence of mucosal continuity with the jejunal lining.

Total pancreatectomy (see pp. 773–782)

The total removal of the pancreas does, of course, avoid the necessity for an anastomosis and should be considered as an alternative to pancreatic duct ligation in patients with a small pancreatic duct and a soft friable gland not suitable for suturing. Total pancreatectomy has also been advocated for the treatment of carcinoma of the head of the pancreas in an attempt to improve long-term survival.

Postoperative care and complications

The management of the postoperative phase of pancreatoduodenectomy is greatly facilitated if the patient is nursed in an intensive care unit where vital signs, fluid balance, blood sugar and changes in serum biochemistry can be monitored at regular intervals.

Vacuum drains should normally be removed after 5 days unless excessive drainage of bile or pancreatic juice persists. On the tenth postoperative day, the biliary T-tube and pancreatic tube are removed if the cholangiogram and pancreatogram demonstrate free flow of bile and pancreatic juice into the jejunal lumen without leakage.

After pancreatoduodenectomy, abut 25 per cent of patients develop significant complications, the most serious of which are related to disruption of the pancreatojejunal anastomosis. The overall incidence of pancreatic fistula is about 15 per cent but most of these are of a temporary nature and close spontaneously in time. While the fistula is open, skin excoriation can be avoided by applying low pressure suction to a catheter inserted into the fistulous track. The pancreatic juice collected in this way can be measured and replaced either directly into a nasogastric tube or intravenously by an equal amount of normal saline if the loss is considerable.

Postoperative haemorrhage may occur from the gastrointestinal tract as a result of stomal ulceration or erosions in the stomach remnant or from the operative site as a result of the corrosive effect of leaking pancreatic juice on local blood vessels. If blood loss is more than minimal, reoperation will be necessary to achieve haemostasis.

Postoperative renal failure in jaundiced patients, diabetes and intra-abdominal sepsis are treated with appropriate measures.

Results

An analysis of 262 patients undergoing pancreatoduodenectomy in the St George's Hospital Unit, has shown that the operative mortality and long-term survival depend to a large extent on the site of the original lesion. For carcinoma of the duodenum and ampulla of Vater the operative mortality was 2.7 per cent but this figure rises to 8.5 per cent for distal common bile duct tumours. For carcinoma of the head of the pancreas the mortality from the operation rises considerably to 20.4 per cent. The overall mortality in the 262 patients was 6.5 per cent[9].

The 5 year survival for cancers of the duodenum and ampulla was 35 per cent; the prognosis for carcinoma of the distal common bile duct was less favourable, with a 19 per cent 5 years survival; while for cancer of the head of the pancreas, only 6 per cent survived for 5 years.

References

1. Halsted, W. S. Contributions to the surgery of the bile passages especially of the common bile duct. Boston Medical and Surgical Journal 1899; 141: 645–654
2. Kausch, W. Das Carcinom der Papilla duodeni und seine radikale entfernung. Beiträge zur Klinischen Chirurgic 1912; 78: 439–486
3. Whipple, A. O., Parsons, W. B., Mullins, C. R. Treatment of carcinoma of the ampulla of Vater. Annals of Surgery 1935; 102: 763–779
4. Brunschwig, A. Resection of head of pancreas and duodenum for carcinoma: pancreatoduodenectomy. Surgery, Gynecology and Obstetrics 1937; 65: 681–684
5. Dam, H. Glavind, J. Vitamin K in human pathology. Lancet 1938 1: 720–721
6. Whipple, A. O. The rationale of radical surgery for cancer of the pancreas and ampullary region. Annals of Surgery 1941; 114: 612–615
7. Evans, H., Torrealba, V., Hudd, C., Knight, M. Effect of preoperative bile salt administration on renal function in jaundiced patients. (In press)
8. Howat, D. D. C. Anaesthesia for biliary and pancreatic surgery. Proceedings of the Royal Society of Medicine 1977; 70: 152–161
9. Smith, R. Cancer of the pancreas. Journal of the Royal College of Surgeons of Edinburgh 1978; 23: 133–150

Hepatic resection

L. H. Blumgart MD, FRCS(Ed.), FRCS(Glas.), FRCS
Professor of Surgery and Director, Department of Surgery,
Royal Postgraduate Medical School and Hammersmith Hospital, London

Introduction

Partial hepatectomy may be necessary for removal of primary or secondary neoplasms of the liver, to allow adequate excision of bile duct tumours at the confluence of the hepatic ducts, for the management of a variety of benign conditions and in selected patients with severe liver injury.

The ability of the surgeon to remove large volumes of liver tissue safely and with expectation of survival depends on a knowledge of the anatomy of the liver and on an appreciation of the extraordinary regenerative capacity of the liver following major resection.

Rapid liver regeneration after resection has long been appreciated and extensively studied. Following resection as extensive as right hepatic lobectomy (at which half the liver mass is removed) liver size is regained within 3–4 weeks[1]. This increase in size is accompanied by histological evidence of regenerative hyperplasia as early as 3 days after resection[2]. During the period of liver regeneration liver function is depressed and the patient may require supportive measures.

Surgical anatomy

A precise knowledge of the surgical anatomy of the liver, its blood vessels and biliary channels is essential for the performance of partial hepatectomy.

1

The division between the right and left lobes of the liver is not at the falciform ligament but follows a line projected through a plane (the principal plane) from the medial margin of the gall bladder bed to the vena cava posteriorly[3]. While excision of portions of the liver had been known to be feasible for many years, Lortat-Jacob and Robert[4] were the first to carry out right hepatic lobectomy based on a knowledge of the principal plane and ligation of the vessels and ducts to the right lobe.

Each of these major right and left lobes is divided into segments. An oblique plane running anteroposteriorly divides the right lobe into anterior and posterior segments, while the left lobe is divided along the line of insertion of the ligamentum teres into left lateral and left medial segments. The portal venous, hepatic arterial and hepatic duct branches conform to the segmental organization and run within the segments, radiating to the periphery from the hilus. Between the segments the draining hepatic veins converge posteriorly towards the vena cava[5,6,7].

The portal vein and hepatic artery divide into major right and left branches outside the liver substance below the hilus. When the overlying peritoneum is incised, it is possible to dissect each major branch beyond the bifurcation. The confluence of the right and left hepatic ducts also occurs outside the liver, although somewhat closer to the liver substance. The right branch of the portal vein is short and its first branch often arises posteroinferiorly close to the bifurcation, where it is easily damaged during dissection. By contrast, the left branch of the portal vein and the left hepatic duct pursue a longer extrahepatic course and are more easily dissected. The ligamentum teres runs sharply into the umbilical fissure of the liver, in the base of which the main vascular and biliary channels branch to the medial and lateral segments of the left lobe. After entering the liver substance the left branch of the portal vein curves caudally just to the left of the falciform ligament; it supplies not only the lateral segment of the left lobe but, together with branches of the left hepatic artery, gives off 'feedback vessels' to the medial segment of the left lobe (quadrate lobe). This feedback blood supply and ductal drainage of the medial segment was described by Goldsmith and Woodburne[7] and is important in dissection for extended right hepatic lobectomy (*see below*).

The liver lies astride the inferior vena cava, immediately below the diaphragm, and the hepatic veins run a short course outside the liver to empty into the vena cava. The right hepatic vein usually enters the vena cava separately but the left hepatic vein is frequently joined by the middle hepatic vein before entering the vena cava. Several smaller veins drain from the posterior surface of the liver and the caudate lobe directly into the vena cava.

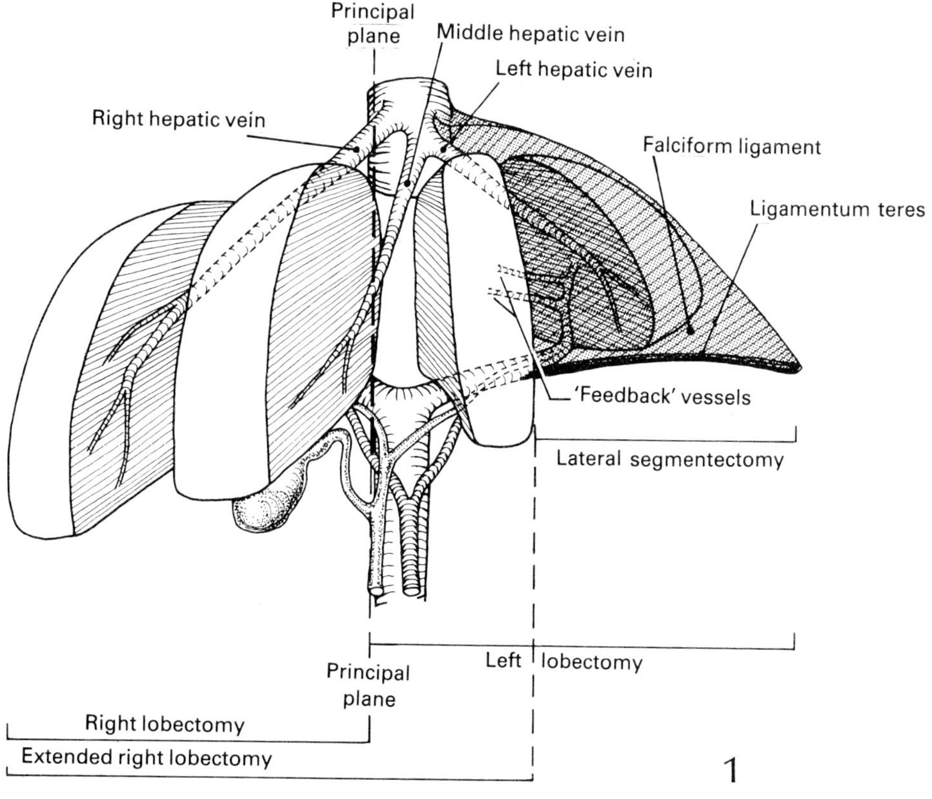

2a & b

Many variations in biliary drainage and in vascular supply to the liver have been described. Hepatic arteriography is useful in displaying these. Thus, in approximately 20 per cent of patients the arterial blood supply to the right lobe arises either in part or totally from the superior mesenteric artery, the vessel then coursing up behind the pancreas and usually lying posterolateral to the common bile duct and common hepatic duct.

The left hepatic artery may arise from the left gastric artery or there may be an accessory left hepatic artery. It should be noted that the left hepatic arterial supply always enters the liver at the base of the umbilical fissure.

The illustration shows selective hepatic arteriography in a case of liver tumour occupying the hilar area of the liver. The right hepatic artery arises from the superior mesenteric trunk and is not involved in the blood supply to the tumour. The left hepatic artery arises independently in association with the left gastric and supplies the central tumour mass.

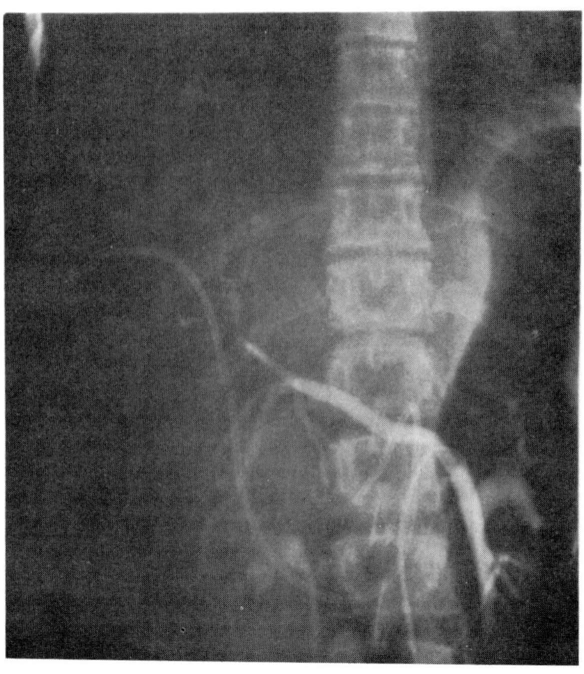

2a

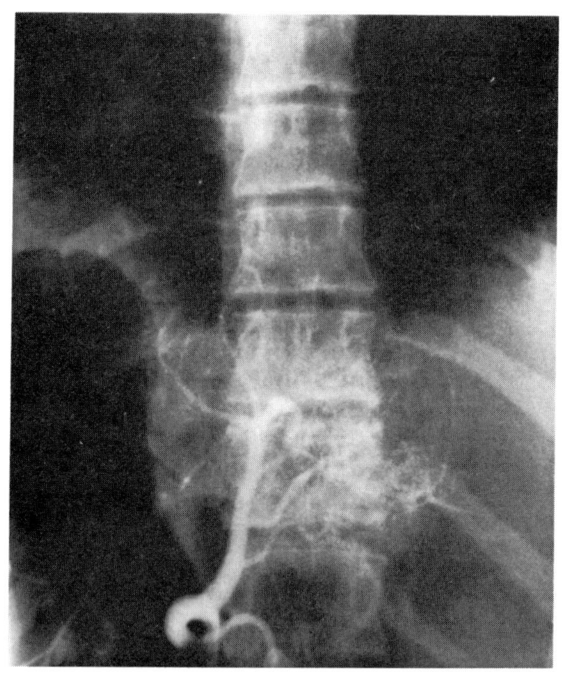

2b

Types of partial hepatectomy

For practical purposes there are four types of partial hepatectomy (*see Illustration 1*).

1. Right or left hepatic lobectomy – the right or left lobes are removed by separating the liver in the principal plane.
2. Left lateral segmentectomy – that portion of the liver to the left of the falciform ligament is removed.
3. Extended right hepatic lobectomy (trisegmentectomy) – the entire right lobe is removed together with the medial segment of the left lobe. The left lateral segment alone remains as a remnant.
4. Quadrate lobectomy – the medial segment of the left lobe (that is, the tissue lying between the principal plane and the falciform ligament) is removed.

The operation of right hepatic lobectomy will be described in detail since this is also the basis for the more radical procedure of extended right hepatic lobectomy and, once understood, the other procedures are readily described, the principles being similar.

Preoperative

Investigations

Preoperative investigation should seek to determine the nature of the lesion and its extent so as to provide information of value to the surgeon. Tests of liver function and coagulation screening should be performed. Australia antigenaemia should be sought and, if primary hepatoma is suspected, alpha fetoprotein measured.

The *major risks* of hepatic resection are as follows.

1. Haemorrhage which may arise at the porta hepatis from branches of the hepatic artery or portal vein or posteriorly from hepatic venous radicles of the inferior vena cava.
2. Biliary stricture or fistula as a result of damage to the biliary apparatus. This is most likely to occur at or about the confluence of the hepatic ducts.

Careful dissection and a knowledge of anatomical variants are essential but should be supplemented by radiological investigation when possible. There is usually no time for this in hepatic resection carried out for trauma but information should be obtained prior to elective operation and especially for tumours close to or involving the hilus of the liver or encroaching on the vena cava posteriorly.

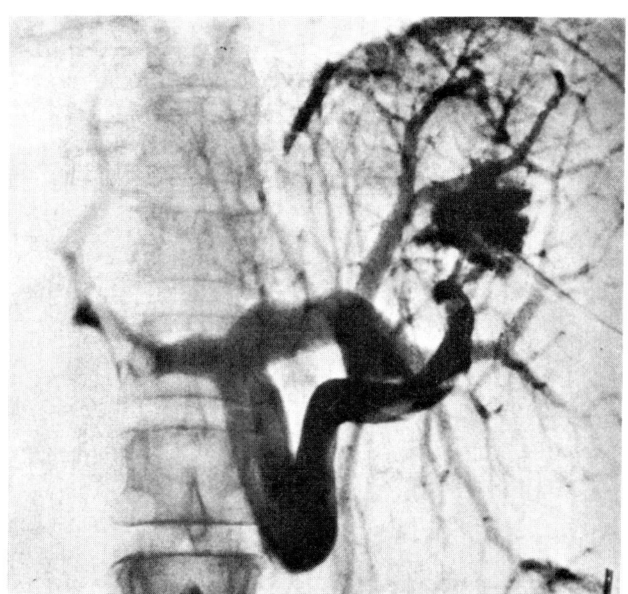

3

Hepatic angiography

3

Hepatic angiography, obtained preferably after selective catheterization, is important. At the time of arteriography late-phase portographic pictures are obtained after injection into the splenic artery or, alternatively, percutaneous splenoportography is carried out.

The illustration shows splenoportography in a patient with a large tumour occupying most of the right lobe of the liver. There was concern that the portal vein might be involved. Note that the splenic vein and main trunk of the portal vein are well displayed and are clear of tumour, as is the left branch of the portal vein. The right branch of the portal vein is involved just beyond its origin and there is almost no portal flow to the right lobe at all. Extended right hepatic lobectomy was possible.

4a & b

For large tumours or lesions close to the midline, inferior vena cavography in anteroposterior and lateral projections will reveal compression or invasion of the inferior vena cava. (*a*) Shows invasion of the inferior vena cava by a large primary hepatocellular carcinoma occupying the right lobe of the liver and extending into the caudate lobe. There are irregular filling defects in the inferior vena cava and a collateral circulation has developed. This case is irresectable. (*b*) Shows extensive displacement of the vena cava to the left by a large tumour occupying the right lobe of the liver, but not directly invading the vena cava. Extended right hepatic lobectomy was carried out in this patient.

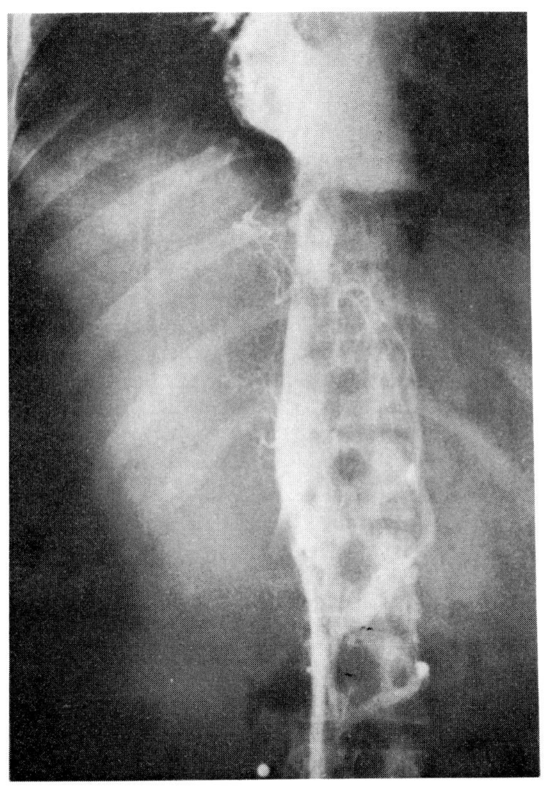

4a

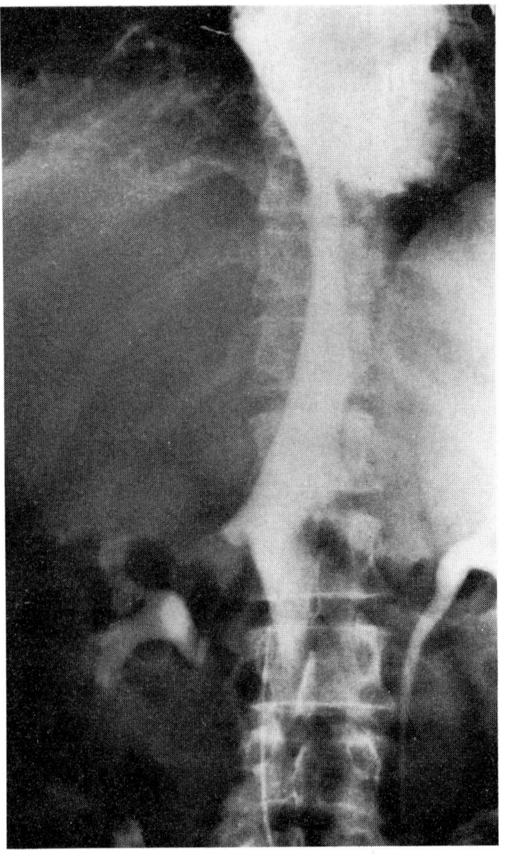

4b

Ultrasonography and CAT

Ultrasonography and computerized axial tomography (CAT) may give valuable preliminary information and may indeed, by demonstrating freedom from involvement, obviate the necessity for some studies (e.g. inferior vena cavography). In patients with hepatic tumours extrahepatic metastases must be sought by means of chest X-ray and bone scanning.

Cholangiography

If biliary tract obstruction is present then preliminary cholangiography, usually obtained by the fine needle percutaneous transhepatic method or by endoscopic retrograde cholangiography, is important. Such studies taken in conjunction with angiographic evidence may indicate irresectability[8]. If jaundice is present, the risks of surgery are increased and a period of preliminary drainage by means of percutaneous transhepatic insertion of a drainage catheter may be indicated[9].

Anaesthesia

Anaesthetic techniques should take into account the possibility of major intraoperative haemorrhage. Suitable monitoring and facilities for rapid transfusion should be set up. The possibility of a thoracoabdominal incision should be allowed for. When surgery is performed transabdominally air embolism is possible, particularly if there is major injury to hepatic venous radicles or the inferior vena cava, and positive pressure respiration should be maintained. During mobilization and manipulation of large tumours, inferior vena caval compression may occur, with a consequent marked fall in venous return, and the anaesthetist should be prepared for this.

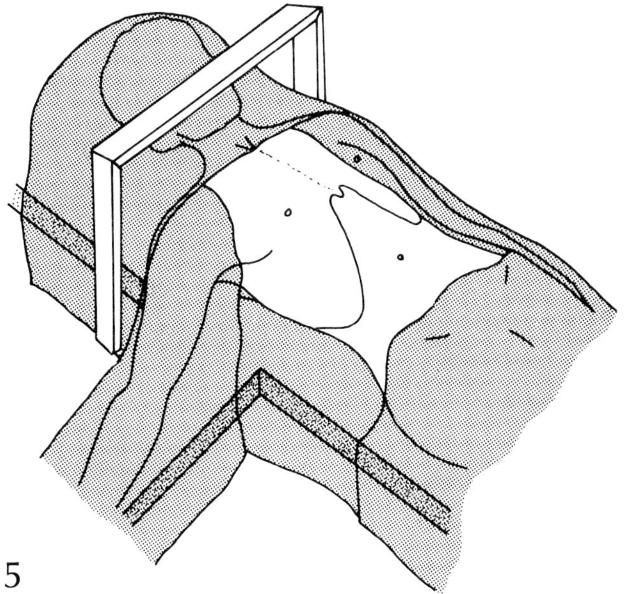

5

5

Position of patient

The patient should be positioned supine with the right arm extended at right angles to the body. It is not necessary to place the patient in a lateral position. Tilting the table allows adequate exposure. ECG leads should be kept clear of the right chest wall and the presternal area. Draping should expose the right chest across the left mid-clavicular line and should extend vertically from the suprasternal notch to the subumbilical area. The abdomen should be widely exposed (from midaxillary line to midaxillary line) so as to allow adequate space for transverse incisions. The cross bar later holds a large retractor used to elevate the costal margin (*see Illustration 8*).

The operation

The incisions

The initial incision depends upon circumstances. There should never be any hesitation to extend or enlarge the wound in order to gain adequate access.

6a

Exploration of the abdomen for *injury* is usually through a right upper paramedian rectus-splitting incision (A to A) or a midline incision (C to B). However if it is already known that a major liver injury requiring possible resection may be present, such as sometimes occurs where there has been a direct blow to the right chest wall or where the patient has been referred following prior laparotomy elsewhere, a subcostal approach is preferable. Initial assessment of the injury is carried out through the laparotomy incision, which should be extended into the thorax either through the 7th interspace with incision of the diaphragm towards the vena cava (C to C) or by means of a median sternotomy (C to D)[10]. In children and young adults a sternal-splitting incision without extension as far as the sternal notch may be adequate.

The sternal-splitting approach is rapid and spares disruption of either pleural cavity. The diaphragm may be split through the central tendon. This gives excellent access to the major hepatic veins. If the pericardium is opened the infracardiac intrapericardial inferior vena cava can be readily controlled.

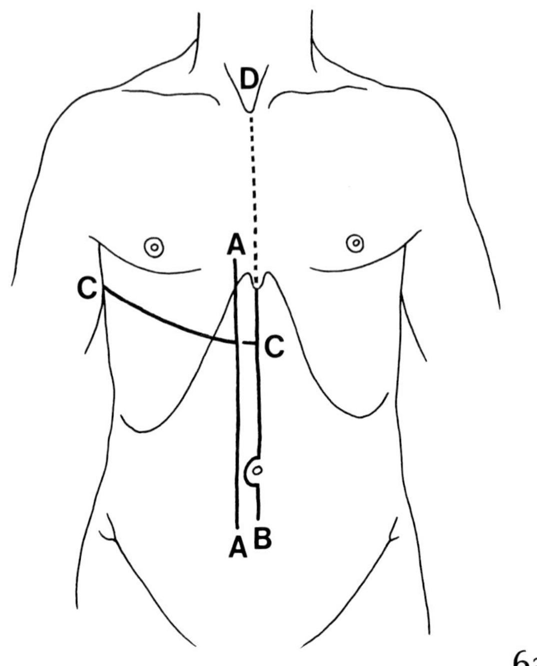

6a

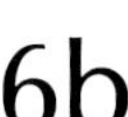

6b

For most other hepatic resections the initial incision should be a bilateral subcostal 'rooftop' incision (E to E). Large tumours of the right lobe of the liver, especially those lying far posteriorly and possibly involving the inferior vena cava, may require extension as a right thoracoabdominal approach (C to C).

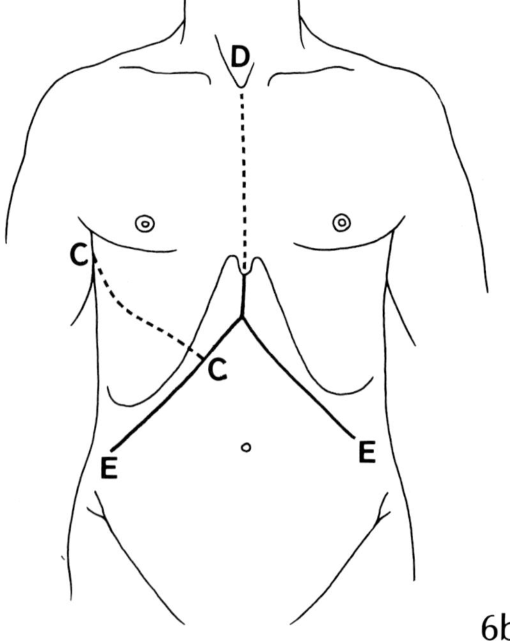

6b

7

Once the abdomen is opened and as a preliminary to exploration, the ligamentum teres is divided and the falciform ligament incised and separated from the anterior abdominal wall. The ligament is divided as far back as the subdiaphragmatic inferior vena cava. Quite large vessels running within the falciform ligament require diathermy or ligation. A stout ligature should be left on the ligamentum teres. This acts as a useful elevator during dissection.

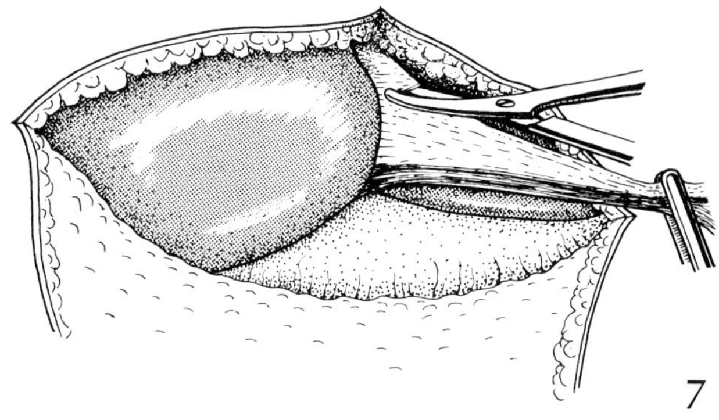

7

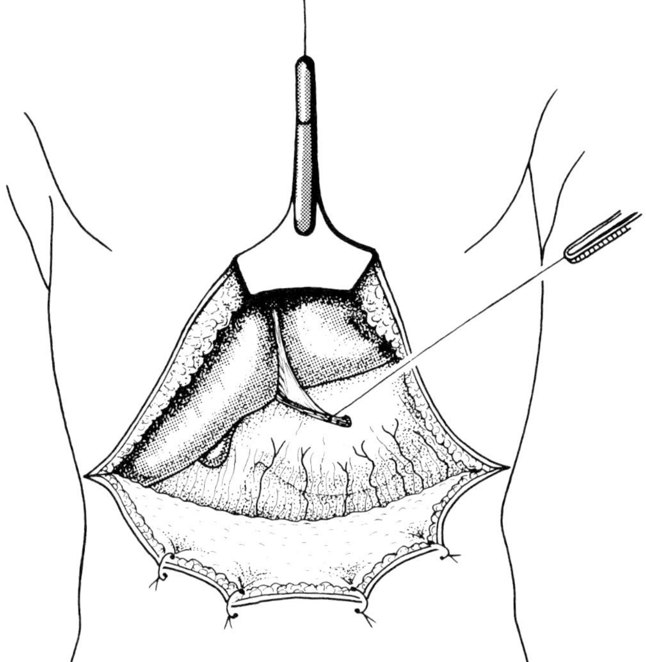

8

8

The lower flap of the transverse rooftop incision is sutured back to the patient's skin and a fixed blade retractor (gallows retractor) is used to elevate the costal margin at the sternal notch.

ABDOMINAL EXPLORATION

In *hepatic injury*, particular attention should be paid to the right posterolateral portion of the liver adjacent to the attachment of the right triangular ligament. It is easy to underestimate damage in this area. Extensive lacerations may be present and yet be missed unless palpation is thorough. The discovery of lacerations on the undersurface of the right lobe of the liver adjacent to the gall bladder should not lull the surgeon into a false sense of security. Such lacerations are often associated with major intrahepatic and posterior damage which may necessitate resection.

9

Exploration of the abdomen for *masses in the liver* should follow adequate division of the falciform ligament and ligamentum teres and, if necessary, division of the triangular ligaments posteriorly. Elevation of the ligamentum teres helps expose the undersurface of the liver and the area of the hilus and umbilical fissure. Both hands should be inserted into the abdomen so as to allow careful bimanual palpation. Unless this is carried out quite large lesions may be missed or underestimated.

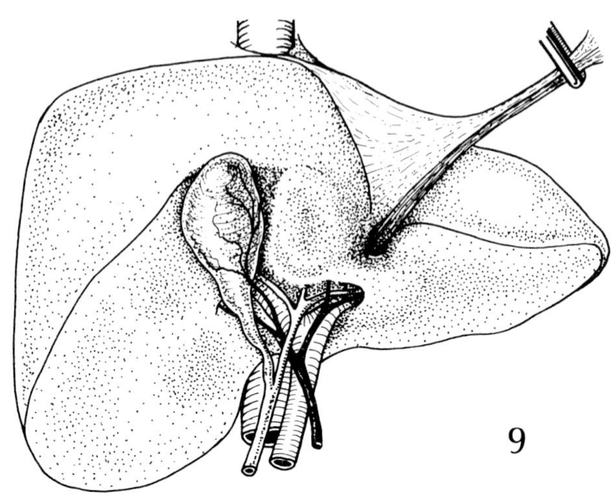

9

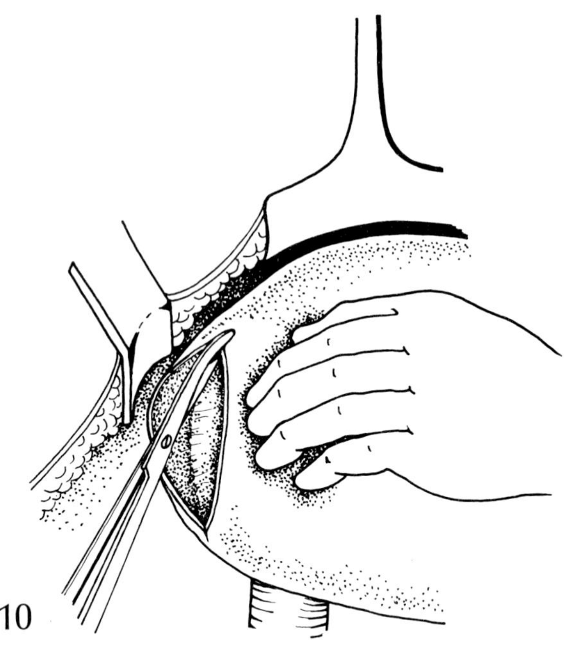

10

10

Complete palpation of the right lobe and particularly assessment of the right side of the vena cava require mobilization of the right lobe of the liver from the diaphragm. The peritoneal reflection at the edge of the right triangular ligament is incised and the incision is developed medially between diaphragm and liver until the entire bare area of the liver on the right side is exposed. This allows the liver to be turned to the left. It sometimes helps in this dissection if the table is rotated a little to the left and the surgeon sits on the right side. Complete exposure of the inferior vena cava and of the right hepatic vein often requires division of a tongue of fibrous tissue, which sometimes obscures the right side of the upper part of the retrohepatic vena cava (*see Illustrations 22, 23*).

Opening of the lesser omentum with passage of a finger posterior to the left lobe of the liver allows palpation of the caudate lobe and of the inferior vena caval area on the left.

In assessing tumours involving the quadrate lobe the tissue that frequently occupies the lower limit of the umbilical fissure, bridging the gap between the quadrate lobe and the left lateral segment, may be easily fractured by squeezing it between forefinger and thumb (*see Illustration 29*). This manoeuvre opens the umbilical fissure and allows adequate exploration for patients with hilar cholangiocarcinoma and is also an essential preliminary manoeuvre in the operation of extended right hepatic lobectomy and left lateral segmentectomy.

RIGHT HEPATIC LOBECTOMY

The liver is elevated to display its inferior surface and the portal structures (see *Illustration 9*).

11

The cystic duct and the cystic artery are exposed, ligated and divided. Division of the peritoneal reflection along the free edge of the lesser omentum exposes the lateral side of the portal vein and the common bile duct.

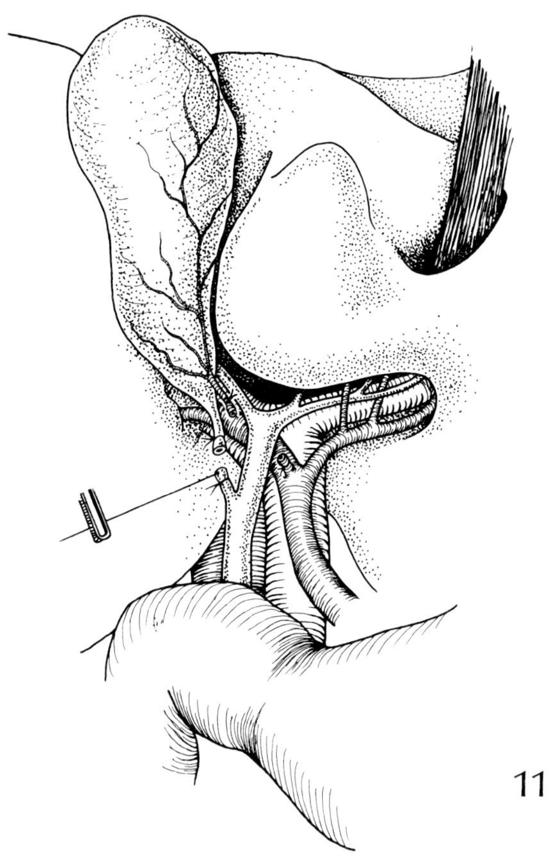

11

12

The right hepatic duct is dissected. It might prove to be small and in cases of injury and particularly if there is coincident haematoma in the region, choledochotomy with insertion of a fine bougie into the right and left ducts may assist in identification.

The confluence of the bile ducts and the origin of the left hepatic duct should be clearly demonstrated.

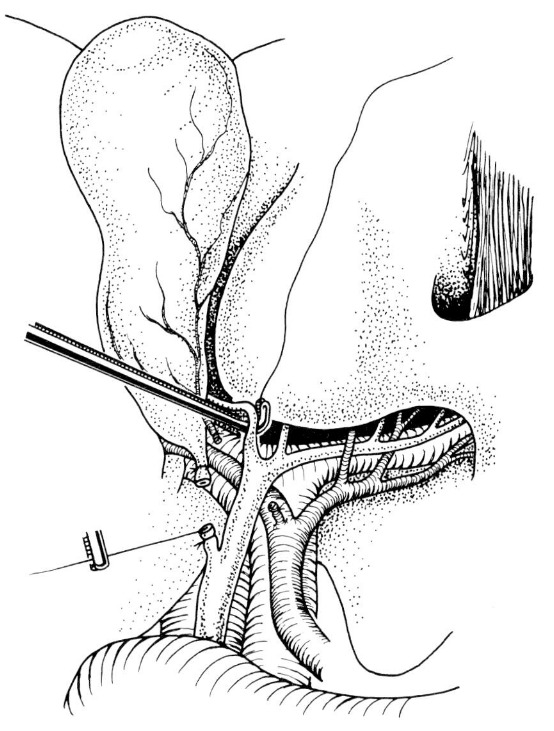

12

13

Traction on catgut ligatures attached to the cystic duct and right hepatic duct stump allow retraction of the common hepatic duct and common bile duct to the left, and assists display of vessels beneath. However, if difficulty is encountered in passing a ligature about the duct, then it may be divided under direct vision and subsequently oversewn with a fine 4/0 catgut suture on an atraumatic needle (*see inset*).

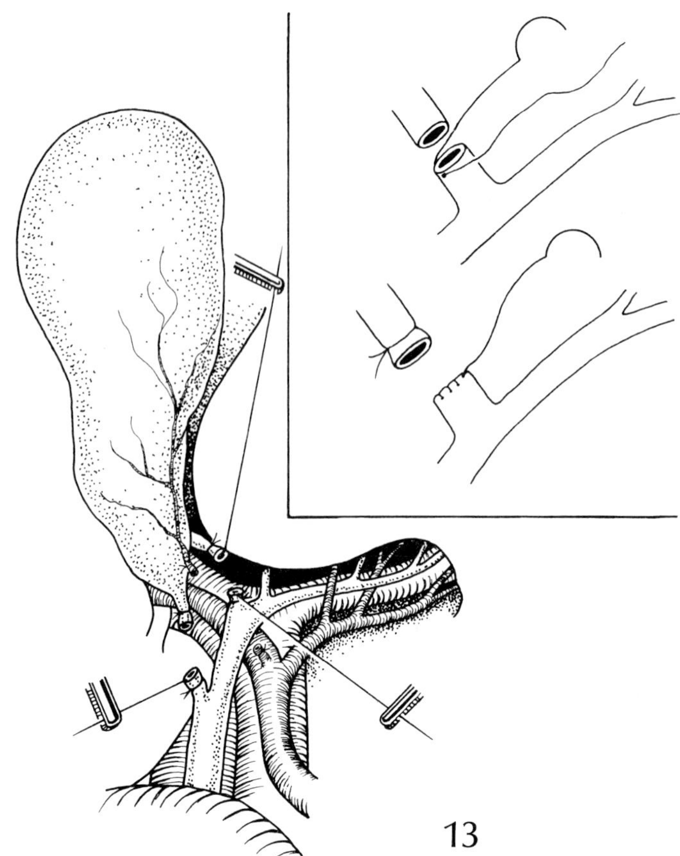

13

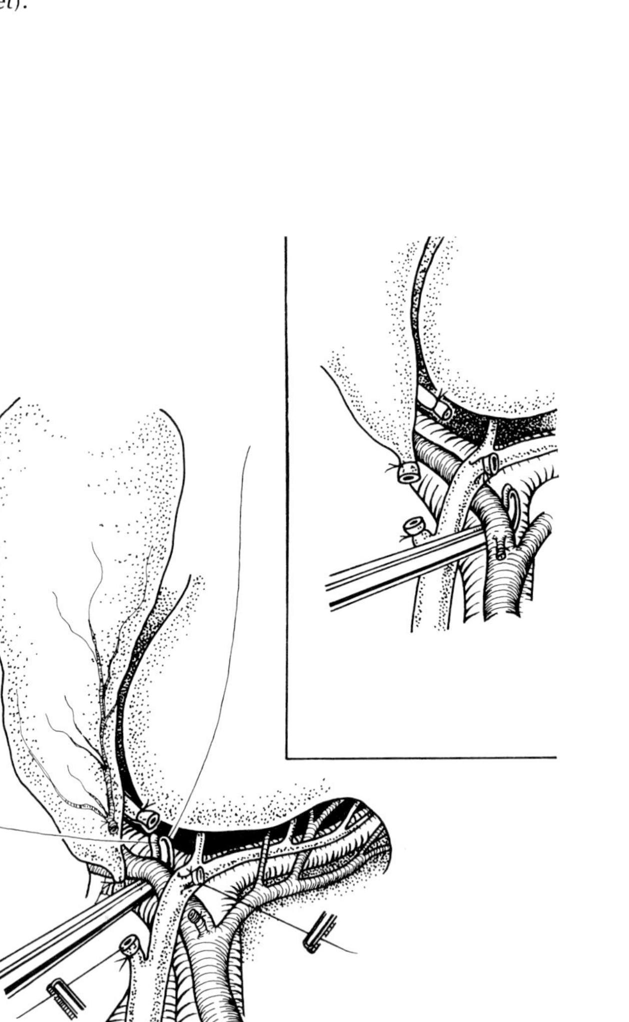

14

14

The right hepatic artery is dissected, ligated and then divided. Prior knowledge of the arterial blood supply is valuable. The right hepatic artery originates from the main hepatic arterial trunk and usually passes posterior to the common bile duct. It may be ligated either to the right or medial to the duct (*see inset*). It is important to be certain by palpation at the umbilical fissure that there is no compromise to the blood supply passing to the left lobe of the liver.

15

The portal vein is exposed. If difficulty is encountered the vein is best approached posterolaterally by retracting the right lobe of the liver anteriorly and to the left, and by gently elevating the common bile duct. Sutures left attached to the cystic duct and right hepatic duct may be useful in this connection. The right branch of the portal vein is carefully dissected and forceps gently passed around it. Special care should be taken not to damage the first branch of the right portal vein which comes off sometimes very early and posteroinferiorly. This branch should be deliberately sought under direct vision and the forceps passed behind the portal vein, taking care to avoid this vulnerable branch.

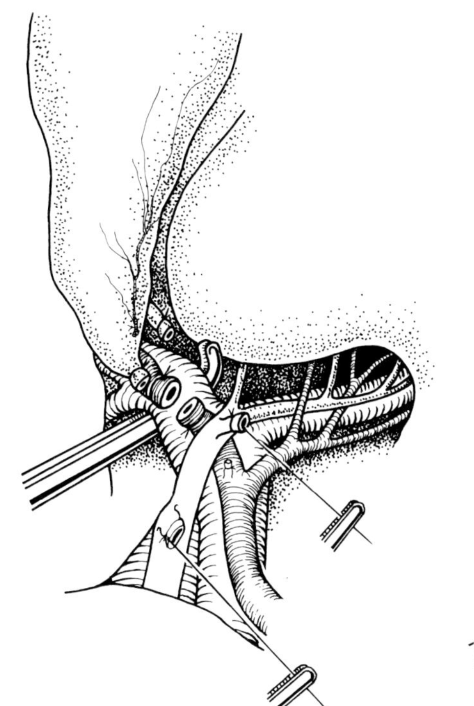

15

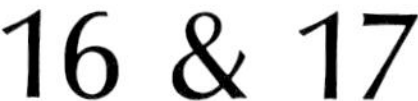

16 & 17

Application of straight-bladed vascular clamps is the safest method of dealing with the right portal vein. It is good practice to pass two retaining sutures to secure the vein before dividing it. These sutures, if left with the needles in place, can be used to oversew the stump once the vein has been divided between the clamps.

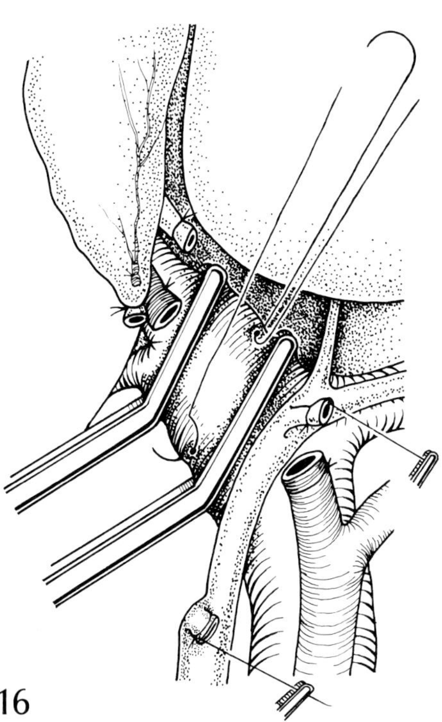

16

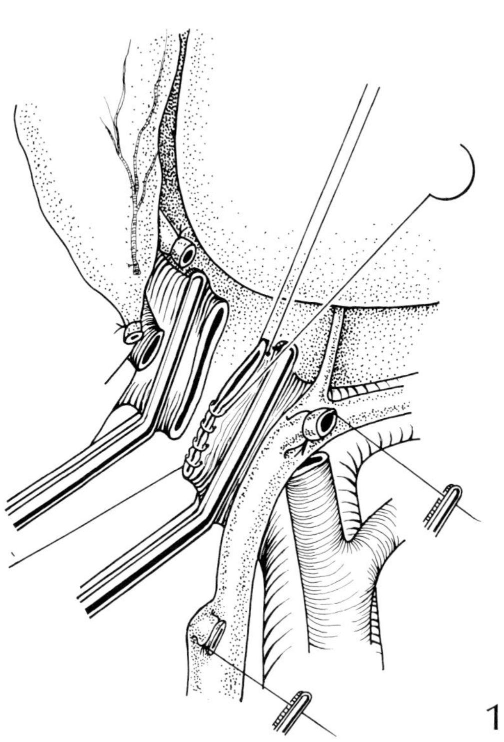

17

18

Division of the right hepatic artery and the right branch of the portal vein is followed by the development of a clear line of demarcation on the liver surface running antero-posteriorly from the gall bladder fossa to the vena cava in the principal vascular plane.

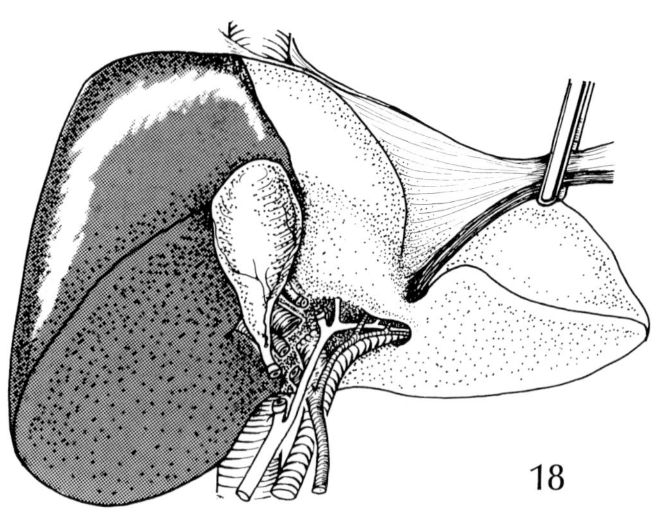

18

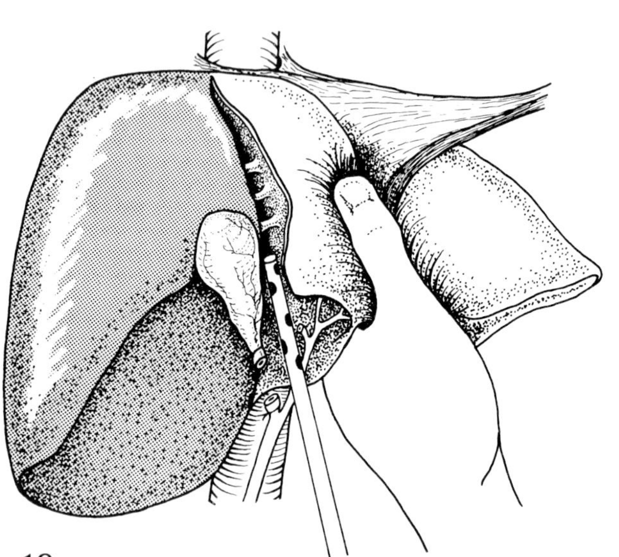

19

Division of liver tissue and hepatic veins

19

Glisson's capsule is opened with scissors along the line of demarcation. The liver tissue is fractured between the finger and thumb. The first assistant compresses the liver tissue with his left hand. Strong suction is applied in the line of division and the blunt end of the suction used to tease the tissues away from the vessels.

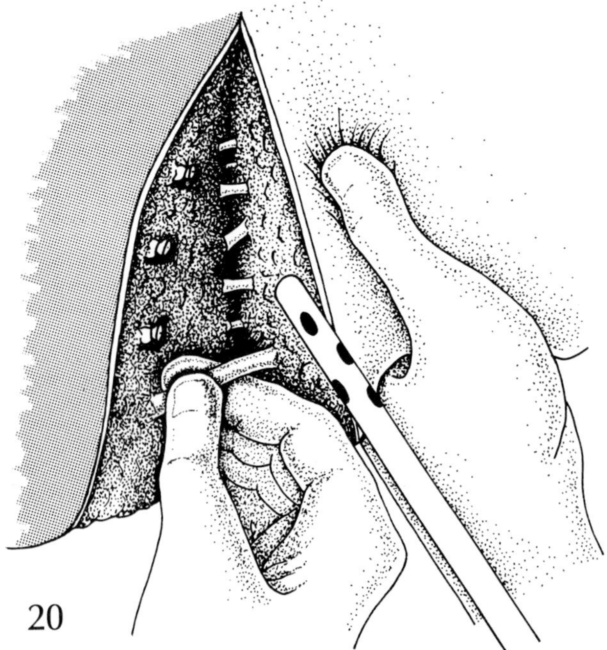

20

20

Once located, vessels and bile ducts are secured and ligated or occluded with metal clips. Large vessels may be either under-run using a 0 catgut suture or ligated, the catgut having been passed around the vessel using an aneurysm needle.

21

As the tissue is divided, the fissure in the liver tissue is opened. The fingers of the operator's left hand are located posteriorly, elevating the right lobe and opening the wound in the liver. At this stage major hepatic veins are identified and secured within the liver substance. This is usually preferable to extrahepatic isolation of the right hepatic vein, which is large and runs a short extrahepatic course. Dissection and division of the vein outside the liver is difficult and more hazardous.

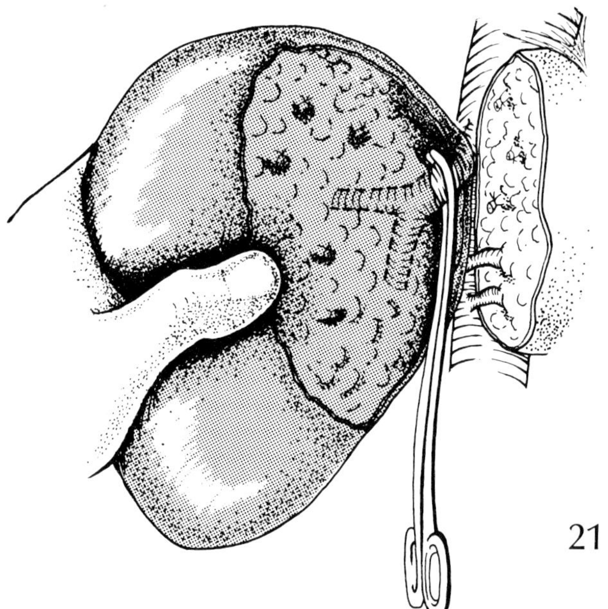

21

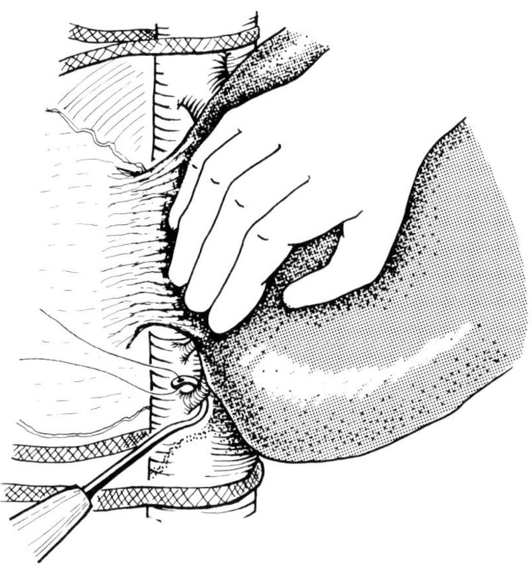

22

22

Control of the hepatic veins from within the liver is, however, not possible for resection of posteriorly lying tumours adjacent to the vena cava. In this instance and prior to commencing finger fracture, the liver must be turned to the left and the hepatic veins serially ligated starting from below where the caudate lobe crosses the vena cava and working upwards. Clips may be used to secure smaller veins but aneurysm needles carrying a fine silk thread are passed around the larger vessels.

23

The main right hepatic venous trunk is short and stubby and requires careful isolation. Complete exposure often requires division of a tongue of fibrous tissue which sometimes obscures the right side of the upper part of the retrohepatic vena cava (*see Illustration 22*). Prior control of the vena cava by passage of slings around the infrahepatic suprarenal vena cava and a further sling around the inferior vena cava above the liver just below the diaphragm, or even within the pericardium, is a wise precaution.

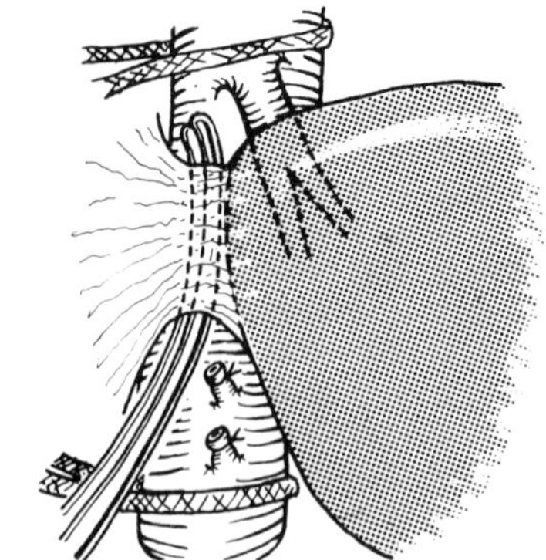

23

24

Once exposed, a vascular clamp is applied on the caval side of the hepatic vein.

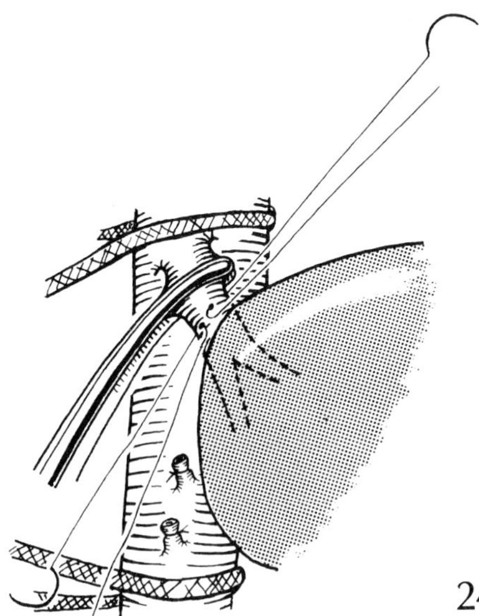

24

25

This allows safe division of the vessel, which is then closed with over-and-over 3/0 vascular suture.

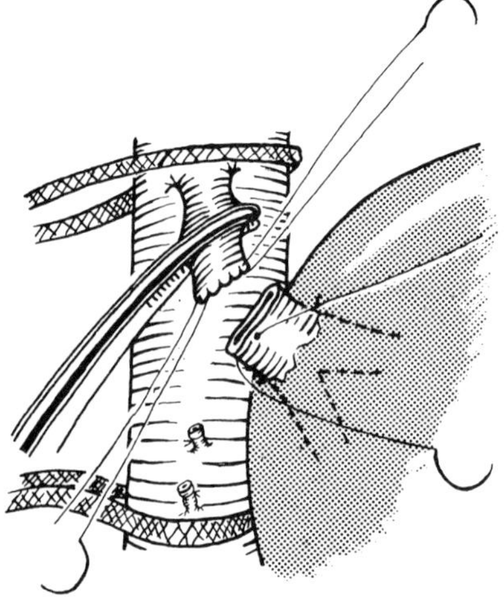

25

26

Haemostasis is secured by a combination of diathermy, suture ligation and finally by passage of a series of large sutures (No. 1 chromic catgut) anteroposteriorly in a mattress fashion.

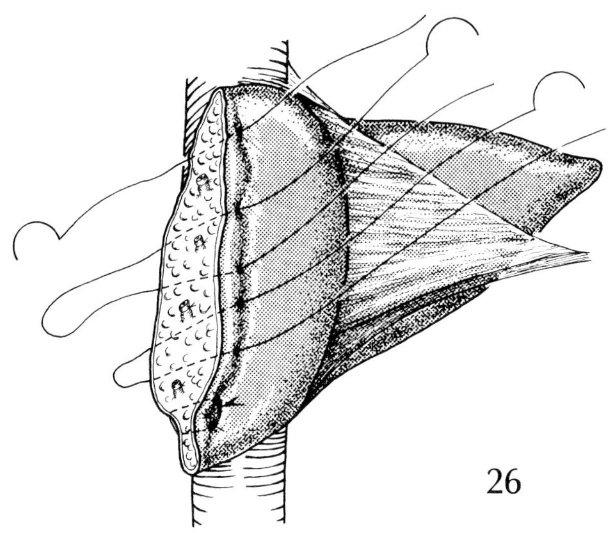

26

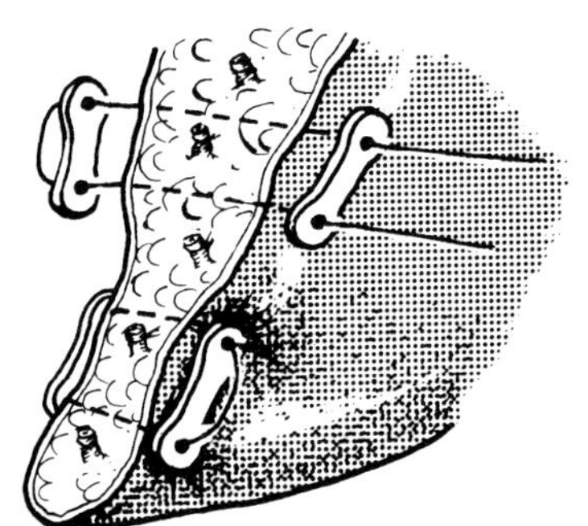

27

27

If the liver tissue is friable, these sutures may be passed through liver buffers[11], to prevent cutting through of liver tissue.

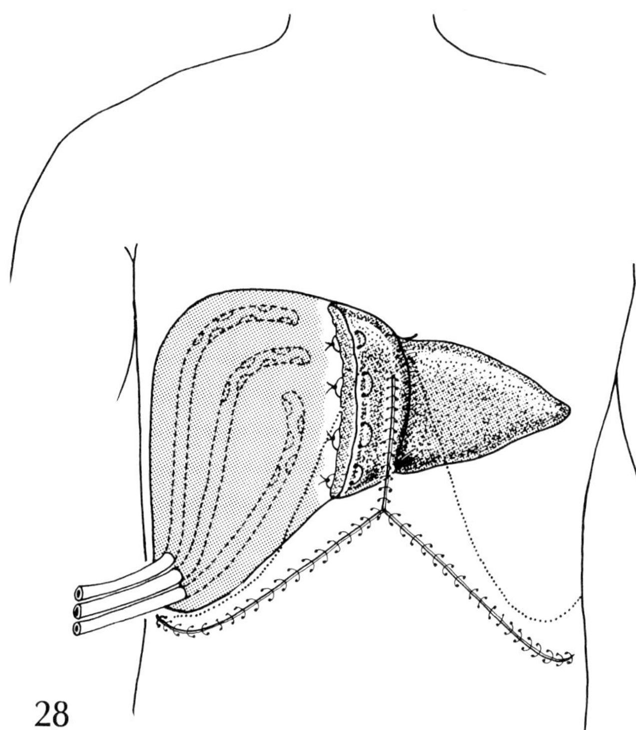

28

Wound closure and drainage

28

If there is a diaphragmatic incision this is closed. Drainage of the large space left in the subdiaphragmatic area must be good. If the field is reasonably dry then two or three large-bore suction drains connected to a closed system are adequate. If there is some concern and oozing, then large sump drains which allow irrigation as well as suction are preferable.

If a choledochotomy has been carried out in order to allow exploration of the biliary tree, or if because of doubt as to the integrity of the biliary tree, then T-tube drainage is instituted but is otherwise not employed.

EXTENDED RIGHT HEPATIC LOBECTOMY

The operation of extended right hepatic lobectomy involves further and continued mobilization, so as to devascularize the quadrate lobe of the liver in addition to the right lobe.

29

The first and essential step is to locate precisely and display the umbilical fissure of the liver[12]. A forceps or strong ligature tied to the ligamentum teres is elevated. In many cases the lower part of the umbilical fissure is concealed by a tongue of liver tissue fusing the inferior part of the lateral segment of the left lobe to the quadrate lobe. This tissue is easily opened by simple fracture between the finger and thumb. No large vessels traverse here and haemostasis is readily secured by diathermy or suture.

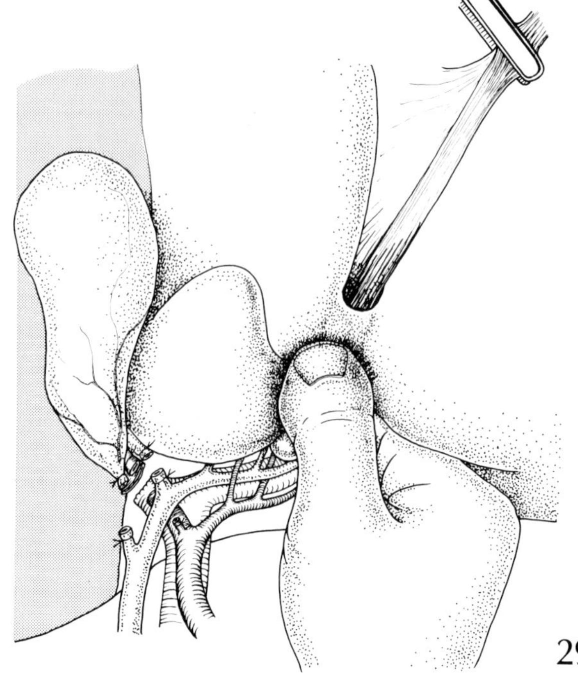

29

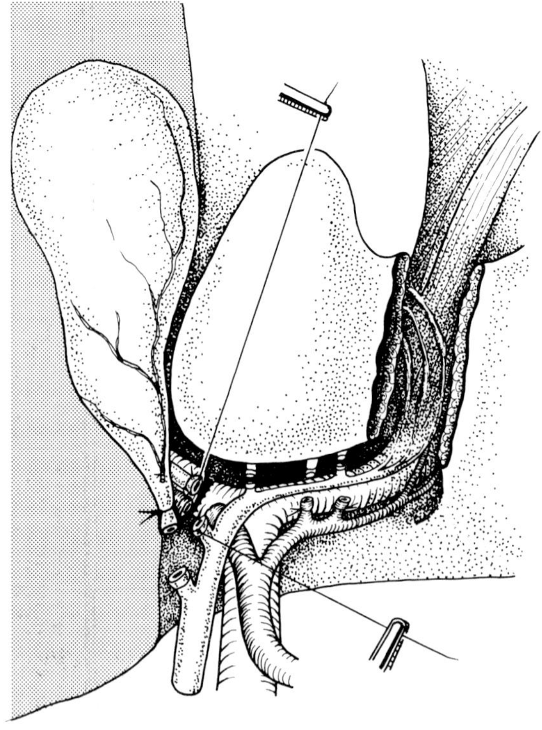

30

30

The medial segment of the left lobe (quadrate lobe) is then clearly seen to be separated from the left lateral segment. The ligamentum teres can now be visualized running down to the base of the umbilical fissure, at which the left triad of portal vein, hepatic artery and hepatic duct enter the left lobe of the liver.

The left branches of the portal triad which are several centimetres in length are now separated from the undersurface of the liver. This involves ligation of any small branches of the portal vein to the quadrate lobe. Similarly, small ducts and arteries running with these branches must be dealt with. A middle hepatic artery arising from the left hepatic artery or sometimes even from the right main trunk is usually present and must be divided. If there is any artery to the left lobe or to the left lateral segment arising from the coeliac axis or from the left gastric artery, this always enters the base of the umbilical fissure and should not be endangered.

It is important to remember that the two last major branches of the left portal tract pass posteriorly to the caudate lobe. Division of these branches will devascularize the caudate lobe which should then usually be removed in its entirety by dissection from the surface of the inferior vena cava. Division of these structures and consequent removal of the caudate lobe is tedious and hazardous and usually not necessary.

The right hepatic vein is now dealt with as described above by division and subsequent oversewing outside the liver substance, or it may be left for intrahepatic dissection at a later stage of the procedure (*see Illustrations 22–25*).

31

Isolation of the medial segment and liver transection

The vital step in the performance of extended right hepatic lobectomy is the division of veins and arteries which originate in the umbilical fissure of the liver and feedback from the main left trunks to the medial segment of the left lobe[12] (*see Illustrations 1 and 30*). It is important not to attempt to divide these structures within the umbilical fissure because the blood supply to the left lateral segment may be damaged. For this reason, the feedback vessels are secured *to the right* of the falciform ligament within the substance of the liver. The dissection is commenced anteriorly and proceeds down to the base of the umbilical fissure. The parenchyma of the liver is opened just to the right of the ligamentum teres by the finger-fracture method. Once these vessels are divided, the medial segment of the left lobe is devascularized and a line of demarcation can be seen extending along the plane of the falciform ligament posteriorly towards the vena cava.

Division of the liver substance is then developed backwards towards the vena cava following exactly the line of demarcation. Several large intersegmental veins are encountered and are preserved if possible, pushing them towards the lateral segment.

Near to the diaphragm the middle hepatic vein is encountered and is sometimes seen entering the main left hepatic vein. Sometimes it enters the inferior vena cava separately. Irrespective of its termination, the middle hepatic vein is secured and ligated.

If the right hepatic vein has not been previously secured, it is now approached from within the liver substance as for right hepatic lobectomy and ligated. The right and quadrate lobes of the liver are now removed.

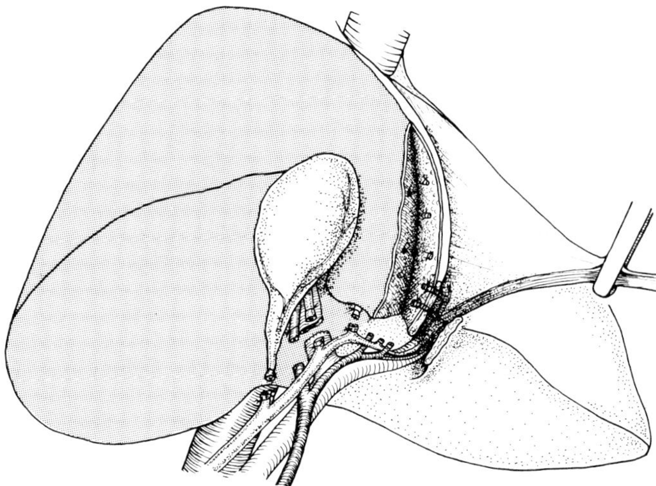

31

HEPATIC LOBECTOMY FOR HILAR TUMOURS

In the case of tumours occupying the hilus of the liver, for which hepatic lobectomy may be necessary, the initial surgical approach differs.

32

The common bile duct is divided early immediately above the duodenum and turned upwards to expose the vascular structures beneath. The gall bladder is also mobilized from its bed. The cystic duct is not divided.

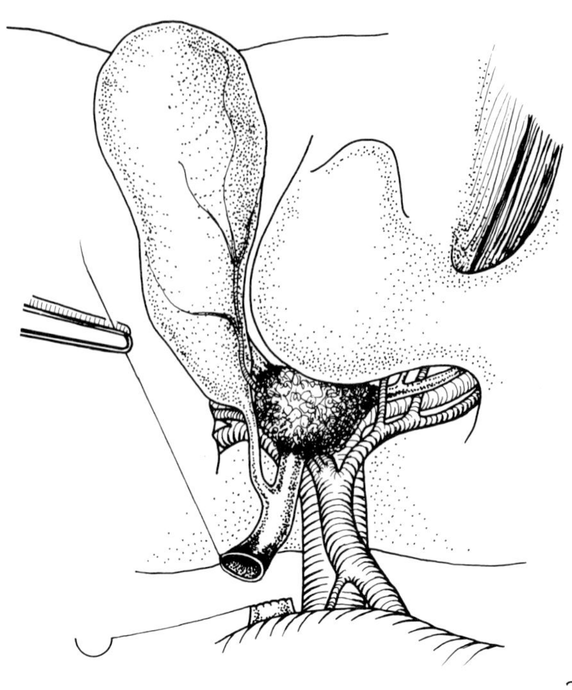

32

33

The bile duct, cystic duct and gall bladder are then turned forward and upward.

The retroductal hepatic artery and portal vein can now be approached and dissected behind the tumour. Preliminary angiography (*see Illustration 3*) should have indicated any involvement of branches of the hepatic artery or of the portal vein by tumour. Involvement of branches of these structures with the lobe to be resected does not necessarily preclude resection, but an intact blood supply to and biliary drainage from the remnant are essential.

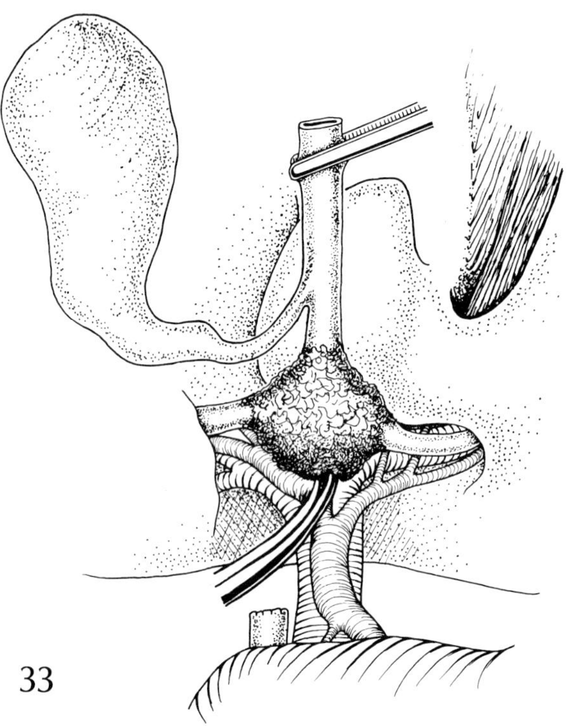

33

34

To assess further such vascular involvement and allow access, the liver may be split (hepatotomy) in the principal plane to the left of the gall bladder fossa, between the right lobe and the medial segment of the left lobe (quadrate lobe) in order to expose structures at the hilus[13, 14, 15]. This approach is particularly useful to allow wide exposure of the confluence of the bile ducts and bifurcation of the vessels in benign or malignant stricture to the liver and may be carried out without vascular control. The liver tissue is split from before backwards, deepening the gap in the liver tissue towards the vena cava and separating the right and left lobes as the dissection proceeds. The middle hepatic vein is pushed laterally and it is usually possible to preserve its main trunk. The approach displays the hilus of the liver well and facilitates application of clamps to the portal vein at its bifurcation with, if necessary, excision of segments of vein and subsequent repair. Performance of such an hepatotomy need not necessarily be followed by subsequent hepatic resection, since the manoeuvre does not devitalize any portion of the liver. However, should hepatic resection prove to be necessary, then the major vessels can be controlled and the initial liver split extended as a partial hepatectomy.

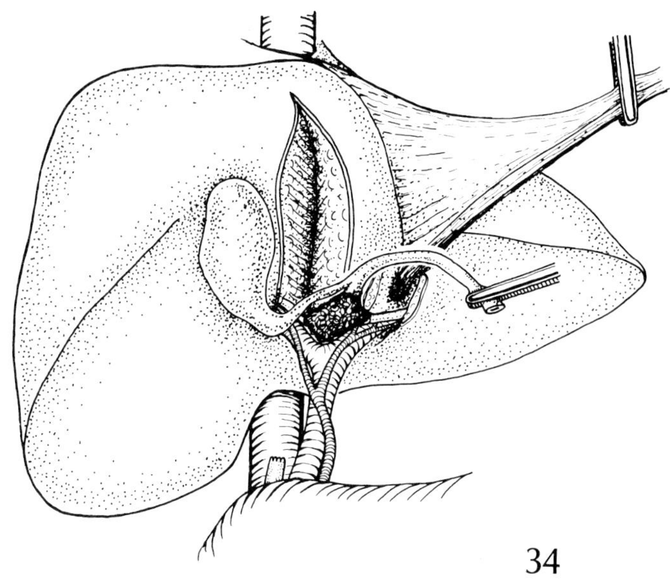

34

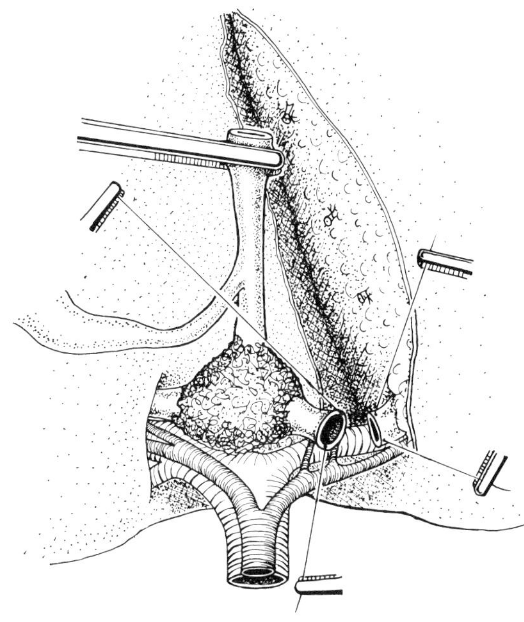

35

35

In carrying out *extended right hepatic lobectomy* for hilar tumours that involve the right hepatic duct, initial dissection should elevate and free the common bile duct and the tumour from the underlying vessels. The left hepatic duct is identified and sectioned distal to the tumour. It may prove more convenient to do this during division of the liver substance to the right of the ligamentum teres.

The margins of the left hepatic duct are marked with stay sutures for subsequent anastomosis. The proximal portion of the left hepatic duct, together with the tumour, is drawn to the right and the remainder of the liver tissue is then divided.

36

After removal of the right and quadrate lobes of the liver, the exposed hepatic duct is anastomosed to a Roux-en-Y loop of jejunum using a single layer of interrupted 3/0 catgut sutures. A silicone tube is placed across this anastomosis, either passed in a transjejunal fashion from below or drawn down in a transhepatic manner through the anterior segmental division of the left hepatic duct.

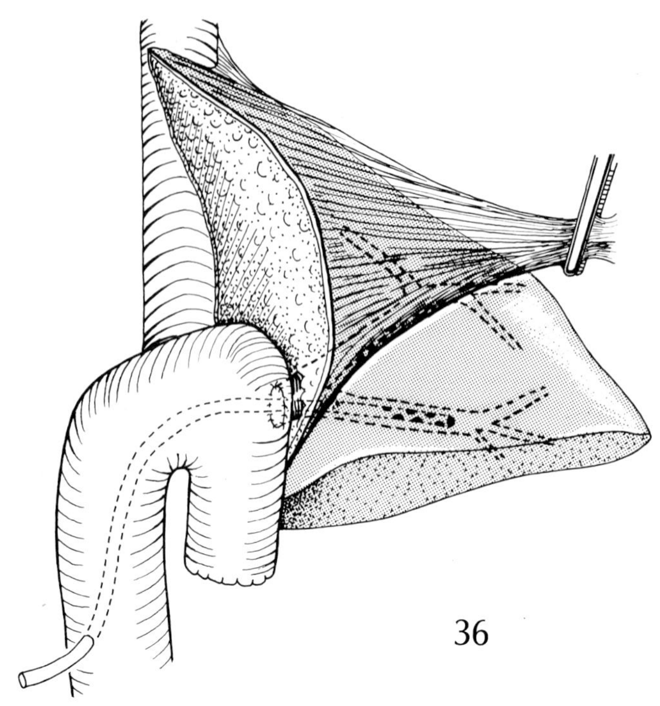

36

LEFT HEPATIC LOBECTOMY

Left hepatic lobectomy involves ligation of the left hepatic artery, left hepatic duct and the left branch of the portal vein. The techniques used are similar to those described above. Any accessory left hepatic artery arising from the left gastric artery or from the coeliac axis should be sought in the lesser omentum at the base of the umbilical fissure.

Once the true left lobe of the liver is devascularized, a line of demarcation will develop to the left of the gall bladder fossa.

The left lobe of the liver is then mobilized by incising the tip of the left triangular ligament and carrying the incision medially as far as the left side of the vena cava. Once the left lobe is mobilized, the left hepatic vein may be visualized as it runs to enter the vena cava and can then be clamped and sutured. If there is any difficulty, this procedure can be delayed until the liver has been split from before backwards. The liver substance is then divided anteroposteriorly. The main trunk of the middle hepatic vein usually enters the left hepatic vein but may enter the vena cava separately.

LEFT LATERAL SEGMENTECTOMY

This operation does not require dissection at the hilus of the liver. The left lobe of the liver is mobilized as described above. The ligamentum teres is clamped and elevated. If present, the bridge of tissue between the left lateral segment and the medial segment of the left lobe is fractured so as to expose the umbilical fissure (*see Illustration 29*). The left lateral segment is now separated either by applying a clamp just to the left of the ligamentum teres and removing the left lateral segment with subsequent suture ligation of exposed vessels, or by splitting the liver tissue anteroposteriorly just to the left of the ligamentum teres. The left hepatic vein is identified posteriorly within the liver substance and secured and the left lateral segment removed.

QUADRATE LOBECTOMY

Removal of the quadrate lobe (medial segment of the left lobe) is seldom justified but is sometimes necessary to allow adequate excision of hilar cholangiocarcinoma or of a small secondary deposit located only within the quadrate lobe.

The structures at the hilus of the liver are isolated. Those vessels and ducts arising from the left portal triad and feeding to the quadrate lobe from below are sacrificed. Once this has been done, the ligamentum teres is elevated and the feedback structures supplying the quadrate lobe are divided to the right of the ligamentum teres of the liver, which is split posteriorly towards the vena cava (*see Illustration 31*).

The liver is then split just to the right of the gall bladder fossa in the principal plane, again progressing posteriorly towards the vena cava (*see Illustration 19*). These manoeuvres isolate the quadrate lobe.

The segment thus isolated is then removed by dividing the liver tissue transversely so as to free the quadrate lobe. During this procedure the middle hepatic vein is ligated. Care should be taken not to damage the left hepatic vein.

Other segmental resections are seldom justified, full lobectomy being safer and easier to perform.

WEDGE RESECTION

For small peripheral lesions a simple wedge excision of liver tissue may be performed. The results for removal of small secondary deposits in the liver are just as good as those for formal lobectomy[16]. A wedge of liver tissue is simply removed between appropriately placed mattress sutures and excised. Further haemostasis may be secured by suture ligation. There is no necessity to approximate the edges of the wound which are simply left open with adequate drainage.

Mortality and morbidity

The mortality of simple wedge resection or a left lateral segmentectomy should be nil. For elective right or left hepatic lobectomy the mortality is probably within the region of 2–5 per cent but should be no higher. By contrast, when lesions involve the hilus of the liver necessitating extended right hepatic lobectomy the mortality rises to about 5–10 per cent, and if division and subsequent reconstruction of major vessels to the remnant is required, mortality reaches 10 or 12 per cent and may be higher in jaundiced patients.

The risks of hepatic resection may be less, particularly for tumours placed peripherally away from major vessels and where the residual liver tissue is normal, but are higher in the following circumstances.

1. Advancing age.
2. Previous operative intervention.
3. Pre-existing infection as a result of bile duct obstruction or as a result of previous surgical interference.
4. Biliary tract obstruction. In cases of biliary tract obstruction requiring hepatic lobectomy (for example, hilar cholangiocarcinoma), hepatic resection is more dangerous because of the general systemic effects of jaundice[13], and also because of the high incidence of pre-existing infection.

   It may be advisable to precede surgery by passage of a percutaneous transhepatic catheter in order to decompress preliminarily the biliary system and allow recovery before proceeding to major surgery at a later date.
5. Cirrhosis of the liver. Liver resection in the presence of established cirrhosis is probably not justified, at least in Western patients[17]. The ability of the liver to regenerate is seriously compromised and liver failure is much more likely to occur[18].

   Similarly, liver resection which leaves a remnant of liver already atrophic as a result of pre-existing disease is likely to result in liver failure.
6. Associated diseases and injuries. Hepatic resection for injury is only necessary for major destructive wounds, and the mortality is high reaching at least 20 per cent and may be much higher in some circumstances[19]. The presence of multiple associated injuries and in particular injury to the chest or head is accompanied by a high mortality. In addition, cases coming late to surgery or where there is associated injury to major hepatic veins or vessels at the porta hepatis carry a high risk. Similarly, judgement as to whether to perform hepatic lobectomy in the presence of severe associated disease (e.g. diabetes) is difficult since the mortality and morbidity of the procedure are undoubtedly higher.

Postoperative care

Total serum protein falls after hepatic resection and administration of intravenous albumin is of value. The serum albumin level will begin to recover about the third postoperative week and reach the normal range within 4–6 weeks of resection[20,21]. Hypoglycaemia is a real risk after resection and should be guarded against. The blood sugar should be monitored regularly. The major risk is within the first 48 h, and infusion of 5 per cent dextrose should be maintained and supplemented by 50 ml 50 per cent glucose solution if necessary.

Jaundice is inevitable but usually mild. On occasion deep jaundice may occur associated with bilirubinuria and retention of conjugated bilirubin. There are many reasons for such jaundice[15], but it is much more likely to occur if there has been hypoperfusion of the liver and the presence of infection. This is due to centrilobular damage and intrahepatic cholestasis and is not a reason for reoperation.

Haemorrhagic problems are recognized after hepatic resection, especially after resection for injury. Careful monitoring of the coagulation status is necessary and coagulation defects can usually be managed by administration of fresh-frozen plasma and Vitamin K.

Conclusion

Major hepatic resections are extensive operations which should not be lightly undertaken, but equally, less effective methods should not be employed when hepatic resection is clearly indicated. Difficulties can be kept to a minimum by adhering to the following rules.

1. Do not operate (unless in the emergency situation) without full preoperative investigation.
2. Knowledge of anatomy and a confident surgeon, good judgement and good assistance are important. Involved techniques and special instruments are not.
3. Good control of vessels and bile ducts at the hilus and precise dissection will minimize haemorrhage and bile duct injury.
4. Liver failure should be minimized by avoiding ischaemia to the liver remnant.
5. Cirrhotic patients should not be submitted to extensive resection.
6. Emergency surgery has to be dealt with by the surgeon on the spot. Elective surgery for tumour or biliary obstruction should be referred to a specialist and dealt with by an experienced team.

References

1. Blumgart, L. H., Leach, K. G., Karran, S. J. Observations on liver regeneration after right hepatic lobectomy. Gut 1971; 12: 922–928
2. Blumgart, L. H. Injuries of the Liver. In: Maingot, R., ed. Abdominal operations, Ch. 51. New York: Appleton-Century-Crofts, 1974
3. McIndoe, A. H., Counseller, V. S. The bilaterality of the liver. Archives of Surgery 1927; 15: 589–594
4. Lortat-Jacob, J. L., Robert, H. G. Hépatectomie droite réglée. Presse Médicale 1952; 60: 549–551.
5. Healey, J. E., Schroy, P. C. Anatomy of the bilary ducts within the human liver. Archives of Surgery 1953; 66: 599–616
6. Healey, J. E. Clinical anatomical aspects of radical hepatic surgery. Journal of the International College of Surgery 1954; 22: 542
7. Goldsmith, N. A., Woodburne, R. T. The surgical anatomy pertaining to liver resection. Surgery, Gynecology and Obstetrics 1957; 105: 310–318
8. Williamson, B. W. A., Blumgart, L. H., McKellar, N. J. Management of tumours of the liver. American Journal of Surgery 1980; 139: 210–215
9. McPherson, G. A. D., Benjamin, I. S., Nathanson, B., Blenkharn, J. I., Bowley, N. B., Blumgart, L. H. The advantages and disadvantages of percutaneous transhepatic biliary drainage as part of a staged approach to obstructive jaundice. Gut 1981; 22: A427
10. Miller, D. R. Median sternotomy extension of abdominal incision for hepatic lobectomy. Annals of Surgery 1972; 175: 193–196
11. Wood, C. B., Capperauld, I., Blumgart, L. H. Bioplast fibrin buttons for the control of haemorrhage of the liver following biopsy and partial resection. Annals of the Royal College of Surgeons of England 1976; 58: 401–404
12. Starzl, T. E., Bell, R. H., Beart, R. W., Putnam, C. W. Hepatic trisegmentectomy and other liver resections. Surgery, Gynecology and Obstetrics 1975; 141: 429–437
13. Blumgart, L. H. Biliary tract obstruction – new approaches to old problems. American Journal of Surgery 1978; 135: 19–31
14. Benjamin, I.S., Blumgart, L. H. Biliary bypass and reconstructive surgery. In: Wright, R., Alberti, K. G. M. M., Karran, S., Millward-Sadler, G. H., eds. Liver and biliary disease: pathophysiology, diagnosis, management, Ch. 54, pp. 1219–1246. London, Philadelphia, Toronto: W. B. Saunders Co. Ltd, 1979
15. Blumgart, L. H. Hepatic resection. In: Talor, S., ed. Recent Advances in Surgery, Vol. 10, Ch. 1, pp. 1–26. Edinburgh: Churchill Livingstone, 1980
16. Wilson, S., Adson, M. A. Surgical treatment of hepatic metastases from colorectal cancer. Archives of Surgery 1976; 3: 330–334
17. Foster, J. H., Berman, M. M. Solid liver tumours. In: Ebert, P., ed. Major problems in clinical surgery, 1. London, Philadelphia, Toronto: W. B. Saunders, 1977: 342
18. Lin, T. Y., Cheng, C.-C. Metabolic function and regeneration of cirrhotic and non-cirrhotic livers after hepatic lobectomy in man. Annals of Surgery 1965; 162: 959–972
19. Walt, A. J. The mythology of hepatic trauma – or Babel revisited. American Journal of Surgery 1978; 135: 12–18
20. Blumgart, L. H., Vajrabukka, T. Injuries to the liver: analysis of 20 cases. British Medical Journal 1972; 1: 158–164
21. Vajrabukka, T., Bloom, A. L., Sussman, M., Wood, C. B., Blumgart, L. H. Post-operative problems and management after hepatic resection for blunt injury to the liver. British Journal of Surgery 1975; 62: 189–200

Bleeding oesophageal varices – a plan of management

R. Shields MD, FRCS, FRCS(Ed.)
Professor of Surgery, University of Liverpool;
Honorary Consultant Surgeon, Royal Liverpool Hospital and Broadgreen Hospital, Liverpool

EARLY MANAGEMENT

The initial management of bleeding oesophageal varices is non-operative. Emergency surgery is attended by such a high mortality that operation should ideally be postponed until the patient's general condition is improved and then it is undertaken to prevent recurrence of bleeding. Obviously, however, if intensive medical treatment fails to staunch the haemorrhage, the surgeon may have to operate to save the patient's life but in these circumstances the patient will only have a one in two chance of surviving the operation and the immediate postoperative period.

In a patient vomiting blood the urgent need is to stop the bleeding and resuscitate him rapidly. Uncontrolled bleeding rapidly leads to a progressive deterioration of the patient whose condition has previously been greatly weakened by underlying liver disease, e.g. cirrhosis, causing impaired clotting of the blood and defective synthesis of protein, especially albumin.

However, before specific medical treatment can be administered, bleeding must be shown to be coming from oesophagogastric varices. In some instances the cause of the haemorrhage is obvious – the patient is jaundiced and oedematous, or in semicoma, with a known history of alcohol abuse. Occasionally disease of the liver is suggested by such stigmata as spider naevi and liver palms. Sometimes the alert physician will suspect the diagnosis because of a slight blurring of the patient's consciousness or a slurring of the speech due to early encephalopathy precipitated by the bleeding. The diagnosis must be confirmed.

Unless indicated otherwise the cross-references in this chapter refer to *Operative Surgery: Alimentary Tract and Abdominal Wall, Volume 2, 4th Edition*

ENDOSCOPY

Endoscopy is preferred because not only can varices be seen but the source of the bleeding, which occasionally may be different, e.g. gastric erosion, duodenal ulcer, can be defined. A thin flexible fibreoptic instrument is preferred and can be passed without difficulty or hazard shortly after the patient's admission to hospital.

1

Rarely varices are seen as large blue, bulging, dilated veins, similar to varicose veins in the leg. They are most often recognized as columns, 3–5 in number, protruding the overlying mucosa, to a variable extent and over a variable length, into the lumen.

An inexperienced endoscopist may miss smaller varices, especially when these are clustered on the gastric side of the cardio-oesophageal junction. The usual error is to miss varices when they are present, rather than to diagnose them in their absence.

Varices can also be seen in the stomach and duodenum where they are not usually the source of bleeding. This is fortunate, because their safe injection with sclerosant can be difficult.

Occasionally there may be some anxiety that the patient had bled from a site other than the varices, especially if the bleeding has stopped. However, if a patient who is known to have portal hypertension is bleeding, the source of the haemorrhage is most likely the varices, especially if there has been a previous episode of haemorrhage from them.

BARIUM SWALLOW

Barium swallow may also demonstrate the varices but this examination is not really suitable in an emergency. Varices are seen as long, wormlike indentations of the mucosa in a dilated oesophagus.

RESUSCITATION

1. Blood should be rapidly transfused through a wide-bore cannula placed in a peripheral vein. Fresh blood is preferred because it will contain factors essential for coagulation. Because fast delivery may be required, the blood should be warmed in a coil. Citrate intoxication is not usually a problem.

   Complete volume replacement of the blood is essential to restore an adequate flow to the liver and the kidney and to ensure that if the patient bleeds again in the near future he will have adequate reserves. The patient should be fully monitored by half-hourly recordings of arterial blood pressure, pulse rate, central venous pressure and urine output, a urethral catheter having been passed.
2. A wide-bore tube is passed into the stomach to empty it of contained blood. The gastric cavity can be washed out with iced isotonic saline but too vigorous lavage should be avoided before endoscopy because mucosal trauma may be misdiagnosed as superficial erosions.

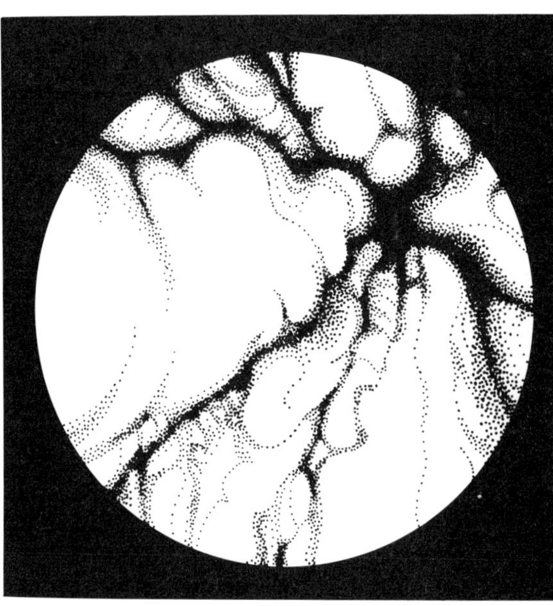

1

STOPPING THE BLEEDING

The two mainstays of emergency medical treatment are vasopressin and balloon tamponade. While some clinicians may prefer one or other treatment, we use them sequentially, proceeding to tamponade if vasopressin fails. Tamponade is the more effective but is uncomfortable, often distressing, to the patient and carries great risk of complications, some of which may be fatal if care is not taken.

Infusion of vasopressin

Through another intravenous catheter, vasopressin is delivered by continuous infusion at a rate of 0.4 u/min. In practice this rate of delivery can be achieved by adding 200 u of vasopressin to 500 ml of a 5 per cent solution of dextrose, which is then infused at a rate of 60 ml/h.

Continuous intravenous infusion over 24 h in this manner is more effective and has fewer side effects than the conventional bolus doses. *Intra-arterial* infusion has largely been abandoned. Owing to the profound cutaneous vasoconstriction the patient looks very pale. Occasionally he may complain of some abdominal cramping, which is caused by the smooth muscle effect of vasopressin. With intravenous infusion, cardiac effects, especially myocardial infarction, are rare.

The infusion of vasopressin at 0.4 u/min should be continued for 24 h. For the next 24 h it should be delivered at 0.2 u/min, and for the succeeding 24 h at 0.1 u/min. If bleeding recurs during the weaning period or after cessation of treatment, the full dosage should be reinstituted.

With this regimen, control of bleeding (defined as cessation of haemorrhage for the succeeding 24 h) can be expected in 60–70 per cent of patients. The patient's response is of some prognostic value – immediate and sustained cessation of bleeding augurs well for the patient. Failure to control bleeding often means that the haemorrhage will continue no matter what medical treatment is given, and surgery, under emergency circumstances, may be necessary.

Balloon tamponade

Balloon tamponade should be instituted if bleeding recurs after, or despite, vasopressin.

2

Several different balloon tubes are available. The Blakemore-Sengstaken tube consists of three channels: the longest one is used for aspirating the stomach, the second for inflating the gastric balloon and the third for inflating the sausage-shaped oesophageal balloon. The oesophagus and hypopharynx above the oesophageal balloon must be kept free of accumulating secretions, which may be aspirated into the lung. For this purpose we use a modification of the Sengstaken tube, the Minnesota tube, in which there is a fourth channel for aspirating the upper oesophagus. If this particular tube is not available, a separate Levin tube is passed after the Sengstaken tube, to aspirate accumulating saliva and secretions.

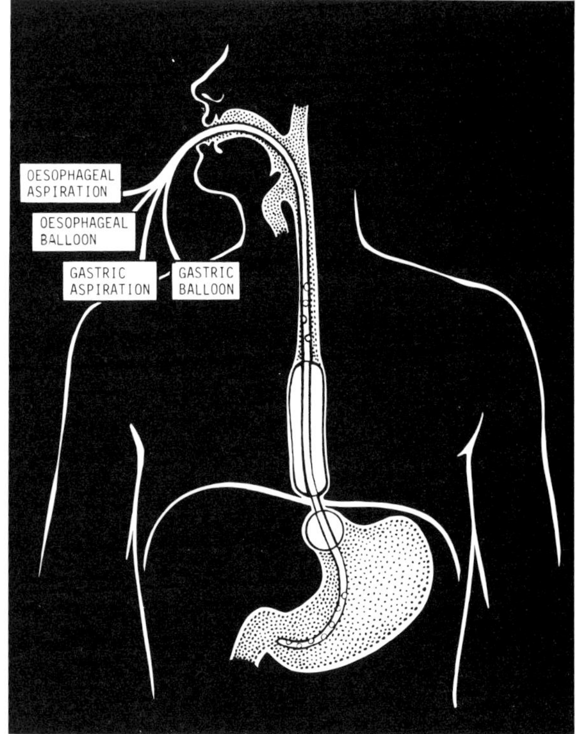

2

Detailed instructions

1. A new tube is used on each occasion. Before use, each balloon is inflated to test for leaks. The balloons are then deflated and coated with a water-miscible, lubricating jelly.
2. A lubricated Levin tube, 18 Fr, is passed by mouth into the stomach, which is then washed with 0.9 per cent iced sodium chloride solution, to remove accumulated blood which may be vomited and aspirated when the Sengstaken tube is passed.
3. The patient is placed, preferably on an operation table whose head end is elevated 45°.
4. The Sengstaken tube should be passed in most instances by mouth to prevent damage and obstruction to the nasal passages and to permit its rapid removal if required.
5. The passage of the tube will be aided by generous lubrication of the tube and careful folding of the oesophageal and gastric balloons. Passage can also be facilitated by encouraging the patient to take sips of water through a straw. The tube should be passed until the 50 cm mark is reached. Its position is checked by X-ray; alternatively, air can be insufflated down the gastric aspiration channel and the epigastrium should be auscultated.
6. Suction is applied to the gastric and oesophageal aspiration channels to reduce the risk of regurgitation of gastric juice, blood and saliva when the gastric balloon is inflated.
7. The gastric balloon is inflated with saline solution containing a small quality of radiopaque contrast medium. After 250–300 ml fluid have been instilled the gastric balloon inlet is doubly clamped with rubber-shod, heavy surgical clamps. Firm traction is applied to the tube until the resistance of the inflated gastric balloon can be felt firmly against the gastro-oesophageal junction. With minimal traction on the tube, its upper end is fixed to the side of the mouth. Alternatively a cord may be tied to the tube and led over pulleys to a 1–2 kg (2.2–4.4 lb) weight.
8. The stomach is washed with isotonic saline solution until the aspirate is clear. If it is evident, however, that bleeding is continuing, the oesophageal balloon should be inflated to 35–40 mmHg as recorded on a mercury manometer attached to the oesophageal channel. The channel leading to the inflated oesophageal balloon is then doubly clamped with rubber-shod heavy clamps.
9. If bleeding continues, a gastrix varix may be the source of the bleeding. Further external traction should be applied to the Sengstaken tube.
10. The stomach should be aspirated at intervals to determine if bleeding is continuing. Continuous aspiration of the oesophagus above the oesophageal balloon is necessary to remove swallowed saliva.
11. The balloons should be kept inflated with the tube on traction for 24 h. The oesophageal balloon is then slowly deflated and, by aspiration through the oesophageal and gastric channels, checks should be made for recurrence of the haemorrhage. If bleeding remains stopped, traction on the tube should be released and the gastric balloon deflated. If bleeding still remains stopped, the tube should be cautiously removed.

If bleeding recurs after these initial deflations, the balloons should be reinflated and traction reapplied for another 24 h. However, during this second 24 h period, the risk of complications is greatly increased and preparation should be made for further treatment.

12. Nursing and medical staff looking after the patient should be completely familiar with the Sengstaken tube. Knowledge and scrupulous care in its use greatly reduce the risk of complications.
    A pair of scissors should always be taped to the head of the patient's bed so that if the oesophageal balloon migrates up into the hypopharynx or if respiratory distress develops, the attendants can cut and remove the tube as rapidly as possible. Only an experienced nurse or clinician should be allowed to remove the tube.
    The traction on the tube and pressures in the oesophageal balloon should be rechecked every 4 h.
13. After removal of the tube, the mouth and posterior pharynx are aspirated using a catheter to remove regurgitated secretions.

Complications of balloon tamponade

1. Aspiration of blood, saliva and secretions into the lungs – these risks can be minimized by great care in passing the tube.
2. Oesophageal laceration and perforation, leading to mediastinitis – the risk of these complications increases greatly during the second 24 h of tamponade.
3. Respiratory obstruction.

PREVENTION OF ENCEPHALOPATHY

Encephalopathy is frequently precipitated because the function of the damaged liver is further impaired by hypovolaemia. The risk of encephalopathy is increased by the presence of a large quantity of blood – a source of protein – in the gastrointestinal tract.

The risk is reduced by:

1. prompt control of bleeding;
2. full replacement of lost blood;
3. correction of electrolyte deficiencies, e.g. hypokalaemia;
4. treatment of associated infections, e.g. pneumonia, infected ascites;
5. irrigation of the colon and rectum by magnesium sulphate enemas;
6. administration of a broad-spectrum non-absorbed antibiotic against faecal flora, e.g. neomycin;
7. avoidance of over-use of sedatives and analgesics, e.g. morphine and pethidine.

FURTHER MANAGEMENT

The further management of the patient's condition will depend upon whether the bleeding has stopped.

Bleeding has stopped

If this is the first episode of bleeding, there is a 50–60 per cent chance that the haemorrhage will recur. If there have been recent previous episodes of bleeding, there will be an 80–90 per cent chance of recurrence. The brief respite is profitably employed:

1. to assess the patient's general condition (to determine the effect upon the patient of the underlying liver disease, e.g. cirrhosis; and of the portal hypertension, e.g. upon the spleen, leading to thrombocytopaenia and leucopaenia);
2. to improve the patient's condition;
3. to determine what further intervention is required, if any.

ASSESSMENT OF PATIENT'S CONDITION

Abnormalities in clotting mechanisms

Prompt identification and correction of abnormalities in clotting mechanisms are essential, partly to reduce the risks and severity of further haemorrhage and partly to determine whether invasive diagnostic procedures, e.g. liver biopsy, can be carried out safely. Expert haematological advice is required.

Liver function

Several methods are available to assess liver function and to define the risks of operation. The simplest is to assign the patient to one of the categories of the Child classification of liver function (*Table 1*) which requires only two simple biochemical tests and three clinical assessments. Patients in Child group C are poor risks for a major operation.

Table 1. Classification of cirrhotic patients in terms of hepatic reserve*

	Group A	*Group B*	*Group C*
Serum bilirubin (μmol/l)	34.0	34.0–51.0	51.0
Plasma albumin (g/l)	35	30–35	30
Ascites	None	Easily controlled	Poorly controlled
Encephalopathy	None	Minimal	Advanced coma
Nutrition	Excellent	Moderate	Poor
Risk of operation	Good	Moderate	Poor

* Modified from Child, C.G. III. Liver and portal hypertension. Philadelphia: Saunders, 1964

Blood tests

Routine blood tests should be carried out, including estimation of hepatic enzymes, serum α-fetoprotein, hepatitis antigen, immunoglobulins and plasma ammonia.

X-rays

Radiology of the chest and abdomen is required, and perhaps barium swallow to confirm the diagnosis if there is any doubt.

Angiography

Angiography may be required, either to determine the cause of the portal hypertension, e.g. to demonstrate portal vein thrombosis, or more usually to decide if the splanchnic veins are patent and suitable for portasystemic shunting.

3 & 4

Splenic venography

The examination should be performed by an experienced radiologist. Under local anaesthesia, a plastic catheter with a metal trocar is inserted through through the skin into the spleen, which has been previously located by percussion. A small volume of contrast material is injected into the spleen.

The intrasplenic pressure is then measured, usually by simple saline manometer, to give an indication of portal vein pressure. The normal range by this technique is 4–22 cmH_2O, using the right atrium as the point of zero reference.

The venogram is performed by attaching the catheter to a syringe full of contrast material. The injection is made using an automatic pressure device, with films being taken at frequent intervals, using an automatic changer.

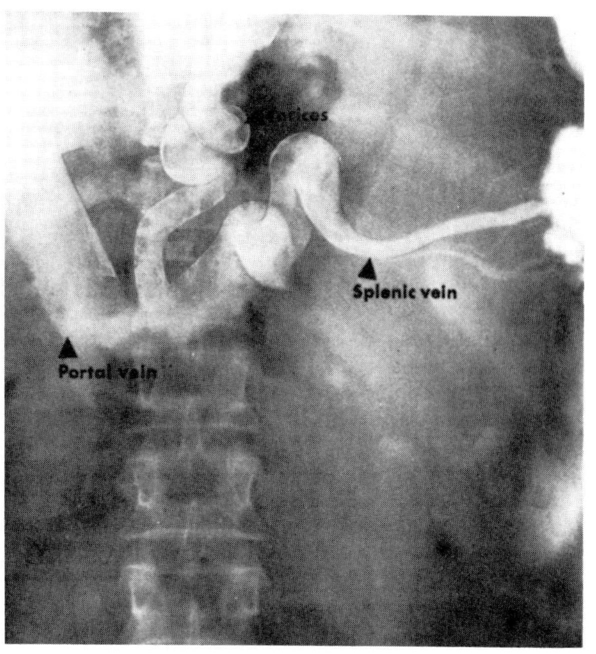

3

Advantages

1. Very accurate in diagnosis of varices.
2. Measurement of splenic pulp pressure, to confirm portal hypertension.
3. Patency of splenic and portal veins confirmed.
4. Display of local anatomy, to show collaterals in operation field.

Disadvantages

1. Potentially hazardous in presence of thrombocytopaenia (less than 45 000/cm^3) and prothrombin deficiency (less than 40 per cent control).
2. Risk of splenic damage (less than 1 per cent).

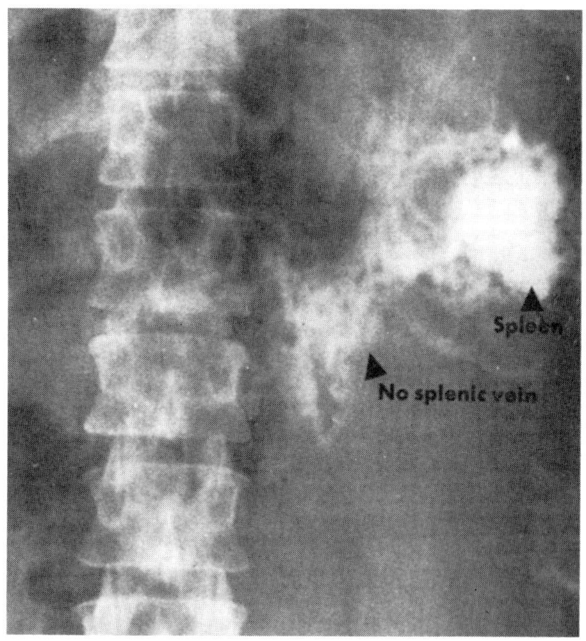

4

Superior mesenteric arteriography

This is often the preferred method of demonstrating the splanchnic circulation and it is the only method if the patient has had a splenectomy.

Advantages

1. Demonstration of vascular anomalies.
2. Determination of patency of portal vein.
3. Demonstration of liver disease, e.g. cirrhosis, hepatoma.
4. Display of local anatomy.

Other radiological investigations

Umbilical vein catheterization requires a minor operation to insert a dilator, and then catheter, into the partially obliterated umbilical vein. The technique not only allows visualization of the portal venous system but direct measurement of portal vein pressure. *Not often used.*

Percutaneous transhepatic catheterization of the portal vein requires considerable expertise and experience. A catheter is passed through the liver into the portal vein to allow direct visualization of the portal vein and measurement of its pressure.

Inferior vena cavagram is essential before a major portasystemic shunt to determine patency of the inferior vena cava.

Intravenous urogram and *left renal venogram* are required before splenorenal shunt.

Hepatic isotope scan and ultrasound examination of the liver

Should be carried out to determine if there is a space-occupying lesion within the liver.

Histology

Should be undertaken to determine the degree of damage to the liver. Major shunting should be avoided in chronic active hepatitis. Normal liver histology suggests a prehepatic cause of portal hypertension.

Electrocardiogram and electroencephalogram

Carried out for baseline investigations.

Wedged hepatic vein pressure

An investigation, which is well established but now performed less often, is the measurement of the wedged hepatic venous pressure. A catheter is passed from an arm vein down the superior vena cava and inferior vena cava into the hepatic vein and into the hepatic venous radicles until it can be inserted no further. The pressure recorded at this stage reflects pressure in the hepatic sinusoids, which is normally 10 cm of saline. When it is used in conjunction with measurement of the splenic pulp pressure, the wedged hepatic vein pressure can help diagnose the cause of portal hypertension. Thus, in obstruction of the main portal vein or in schistosomiasis the splenic pulp pressure is increased but hepatic sinusoidal pressure – and therefore wedged hepatic pressure – remains normal. However, in cirrhosis both the splenic pulp pressure and the wedged hepatic vein pressure are elevated.

IMPROVEMENT OF THE PATIENT'S CONDITION

There is good evidence that improvement of the patient's condition will reduce the risks of operation and improve the patient's chances of surviving another haemorrhage.

1. Hypovolaemia should be fully corrected by transfusion of fresh blood. Half-hearted and incompleted attempts at resuscitation must be avoided.
2. Methods for preventing and reducing encephalopathy (see p. 523) should be continued.
3. If the plasma albumin is less than 30 g/l, a high protein diet should be given (beware of the risks of encephalopathy). Albumin may have to be infused intravenously.
4. Abnormalities in the clotting mechanism should be corrected by the intramuscular administration of vitamin K1, the infusion of platelet concentrates and the replacement of specific clotting deficiencies.
5. Ascites should be vigorously treated with the use of a salt-free diet. Diuretics should be administered but care should be exercised because their too vigorous use may lead to renal failure.
6. Renal function should be carefully monitored to detect early failure.
7. The malnourished patient, especially the alcoholic, should be treated appropriately by diet and vitamins.
8. A search should be made for underlying infection by systematic bacteriology of ascitic fluid, urine, etc. Blood should be cultured.

TO OPERATE OR NOT TO OPERATE – TIMING AND TYPE OF SURGERY

If this is the patient's first haemorrhage, there is a 40 per cent chance that bleeding will not recur in the near future. There is therefore an argument to delay further operative treatment until there is a recurrent haemorrhage. This is a wise decision if a major operation, e.g. portacaval shunt or porta-azygos disconnection, were being contemplated. However, the hazards of lesser procedures, e.g. injection sclerotherapy, are so minor, that even after the first haemorrhage treatment should be instituted to obliterate the varices and reduce the risk of recurrent haemorrhage.

The probability that bleeding will recur is increased if the patient has had previous episodes of haemorrhage; the risks of massive catastrophic haemorrhage are great if the bleeding recurs after operative treatment.

Portal hypertension

An attempt should be made to determine the cause of the portal hypertension because further strategy rests on this decision.

Prehepatic cause; patient under 15 years

If a patient has a prehepatic cause of portal hypertension, e.g. portal vein thrombosis, and is under the age of 15 years (the thrombosis is often secondary to neonatal umbilical sepsis), an adequate collateral circulation usually develops. These young patients have good hepatic function and are able to 'ride out' repeated haemorrhages because of their youth, good general health and absence of underlying liver disease. Radical surgery should therefore be delayed. Each haemorrhage should be treated by vigorous resuscitation and transfusion.

Prehepatic cause; patient over 15 years

If the bleeding continues despite the above measures, or if the patient is above the age of 15 years, it becomes increasingly unlikely that further collaterals will develop and operative intervention is required. The portal and splenic veins are usually thrombosed and therefore not available for major portasystemic shunts. The superior mesenteric vein may be patent and a mesocaval shunt is possible. In children under the age of 15 years, a Clatworthy shunt (*see* p. 587) should be considered because interruption of the inferior vena cava in such young children is not followed by oedema of the lower limb, as in the adult. In older patients interposition mesocaval shunt is a possibility (*see* pp. 581–586).

Sometimes other shunts are possible, for example, a coronary-caval shunt, that is, an anastomosis between the left gastric vein and the inferior vena cava, using a segment of autogenous vein. Makeshift shunts, that is, shunts between dilated collaterals and the systemic veins, should be avoided because the venous wall is extremely flimsy, tears easily and kinking of the veins at the anastomosis is very common.

Alternatively, and more commonly, the varices are tackled directly. The present fashion, which shows reasonable success in the short term, is injection sclerotherapy (*see* pp. 406–412 in this volume). Usually the bleeding can be brought under control and with repeated injection the varices obliterated. Early reports are encouraging but time is required to find how successful this treatment will be in the long term.

If bleeding recurs or if the varices are not controlled with this treatment, major intervention is required. The following operations are available.

Transection and stapling of the oesophagus with the Russian or American stapling instrument (*see* pp. 399–405 in this volume) has the advantage of requiring only a simple abdominal operation. The long-term results are not known.

Boerema-Crile operation, in which the varices in the thoracic oesophagus are individually ligated, is followed commonly by recurrent bleeding.

Milnes-Walker oesophageal transection has the merit of simplicity but, since it is an entirely thoracic operation, the abdominal contents cannot be explored to determine other causes of bleeding. The rate of recurrent bleeding is high.

Porta-azygos disconnection by gastric transection (Tanner operation) is a formidable procedure involving a thoracoabdominal approach and frequently removal of an enlarged spleen to give access. The incidence of rebleeding is high. This is too formidable an operation for severely ill patients.

Ligation and division of the extrinsic venous drainage at the lower end of the oesophagus and the upper end of the stomach is not particularly effective in these patients, but does enjoy popularity in the treatment of schistosomiasis.

If the above attempts at directly ablating the varices are unsuccessful, *oesophagogastrectomy* must be considered. The upper end of the stomach and the lower end of the oesophagus are resected and the oesophagus is then anastomosed to the gastric remnant. Often the spleen is removed. This is a formidable procedure but is reasonably successful in young patients with persistent haemorrhage caused by portal vein thrombosis.

Underlying liver disease

If the cause of the portal hypertension is underlying disease of the liver, further treatment will depend on the type of liver disease and its severity.

Presinusoidal

If the patient has a presinusoidal form of portal hypertension, e.g. hepatic fibrosis, *shunting operations*, e.g. portacaval shunt, are often successful and recurrent bleeding is rare. Encephalopathy is usually not a problem. However, this statement does not hold true for schistosomiasis, which is also a presinusoidal form of portal hypertention. There seems to be a remarkably high incidence of postoperative encephalopathy in these patients and direct attack procedures, e.g. injection, devascularization, etc., are preferred. Good results have also been obtained in patients with schistosomiasis, using a selective shunt, e.g. distal splenorenal (Warren) shunt (*see* pp. 393–398 in this volume).

Postsinusoidal

Patients with postsinusoidal liver diseases, e.g. cirrhosis, have an associated impairment of liver function. The Child classification is of good predictive value in assessing the risks and outcome of operation.

Patients belonging to Child groups A and B should actively be considered for a major portasystemic shunt. Provided that the major vessels are patent, the following shunts should be considered.

An *end-to-side portacaval shunt* does not present great technical difficulty in its performance. The operation is usually successful in the sense that recurrence of bleeding is rare. However, late liver failure and hepato-portal encephalopathy occur in about 20 per cent of the patients. These sequelae are related partly to the progression of the underlying liver disease, as well as to the shunt itself, producing an abrupt venous deprivation of the liver. Recent controlled trials have deprecated the use of major shunts, but these trials were conducted mainly in older male alcoholics, in whom any operative intervention is associated with grave sequelae. Portacaval shunt gives good, well-sustained control of bleeding, with minimal side-effects when it is carried out in the young, non-alcoholic patient with liver disease.

While *interposition mesocaval shunt* (see pp. 581–588) is probably easier to perform, and is therefore an attractive operation in emergency circumstances, it does not seem to possess any other advantages, particularly in the context of postoperative encephalopathy. Indeed there is increasing evidence that the rate of occlusion of the graft is becoming unacceptably high in the months and years after operation.

The *distal splenorenal (Warren) shunt* (see pp. 393–398 in this volume) has been advocated to decompress the splanchnic circulation with a low risk of recurrent bleeding, but at the same time preserving some degree of venous blood flow to the liver. Although this operation is technically demanding to perform, especially in the chronic alcoholic who may have associated chronic pancreatitis, encephalopathy seems to be less common and recurrence of bleeding infrequent.

Patients in Child group C should, in general, not be submitted to a major portasystemic shunt, or indeed any other major operation because of the high mortality and morbidity rate. Repeated injection scleropathy, or transection using a stapling instrument, if the bleeding tends to recur, is advocated.

Bleeding continues or recurs

The patient's condition is usually not good because of continuing repeated bleeding and because of the underlying disease and its consequences. If at all possible, major operations should be avoided. Portasystemic shunts or major attacks directly upon the oesophageal varices should only be undertaken as a last resort after lesser procedures have been tried and found wanting. Considerable judgement is required in choosing the best course for the patient. Thus, in a young patient with good liver function who continues to bleed, the surgeon must be prepared to carry out an oesophagogastrectomy if the underlying cause of the portal hypertension is portal vein thrombosis, or an emergency shunt if the major veins are patent. By contrast there is little place for these major operations in the older alcoholic with poor liver function who is jaundiced, oedematous and advanced in encephalopathy.

Current practice is to employ lesser procedures initially. Injection sclerotherapy should be attempted on at least two occasions with balloon tamponade between sessions to control the haemorrhage. If bleeding continues despite apparently adequate treatment, transection and stapling are indicated. With these treatments bleeding is usually controlled, at least in the short term. The patient's condition can be greatly improved and decisions can be taken about further procedures, particularly major portasystemic shunts.

In selected centres, the varices may be treated by embolization but haemorrhage often recurs after 6–8 weeks.

Acknowledgements

In devising the plan of the initial management of patients with oesophageal varices, I have been greatly helped by the medical and nursing staff at the Royal Liverpool Hospital and Broadgreen Hospital. In particular I should wish to acknowledge my indebtedness to Mr Peres Devitt, FRCS, Mr Shanti Sagar, FRCS and Mr Alan Taylor, FRCS who, as senior registrars in our unit, have played an important part in the management of these ill patients.

Portal hypertension: distal splenorenal (Warren) shunt

R. Shields MD, FRCS, FRCS(Ed.)
Professor of Surgery, University of Liverpool;
Honorary Consultant Surgeon, Royal Liverpool Hospital and Broadgreen Hospital, Liverpool

P. Devitt MS, FRCS
Lecturer in Surgery, University of Liverpool;
Honorary Senior Registrar, Royal Liverpool Hospital

Preoperative

Indications

A technically exacting operation, the distal splenorenal shunt (Warren operation) is finding increasing popularity in the definitive treatment of bleeding oesophageal varices and portal hypertension, because postshunt encephalopathy seems less common than after other conventional shunt operations, e.g. portacaval shunt. However, this benefit may only be obtained in the short term: there is some evidence that, with the passage of time, the diversion of blood from the liver becomes total.

The indications for operation are similar to those already described in the chapter on 'Bleeding oesophageal varices – a plan of management' (*see* pp. 385–392 in this volume). The operation should only be performed electively, when variceal haemorrhage has been brought under control and the patient's general condition, especially hepatic function, has been improved as far as possible. The operation is not suitable as an emergency procedure because several preoperative investigations are required before it is undertaken. Moreover, the duration of the operation owing to its greater technical difficulty makes it unsuitable for an emergency.

The objectives of the operation are: (*1*) to reduce pressure in the splanchnic venous circulation by anastomosing the distal (splenic) end of the splenic vein to the side of the left renal vein; (*2*) to preserve direct venous connections between the spleen and the stomach (short gastric veins) to decompress the critical area at the gastro-oesophageal junction; (*3*) to maintain a selective portal venous flow to the liver to prevent further deterioration in its function.

Unless indicated otherwise the cross-references in this chapter refer to *Operative Surgery: Alimentary Tract and Abdominal Wall, Volume 2, 4th Edition*

Contraindications

These are described on p. 581.

An additional, and absolute, contraindication is the absence, or thrombosis, of the splenic vein, or absence, thrombosis or congenital anomaly of the left renal vein.

The operation can be difficult in the presence of gross obesity or massive splenomegaly.

Preoperative evaluation

The preoperative evaluation of a patient with portal hypertension has already been described (*see* pp. 385–392 in this volume). The following specific investigations should also be performed.

1. Preoperative angiography, to establish the patency of the splenic vein, usually by splenoportography.
2. Left renal venography, by means of a catheter passed percutaneously up the inferior vena cava from a femoral vein, to demonstrate the presence, and normality, of the renal vein. The operation may be rendered difficult, or impossible, by thrombosis or congenital duplication, or even triplication, of the left renal vein. The combination of splenoportography and left renal venography permits a preoperative assessment of the relative positions of the renal vein and the splenic vein. Occasionally, if these veins are too far apart, the operation may not be feasible and another type of shunt may have to be undertaken.
3. Intravenous urogram, to determine the presence and function of the kidneys.

The operation

Position of patient and incision

The patient is placed in a supine position with the left side slightly elevated. The abdomen is open through a long, midline incision. However, a transverse incision in the upper abdomen can be used with advantage in grossly obese patients.

Wide abdominal exploration should be avoided because of the risk of haemorrhage from the tearing of vascular adhesions between the abdominal viscera and parietes. The abdominal viscera are carefully examined and, if the portal pressure has not been hitherto measured, or if splanchnic venography is considered essential, a fine catheter may be inserted into a small branch of a jejunal mesenteric vein and advanced into a major trunk.

1

(This, and all subsequent illustrations, are shown as if the viewer were standing in the position of the surgeon, on the patient's right-hand side.)

The illustration shows a cirrhotic liver and the stomach with attached greater omentum.

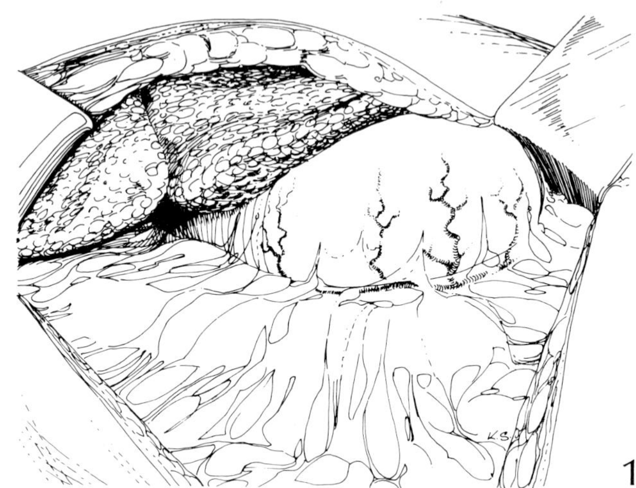

1

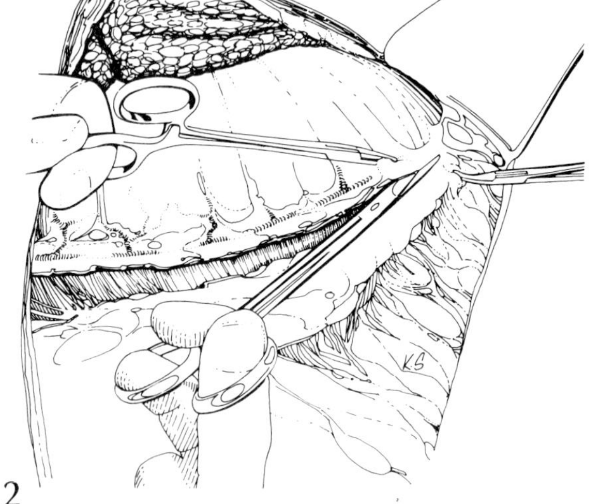

2

2

The lesser sac is opened by dividing the gastrocolic omentum between clamps, outside the arcade of the gastroepiploic vein which is separately identified, ligated and cut.

3

The division of the gastrocolic omentum continues to the left, until the short gastric (gastrosplenic) veins are reached. In this illustration, the spleen (which is shown small for the purpose of clarity) can be clearly seen in front of the retractor. The stomach has been drawn to the right and large gastrosplenic veins are seen crossing from the upper part of the greater curvature of the stomach to the splenic hilum.

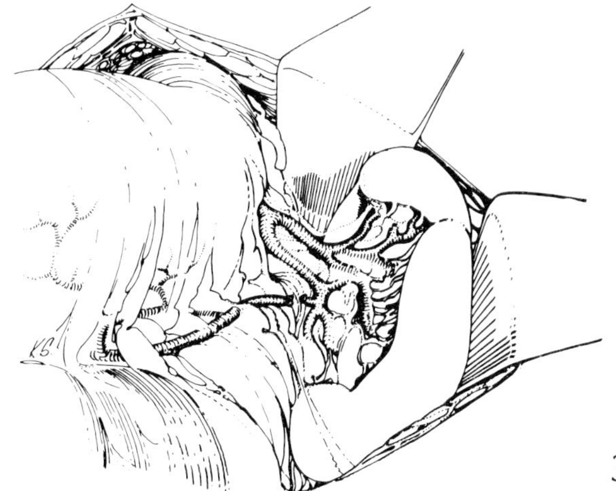

3

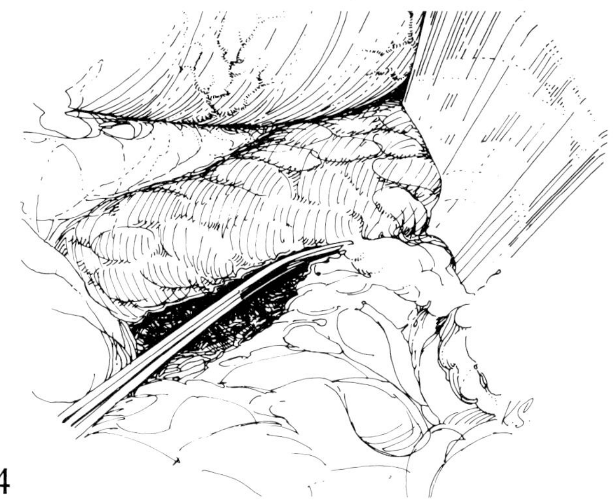

4

4

The stomach is lifted cranially and the transverse colon caudally to open the lesser sac. Any adhesions crossing the lesser sac between the stomach and the posterior abdominal wall should be identified, separately ligated and cut.

In the posterior wall of the lesser sac the pancreas is identified and the peritoneum along its inferior border incised, so that the pancreas, over a distance of 10 cm, can be reflected cranially.

5

After sufficient length of the pancreas has been mobilized, the splenic vein is identified. The splenic vein can usually be seen as the inferior border of the pancreas is reflected cranially, because it lies attached to, or adjacent to, the posterior surface of the pancreas near its inferior border. The inferior aspect of the splenic vein is the easiest to dissect because only a few vessels join this surface, which should be cleared over a distance of 8–10 cm. Dissection of the splenic vein should be continued medially, that is to the right. The inferior mesenteric vein is ligated and divided close to the junction of the splenic vein with the superior mesenteric vein.

The mobilization of the splenic vein from the posterior surface of the pancreas may be a difficult and tedious part of the operation, because of the fragile, short and stumpy pancreatic veins which join the splenic vein. These vessels should be carefully identified, ligated doubly and divided between ligatures. Clamps should not be applied because they can easily be torn off with troublesome, and occasionally catastrophic, bleeding.

In this way the splenic vein is mobilized over a sufficient length, that is 8–10 cm, for subsequent anastomosis to the renal vein. The vein is not divided at this stage, because the consequent venous congestion may produce a troublesome ooze.

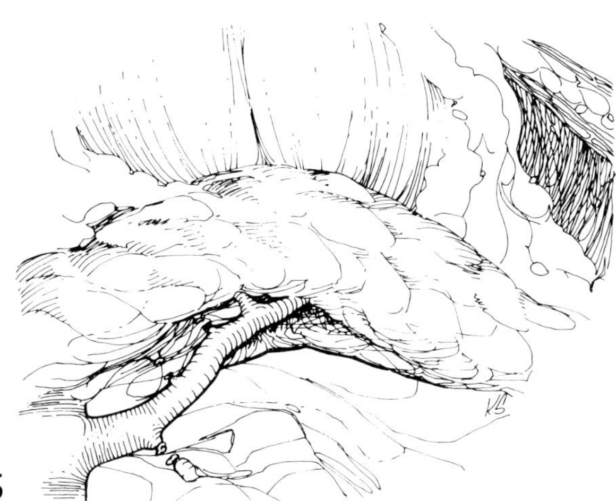

5

6

The left renal vein should now be identified. Its position relative to the splenic vein should have been suggested by preoperative splenoportography and left renal venography. The renal vein often lies more deeply than suspected, particularly in obese patients, and indeed is frequently covered by 3–4 cm of dense retroperitoneal tissue. Certain fixed landmarks are helpful in exposing the left renal vein[1]. A triangular area should be identified, bounded medially by the superior mesenteric artery, laterally by the left border of the superior duodenal fold (or duodenojejunal fold) and inferiorly by the fourth part of the duodenum where it joins the jejunum. The left renal vein usually crosses deep in the retroperitoneal space opposite this triangle.

Great care should be taken to avoid injury to the left renal vein. Venous collaterals nearby may be the source of troublesome bleeding if accidentally damaged. Dissection of the renal vein into the hilum of the left kidney should be avoided because major haemorrhage may result, perhaps necessitating nephrectomy.

Occasionally the veins draining the left suprarenal gland and the left testicular, or ovarian, vein have to be divided to provide better exposure and more mobility of the left renal vein.

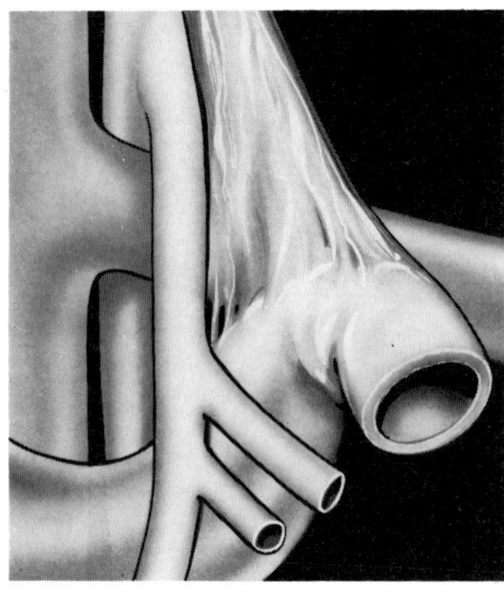

6

7

When the two veins are completely dissected, the splenic vein is divided between clamps close to its junction with the superior mesenteric vein. In this illustration the pancreas is held up cranially by tissue forceps. The left renal vein is seen in the depth of the wound.

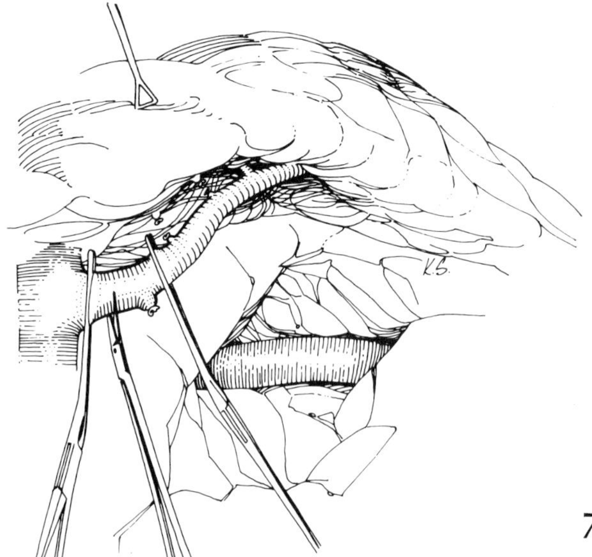

7

8

The stump of the splenic vein, where it joins the superior mesenteric vein, is then closed with a continuous 5/0 arterial suture.

At this stage the left gastric vein may easily be identified and, if desired, can be ligated above its junction with the portal vein.

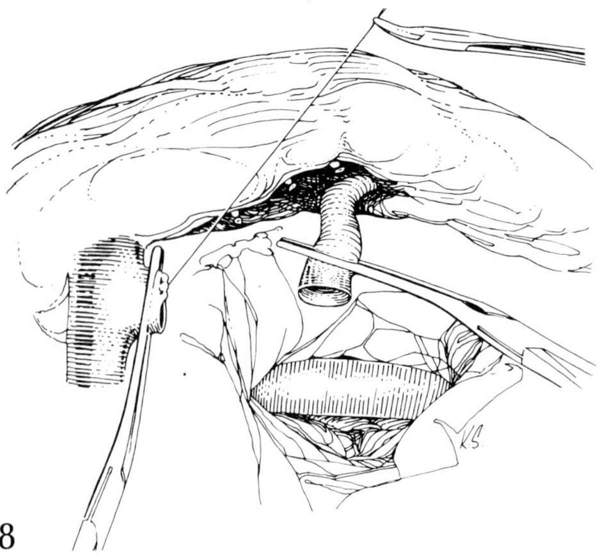

8

9

The site of anastomosis of the splenic vein to the renal vein should now be selected. Kinking or twisting of the vessels should be avoided. A simple anterior venotomy of the renal vein is not sufficient. A partially occluding clamp is applied to the renal vein and a small segment of its superior surface is excised.

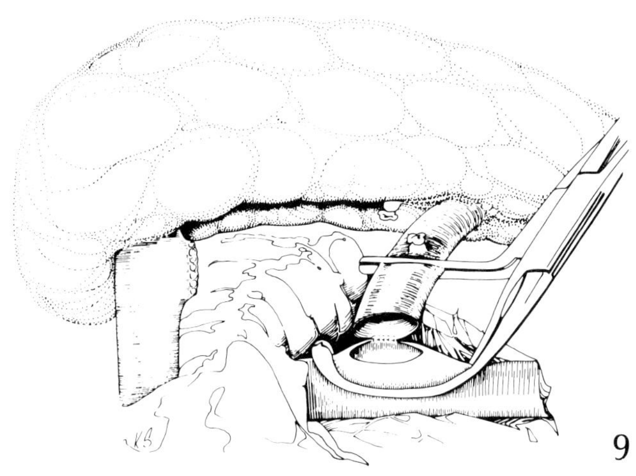

9

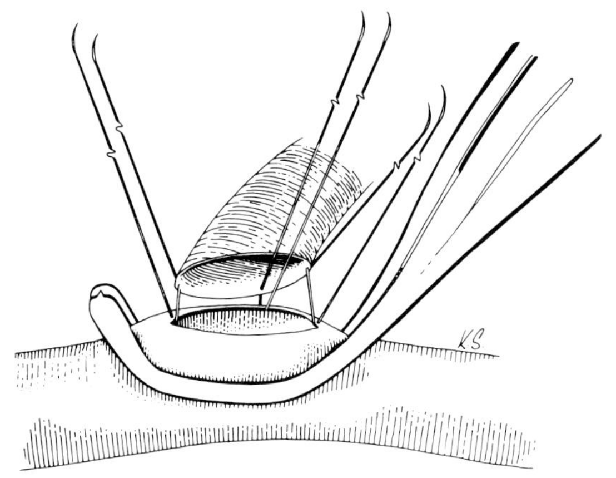

10

10

Great care should be taken to avoid rotation or twisting of the splenic vein. The splenic vein should be trimmed obliquely to ensure a long anastomosis, after marking its inferior border which becomes the left angle of the anastomosis. An end-to-side anastomosis is begun using continuous 5/0 arterial suture.

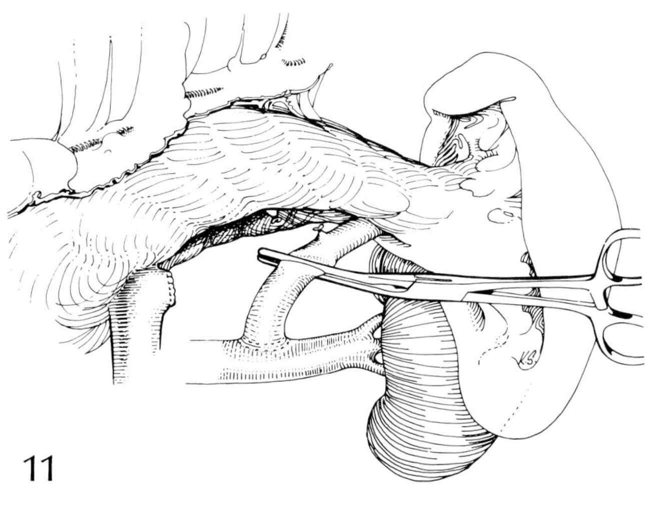

11

11

The anterior row of sutures is then applied, either continuously or in an interrupted fashion. The anastomosis is thus completed, and clamps removed. The fall in portal pressure is measured either by direct puncture of the splenic vein or by means of the catheter previously inserted into a jejunal mesenteric vein. The fall in the portal pressure is usually not so marked as after an end-to-side portacaval shunt.

12

Attention is now directed to the completion of the porta-azygos disconnection. The lesser omentum is divided and the left gastric vein is freed from surrounding structures, doubly ligated and divided.

During the course of this disconnection, the splenic artery and the hepatic arteries should be preserved. The right gastric artery should not be divided. The vagus nerves should also be preserved.

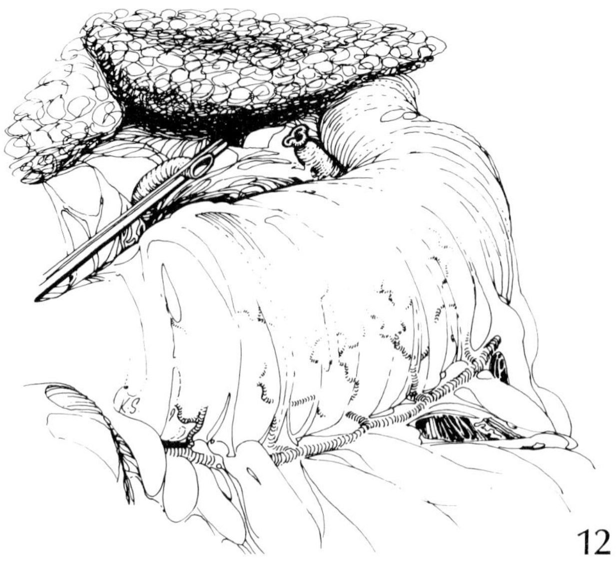

12

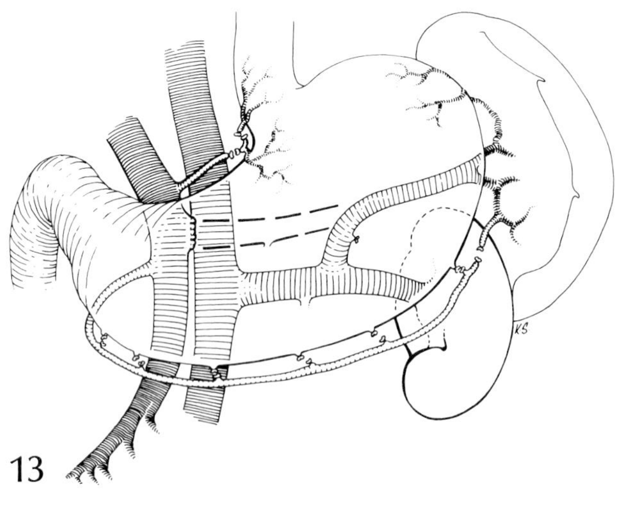

13

13

This diagram shows the completed operation.

Wound closure

The wound is closed in the usual fashion, using non-absorbable sutures for the linea alba or rectus sheath.

Postoperative care

Hyperbilirubinaemia and transient postoperative ascites are common. The postoperative care described on p. 586 should be followed.

Reference

1. Warren, W. D., Salam, A. A., Faraldo, A. Hutson, D., Smith, R. B. End renal vein-to-splenic vein shunts for total or selective portal decompression. Surgery 1972; 72: 995–1006

Transabdominal oesophageal transection

George W. Johnston MCh, FRCS
Consultant Surgeon, Royal Victoria Hospital, Belfast;
Honorary Lecturer in Surgery, Queen's University, Belfast

Introduction

In patients with one episode of proven bleeding from oesophageal varices, the risk of rebleeding within the next 6 months is very high. Unfortunately, the majority of these patients are not suitable candidates for shunt surgery and a devascularization procedure offers a reasonably satisfactory alternative. Since Boerema[1] and Crile[2] first described a technique of direct ligation of the varices, there have been many modifications of the method. The most exciting change has been the application of a circular stapling apparatus for the anastomosis[3,4,5]. This allows oesophageal transection to be performed via the abdomen and provides full-thickness division of the oesophageal wall with safe anastomosis. However, it is probably wise to use one of the forms of injection sclerotherapy (*see* pp. 406–412 in this volume) for the emergency control of bleeding, reserving transection until after recovery from the acute episode.

The operation

Position of patient and incision

The patient is placed supine on the operating table and a midline supraumbilical incision is normally used. However, if splenectomy is considered necessary because of severe hypersplenism, a left subcostal incision gives better exposure. Exploration of the abdomen is carried out to confirm the diagnosis and exclude other relevant disease such as peptic ulceration, gall stones or hepatoma. Generally, the main channel transmitting the high portal pressure to the oesophageal varices is a large left gastric vein which must be ligated.

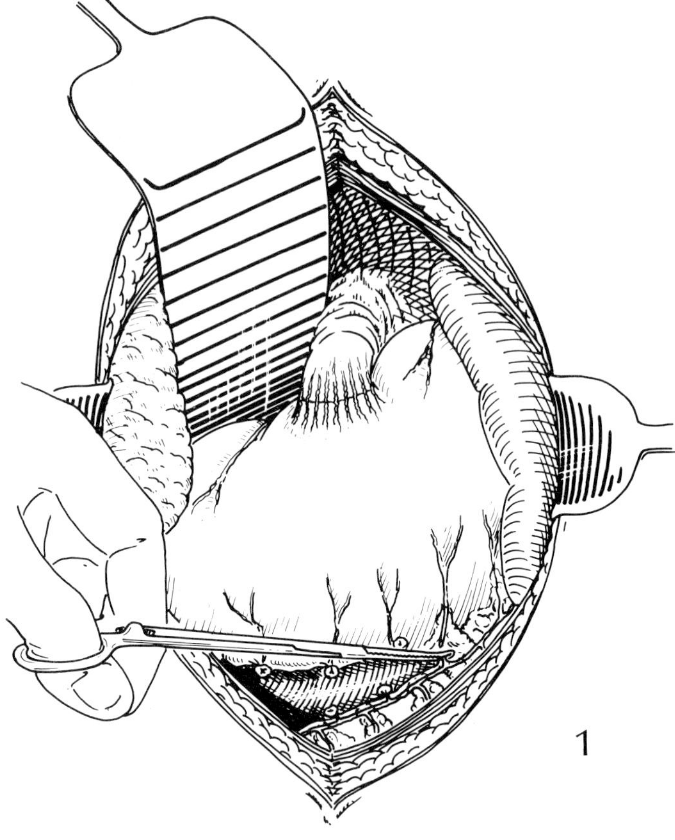

1

1

Exposure of left gastric pedicle

The left gastric pedicle can be approached from the lesser curvature of the stomach through the gastrohepatic omentum, but the approach via an opening in the gastrocolic omentum at the greater curvature is easier and allows a better view. Individual gastroepiploic vessels are ligated, making an opening into the lesser sac large enough to allow easy vision of the left gastric pedicle at the upper border of the pancreas. If the window is too small, further tearing of the gastroepiploic arcade is almost inevitable, causing unnecessary blood loss. One or two packs may be inserted to protect the large spleen and also to retain the viscera inferiorly.

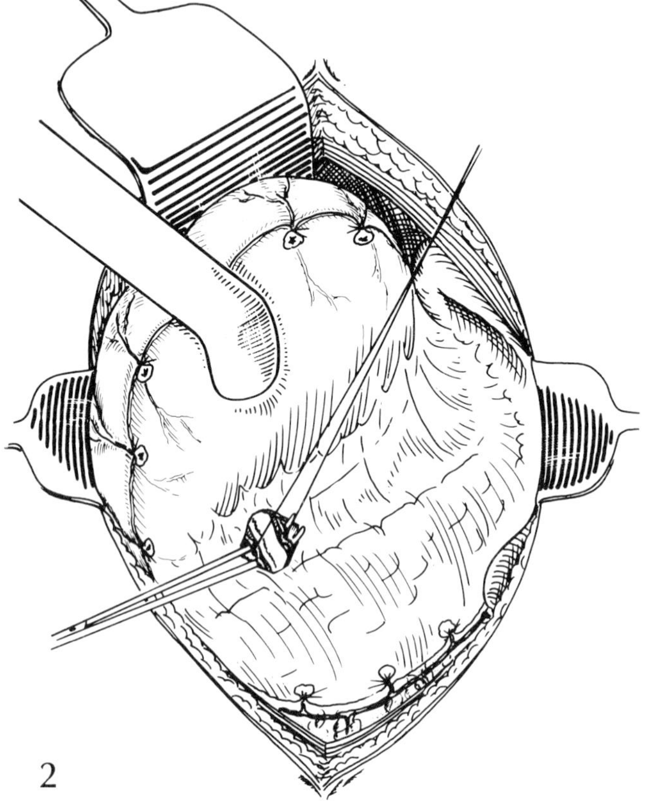

2

Ligation of left gastric pedicle

2

The mobilized stomach is retracted upwards and any adhesions in the lesser sac divided until the left gastric pedicle is reached at the upper border of the pancreas. Even in portal hypertension, these adhesions are generally not very vascular and diathermy is sufficient to control bleeding. The pedicle of left gastric vessels is cleared sufficiently inferiorly to allow vision of the main left gastric vein. It is not necessary to dissect out the individual vein as it is best to ligate all the vessels in the pedicle and not merely the main left gastric vein. Using fine right-angled forceps, a No. 0 linen or other non-absorbable ligature is passed around the whole pedicle and tied in continuity; care must be taken not to tear any branches with the clamp. A second ligature should be applied or, alternatively a large metal clip can be used; it is not necessary to divide the pedicle.

3

Mobilization of oesophagus

Attention is now turned to the region of the oesophago-gastric junction. In portal hypertension the peritoneum on the front of the oesophagus generally contains multiple fine spidery venules. In spite of this extra vasculature, it is usually possible to visualize the 'white line' underneath the peritoneum, marking the position of the phreno-oesophageal ligament (i.e. the peritoneal reflexion from diaphragm to oesophagus). A transverse incision is made in the peritoneum at this level. Bleeding from small peritoneal vessels is easily controlled by diathermy. When the phreno-oesophageal ligament has been exposed, it is brushed upwards using a small gauze dissector. This exposes the oesophagus and the large perioesophageal collateral veins which lie deep to the peritoneum.

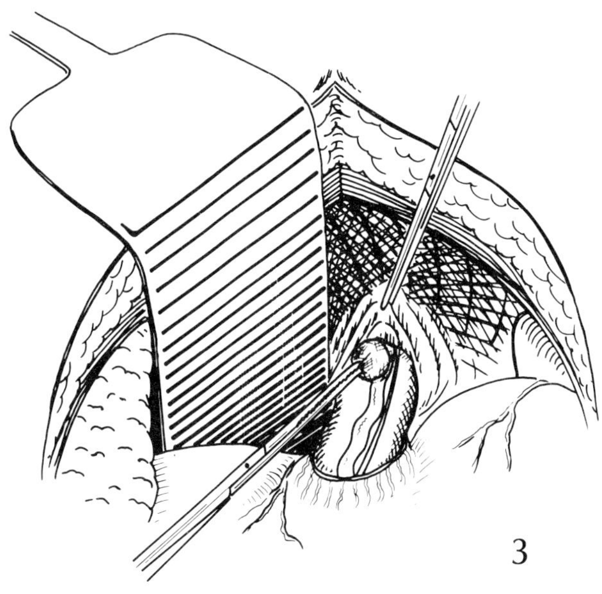

3

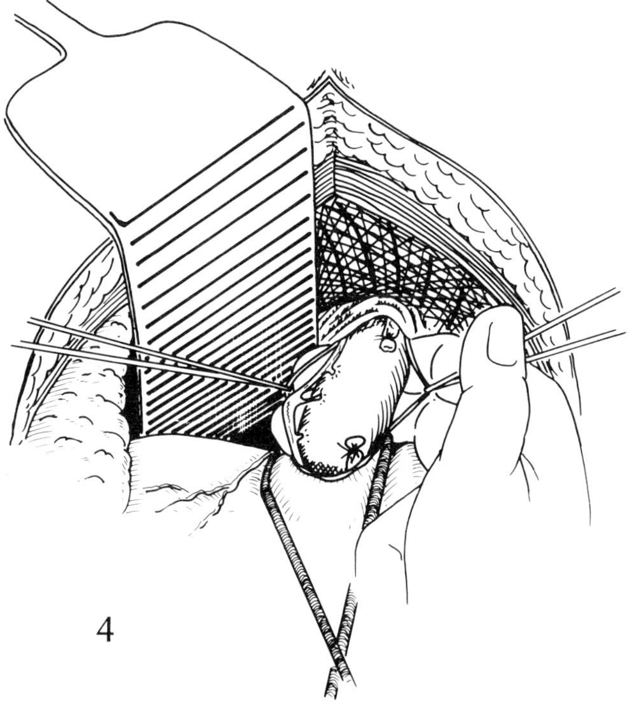

4

Devascularization of lower oesophagus

4

Usually, one or two large channels run with the anterior vagus and a number of even larger vessels run with the posterior vagus. It is usually possible to free these vessels from the anterior and posterior vagus nerves which are then protected in Silastic slings. At this stage it is helpful to place a rubber catheter sling around the oesophagus to aid in its future manipulation. With the fingers positioned behind the oesophagus, the posterior veins are displaced forwards to facilitate separation from the posterior vagus. If there is difficulty in separating the vessels from the vagi, one or other vagus nerve, but not both, may be sacrificed. The vessels should then be separated from the oesophageal wall for a distance of 5 or 6 cm, ligated and divided.

5

Branches passing directly into the oesophagus from these vessels require individual ligation or diathermy coagulation on the oesophageal side. Usually, there are only one or two branches on the front, but three or four such veins penetrate the oesophagus from the posterior vessel or vessels. It is often stated that dissection around the hiatus carries a high risk of serious haemorrhage in patients with portal hypertension but this is rarely the case. However, mobilization of the oesophagus can be more difficult in patients who have had previous injection sclerotherapy or who have perioesophagitis from an associated hiatus hernia.

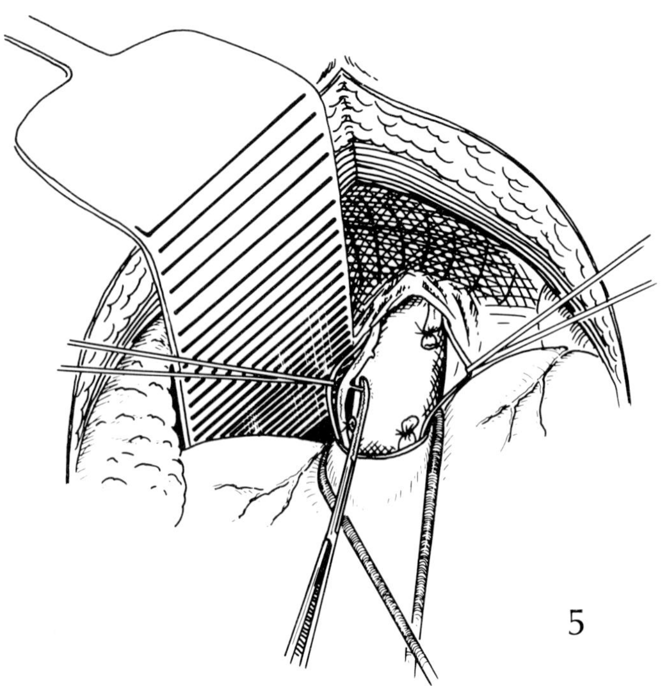

5

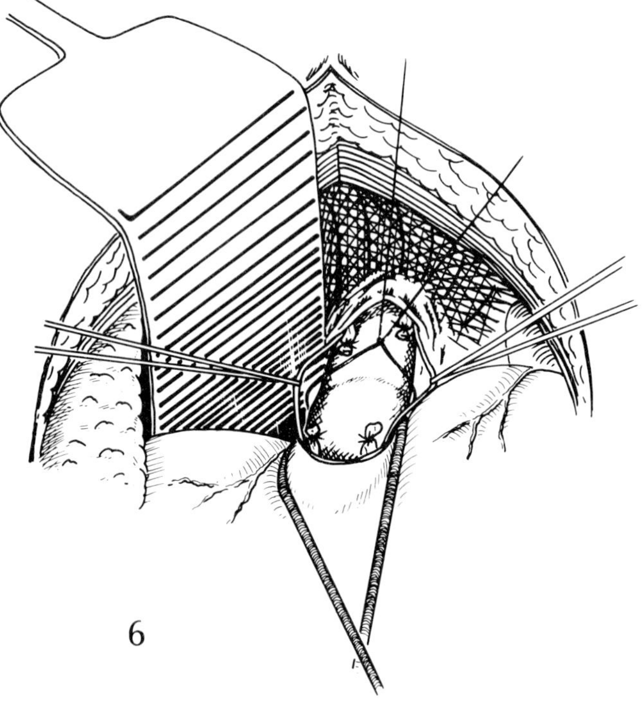

6

6

Placement of encircling ligature

A No. 0 linen ligature is passed around the now cleared oesophagus and loosely tied. It is important to place this ligature in position before insertion of the stapling device; with the device in place it is technically much more difficult and also increases the risk of damage to the oesophageal wall.

Insertion of the stapler

A number of circular stapling guns are now available and more are being produced. The American-produced EEA stapler is supplied with disposable heads of 25, 28 and 31 mm diameter, respectively. The Russian-produced SPTU gun is supplied with four interchangeable rechargeable staple-bearing heads of 21, 26, 29 and 32 mm diameter, respectively. The Ethicon 'Proximate' ILS has an approximately similar configuration. In large male patients it may be possible to use the largest diameter head but often a smaller size is required; a sizer can be introduced into the oesophagus to assess which head will fit comfortably without risk of oesophageal splitting.

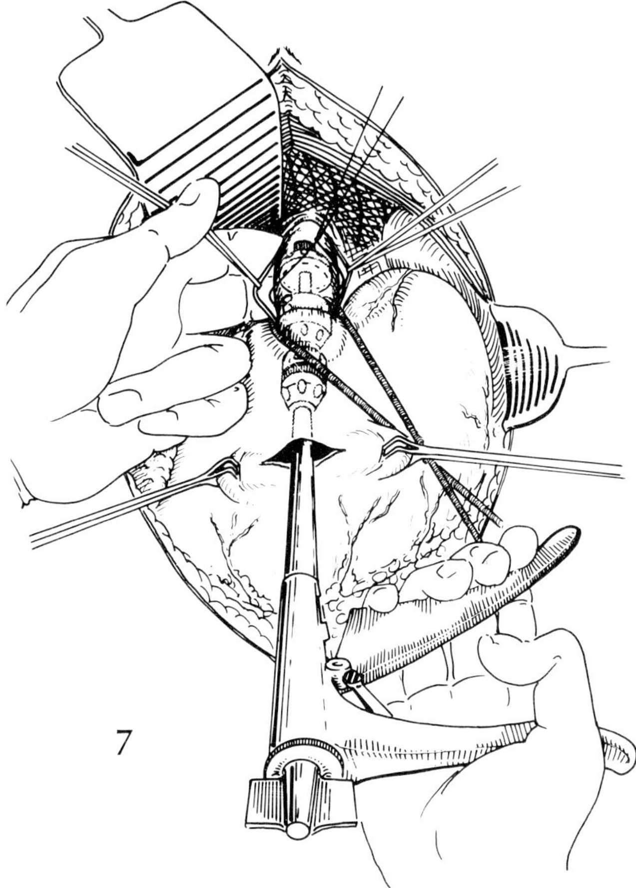

7

7

A small gastrotomy is made in a relatively avascular part of the anterior wall of the stomach. The gun is then advanced through the gastrotomy into the lower oesophagus, making sure that neither the linen ligature nor the rubber catheter is causing obstruction by constricting the oesophagus from the posterior aspect. When the gun has been advanced into the oesophagus for 5 or 6 cm, the gap in the head of the gun is opened up by adjusting the nut in its handle; a gap of about 3 cm should be produced between the two portions of the head. The gun is then carefully withdrawn down the oesophagus until digital palpation confirms that the lowest part of this gap in the head lies immediately above the gastro-oesophageal junction. The assistant must support the handle of the gun and prevent it slipping backwards too far towards the stomach. Traction on the rubber sling around the oesophagus is helpful at this point.

Technique of transection

8

The previously placed linen ligature is now tied, thus invaginating a flange of full-thickness oesophageal wall between the two portions of the head of the gun. The gap is reduced to less than 2 mm, care being taken not to include the rubber oesophageal sling.

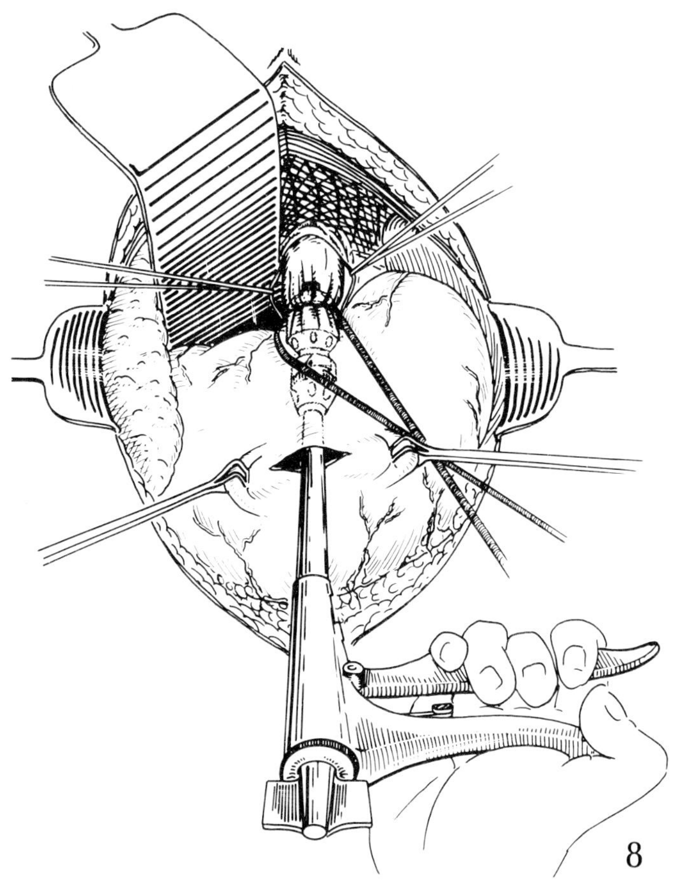

8

9

In the American EEA gun it is only necessary to align the black mark (A) on the spindle of the gun within the marker (B) on the body. In the Russian SPTU gun the 2 mm distance is assessed on the micrometer scale (B) after the hole (A) in the spindle of the gun becomes totally visible beyond the micrometer screw. A similar technique is used for the ILS. When the trigger is pulled, a circular guillotine cuts off a ring of full-thickness oesophagus and one (SPTU gun) or two (EEA gun; ILS gun) rows of staples are inserted.

Where the anastomosis has only one row of staples, it is probably advisable to insert a few reinforcing muscular sutures anteriorly. Before withdrawing the gun through the newly formed anastomosis, it is necessary to reopen the gap in the head of the gun to about 3 cm. The head of the gun is then eased through the anastomosis and withdrawn.

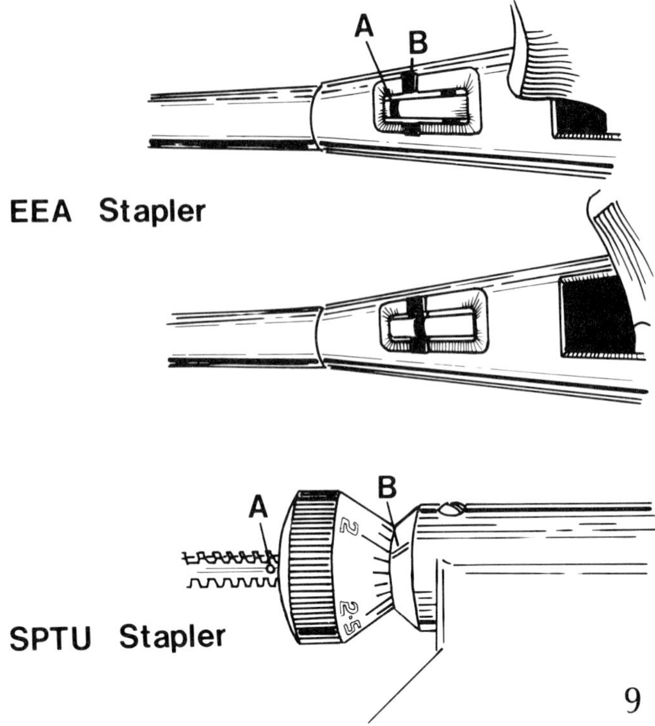

9

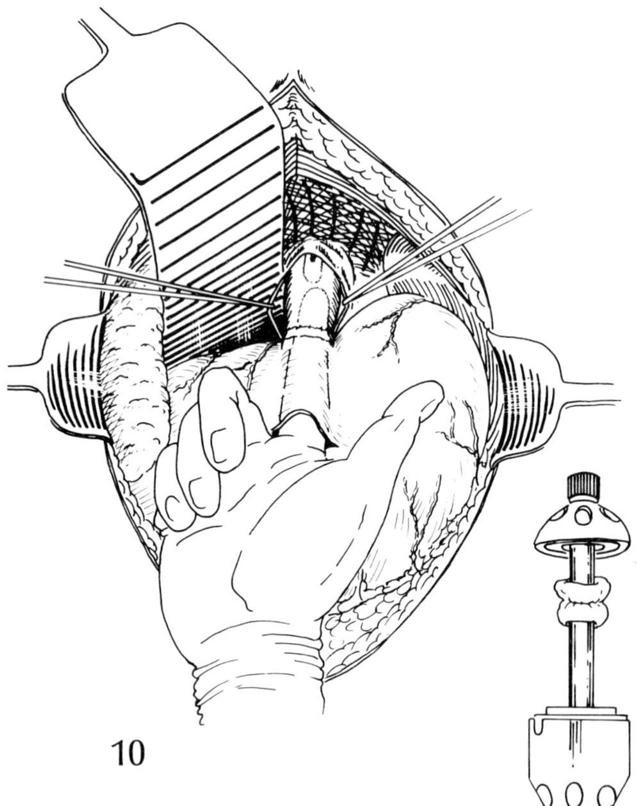

10

10

The ring of tissue in the gun is inspected: a complete 'doughnut' of full-thickness oesophageal wall indicates a satisfactory transection. A finger is introduced through the gastrotomy wound to confirm the satisfactory nature of the suture line and to direct a nasogastric tube into the stomach for postoperative decompression.

Closure

The gastrotomy wound is closed in two layers using a polyglycolic acid (Dexon; Vicryl) suture. A number of needle biopsies or a wedge biopsy of liver should be obtained before closing the abdomen in layers. Because ascites can form in the postoperative period, it is wiser not to drain the abdomen in order to prevent significant protein loss.

Postoperative care

Postoperatively, nasogastric aspiration continues for 24–48 h but all oral fluids are withheld until the fifth postoperative day, after which the patient is gradually introduced to a normal diet.

Additional procedures

The abdominal approach allows additional procedures to be carried out where indicated. For example, where splenectomy is indicated because of hypersplenism, it is advisable to do this before the ligation of the left gastric pedicle in that splenectomy greatly facilitates the approach to this vessel in the lesser sac. Where a patient has a concomitant peptic ulcer, the gastrotomy for the introduction of the gun can be made in the most dependent part of the stomach and subsequently used for gastrojejunostomy in conjunction with vagotomy.

Results

Since January 1976 we have used this method in 79 patients with bleeding oesophageal varices; all were considered unsuitable for shunt surgery. The Russian SPTU gun was used in 64 patients and the American EEA stapler in 15. Of the 79 patients, 69 had cirrhosis and 10 had extrahepatic block; 40 per cent of the cirrhotics were alcholics. The average age in the series was 55 (range 14–81) and there were 42 males in the group. Using Child's classification, there were 33 Grade A patients, 15 B, and 31 with Grade C hepatic dysfunction. The fact that 33 Grade A patients were considered shunt rejects is due to the high age of many of the patients (17 were over 70), the 19 operations for acute bleeding, and the inclusion of 10 patients with extrahepatic block and no veins suitable for shunting. The overall hospital mortality for the series was 14 per cent. In the 19 emergency transections the mortality rose to 31 per cent while in the remaining non-emergency operations it was only 8 per cent. Most of the deaths were due to liver failure, often progressing to multiple organ failure. No patient developed a leak from the oesophageal suture line but one had an iatrogenic perforation of the oesophagus 2 cm above the transection line – the result of dilatation of a pre-existing stricture caused by previous injection sclerotherapy. Many patients developed minor dysphagia for a few weeks after starting on solid food, but in the majority this settled spontaneously. However, 11 of the 68 survivors (16 per cent) required one or more oesophageal dilatations with Eder-Puestow dilators. Dysphagia was more of a problem in the early part of the series when the transection was done 2 or 3 cm above the cardia; we now do the transection immediately above the oesophagogastric junction.

Obviously, this operation is not as effective as a portacaval shunt in preventing recurrent bleeding but it has the advantage of not predisposing to portal systemic encephalopathy. Only 4 patients have had postoperative encephalopathy and the episodes have been transient. Of the 68 patients who survived to leave hospital, 13 have had further bleeding episodes but in only 4 were varices shown to be the source of haemorrhage. One patient with recurrent variceal bleeding died and 3 of the others, who bled from other sites, also died. In all, there have been 12 late deaths in the series, occurring after an average of 19 months; thus, of the original 79 patients, 56 (71 per cent) still survive after a mean follow-up of almost 3 years.

It is felt that in patients unfit for shunt surgery, or where the risks of postshunt encephalopathy are high, oesophageal transection offers a useful alternative technique.

References

1. Boerema, I. Bleeding varices of the oesophagus in cirrhosis of the liver and Banti's syndrome. Archivum Chirurgicum Neerlandicum 1949; 1: 253–260
2. Crile, G. S. Transesophageal ligation of bleeding esophageal varices: a preliminary report of 7 cases. Archives of Surgery 1950; 61: 654–660
3. Van Kemmel, M. Résection-anastomose de l'oesophage sus-cardial pour rupture de varices oesophagiennes. Nouvelle Presse Médicale 1976; 5: 1123–1124
4. Johnston, G. W. Treatment of bleeding varices by oesophageal transection with the SPTU gun. Annals of the Royal College of Surgeons of England 1977; 59: 404–408
5. Johnston, G. W. Bleeding oesophageal varices: the management of shunt rejects. Annals of the Royal College of Surgeons of England 1981; 63: 3–8

Sclerosant injection of oesophageal varices

John Terblanche ChM, FRCS, FCS(SA)
Professor and Head, Department of Surgery, University of Cape Town and Groote Schuur Hospital;
Co-Director, Medical Research Council Liver Research Group, University of Cape Town, South Africa

History

Crafoord and Frenckner first used injection sclerotherapy in 1936 in Scandinavia and published their case report in 1939[1]. Moersch of the Mayo Clinic reported one case in 1940 and by 1947 had accumulated 22 patients using sodium morrhuate as sclerosant[2]. The same solution was used by the British pioneer, Macbeth, of Oxford, whose major publication in 1955 restimulated interest in the technique[3]. Despite early enthusiasm and success, the widespread introduction of portacaval shunting tended to overshadow injection sclerotherapy, which was infrequently used for the next three decades. Notable exceptions were Johnston and Rodgers of Belfast, who used ethanolamine oleate as the sclerosant[4], and Continental workers, including Wodak[5] and Pacquet[6], who built up considerable experience. Renewed interest has arisen as a result of recent dissatisfaction with conventional portacaval shunting.

Principles and alternative techniques

Of all the definitive procedures available today, peroesophageal injection sclerotherapy is the only simple technique that deals directly with the fundamental problem in patients who have had a variceal haemorrhage, namely, the submucosal oesophageal varices themselves.

Intravascular injection: rigid oesophagoscope

We inject ethanolamine oleate intravascularly directly into the varices at the oesophagogastric junction using a rigid oesophagoscope under general anaesthesia. The aim is to thrombose the varices and the technique has proved highly successful[4,7–9]. Although ethanolamine oleate is not freely available in the United States, sodium morrhuate 5 per cent appears to be a satisfactory alternative sclerosant.

Intravascular injection: fibreoptic oesophagoscope

The Kings College Hospital group have developed a sheath with a window, which is passed over the fibreoptic scope to simulate the rigid scope technique[10]. However, they use general anaesthesia, which removes one of the major advantages of using the fibreoptic scope. Other workers have incorporated balloons, either attached to the scope[11] or distal to the scope[12], to compress the varices. These procedures should be applicable without an anaesthetic. There are also groups who inject various sclerosants directly into the varices without subsequent compression. All require controlled trials comparing them with the established rigid scope technique.

Submucosal injection

Submucosal injection has been widely practised in Europe with good results[5,6]. The injections are placed submucosally adjacent to the varices, with the aim of thickening the mucosa and thereby preventing bleeding. Originally a rigid oesophagoscope was used with general anaesthesia, but the procedure can be easily performed with a fibreoptic scope without anaesthesia. Although local oedema is said to prevent recurrent acute bleeding, it is difficult to conceive how it can be as effective as intravascular injection. Only a controlled trial will answer this question.

Indirect percutaneous transhepatic sclerotherapy

Here the coronary vein with or without the short gastric veins is sclerosed or occluded via the portal vein using the indirect percutaneous transhepatic route. Good results have been reported by a number of groups, particularly Viamonte *et al.* of Miami[13]. However, the originators of the technique from Lund, Sweden have emphasized the problems and no longer utilize the procedure for acute variceal bleeding[14]. Major problems include portal vein thrombosis in 36 per cent of patients, a 55 per cent rebleed rate and difficulty in repeating the technique in long-term management (*see also* p. 392 in this volume).

Preoperative

Preoperative preparation in acute variceal bleeds

Patients are admitted to hospital, resuscitated and, if variceal bleeding is suspected, vasopressin (Pitressin) is administered intravenously. Although we originally used bolus doses[7,9], continuous intravenous infusion at the rate of 0.4 u/min is preferred[15,16] (*see also* p. 386 in this volume). Emergency endoscopy is mandatory to confirm that the patient has oesophageal varices and that a varix, rather than another lesion, is the site of bleeding[7,9]. Sengstaken tube tamponade is reserved for those patients in whom initial conservative management fails and who are still actively bleeding from varices at the time of endoscopy. Correct use of the Sengstaken tube is essential to prevent complications. The technique is described in detail elsewhere[17] (*see also* p. 387 in this volume). A properly sited Sengstaken tube will invariably control bleeding, even if only temporarily[7,9]. Unfortunately, the rebleed rate is high after removal of the tube. Patients should thus proceed to injection sclerotherapy for definitive control of bleeding[7,9]. Emergency injection sclerotherpy is only required in the difficult group of patients who continue to bleed and who are initial Sengstaken tube tamponade.

Once the Sengstaken tube has been inserted the patient is prepared for theatre. Energetic resuscitation is continued until the patient is stable, clotting defects are corrected and the patient rendered as fit as possible for a general anaesthetic. Emergency injection sclerotherapy is performed 6–24 h later, at a convenient time. A major advantage of preliminary Sengstaken tube tamponade is that bleeding will have been controlled by the time sclerotherapy is performed, and rigid endoscopy is not undertaken in the extremely dangerous setting of active variceal bleeding.

Anaesthesia

In Cape Town a standard anaesthetic regimen has been used as part of the trial protocol and has proved satisfactory. Premedication is with atropine (0.6 mg) and diazepam (5–10 mg) unless the patient is stuporous or unconscious. The drugs are frequently given in the operating theatre. Thiopentone sodium and suxamethonium are used for induction of anaesthesia, and anaesthesia is maintained with nitrous oxide/oxygen, intermittent thiopentone plus intermittent suxamethonium or alloferrin.

The operation

Removal of Sengstaken tube

With injections for acute variceal bleeds the Sengstaken tube will be *in situ*. It should not be removed until the patient is anaesthetized and intubated and the surgeon ready to insert the oesophagoscope immediately after withdrawal of the tube. In chronic injections to eradicate varices the patient will not have a Sengstaken tube *in situ* but the procedure is otherwise the same.

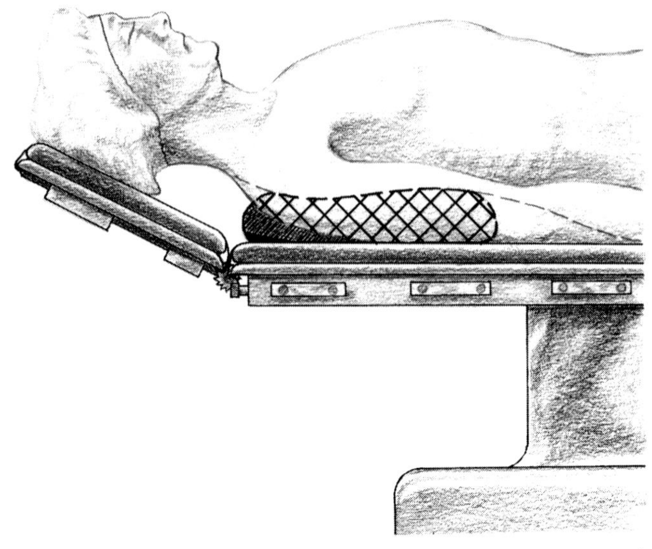

1

1

Position of patient

The patient is carefully positioned on an operating table with a movable headpiece so that the head can be flexed or extended. To facilitate insertion of the oesophagoscope and prevent bronchial compression, a small sandbag is placed between the shoulder blades. The operator sits at the head of the table with the anaesthetist on his left and the theatre sister on his right.

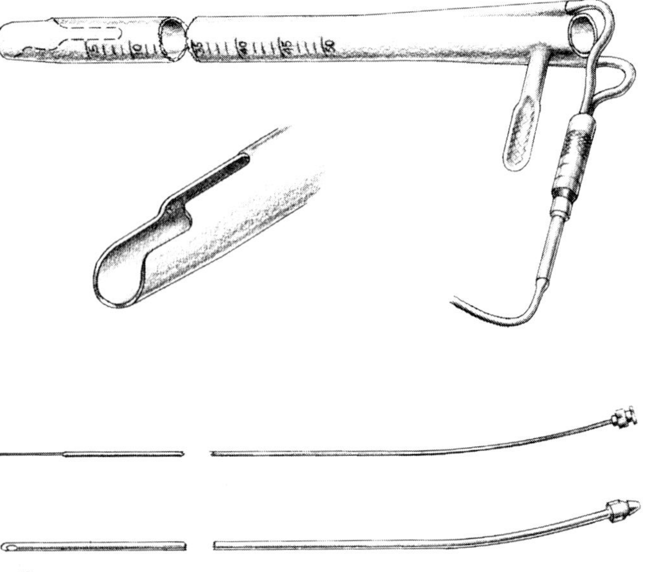

2

2

The oesophagoscope

A 50 cm rigid Negus oesophagoscope with proximal fibre lighting is modified by cutting a slot (4 cm × 0.5 cm) at the distal end opposite the beak[18]. A long wide-bore sucker is required to remove blood and secretions. The modified Macbeth or Roberts needle, which is longer than the oesophagoscope, has a 21 or 22 gauge tip and a secure syringe fitting at the other end. Both should be off-set at the proximal end so that they do not obscure vision.

3

Insertion of the oesophagoscope

The upper teeth are protected with a lubricated gauze swab or a Silastic tooth or gum guard. The neck is partially flexed and the endotracheal tube moved to the left. The beak of the scope is passed over the dorsum of the tongue into the pharynx, at the same time sweeping the scope gently backwards. As the larynx is reached, the scope is directed to the right into the pyriform sinus and advanced 2–3 cm. It is then brought back into the midline and lifts the larynx forwards. The cricopharyngeal sphincter is then visualized and the oesophagoscope passed into the upper oesophagus. At times difficulty is experienced and it is necessary further to flex the neck to facilitate passage of the wide-bore scope through the thoracic inlet.

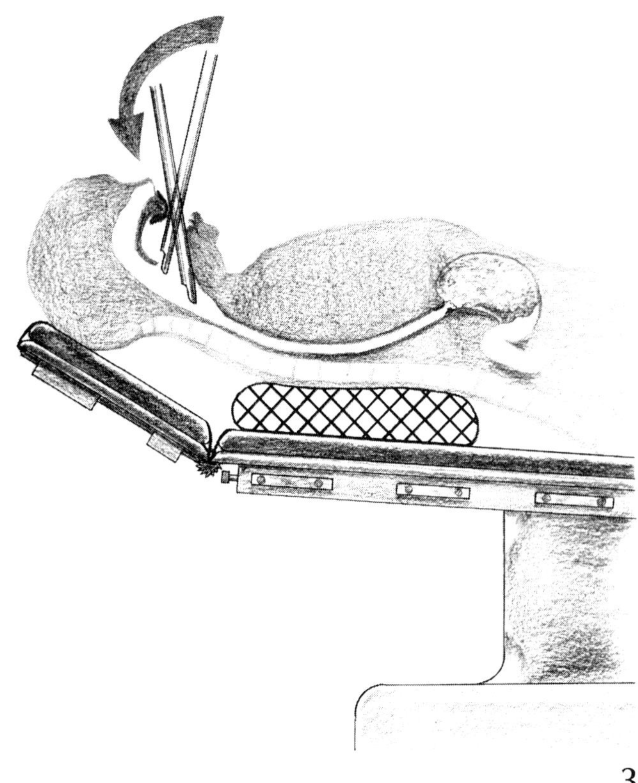

3

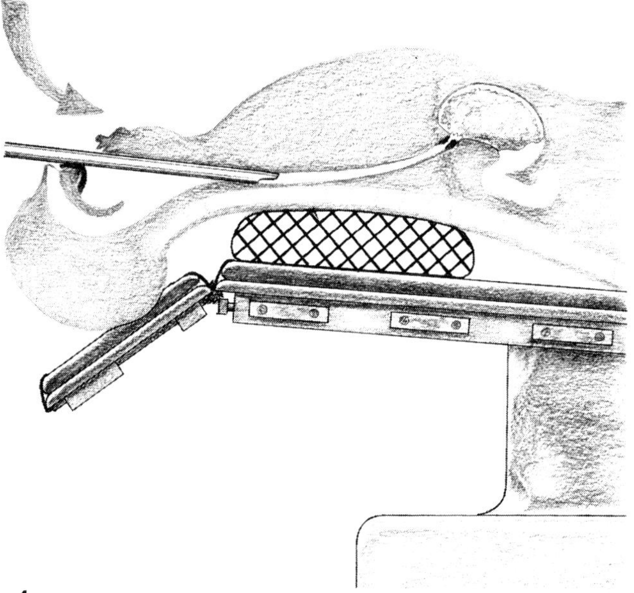

4

4

The neck is extended and the scope passed gently and steadily down the oesophagus, visualizing the lumen at all times. The operating table is readjusted as necessary by a combination of raising and tilting to a footdown position to keep the proximal end of the oesophagoscope at the operator's eye level.

5

Near the oesophagogastric junction it is frequently necessary to extend the neck further. This can be difficult in older patients when extension is limited by fixity of the cervical spine. The scope should ultimately be sited with the beak protruding slightly into the stomach as the planned site of injection is immediately above the oesophagogastric junction. Should bleeding occur at this time, it is easily controlled by rotating the scope to compress the bleeding site while the other varices are injected first.

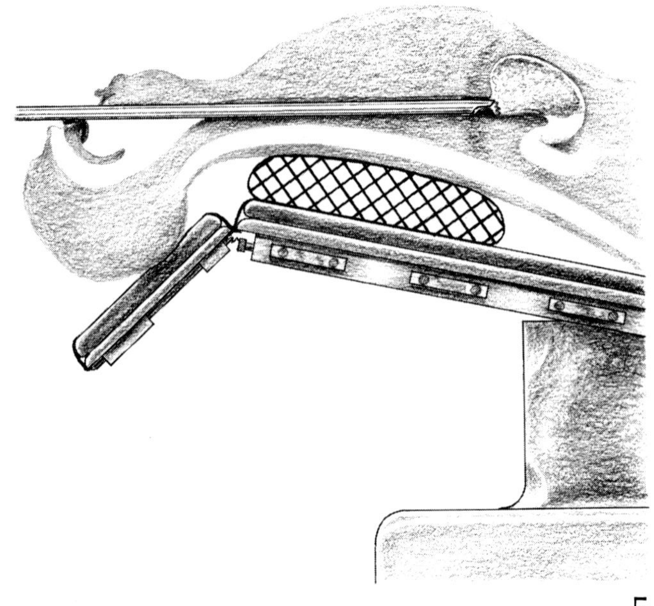

5

6

Injection of varices

6

A single varix protrudes into the slot of the scope at 6 o'clock. Any secretions or blood are sucked away and the sucker removed. A syringe containing 8–10 ml of ethanolamine oleate is securely attached to the needle and the needle filled with sclerosant. The needle is passed down the scope and directly into the varix, and 6–8 ml of sclerosant are injected intravascularly. If sodium morrhuate 5 per cent is used the amount should probably be limited to 4–6 ml. The varix will be noted to distend down into the stomach and become a paler colour. Inadvertent submucosal injection is more difficult and causes a local bleb. If a thrombosed varix presents in a repeat injection patient, it will feel thickened and injection is difficult. Once recognized, injection is discontinued. If sclerosant leaks out of the varix, the lumen of the oesophagus will fill with whitish-red fluid (blood plus sclerosant) which has a distinctive colour. This varix should be compressed by rotating the oesophagoscope and injected later.

7

At the end of the injection, the needle is withdrawn and the oesophagoscope immediately rotated. The injected varix and the injection site is thereby compressed, promoting sclerosis and preventing loss of both blood and sclerosant from the needle puncture site. At the same time the next varix presents in the slot for injection and is similarly injected. Usually three varices present for injection and are situated at approximately the 6, 10 and 2 o'clock positions. A relatively rigid needle, with the needle point bent slightly towards the varix, facilitates injection of the 10 and 2 o'clock variceal channels which is accomplished against gravity. After injection of the last varix, the oesophagoscope is rotated again and advanced (if possible) to compress all varices for a further arbitrary 5 min.

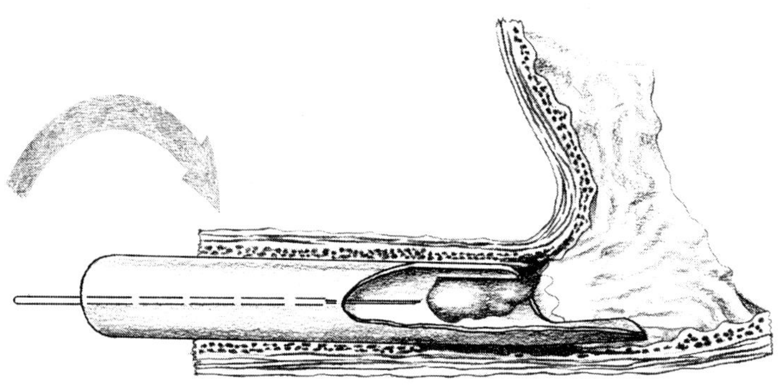

7

Removal of the oesophagoscope

The oesophagoscope is gently removed, flexing the neck if necessary. Even after an injection for an acute variceal bleed, a Sengstaken tube should *not* be reinserted at the end of the procedure as it is unnecessary and may be hazardous. The anaesthetist should prevent the patient coughing or straining during extubation as a Valsalva manoeuvre will increase the pressure in the varices and might precipitate bleeding.

Postoperative care

The patient is returned to an intensive care unit for 24–48 h post injection. Unless the patients are stuporous or in coma they are allowed oral fluids for the first 24 h and thereafter full feeding is recommended. Prophylactic antibiotics are not administered. Hepatic encephalopathy is treated with standard therapy. A post-injection chest X-ray is performed to check the lung fields and to look for mediastinal widening. Mild retrosternal discomfort and moderate pyrexia is usual for 24–48 h. If either is excessive, or if the patient has dysphagia, a gastrografin contrast swallow is obtained to exclude an injection site leak[9].

Subsequent management

After injection for an acute bleed

No further bleeding will occur in 70 per cent of the patients[9]. If bleeding does recur, vasopressin (Pitressin) is infused intravenously; and if bleeding continues, the Sengstaken tube should be reinserted and the patient reinjected to achieve definitive control of bleeding.

Subsequent management depends on the policy of the institution. The regimen for chronic injections is presented below. If a portosystemic shunt is to be performed, this can be delayed until the patient's condition has improved, as bleeding will have been controlled in 95 per cent of patients[9].

After chronic injection

If injections are being performed with the aim of eradicating varices, injections should be repeated at weekly or fortnightly intervals until the varices have been eradicated, as assessed on fibreoptic endoscopy. Subsequent assessment is at 6 months then annually for life. Any recurrent variceal channels noted on fibreoptic endoscopy require further injection sclerotherapy.

Results

Acute variceal bleeding

The technique described has been assessed in a 5 year prospective study of patients with endoscopically diagnosed acute oesophageal variceal bleeding who failed to respond to initial conservative measures. In the study period 66 patients had 137 such episodes of variceal bleeding during 93 admissions. Definitive control of variceal bleeding was achieved on 95 per cent of hospital admissions[9]. Mortality was related to the underlying liver disease and patients no longer die of continued variceal haemorrhage. The combined use of Sengstaken tube tamponade followed by injection sclerotherapy has markedly simplified the management of this difficult group of patients.

Long-term management

Repeated injection sclerotherapy in the long-term management of patients after oesophageal variceal bleeding has been evaluated in a prospective randomized controlled clinical trial comparing this technique with conventional medical management. By 5 years 75 patients had been randomized. The results at 2 years have been published[8] and the 4 year data presented in abstract form[19]. In this analysis eradication of varices was achieved in 90 per cent of patients after an average of 3.6 injections. Attention has been drawn to the complete disappearance of both gross oesophageal and gastric varices with injections localized to the oesophagogastric junction only. Varices recurred after an average of 15 months and were easily re-eradicated by further injection sclerotherapy. Annual follow-up with fibreoptic endoscopy thus appears to be adequate. Furthermore, after eradication of varices recurrent variceal bleeding has been prevented for as long as 4 years. Although survival was the same in both groups, the control medical management group was favoured because ethical considerations prevented withholding emergency injection sclerotherapy for acute life-threatening bleeds. It was concluded that repeated injection sclerotherapy is a viable alternative form of therapy for patients who have bled from oesophageal varices[19].

Acknowledgements

The study was supported by grants from the South African Medical Research Council and the Staff Research Fund of the University of Cape Town.

References

1. Crafoord, C., Frenckner, P. New surgical treatment of varicose veins of the oesophagus. Acta Oto-laryngologica 1939; 27: 422–429
2. Moersch, H. J. Treatment of esophageal varices by injection of a sclerosing solution. Journal of the American Medical Association 1947; 135: 754–757
3. Macbeth, R. Treatment of oesophageal varices in portal hypertension by means of sclerosing injections. British Medical Journal 1955; 2: 877–880
4. Johnston, G. W., Rodgers, H. W. A review of 15 years' experience in the use of sclerotherapy in the control of acute haemorrhage from oesophageal varices. British Journal of Surgery 1973; 60: 797–800
5. Wodak, E. Akute gastrointestinale Blutung; Resultate der endoskopischen Sklerosierung von Ösophagusvarizen. Schweizerische Medizinische Wochenschrift 1979; 109: 591–594
6. Paquet, K.-J., Oberhammer, E. Sclerotherapy of bleeding oesophageal varices by means of endoscopy. Endoscopy 1978; 10: 7–12
7. Terblanche, J., Northover, J. M. A., Bornman, P. *et al.* A prospective evaluation of injection sclerotherapy in the treatment of acute bleeding from esophageal varices. Surgery 1979; 85: 239–245
8. Terblanche, J., Northover, J. M. A., Bornman, P. *et al.* A prospective controlled trial of sclerotherapy in the long term management of patients after esophageal variceal bleeding. Surgery, Gynecology and Obstetrics 1979; 148: 323–333
9. Terblanche, J., Yakoob, H. I., Bornman, P. C. *et al.* Acute bleeding varices. A 5-year prospective evaluation of tamponade and sclerotherapy. Annals of Surgery 1981; 194: 521–530
10. Clark, A. W., Macdougall, B. R. D., Westaby, D. *et al.* Prospective controlled trial of injection sclerotherapy in patients with cirrhosis and recent variceal haemorrhage. Lancet 1980; 2: 552–554
11. Brooks, W. S. Adapting flexible endoscopes for sclerosis of oesophageal varices. Lancet 1980; 1: 266
12. Lewis, J., Chung, R. S., Allison, J. Sclerotherapy of esophageal varices. Archives of Surgery 1980; 115: 476–480
13. Viamonte, M., Pereiras, R., Russell, E., Le Page, J., Hutson, D. Transhepatic obliteration of gastroesophageal varices. Results in acute and nonacute bleeders. American Journal of Roentgenology 1977; 129: 237–241
14. Bengmark, S., Börjesson, B., Hoevels, J., Joelsson, B., Lunderquist, A., Owman, T. Obliteration of esophageal varices by PTP. A follow-up of 43 patients. Annals of Surgery 1979; 190: 549–554
15. Sagar, S., Harrison, I. D., Brearley, R., Shields, R. Emergency treatment of variceal haemorrhage. British Journal of Surgery 1979; 66: 824–826
16. Chojkier, M., Groszmann, R. J., Atterbury, C. E. *et al.* A controlled comparison of continuous intraarterial and intravenous infusions of vasopressin in hemorrhage from esophageal varices. Gastroenterology 1979; 77: 540–546
17. Terblanche, J. Treatment of esophageal varices by injection sclerotherapy. In: MacLean, L. D. ed. Advances in surgery, Vol. 15. Chicago: Year Book Medical Publishers, 1981: 257–281
18. Bailey, M. E., Dawson, J. L. Modified oesophagoscope for injecting oesophageal varices. British Medical Journal 1975; 2: 540–541
19. Terblanche, J., Bornman, P. C., Yakoob, H., Bane, R., Wright, J., Kirsch, R. E. Prospective randomised controlled trial of sclerotherapy after esophageal variceal bleeding. Gastroenterology 1980; 79: 1128

Portal hypertension: portacaval anastomosis

Marshall J. Orloff MD
Professor and Chairman, Department of Surgery,
School of Medicine, University of California, San Diego

Introduction

Portal hypertension is a manifestation of various diseases of the liver and its circulation and is the complication of hepatic disease that most frequently requires surgical treatment. Clinically important portal hypertension exists when the pressure in the portal vein and its major tributaries is at least 150 mm saline *higher than* the pressure in the inferior vena cava. The elevated pressure in the portal venous system is almost always the result of obstruction to portal blood flow, usually within the liver (90 per cent of patients) but occasionally at an extrahepatic site (10 per cent of patients). The only definitive treatment of portal hypertension is decompression of the portal system by a bypass anastomosis between the portal and systemic circulations.

Preoperative

Inidications for portacaval anastomosis

The most frequent indication for portacaval anastomosis is *bleeding oesophageal varices* caused by intrahepatic obstructive disease. Other, uncommon indications are intractable ascites, severe hypersplenism, Budd-Chiari syndrome and two rare metabolic disorders unassociated with portal hypertension: glycogen storage disease and type II hyperlipoproteinaemia. Bleeding from oesophageal varices caused by intrahepatic obstructive disease is the most lethal form of gastrointestinal haemorrhage. Moreover, if a patient recovers spontaneously from an episode of variceal bleeding he is almost certain to bleed again and to die of either the complications of bleeding or the underlying liver disease within a few years, unless the portal hypertension is corrected.

There are three circumstances in which the portacaval shunt operation has been used in patients with oesophageal varices and liver disease.

1. *Prophylactic portacaval shunt* has been advocated to prevent bleeding in patients with demonstrable oesophageal varices who have never bled. However, there is nothing to suggest that the mere demonstration of varices permits a prediction regarding the likelihood of variceal rupture and, in fact, recent statistics indicate that no more than one-third of patients with oesophageal varices who have no history of bleeding will subsequently develop variceal haemorrhage. Thus, two-thirds or more of patients subjected to prophylactic portacaval shunt undergo an operation to prevent a complication that would not have developed. Not surprisingly, three prospective, controlled clinical trials of prophylactic portacaval shunt demonstrated that it did not prolong life. The prophylactic operation is clearly not indicated.
2. *Elective therapeutic portacaval shunt* is indicated in patients who have recovered from an episode of bleeding oesophageal varices unless they have little chance of surviving the operation because of hepatic decompensation. There are no clear-cut criteria for determining which patients have less chance of surviving with elective operative treatment than with non-operative therapy, which almost invariably is unsuccessful. The presence of persistent jaundice, of ascites that cannot be stabilized, of repeated bouts of encephalopathy, of advanced muscle wasting and of a poor appetite indicate that the elective operation has little chance of success, particularly when these manifestations of end-stage liver disease exist together. Because of the high mortality rate associated with the first episode of variceal haemorrhage, only approximately 10–20 per cent of bleeding cirrhotic patients survive the bleeding episode *and* recover sufficient hepatic function to become eligible for elective therapeutic portacaval shunt.
3. *Emergency therapeutic portacaval shunt* is indicated at the time of bleeding in most patients with liver disease and variceal haemorrhage. Our prospective studies over the past 20 years have demonstrated that in our hands the emergency operation is applicable to the vast majority of bleeding cirrhotic patients and provides the best chance, by far, of long-term survival and useful life. The only type of patient in whom emergency portacaval shunt may not be of value is the one who presents with *concurrent* bleeding, ascites, jaundice, encephalopathy and severe muscle wasting, and even some of these patients have survived for more than 5 years after undergoing portacaval shunt.

Diagnosis of bleeding oesophageal varices due to liver disease

In most patients who enter the hospital with upper gastrointestinal haemorrhage, the diagnosis of bleeding oesophageal varices depends on affirmative answers to three questions. Does the patient have liver disease? Does the patient have portal hypertension and oesophageal varices? Are the varices the site of the bleeding, rather than some other lesion such as duodenal or gastric ulcer, gastritis or hiatus hernia? Information sufficient to answer these questions usually can be obtained within a few hours of the patient's admission to the hospital by means of an organized diagnostic plan that usually includes the following five steps.

History and physical examination

A history of chronic alcoholism, hepatitis, jaundice, previous bleeding episodes, melaena, abdominal swelling, oedema and mental abnormalities, and the absence of symptoms of peptic ulcer suggest the diagnosis of chronic liver disease. The most important physical findings are hepatosplenomegaly, spider angiomas, palmar erythema, collateral abdominal veins, muscle wasting, jaundice, ascites, oedema, and neurological signs such as tremor and asterixis. In many patients, not all these classic signs are present. Confirmation of gastrointestinal bleeding by aspiration of the stomach through a nasogastric tube and by gross and chemical examination of the stool is an essential early measure and should really be considered part of the physical examination. A nasogastric tube is inserted in all patients.

Blood studies

Blood samples for typing and crossmatching and for studies are drawn immediately on admission. The initial studies include a complete blood count, liver function tests (Bromsulphalein or indocyanine green dye excretion, prothrombin, bilirubin, alkaline phosphatase, albumin, globulin, glutamic oxalacetic transaminase, glutamic pyruvic transaminase), urea nitrogen, electrolytes, pH, blood gases, and blood alcohol. The liver tests that are most consistently abnormal and of greatest value are the Bromsulphalein or indocyanine green dye excretion, if performed in the absence of marked jaundice and after hypovolaemic shock has been corrected, and the prothrombin and serum bilirubin. It is not unusual for the other liver function tests to be normal in the presence of advanced cirrhosis.

Oesophagogastroduodenoscopy

With the development of the flexible fibreoptic oesophagogastroscope, endoscopy has become a well tolerated, relatively simple procedure that can be performed rapidly at the bedside in the emergency room. It is the best diagnostic measure for determining with certainty the presence or absence of gastritis and of Mallory-Weiss syndrome, and it makes possible the diagnosis of oesophageal varices with a high degree of confidence.

Upper gastrointestinal X-rays

As soon as shock has been corrected and the patient's condition stabilized, a barium contrast upper gastrointestinal series is obtained. Parenteral fluid therapy and monitoring should continue throughout this procedure, and the physician in charge of treatment should accompany the patient to the radiology department and remain in constant attendance. When this is done, X-ray studies can be performed safely in almost all patients. It is to be emphasized that roentgenographic studies are directed at determining the presence or absence not only of oesophageal varices, but also of other lesions such as a duodenal ulcer, gastric ulcer or hiatus hernia. The literature contains many statements that suggest that oesophageal varices are demonstrated in only 50–60 per cent of patients who have them. Our experience indicates that a skilful and interested radiologist can accurately demonstrate varices at the time of bleeding in more than 90 per cent of patients.

Hepatic vein catheterization

This relatively simple procedure has become a routine diagnostic measure in our institution. It is used to determine wedged hepatic vein pressure, free hepatic vein pressure and inferior vena caval pressure. Hepatic venography is usually added to the studies, although it is not essential and does not yield information that is as important as that obtained from the pressure measurements. The main purpose of venography is to determine the direction of flow in the portal vein. Wedged hepatic vein pressure accurately reflects portal pressure in the common forms of cirrhosis and establishes the diagnosis of portal hypertension with certainty.

Angiographic studies are usually not required for diagnosis of variceal haemorrhage in patients with liver disease. However, in the small number of patients with normal liver function who are suspected of having extrahepatic portal obstruction, splanchnic angiography provides crucial information about the site of obstruction and patency of the portal venous system. Percutaneous selective catheterization and visualization of the splenic artery or superior mesenteric artery usually provides delayed visualization of the portal vein and its collateral connections, a technique known as indirect portography. An alternative procedure that carries a slightly higher risk is percutaneous splenoportography which provides visualization of the portal venous system by direct injection of contrast media into the spleen.

Preoperative preparation

There are certain general principles of treatment that apply to all patients with liver disease and bleeding varices, regardless of the specific therapeutic measures used to control portal hypertension.

Stopping the haemorrhage

Temporary haemostasis can be obtained in most patients by systemic intravenous administration of vasopressin (posterior pituitary extract, Pituitrin). The agent is administered intravenously over a period of 15–20 min in a dose of 20 u of Pituitrin diluted in 200 ml of solution. It has been demonstrated clearly that systemic intravenous administration of vasopressin is as effective as continuous infusion of vasopressin into an indwelling catheter inserted in the superior mesenteric artery, and is both simpler and less hazardous. Every patient with bleeding oesophageal varices is given vasopressin soon after admission to our emergency room, and this measure of therapy has largely replaced oesophageal balloon tamponade as our means of obtaining immediate control of haemorrhage. However, in the few patients who do not respond to vasopressin (approximagely 5 per cent), the Sengstaken-Blakemore oesophageal balloon tube, or one of its variants, is used for temporary haemostasis.

Prompt restoration of the blood volume

Vigorous replacement of blood loss with whole blood transfusion is an essential intitial step in therapy. Large-bore intravenous catheters should be inserted in each arm at the start of therapy. Every effort is made to obtain fresh blood less than 12 h old for administration because of the serious defects in coagulation associated with liver disease plus those superimposed by multiple transfusions. Bleeding cirrhotic patients usually have thrombocytopenia in addition to abnormalities of the protein blood-clotting factors. In addition, recent evidence indicates that the red blood cells of cirrhotic patients are deficient in 2,3-diphosphoglyceric acid, a substance that influences the dissociation of oxygen from haemoglobin. It has been proposed that this deficiency impairs the delivery of oxygen to the tissues. Since there is progressive decline in 2,3-DPG levels in blood during storage, the use of fresh blood has been recommended to correct the abnormality in oxygen transport. If fresh whole blood is not available, a satisfactory substitute is the combined administration of packed red blood cells, fresh frozen plasma and packs of platelets.

Prevention of hepatic encephalopathy

Though the nervous disorders associated with liver disease are diverse and poorly understood, the encephalopathy observed in patients with bleeding oesophageal varices sometimes appears to be the result of the absorption of large quantities of ammonia directly into the systemic circulation via portasystemic collaterals. For this reason, measures directed at destroying ammonia-forming bacteria and eliminating all nitrogen from the gastrointestinal tract are initiated promptly. These include removal of blood from the stomach by lavage with iced saline through a nasogastric tube, instillation of cathartics (60 ml magnesium sulphate) and neomycin (4 g) into the stomach, and thorough and repeated cleansing of the colon with enemas containing neomycin (4 g/litre of water). The fear that insertion of a nasogastric tube will perforate the varices is unfounded, and such a tube should be placed at the start of the diagnostic work-up. Although ammonia-binding agents, such as sodium glutamate and arginine, and ion exchange resins have been used, we have obtained no evidence that agents of this sort have been of value.

Support of the failing liver

Parenterally administered hypertonic glucose solutions containing therapeutic doses of vitamins K, B and C are included in the initial treatment regimen. Appropriate amounts of electrolytes are added to the parenteral fluids. In general, administration of sodium is avoided because patients with advanced cirrhosis usually have an increase in total-body sodium and a tendency to retain salt and water.

Correction of hypokalaemia and metabolic alkalosis

The vast majority of the many bleeding cirrhotic patients that we have studied have been found to have significant hypokalaemia and a metabolic alkalosis preoperatively or immediately postoperatively. The deleterious effects of hypokalaemia are well known. In addition, alkalosis has a number of harmful consequences that include: (*1*) interference with the release of oxygen to the tissues by shifting the oxyhaemoglobin dissociation curve to the left; (*2*) in combination with hypokalaemia, precipitation of cardiac arrhythmias, particularly in patients taking digitalis; (*3*) potentiation of ammonia toxicity by elevating the tissue concentration of ammonia and increasing the passage of ammonia across the blood–brain barrier; and (*4*) production of tetany by lowering the level of ionized calcium in extracellular fluid. Correction of hypokalaemia and metabolic alkalosis is undertaken soon after admission to the hospital and consists of parenteral administration of large quantities of potassium chloride supplemented, occasionally, by infusion of an acidifying agent such as arginine hydrochloride or hydrochloric acid, or ammonium chloride. Administration of potassium is usually required for several days in amounts occasionally as high as 500 mmol per day.

Frequent monitoring of vital functions

The usual techniques are used to determine the magnitude of bleeding and adequacy of blood volume replacement. These include measurements of vital signs, of urine output by way of an indwelling catheter, of central venous pressure via a polyethylene catheter threaded through an arm cutdown into the superior vena cava, of haematocrit and of rate of blood loss by continuous suction through a nasogastric tube. Serial measurements of arterial pH and blood gases are facilitated by insertion of an indwelling catheter into the radial artery, which also makes possible continuous recordings of blood pressure. Because of the systemic circulatory abnormalities and hyperdynamic state that frequently exist in bleeding cirrhotic patients, we have added serial determinations of cardiac output by the dye dilution technique, using indocyanine green, to our monitoring regimen, and occasionally perform measurements of pulmonary artery wedge pressure by percutaneous insertion of a Swan-Ganz pulmonary artery catheter.

CHOICE OF PORTASYSTEMIC SHUNT

Because the portal venous system contains no valves it is possible to decompress it at various points, provided the anastomosis with the low-pressure systemic venous system is of sufficient size to accomodate a large flow of blood. The portasystemic shunts most commonly used for relief of portal hypertension are shown, and some brief comments on each follow.

1

End-to-side portacaval shunt

This anastomosis accomplishes splanchnic decompression by shunting all splanchnic venous blood into the inferior vena cava and, at the same time, it decompresses the liver sinusoids by eliminating the contribution of portal venous blood to hepatic inflow and pressure. However, it rarely lowers hepatic sinusoidal pressure to normal, and sinusoidal hypertension often persists because hepatic arterial blood continues to encounter difficulty in leaving the liver through the obstructed hepatic venous outflow system.

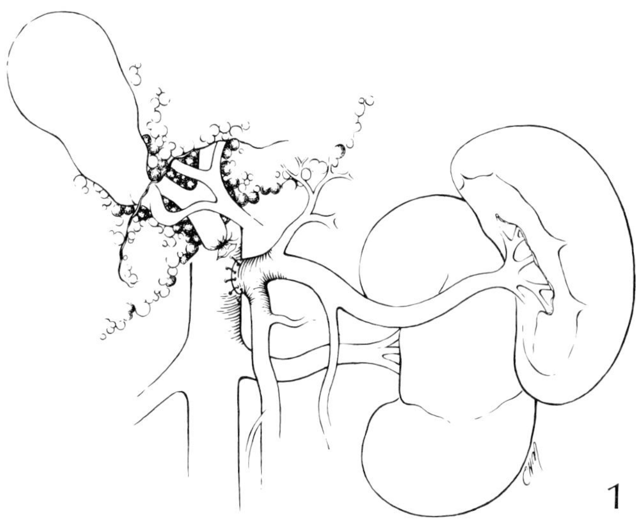

1

2

Side-to-side portacaval shunt

This other type of direct anastomsis between the portal vein and inferior vena cava produces splanchnic decompression equivalent to the end-to-side anastomosis, but it accomplishes significantly greater hepatic decompression by allowing egress of liver blood in a retrograde direction through the portal vein into the low-pressure vena cava. The side-to-side shunt converts the portal vein into an outflow tract, and portal blood does not continue to perfuse the liver in substantial amounts, if at all.

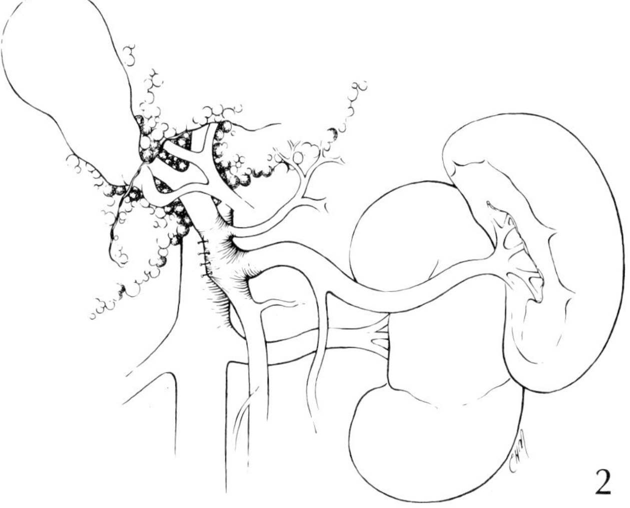

2

Although the two types of direct portacaval shunt produce similar splanchnic decompression and are equally effective in relieving and preventing variceal haemorrhage, the overall haemodynamic effects of the two procedures are distinctly different. Hence, there has been a continuing controversy regarding the comparative advantages and disadvantages of the end-to-side and side-to-side anastomoses. In a series of studies, we have compared the effects of the two types of shunt on hepatic blood flow, liver function, liver morphology and ammonia tolerance in dogs with experimental cirrhosis; and on hepatic function, ammonia tolerance, the 5 year incidence of encephalopathy and the 5 year survival rate in cirrhotic humans who were operated on for bleeding oesophageal varices. There were no significant differences between end-to-side and side-to-side portacaval shunt in any of the parameters that were evaluated. We have concluded that there is no demonstrable advantage of one type of direct portacaval shunt over the other in most circumstances. The one exception may be the unusual patient with severe hepatic outflow obstruction manifested by a pressure on the hepatic side of a clamp occluding the portal vein (HOPP) that is higher than the free portal pressure (FPP). Such patients may have a reversal of portal flow, and they have been known to develop intractable ascites following an end-to-side portacaval shunt, which eliminates the portal vein as an outflow track and, thereby, may increase sinusoidal hypertension. Although clear documentation of this phenomenon does not exist, a side-to-side portacaval shunt would seem to be the procedure of choice in such cases.

3

Mesocaval shunt

This operation consists of an anastomosis between the upper end of the divided inferior vena cava and the side of the superior mesenteric vein. In principle, it is haemodynamically similar to the side-to-side portacaval shunt. In patients with extrahepatic portal hypertension due to occlusion of the portal vein, this type of shunt is very effective. However, in adult cirrhotic patients it is doubtful that this procedure represents a first choice. Cirrhotic patients have a tendency to retain salt and water, and division of the inferior vena cava may lead to intractable oedema of the lower extremities.

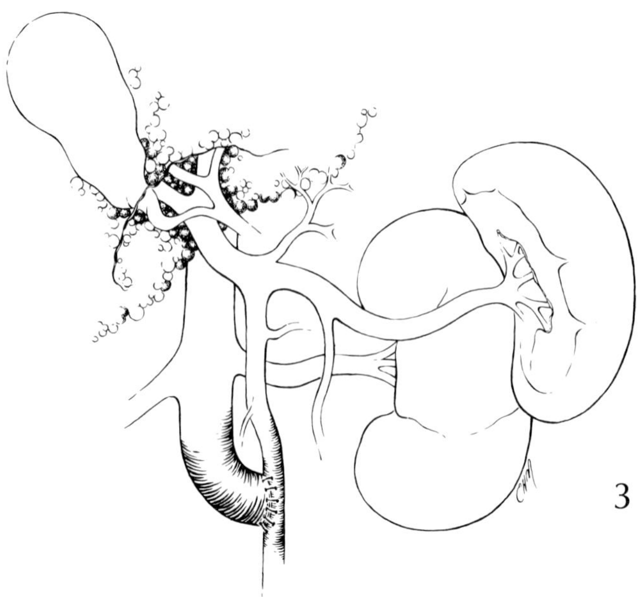

3

4

Interposition mesocaval H-graft shunt

The use of H-grafts between the intact portal or superior mesenteric vein and inferior vena cava, introduced 25 years ago, has recently attracted renewed interest. Synthetic prostheses of Dacron and Teflon, autogenous jugular vein, and homologous vena cava have been used for this purpose. The interposition mesocaval or portacaval H-graft is a relatively minor technical variation of the direct side-to-side portacaval shunt and, despite claims to the contrary, the two procedures are haemodynamically identical. The major advantage claimed for the H-graft procedure is that it is technically less difficult to perform than conventional shunts. The major potential disadvantage is the possibility of thrombosis, particularly of the synthetic prostheses.

Short-term results of interposition shunts involving a collective total of some 240 patients have been reported from 10 centres. The operative mortality rate in this heterogenous collection of patients has been about 15 per cent, which is not different from that associated with conventional portacaval shunts. The short-term incidence of thrombosis has ranged from 5 to 20 per cent which is unacceptable when compared with the less than 2 per cent long-term occlusion rate of direct portacaval anastomoses in experienced hands.

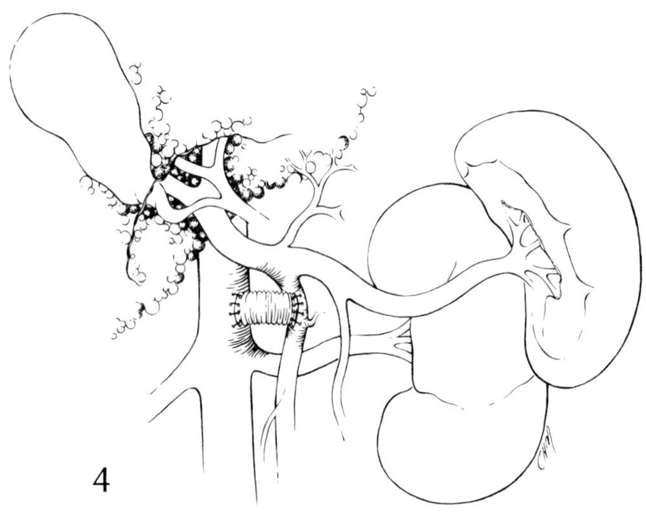

4

5

Splenorenal shunt (conventional)

The conventional splenorenal anastomosis is a variant of the side-to-side, in-continuity shunt. It utilizes tributaries of the portal vein and vena cava which, obviously, are of smaller size than the parent vessels. It is followed by a lower incidence of protein-related portasystemic encephalopathy than the direct portacaval anastomosis because it shunts a small volume of nitrogen-containing portal blood into the systemic circulation. At the same time, it does not decompress the portal bed as effectively as the direct portacaval shunt, is associated with a significant incidence of variceal rebleeding and has a high incidence of thrombosis. In the author's opinion it is the procedure of choice only in rare instances when severe and intractable hypersplenism complicates portal hypertension and requires splenectomy.

The most commonly used type of splenorenal shunt involves removal of the spleen and anastomosis of the end of the splenic vein to the side of the left renal vein. However, a central side-to-side splenorenal shunt can be done in continuity, without splenectomy. It has been proposed that the latter operation permits continued portal venous perfusion of the liver, but it is doubtful that such is the case because the principles that govern the haemodynamics of a valveless system dictate that flow is in the direction of the area of lowest pressure, i.e. the splenorenal anastomosis.

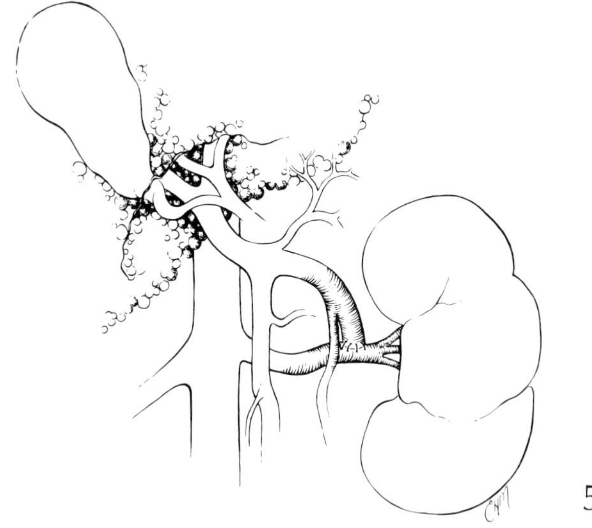

5

6

Selective distal splenorenal shunt

This procedure is designed selectively to decompress oesophageal varices while at the same time preserving blood flow to the liver and avoiding systemic shunting of intestinal blood. The operation involves anastomosis of the splenic stump of the divided splenic vein to the intact left renal vein, and is combined with gastrosplenic isolation aimed at diverting the gastro-oesophageal venous flow through the shunt. Gastrosplenic isolation is accomplished by ligation of the coronary vein, right gastric vein and right gastroepiploic vein and division of the gastrohepatic, gastrocolic and splenocolic ligaments. The operation is applicable to a relatively small segment of the bleeding cirrhotic population which does not have ascites, has good liver function and is eligible for elective treatment. It is technically the most difficult of all the shunt procedures. Since its introduction over 10 years ago, selective distal splenorenal shunt has been used rather widely and the results have led to the following impressions when compared with direct portacaval shunt performed electively in similar patients. (*1*) Distal splenorenal shunt appears to be associated with a higher operative mortality rate and higher incidences of shunt occlusion, persistence of varices and recurrent varix haemorrhage. (*2*) The 5 year survival rate does not appear to be different. (*3*) The incidence of encephalopathy during the first few years postoperatively appears to be lower and encephalopathy tends to be milder. However, with passage of time the incidence of encephalopathy apears to increase along with evidence of development of collateral vessels connecting the portomesenteric and gastrosplenic sides of the portal circulation, and evidence of loss of portal perfusion of the liver. Furthermore, there appears to be a substantial incidence of late thrombosis of the portal vein, which eliminates the possibility of continued portal perfusion of the liver.

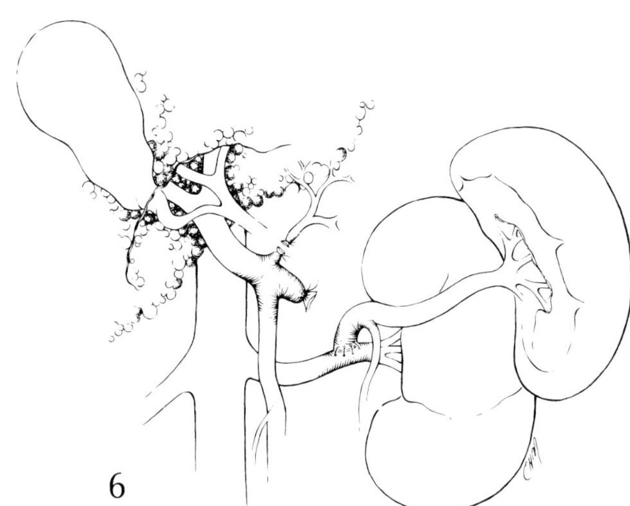

6

Technique of direct portacaval anastomosis

Anaesthesia

During the past 25 years we have systematically evaluated a variety of anaesthetic regimens and have come to the conclusion that the technique of 'balanced anaesthesia' gives the best results. This technique entails giving a nitrous oxide-oxygen mixture by endotracheal inhalation with intravenous administration of an analgesic such as meperidine and a muscle relaxant. Parenteral fluid therapy consists of a solution of 10 per cent dextrose in water in addition to whole blood transfusion to replace blood loss. Because patients with liver disease usually have an excess of total body sodium and water, solutions containing sodium are avoided. However, potassium is added to the parenteral fluids to repair the almost invariable deficit in body potassium. Performance of an emergency portacaval shunt usually requires 2½ to 5 h and 1000–3000 ml of whole blood transfusion.

Positioning the patient

7

The patient is placed on the operating table with the right side elevated at an angle of 30° to the table. The costal margin is at the level of the flexion break of the table, the right arm is suspended from an ether screen with towels, and the left arm is extended on an arm board cephalad to the ether screen. Monitoring and sampling devices include:

1. Nasogastric tube placed on intermittent suction;
2. Naso-oesophageal temperature probe for continuous recording of body temperature;
3. Left radial artery catheter for continuous recording of arterial blood pressure via a transducer and polygraph;
4. Large-bore intravenous catheter inserted through a cutdown in the left arm for administration of blood transfusions and parenteral fluids;
5. Large-bore intravenous catheter inserted into the superior vena cava through a cutdown in the right arm for continuous recording of central venous pressure (via a transducer and polygraph), blood sampling and administration of parenteral fluids;
6. Blood pressure cuff on the right arm for intermittent determination of arterial blood pressure as a reserve alternative to direct intra-arterial recordings;
7. Three ECG leads on chest for continuous recording of electrocardiogram;
8. Indwelling Foley bladder catheter attached by tubing to a collecting bag at the head of the table for continuous monitoring of urine output;
9. Ground plate for electrocautery fixed to the right thigh.

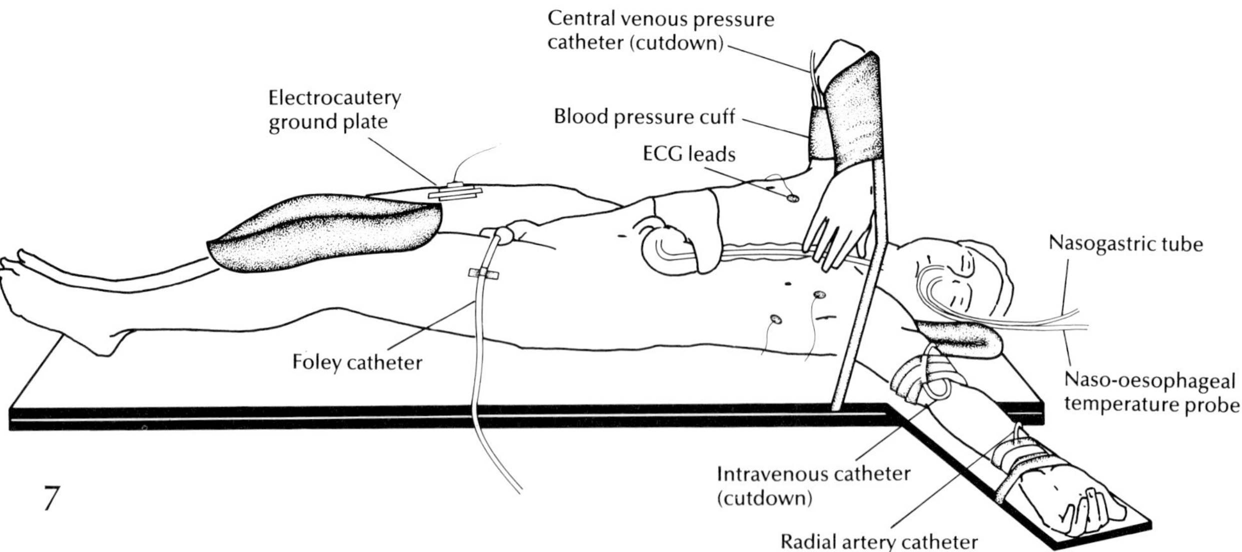

7

8

View of the initial position of the patient from the right side of the table where the operating surgeon stands. The right side of the body is elevated at an angle of 30° by two sandbags placed underneath the patient. The patient is secured to the table by a large strap placed over a towel across the iliac crest. A large pillow is positioned between the lower extremities.

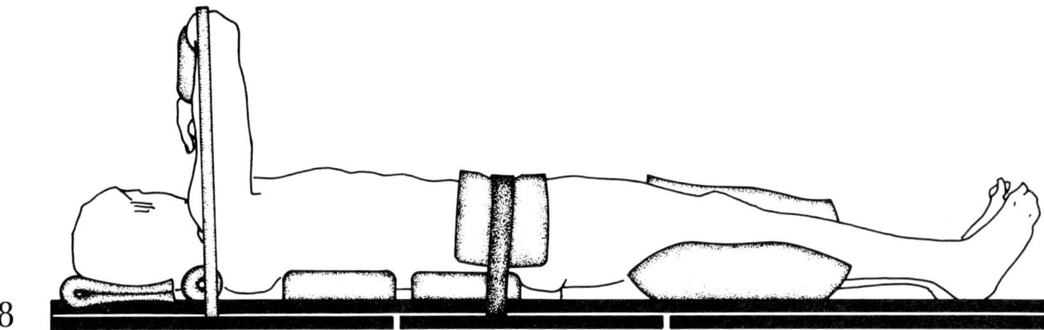

8

9

The head-down position is next adopted in preparation for breaking the table.

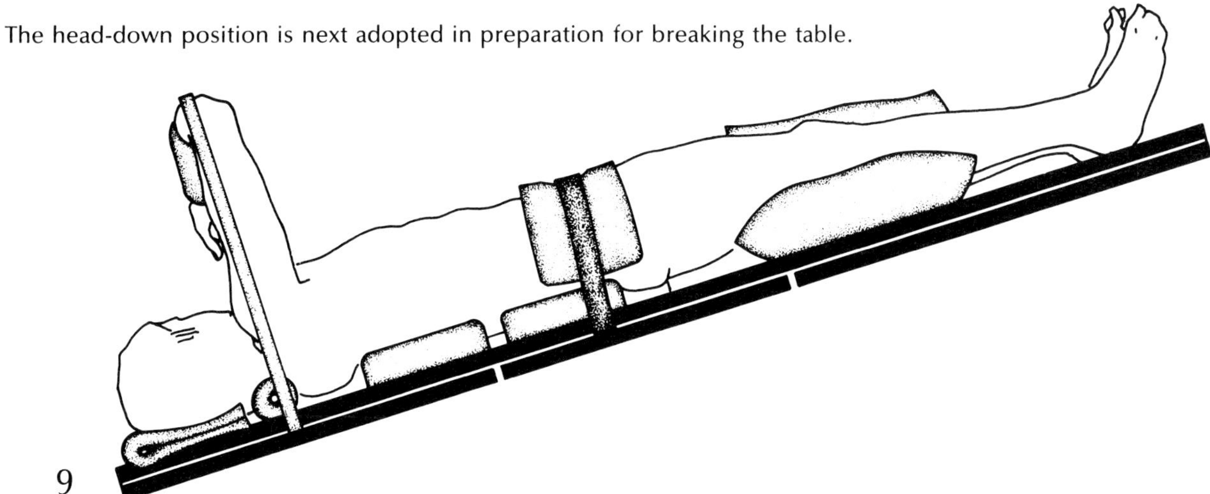

9

10

The table is then 'broken' at the level of the costal margin. The objective is to widen the space between the right costal margin and right iliac crest so that the operation can be performed easily through a right subcostal incision.

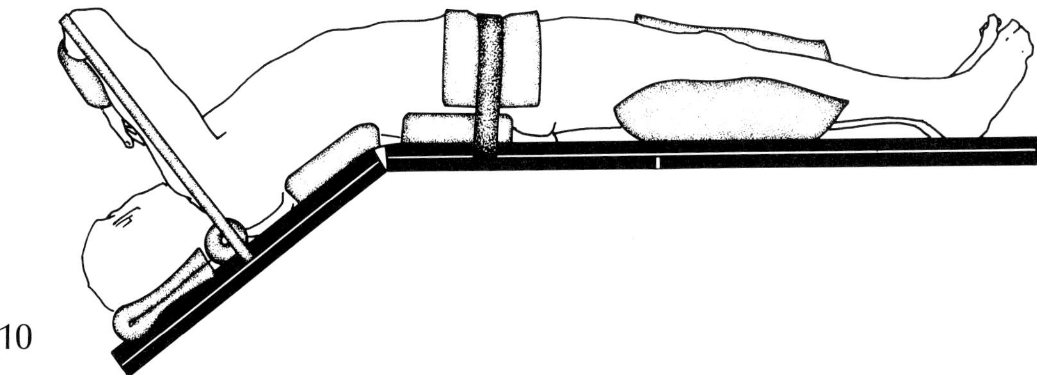

10

11

The final step involves breaking the table at the level of the knees by dropping the leg support section about 20°.

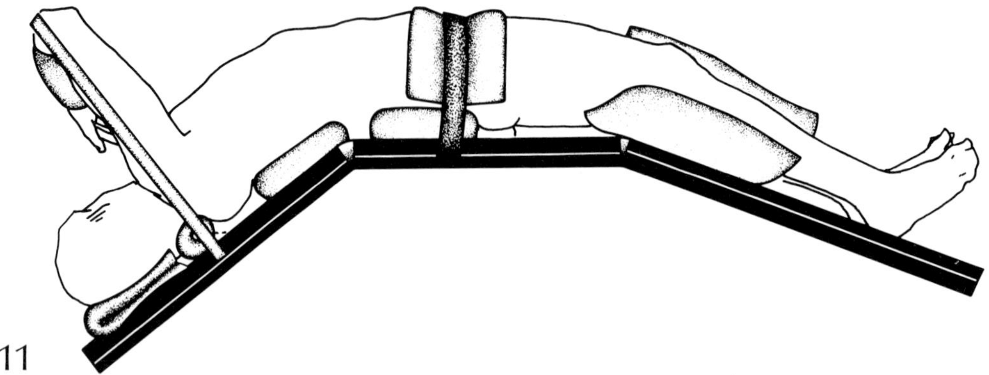

11

12

The incision

A long right subcostal incision extending from the xiphoid to well into the flank is made two fingers' breadths below the costal margin. We have used this incision in every operation during the past 25 years; it is associated with many fewer postoperative complications than the previously popular thoracoabdominal incision. The skin is incised superficially with the scalpel and the other layers with the electrocautery, which greatly reduces the blood loss and shortens the operating time. When the electrocautery is used it is usually unnecessary to clamp any blood vessels with haemostats. The right rectus abdominis, external oblique and transversus abdominis muscles are completely divided and the medial 3–4 cm of the latissimus dorsi muscle is often incised. The peritoneum often contains many collateral blood vessels and is incised with the electrocautery to obtained immediate haemostasis.

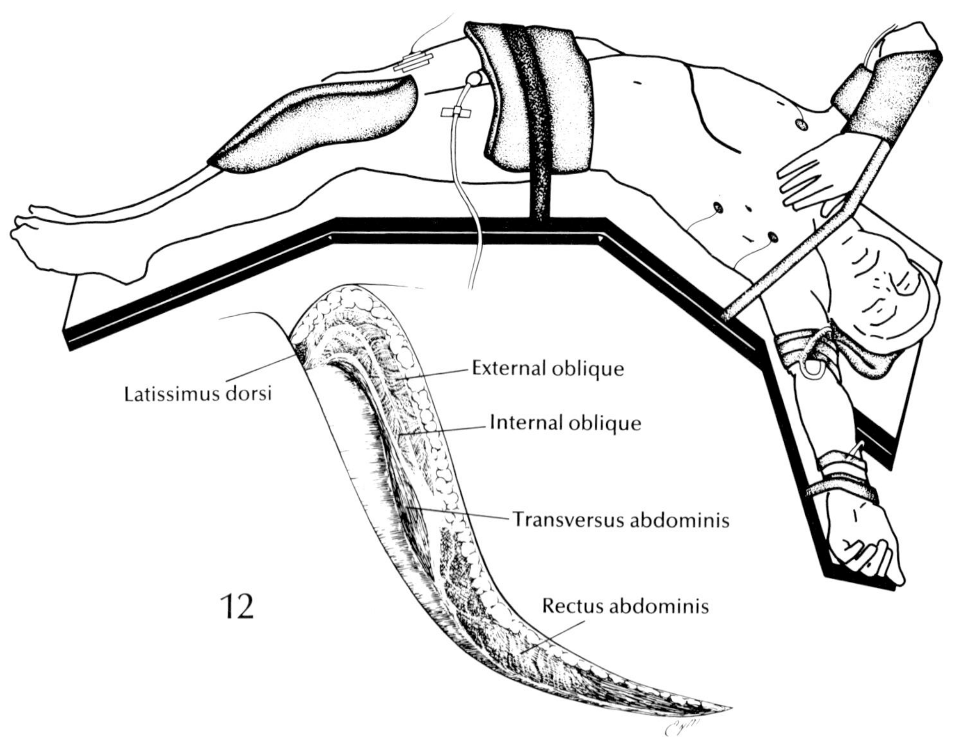

12

13

Exposure of operative field

The operative field is exposed by retraction of the viscera with three Deever retractors positioned at right angles to each other. The inferior retracts the hepatic flexure of the colon toward the feet, the medial displaces the duodenum medially and the superior retractor retracts the liver and gall bladder toward the head. The posterior peritoneum is often intensely 'stained' with portasystemic collateral vessels.

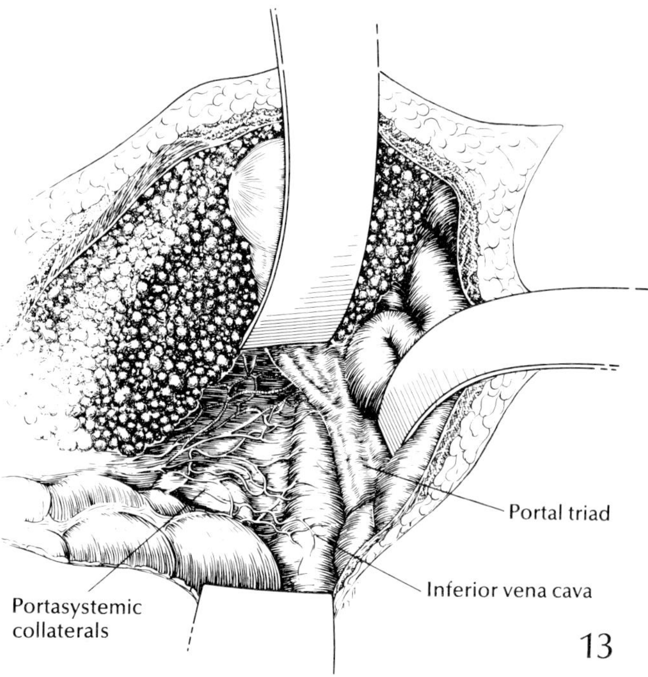

13

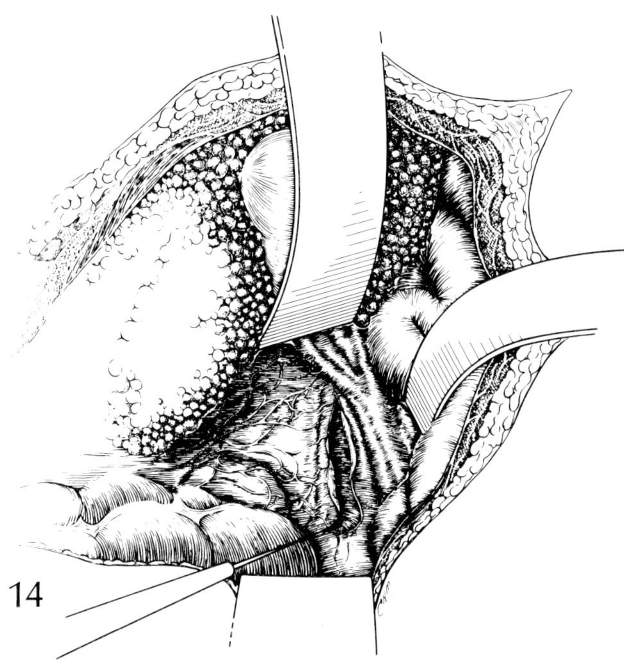
14

14

Incision of posterior peritoneum by an extended Kocher manoeuvre

The posterior peritoneum overlying the inferior vena cava is incised with the electrocautery by an extended Kocher manoeuvre just lateral to the descending duodenum. The peritoneum often is greatly thickened and contains many collateral blood vessels. Bleeding usually can be controlled with the electrocautery but sometimes requires suture ligatures.

15

Exposure of anterior surface of inferior vena cava

The medial retractor is repositioned to retract the head of the pancreas as well as the descending duodenum medially, thereby exposing the inferior vena cava which lies behind the duodenum. The inferior retractor is repositioned to retract the right kidney as well as the hepatic flexure of the colon towards the feet. The anterior surface of the inferior vena cava is cleared of fibroareolar tissue by sharp and blunt dissection.

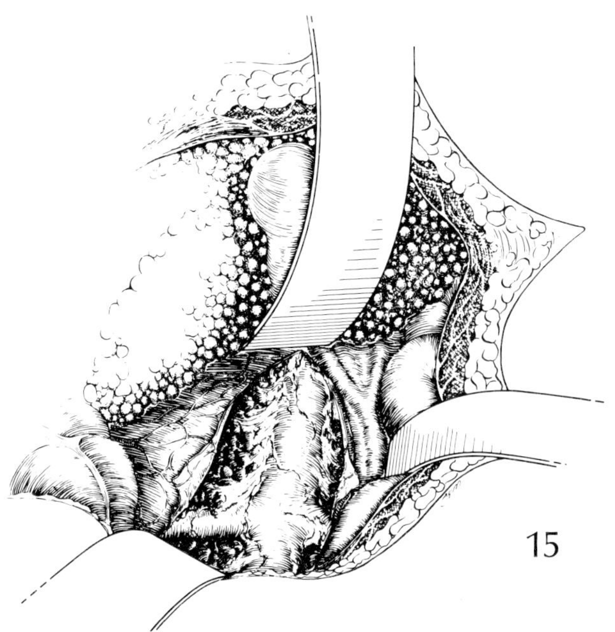
15

Isolation of inferior vena cava between renal veins and liver

16

The inferior vena cava is isolated around its entire circumference by blunt and sharp dissection from the entrance of the right and left renal veins below to the point where it disappears behind the liver above, and it is surrounded with an umbilical tape. To accomplish the isolation several tributaries must be ligated in continuity with fine silk ligatures and then divided. These include the right adrenal vein, one or two pairs of lumbar veins that enter on the posterior surface, and the caudal pair of small hepatic veins that enter on the anterior surface of the vena cava directly from the liver.

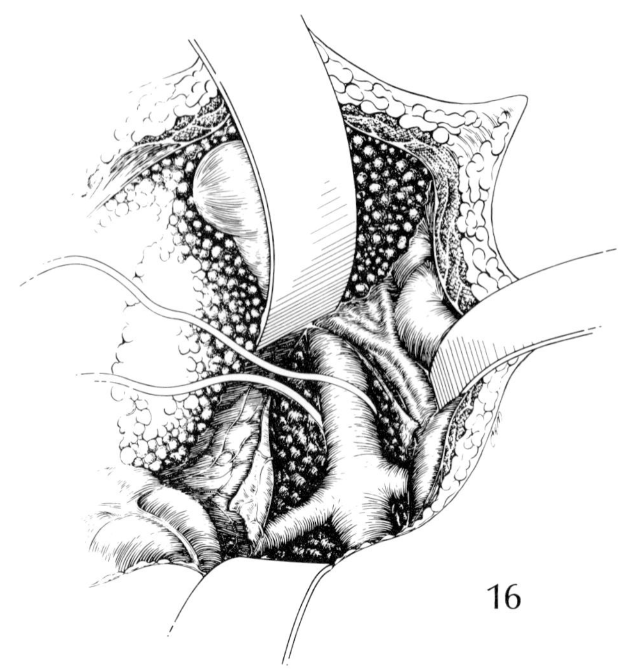

16

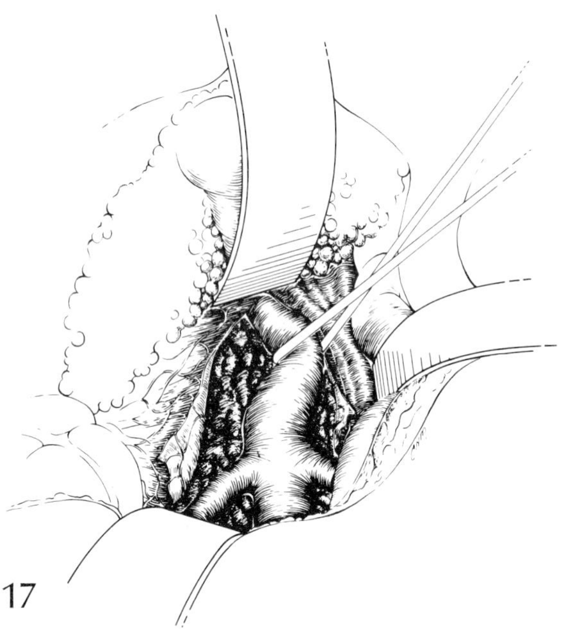

17

17

When the inferior vena cava has been mobilized completely it can be lifted up toward the portal vein. Failure to isolate the vena cava circumferentially is one major reason for the erroneous claim that the side-to-side portacaval shunt often cannot be performed because the portal vein and inferior vena cava are too widely separated.

Exposure of portal vein

18

The superior retractor is repositioned medially so that it retracts the liver at the point of entrance of the portal triad. The portal vein is located in the posterolateral aspect of the portal triad and is approached from behind. The fibrofatty tissue on the posterolateral aspect of the portal triad, which contains nerves, lymphatics and lymph nodes, is divided by blunt and sharp dissection. This is a safe manoeuvre because there are no portal venous tributaries on this aspect of the portal triad. As soon as the surface of the portal vein is exposed, a vein retractor is inserted to retract the common bile duct medially.

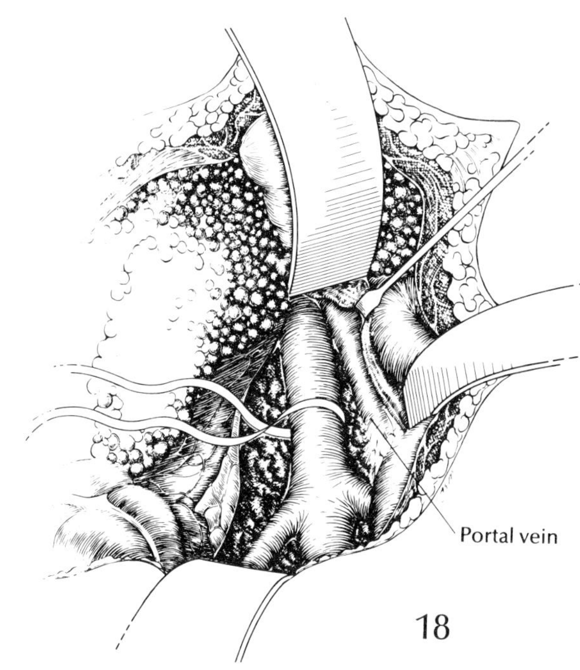

18

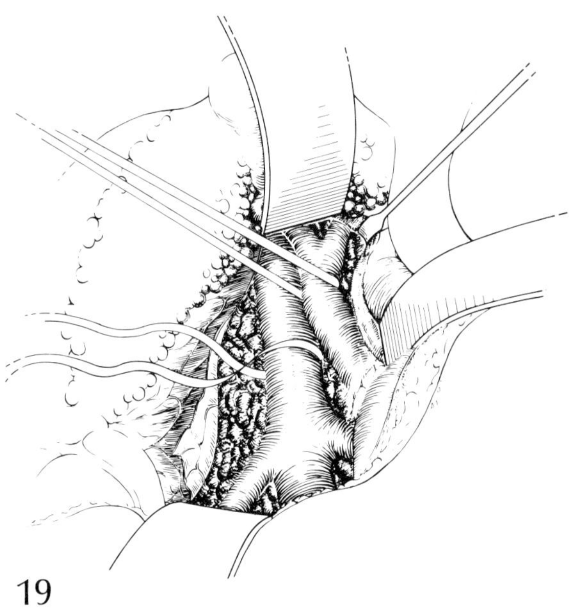

19

19

The portal vein is mobilized circumferentially at its mid-portion and is surrounded with an umbilical tape. It is then isolated up to its bifurcation in the liver hilum. Several tributaries on the medial aspect are ligated in continuity with fine silk and divided.

Mobilization of portal vein behind the pancreas

20

Using the umbilical tape to pull the portal vein out of its bed, the portal vein is cleared to the point where it disappears behind the pancreas. The tough fibrofatty tissue that binds the portal vein to the pancreas must be divided. Several tributaries that enter the medial aspect of the portal vein and one tributary that enters the posterolateral aspect are divided. It is usually not necessary to divide the splenic vein. Wide mobilization of the portal vein is essential for performance of a side-to-side portacaval anastomosis. Failure to mobilize the portal vein behind the pancreas is a second major reason for difficulty in accomplishing the side-to-side shunt.

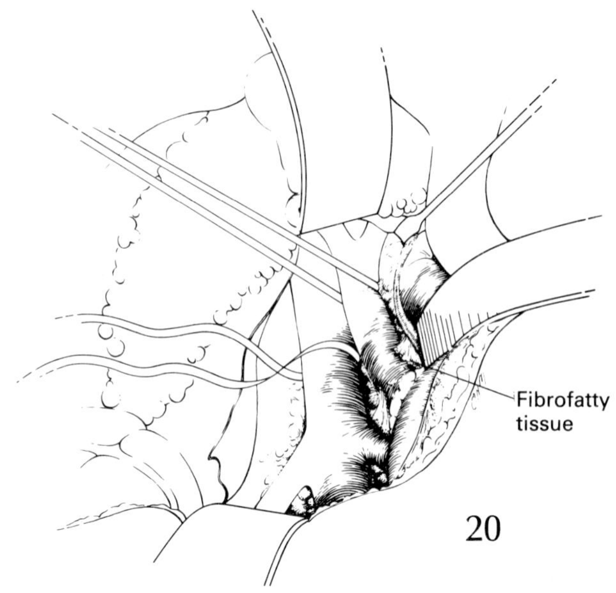

20

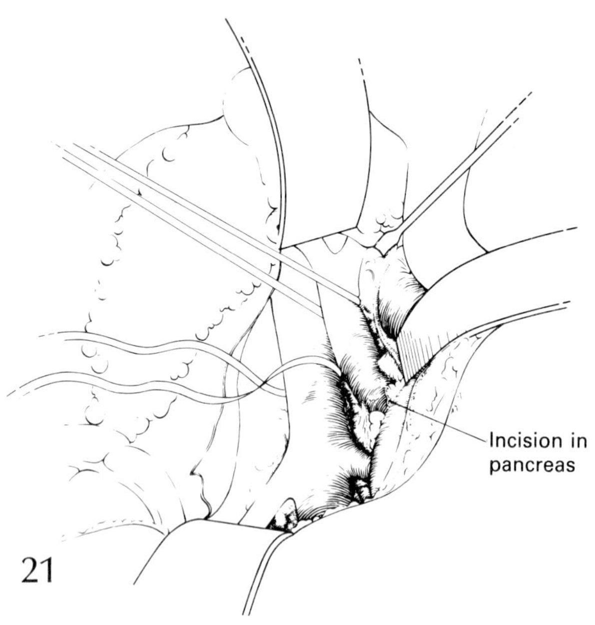

21

21

In some patients it is necessary to divide a bit of the head of the pancreas between right-angled clamps to obtain adequate mobilization of the portal vein. Bleeding from the edges of the divided pancreas is controlled with suture ligatures. Division of a small amount of the pancreas is a very helpful manoeuvre and we have never observed postoperative complications, such as pancreatitis, from its performance.

22

Determination of adequacy of mobilization of inferior vena cava and portal vein

To determine the adequacy of mobilization of the inferior vena cava and portal vein, the two vessels are brought together by traction on the umbilical tapes that surround them. It is essential to determine that the two vessels can be brought together without excessive tension. If this cannot be done it is almost always because the vessels have not been adequately mobilized, and further dissection of the vessels should be undertaken. Resection of part of an enlarged caudate lobe of the liver, recommended by some surgeons to facilitate bringing the vessels together, is associated with many difficulties and, in our opinion, is neither necessary nor advisable.

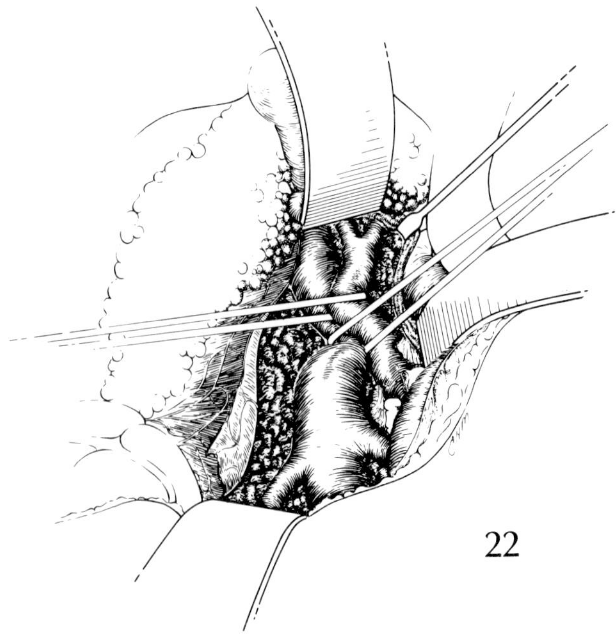

22

23

Measurement of venous pressures

Pressures in the inferior vena cava and portal vein are measured with a saline (spinal) manometer by direct needle puncture. For all pressure measurements, the bottom of the manometer is positioned at the level of the inferior vena cava, which is marked on the skin surface of the body with a towel clip. All portal pressures are *corrected* by subtracting the inferior vena caval pressure from the portal pressure. A corrected free portal pressure of 150 mm saline or higher represents clinically significant portal hypertension, and most patients with bleeding oesophageal varices have a corrected free portal pressure of 200 mm saline or higher. The pressure measurements include:

IVCP – inferior vena caval pressure (*b*)
FPP – free portal pressure (*c*)
HOPP – Hepatic occluded portal pressure, obtained on the hepatic side of a clamp occluding the portal vein (*d*)
SOPP – splanchnic occluded portal pressure, obtained on the intestinal side of a clamp occluding the portal vein (*e*).

In normal humans HOPP is much lower than FPP, and SOPP is much higher. In patients with portal hypertension, the finding of a HOPP that is higher than the FPP suggests the possibility that blood flow in the portal vein is reversed because of severe hepatic outflow obstruction.

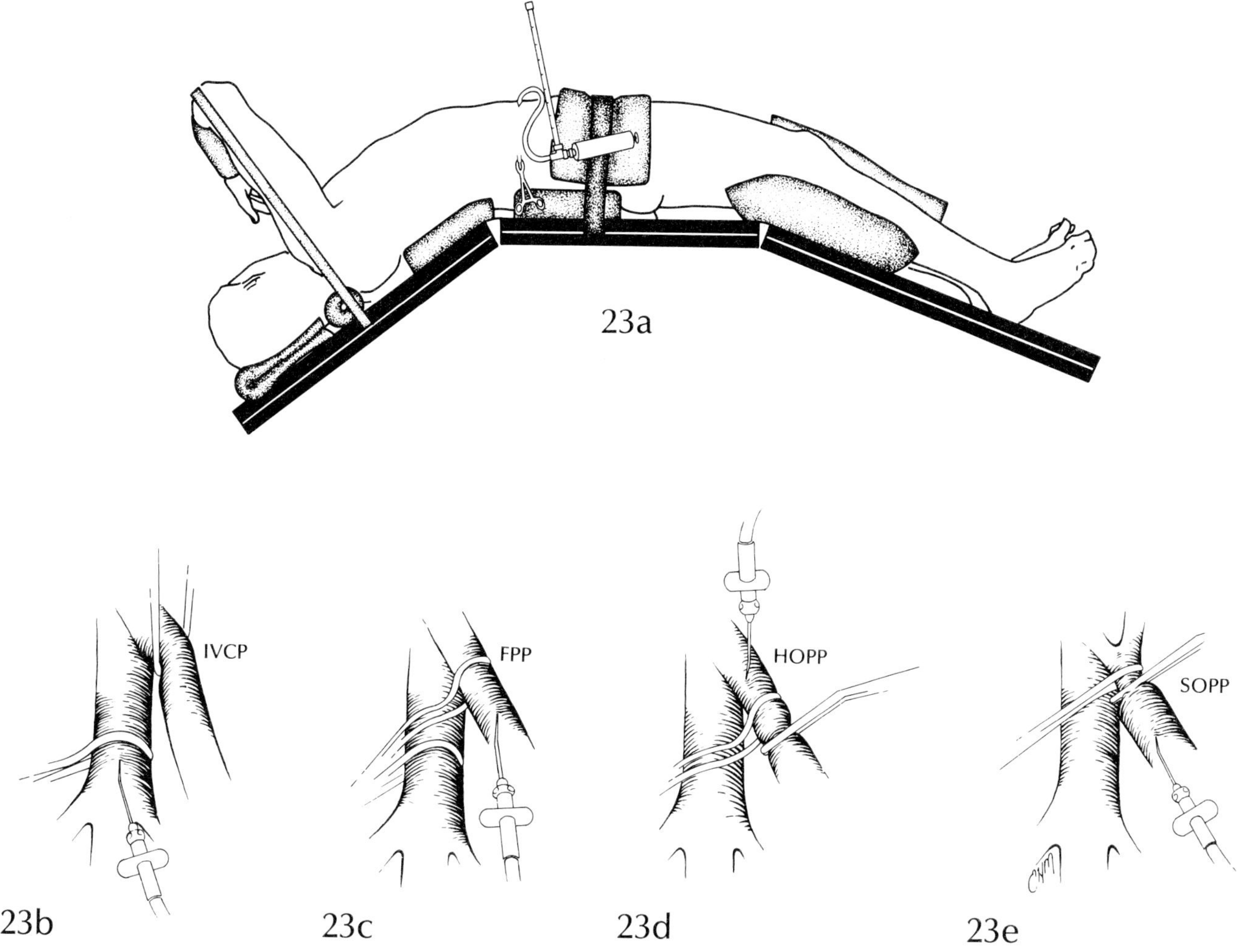

23a

23b 23c 23d 23e

Side-to-side portacaval anastomosis

24

A Satinsky clamp is placed obliquely across a 5 cm segment of the anteromedial wall of the inferior vena cava in a direction that is parallel to the course of the overlying portal vein and the vena cava is elevated towards the portal vein. A 5 cm segment of the portal vein is isolated between two angled vascular clamps, and the portal vein is depressed towards the vena cava, bringing the two vessels into apposition.

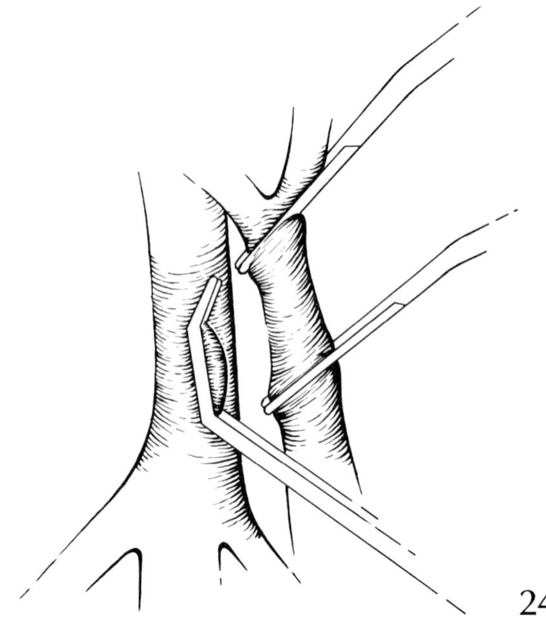

24

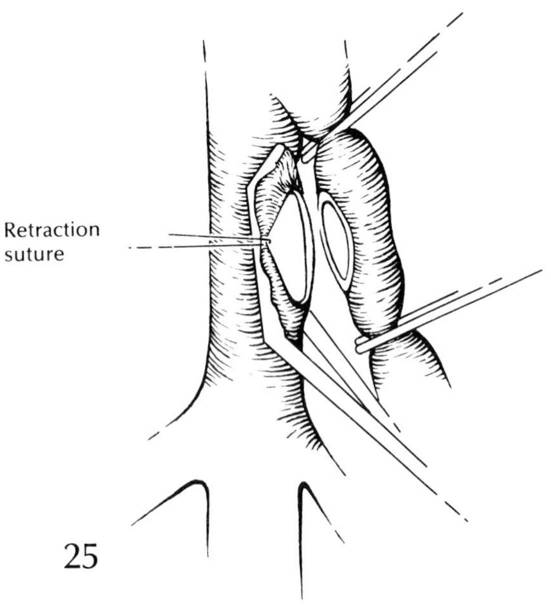

25

25

A 2.5 cm long strip of the inferior vena cava and a 2.5 cm long strip of the portal vein are excised with the scissors. It is important to excise a longitudinal segment of the wall of each vessel rather than simply to make an incision in each vessel. A retraction suture of 5/0 silk is placed in the lateral wall of the vena caval opening and is weighted by attachment to a haemostat to keep the vena caval orifice open. The clamps on the portal vein are momentarily released to flush out any clots and then the openings in both vessels are irrigated with saline.

26

The anastomosis is started with a posterior continuous over-and-over suture of 5/0 vascular silk or other vascular suture material. The posterior continuous suture is tied at each end of the anastomosis.

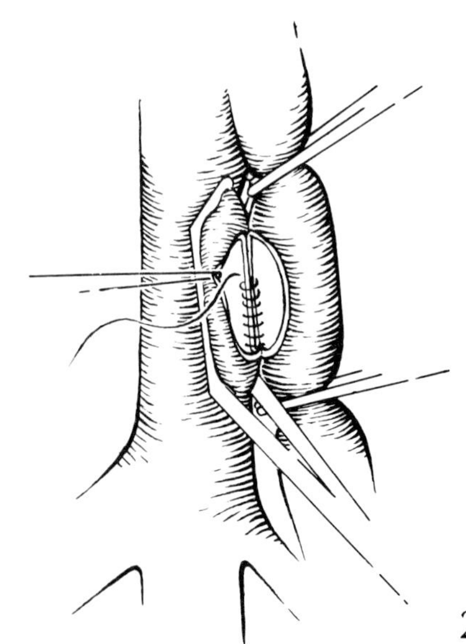

26

27

The anterior row of sutures consists of an everting continuous horizontal mattress stitch of 5/0 vascular material started at each end of the anastomosis. The suture started at the inferior end of the anastomosis is discontinued after three or four throws and is deliberately left loose so that the interior surface of the vessels can be visualized as the anastomosis is completed. In this way, inadvertent inclusion of the posterior wall in the anterior row of sutures is avoided. The suture started at the superior end of the anastomosis is inserted with continuous tension until it meets the inferior suture, at which point the inferior suture is drawn tight and the two sutures are tied to each other. Before drawing the inferior suture tight, the clamps on the portal vein are momentarily released to flush out any clots, and the anastomosis is thoroughly irrigated with saline.

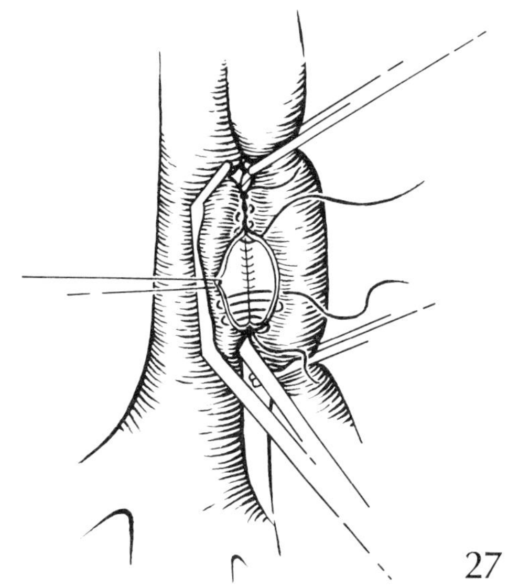

27

28

28

Upon completion of the anastomosis, a single interrupted tension suture is placed just beyond each end of the anastomosis to take tension off the anastomotic suture line. The clamp on the inferior vena cava is removed first, the clamp on the hepatic side of the portal vein is removed next, and finally the clamp on the intestinal side of the portal vein is removed. Bleeding from the anastomosis infrequently occurs; it can be controlled by one or two well placed interrupted sutures of 5/0 vascular material.

Pressures in the portal vein and inferior vena cava must be measured after the anastomosis is completed. Usually the postshunt pressures in the portal vein and vena cava are identical. A pressure gradient of greater than 50 mm saline between the two vessels indicates that there is an obstruction in the anastomosis, even when no obstruction can be palpated. In such circumstances, the anastomosis should be opened to remove any clots and, if necessary, the entire anastomosis should be taken down and done again. It is essential that there be no more than a 50 mm saline gradient between the portal vein and inferior vena cava to achieve permanently adequate portal decompression and avoid ultimate thrombosis of the shunt. Only two of the shunts that we have performed during the past 25 years have closed (both of them end-to-side anastomoses).

End-to-side portacaval anastomosis

The end-to-side portacaval anastomosis is a satisfactory alternative to the side-to-side shunt in most cases, and some surgeons believe that it is somewhat less difficult to perform. It is not essential to isolate the inferior vena cava around its entire circumference, and it is often not necessary to clear as long a segment of the portal vein as in the lateral anastomosis.

29

The Satinsky clamp on the inferior vena cava is placed obliquely on the anteromedial wall in a direction that will receive the end of the portal vein at an angle of about 45°. A 2 cm long strip of the inferior vena cava is excised and a retraction suture is placed in the lateral wall. The portal vein is doubly ligated with a free ligature and a suture ligature of 2/0 silk just before its bifurcation in the hilum of the liver. An angled vascular clamp is placed across the portal vein near the pancreas, and the portal vein is divided obliquely just proximal to the ligation site.

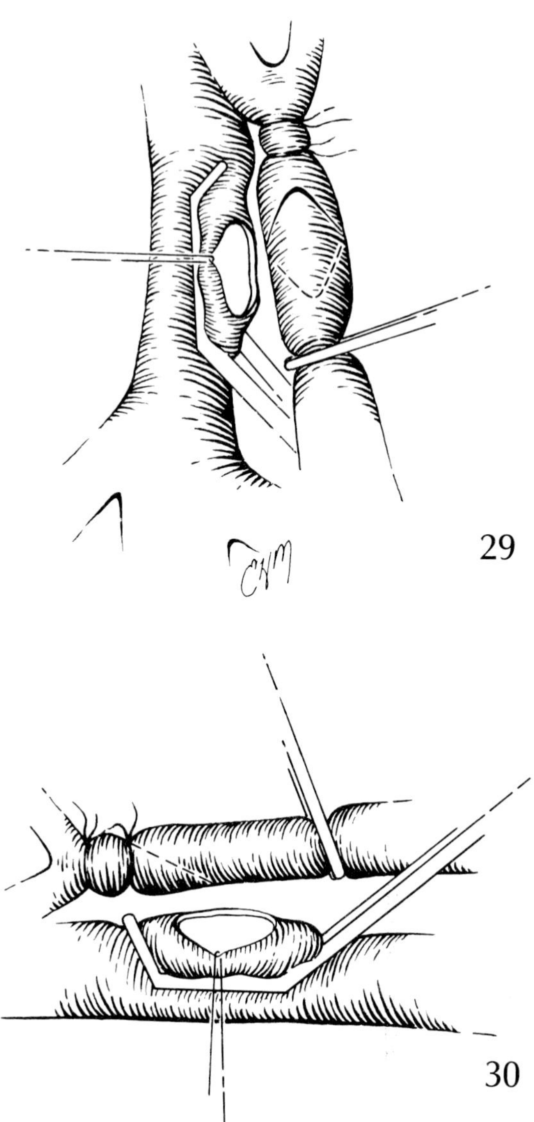

29

30

30

In order to maximize the size of the anastomosis, the portal vein is transected tangentially so that the anterior wall is longer than the posterior wall at the transected end. After transection, the clamp on the portal vein is momentarily released to flush out any clots before starting the anastomosis. This manoeuvre is repeated just before the final sutures in the anterior row of the anastomosis are placed.

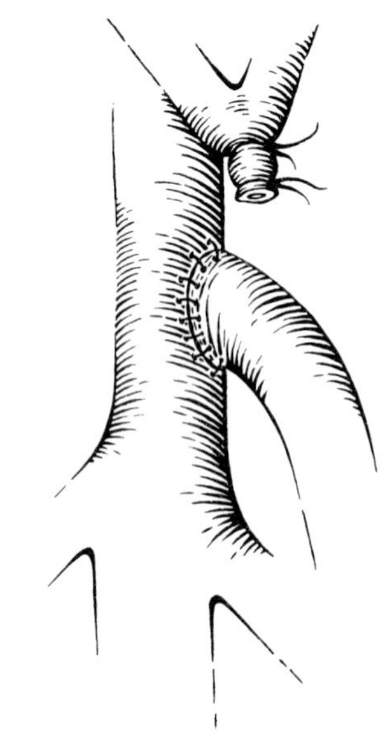

31

31

The end-to-side anastomosis is performed with a continuous, over-and-over 5/0 vascular suture in the posterior row and then a second 5/0 vascular suture in the anterior row. It is important that the portal vein describe a smooth curve in its descent toward the vena cava and that it be attached to the vena cava at an oblique angle. Twisting and kinking of the portal vein are the most common causes of a functionally unsatisfactory anastomosis. After the anastomosis is completed, pressure measurements are performed according to the guidelines described for the side-to-side shunt.

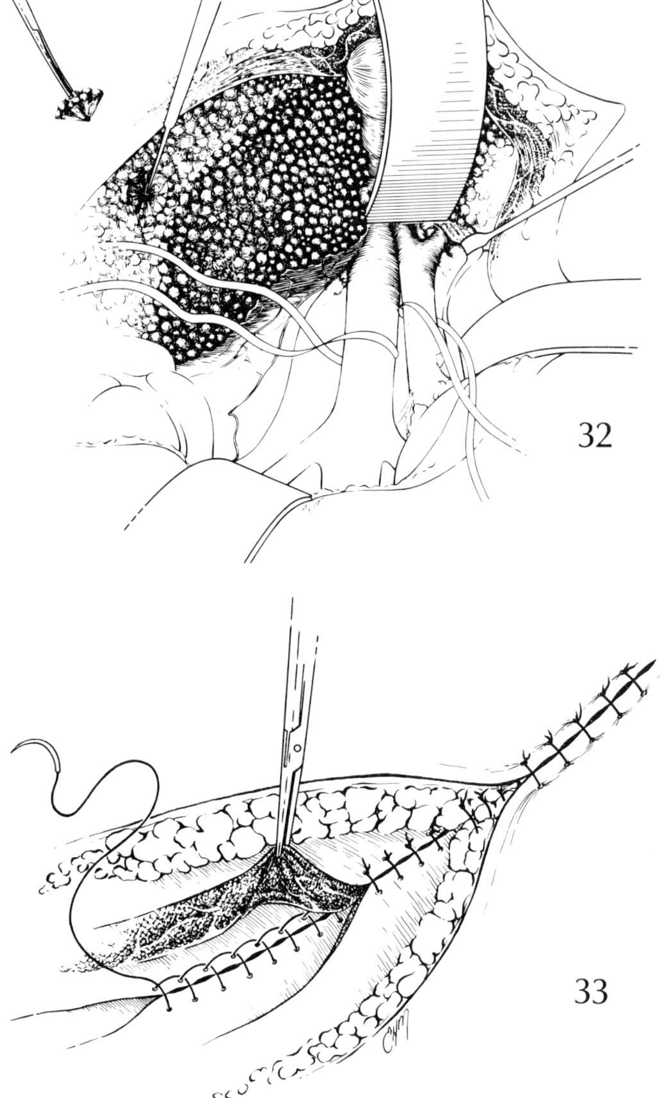

32

Liver biopsy

A wedge liver biopsy is always obtained. The wedge of liver is excised with the scalpel and the excision site is cauterized with the electrocautery. No sutures are required in this rapid and effective method of liver biopsy which we have used in over 2000 patients without a complication.

33

Closure of the incision

The peritoneum is closed with a continuous locking suture of No. 1 chromic catgut. The muscles are closed in layers with interrupted sutures of No. 28 (2/0) braided stainless steel wire. The subcutaneous tissues are approximated with interrupted sutures of 3/0 plain catgut, and the skin edges are approximated with interrupted sutures of 4/0 nylon. No drains are used. Drainage of the peritoneal cavity often leads to continuous and substantial losses of ascitic fluid and creates problems in fluid and electrolyte balance.

Summary of important technical features

1. The position of the patient on the operating table is crucial and can make the difference between an easy and difficult operation.
2. A long right subcostal incision is associated with many fewer postoperative complications than a thoraco-abdominal incision and is much to be preferred.
3. Use of the electrocautery throughout the operation substantially reduces the operating time and the blood loss.
4. Bleeding from the many portasystemic collateral vessels is best managed by pressure with gauze sponge packs, particularly as most of the bleeding stops as soon as the portacaval anastomosis is completed and the portal hypertension is relieved. Attempts to control each of the bleeding collaterals with ligatures and sutures prolongs the operation and increases the blood loss. The objective is to decompress the portal system as rapidly as possible.
5. Circumferential mobilization of the inferior vena cava between the entrance of the renal veins and the liver is essential for the side-to-side anastomosis and is neither hazardous nor difficult to perform. Apposition of the two vessels is greatly facilitated by elevation of the vena cava towards the portal vein.
6. Mobilization of a long segment of portal vein, which includes division of the tough fibrofatty tissue that binds the portal vein to the pancreas and sometimes includes division of a bit of the head of the pancreas, is essential for the side-to-side anastomosis and sometimes for the end-to-side anastomosis.
7. Resection of an enlarged caudate lobe of the liver to facilitate apposition of the two vessels is hazardous and unnecessary.
8. Pressures in the inferior vena cava and portal vein should always be measured after completion of the portacaval shunt. A pressure gradient of greater than 50 mm saline is unacceptable and requires revision of the anastomosis.

Postoperative care

Patients with liver disease who bleed from oesophageal varices are among the most seriously ill patients in any hospital, regardless of the specific therapy used to control the bleeding. In those who undergo emergency portacaval shunt, the expertise of the postoperative care is a major factor in determining survival. All such patients should be admitted to an intensive care unit with equipment and personnel geared to managing the complicated problems associated with hepatic disease. A description of specific prophylactic and therapeutic aspects of postoperative care follows.

Monitoring

Careful monitoring of vital signs, central venous pressure, urine output, arterial pH, arterial and alveolar gases, fluid balance, body weight and abdominal girth is essential. Serial electrocardiograms and determinations of cardiac output and peripheral resistance are often very helpful. Measurement of pulmmonary artery wedge pressure with a Swan-Ganz catheter occasionally is indicated. Serial measurements of liver function, of the formed elements in the blood (including platelets), of blood coagulation, of serum electrolytes, and of renal function, must be done.

Parenteral fluid therapy

Patients with liver disease are often waterlogged before the onset of bleeding from varices, and they have a markedly impaired capacity to excrete water loads. The bleeding episode and the operation intensify renal sodium and water retention and exaggerate the already existing fluid intolerance. Parenteral fluid therapy should be calculated to maintain such patients on the dry side. Fluid losses are replaced by a solution of 10 per cent dextrose in water containing all the B vitamins as well as C and K. The total volume usually amounts to 1500–2000 ml/day, based on daily losses of 500 ml of nasogastric aspirate, 500–1000 ml of urine, 800–1000 ml of insensible water, and a gain of 250–500 ml from endogenous water formation. Sodium is given only to replace nasogastric losses, which rarely exceed 30–40 mmol/day. Parenteral potassium therapy is started as soon as the urine output is adequate and is given in whatever amounts are necessary to maintain the serum potassium concentration between 4 and 5 mmol/litre. Usually, the requirement is 150–200 mmol/day but amounts as high as 500 mmol/day may be necessary. If a metabolic alkalosis develops, it usually responds to repletion of potassium with large quantities of parenteral potassium chloride. If the alkalosis fails to respond, an acidifying agent such as arginine hydrochloride or hydrochloric acid should be administered slowly so as to lower the arterial blood pH below 7.5. In addition to crystalloid fluid therapy, it is often necessary to add colloid therapy to replace continuing losses of blood and plasma. Transfusions of fresh blood are given for blood loss or a haematocrit below 30 per cent. Type-specific, single-donor plasma, fresh-frozen plasma, or salt-poor concentrated albumin is given for losses of fluid into the operation site and peritoneal cavity (acute ascites), as determined by the combined measurements of abdominal girth, central venous pressure, urine output, body weight and a haematocrit showing haemoconcentration.

Pulmonary therapy

Pulmonary complications, particularly infection and wet lung, are a major cause of morbidity and mortality in patients with cirrhosis and bleeding varices. In about 5 per cent of our cases it has been necessary to maintain the patient on a respirator for several days postoperatively. In such cases, mechanical ventilatory support usually can be provided through an endotracheal tube that may be left indwelling for 48–72 h. Occasionally it is necessary to perform a tracheostomy for ventilation and tracheobronchial toilet, but it should be recognized that complications of tracheostomy, particularly bleeding, are more frequent in cirrhotic patients. Portable chest X-rays are obtained daily in patients on respirators or those having pulmonary problems. The decision to taper off and then discontinue mechanical ventilatory support is based on measurements of arterial blood and alveolar gases, ventilatory volumes, chest X-rays and physical findings.

All patients not on a respirator are given continuous oxygen therapy by nasal catheter or mask for 5–7 days postoperatively because of the frequent cardiovascular abnormalities and arteriovenous shunting that exist in cirrhosis. From the start, all patients receive intensive respiratory therapy that consists of intermittent tracheobronchial aspiration, postural drainage, chest physiotherapy, intermittent positive-pressure respiration, frequent turning, encouragement to cough and breathe deeply, and the use of blow bottles and a humidifier. Diuretics may be of value in the treatment of pulmonary oedema caused by left heart failure or infection.

Hyperdynamic circulation

Numerous studies have shown that patients with cirrhosis and portal hypertension frequently have a hyperdynamic state that consists of a decrease in vascular tone and peripheral resistance, an increase in cardiac index, an increase in venous oxygen saturation with widespread peripheral arteriovenous shunting, and marked pulmonary arteriovenous admixture. These abnormalities are sometimes intensified by bleeding from oesophageal varices or performance of a portacaval shunt, and high-output cardiac failure may develop, particularly in older patients and those with far advanced liver disease. It is for this reason that we perform serial measurements of cardiac output in all patients both preoperatively and postoperatively. Patients with hyperdynamic state are digitalized immediately postoperatively before there are any signs of cardiac failure. Vigorous correction of hypovolaemia is undertaken simultaneously. Once blood volume is restored, fluids are restricted to avoid circulatory overload, and diuretics are used if there are any signs of overhydration. Inotropic drugs are used when appropriate.

Delirium tremens

Alcoholic cirrhotic patients frequently have delirium tremens following haemorrhage alone or in combination with a portacaval shunt or other operation. There is not always a close temporal correlation between alcohol withdrawal and the development of this serious disorder; we have observed postoperative delirium tremens weeks and months after ingestion of alcohol was stopped. Delirium tremens by itself, in the absence of bleeding or an operation, is associated with a mortality rate of 15–20 per cent. When added to the stress of haemorrhage or major surgery, the mortality rate climbs to 50–60 per cent. Initial treatment consists of administration of a central nervous system depressant. We prefer intramuscular magnesium sulphate in doses of 2 g every 2–4 h. If magnesium sulphate therapy is not rapidly effective, chlordiazepoxide hydrochloride (Librium) is added in a dose of 25–50 mg intramuscularly every 4 h.

Supportive treatment in the form of adequate parenteral fluids containing concentrated glucose and vitamins, antipyretic agents, and pulmonary therapy is important. This hyperactive, hypermetabolic disorder must not be confused with hepatic encephalopathy, because the use of a central nervous system depressant in hepatic encephalopathy may be lethal. Intravenous alcohol is a severe hepatotoxin, and there is no basis for its use in cirrhotic patients with postoperative delirium tremens. Parenteral paraldehyde has no advantages over other hypnotic drugs and, in the author's opinion, should not be used because of the frequent soft tissue abscesses and noxious odour it produces.

Hepatic failure

The majority of patients appear to be in surprisingly good condition immediately following an emergency portacaval shunt. However, by the second or third postoperative day there is evidence of some deterioration of liver function in almost all patients. In many patients the liver dysfunction stabilizes and then improves, but in some it progresses to hepatic coma and the full syndrome of hepatic failure, with jaundice, severe abnormalities of blood coagulation, ascites and renal insufficiency. Liver failure is the most frequent cause of death in cirrhotic patients who bleed from oesophageal varices, whether or not they have had a portacaval shunt.

It should be emphasized that the hepatic coma that occurs during the immediate postoperative period is due to liver cell failure and is *not* related to ammonia intoxication or systemic shunting of nitrogenous substances absorbed from the intestines. Unfortunately, there is no specific therapy for hepatic failure, and all that can be done is to provide parenteral nutritional support and symptomatic therapy of the individual abnormalities that arise. There is no evidence that exchange transfusion, haemodialysis or extracorporeal perfusion of the blood through a pig, baboon or human liver is of value in this situation. Spontaneous recovery sometimes occurs.

Because it is rarely possible to remove all of the blood from the gastrointestinal tract preoperatively, neomycin therapy (1 g every 6 h via the nasogastric tube), cathartics (60 ml magnesium sulphate per day via the nasogastric tube), and a daily neomycin enema (4 g in 1.5 litres of water) are continued for 3 days postoperatively. If continued beyond 3 days, troublesome diarrhoea usually follows. With this regimen, significantly elevated blood ammonia levels or signs of nitrogen-related encephalopathy rarely occur within the first postoperative week.

Gastric acid hypersecretion

Inconclusive evidence suggests that, following portacaval shunt, gastric acid hypersecretion develops and is associated with an increased incidence of peptic ulcer. To protect against this potential complication, nasogastric suction is continued for 3 to 4 days postoperatively and the patient is given cimetidine parenterally. As soon as the nasogastric tube is removed, the patient is started on hourly antacid therapy until his oral dietary intake is good and then the antacid schedule is changed to between meals and at bedtime. An antacid that does not contain sodium is used. Antacid and cimetidine therapy are discontinued 3 months postoperatively.

Renal failure

There are two common forms of renal dysfunction following variceal haemorrhage and portacaval shunt. The first is acute tubular necrosis which results from a period of hypotension and consequent renal ischaemia. It is manifested by oliguria, uraemia, hyperkalaemia, a low, fixed urine specific gravity and osmolality, substantial quantities of sodium in the urine, and a urine sediment containing casts and red blood cells. Treatment consists of stringent fluid restriction, measures to reduce serum potassium, and, if necessary, haemodialysis.

The second renal disorder is *spontaneous renal failure* associated with hepatic decompensation, the so-called 'hepatorenal syndrome'. It is more insidious in onset than acute tubular necrosis and is manifested initially by progressive uraemia without striking oliguria. In contrast to acute tubular necrosis, the urine specific gravity is variable and ranges up to 1.020. There is almost no sodium in the urine, the osmolality of the urine is high and the urine sediment is normal. There is no specific treatment for spontaneous renal failure and therapy is directed at reversing the hepatic decompensation, minimizing dilutional hyponatraemia and correcting problems as they appear. There is no indication for the use of diuretics and, in fact, they may intensify the renal abnormality. Numerous vasoactive agents have been used for the purpose of improving renal blood flow, but none has influenced the outcome significantly. Haemodialysis has created more problems that it has solved. The mortality rate of the combined syndrome of hepatic and renal decompensation is very high.

Infection

Substantial evidence indicates that patients with cirrhosis have a high incidence of infection, perhaps because of their debilitated general condition. Surprisingly, wound and intraperitoneal infections following emergency portacaval shunt have been uncommon in our experience.

However, pulmonary infections have been common and urinary tract infections not infrequent. The value of prophylactic antibiotic therapy in this condition is uncertain. Appropriate antibiotics are given for proven infections, always on the basis of bacterial cultures and antibiotic sensitivity tests. We routinely obtain cultures of tracheal aspirates and urine during the early postoperative period to avoid delays in therapy should infection develop.

Nutrition

Nutritional therapy is very important in liver disease. Oral diet is started as soon as the patient tolerates removal of the nasogastric tube for 24 h, usually on the fifth or sixth postoperative day. Initially, 10 mmol sodium, 4000 calorie (16.8 kJ), high carbohydrate, regular fat, 20 g protein, bland diet is introduced. There is no basis for restricting fat and doing so only serves to make the diet unpalatable. The protein content of the diet is increased in 20 g increments every 3 days up to 80 g and the patient is carefully observed for signs of encephalopathy. If the patient tolerates 80 g of protein per day, he is discharged on a 60 g protein diet after having received a diet list and specific instructions from a dietician. Rigorous sodium restriction is continued for several months and, even after a year has elapsed, sodium intake is not allowed to advance above 50 mmol per day. Daily therapeutic doses of vitamins B and C are added to the diet.

Alcoholism

Perhaps the major factor that determines long-term survival following portacaval shunt is abstinence or failure to abstain from alcohol. It is vitally important that a frank discussion be held with the patient regarding the extremely serious dangers of further ingestion of alcohol. The help of psychiatrists and social workers should be obtained while the patient is in the hospital and continued after discharge. It is incumbent upon the surgeon to exploit his special relationship with the patient in a long-term effort to cure the underlying cause of the patient's liver disease.

Follow-up

A lifelong programme of follow-up evaluation and treatment is a crucial part of the care of cirrhotic patients who have undergone portacaval shunt. The liver disease cannot be cured, but it can be stabilized to the point of permitting a long and productive life in reasonable comfort. After discharge from the hospital, outpatient visits are schedule weekly for the first 8 weeks, monthly for the remainder of the first postoperative year and every 3 months thereafter for the remainder of the patient's life.

Results

Between 1958 and 1982 we performed 1117 portal-systemic shunts for portal hypertension. In 128 of these patients the shunt was performed electively for bleeding oesophageal varices due to extrahepatic portal obstruction and there were no operative deaths. An additional 712 patients had elective therapeutic portacaval shunts for portal hypertension due to liver disease, and the operative mortality rate in this group was 2 per cent. The remaining patients in our series underwent emergency therapeutic portacaval shunt.

Between 1960 and 1978 we conducted a prospective study of emergency treatment of bleeding oesophageal varices in unselected patients with alcoholic cirrhosis. At first we compared emergency medical therapy and emergency transoesophageal variceal ligation, both followed by elective portacaval shunt, in a randomized clinical trial. Later we evaluated emergency portacaval shunt. Every patient admitted to our hospital with bleeding varices was included in these studies regardless of condition, and all operations were performed within 8 hours of admission to our emergency room. Follow-up study has been conducted in a special clinic, and the current status of 97 per cent of the patients is known. The results are shown in *Table 1* and *Figure 1*.

The early survival rate following emergency portacaval shunt was 58 per cent, compared to 54 per cent for variceal ligation and 17 per cent for medical therapy. The 12 year survival rate, calculated according to the actuarial method, was 30 per cent, compared to 11 per cent for variceal ligation and 0 for medical treatment. Portacaval shunt controlled the bleeding promptly and permanently in 98 per cent of the patients. Encephalopathy of any degree developed at some time in 31.5 per cent of the survivors. It

Table 1 Comparison of results of emergency portacaval shunt, transoesophageal varix ligation and medical treatment in unselected patients with cirrhosis and bleeding varices

	*Medical treatment**	*Varix ligation**	*Emergency shunt*
Number of patients	59	28	180
Jaundice on admission (%)	42	57	49
Ascites on admission (%)	41	50	53
Encephalopathy on admission (%)	25	25	19
Mean liver index on admission	2.8	2.8	2.4
Admission haemoglobin 11 g/100 ml or less (%)	70	71	71
Varices demonstrated (%)	95	100	100
Mean volume of blood transfused (litres)	7.2	4.2	5.0
Early (30 day) survival (%)	17	54	58
Twelve-year survival (%)	0	11	30

* Followed by elective portacaval shunt when possible

is noteworthy that one-third of the patients had encephalopathy before the shunt operation. In 7 per cent of the survivors, encephalopathy was severe and required chronic dietary protein restriction; in 12 per cent it required transient protein restriction, usually for a single episode of neurological disturbance; and in 13 per cent it was mild and did not require protein limitation. Forty-eight per cent of the survivors abstained from alcohol permanently and 60 per cent resumed gainful employment or full-time housekeeping.

As our experience with emergency portacaval shunt has increased, the results have improved. *Figure 2* shows the cumulative survival curve of 86 unselected, consecutive patients who underwent emergency shunt during the recent 5 year period from 1977 to 1982. The survival curve of the previous series of 180 patients is included for comparison. The early survival rate of the recently treated group was 81 per cent, and the 5 year actuarial survival rate is 70 per cent. The long-term survival rate in this group of unselected patients, all comers included, is as least as high as that reported by other surgeons for elective portal-systemic shunt in highly selected patients. The results of our studies indicate that emergency portacaval shunt has produced a significant improvement in immediate and long-term survival of cirrhotic patients with bleeding oesophageal varices. As is true of survival statistics for cancer and other lethal disorders, the absolute survival rate is of limited meaning unless it is viewed in the context of the natural history of the disease. The 12 year survival rate in our experience to date is many times greater than that associated with emergency medical therapy followed, in the few patients who survive, by elective portacaval shunt.

Some results of elective therapeutic portal-systemic shunt are shown in *Table 2*. It should be recognized that the statistics reflect operations on highly selected patients, all of whom survived one or more episodes of bleeding varices and had sufficiently good hepatic function to qualify for elective surgical therapy.

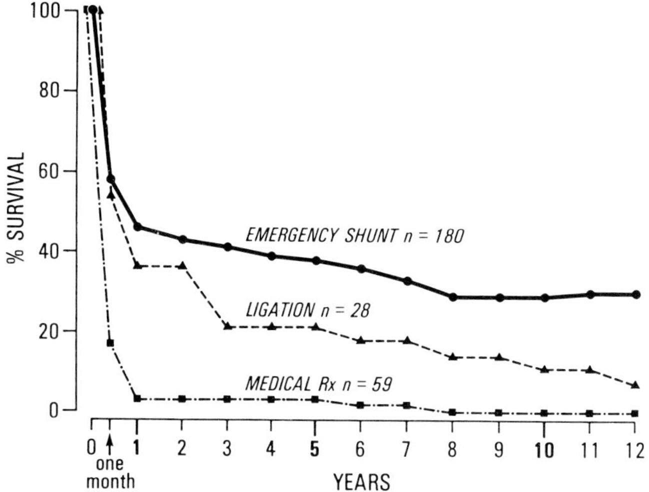

Figure 1 Cumulative 12 year survival rates of unselected patients with cirrhosis and bleeding oesophageal varices following emergency portacaval shunt, transoesophageal variceal ligation and medical treatment

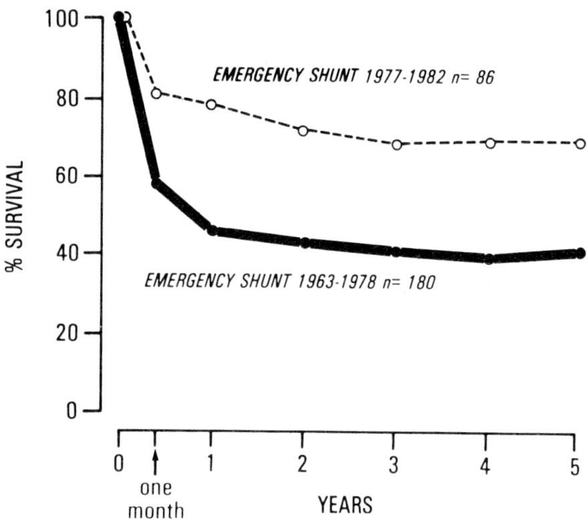

Figure 2 Cumulative 5 year survival rate of 86 unselected patients with cirrhosis who underwent emergency portacaval shunt during the period 1977–1982, compared with the cumulative survival rate of 180 patients who were operated upon from 1963 to 1978

Table 2 Results of elective portal-systemic shunt in highly selected patients with cirrhosis

Authors	*No. of Patients*	*Type of shunt*	*Operative mortality (%)*	*Varix rebleeding (%)*	*5 Year survival (%)*
Voorhees, Price and Britton	404	324 portacaval, 80 splenorenal & other	12	7	51
McDermott *et al.*	237	166 splenorenal, 71 portacaval	23	15	54
Barnes *et al.*	173	103 portacaval, 70 splenorenal	13	14	39
Mikkelsen, Turrill and Pattison	173	All portacaval	12	7	44
Linton, Ellis and Geary	169	129 splenorenal, 47 portacaval	12	19	50
Turcotte and Lambert	147	All portacaval	21	—	35
Bismuth, Franco and Hepp	120	72 central splenorenal, 48 portacaval	2	3	66
Wantz and Payne	97	All portacaval	11	5	68 (4 year)
Walker	50	All portacaval	6	12	70
Orloff	612	All portacaval	2	0.5	60

References

1. Orloff, M. J., Bell, R. H., Hyde, P. V., Skivolocki, W. P. Long-term results of emergency portacaval shunt for bleeding esophageal varices in unselected patients with alcoholic cirrhosis. Annals of Surgery 1980; 192: 325–340

2. Orloff, M. J. Emergency portacaval shunt: A comparative study of shunt, varix ligation and nonsurgical treatment of bleeding esophageal varices in unselected patients with cirrhosis. Annals of Surgery 1967; 166: 456–478

3. Orloff, M. J., Chandler, J. G., Charters, A. C., Condon, J. K., Grambort, D. E., Modafferi, T. R., Levin, S. E. Emergency portacaval shunt for bleeding esophageal varices. Prospective study in unselected patients with alcoholic cirrhosis. Archives of Surgery 1974; 108: 293–299

4. Orloff, M, J., Duguay, L. R., Kosta, L. D. Criteria for selection of patients for emergency portacaval shunt. American Journal of Surgery 1977; 134: 146–152

5. Charters, A. C., Brown, B. N., Sviokla, S. C., Knox, D. G., Orloff, M. J. The influence of portal perfusion on the response to portacaval shunt. American Journal of Surgery 1975; 130: 226–232

6. Orloff, M. J., Chandler, J. G., Charters, A. C., Condon, J. K., Grambort, D. E., Modafferi, T. R., Levin, S. E. Comparison of end-to-side and side-to-side portacaval shunts in dogs and human subjects with cirrhosis and portal hypertension. American Journal of Surgery 1974; 128: 195–201

7. Orloff, M. J. Effect of side-to-side portacaval shunt on intractable ascites, sodium excretion, and aldosterone metabolism in man. American Journal of Surgery 1966; 112: 297–298

8. Orloff, M. J., Johansen, K. H. Treatment of Budd-Chiari syndrome by side-to-side portacaval shunt: experimental and clinical results. Annals of Surgery 1978; 188: 494–512

9. Orloff, M. J. The liver. In: Sabiston, D. C., ed. Davis-Christopher textbook of surgery. 12th ed. Philadelphia: Saunders, 1981: 1131

End ileostomy

Victor W. Fazio MB, BS, FRACS, FACS
Chairman, Department of Colon and Rectal Surgery,
The Cleveland Clinic Foundation, Cleveland, Ohio;
Medical Director, Rupert B. Turnbull Jr School of Enterostomal Therapy,
The Cleveland Clinic Foundation, Cleveland, Ohio

Preoperative

Indications

An end ileostomy is made at the completion of abdominal colectomy or proctocolectomy for inflammatory bowel disease. Some surgeons favour proctocolectomy and ileostomy for patients with familial polyposis. Others will reserve it for patients with this disease where either a rectal carcinoma or a diffuse 'sea' of sessile polyps will make future attempts at polyp control difficult. The operation may also be required in the rare circumstances where multiple synchronous cancers are present in the large bowel. A 'temporary' end ileostomy is sometimes made in patients following ileal or ileocaecal resection for perforating Crohn's disease, ileocaecal trauma or obstructing right colonic lesions. A 'take down' of the end ileostomy and an ileocolic anastomosis may be carried out subsequently. On rare occasions an end ileostomy is made without colectomy; this has been used in inflammatory bowel disease to allow the patient's general condition to improve before elective colectomy but is seldom advised today. An end or loop ileostomy may also be used when constructing an ileal conduit.

Preoperative preparation

This largely depends upon the underlying condition for which a colectomy and ileostomy is planned. The surgeon must spend time discussing the implications of surgery with the patient *and* his family. This discussion is complemented by further contact with the enterostomal therapist and usually with a visit by a trained 'lay' ostomy visitor. Many patients may request pertinent literature, available from the local cancer society, ostomy association or one's own institution. Reassurance and encouragement are given to the patient; the more ill the patient the less a surgeon should dwell on the technical aspects of the surgery.

1

Siting the stoma

Rehabilitation of the patient begins at this point, *before* the operation, with the accurate selection of the optimal stoma site. The author's own experience of having patients wear a bag preoperatively to see 'if the fit is right' has been unhelpful; patients really don't know what a 'right fit' is; the author prefers to mark a stoma site with the patient in the sitting position when any crease or fold of skin will become more prominent, and then check the position with the patient supine.

The following rules apply.

1. Use the summit or apex of the infraumbilical fat mound.
2. The mark should be in the middle or at least within the surface marking of the rectus abdominis muscle.
3. The mark should be at least 5 cm from the planned incision line.
4. Using a preoperative standard-sized face plate, the stoma site and adjacent skin should be away from creases, scars, the umbilicus, bony prominences and future incisions.
5. A site where the skin has been injured, e.g. from a skin graft or radiotherapy, must be avoided.

Once the stoma site has been selected, a vertical line is marked downwards from the umbilicus and a horizontal line is marked outwards from the lower border of the umbilicus.

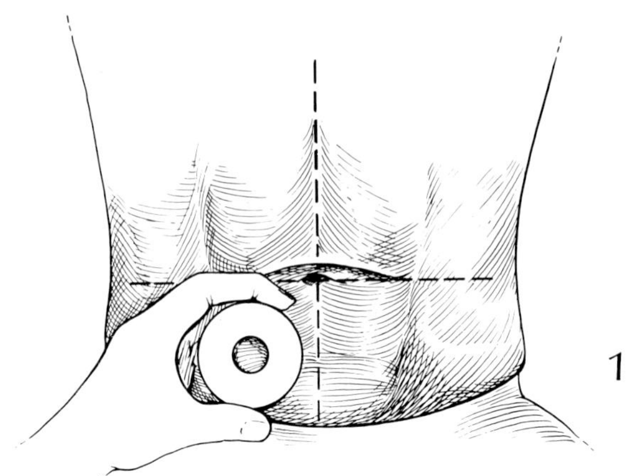

1

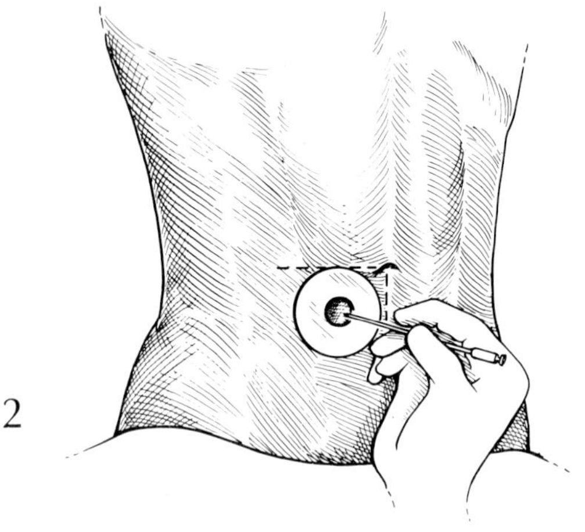

2

2

Marking the stoma

The plate is positioned to fit within these boundaries. An indelible mark is made by placing a drop of India ink or methylene blue over the stoma site, and a needle prick produces a tattoo which cannot be washed away, like other surface markers, during preoperative bathing or when painting the abdominal wall with antiseptic solution.

Anaesthesia and position of patient

General anaesthesia with relaxant agents and endotracheal intubation is used. A nasogastric tube is inserted after induction of anaesthesia and the bladder is catheterized if bowel resection is contemplated. A supine or modified lithotomy-Trendelenburg position is used depending on whether or not a combined abdominoperineal proctectomy is to be part of the procedure.

The operation

The incision is made in the midline, skirting to the left side of the umbilicus. If colectomy is planned, the incision is carried to the upper epigastrium to a point where the surgeon judges that safe mobilization of the splenic flexure can be carried out. Because of the future possibility of stoma revision and relocation (especially when operating for Crohn's disease) it seems wise to use a midline incision rather than a left paramedian so that the left lower abdomen is left intact.

3

Division of the terminal ileum

In the absence of ileal disease, the ileum is transected 7–10 cm from the ileocaecal valve. One occasionally sees very thick ileostomy effluent, capable of pushing an appliance off when the division has been made at the ileocaecal junction. To minimize contamination in the course of delivery of the end of the ileum through the abdominal wall, a GIA Auto Suture is used.

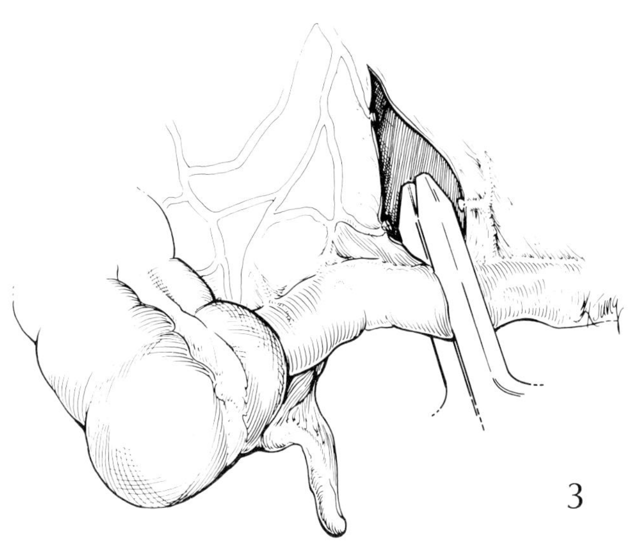

3

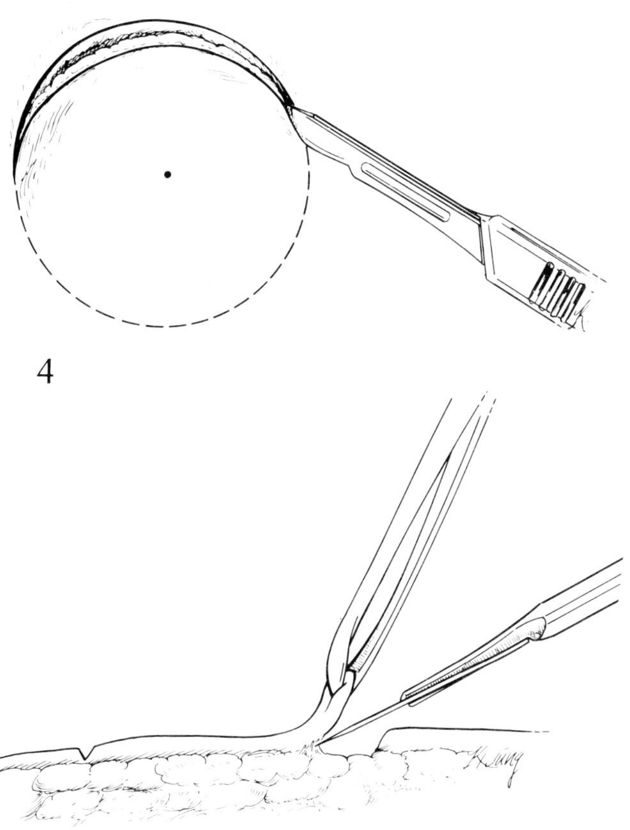

4

5

The ileostomy aperture and the fashioning of the stoma

4 & 5

A circumferential incision is made around the previously marked stoma site, about 3.5 cm in diameter. No trephine is made, rather the subcutaneous fat is preserved to minimize the chances of a dead space and accumulation of a parastomal seroma or abscess. The sagittal view shows excision of the skin disc and preservation of the fat.

6

A vertical incision is made with the cutting cautery. Any bleeding from the skin edge is left to stop spontaneously. Coagulation here can severely traumatize the skin with subsequent mucocutaneous separation.

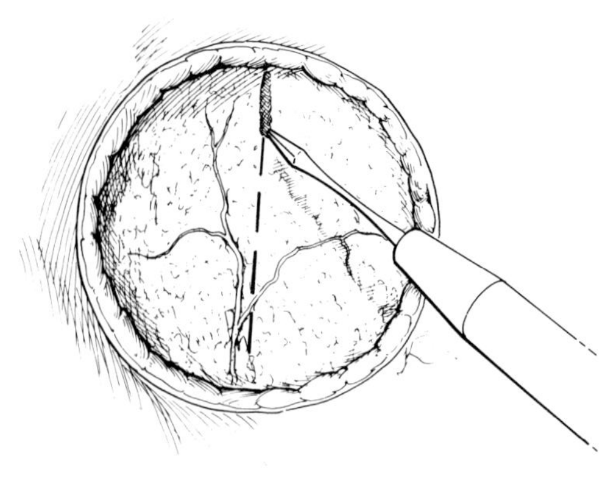

6

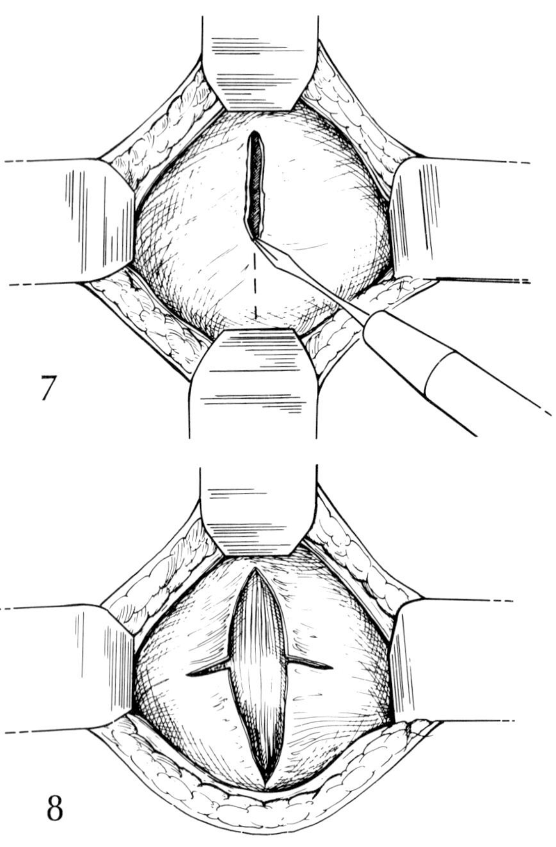

7

8

7 & 8

After incising Scarpa's layer of fascia, short right-angle retractors are positioned to display the anterior rectus sheath. The cutting cautery incises the sheath for 3.5 cm in a vertical direction. If the fascial aperture is considered too snug, lateral cruciate incisions may be added.

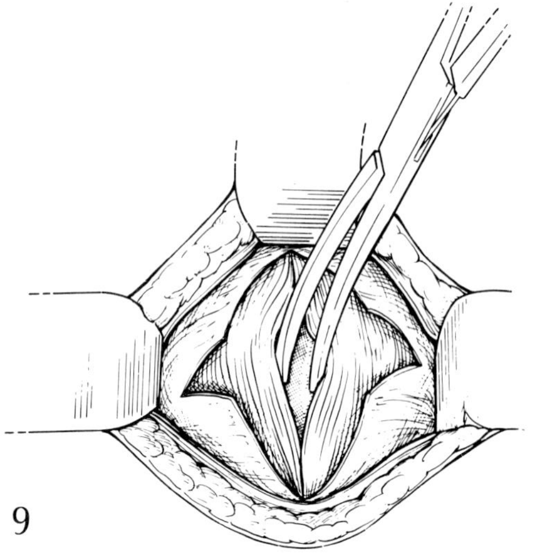

9

9

An artery forceps is inserted in a perpendicular fashion right down to the posterior sheath and the jaws are gently opened in the horizontal plane, minimizing the risk of injury to the inferior epigastric vessels. Before withdrawing the instrument, medial and lateral retractors are placed as the vertical fibres of the muscle spring back, making identification of the site of the rectus split quite difficult. A muscle split, rather than a muscle-cutting procedure, is done to minimize the risk of postoperative hernia or prolapse of the ileostomy.

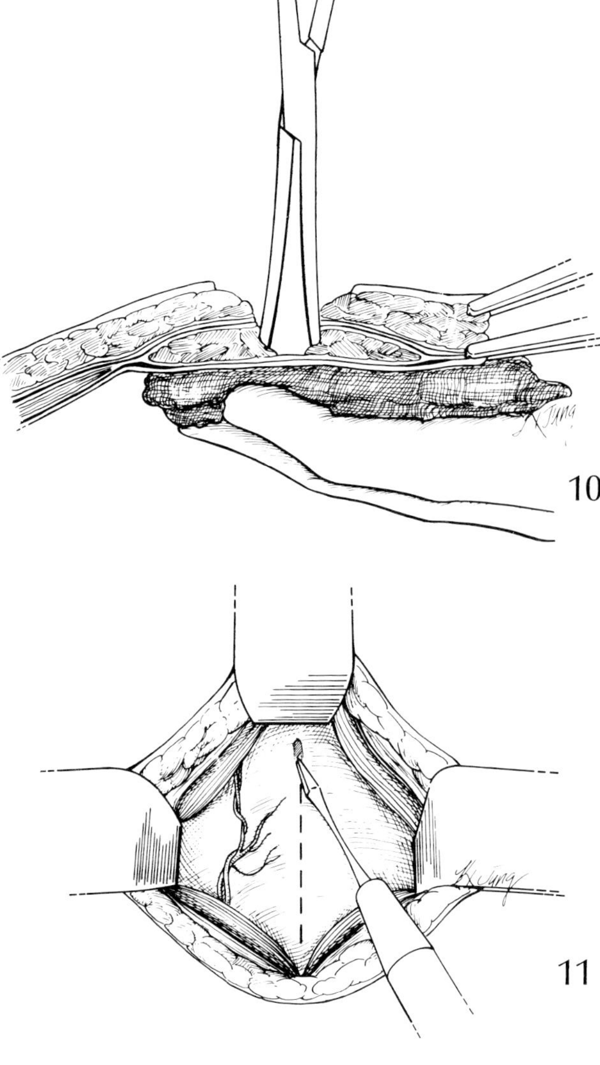
10

11

10 & 11

Kocher clamps placed on the subcutaneous fat and fascia of the wound opposite the stoma site provide retraction medially, so that the rectus muscle is not allowed to slip laterally during the course of fashioning the ileostomy aperture.

The manoeuvre is facilitated by the operator's hand pushing upwards from inside the abdomen over the area of the ileostomy aperture using a sponge to protect the operator's left hand. An incision of the posterior sheath and peritoneum is made using cutting cautery.

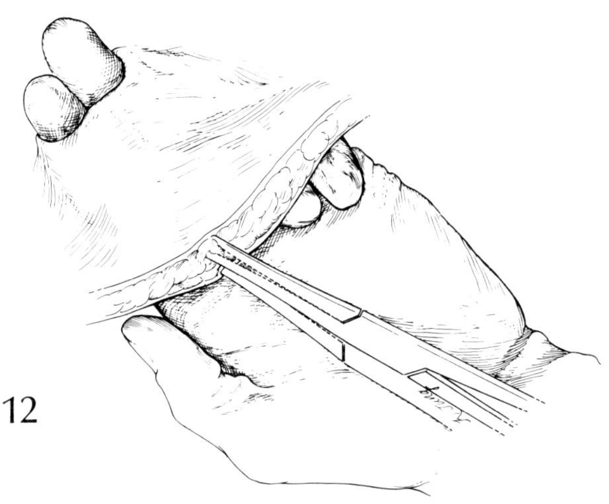
12

12

The operator tests the aperture for size. For the surgeon who uses Size 7 or 8 gloves, this corresponds to a snug two-finger aperture such that the distal interphalangeal joint of the middle finger and the pulp of the index finger can be seen. This minimizes the chances of occurrence of prolapse or parastomal hernia (too large an aperture) and of obstructive symptoms (too narrow an aperture).

13

With manipulation of the aperture, bleeding may occur from the rectus muscle or tributaries of the inferior epigastric vessels. A useful manoeuvre is to pass a large Kelly forceps through the aperture and use it as a retractor to check for any bleeding.

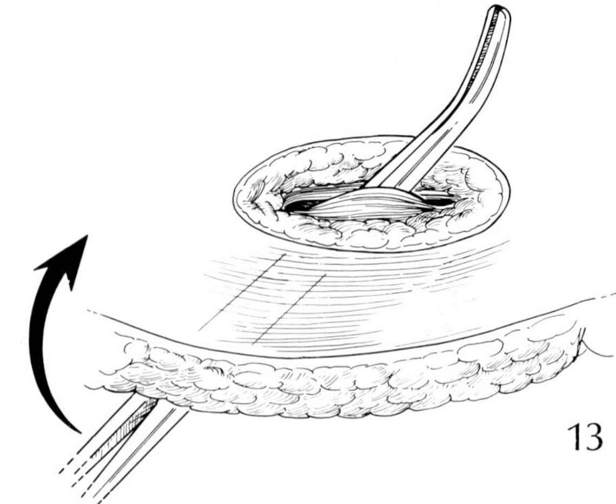

13

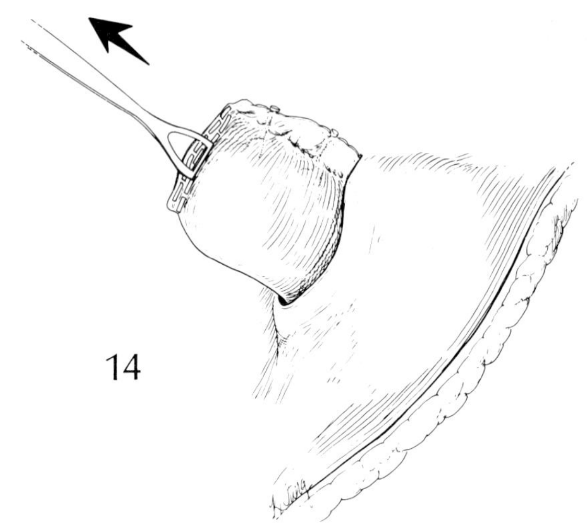

14

14

A Babcock clamp is passed through the aperture and the stapled end of the ileum is grasped. The ileum is drawn through the abdominal wall so that the ileal mesentery lies in a *cephalad* direction to facilitate obliteration of the mesenteric defect. A 6 cm length of exteriorized ileum seems best.

15

Although after colectomy some surgeons prefer to obliterate the mesenteric defect by suturing the cut edge of the mesentery to the lateral abdominal wall, this can be difficult especially in a fat patient. Others will prefer to fashion an extraperitoneal ileostomy[1]. The author's own preference, after completion of the colectomy, is to suture the cut edge of the mesentery to the anterior abdominal wall. The cephalad suture of 0 chromic catgut is placed between the most superior part of the falciform ligament and the cut edge of the mesentery over the head of the pancreas. Residual transverse mesocolon or redundant lesser omentum can be included in the stitch. One then proceeds in a caudad direction with interrupted 0 chromic sutures, keeping about 2.5 cm lateral to the wound edge down to the ileostomy aperture. If the mesentery is fat laden, or if there is a hazard of traumatizing a significant vessel in the mesentery, injection of normal saline with syringe and needle into this cut edge will displace the vessel allowing the cut edge to be picked up safely.

Stabilizing sutures (4/0 chromic catgut) are usually placed between the seromuscular layer of the ileum and the peritoneum around the internal aperture. Some surgeons consider these sutures hazardous and prone to fistula formation, but if they are inserted carefully *without* taking deep bites into the bowel, then they are safe and probably add another measure against the occurrence of ileal prolapse. When ileostomy is done without total colectomy (i.e. after ileostomy alone or after segmental resection of ileum or right colon) the paraileal gutter is left unclosed and the small risk of volvulus accepted until definitive colectomy or bowel anastomosis is carried out.

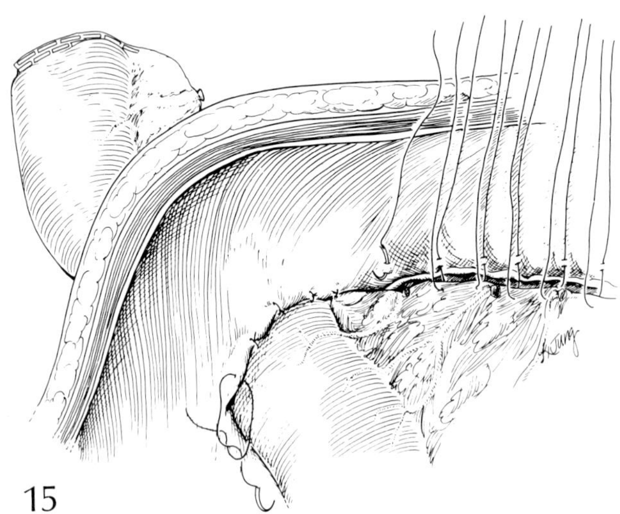

15

16 & 17

The ileum will have a natural curvature concave in a cephalad direction because of the shortening effect of the exteriorized mesentery. If this is not prominent, then nothing needs to be done to straighten the bowel. However, usually a considerable curve is noted which is released by clamping the mesentery (not all the way to the bowel edge) and suture-ligating the vessel. The needle of this suture may also be used to pick up subcutaneous fat or anterior rectus sheath of the cephalad part of the aperture for further fixation of the mesentery. Redundant fat and mesentery can be trimmed distal to this tie (about 3–4 cm) provided one does not encroach too closely on the bowel wall. Arterial bleeding from the distal mesenteric attachment is sought to confirm a good blood supply to the stoma.

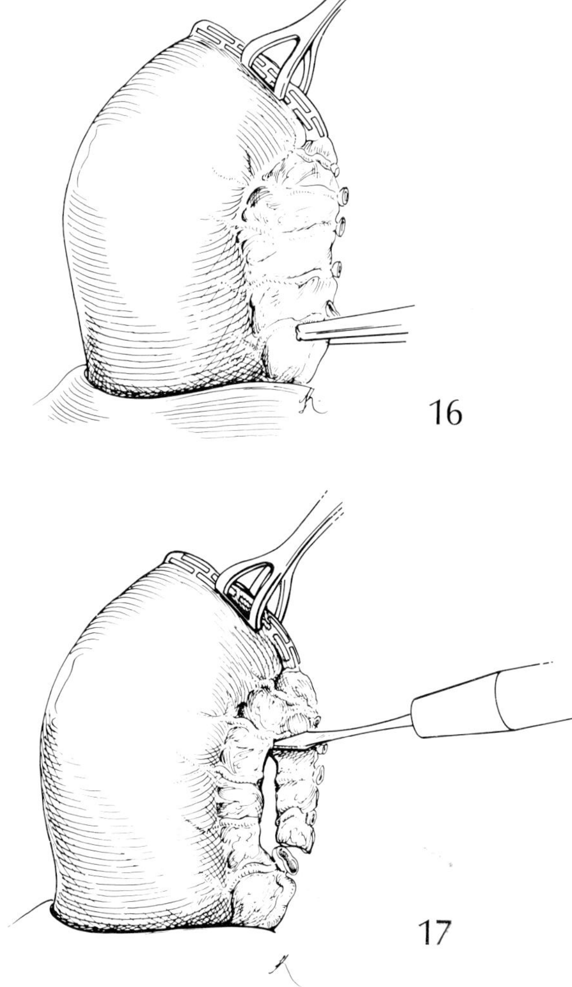

16

17

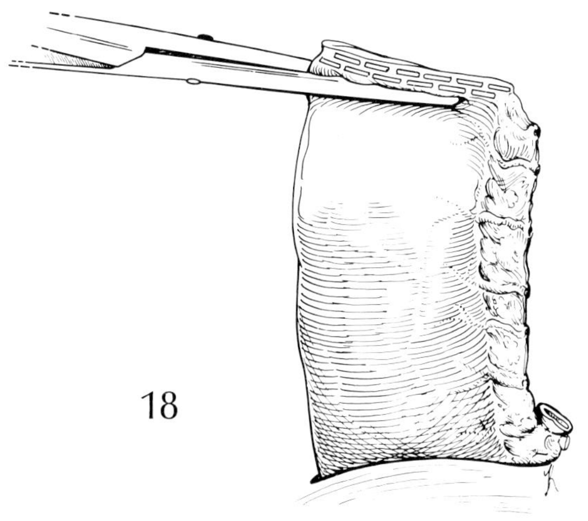

18

18

The end of the ileostomy is opened *after* the main incision has been closed and isolated with drapes to minimize bacterial wound contamination. Again, arterial or 'nuisance' bleeding from the cut end of bowel is a useful sign of bowel viability.

19

One of the problems that confronts the surgeon and the stomatherapist is the late occurrence of a gully or 'moat' at the mucocutaneous junction of the stoma. This tends to occur as the patient gains weight, notwithstanding the initial satisfactory placement of the stoma. To minimize this effect, the skin edge can be everted a little more by placing radial sutures of 4/0 chromic between the bowel wall and subcutaneous fat. The seromuscular bowel stitch is placed about 1 cm above skin level and is sutured to the most superficial part of the subcutaneous fat, bringing the suture out at the fat–epidermis junction. As the suture is tied a slight concertina effect is produced which eliminates any tendency for formation of a parastomal gully.

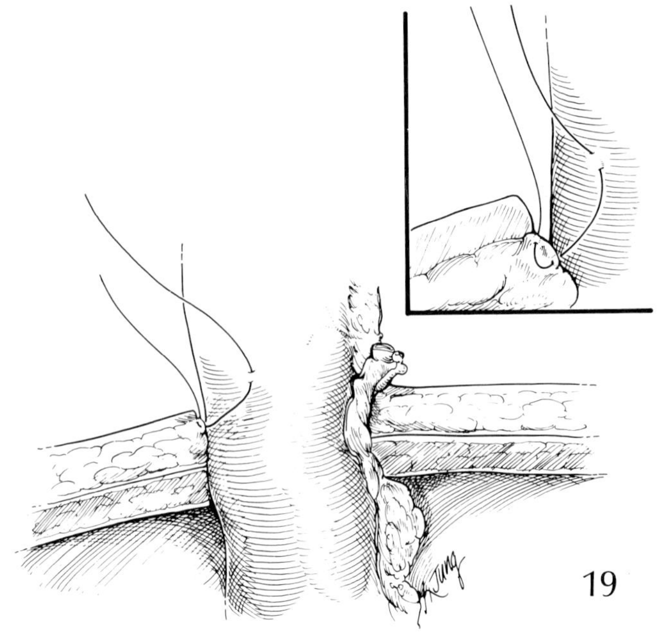

19

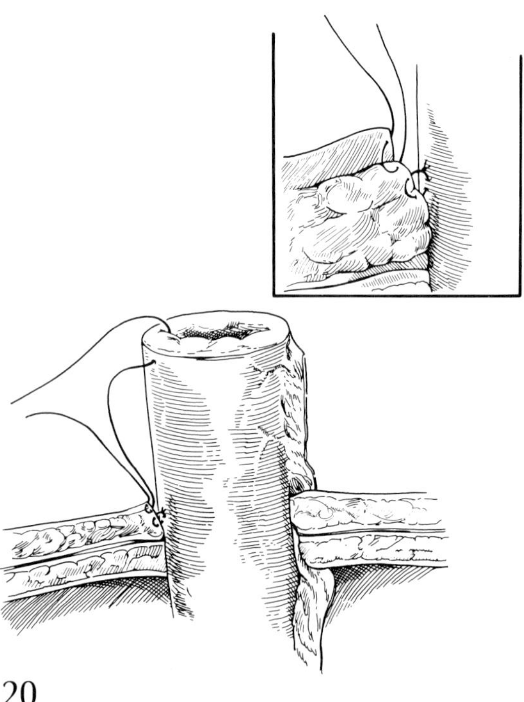

20

20

Radial sutures of 4/0 chromic catgut are placed at the four compass points of the stoma, through full-thickness bowel edge and sutured to the subcuticular skin. They should be placed vertically rather than tangentially or horizontally through the subcuticular skin, because minor degrees of vascular compromise here may cause later separation of the mucosa and serositis of the exposed ileum. The sutures should not go through the external skin, because of the risk of ileal mucosa island implantation which may cause early separation of the face plate from most skin barriers (Stomahesive R is the exception).

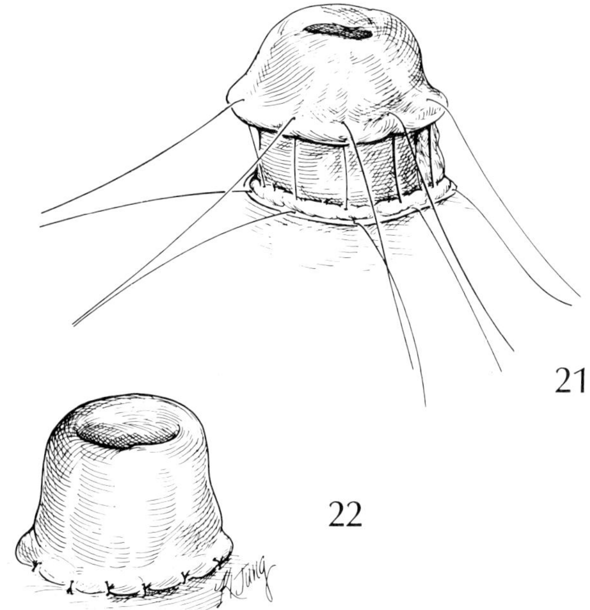

21 & 22

The sutures are then tied down, producing eversion of the stoma.

23

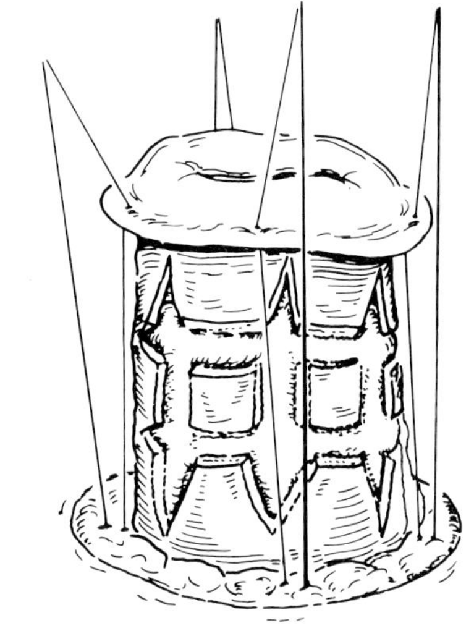

23

An alternative method of constructing the end ileostomy is to add a two-directional myotomy to the spout. This minimizes the risk of stoma recession and is appropriate for short stomas or those patients with a thick abdominal wall[2].

Ileostomy care

Stoma

The stoma is unlikely to function for 36–72 h. A skin barrier is applied postoperatively; the author prefers a large karaya disc which is applied to an open-ended transparent postoperative pouch with adhesive backing, e.g. Marlen or Hollister pouch. Hypoallergenic paper tape is used to secure the periphery of the pouch to the skin. A clear pouch is used to allow easy inspection of the stoma in the postoperative period – colour, skin separation and oedema are checked for. The United and Atlantic postoperative pouches have the advantage of extra length allowing the filled pouch to rest in the bed alongside the patient so that the weight of the contents does not cause separation of the pouch from the skin. The Hollister pouch, being a one-piece unit, has the advantage that it can be used by personnel less highly trained in stoma management.

Instruction

Starting 5–7 days after surgery, instruction of the patient in the care of the ileostomy is begun. Until that time the stoma therapist or nurse has checked the pouch daily once the stoma has started to function. The skin barrier, Stomahesive R, is used. Usually 3–4 days of careful instruction are required before the patient can assemble and apply the pouch to the stoma with confidence.

Homegoing equipment

At the time of discharge from the hospital, and if there is some swelling of the stoma, a Hollister pouch may be used. Once this has settled, our preference is for 'permanent' equipment, which is a semidisposable pouch that lasts about 2 weeks. The Marlen[4] double-lumen vinyl pouch comes with a gas valve and has a liner which acts as a gas barrier, making it especially useful for patients with a large output of flatus.

Application of the pouch

Preparation of the skin

The skin is prepared with a fat solvent, e.g. non-medicated soap. The stoma diameter is measured with calipers and a hole is cut in the skin barrier to size. A small karaya washer is placed over the skin barrier to seal the ileostomy gap at the base of the stoma. The barrier and washer are placed over the stoma.

Preparation of the pouch

A double-sided adhesive disc is applied to the mounting ring of the pouch (without wrinkling). Peeling the cover from the other side of the disc activates the adhesive and this is then guided accurately over the stoma to adhere to the skin barrier. A dissolvable paper guide-strip facilitates this manoeuvre. The surrounding skin is then painted with a skin protector (United Skin Prep) and the mounting ring is taped to the skin with microporous tape. A pouch cover (cotton) is useful for patients with vinyl sensitivity or in hot weather.

Accessories

Modern skin barriers (e.g. Stomahesive, Relia-Seal, Skin-Seal) allow for minimal skin problems with a well constructed stoma. However, skin irritation may occur and an application of a steroid spray (e.g. Kenalog) followed by lightly applied antifungal agents (e.g. Mycostatin) may be of value. Several deodorants can be placed in the pouch.

Follow-up

The patient is seen in the follow-up clinic at regular intervals to remeasure the stoma diameter, as shrinkage may occur, especially in the first month. The patient's skin is checked, problems discussed, and encouragement given.

Complications of ileostomy

High output

Early in the postoperative period, a watery, green effluent may be noted. One should be cautious before interpreting this as a sign of return of normal bowel function because a pseudo-obstruction or ileus may exist. This may be recognized by finding clumps or strands of particulate matter, gray-white in appearance, that are in fact clumps of mucus. Oral intake should then be withheld until a more brownish, thicker effluent is noted.

Afterwards the effluent may still be high in volume and codeine, Lomotil, loperamide, tincture of laudanum or combinations of these are used to reduce the output to 700–1000 ml per day. Augmenting oral salt intake is usually of value.

Parastomal irritation

The many causes of this include leakage from a poor seal; candidiasis; parastomal ulceration; allergy to the pouch material, adhesive tape; folliculitis; trauma to the skin from frequent pouch changes; pressure ulcers; psoriasis.

Ileostomy recession

This may be treated by good enterostomal therapy techniques if leakage is the problem. If this is unsuccessful, stomal revision (usually without laparotomy) is required.

Ileostomy prolapse and hernia

Fixation of the mesentery and limiting the abdominal wall aperture will usually prevent prolapse. Treatment necessitates relocation of the ileostomy, as is the case with paraileostomy hernia.

Mucosal slough

This occurs as the result of ischaemia or excessive tension, and if minor in nature, requires no treatment. Slough of part of the everted muscle as well, or mucocutaneous separation, may leave exposed the serosa of the non-everted part of the ileostomy, resulting in delayed stoma maturation.

Degrees of pseudo-obstruction may be encountered and even late stenosis (Bishop's collar deformity) may be seen if the defect is significant. Usually early surgery is not indicated except for the obviously necrotic stoma.

Ileostomy fistula

This may occur early, as the result of suturing the bowel wall to the rectus fascia (as opposed to peritoneum or subcutaneous fat) or as a late event secondary to face plate trauma or recurrent disease. If it is symptomatic, surgical revision is required.

Paraileostomy ulceration

When extensive debridement of the ulcer is done and a non-seal appliance of the Perry 51 type is used, the pouch is changed three or four times a day until the ulcer is small enough to allow a conventional pouch to be applied.

Ileostomy obstruction

Bowel obstruction after fashioning of an ileostomy may occur at any time because of adhesions, volvulus or entrapment of bowel in the fascial closure. Food bolus obstruction is also seen after this operation. Ingestion of poorly digested foods (stringed vegetables, corn, popcorn, peanuts, fruit skins) may produce a picture of bowel obstruction, especially within the first 3 months of surgery. Predisposing causes such as low grade adhesive obstruction or Crohn's disease may exist. This condition should be treated conservatively; irrigation of the ileostomy by gentle lavage with 50–100 ml of saline is carried out, and repeated at intervals until an adequate return is seen. The bolus should then break up and this is recognized by the presence of vegetable fibre in the returned irrigation fluid.

References

1. Goligher, J. C., ed. Ulcerative colitis. In: Surgery of the anus, rectum and colon, 4th ed. London: Baillière-Tindall, 1980: 755–757

2. Turnbull, R. B., Jr., Fazio, V. Advances in the surgical technique of ulcerative colitis surgery. Endoanal proctectomy and two-directional myotomy ileostomy. Nyhus, L. M. Surgery Annual 1975; 7: 315–329

Loop ileostomy and loop-end ileostomy

Victor W. Fazio MB, BS, FRACS, FACS
Chairman, Department of Colon and Rectal Surgery,
The Cleveland Clinic Foundation, Cleveland, Ohio;
Medical Director, Rupert B. Turnbull Jr School of Enterostomal Therapy,
The Cleveland Clinic Foundation, Cleveland, Ohio

Indications

The major advantage of the loop is that the mesenteric vessels are not divided in its construction, so that ischaemia is virtually impossible. The major disadvantage is that the amount of ileal protrusion above skin level is limited and with the passage of time is more prone to ileostomy recession than an end stoma.

The loop ileostomy is used above an ileorectal anastomosis for inflammatory bowel disease; above an ileoanal pull-through anastomosis with or without internal reservoir; for diversion above a continent ileal reservoir; above enterocutaneous fistulae especially in the postoperative period; proximal to colorectal anastomoses where a loop colostomy is judged to be technically difficult; in certain cases of ileocaeco-appendiceal sepsis, e.g. perforating Crohn's disease; to complement colonic decompression in certain cases of toxic megacolon; proximal to any distal bowel anastomosis where the anastomosis is tenuous or lies in proximity to a septic inflammatory 'nest'; for certain cases of Crohn's disease or ulcerative colitis where there is associated major debility of the patient.

A loop-end ileostomy may be used as a primary procedure for the definitive stoma with ileal conduits or ileostomies in obese patients. On occasion, where a loop ileostomy has been performed previously, this can be converted to a loop-end stoma by transection and closure of the efferent limb of ileum just inside the peritoneal cavity. In these patients obliteration of the mesenteric defect is not done unless a loop-end ileostomy is made during a primary procedure.

The cross-reference in this chapter refers to *Operative Surgery: Alimentary Tract and Abdominal Wall, Volume 3, 4th Edition*

LOOP ILEOSTOMY

The operation

1

The ileostomy site is chosen and marked out preoperatively as for end ileostomy. A midline incision is used.

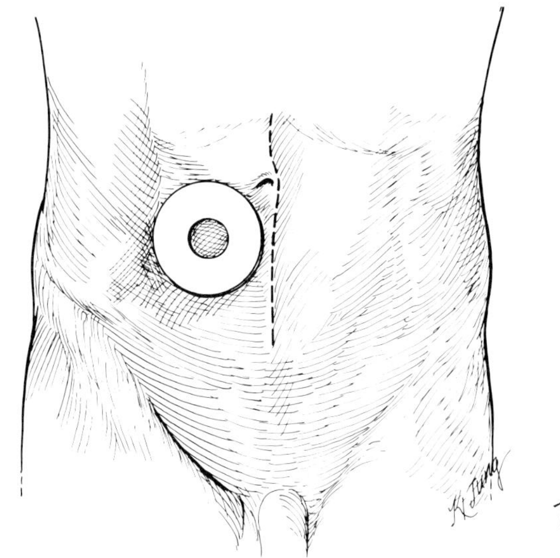

1

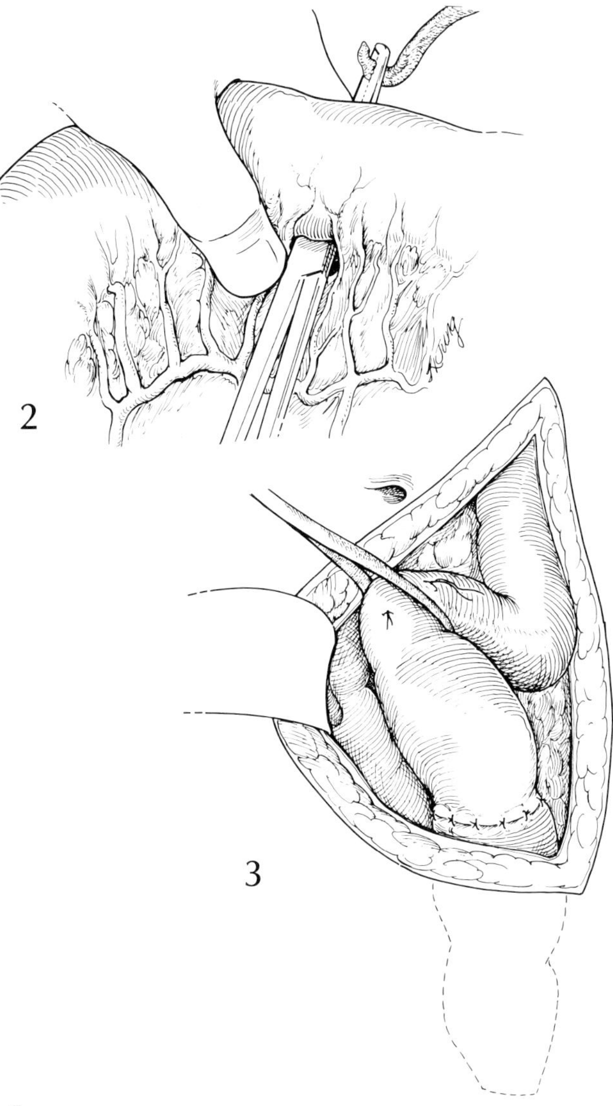

2

3

2 & 3

For a loop ileostomy placed proximal to an ileorectal anastomosis, a tape is brought through a small window made in the small bowel mesentery, to act as a retractor. Depending upon the thickness of the abdominal wall, the tape is placed 15–20 cm above the anastomosis. It is important to be able to differentiate the proximal side of the loop from the distal because, as the loop is brought through the abdominal wall aperture, rotation may occur and not be recognized. Therefore, each side is tagged, adjacent to the apex of the loop, with an identifying suture.

4

A disc of skin is excised, the fat and fascia are incised and the rectus abdominis muscle is separated. In the case shown, lateral fascial incisions have been made but these are optional. The ileostomy aperture is then completed.

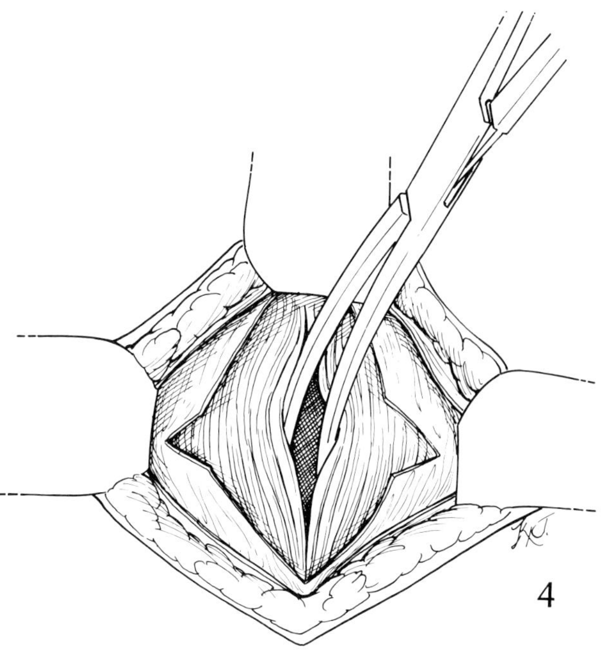

4

5–9

A curved forceps is passed through the abdominal wall aperture and the ends of the tape are grasped. The ileostomy loop is then brought through the abdominal wall aperture, checking the orientation of the loop so that the *proximal end is cephalad* and the *distal end of the loop is caudad*. An ileostomy rod is placed under the loop. In doing so, injury to the mesenteric vessels is possible. This can be minimized by placing a Kocher clamp on one end of the tape and making several twists in the tape. As the tape is pulled through the mesentery, detorsion or rifling of the Kocher clamp will lessen the risk of mesenteric vascular damage by the clamp. The rod is grasped by one of its eyelets and gently brought through the mesentery to support the loop.

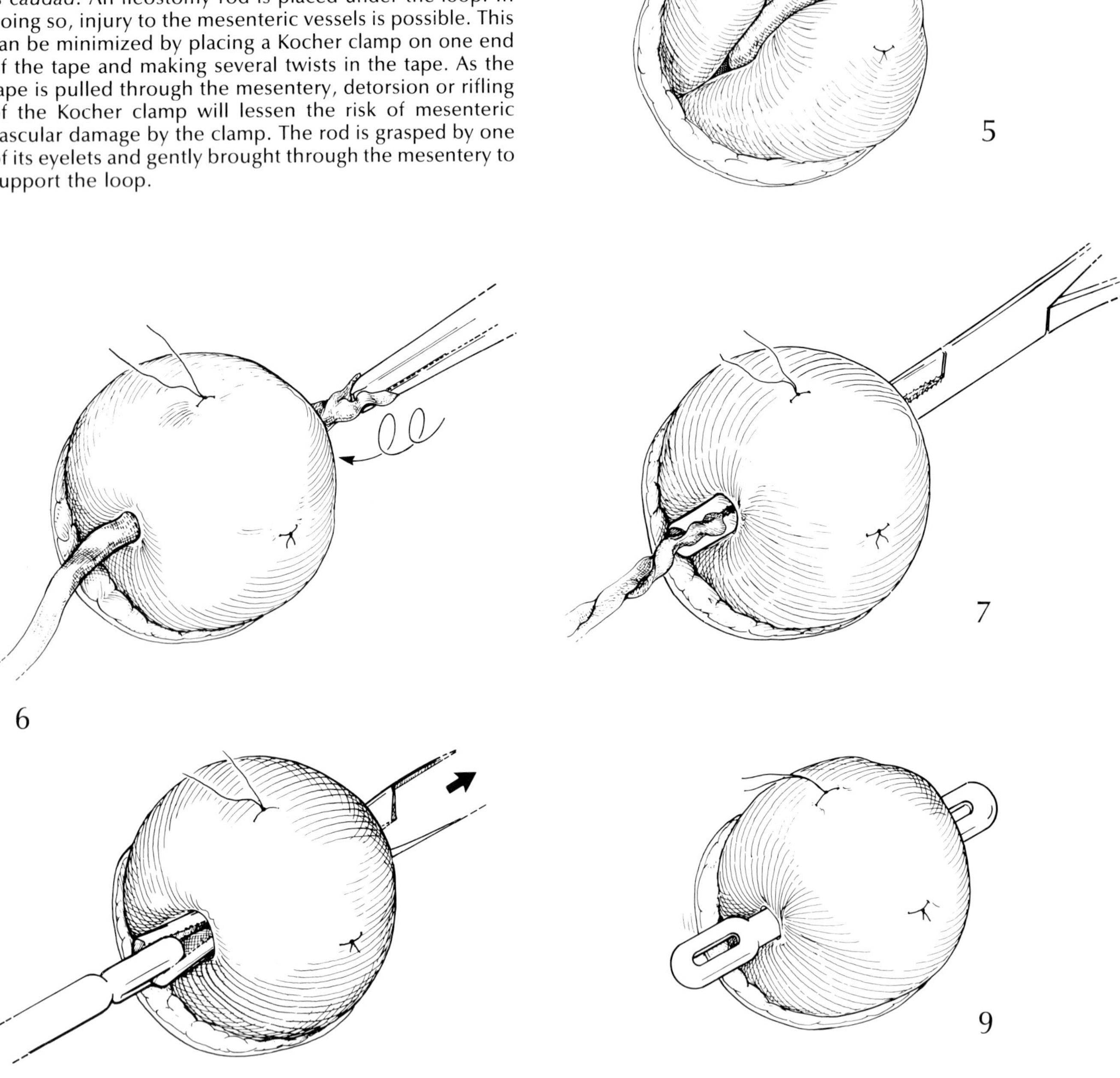

10

The abdomen is then closed and the main incision is isolated from the ileostomy with drapes. The identifying tags may now be removed. An incision is made in the loop on its *caudad and distal side across four-fifths of its circumference*. This will allow the distal, recessive limb to 'escape' from the proximal limb. It is useful to make the enterotomy about 1 cm above skin level. If it is made flush with the skin mucus may escape from the recessive limb and cause a faulty seal with the appliance.

As the enterotomy is extended towards the mesenteric edges bleeding may occur, so the incision is stopped about 5 mm short of the mesentery on both sides. A useful technique to minimize bleeding is to make an initial seromuscular incision with scissors, allowing the submucosa to pout out. Selective light electrocoagulation of the visible submucosal vessels can then be done before the enterotomy is completed.

If diversion is required for a prolonged period (e.g. greater than 3 months), then 4/0 chromic catgut sutures are placed between the serosa of the bowel and subcutaneous fat.

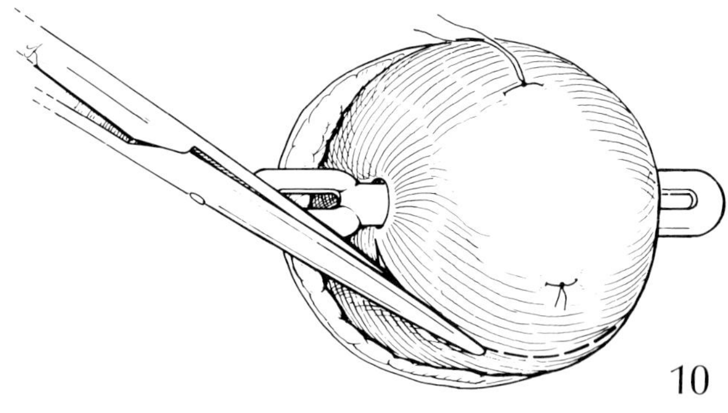

10

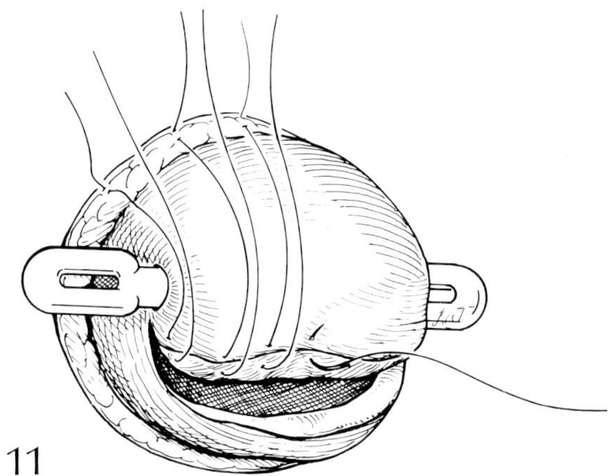

11

11

Sutures of 4/0 chromic catgut are placed for both loops through full-thickness bowel edge and then through the subcuticular layer of skin. The sutures are tagged and not tied down until all have been inserted, as it is difficult to place them alongside the rod with accuracy.

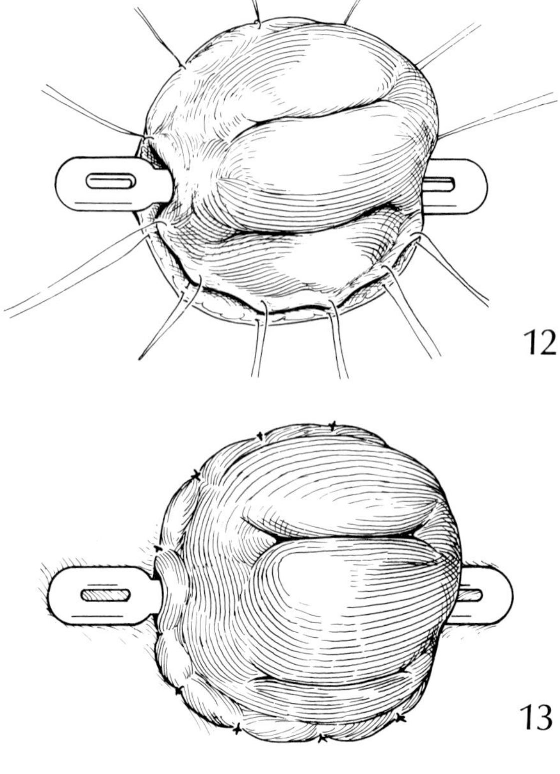

12 & 13

The sutures are then tied down.

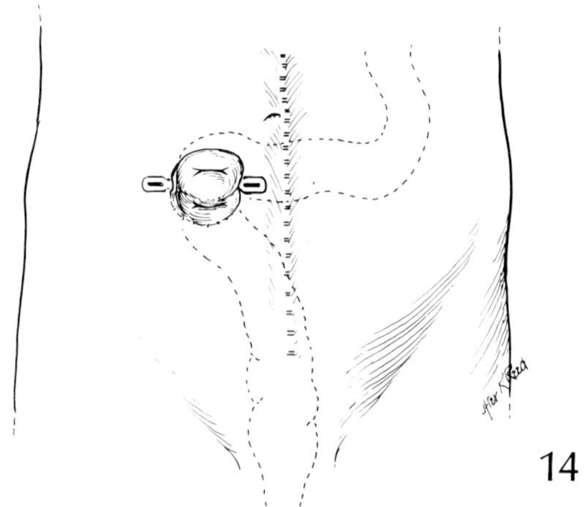

14

The completed loop ileostomy to divert the faecal stream above an ileorectal anastomosis is shown.

Postoperative care

The care of the ileostomy is as for the patient with an end ileostomy with few exceptions. The postoperative skin barrier is placed over the rod, not under it; as otherwise an inexperienced attendant could, in changing the postoperative pouch, dislodge the rod or, worse, injure the stoma. The rod is removed on the seventh postoperative day.

A loop ileostomy may be closed after 2–3 months, after the integrity of the distal anastomosis has been checked with a barium enema. When the ileostomy has been made for inflammatory bowel disease, there is always a potential need for making another, permanent ileostomy. It is important, therefore, to take the ileostomy loop down without taking a cuff of adjacent skin (as for closure of a loop colostomy), as this leaves a large wound that may exclude that site from future use. The site is left open to heal by secondary intention and the disc of new skin can be excised again. For the same reason the fascial defect is closed with an absorbable suture, such as Dexon.

LOOP-END ILEOSTOMY

This may be done at the time of colectomy or by conversion of a loop to a loop-end ileostomy. In the latter instance, the distal limb is transected and oversewn just inside the peritoneal cavity. The accompanying diagrams show the technique for construction of the loop-end stoma at the time of colectomy (or for constructing an ileal conduit in an obese patient).

The operation

15 & 16

The line of transection of the ileum is chosen close to the ileocaecal valve. The proximal segment may be closed with a continuous absorbable suture of 4/0 chromic catgut, reinforced by an outer layer of interrupted 4/0 Ethibond sutures. However, the author prefers to use the GIA stapler. A moist linen tape is placed around the ileum about 7–10 cm above the transected bowel, after judging the amount needed to traverse the thickness of the abdominal wall.

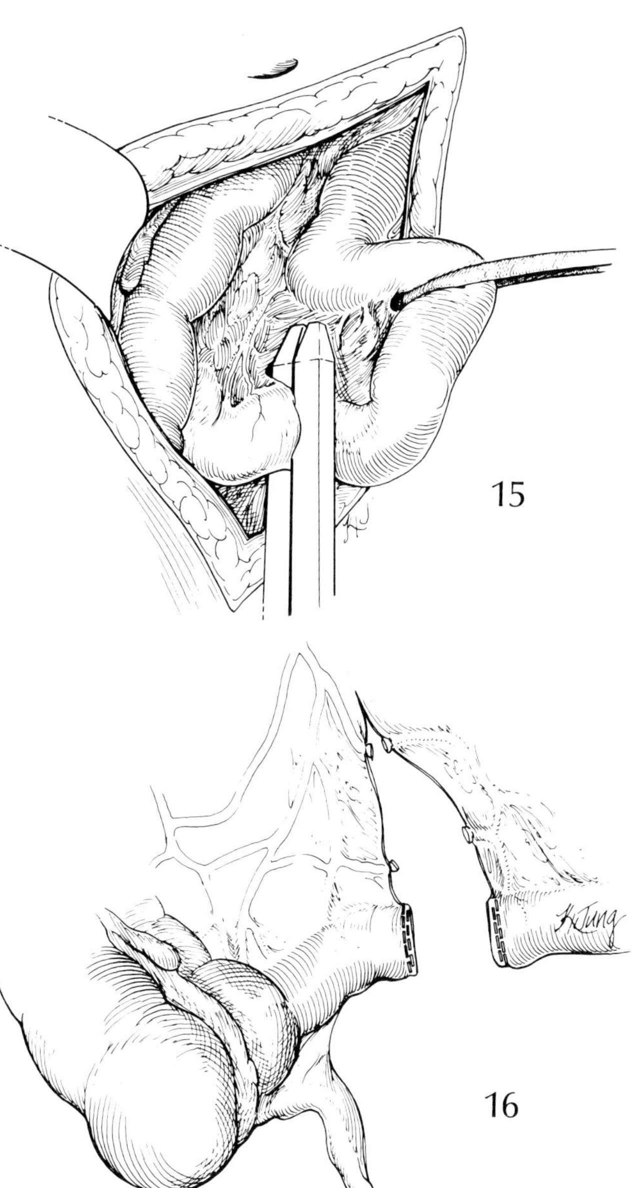

15

16

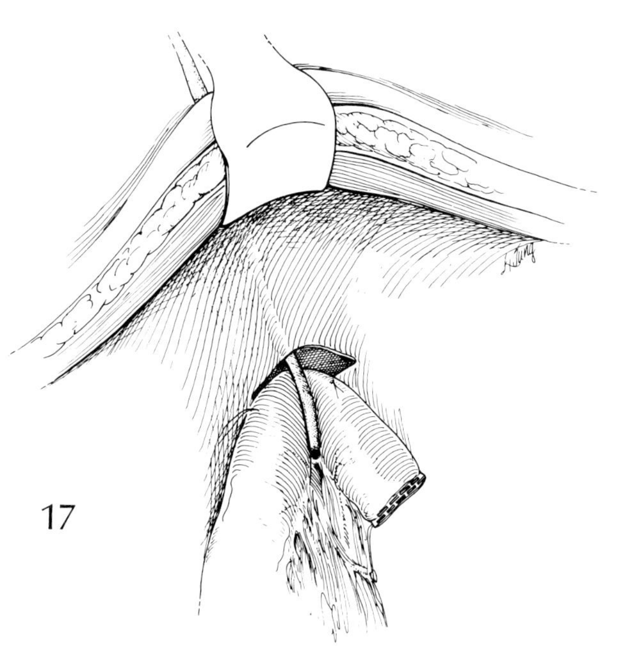

17

17

The abdominal wall aperture is made as for the conventional ileostomy and the loop is drawn through. The proximal and distal ends are tagged. Because the mesenteric defect is to be obliterated when making a permanent ileostomy, the proximal functional end lies in a caudad direction and the non-functional end in a cephalad direction. This allows the cut edge of the small bowel mesentery to be aligned with the anterior abdominal wall with considerable ease.

18

After a sufficient amount of the loop is protruding beyond the skin edge, the mesentery is sutured to the anterior abdominal wall about 2–3 cm lateral to the main incision. This is carried in a cephalad direction up to the falciform ligament and in a caudad direction to the internal aspect of the abdominal wall aperture. Seromuscular sutures may be applied between the limbs of the loop and the peritoneum of the ileostomy aperture.

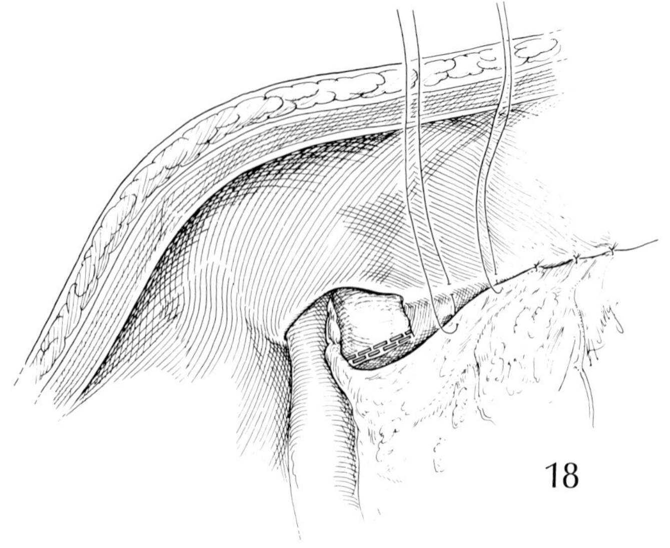

18

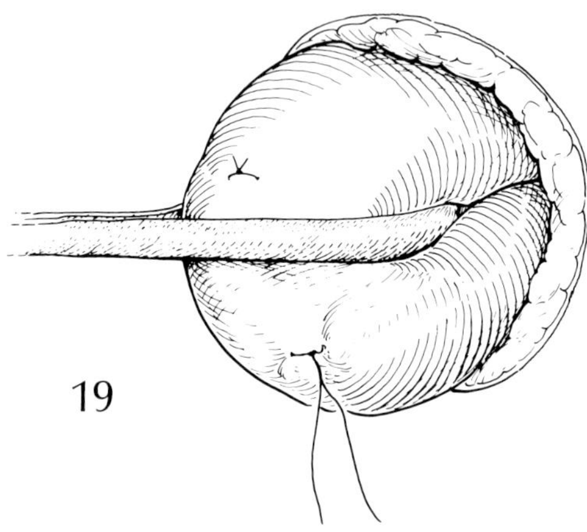

19

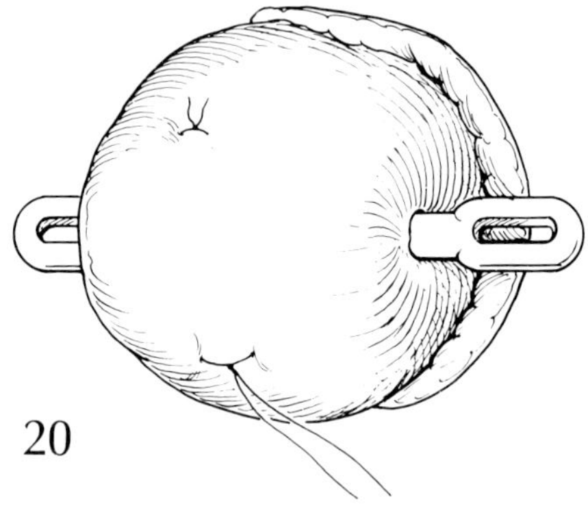

20

19 & 20

The loop protrudes about 2–3 cm beyond the skin level. The tape is replaced by a short plastic ileostomy rod. Stabilizing sutures of 4/0 chromic catgut may then be placed between the seromuscular layer of the loop and the subcutaneous fat, especially if there is a downturning of the skin of the aperture. This manoeuvre facilitates further eversion of the skin and a future improved ileostomy seal with pouching of the stoma.

21

An enterotomy is made on the cephalad side of the loop across four-fifths of the circumference of the ileum, about 1 cm above skin level.

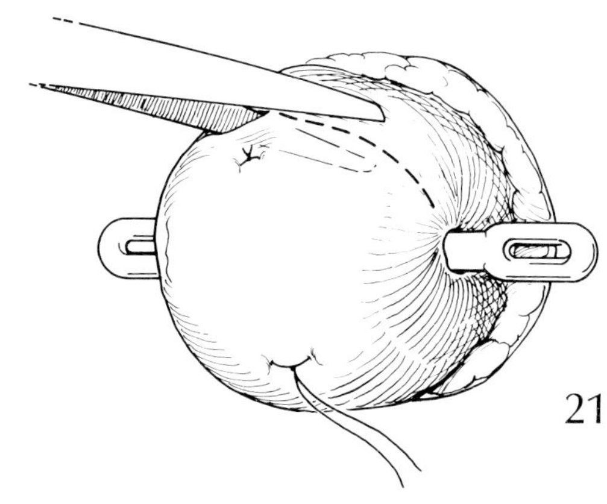
21

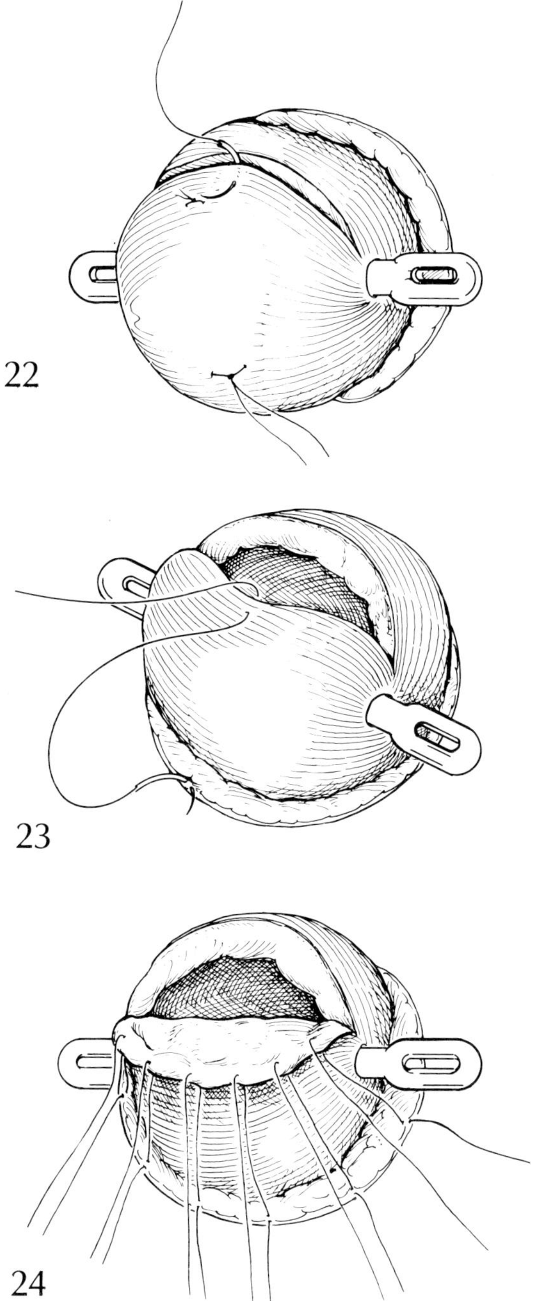
22

23

24

22–25

Using 4/0 chromic catgut, a suture is placed through the full thickness of the cut edge of the ileum and sutured to the subcuticular layer of skin. As described for loop ileostomy, sutures are placed but not tied until all have been inserted. Using the blunt end of tissue forceps is less traumatic in obtaining eversion of the ileostomy spout than using Babcock forceps inside the bowel lumen.

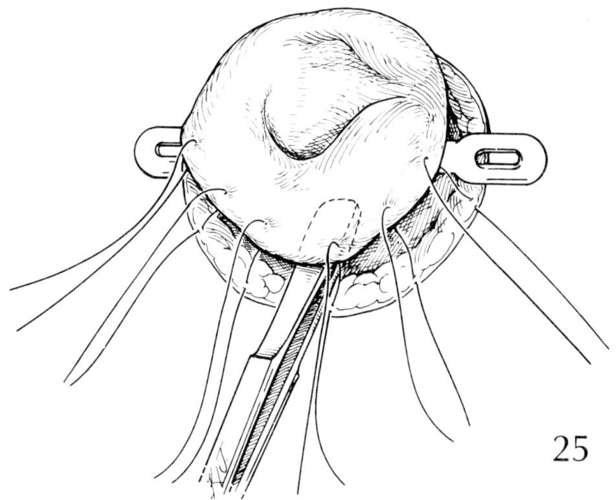
25

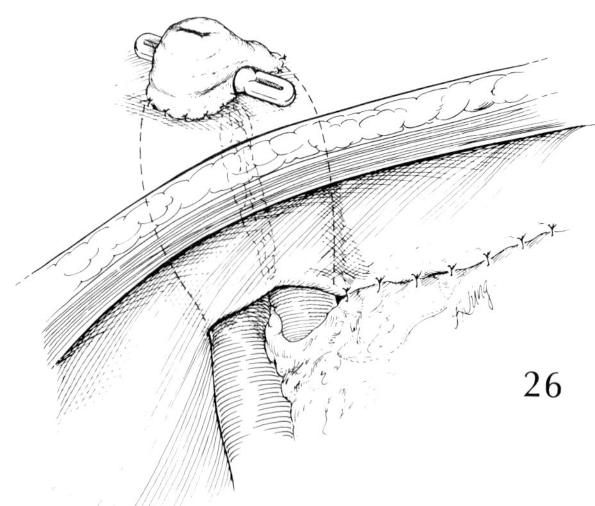

26

26 & 27

As with other types of ileostomy construction, the main incision is closed before breaching the ileal lumen; but for clarity, the completed stoma is shown in *Illustration 26* with the incision still unclosed.

When operating for inflammatory bowel disease, particularly Crohn's disease, the bowel specimen is opened and examined carefully, especially the distal ileum, before proceeding with the ileostomy. If there is evidence of disease at the line of proximal resection, the surgeon may judge that further resection is necessary.

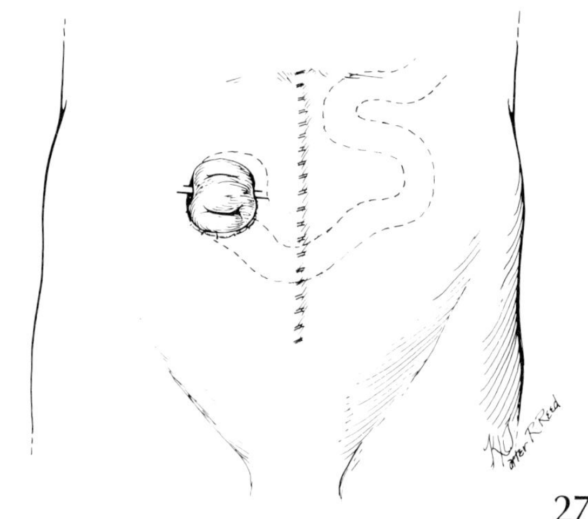

27

Addendum

In certain cases of extreme obesity, the fashioning of an ileostomy, even a loop ileostomy, may be extraordinarily difficult. A technique similar to that used in construction of an end colostomy in the obese patient may be used. Here a generous 8–10 cm incision is made in the peritoneum and posterior rectus sheath of the internal aperture such that the bowel can be brought through the abdominal wall, but before delivering the bowel through the aperture, sutures (No. 1 Prolene) are placed on both sides of the extended incision and left untied. After the bowel is delivered to a length that satisfies the surgeon, the sutures may then be tied, partly closing the defect; any ischaemic effects on the bowel produced by these ties are watched for. This will help reduce the possibility of parastomal hernia formation.

Colostomy: end iliac and loop transverse

James P. S. Thomson MS, FRCS
Consultant Surgeon and Dean of Postgraduate Studies, St Mark's Hospital, London;
Consultant Surgeon, Hackney Hospital; Honorary Lecturer in Surgery,
The Medical College of St Bartholomew's Hospital, London

Types of colostomy

1. *Loop colostomy*, which is usually temporary and therefore constructed with a view to eventual closure.
2. *Terminal colostomy*, which is usually permanent.
3. A *divided colostomy* is less commonly performed – the two ends of the colon are separated by a skin bridge of varying size. This is usually a temporary stoma but is more difficult to close than a loop colostomy.
4. A *double-barrelled colostomy* is constructed as part of the rarely used Paul-Mikulicz operation. A spur is fashioned between the two limbs of the colostomy which can subsequently be necrosed by the application of a crushing enterotome. Theoretically this type of colostomy should close spontaneously after the spur is crushed, but usually a formal closure is required. Whilst this operation was originally described for treating patients with complicated diverticular disease or carcinoma of the colon, its use now is almost confined to the treatment of patients with acute sigmoid volvulus.

The cross-reference in this chapter refers to *Operative Surgery: Alimentary Tract and Abdominal Wall, Volume 3, 4th Edition*

LOOP COLOSTOMY

A loop colostomy may be fashioned in any part of the colon that can be brought to the surface of the anterior abdominal wall without tension. The most commonly selected sites are the transverse and sigmoid colon.

In principle a loop of colon is brought to the surface and held in place by a rod or tube. In addition, it is now usual for these colostomies to be opened at the time of operation and for a mucocutaneous suture to be performed. As most loop colostomies are constructed during an emergency laparotomy the colon is usually unprepared. However, if the operation is being performed electively the colon should be prepared in the same way as for anterior resection.

A transverse loop colostomy may readily be raised through a small incision as this part of the colon is very mobile and the size of the lumen is such that subsequent closure presents few problems. By contrast a sigmoid loop colostomy is more difficult to fashion because the bowel may be tethered by the congenital adhesion in the left iliac fossa. A small subumbilical midline incision may be required to facilitate mobilization but the sigmoid colon may be the site of diverticular disease and this, together with the smaller lumen, may make closure more difficult than in a transverse colostomy. However, an advantage of a sigmoid loop colostomy is that the effluent is firmer and thus is easier for the patient to manage.

Indications

The indications for constructing a loop colostomy may be subdivided into two groups – those employed in the emergency situation and those used as part of an elective procedure.

Emergency

1. *Large bowel obstruction*. In the adult this is most commonly due to a carcinoma, although occasionally diverticular disease is the cause. The presence of a defunctioning loop colostomy permits some mechanical bowel preparation before the definitive bowel resection. It is important to remember that the loop colostomy should be sited well to the right of the transverse colon so that during the definitive operation, once the splenic flexure is mobilized, there is adequate colon to restore the continuity of the bowel without tension on either the anastomosis or the colostomy (*see* chapter on 'Management of the obstructed bowel', pp. 210–229).
2. *Anastomotic dehiscence* (*see* chapter on 'Surgical management of anastomotic leakage and intra-abdominal sepsis' pp. 185–192).
3. In children with Hirschsprung's disease or an imperforate anus (*see* chapter on 'Hirschsprung's disease', pp. 617–628).

Elective

1. *Anterior resection*. A loop colostomy may be constructed in association with a left-sided anastomosis – particularly a difficult colorectal or endoanal anastomosis. There is no evidence that such a defunctioning stoma enhances the chance of primary anastomotic union, but its presence will reduce the severity of the sequelae of an anastomotic leak. (*Editors' comment*: The possible effects of 'routine' transverse colostomy in this situation are not known and are currently being investigated.)
2. *Colonic fistulae*. In patients with established fistulae from the colon, often the result of diverticular disease, local sepsis can be considerably reduced before definitive surgery if a proximal loop colostomy is established.
3. *Anal operations*. Certain anal operations, such as those for complex fistulae or to repair the sphincter mechanism, are more likely to succeed if the faecal stream is diverted. It is the author's preference to use a left-sided transverse colostomy rather than a sigmoid colostomy.

Anaesthesia

General anaesthesia is to be preferred as traction on the mesentery causes pain and nausea. However, it is possible to undertake these operations under local field anaesthesia.

The operation

1

The incision

The sites of the incision for a transverse colostomy and a left iliac fossa sigmoid colostomy are shown. The ideal siting for a transverse colostomy is in the right upper abdomen mid-way between the umbilicus and the costal margin placed over the rectus abdominis muscle and extending just lateral to the lateral border of the rectus abdominis muscle. It is usually about 6 cm in length.

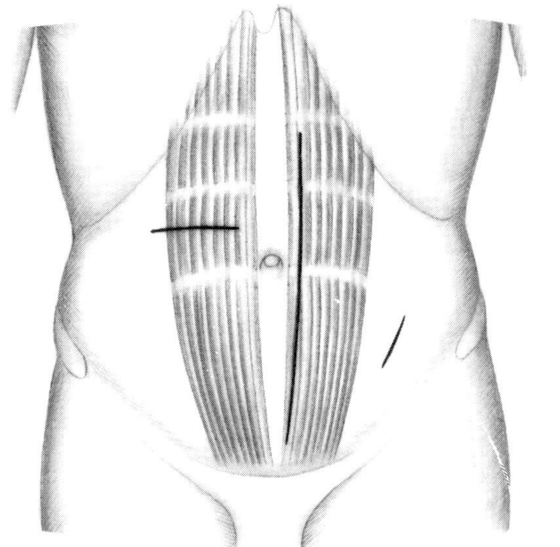

1

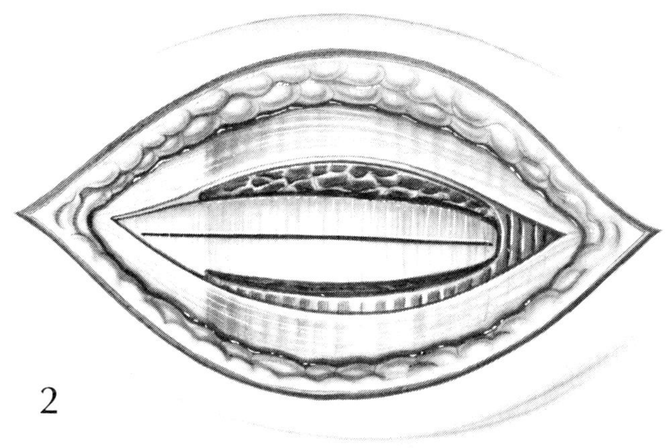

2

2

Division of rectus abdominis muscle

The incision is deepened through all the layers of the anterior abdominal wall. The muscle fibres of the rectus abdominis are divided.

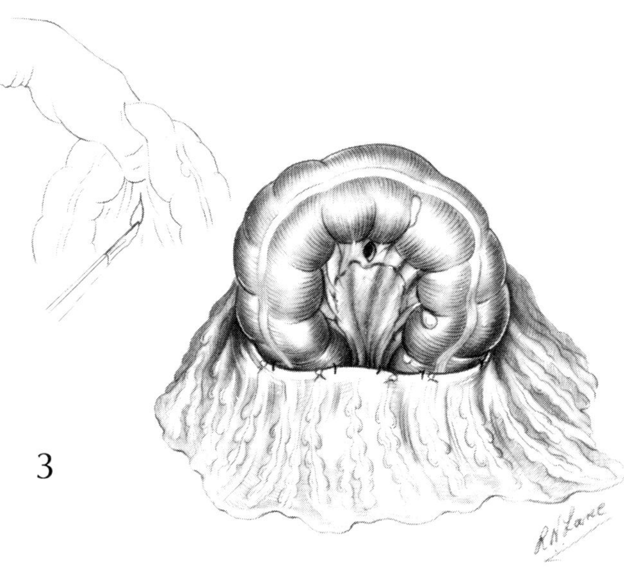

3

3

Preparation of the colon

The transverse colon is prepared for delivery through the anterior abdominal wall, either by incising the greater omentum, as shown, or by bringing it below the free border of the greater omentum. A small hole is made in the transverse mesocolon by the edge of the bowel wall and a rubber tube placed through it to facilitate delivery of the colon through the anterior abdominal wall.

If a sigmoid loop colostomy is to be made, the sigmoid colon must be carefully identified. It has no omentum, but has appendices epiploicae and taeniae.

4

Securing the colostomy

Once the colon has been delivered through the anterior abdominal wall it is held on the surface with the aid of a rod, or as illustrated with tubing, the ends of which have been turned back and tied. This latter method allows easier application of the colostomy appliance.

Other methods of supporting the loop include the use of a subcutaneous plastic rod, an ox-fibrin (Biethium) bar, or a skin bridge.

The colon may be opened longitudinally as indicated, but some surgeons prefer to open the colon transversely as this damages fewer of the encircling vessels in the colonic wall.

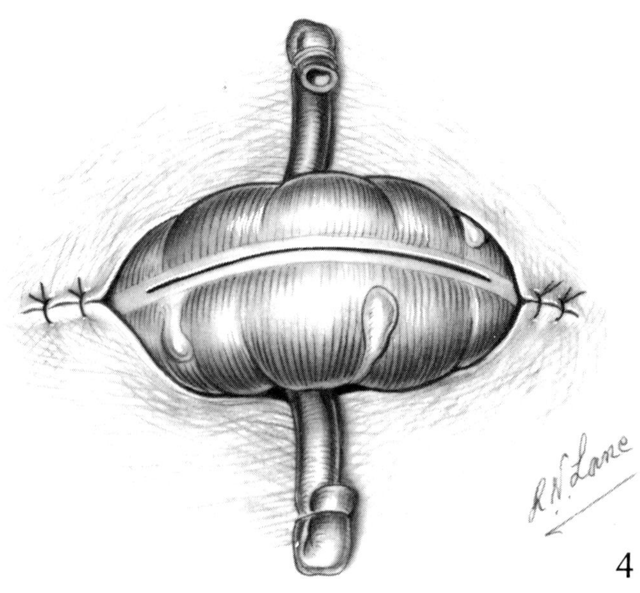

4

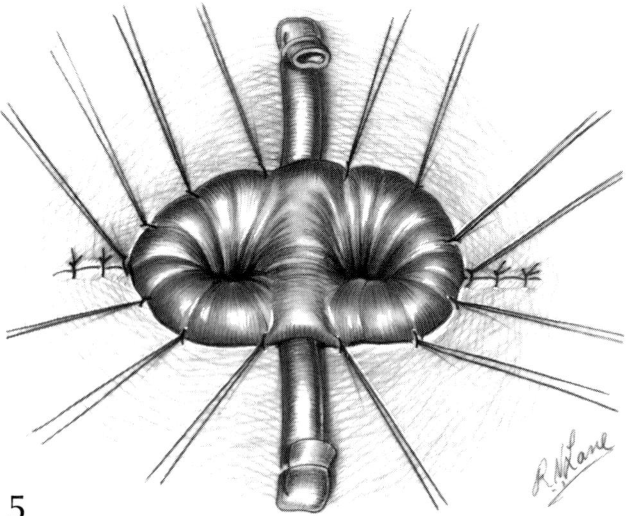

5

5

Mucocutaneous suture

Once open the colostomy is sutured to the skin using a chromic 3/0 catgut suture. Tincture benzoin co. or Stomahesive is then applied to the skin around the colostomy and an appliance immediately fitted.

SKIN BRIDGE

6

If a skin bridge is used to support a loop sigmoid colostomy, the skin flap, together with its subcutaneous fat, is fashioned from the skin surrounding the proximal limb of the loop. This allows the incision in this area to become rounded rather than elliptical.

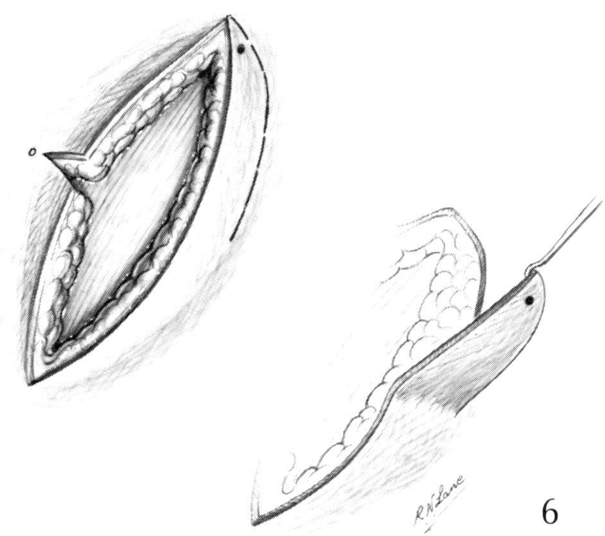

6

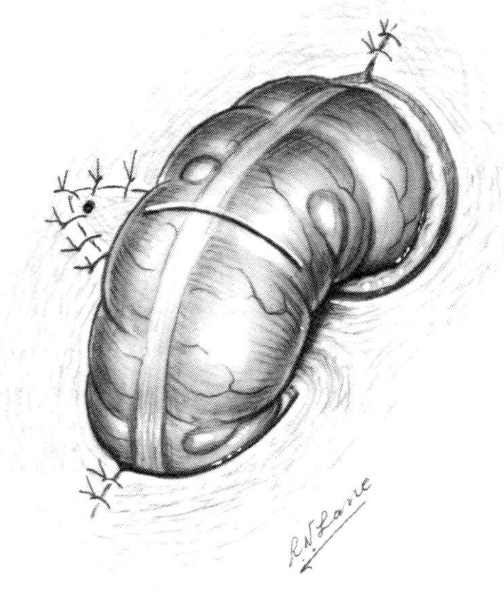

7

7

The flap is passed through the mesentery and sutured into a V-cut on the opposite side of the incision. A rod may be used, in addition, if desired.

8

After 1 week when the stoma is stable the loop of colon may readily be divided, employing a diathermy needle without anaesthesia.

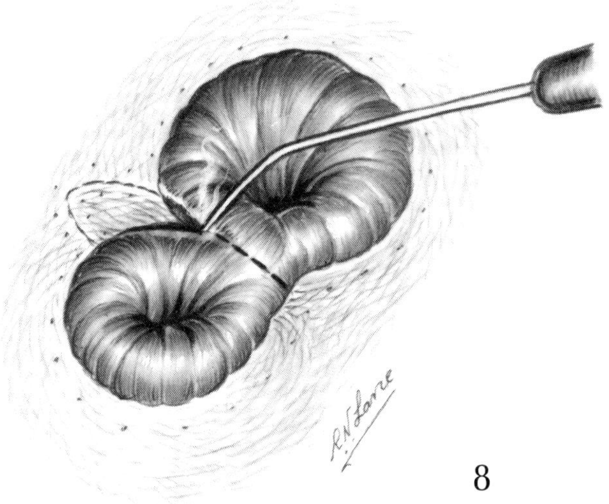

8

TERMINAL COLOSTOMY

A terminal colostomy is constructed in association with operations to excise the rectum or Hartmann's procedure. The colostomy is usually formed from the sigmoid or lower descending colon, which is brought to the surface through a trephine in the left side of the anterior abdominal wall. At the conclusion of the operation a direct mucocutaneous suture is performed.

There is some debate as to whether the trephine should be made through the left rectus muscle, with the operation being performed through a right paramedian incision or through the oblique muscles in association with a left paramedian incision. With the latter situation the colon may be placed either intraperitoneally or extraperitoneally. If the intraperitoneal position is chosen then the space between the colon and the abdominal wall (lateral space) will need to be closed as this is a potential site for internal herniation of the small intestine.

This procedure will be referred to only briefly in this chapter as it is also dealt with in the chapters on 'Abdominoperineal excision of the rectum', (*see* pp. 327–352).

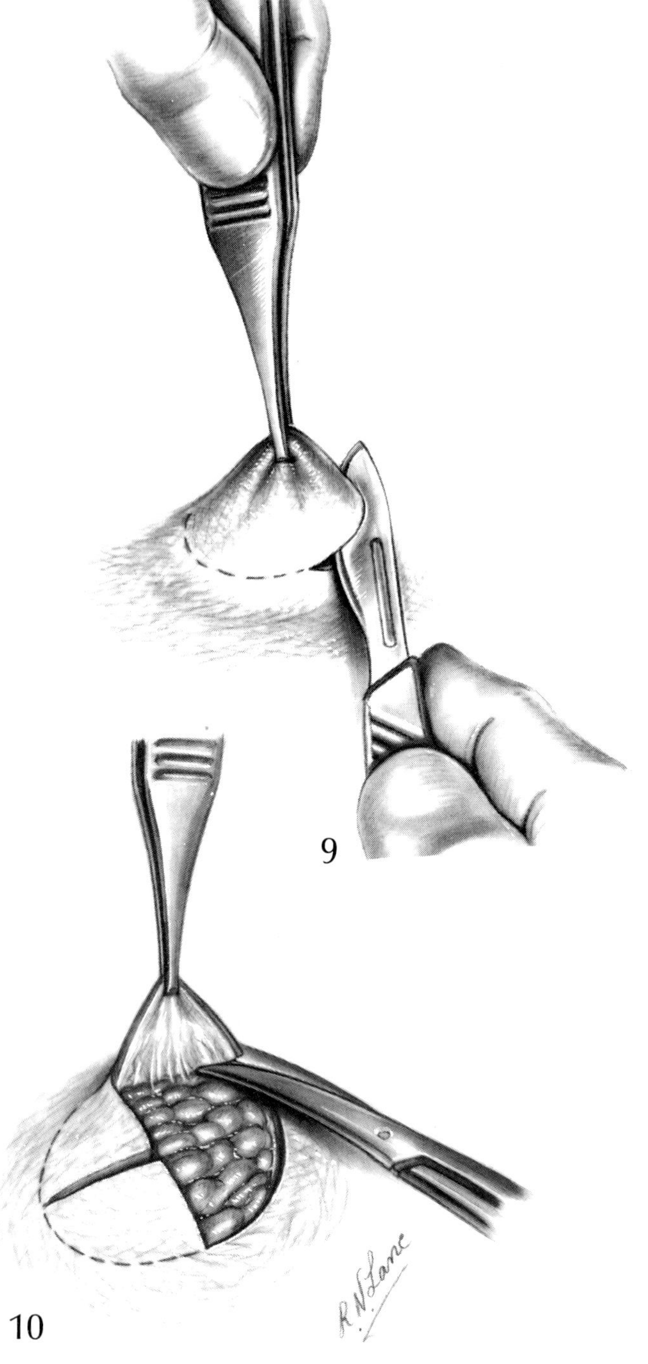

9

10

The operation

9 & 10

Removal of skin disc

The exact site for the colostomy, whether it is to be made in the region of the left abdominis rectus muscle or the oblique muscles, should be selected to ensure that an appliance will fit satisfactorily away from the umbilicus, the anterior superior iliac spine, the groin crease and any pre-existing scars. A disc of skin approximately 2 cm in diameter is excised. This may be done by holding up the skin with tissue forceps and excising the circle so formed or by using a cruciate incision and excising the four pieces of skin with curved scissors.

11

Removal of a cylinder of superficial fascia

A cylinder of superficial fascia and fat is removed, care being taken to obtain good haemostasis.

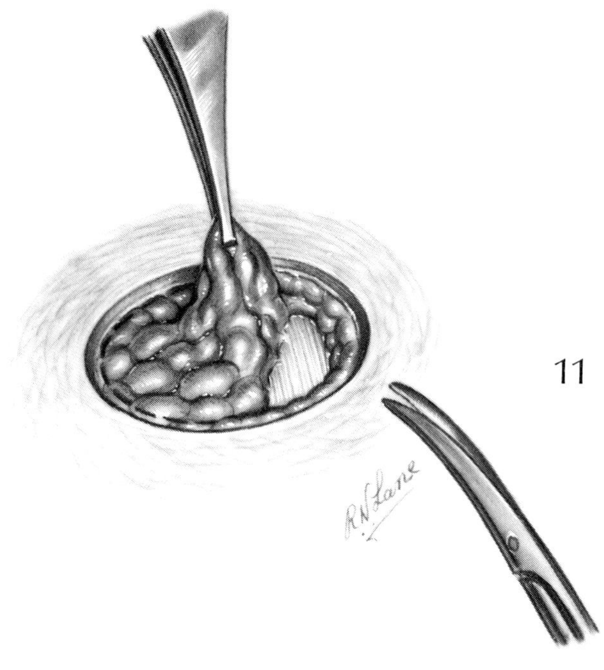

11

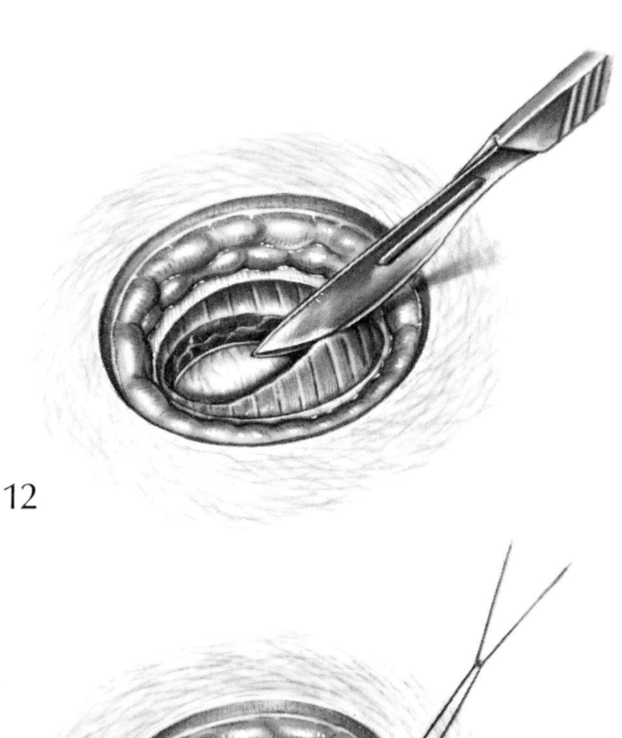

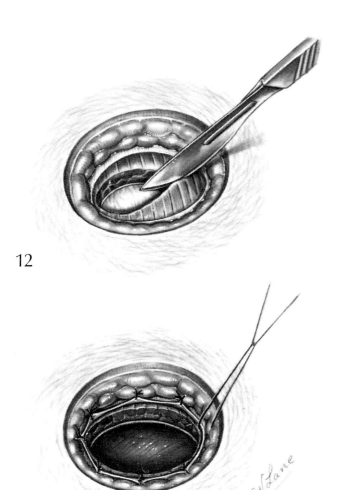

12

13

12 & 13

Division of muscle layers

A disc of the external oblique or anterior rectus sheath is excised in the line of the skin hole and the underlying muscle divided. The peritoneum is also divided. There is a potential space between the fibrous layer of the superficial fascia and the external oblique or anterior rectus sheath. It is in this space that the considerable bulge of a colostomy hernia occurs. This space may be obliterated by a series of 2/0 chromic catgut sutures joining the two layers.

14

Delivery of colon through abdominal wall

The colon is delivered through the anterior abdominal wall. If it remains totally intraperitoneal it is desirable for the space between the mesocolon and the abdominal wall (the lateral space) to be closed using nonabsorbable sutures. This prevents the possible complication of internal herniation of the small intestine. Alternatively, the colon may be brought to the surface extraperitoneally.

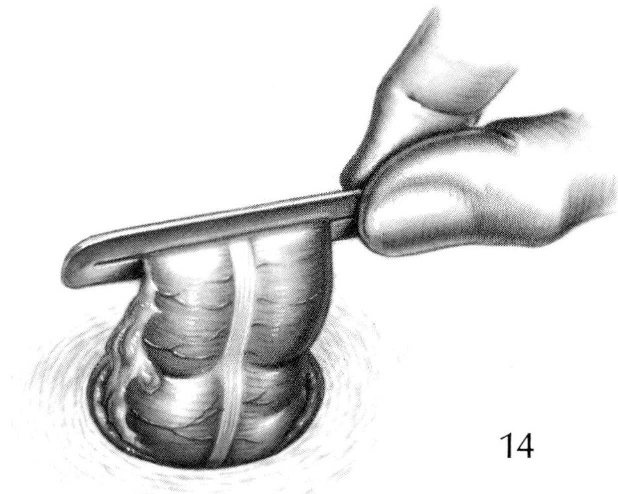

14

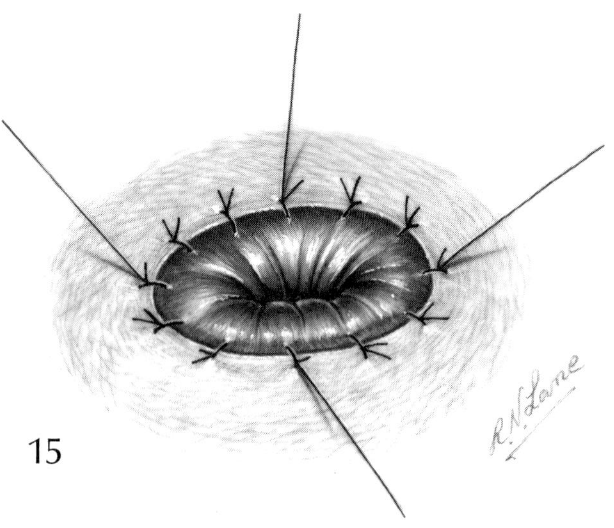

15

15

Mucocutaneous suture

Once the main abdominal incision has been sutured and dressed, the clamp on the distal colon is removed and a mucocutaneous suture performed with 3/0 chromic catgut. Before the main abdominal incision is closed it is important to ensure, by adequate mobilization of the colon, that there is no tension on the mucocutaneous suture line.

Postoperative care

General management

The general care of the patient will be largely determined by the indication for performing the colostomy or the injuries sustained. It is wise for the patient to be maintained on intravenous liquids until the colostomy has discharged some flatus and bowel sounds are well established.

It is important to examine the viability of the colostomy after the operation and also to make certain that it has not become detached.

Care of the colostomy

An appliance should be put on as soon as the stoma has been fashioned. Because the effluent from a transverse colostomy is semiliquid some protection of the skin should be provided, and Stomahesive or a karaya gum washer is very useful in this respect because it can be shaped to the colostomy. If the colostomy effluent is very liquid, the oral administration of hydrophilic substances such as methyl cellulose (Isogel) or codeine phosphate usually results in reduction in colostomy activity.

Complications

Loss of viability

This occurs early after the operation if the blood supply to the colon has been compromised. The operation has to be repeated with viable colon.

Separation of the colostomy

This is caused by tension at the mucocutaneous junction and if it occurs the colostomy may have to be re-established. Partial separation may also occur either because of tension or infection but will usually heal spontaneously provided that less than half the circumference is involved.

Infection

Although established in a potentially septic field it is very rare for sepsis to complicate the construction of a colostomy. Occasionally it may happen with surrounding cellulitis and some separation of the edge of the colostomy. A haematoma surrounding the stoma is a predisposing factor and emphasizes the importance of good haemostasis in the colostomy wound. Provided that there is adequate drainage the colostomy will heal but subsequent scarring may lead to some stenosis at the mucocutaneous junction.

Stenosis

Stenosis of a stoma usually occurs at the mucocutaneous level but, provided that there has been no sepsis, it is rare when direct mucocutaneous suture has been performed. To correct this complication the colostomy needs to be refashioned by excising a ring of skin and any scar tissue that may be present. While this can be carried out under general anaesthesia it may be performed equally well under local anaesthesia.

Hernia

Some degree of herniation is very common after a terminal colostomy. It usually takes the form of an interstitial bulge between the muscle layer and the superficial fascia. Occasionally it results from considerable widening of the hole in the muscle layer. The former is usually best treated initially by wearing a belt. If, however, it is large or the belt is unsatisfactory, the excess colon may be excised after mobilizing it at the stoma. The space between the muscle layer and the superficial fascia will also need to be closed.

The latter type of colostomy hernia is best treated by resiting the stoma and closing the defect by direct suture or by inserting a piece of synthetic material.

Prolapse

Prolapse may occur with either a transverse colostomy, when it more commonly involves the distal limb, or a terminal colostomy. Because transverse colostomy is usually a temporary measure, prolapse is relatively unimportant, although occasionally, if the viability of the prolapse is in question, reoperation may be needed. If prolapse of a terminal colostomy troubles the patient and causes dysfunction, reconstruction, usually at a new site, is required.

Closure of loop colostomy

James P. S. Thomson MS, FRCS
Consultant Surgeon and Dean of Postgraduate Studies, St Mark's Hospital, London;
Consultant Surgeon, Hackney Hospital; Honorary Lecturer in Surgery,
The Medical College of St Bartholomew's Hospital, London

Preoperative

Indications

A temporary loop colostomy is closed when there is no longer a need to defunction the distal bowel. If a colostomy has been constructed to cover a healing anastomosis then it is essential that total healing of the anastomosis has occurred before undertaking the colostomy closure. This may be assessed either endoscopically with the sigmoidoscope or radiologically using a water-soluble contrast enema (e.g. Gastrografin), when two films in planes at right angles (anteroposterior and lateral) should be taken. The position of the anastomosis is more readily judged on the radiographs if two silver clips have been placed on the outer layer of sutures at the time the anastomosis was performed. In addition, the colostomy itself must be suitable for closure in that it should be pink in colour and not cyanosed or oedematous. It is unlikely that the local conditions for closure will be ideal until 3–4 weeks after colostomy construction.

Preparation of patient

The proximal bowel is prepared by placing the patient on clear fluids for the 2 days before the operation and by proximal colonic wash-outs. Oral purgatives such as magnesium sulphate in small doses may assist the preparation but as diarrhoea may be marked it is important to ensure that the appliance is firmly adherent and readily drainable.

The distal bowel is washed through with normal saline. This is especially important if a barium enema has been performed because barium remaining in the bowel will solidify and may act as an intraluminal obstruction after reconstruction; a water-soluble contrast enema is preferable.

Anaesthesia

The operation is best performed under general anaesthesia. Intravenous antibiotics such as an aminoglycoside and metronidazole are usually given on induction and repeated at 6 and 12 h.

Principles of technique

A loop may be closed using one of two techniques.

1. *Simple closure* – after mobilization of the colon the opening is sutured (half-anastomosis).
2. *Excision of the colostomy and anastomosis* – the site of the colostomy is excised and the continuity of the colon is restored by end-to-end anastomosis.

In both these instances the operation is conducted so that the colon is returned to within the peritoneal cavity. So-called extraperitoneal closure of the colostomy is seldom performed and is unsatisfactory because there is inadequate colonic mobilization. This may result in anastomotic dysfunction or breakdown.

The operation

1

Mobilization of the colostomy

Eight strong silk sutures are placed around the mucocutaneous junction of the colostomy. This allows good control of the colon during mobilization. The incision is made around the edge of the colostomy taking a small fringe of skin approximately 2 mm wide. If necessary the incision may be enlarged at either end of the colostomy in the transverse plane.

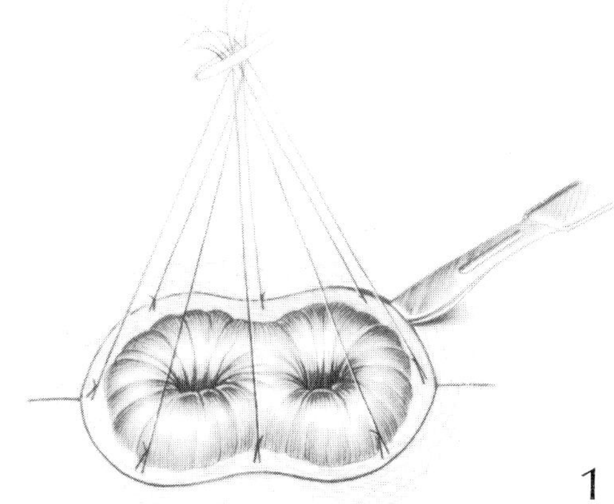

1

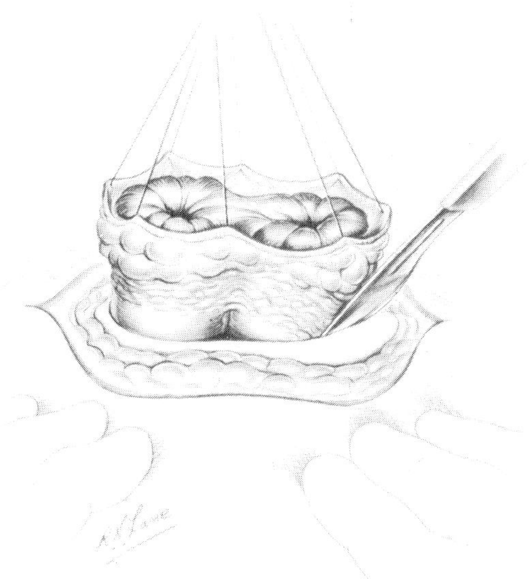

2

2

Separation from the anterior abdominal wall

With traction applied to the colostomy using the stay sutures the tissue of the anterior abdominal wall is freed from the colon. Great care must be exercised to remain in the correct plane and avoid damage to the colon. There is usually little blood loss during this procedure. If there is haemorrhage this suggests the surgeon is in an incorrect plane.

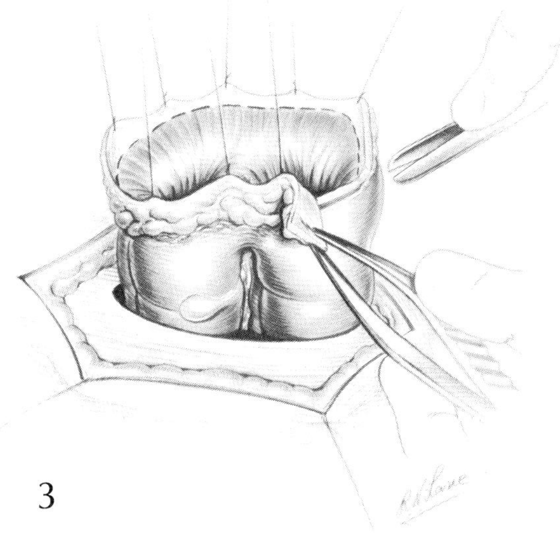

3

3

Removal of the skin edge and unrolling of the colostomy edge

The rim of skin is removed and the edge of the colostomy unrolled. When all the scar tissue has been removed the colon is then ready for closure.

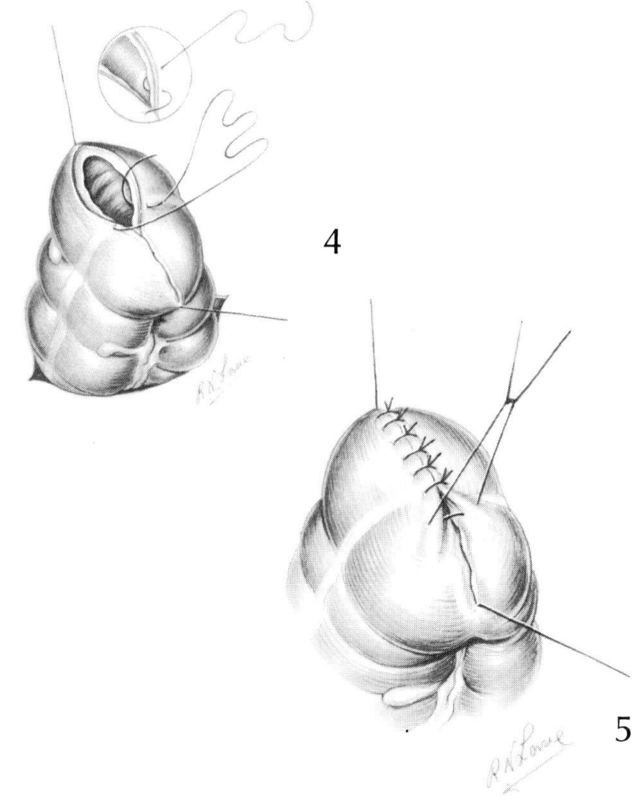

4

5

4 & 5

Simple closure of the colon

This is usually done in two layers. A layer of chromic catgut sutures is inserted first, often using the Connell stitch, and taking all layers. Then an outer layer of interrupted fine silk seromuscular Lembert sutures is inserted. If the colostomy has been excised an end-to-end anastomosis is performed in the same way as it would be during a transverse colectomy.

Some surgeons advocate using a single layer of sutures for this closure.

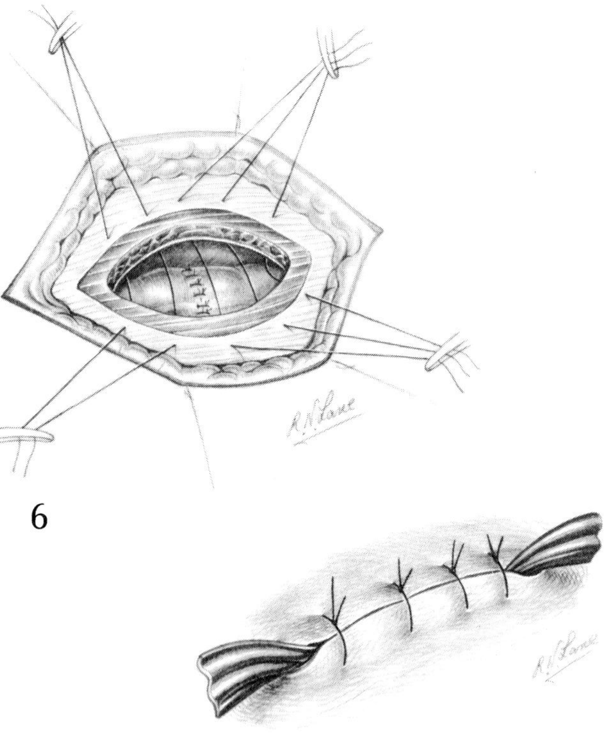

6

7

6 & 7

Closure of the abdominal wound

A single layer of monofilament nylon sutures is inserted into all layers taking large bites of tissue on either side of the wound. After all the sutures have been placed they are tied so that the edges of the abdominal wall are closely, but not tightly, apposed. The skin wound is loosely closed over a corrugated drain which is placed from one end of the wound to the other. This technique will allow any haematoma to drain and thus prevents wound infection.

Postoperative care

It is unusual for the patient to need a nasogastric tube but intravenous fluids should be maintained until good bowel sounds are established and the patient has passed flatus. Oral fluids are then started and gradually increased. Milk of magnesia is a useful laxative if there is some delay in the establishment of the bowel movements once oral feeding has begun. The drain is removed after 48 h.

Complications

At the site of colostomy closure

Wound infection is usually avoided if the skin has been loosely sutured and a wound drain used.

There is an incidence of *hernia* in these wounds which is occasionally complicated by strangulation.

Breakdown of the colonic suture line results in a faecal fistula, which usually closes spontaneously, or peritonitis which will require further vigorous treatment and re-establishment of the colostomy (see chapter on 'Surgical management of anastomotic leakage and intra-abdominal sepsis', pp. 185–192).

At the site of the distal anastomosis

If the colostomy is closed before satisfactory healing of the anastomosis has occurred then an abscess may develop at this site. This may necessitate re-establishment of the colostomy. However, if the proper indications for performing colostomy closure have been observed this complication should not occur.

Further reading

Thomson, J. P. S., Hawley, P. R. Results of closure of loop transverse colostomies. British Medical Journal 1972; 3: 459–462

Rosen, L., Freidman, I. H. Morbidity and mortality following intraperitoneal closure of transverse loop colostomy. Diseases of the Colon and Rectum 1980; 23: 508–512

Thomson, J. P. S. Caecostomy and colostomy. Clinics in Gastroenterology 1982; 11: 285–296

Panproctocolectomy and ileostomy

Miles Irving MD, ChM, FRCS
Professor of Surgery and Consultant Surgeon, Hope Hospital,
University of Manchester School of Medicine, Salford

Introduction

Panproctocolectomy and ileostomy – the simultaneous removal of all the colon and rectum and the construction of a spout ileostomy on the anterior abdominal wall – was, until recently, the standard treatment for many large bowel diseases that had progressed beyond effective medical treatment.

There is worldwide confirmation of its value in the treatment of ulcerative colitis and Crohn's colitis, polyposis coli and multiple colonic carcinomas. There is no doubt that the operation cures all the above conditions, apart from Crohn's disease, but always at the price of a permanent ileostomy. It is the necessity for a stoma that has led to the place of the operation being challenged by other procedures designed to preserve anal sphincter function and thus avoid a stoma. Therefore, it is reasonable before recommending proctocolectomy that every patient with one of the above conditions should be carefully considered for a sphincter-saving procedure – an ileorectal anastomosis or, where the necessary experience is available, an ileoanal anastomosis with or without a pelvic reservoir, except for patients with Crohn's disease.

Panproctocolectomy is now recognized to be inappropriate in patients with toxic dilatation of the colon, where colectomy has become inevitable. In such patients the correct procedure is total colectomy and ileostomy with exteriorization of the proximal end of the rectum as a mucous fistula. The preserved rectum can be excised or otherwise dealt with when the patient has recovered from the crisis.

Panproctocolectomy remains the operation of choice for the elective treatment of total Crohn's colitis. It is also indicated in other conditions when the patient wants a well tried operation which will rid him permanently of his diseased large bowel with minimal chance of postoperative complications. The price is a permanent ileostomy of either the spout or the reservoir type.

The cross-reference in this chapter refers to *Operative Surgery: Alimentary Tract and Abdominal Wall, Volume 3, 4th Edition*

Preoperative preparation

The patient should be generally assessed to see that he is fit enough for this major procedure. If not it should be staged. The nature of the operation must be fully discussed with the patient beforehand. In particular the problems associated with an ileostomy must be made clear. In this respect the counselling provided by a stoma care nurse and a patient who has already undergone the operation can be invaluable.

The proposed site of the stoma should be discussed with the patient and a position agreed that takes into account the patient's shape, occupation and usual clothing habits.

The site will usually be in the right iliac fossa over the outer third of the rectus abdominis muscle. It should normally be below the belt line and far enough away from the anterosuperior iliac spine to allow accurate fitting of an appliance. Particular care should be taken in obese patients and those with scars in the area. On the morning of the operation, the site of the stoma should be clearly marked with an indelible skin marker.

Preoperative preparation

Preoperative mechanical bowel preparation is not absolutely necessary as there is no anastomosis, and in any case the bowel is usually empty because of the diarrhoea associated with colitis. However, in cases of polyposis or multiple carcinomas, or where there is considerable faecal residue the bowel can be emptied by whole gut irrigation or enemas.

As with all colon surgery an antibiotic combination (dictated by local antibiotic policy), such as gentamicin and metronidazole, should be administered with the premedication and repeated on one occasion 12 h after operation.

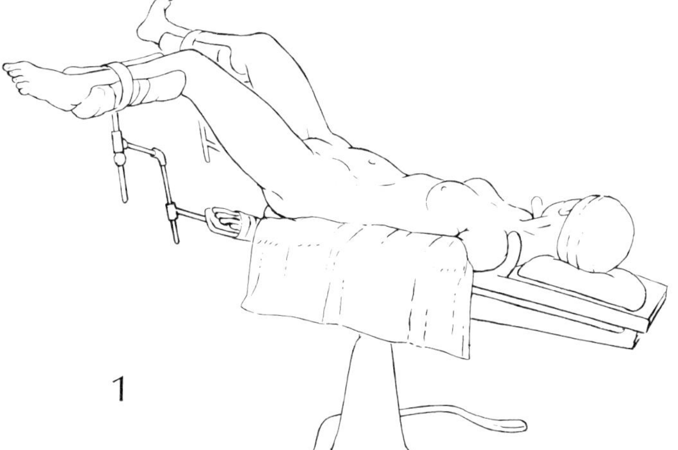
1

1

The operation

The patient should be positioned in the lithotomy-Trendelenburg position under general anaesthetic. A nasogastric tube and bladder catheter should be passed. In the male, the genitalia should be strapped to one thigh in order to keep the scrotum out of the way of the perineal surgeon. Before the skin drapes are applied the anus should be thoroughly swabbed with chlorhexidine skin preparation and then occluded by a double purse-string suture of 2/0 black silk inserted through the skin around the anal margin. The whole of the abdominal wall from the nipples to the midthighs should be prepared and towelled as should the perineum and buttocks to the midthighs.

ABDOMINAL OPERATION

2

The incision

A long midline incision curving to the left around the umbilicus gives good easy access to the whole of the abdominal contents. The contents are inspected to assess the state of the large bowel and to ascertain whether any other disease is present.

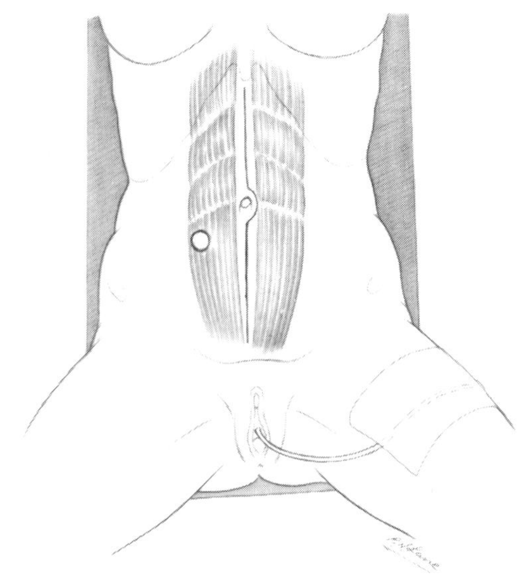

2

3

Mobilization of the colon

There are several ways of approaching this problem. The author prefers to undertake the pelvic dissection after having mobilized the colon, which does not take long. He therefore commences by dissecting the greater omentum off the transverse colon, thereby leaving it attached to the greater curve of the stomach where subsequently it can be used as an omental pedicle.

In cases where perforation of the colon has occurred and been sealed off by omentum or peritoneum, the involved area should be mobilized last. The omentum and peritoneum sealing the perforation should be divided in a manner that avoids breaking the seal.

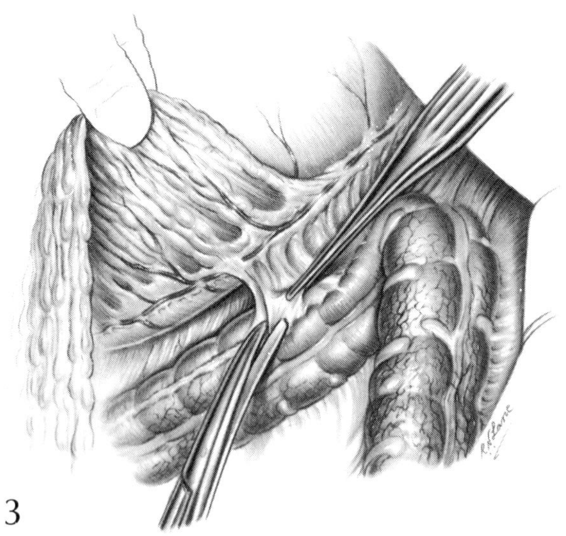

3

Mobilization of the left hemicolon

4

The sigmoid colon is mobilized by dividing the peritoneum in the left paracolic gutter. The gutter is demonstrated by pulling the sigmoid colon over to the patient's right, revealing the congenital peritoneal reflection visible as a white line. This is breached by the point of the scissors and incised down to the pelvic brim and up as far as possible towards the splenic flexure.

In inflammatory bowel disease the peritoneal gutter may be very vascular and vessels may need to be coagulated with the diathermy or occluded with haemostatic clips.

The sigmoid mesentery is swept medially by gauze dissection, an easy and bloodless procedure, to reveal the ureter, which must be identified and safeguarded down to the pelvic brim.

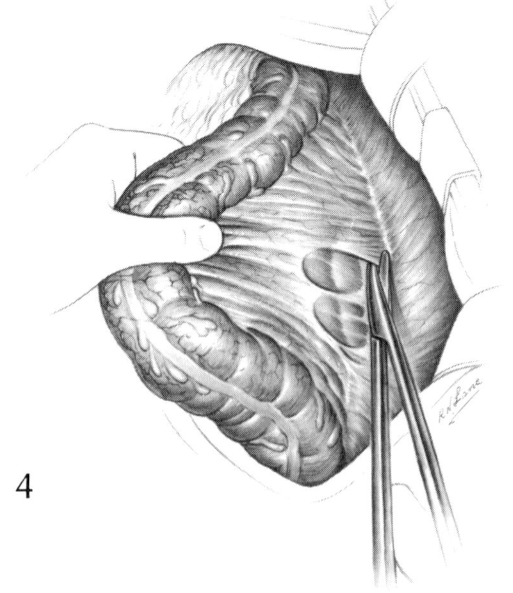

4

5

The left colon is then mobilized in the same fashion up towards the splenic flexure. As the splenic flexure is approached gentle traction is put on both the left half of the transverse colon and the descending colon.

This will reveal the lower pole of the spleen. Care must be taken not to tear this, but if the capsule is torn the surgeon should not remove the spleen but complete the mobilization of the splenic flexure, cover the torn capsule with an absorbable haemostatic gauze and leave a pack on it until the end of the operation when reinspection will almost invariably show that bleeding has stopped. If not, a few lightly tied sutures of 2/0 Dexon inserted through the splenic tear on a round-bodied needle will usually control the haemorrhage.

In many cases of chronic colitis, mobilization of the splenic flexure will be easy because of the contraction of the colon which pulls it down but in others where access is difficult it can be tedious. In these circumstances the use of haemostatic clips helps to occlude vascular elements of the phrenicocolic ligament and remnants of the greater omentum. With persistent and gentle dissection the splenic flexure can be brought down sufficiently to enable a hand to be placed behind the mesentery and sweep the whole down into the wound.

In patients with toxic dilatation this mobilization is associated with the risk of colonic perforation and in such circumstances the rest of the abdominal contents should be covered by large abdominal packs.

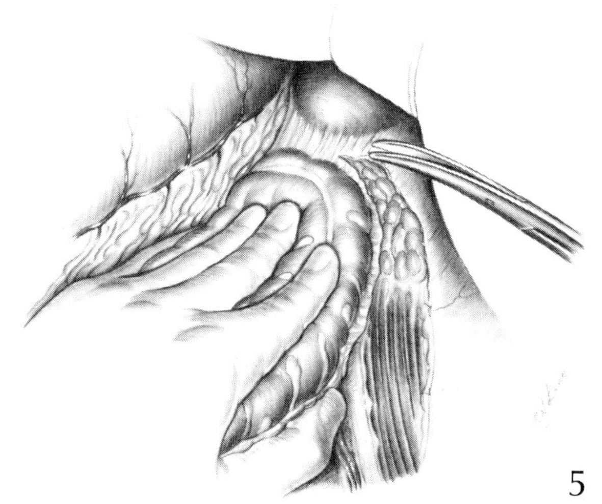

5

Mobilization of the right hemicolon

6

This is usually easy, but if access is difficult the surgeon can change sides in order to operate from the patient's left, or ask the assistant to undertake the mobilization.

The peritoneum in the right gutter is incised in the same manner as that described for the left gutter, the caecum, terminal ileum and ascending colon being swept forward to identify and preserve the ureter.

Freeing the hepatic flexure is undertaken in a similar manner to freeing the splenic flexure but care must be taken not to damage either the gall bladder or the duodenum which lies beneath the hepatic flexure.

The whole colon is now mobilized down to the pelvic brim and is ready for division from its mesentery.

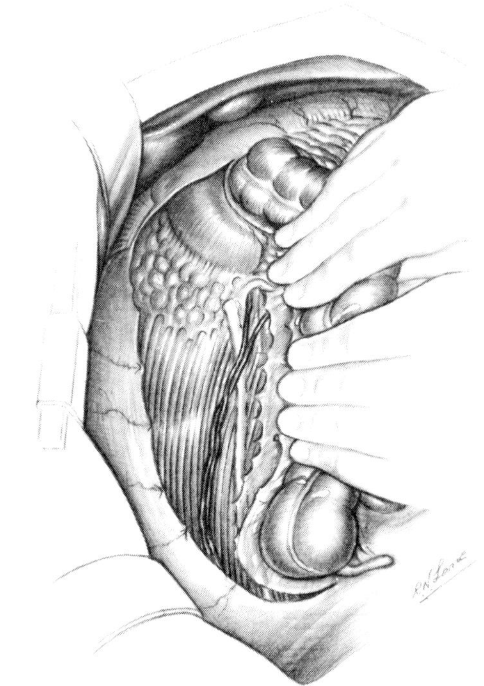

6

7

Except in cases where the operation is being undertaken for carcinoma, the mesentery is divided close to the bowel wall to avoid risk of damage to retroperitoneal structures. This procedure is aided by elevating the mesentery so that it can be transilluminated to demonstrate the vessels and thus ensure their accurate isolation and division. In the region of the terminal ileum the vessels are divided in a manner which ensures a good blood supply to the terminal ileum yet narrows the mesentery to allow eversion of the stoma. This can be difficult when the mesentery is thickened as in obesity or Crohn's disease. In such circumstances the priority is to preserve the blood supply, even if this makes eversion of the stoma difficult.

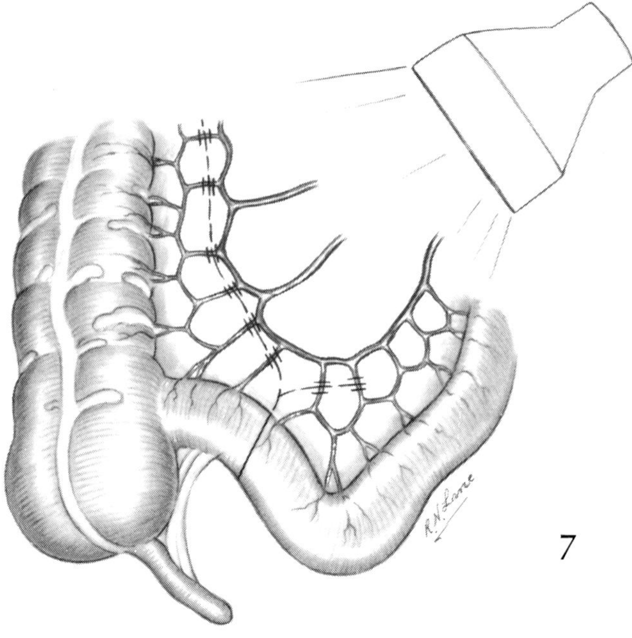

7

8

Once the mesentery to the right colon and terminal ileum is divided the terminal ileum can be transected, which should be done as close to the caecum as possible though this may have to be modified where the terminal ileum is involved with Crohn's disease or backwash ileitis.

It is useful to divide the ileum with a Zachary-Cope clamp. The proximal end is carefully covered with a pack and dropped back into the abdominal cavity. The distal end and the caecum are then placed in a plastic bowel bag and the remainder of the bowel is fed into it as the mesentery is divided.

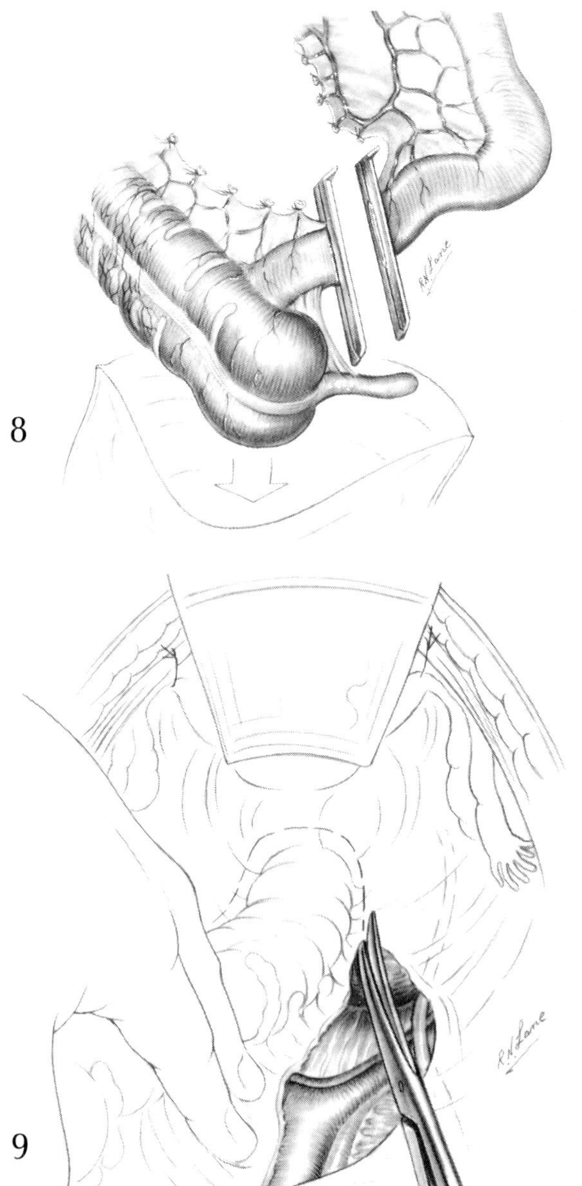

8

9

9

Mobilization of the rectum

Attention is then turned to the pelvis. A deep retractor is placed in the rectovesical or rectouterine pouch. If the uterus is bulky it can be pulled out of the way by inserting sutures around the Fallopian tubes and round ligaments on each side and tying them up to the lower end of the abdominal incision.

Incisions in the peritoneum are commenced at the lower ends of the right and left hemicolon and carried down on either side of the rectum to be joined anteriorly in the depths of the rectovesical or rectouterine pouch. Care must be taken to divide only the peritoneum; the ureters are at particular risk during this manoeuvre.

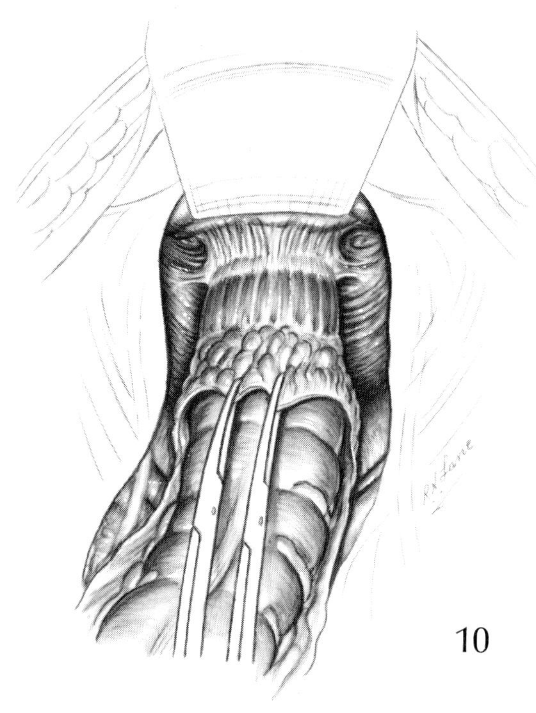

10

10

The aim of the rectal mobilization is to avoid damage to the pelvic nerves. Because of this the superior rectal vessels, the mesorectum and the lateral ligaments must be divided close to the rectum at the point where the vessels pass from the mesentery into the bowel wall. Thus, this technique is different from that for the treatment of patients with cancer and is, inevitably, a more time-consuming and bloody technique; but once again haemostatic clips are of considerable help. (This approach must not be used where the operation is being undertaken for cancer of the colon or rectum.)

The seminal vesicles are identified and dissected forward from the anterior surface of the rectum. The fascia of Denonvillier is divided and the dissection carried down to the apex of the prostrate.

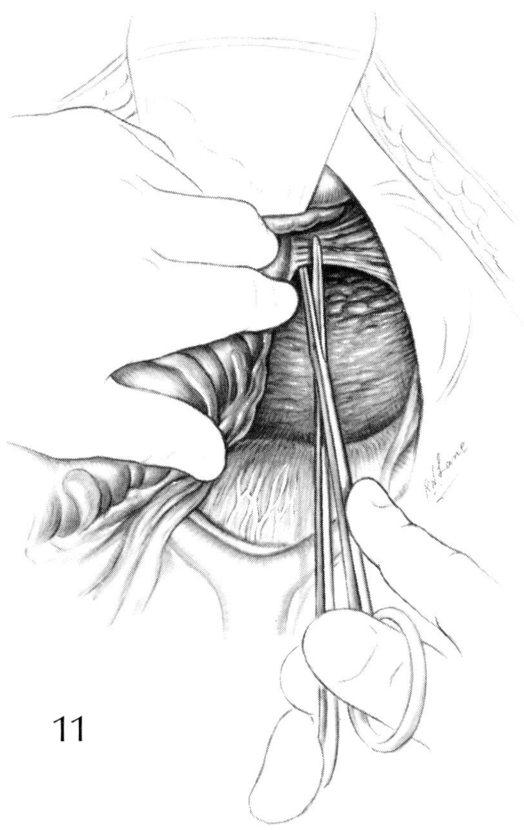

11

11

The rectum can now be pulled up and the lateral ligaments divided close to the bowel wall. The abdominal surgeon will at this stage meet the perineal surgeon dissecting upwards.

When the perineal dissection is complete the whole large bowel can be removed through the perineum, but in bulky colons or those with toxic dilatation this can be difficult and the abdominal surgeon, after packing off the rest of the abdominal contents, should not hesitate to pull the bowel upwards and place it in the intestinal bag for removal. A warm moist pack is placed in the pelvic cavity for 2–3 min and then removed to allow bleeding points to be coagulated or clipped. The author then normally irrigates the pelvis with a litre of warm saline to remove clot and debris.

Closure of the pelvic peritoneum

This is a controversial topic with strongly held individual views. In proctocolectomy, where there has not been wide dissection or excision of the pelvic peritoneum, the author prefers to close the peritoneum with a continuous suture of 0 Dexon.

THE PERINEAL DISSECTION

12

In colitis and polyposis coli the aim of the perineal dissection is to remove only the bowel wall and not the perirectal tissues. This dissection leaves the pelvic nerves intact and ensures, by maintaining the levator ani, a strong pelvic floor. In both males and females this is achieved by an intersphincteric dissection commencing between the internal and external sphincters. Although this can usually be accomplished without difficulty, in Crohn's disease with gross perianal lesions it can be technically difficult.

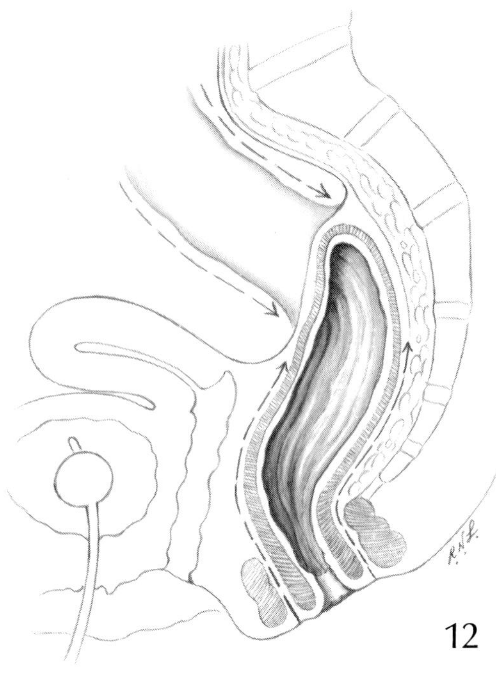

12

13

The perineal dissector can begin at the same time as the abdominal operator and take his time to achieve an anatomically accurate dissection with minimal blood loss. The dissection commences with a circumferential incision over the intersphincteric groove.

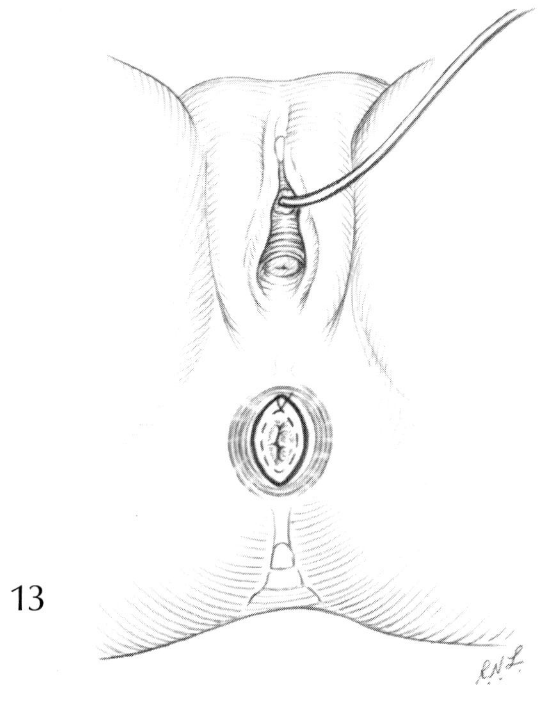

13

14

The pale fibres of the internal sphincter are identified and dissection carried out in the plane between the internal and external sphincter. The plane is usually easy to develop and with a combination of blunt and sharp dissection with McIndoe's scissors can be carried up towards the pelvis.

It is easiest to start on the lateral sides, continue the dissection anteriorly and then complete it posteriorly. Retraction is accomplished by the assistant using two Langenbeck retractors or a small self-retaining retractor.

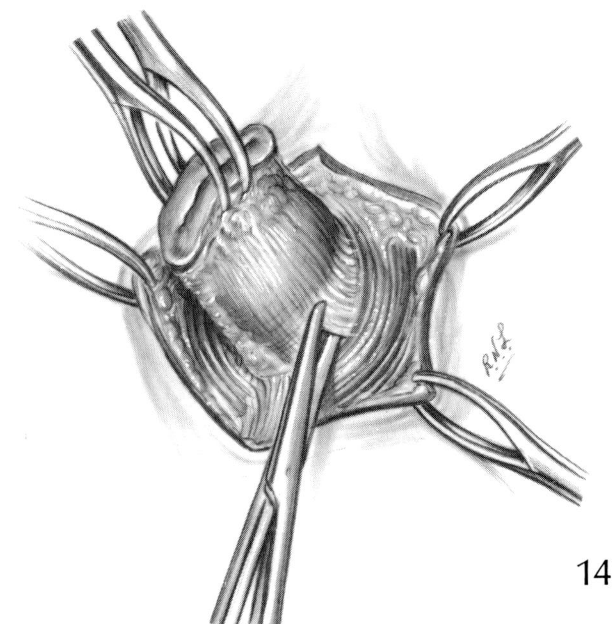

14

Completion of the perineal dissection

15

Anteriorly the external sphincter decussates in the midline and becomes attached to the fibres of the rectourethralis. It is thus necessary to cut through the external sphincter in this plane to expose the posterior surface of the prostate.

As dissection proceeds higher, the fascia on either side is divided until the lower end of the lateral ligaments not divided by the abdominal operator are reached and these are then cut. The fascia overlying the prostate is divided and the lower end of the seminal vesicles exposed and dissected free up to the point exposed by the abdominal operation.

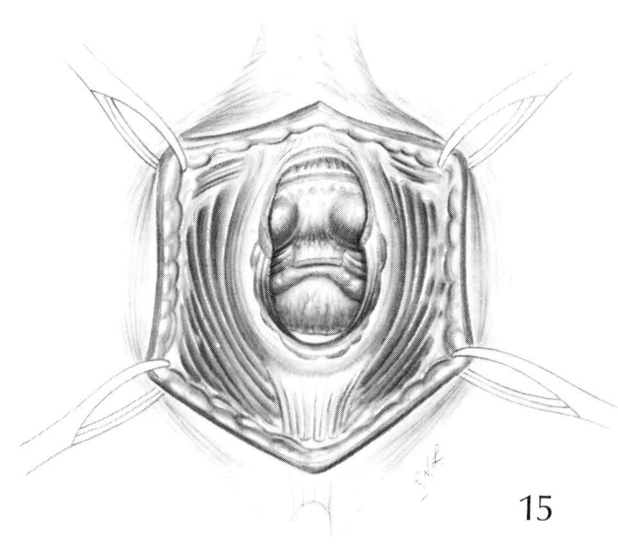

15

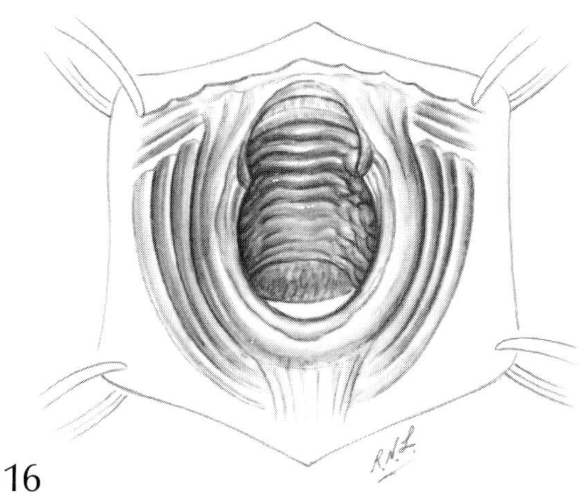

16

16

In the female it is necessary to dissect the vagina forwards off the anal canal and lower rectum until the plane opened from above through the rectouterine pouch is reached.

The bowel is then free and is removed.

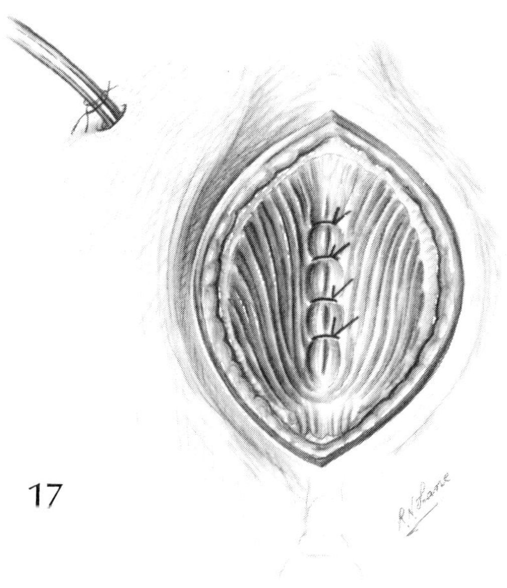

17

Closure of the perineal wound

17

A closed low pressure suction drain catheter is inserted through a lateral stab incision and is positioned above the levator ani and below the pelvic peritoneum. The puborectalis and levator ani muscles are then approximated with interrupted 0 Dexon sutures. The skin is closed with interrupted vertical mattress sutures of 2/0 black silk or a continuous subcuticular suture of 2/0 Dexon. A gauze dressing and pad are applied. Suction is continued for 5 days and the skin sutures removed at 10 days.

Some surgeons strongly favour closure of the perineal wound over a double lumen catheter placed in the presacral space with irrigation using isotonic saline at a rate of 80 ml/h for 5 days. The irrigating fluid is removed by continuous suction down the second lumen[1].

Occasionally, such as in Crohn's disease where a perineum is a mass of fistulae and active sepsis, it is reasonable to pack the cavity with gauze soaked with an antiseptic solution.

If the perineum is very septic, it is probably wise to bring the drain through the centre of the suture line.

CONSTRUCTION OF THE ILEOSTOMY

Ideally the ileal stoma should be brought to the surface through an extraperitoneal tunnel before penetrating the abdominal wall. However, this method is contraindicated where the terminal ileum is involved with active Crohn's disease and a standard approach should be used in these circumstances (*see* chapter on 'End ileostomy II', pp. 65–69).

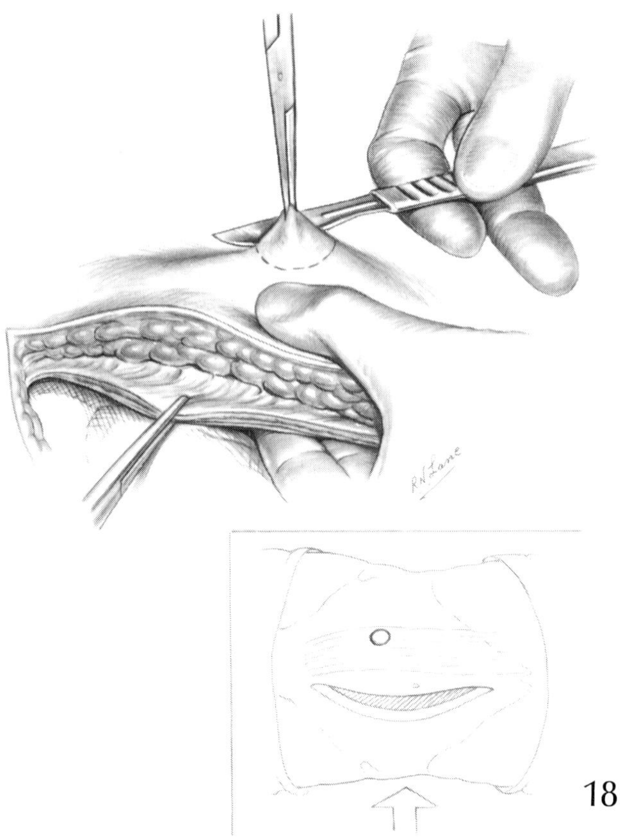

18

18

In either case creation of the stoma commences by cutting a disc of skin 2 cm in diameter from the previously marked site. This is achieved by pinching up the skin in the centre of the disc with a pair of artery forceps and cutting horizontally across the base with a scalpel.

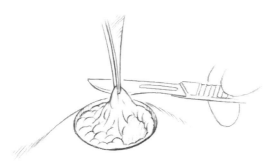

19

The procedure is repeated with the subcutaneous tissue until the aponeurosis of the external oblique, where it becomes the anterior wall of the rectus sheath, is reached. At this stage, because of lateral retraction of the abdominal muscles, the edge of the midline incision, the linea alba and the peritoneal edge are grasped in artery forceps and drawn to the midline.

19

20

A cruciate incision is made in the aponeurosis of the external oblique (anterior rectus sheath).

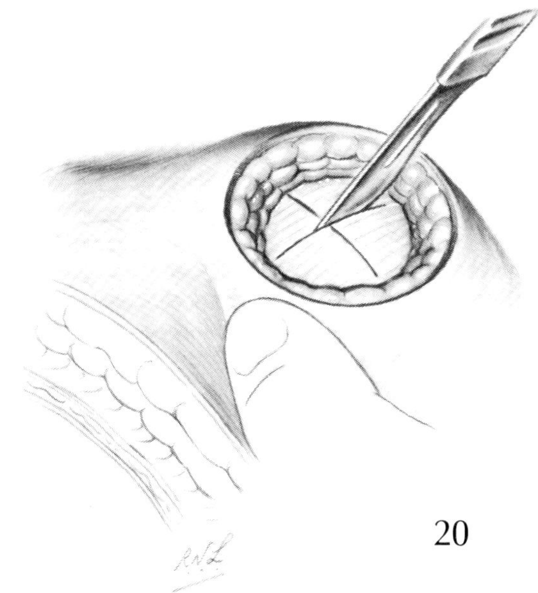

20

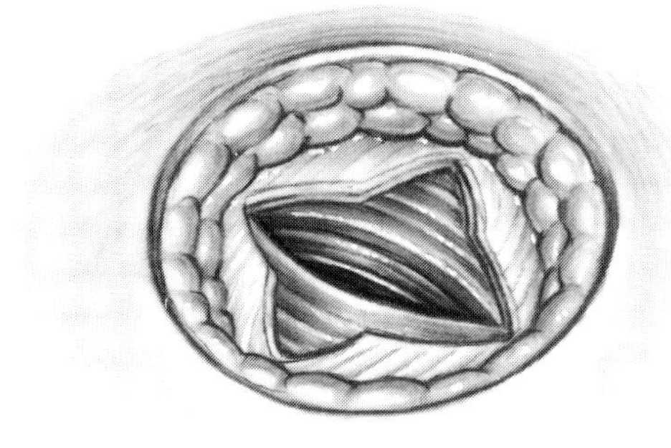

21

21 & 22

The rectus muscle is split and the peritoneum exposed. This is incised and two fingers inserted through the defect created. Where the abdominal wall is thin, and it is intended to create an extraperitoneal ileostomy, the peritoneum can be left intact.

The defect created is stretched to a width where it will easily admit two fingers.

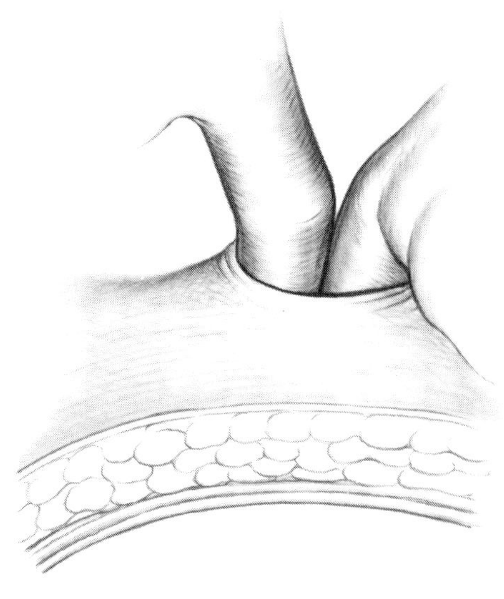

22

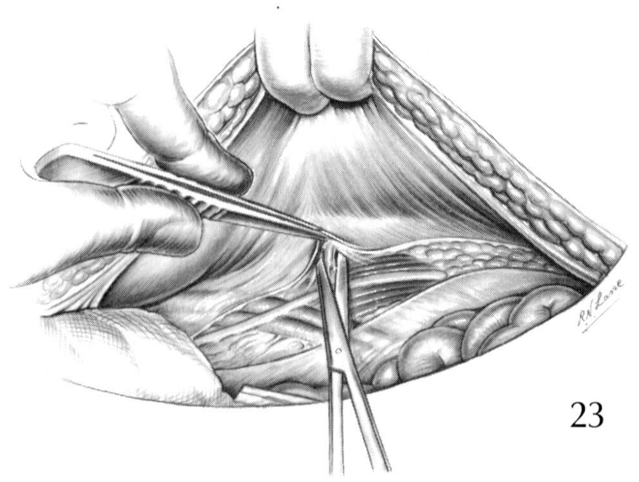

23

Extraperitoneal ileostomy

23 & 24

The peritoneum on the right lateral wall of the abdomen is lifted up at the point where it was incised in the paracolic gutter. Two fingers are introduced into the retroperitoneal space and pushed easily up to the defect created in the muscles in the right iliac fossa.

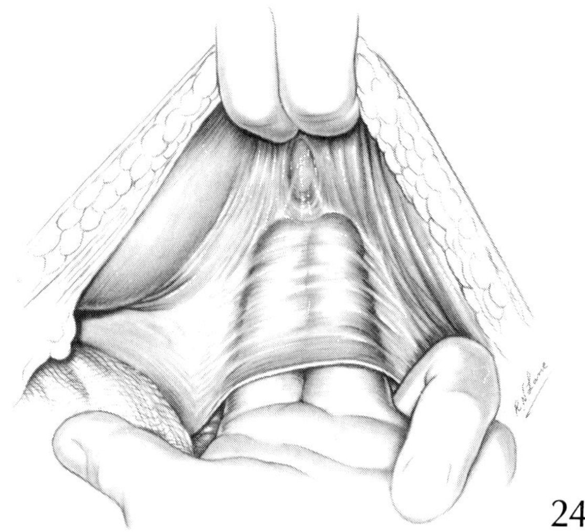

24

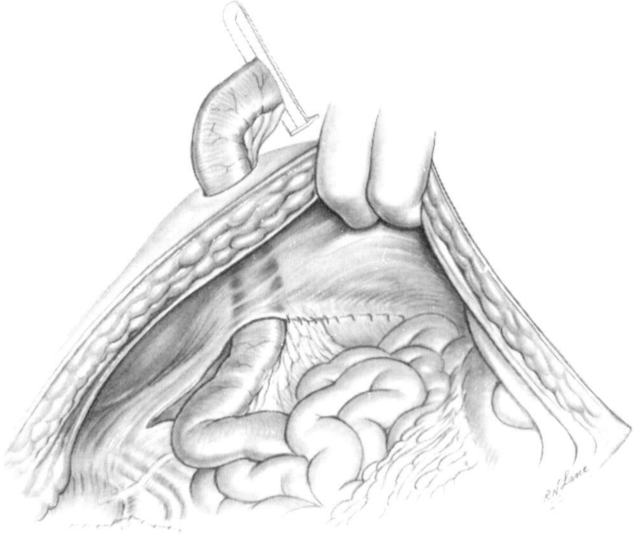

25

25

The terminal ileum is then passed through this space to emerge on the anterior abdominal wall. To enable this to be easily everted 10 cm of bowel should protrude – this allows for some sagging into the subcutaneous tissue.

Care is taken to ensure that the mesentery is not twisted. The peritoneum is then sutured to the leaf of the mesoileum to obliterate the potential space. If the peritoneum below the stoma was opened when creating the passage through the abdominal wall, this too is closed with interrupted sutures.

Conventional ileostomy

26

Where the experitoneal technique is not indicated mesoileum is laid against the lateral abdominal wall and the ileum passed through the defect in the peritoneum and muscles to the surface.

Using either a purse-string suture or multiple interrupted sutures the defect between the mesoileum and the lateral abdominal wall is closed so that nothing can prolapse through and become strangulated. The author normally inserts a few sutures of 2/0 Dexon between the point of exit of the ileum and the peritoneum.

At the end of the operation the peritoneum is checked to ensure there are no bleeding points. The omentum is laid over the anterior surface of the small bowel and positioned in the pelvis. If for any reason there has had to be extensive pelvic dissection and the peritoneum has not been closed the author creates a pedicle of omentum on the left gastroepiploic artery and fills the pélvic cavity with it, fixing it in position with a few Dexon sutures.

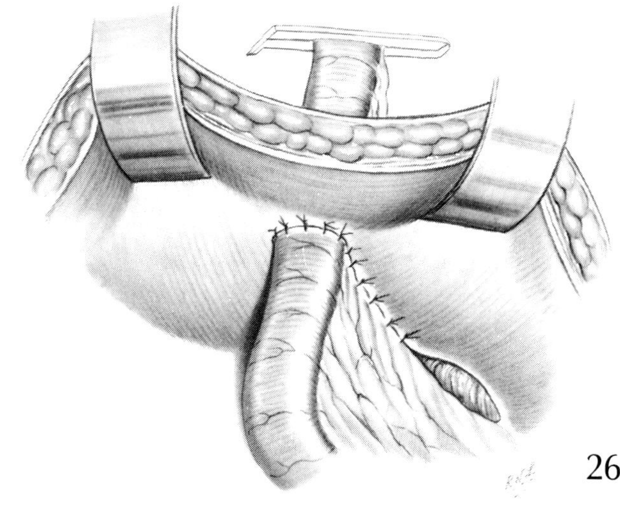

26

Closure

The abdominal wall is closed in layers with 0 Dexon to the peritoneum and 1 Prolene to the linea alba, taking many large bites of the muscle on either side. No abdominal drainage is needed. Clips or silk can be placed in the skin.

Making the spout of the ileostomy

The spout ileostomy is constructed by everting the mucosal surface.

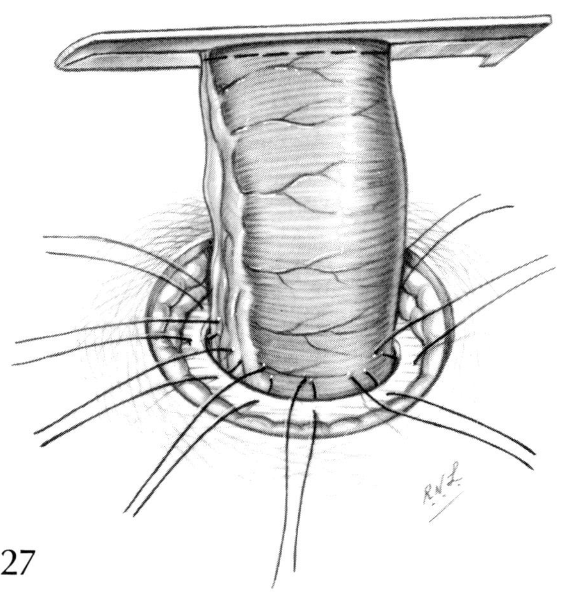

27

27

To accomplish this about 8–10 cm of bowel should have been brought through beyond the abdominal skin. The clamp is excised to remove the crushed bowel. The stoma is then fixed by sutures of 2/0 chromic catgut on a round bodied needle that passes through the anterior rectus sheath and the serosa of the bowel wall with a superficial bite. Care should be taken not to transfix the mesentery of the small bowel.

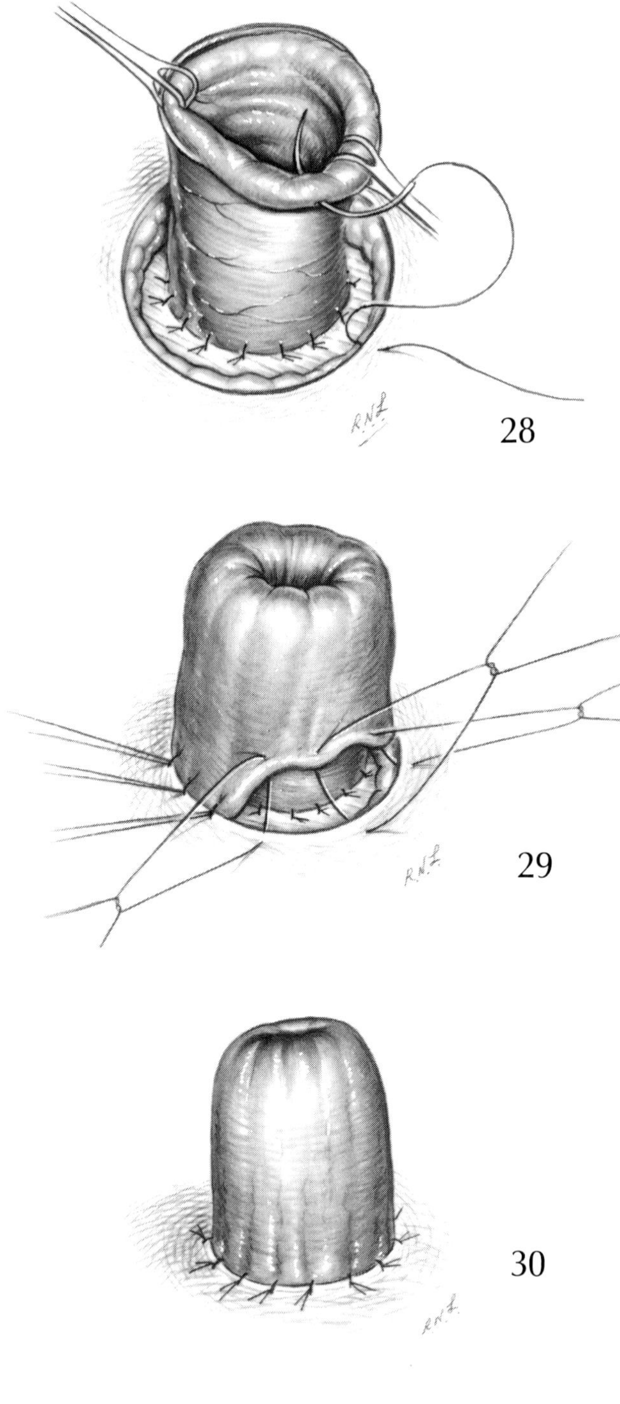

28, 29 & 30

The bowel is then everted to form a spout, the edge of the everted bowel being sutured to the skin with sutures of 0 catgut on a cutting needle. When completed the stoma is inspected to ensure it is pink and healthy. A transparent drainable stoma bag is applied immediately.

Postoperative care and complications

The stoma is inspected through the transparent stoma bag every hour for the first 12 h. Any change in colour or retraction is reported immediately to the surgeon.

Intermittent nasogastric suction and intravenous infusion are maintained until the ileostomy works continuously. This is usually within 48 h. Ileostomy output can become very large at this point and patients have difficulty in keeping up the necessary oral intake. In these cases the intravenous infusion should be continued until the output slows down.

The urinary catheter can be removed on the third postoperative day and the skin sutures or clips at 1 week. The perineal suction drain should be left for 5 days before removal.

When correctly carried out this operation is rarely associated with complications in the early postoperative period. It is however dangerous to attribute to 'ileus' failure of the ileostomy to function. Abdominal distension, high nasogastric aspirates, an empty ileostomy bag after 72 h, even the absence of colicky pain, should stimulate the surgeon to consider the need for re-exploration of the abdomen. Such a course of events is nearly always the result of intestinal obstruction caused by angulation or entrapment of the small bowel and will only respond to relief of the obstruction.

The only other recurring problem associated with this operation is failure of the perineal wound to heal. This is not usually the case when the operation is undertaken for ulcerative colitis or neoplasm but is a problem in Crohn's disease. Where the wound continues to discharge the sutures should be removed and an attempt made to create a conical cavity. This is then irrigated twice daily with saline and packed with ribbon gauze soaked with an antiseptic solution. Healing of such cavities can take many months but nearly always occurs eventually.

Reference

1. Beart, R. W., McIlrath, D. C., Kelly, K. A. *et al*. Surgical management of inflammatory bowel disease. Current Problems in Surgery 1980; 17: 533–584

Ileorectal anastomosis for inflammatory bowel disease

John Alexander-Williams MD, ChM, FRCS, FACS
Consultant Surgeon, The General Hospital, Birmingham

Preoperative

Indications

When the colon has to be removed for severe inflammatory bowel disease it is always desirable to retain the rectum providing it is not severely diseased, has relatively normal function particularly regarding distensibility and does not have a prohibitively high risk of early recrudescence of the disease within it.

The two principal types of ileorectal anastomosis are as follows.

1. A primary ileorectal anastomosis at the time of colectomy. This is more likely to be performed in Crohn's colitis and rarely in ulcerative colitis, the indication for operation being severe colonic disease of the colon with relative sparing of the rectum.
2. A secondary ileorectal anastomosis after emergency colectomy for fulminating colitis.

In Crohn's colitis, the disease is often maximal on the right side and sometimes the rectum is relatively normal though in some cases there may be associated perianal disease. In ulcerative colitis the rectum is usually the maximal site of the disease. However, in approximately 10 per cent of patients with ulcerative colitis the rectum is relatively spared. In patients with a first fulminating attack of colitis the maximum disease may be in the transverse colon and splenic flexure and the rectum may not have time to become severely affected. For this reason whenever surgery becomes inevitable for fulminating colitis with risk of toxic dilatation or perforation, it is best to confine the operation to total colectomy with preservation of the rectum either as a mucous fistula or as a Hartmann's procedure because it may be possible subsequently for an ileorectal anastomosis to be carried out if the rectum has not been irrevocably destroyed by severe disease.

Preoperative assessment

The success of ileorectal anastomosis depends particularly on the lack of disease in the rectum. This disease can be: acute inflammation or ulceration of the mucosa; chronic fibrosis and lack of distensibility of the wall; sometimes severe destructive perianal disease will also be present.

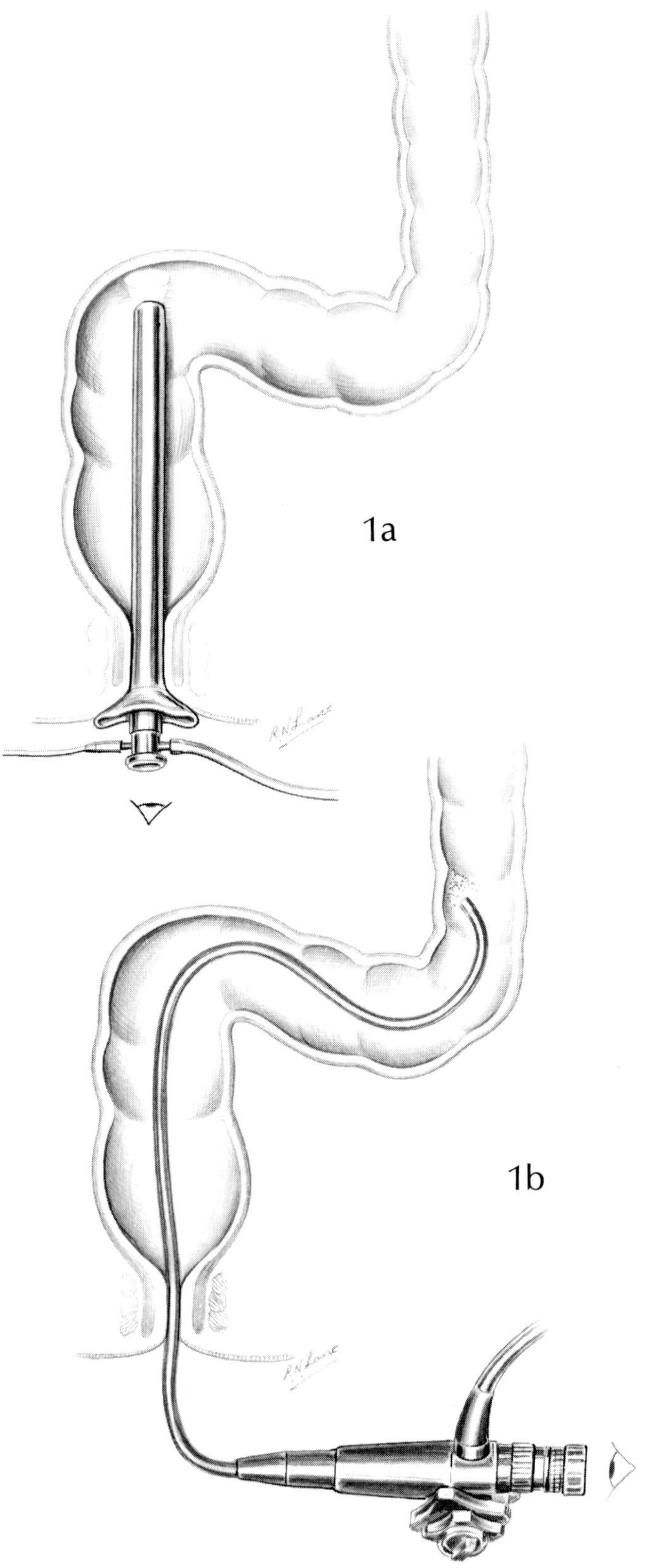

1a & b

Sigmoidoscopy

Before a planned ileorectal anastomosis it is only the state of the distal 15 cm of the rectum that is being assessed and a rigid sigmoidoscope (*a*) is preferable to a flexible colonoscope (*b*) because it is easier to assess the rigidity and distensibility of the rectal wall with the rigid instrument. Visual inspection is very important in this assessment and careful cleaning of the mucosa is required; the examination must be gentle to avoid the mucosa becoming obscured by bleeding due to trauma. Multiple biopsies should be taken for documentation.

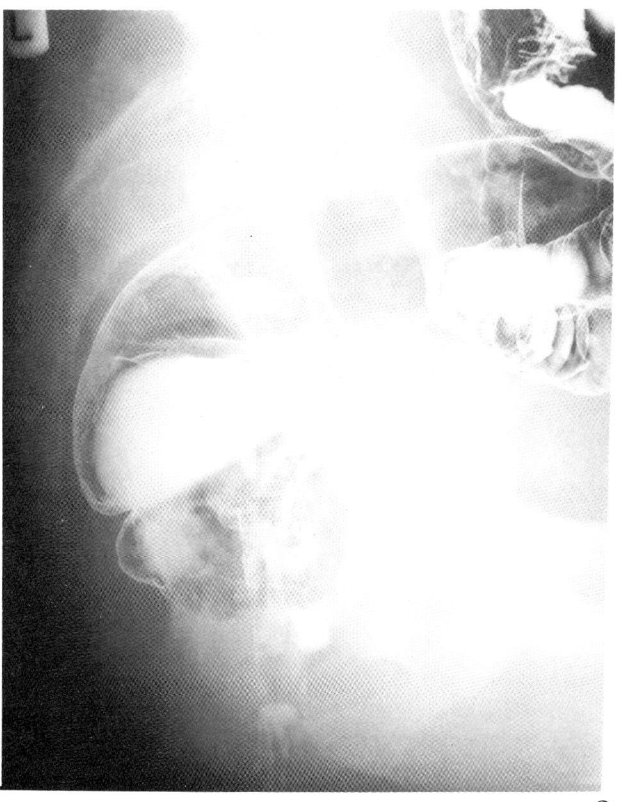

2

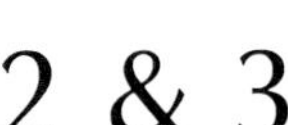

2 & 3

The capacity of the rectum can be assessed, to some extent, by its distensibility as seen on the lateral radiograph of the pelvis on barium enema (illustrated) or by assessing the distensibility on inflation during sigmoidoscopy.

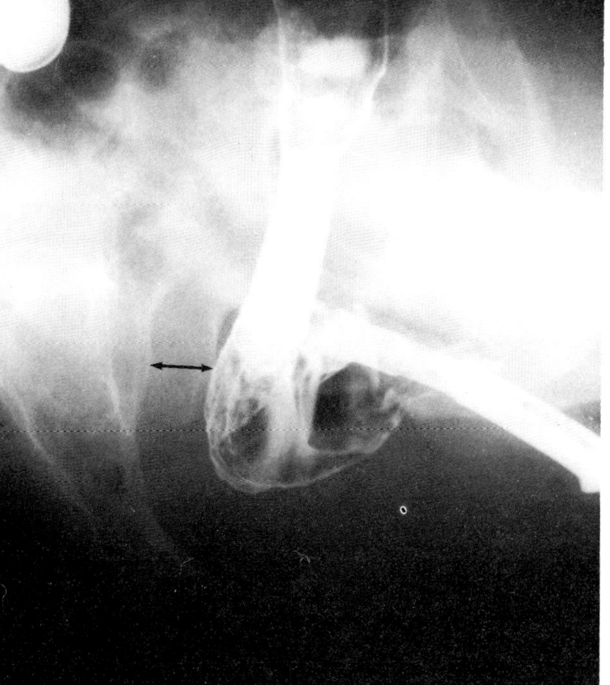

3

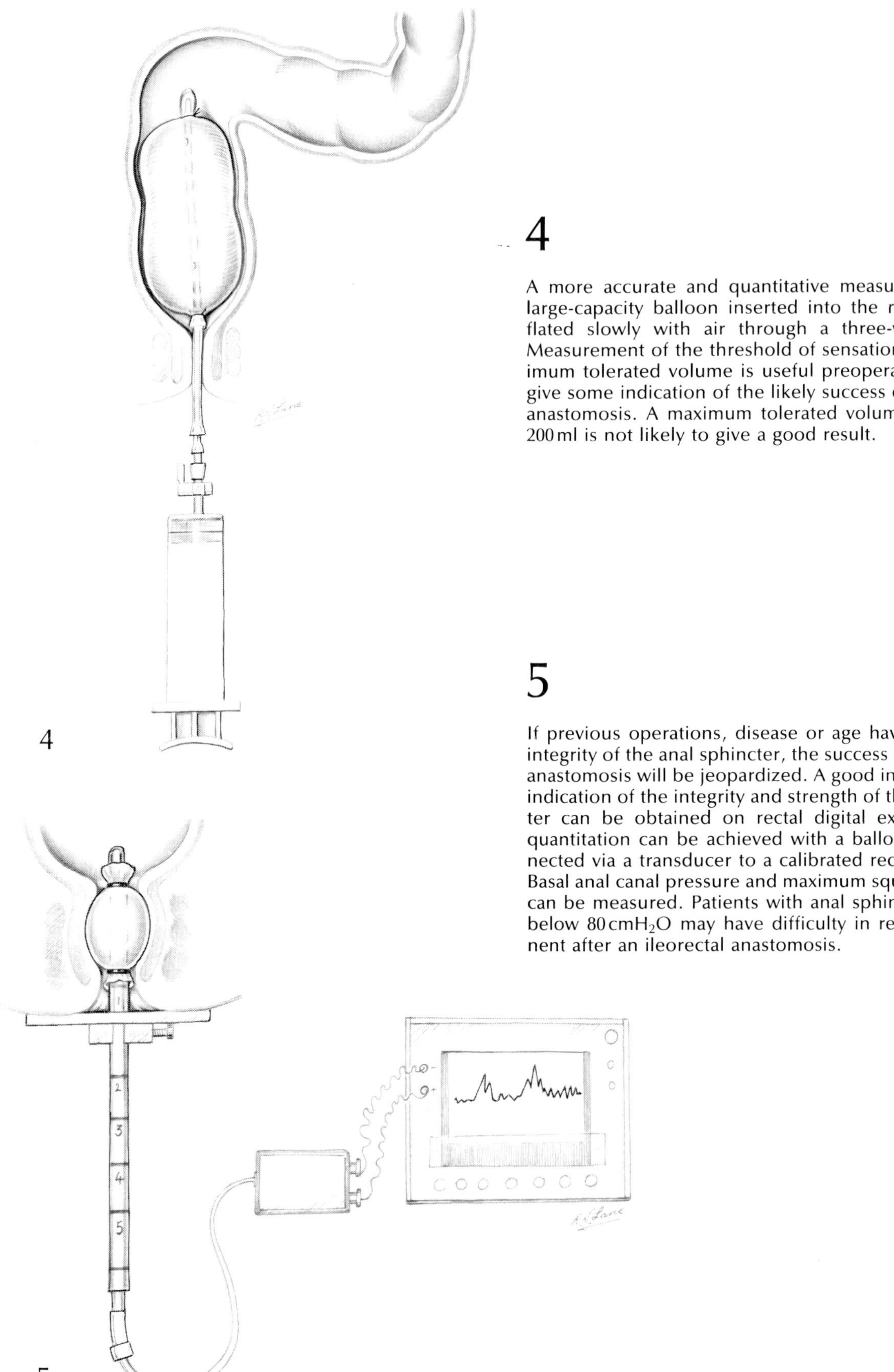

4

5

4

A more accurate and quantitative measure is to use a large-capacity balloon inserted into the rectum and inflated slowly with air through a three-way stopcock. Measurement of the threshold of sensation and the maximum tolerated volume is useful preoperatively and will give some indication of the likely success of an ileorectal anastomosis. A maximum tolerated volume of less than 200 ml is not likely to give a good result.

5

If previous operations, disease or age have affected the integrity of the anal sphincter, the success of an ileorectal anastomosis will be jeopardized. A good indication of the indication of the integrity and strength of the anal sphincter can be obtained on rectal digital examination but quantitation can be achieved with a balloon probe connected via a transducer to a calibrated recording device. Basal anal canal pressure and maximum squeeze pressure can be measured. Patients with anal sphincter pressures below 80 cmH_2O may have difficulty in remaining continent after an ileorectal anastomosis.

The operation

6

The incision

A midline incision extending from the xiphisternum to the symphysis pubis is best and ensures that if stomas are needed at the time of operation or subsequently the iliac fossae will be clear of scars.

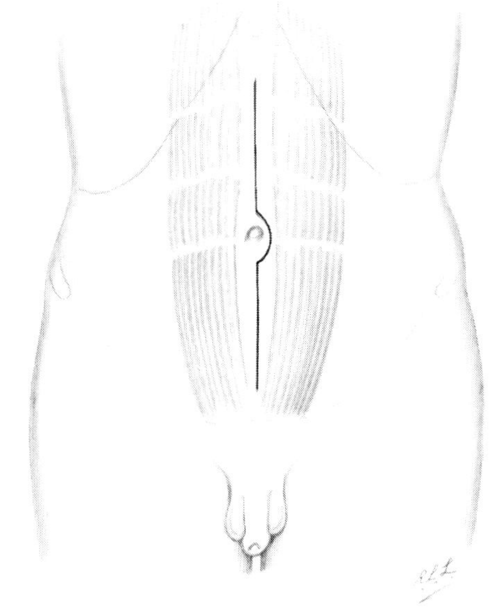

6

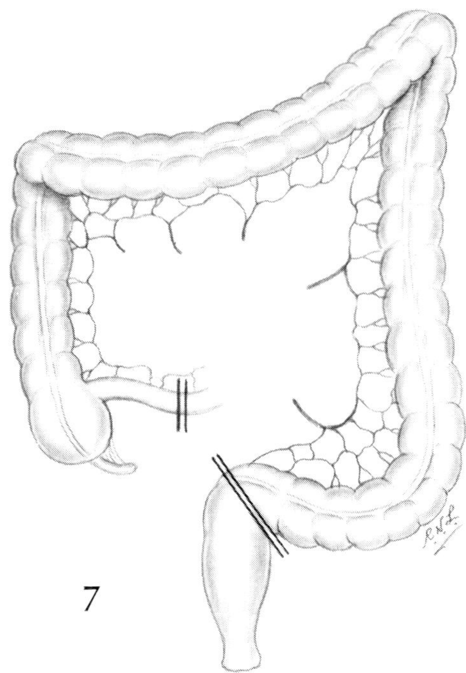

7

7

Colectomy

A total colectomy is performed, with the blood vessels being divided at the most convenient site, often close to the bowel, unlike the technique employed in cancer surgery. The omentum is removed only if it is closely bound to the transverse colon. It is almost always possible to preserve most of the omentum which has the theoretical advantage of a protective capacity against postoperative sepsis or anastomotic leakage. The spleen is also preserved.

The rectum is divided at a point determined by the previous sigmoidoscopy and by the external appearance of the bowel. Usually it is not necessary to resect below the sacral promontory, so the subsequent anastomosis is not technically difficult or performed under tension.

The terminal ileum is divided proximal to macroscopical disease (in Crohn's disease) or close to the ileocaecal valve (in ulcerative colitis).

The ileorectal anastomosis

There are many options available in choosing the method of ileorectal anastomosis. Inevitably, there is a size discrepancy with the rectal diameter being much larger than the ileal. For this reason some surgeons prefer to anastomose the side of the ileum to the end of the rectum or even to perform a side-to-side ileorectal anastomosis. Some advocate an end-to-end stapled anastomosis. The author has used all of these techniques but now prefers an end-to-end anastomosis: it is always possible to achieve this neatly and securely and the principal reason for favouring it is that it facilitiates subsequent regular follow-up by sigmoidoscopy on X-ray whereas a blind end may make sigmoidoscopy confusing or even hazardous.

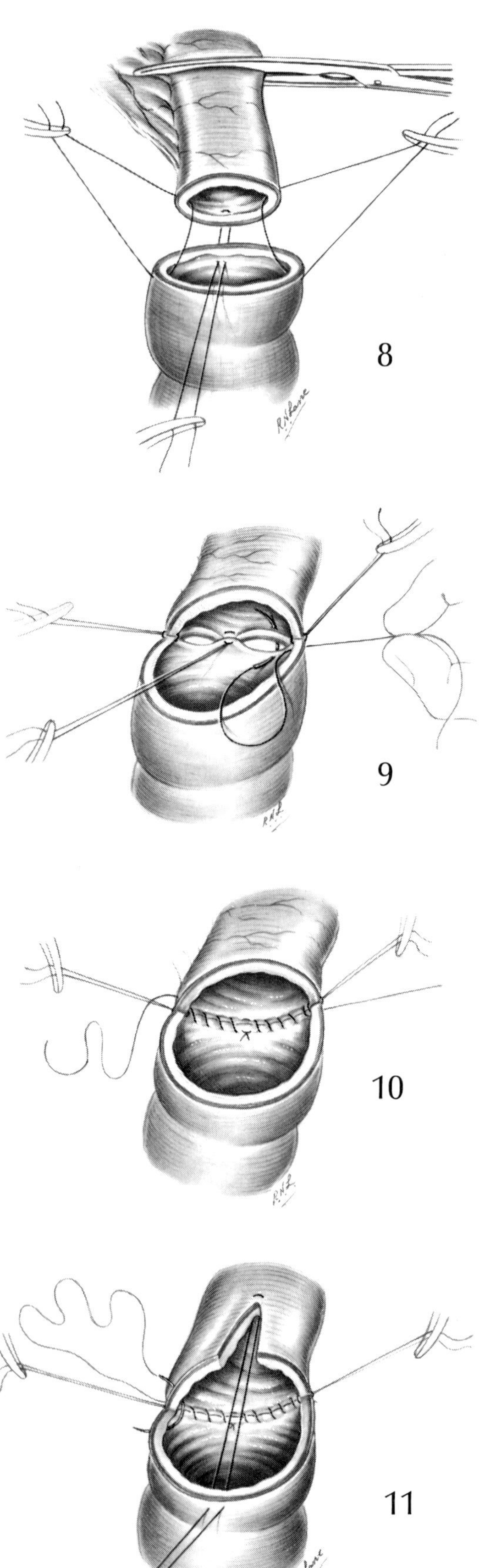

8–12

As the anastomosis is usually made at the level of the sacral promontory there is no difficulty in achieving a good hand-sewn anastomosis and as there is usually size discrepancy a circular stapled anastomosis is not ideal. The author's technique is to perform an open anastomosis with a proximal soft clamp to prevent ileal content being discharged during the anastomosis. The posterior layer is secured with two lateral sutures and a central stay suture; the back row is then completed with a running suture of smooth absorbable synthetic material (Vicryl). If there is a large size discrepancy between the two diameters a small vertical incision on the antimesenteric border of the ileum enables the continuous suturing to be continued around the diameter of the bowel with approximately equal 'bites' on the ileal and rectal side. One central stay suture anteriorly helps to guide the continuous running suture. Previously, the author has used single-layer interrupted thread sutures or a continuous inner catgut haemostatic suture with outer inverting interrupted thread sutures. The advantage of the continuous absorbable suture is that it is quick strong, non-reactive and does not produce stitch granulomas that tend to look like recurrent disease at follow-up sigmoidoscopy. There is, however, little to choose between the methods.

The gap between the cut edge of the ileal mesentery and the peritoneum of the posterior wall of the pelvis is closed to prevent small bowel herniation behind the anastomosis.

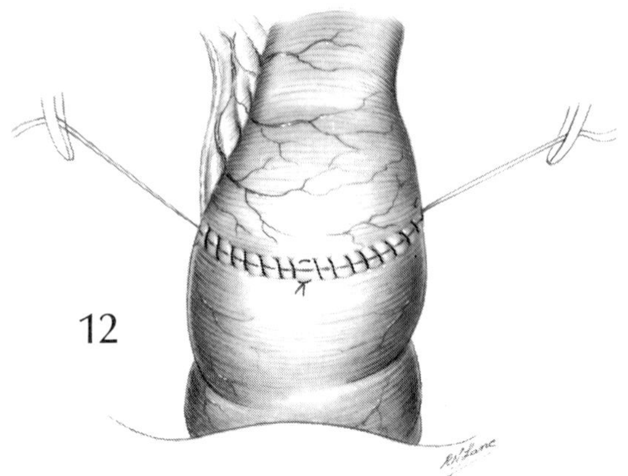

Protecting ileostomy

It used to be the author's custom to use a diverting ileostomy to 'protect' an ileorectal anastomosis in inflammatory bowel disease, particularly if the rectum was so diseased as to compromise the integrity of the anastomosis. However, he now feels that if an ileorectal anastomosis cannot be performed safely as a primary procedure then it probably should not be performed at all because this implies that the rectum is so severely diseased that a good functional result is unlikely.

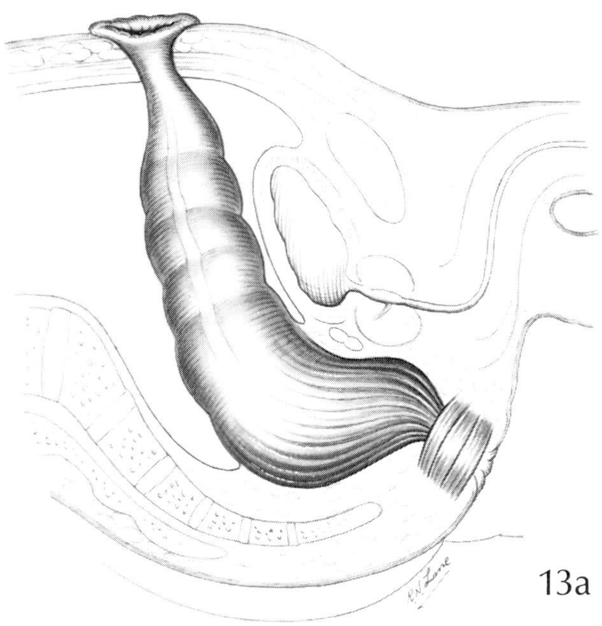

13a

Secondary ileorectal anastomosis

13a & b

When the first operation was a total colectomy with either (*a*) a mucous fistula or (*b*) a Hartmann's procedure, secondary ileorectal reconnection can be achieved once the patient's condition has improved. This is usually delayed until the mucosa of the retained rectum has reverted to normal or nearly so. A certain amount of inflammation and pus usually remains within the defunctioned rectum. It is advisable not to leave reconnection too long or the defunctioned rectum will contract. Three months after the original colectomy is often an ideal time to restore continuity.

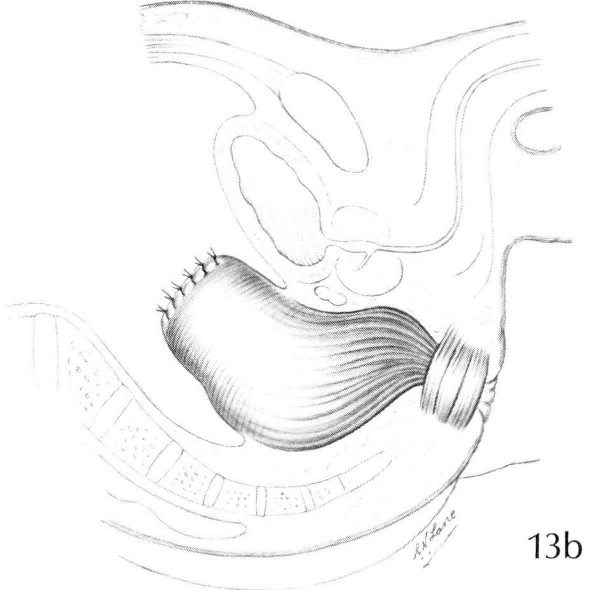

13b

14

A laparotomy is required for the reconnection and is performed by reopening the original incision. If there is a mucous fistula this is disconnected from the skin and the stump trimmed back until the mucosa appears healthy and the bowel wall is pliable; it is usually not necessary to trim it back further than the sacral promontory. The secondary anastomosis is then performed in the same way as the previous primary anastomosis already described.

If a Hartmann's procedure has been performed an alternative technique is employed. Instead of dissecting out and mobilizing the rectal stump from above, the pelvis is simply cleared of any adherent small bowel and an appropriate instrument (an obturator of a sigmoidoscope) passed through the anus and pushed upwards to demonstrate to the abdominal surgeon where the closed end of the bowel is buried.

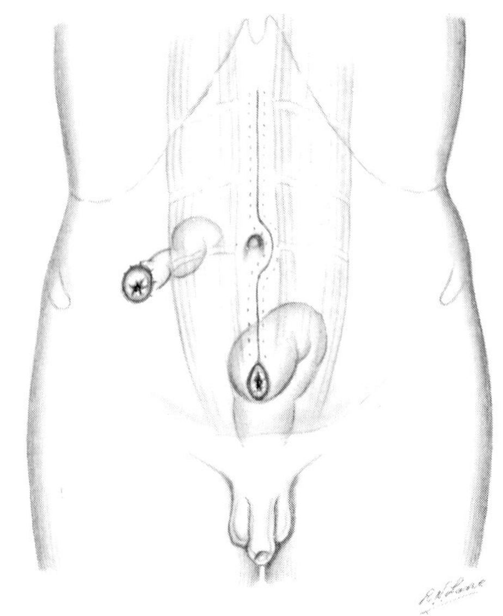

14

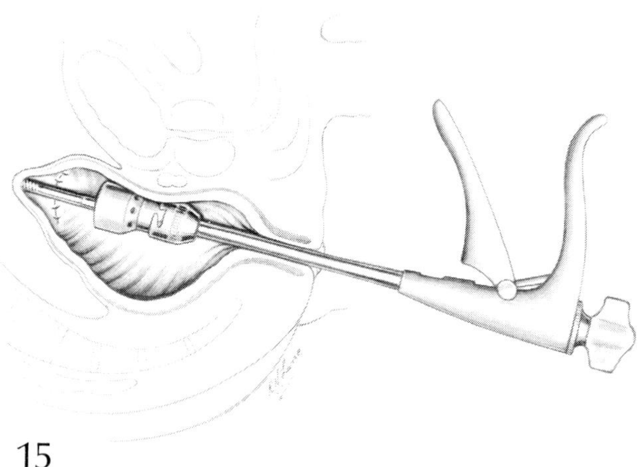

15

15

An end-to-end stapling gun is prepared by removing the anvil/head with the wing nut screwed up to give maximal projection to the shaft. This is then introduced gently into the rectal stump in the same direction as the original guiding instrument and pushed up until it shows through as a projection in the rectal stump. This point is then adjusted so that it is away from the original suture line if this can still be seen. It is usually most convenient to site this anterior to the suture line but it may be posterior. It is better to avoid the suture line itself as the tissue is often thicker and fibrous at this point. Although some surgeons claim that they can perform this type of stapled anastomosis even if the rectal stump was closed with staples the author does not advise this and prefers to close the rectal stump with an absorbable synthetic suture (Vicryl) when doing a Hartmann operation.

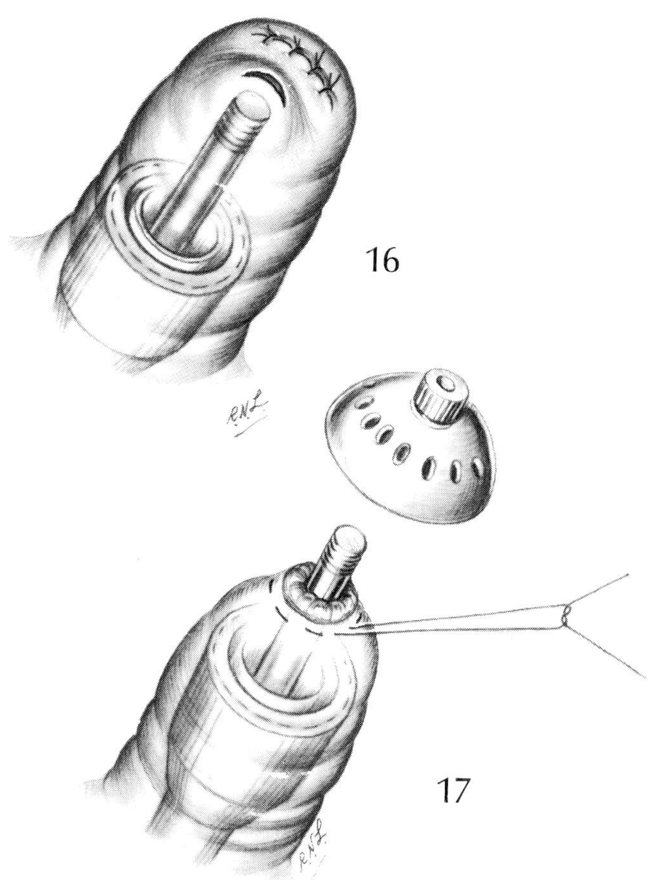

16 & 17

When the shaft can be seen pressing up through the rectal wall a small incision surrounded by a small 0 Prolene purse-string suture is made to allow the shaft to project into the pelvis. The author prefers to use a purse-string suture although some claim it is unnecessary.
The anvil/head is then screwed onto the projecting shaft. The ileum, with the purse-string suture at its end, is brought down into the pelvis and inserted over the anvil. The purse-string is pulled tight and knotted.

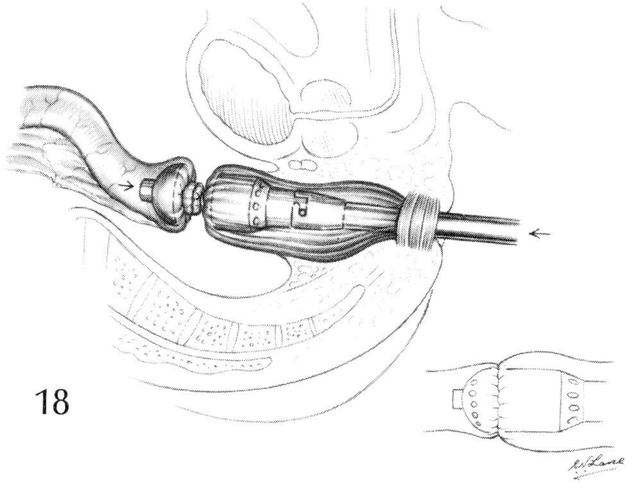

18

The anvil and head of the stapling machine are screwed together until the marks on the shaft of the instrument are aligned, the safety catch is removed and the stapling and cutting with a circular knife are then performed in the standard manner.

If the ileum appears to be too small to insert over the head of the machine it can be stretched gently by the insertion of a dilator or by the surgeon's fingers.

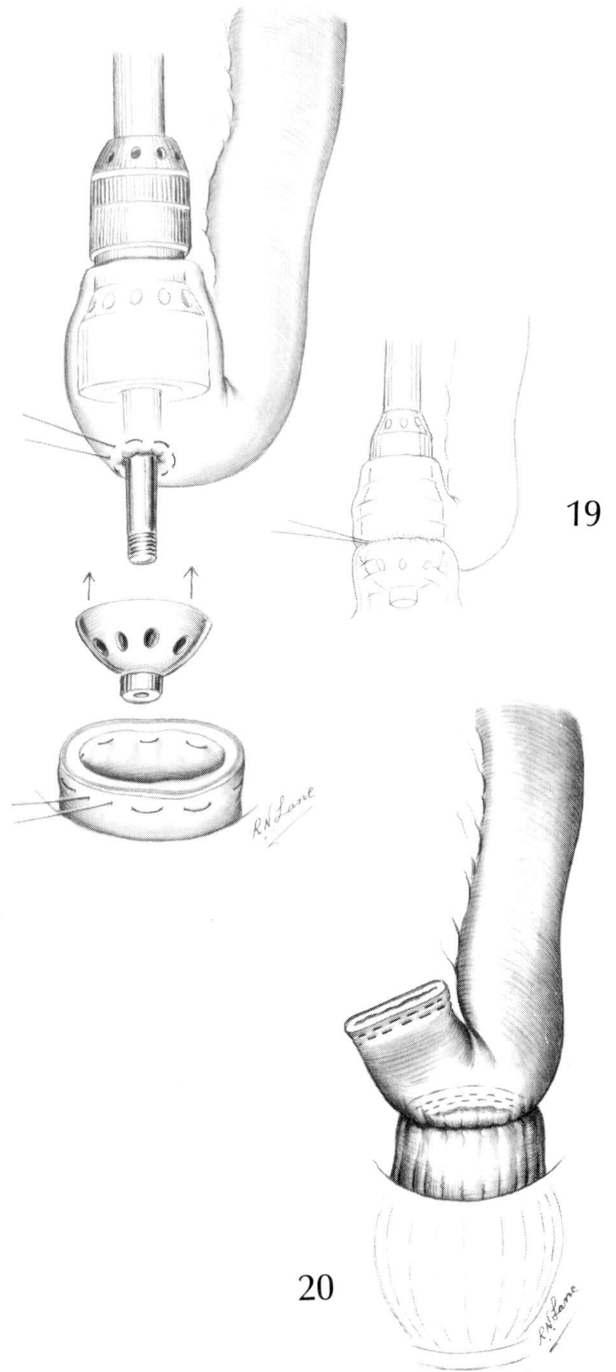

19 & 20

It is sometimes difficult to insert the stapler via the anus. An alternative method of carrying out a stapled side-to-end anastomosis is shown. The end of the ileum is closed with a TA 55 stapling device.

Postoperative care

Bowel function does not usually return until the second to fourth postoperative day. During this time the patient is given parenteral fluids. A nasogastric tube is used until bowel function returns. As patients are often potassium depleted, parenteral potassium 80–120 mEq/day is given once adequate urinary output is established.

It is our practice to cover the operation with a short course of parenteral antibiotics, effective against aerobic and anaerobic organisms (metronidazole and gentamicin or a cephalosporin).

As soon as bowel function returns, the patient is allowed to take fluid by mouth. There is almost invariably an initial diarrhoea (particularly in those patients suffering from Crohn's disease). If this amounts to more than 1.5 litres/day the parenteral fluid and electrolyte regimen is maintained. Codeine phosphate, loperamide or diphenoxylate (Lomotil) may be effective in reducing the diarrhoea and are used frequently. If the patient's recovery is uninterrupted the faecal output begins to thicken by the fifth or seventh day, intravenous feeding is stopped and a light diet begun.

Conservative intersphincteric excision of the rectum in inflammatory bowel disease

P. R. Hawley MS, FRCS
Consultant Surgeon, St Mark's Hospital and King Edward VII Hospital for Officers, London

Preoperative

Indications

This procedure is adopted in patients undergoing proctocolectomy for ulcerative colitis in the absence of carcinoma of the rectum. It can also be carried out in many patients with Crohn's disease without extensive destruction of the sphincters by abscess or fistula formation. Even in these patients, when it is difficult to find the intersphincteric plane, it is surprising how often most of the external sphincter and the levators can be preserved.

This method of excision guarantees the preservation of the presacral sympathetic nerves and the nervi erigentes, thus preventing urinary and sexual problems postoperatively. As the levators and external sphincter muscles are intact and can be approximated at the end of the operation a sound pelvic floor results. The perineal wound is small and most will complete primary healing. This not only decreases the period of hospitalization but is much more comfortable for the patient.

The operation

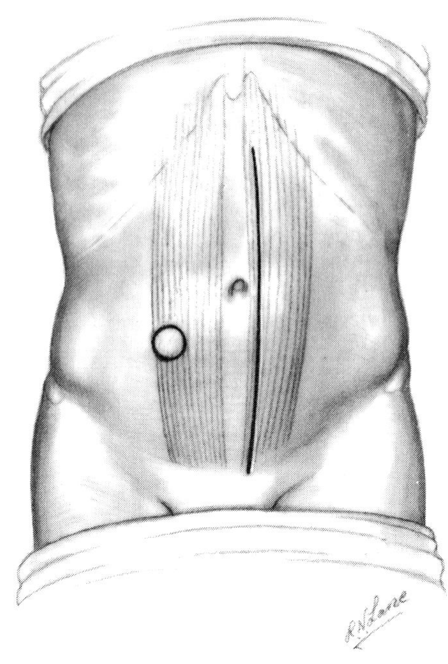

1

1

Position of patient and the incision

The patient is placed in the lithotomy-Trendelenburg position using the Lloyd-Davies stirrups as described in the Chapter on 'Abdominoperineal excision of the rectum II', p. 339. The abdomen is opened through a long left paramedian incision and the site of the ileostomy is shown. The colon is removed as described in the chapter on 'Panproctocolectomy and ileostomy', pp. 470–482 in this volume.

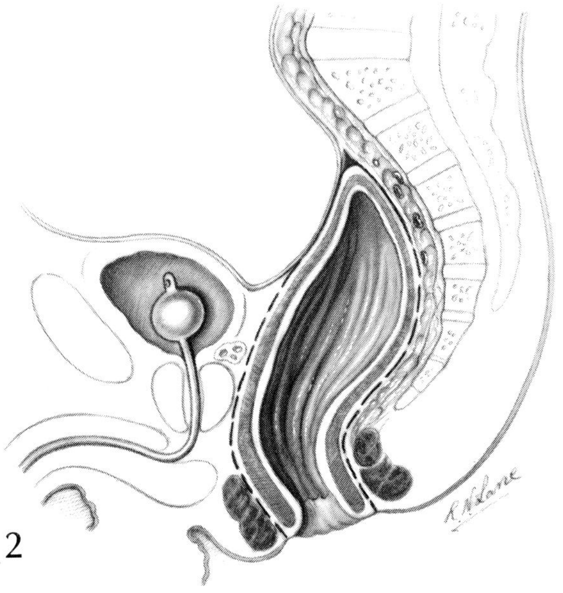

2

2

Extent of rectal excision

This diagram shows the extent of the rectal excision. The perineal operator commences the excision in the intersphincteric plane, leaving the external sphincter and the levator muscles intact. The abdominal operator should preserve the superior mesenteric vessels and as much of the presacral fat as possible. The dissection is at all times close to the rectal wall. A solution of 1:300000 adrenaline in saline may be injected into the intersphincteric plane to facilitate the dissection.

3

Abdominal excision

After the proximal colon has been mobilized the abdominal surgeon commences the excision of the rectum. Incisions are made in the pelvic peritoneum close to each side of the rectum and joined anteriorly at the lowest point of the rectovesical pouch. The sigmoid colon is mobilized, the sigmoid arteries and veins being individually ligated close to the colonic wall. The posterior dissection extends downwards behind the rectum which is mobilized from the underlying mesentery by ligating the vessels as they pass into the rectal wall. The vesicles are dissected and held forwards with a St Mark's lipped retractor. The fascia of Denonvilliers is divided and the dissection is carried down to the apex of the prostate. The lateral ligaments are divided close to the rectal wall. At this stage the operation by the perineal dissector will be complete and the specimen can be removed from the perineal wound. The pelvic peritoneal floor is usually closed by continuous 2/0 catgut without tension and the abdomen is then closed without drainage.

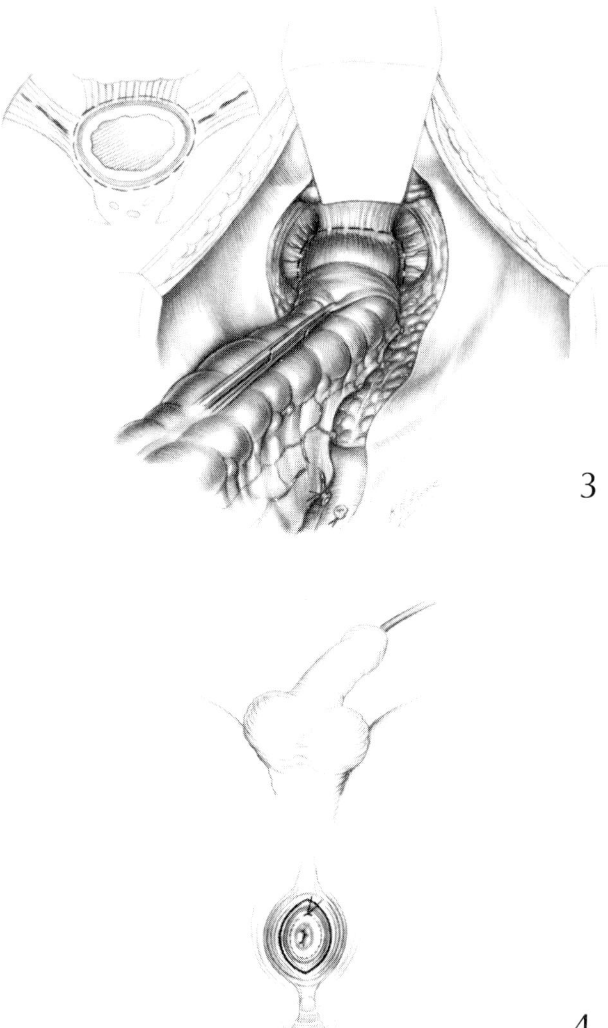

3

4

4

Perineal dissection

The anus is closed with a strong purse-string suture close to the anal margin. A circumferential incision is made over the intersphincteric groove.

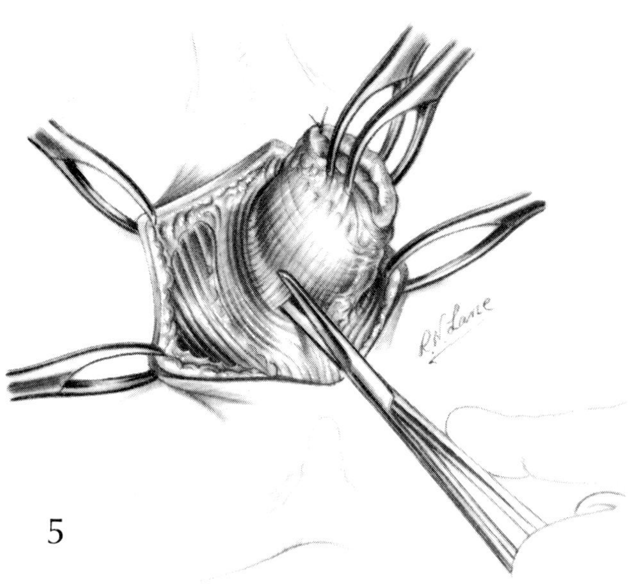

5

5

The intersphincteric plane

The pale fibres of the internal sphincter muscle are identified on each side of the anus and the intersphincteric plane developed by blunt and sharp dissection. The longitudinal fibres passing through to the internal sphincter need to be divided. The plane can thus easily be developed with blunt dissection into the pelvis. Following mobilization of each lateral quadrant the posterior aspect is dissected out.

6

Completion of the perineal dissection

Anteriorly the external sphincter decussates in the midline and becomes attached to the fibres of the recto-urethralis muscle. Part of the external sphincter is therefore cut in this plane to expose the posterior aspect of the prostate. Because the wound is small it may be impossible to insert a Travers self-retaining retractor. If so, the assistant should use a Langenbeck, Landon or Lockhart-Mummery retractor. Visibility may be difficult and good retraction and careful haemostasis are necessary.

The perineal part of the operation is then completed by dividing the visceral pelvic fascia laterally on each side, and anteriorly where it is condenses on to the lateral lobes of the prostate. The vesicles are seen and the lower part of the lateral ligaments divided close to the rectum. At this stage the abdominal and perineal operators will have completed the excision and the whole specimen can be drawn downwards through the perineal wound. In the female, the dissection is carried out in a similar way in the intersphincteric plane, the vagina being left intact anteriorly.

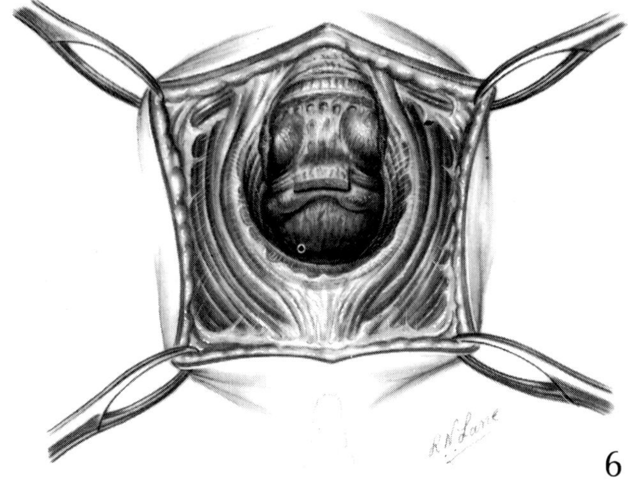

6

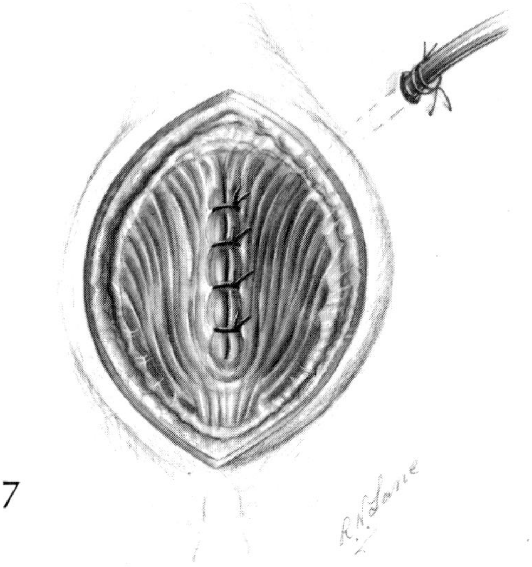

7

7

Wound closure

One or two suction catheters of the Shirley sump type are inserted through a lateral stab wound and placed above the levator muscles. The puborectalis and levators are then approximated loosely with interrupted catgut sutures. The skin is closed with interrupted mattress sutures of Dexon or Vicryl. Continuous suction drainage is started immediately by connecting the catheter to a vacuum pump. The wound is sealed with Whitehead's varnish and gauze dressings which are left undisturbed until the sutures are removed. When the perineal wound is closed in this way a broad-spectrum antibiotic is administered intravenously at operation and for 5 days afterwards. The small pelvic wound heals rapidly. Continuous suction drainage is maintained until drainage ceases and then the catheter is removed. The sutures are kept in place for 10 days.

Complications

The complications of excision of the rectum as part of the proctocolectomy are similar to those described in the chapter on 'Abdominoperineal excision of the rectum, p. 569 in this volume.

Elective operation for sigmoid diverticular disease

Mark Killingback FRCS, FRCS(Ed.), FRACS
Surgeon, Edward Wilson Colon and Rectum Unit, Sydney Hospital, Sydney

Introduction

Patients may have significant clinical problems attributable to diverticular disease caused by functional colon muscle abnormalities without local inflammation of the colon being present[1]. This concept has led to a better understanding of the indications for surgical treatment. Furthermore there may be a discrepancy between the clinical and radiological assessments in these patients – a barium enema may underestimate or exaggerate the apparent significance of the diverticular disease.

In recent years there has been a better appreciation of the response of symptoms to dietary manipulation – the effect of increasing food residue with unprocessed bran has greatly reduced the number of patients requiring surgery for 'failed medical treatment'.

Caution must be exercised in attributing abdominal and bowel symptoms to diverticular disease, particularly in those patients whose principal complaint is chronic abdominal pain. The irritable bowel syndrome may be indistinguishable from the symptoms of non-inflammatory functional chronic diverticular disease. The author does not believe that there is any pathological relationship between these two conditions.

Prophylactic resection of sigmoid diverticular disease is not justified in the early stage of the disease to prevent complications such as perforation and fistula formation. Their development is largely unpredictable and is often the first manifestation of the disease.

If, however, symptoms have become refractory to treatment, surgery is indicated because repeated attacks of inflammation cause progressive pericolic and mesenteric fibrosis and may lead to technically difficult surgery.

Most elective resections are performed for complicated disease such as chronic phlegmonous diverticulitis, chronic pericolic or pelvic abscess and fistulae. Some of these patients will present for a second-stage elective procedure after a previous laparotomy for acute diverticulitis, drainage of an abscess or frank peritonitis.

Preoperative

Indications

Persistent symptoms despite conservative management with a high-residue diet and unprocessed bran may warrant elective surgery. In this group, patients with irritable bowel syndrome should be diagnosed and excluded.

Repeated attacks of acute diverticulitis of significance with evidence of peritoneal irritation, fever and systemic effects. Such attacks usually settle with antibiotic therapy in a few days but often leave a focus for subsequent attacks. Two or three such episodes in a fit patient is a sufficient indication for elective surgery, but this advice may have to be modified in the elderly or unfit. The patient with recurrent acute attacks may be more likely to develop a serious complication.

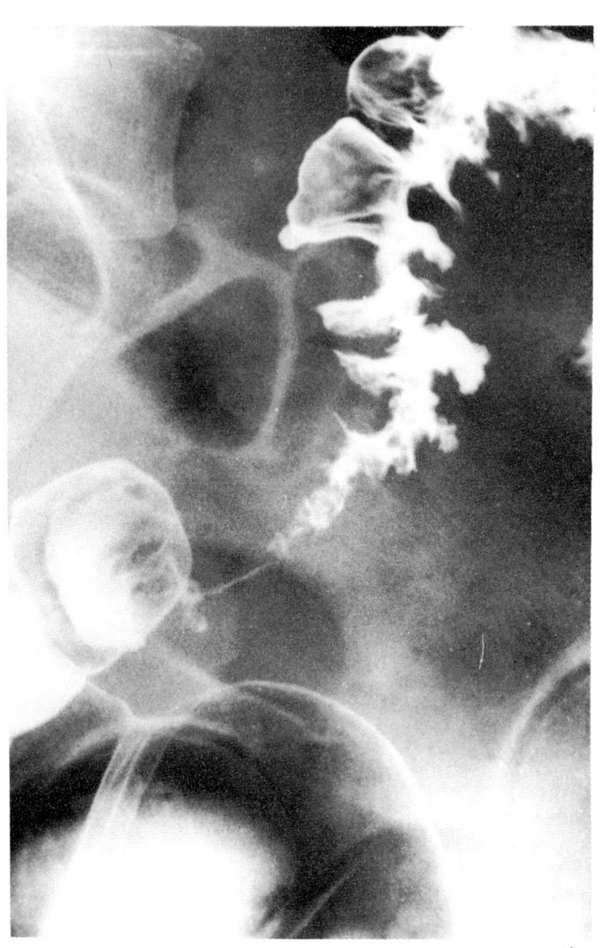

1a

1a & b

A persistent inflammatory mass for more than 4–6 weeks is an indication for resection in the fit patient. Invariably it will be associated with a stricture on X-ray (*a*) and this in turn will raise the possibility that a carcinoma is present. Although the inflammatory stricture usually shows mucosal continuity (*b*), indicating its benign nature, the X-ray can appear indistinguishable from a carcinoma.

Flexible sigmoidoscopy or colonoscopy can differentiate some of these lesions but not all because stenosis, fibrosis and angulation of the colon may impede the passage of an endoscope. In this situation there will be a combination of indications for surgery. Clinically it should be possible to distinguish the oedematous inflammatory mass by rectal examination from the thickened sigmoid colon with palpable diverticula which may be felt lying in the pelvis.

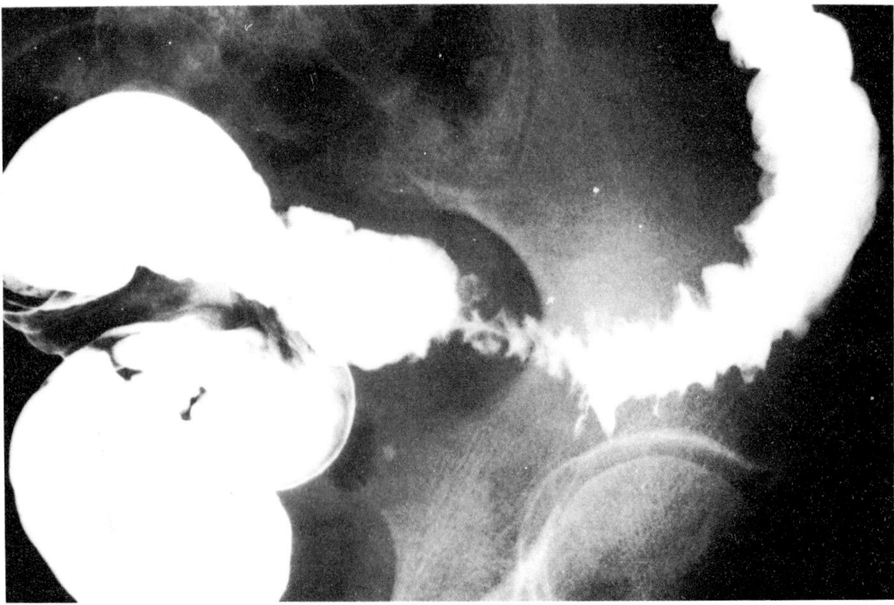

1b

2

A barium enema may show *extravasation beyond the wall of the colon* indicating localized perforation. There may or may not be an associated stricture and it is likely that there is an associated inflammatory mass. Whilst this situation may be tolerated in the unfit patient without symptoms, the colon is best resected.

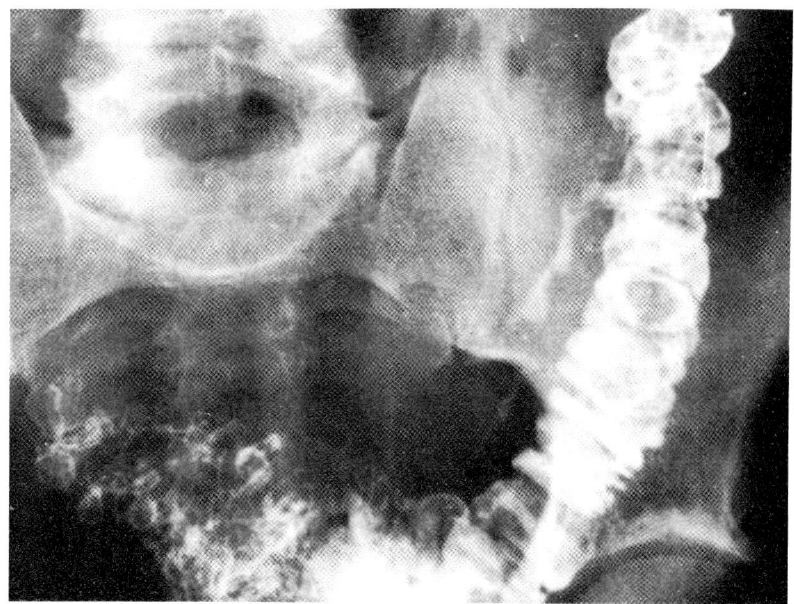

2

Colovesical and colocutaneous fistulae are common and may complicate sigmoid diverticulitis. Less common fistulae are colovaginal, coloenteric and colofallopian, but diverticular disease can form a fistula into any organ and many bizarre fistulae have been described. Such fistulae are usually an absolute indication for resection of the sigmoid disease but in some elderly patients in whom the fistula is not associated with an active, perisigmoid abscess (which can be almost completely quiescent) the risk for the patient of surgery may be greater than that of conservative treatment.

A resection is usually indicated as a secondary procedure *if emergency surgery of acute diverticulitis with peritonitis has previously been carried out*. Such patients may have an associated fistula and a proximal stoma may be present. Patients in whom a Hartmann operation was performed as an emergency will need careful assessment to see if a further resection of proximal and/or distal residual disease is needed before an anastomosis is carried out.

Rarely interval elective surgery is indicated between persistent episodes of profuse colonic bleeding. Whilst most bleeding of this type is due to vascular dysplasia (most often from the right colon), bleeding from diverticula has been demonstrated by angiography and histology. If angiography has demonstrated the bleeding site, then a segmental resection can be performed. If the episodes of bleeding recur significantly without localization, then colectomy and ileorectal anastomosis should be considered as an elective treatment.

Preoperative preparation

The preparation for the patient with diverticular disease is the same as for any major colorectal operation and will include a full blood count, blood biochemistry, chest X-ray and ECG. An intravenous pyelogram is a preferred investigation before sigmoid resection for uncomplicated disease but is essential if complicated diverticulitis is present. It may reveal incidental urinary tract abnormality such as ureteric duplication, deviation of the ureter, non-functioning of one kidney or obstruction of the ureter by the inflammatory disease in the pelvis.

Bowel preparation is carried out over a 48 h period: the patient is given clear fluids and two separate doses of magnesium sulphate (30 ml) are administered each day. A 1.5 litre saline enema is administered on each of the two preoperative days. A 48 h oral antibiotic preparation with metronidazole (400 mg 4 hourly) and kanamycin (four doses of 1000 mg given hourly then 1000 mg, 4 hourly) has been satisfactory. More recently two doses 6 h apart of metronidazole (500 mg intravenously) and kanamycin (1000 mg intravenously) have been used and are associated with a lower incidence of postoperative sepsis.

Ureteric catheterization

In patients in whom a large pelvic inflammatory mass is evident on rectal examination, considerable extraperitoneal pelvic fibrosis is likely. In such patients the introduction of ureteric catheters before operation is most helpful.

The operation

Position of patient

The Lloyd-Davies position (modified lithotomy-Trendelenburg position) with the Lloyd-Davies stirrups is preferred. This allows better retraction by the second assistant standing between the patient's legs, vaginal examination which may assist in a difficult anterior dissection (particularly after a hysterectomy) and is necessary for the use of the intraluminal stapling instrument which is the author's preferred method of anastomosis.

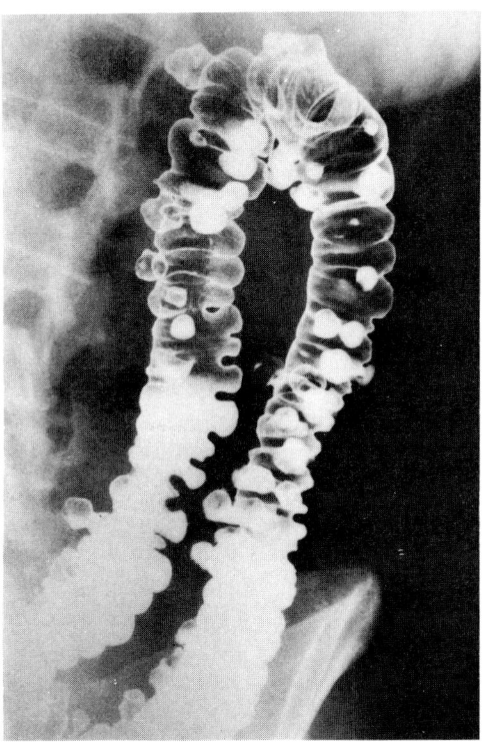

3

Incision and laparotomy

A midline incision is made from the pubis to as far above the umbilicus as necessary to gain wide exposure. A thorough laparotomy is performed to assess the diverticular disease, its complications and any other intra-abdominal pathology

In assessing the diverticular disease the possibility that a carcinoma may coexist must be considered. If there is doubt about such a diagnosis, the problem is usually diverticular disease. Any attachment of the diverticular disease to adjacent organs should be noted. The extent of the diverticula along the colon proximally must be assessed as well as any abnormal muscular thickening. A similar examination of the rectosigmoid and upper rectum is important to assess possible inflammatory disease and associated muscle changes with diverticula.

3

In deciding the proximal extent of resection several aspects are important. Obviously, active chronic infection in the colon and mesentery must be included. Muscle-thickening, which may be proximal to the sigmoid colon, is best removed, and it is preferable to remove colon which contains many diverticula. In the fit patient it is reasonable to include the descending colon and distal transverse colon in order to remove diverticulosis. More proximal excision of the colon requiring division of the middle colic vessels is not recommended.

In older patients, a compromise is reasonable and residual diverticula in the proximal colon are preferable to extending the scope of surgery.

4 & 5

The distal level of excision is also determined by the site of inflammation in the wall and mesentery of the bowel. It is important to remove distal diverticula which may be obscured in the pericolic and perirectal fat just above or below the rectosigmoid junction. Careful examination of the barium enema may also help to localize the distal limit of diverticula formation. The longitudinal muscle coat is usually thickened in the rectosigmoid region and sometimes in the upper rectum and it is preferable to remove this abnormality also. Therefore, the distal level of resection is usually below the promontory of the sacrum and frequently through the upper third of the rectum.

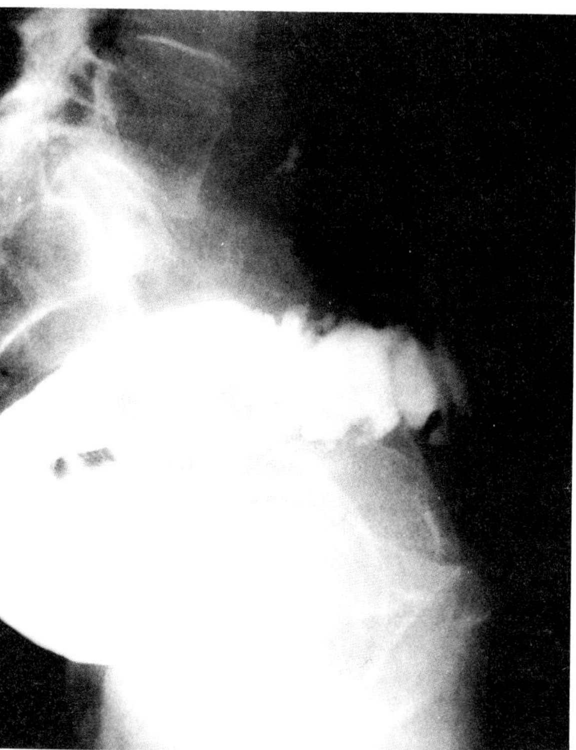

4

The diverticular disease has not involved the rectosigmoid junction or upper rectum

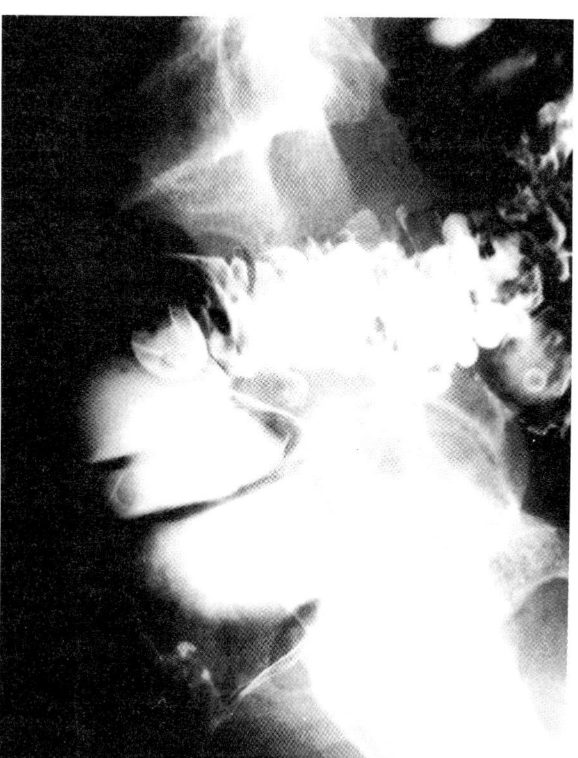

5

The X-ray shows marked disease in the upper third of the rectum

6

It may be necessary to extend the distal line of excision in complicated diverticular disease even further when it is associated with a chronic pelvic abscess causing secondary inflammatory changes in the upper third of the rectum and pelvic peritoneum. Even though the primary focus may be in the sigmoid colon, it is safer to dissect below the pelvic peritoneum and obtain healthy bowel at the midrectal level which will necessitate a low extraperitoneal anastomosis.

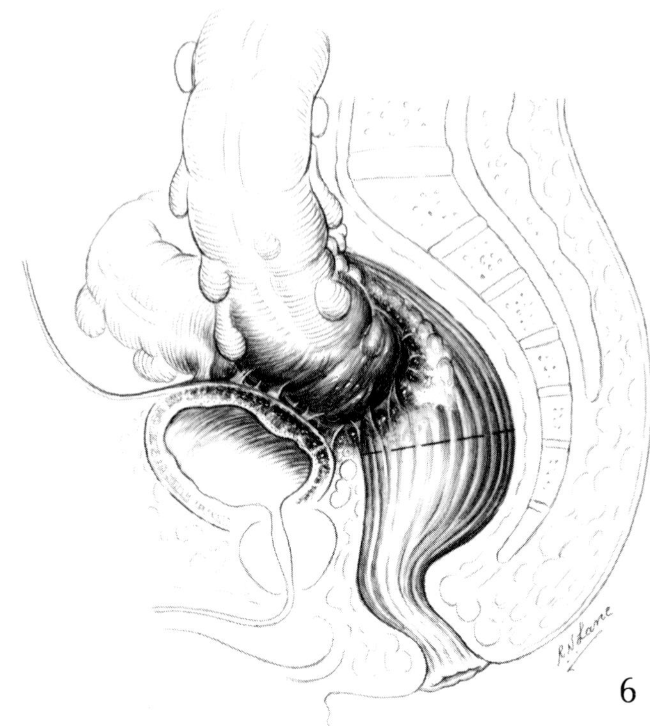

6

Mobilization of the sigmoid and descending colon

1. After placement of a plastic ring wound protector in the abdominal wound, incision of the parasigmoid peritoneum along the line of mesenteric and parietal fusion will expose the gonadal vessels and lower part of the ureter.
2. Careful identification of the mesenteric layer of the left colon will ensure the correct anatomical plane.
3. Gentle hand dissection medially and upwards is needed to push the colon mesentery forwards with the right hand and the gonadal vessels, ureter and perinephric fat posteriorly with the left hand. The left hand gently dissects in this plane until a level above the left kidney is reached and at this point the fingertips are close to the lower border of the pancreas and the lower pole of the spleen.
4. Lateral spreading of the dissection with the left hand will define a thin layer of paracolic peritoneum and fascia almost to the splenic flexure.
5. More digital and hand dissection medially to the aorta will reveal the ureter from the lower pole of the kidney to the iliac vessels.
6. Incision of the paracolic peritoneum is performed to the splenic flexure.

Cancer or diverticulitis? – extent of local excision

Despite preoperative investigations and careful intraoperative assessment, real doubt may exist that cancer is present. Therefore, it is important that an adequate 'cancer' operation be performed at this stage with reference to the local disease. Adjacent small bowel, uterus, ovary and fallopian tube may need excision *en bloc* with the specimen. If attachment to the bladder has occurred, then a segment of bladder wall should be excised in continuity. Should the attachment to the bladder wall be more posterior and deeper in the pelvis than the usual attachment to the vault, dissection can be facilitated by instilling saline into the bladder to lift the attached sigmoid from the pelvis as the bladder distends.

Diverticulitis – difficulties of local excision

The apex of the sigmoid colon is frequently fixed into the pelvis by adhesion to a deep, chronic pelvic abscess and until this is mobilized adequate dissection of the sigmoid colon is not possible. Frequently this pelvic dissection can be achieved by careful, 'pinching off' manoeuvres. In other instances, however, sharp scalpel dissection (too tough for scissors) is required to cut through the very hard fibrosis that may join the sigmoid colon to the parietal peritoneum or other pelvic structures. It is in this circumstance that ureteric catheters which can be palpated (and visualized if divided!) are most helpful.

7

Splenic flexure mobilization

1. Preliminary clipping and division of small splenic-omental adhesions should prevent trauma to the splenic capsule.
2. Separation of the splenic flexure and spleen by sharp dissection and paring movements with the finger to the fascial and peritoneal attachments close to the spleen.
3. Division of the fascia between the colon and mesentery in the 'splenic corner' and the perinephric fascia posteriorly.
4. Separation of the greater omentum from the upper border of the transverse colon (often to the midpoint of the transverse colon).
5. Identification of the left limit of the lesser sac which is opened if this has not already been done.
6. Division of the posterior wall of the lesser sac just beneath the body and tail of the pancreas until medially the inferior mesenteric vein is reached.

The need for splenic flexure mobilization will vary according to the selection of the optimal site for distal as well as proximal bowel section. It is also influenced by the use of staplers in surgery of diverticular disease (*see below*).

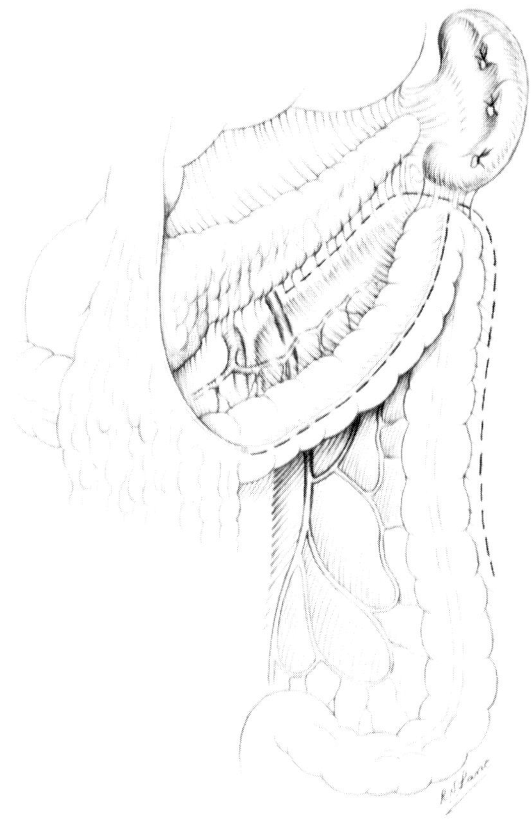

7

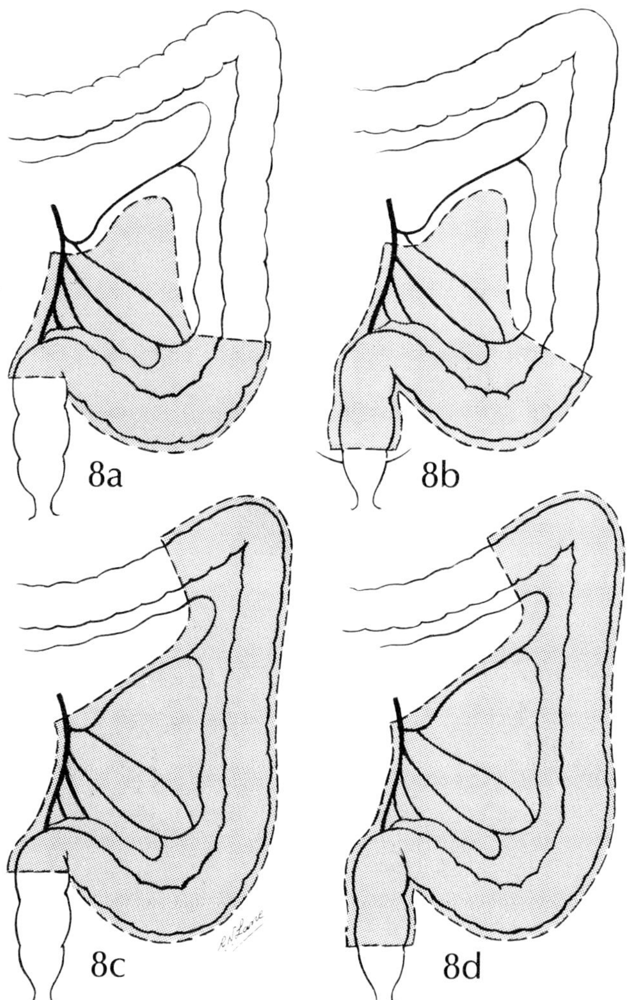

8a–d

Proximal vascular ligation

The vascular ligation pattern will also depend on the amount of bowel removed. The vascular ligation is performed in a 'radical' fashion as for carcinoma because this is a simpler technical approach than dividing multiple vessels in the mesentery close to the bowel wall. Dissection *immediately posterior* to the inferior mesenteric artery as it lies on the aorta (with the left colon drawn over to the right) will ensure that the preaortic sympathetic nerves are not damaged; this plane followed distally will keep the surgery close to the posterior limit of the mesorectum and again avoid damage to the presacral nerves and veins. This becomes more important in the lower resections which occasionally are necessary to the midrectum. The transverse 'take-off' of the left colic artery from the inferior mesenteric artery is identified and seen to join with the inferior mesenteric vein as it passes upwards. As the usual proximal level of resection will be at the sigmoid–descending colonic junction, the descending marginal artery and vein must be carefully preserved (*a* and *b*).

The left colic artery is preserved unless an extended proximal resection is being performed to include the splenic flexure (*c* and *d*), when the inferior mesenteric artery and the inferior mesenteric vein will be divided.

Preparation of the colon

9

It is preferable to 'overshoot' on the mesentery level of resection (compared with the colon level of division) to ensure the marginal vessels and related vasa longa and vasa breva are preserved to the site of bowel wall for anastomosis. When the marginal vessel is divided the proximal end should be allowed to bleed to ensure that the arterial flow is pulsatile. Mere flow must be carefully checked to exclude passive 'backflow' which is unacceptable, requiring further resection to obtain better bleeding from the marginal vessel. Although one or two obtrusive appendices epiploicae may be excised (with preservation of the vasa within them if possible) clearing of pericolic fat is best avoided.

For sutured anastomosis 0.5 cm of 'naked' colon is all that is required. For a stapled anastomosis 1.5 cm of colon should be available distal to the pericolic fat for the application of the purse-string clamp and the formation of the staple 'doughnut'. If one or two small diverticula have been incidentally left on the bowel wall close to the site for anastomosis they can be inverted with a single suture. They can be ignored for a sutured anastomosis but could be a vulnerable area in a stapled anastomosis if left near the staple line. Nylon tape is tied around the bowel wall (without compression of the marginal vessels) 10 cm from the end of the proximal colon.

For sutured anastomosis the colon is transected proximal to a bowel clamp which leaves 0.5 cm of colon wall clear of pericolic fat for sutures.

10

For stapled anastomosis the purse-string clamp is placed across the bowel wall leaving 1.0 cm of colon between the clamp and the pericolic fat. A 0 Prolene suture on a straight round-bodied needle is passed through the clamp to insert the purse-string. This clamp is removed after division of the colon is performed 0.2 cm distal to the clamp.

11

Proximal colon irrigation

Babcock forceps are used to suspend the colon which is then irrigated meticulously with water to clear away all the faecal debris.

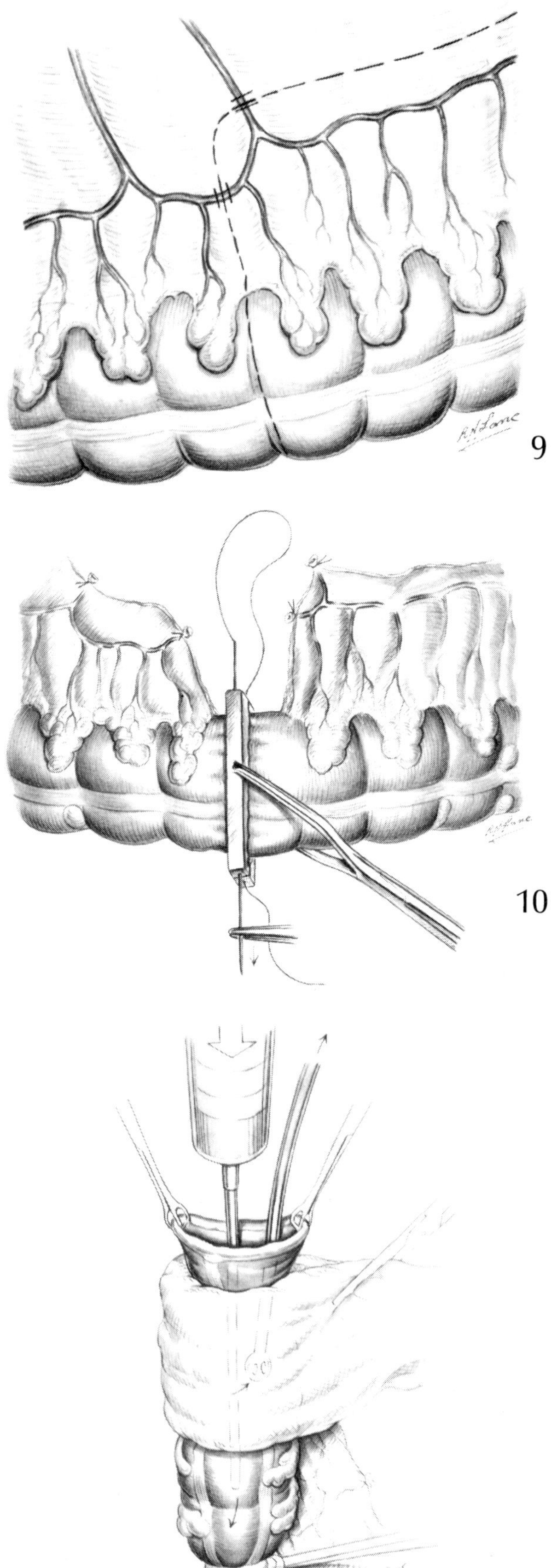

9

10

11

Stay sutures for control of the colon stump

For sutured anastomosis two 3/0 silk stay sutures are inserted (mesenteric and antimesenteric).

12

For stapled anastomosis four 3/0 silk stay sutures are inserted and tied as illustrated. Each of the antimesenteric stay sutures should be placed to lock the taeniae with the purse-string to prevent eversion during the final apposition of the bowel ends. A locking suture should be inserted around the mesenteric taenia which especially tends to retract and escape the purse-string. Any 'jumps' in the purse-string suture can be similarly locked in place by individual 3/0 silk sutures.

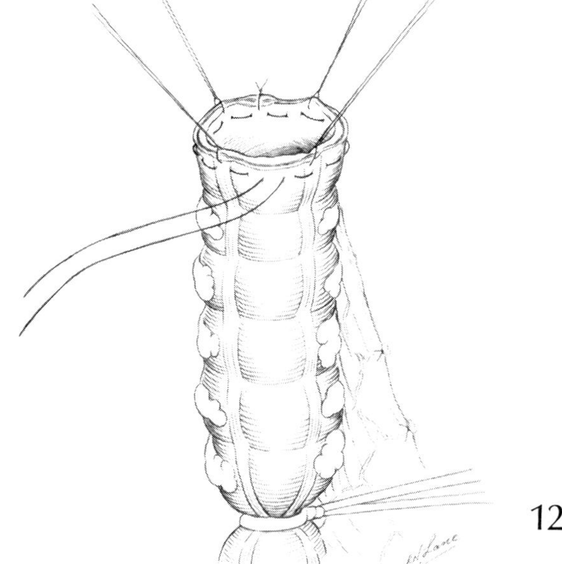

12

Preparation of distal rectal stump

Usually the distal line of resection will pass through the upper third of the rectum and it will not be necessary to dissect fully the presacral space, incise pelvic peritoneum, divide lateral ligaments of the rectum or separate rectum from anterior pelvic structures. The necessity for a low extraperitoneal anastomosis under certain circumstances has been referred to but this technique will not be described in detail. In the upper third of the rectum the mesentery is predominantly posterior. The anterior peritoneum is divided transversely at the selected level and with the left index finger and thumb defining the bowel wall by palpation artery forceps are used to dissect and clamp the mesorectum. As this posterolateral clearing of the rectum occurs the released rectal wall stretches to reveal at least 2 cm of cleared rectal wall suitable for anastomosis. It is not necessary to ligate and clear the small vessels which penetrate the rectum from the mesorectal fat.

For a sutured anastomosis a Hayes angled rectal clamp is applied from right to left transversely across the bowel wall immediately below the proximal divided mesorectum.

For a stapled anastomosis the Hayes clamp is applied more proximally to leave more space for the purse string clamp to be applied to the 'bare area' of the rectal wall.

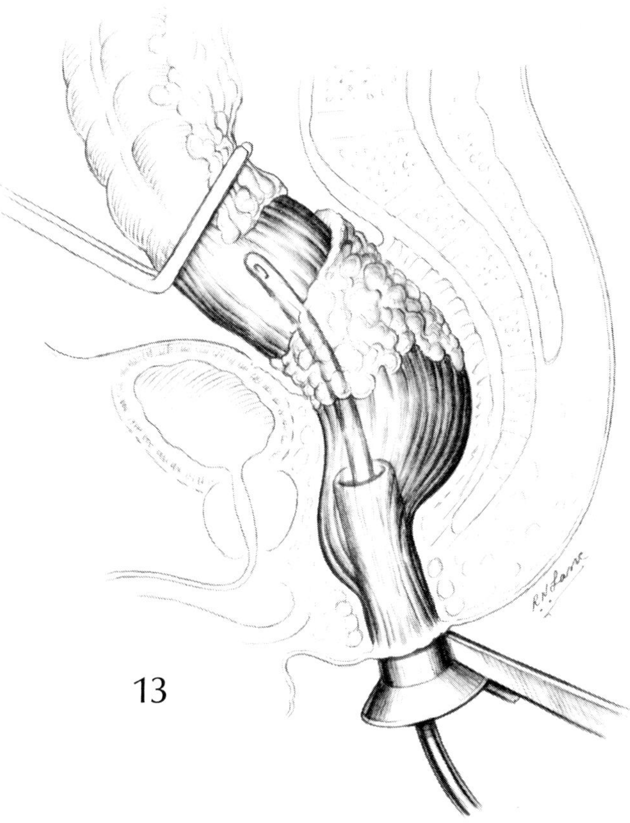

13

13

Irrigation of the rectum

The rectal stump is now thoroughly irrigated via a rectal catheter through a proctoscope *per anum* using water delivered by a hand pump. Again meticulous cleansing and drying is required, particularly for the stapled anastomosis technique or faecal debris will be pushed into the pelvis by the advancing anvil.

14

For a stapled anastomosis the purse-string clamp is applied transversely immediately below the proximal divided mesorectum. A 0 Prolene suture is passed on a straight needle from and returning to the left side. The rectum is divided 0.2 cm above the clamp and the resected specimen is removed. The purse-string clamp is removed and the purse-string suture inspected for faults. Four stay sutures (3/0 silk) are used to control the rectal stump and any 'jumps' in the purse-string locked with individual 3/0 silk sutures.

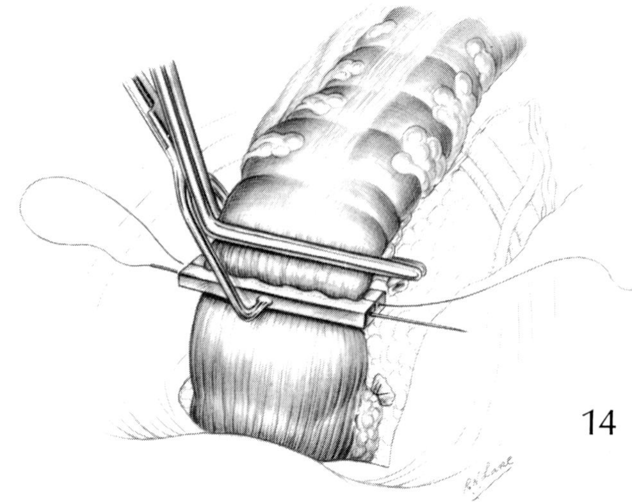

14

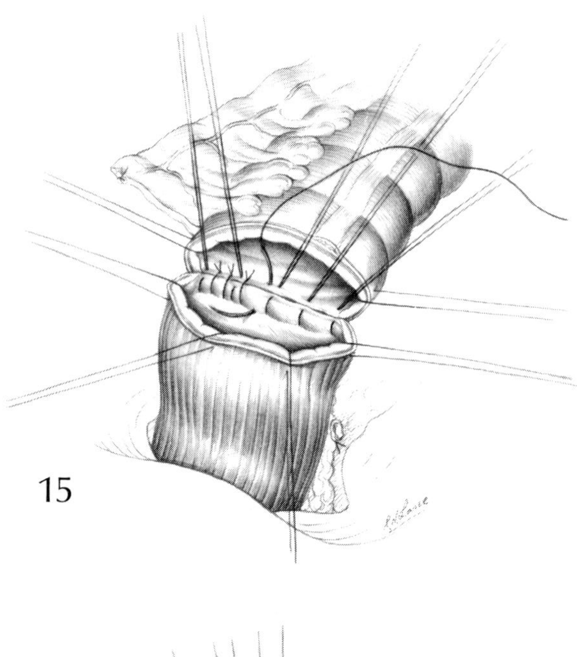

15

15 & 16

The sutured anastomosis

For a sutured anastomosis the bowel is divided immediately below the Hayes clamp and four 3/0 silk sutures placed to control and suspend the rectal stump. An open anastomosis is performed with a single layer of inverting 3/0 absorbable sutures of polyglycolic acid (Dexon) or polyglactin 910 (Vicryl). Five vertical mattress sutures are placed with the bowel ends separated. The posterior wall of the colon is then approximated to the posterior wall of the rectum and the five sutures tied and left long for traction. This suspension of the posterior wall of the bowel ends by traction creates a ridge of the apposed colon and rectal muscle and facilitates the placement of one or two sutures between the mattress sutures to complete the posterior layer. The anterior layer is completed with interrupted/inverting mattress sutures (two loops on the mucosa) also known as the Gambee suture. At least 0.4 cm of bowel wall is included in the sutures placed 0.3–0.4 cm apart. The anterior layer is not tied until all the sutures have been placed in the colon and rectum. The tension on all anastomotic sutures must only be sufficient for comfortable, firm apposition without compression of the bowel wall which might induce local ischaemia.

If the descending colon is being suture-anastomosed to the mid or low rectum then a Cheatle slit on the antimesenteric aspect may be helpful to enlarge the colon.

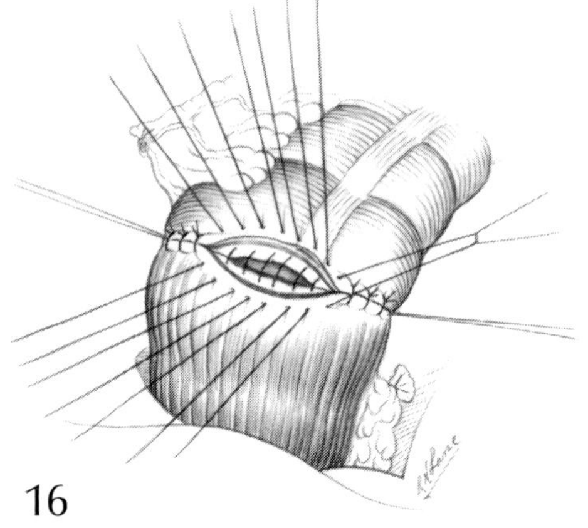

16

The stapled anastomosis

1. After checking the stapling instrument the anvil is lubricated.
2. The anal operator (AO) examines the anal sphincter and gently dilates it if there is any anal stenosis.

17 & 18

3. The pelvic operator (PO) aspirates the rectal stump to remove residual irrigating fluid or mucus and places the right index finger into the rectal stump to guide the AO advancing the stapler.
4. As the anvil appears the advance ceases and the anvil is separated fully from the staple cartridge by the AO.
5. The PO ties the distal rectal purse-string around the central rod.
6. The proximal colon, if in spasm, can be gently dilated by an index finger immediately before placement of the colon over the anvil by the PO and the assistant using the four stay sutures, slipping the colon first over the posterior lip of the anvil.
7. The proximal colon purse-string is tied, cut and the colon drawn back over the anvil until only the optimal slack is taken up to avoid excess tissue in the proximal 'doughnut'.

8. The cartridge and anvil are approximated by the AO while the PO ensures that no pelvic structures or appendices epiploicae are drawn into the staple approximation.
9. As the tissues 'snug together' the final approximation should be in stages (AO) to compress gently the bowel wall for stapling and avoid fragmentation of thickened muscle which is occasionally present after resection of diverticular disease.
10. After 'firing' of the stapling instrument, separation of the cartridge and the anvil is performed (1.0 cm) and 360° rotation is carried out twice to check that the staple line is free (AO).
11. By tilting and rotating, the stapler is withdrawn (AO) while the rectal stump is supported (PO).
12. The 'doughnuts' are carefully checked (AO).
13. If the anastomosis can be checked visually (PO), which it usually can be at this level of resection, then the peranal injection of Betadine (povidone-iodine) into the rectum is not used to test for staple line leak.
14. Bleeding from the anastomosis on the serosal aspect invariably ceases spontaneously.

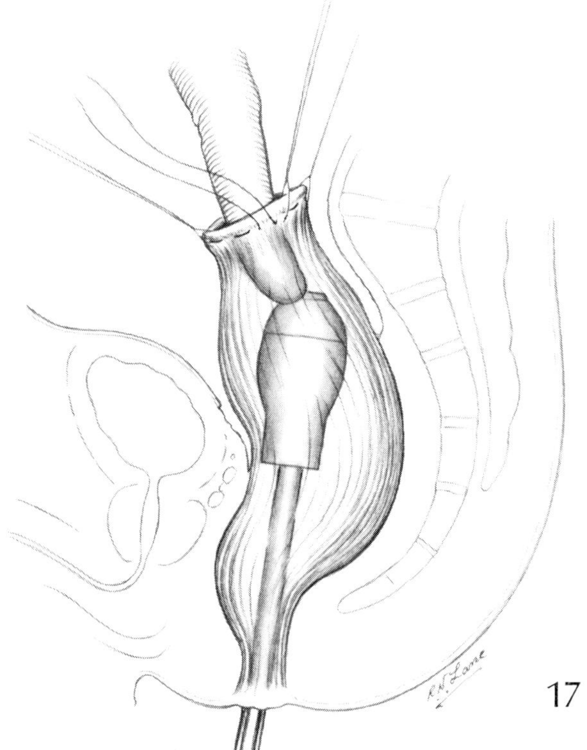

17

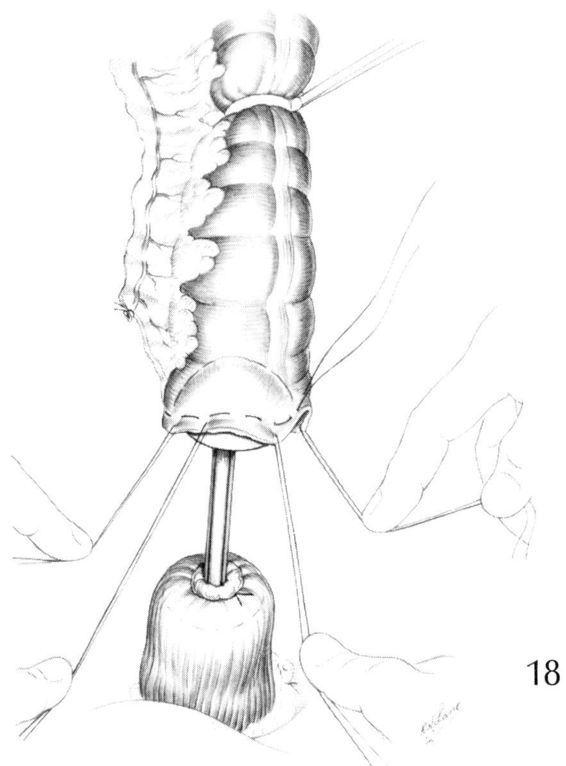

18

Contraindications to the use of the stapling instrument in diverticular disease

1. If the surgeon chooses to perform a conservative resection then residual muscle thickening in the recto-sigmoid and the descending colon proximally may cause difficulty as this muscle tends to fragment and can be thicker than optimal for the size of the staples.
2. The colon which has been defunctioned prior to resection will be contracted and may not dilate without damage to the bowel wall. The bowel muscle wall is thickened also in these circumstances.

On completion of the anastomosis pelvic haemostasis is achieved by thorough 'spot' diathermy. The pelvis is generously irrigated by warm saline. The proximal colon tape is removed. The splenic flexure region is checked for haemostasis.

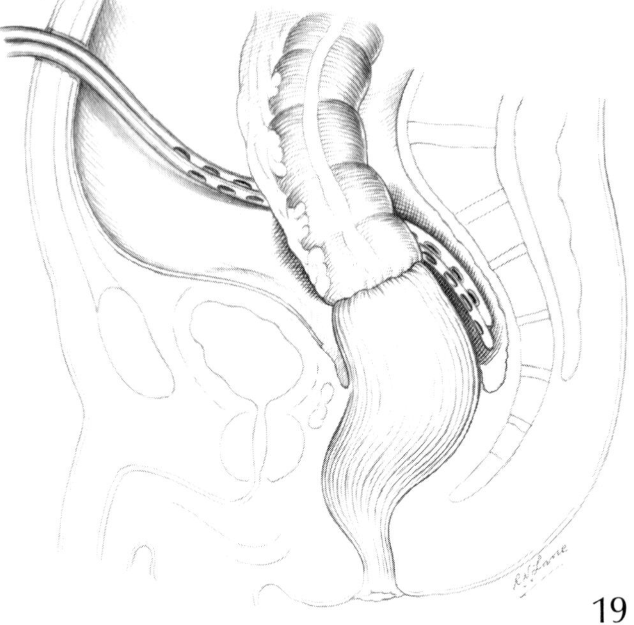

19

Drains

Anastomostic drains are not recommended but if the presacral space is fully dissected then two Shirley drains are placed in this area for suction and irrigation drainage for 24h. This drainage may also be used if haemostasis in the pelvis is difficult to achieve.

19 & 20

If after resection the wall of a chronic pelvis abscess remains (the inflammatory 'nest' referred to by Turnbull[2]) then prolonged pelvic drainage (PPD) helps to nullify delayed postoperative pelvis sepsis which could adversely affect the anastomosis. Two Shirley drains are placed in the pelvis and the following regimen is followed.

Prolonged pelvic drainage (PPD) with saline

Day	*Irrigation*	*Suction*
0–1	6 litres/24 h	−50 mmHg
2–12	1 litre/24 h	Suspend day 4–6
12	Remove drain Small catheter Sinogram*	Remove drain
13–18	Shorten daily	

* *See Illustration 20* showing minimal drain space achieved by day 12

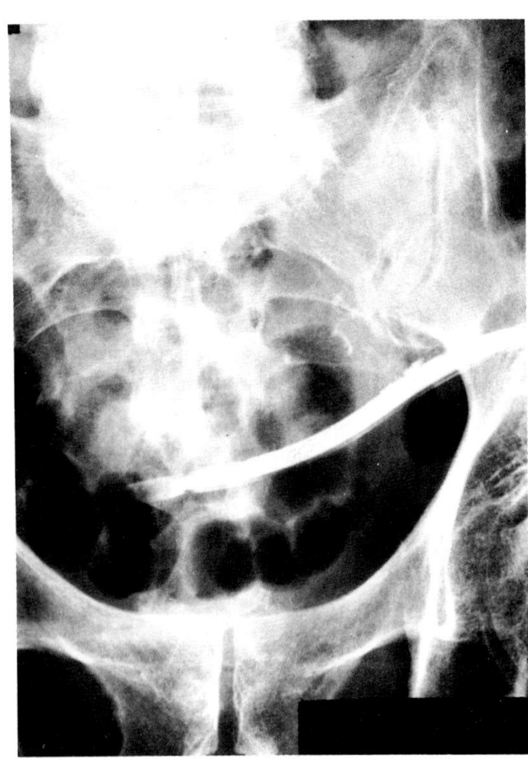

20

Colovesical fistula

The management of a colovesical fistula is principally that of the diseased colon with all its implications. The fistula in the bladder wall is usually not a difficult technical problem and may not be identifiable. The operation is usually performed in the chronic phase of diverticulitis and a preliminary colostomy followed by a second-stage resection is usually unnecessary. Blunt digital dissection will usually separate the colon from the bladder and if a small defect is noted in the vault of the bladder (usual site) it can be closed with a single layer of 2/0 chromic catgut. On rare occasions a larger defect in the bladder wall is present with fibrotic margins and in these circumstances excision of the defect in the wall of the bladder is preferable with a two-layer closure, the inner with continuous 2/0 plain catgut and an an outer layer of interrupted 0 chromic sutures. It is important to separate the bladder repair from the colorectal anastomosis, particularly in the presence of chronic residual pelvic granulation tissue which could suppurate subsequently. If omentum is available it can be placed between the intestinal anastomosis and the bladder. The use of the PPD technique previously described will prevent the sequence of sepsis-anastomotic defect and possible anastomotic-vesical fistula.

The indications for a complementary transverse colostomy are those referred to when resecting diverticulitis and are not specifically related to the problem of the colovesical fistula (*see below*).

The bladder is drained with a urethral catheter for 10 days, during which period urinary drainage is checked to ensure blockage of the catheter does not go undetected. It is in this circumstance that the use of the new smaller suprapubic catheters may be preferable to that of urethral catheter drainage. Whichever method is used the bladder should be drained for 10 days.

Indications for proximal stoma

Editors' comment: This is a controversial subject and there are considerable differences in the use of the so-called 'complementary transverse colostomy' (*see* chapter on 'Management of the obstructed bowel', pp.210–229 for further discussion).

Approximately one-third of patients undergoing resection will have an associated proximal stoma and these stomas will be evenly distributed between pre-existing stomas and complementary stomas performed at the time of resection. Although a loop ileostomy may be used, a right transverse loop colostomy initially over a plastic Marlin colostomy rod is preferred. Almost all patients whose resection is associated with a proximal stoma have suffered the more severe inflammatory complications with local abscess formation beyond the colon.

The indications which are not absolute and often present in combination are as follows.

1. Residual inflammatory changes in the rectal stump if it is not possible (rarely) to resect to a lower level and obtain healthy rectal wall.
2. Equivocal circulation in the colon stump (particularly) despite technical steps to ensure a good blood supply.
3. The presence of proximal colon obstruction with secondary changes of muscle hypertrophy or bowel dilatation.
4. Deficient bowel cleansing due to the stricture with a loaded colon remaining.
5. Trauma to the area of rectal anastomosis, such as muscle separation or fragmentation, submucosal or intramural haematomas. These problems may arise in fragile tissues in the elderly or result from a difficult and prolonged pelvic dissection.
6. A less than 'perfect' closure of the suture line in a sutured anastomosis or problems with staple technique that cannot be satisfactorily overcome with supporting sutures.
7. A prolonged operation with unusual blood loss in a patient whose general health is not optimum may benefit from a proximal colostomy.

Specific postoperative care

1. Intravenous therapy continues for 7 days.
2. Feeding is commenced with a soft diet on the seventh day but only if there is no abdominal distention, flatus has passed per rectum and there is no nausea or vomiting.
3. Nasogastric aspiration is not used as a routine but is promptly instituted if the patient has severe nausea, hiccoughs, vomits significant amounts of fluid or has a significantly distended abdomen.
4. The urinary catheter is kept on continuous drainage and is usually removed on the fourth day.
5. Proper stomal care is essential for these patients with a defunctioning colostomy or ileostomy. The plastic Marlin stoma rod is removed on the tenth day. Closure of the stoma is preferred at 8–10 weeks after resection to allow the patient full recovery. Modern stomal care has greatly facilitated the patient's comfort in the interval between the two stages of surgery.
6. A limited Gastrografin enema is routinely performed 12–14 days after operation to evaluate the anastomosis.
7. If a defect has ocurred in the anastomosis, demonstrated by extravasation of Gastrografin, the stoma is not closed until the defect is healed. Serial X-rays are performed to assess this problem at intervals depending upon the size of the defect in the anastomosis. Rarely patients may develop a small, stable para-anastomotic cavity and if the healing appears to be static it is usually safe to close a defunctioning stoma without waiting for final resolution.

References

1. Morson, B. C. The muscle abnormality in diverticular disease of the sigmoid colon. British Journal of Radiology 1963; 36: 385–392

2. Turnbull, R. B. Operations for sigmoid diverticulitis. In: Rob, C., Smith, R., eds. Operative surgery: abdomen and rectum and anus, Part II, 2nd ed. London: Butterworths, 1969: 681–688

Colectomy for malignant disease

Sir Hugh Lockhart-Mummery KCVO, MD, MChir, FRCS
Consulting Surgeon, St Thomas' Hospital and St Mark's Hospital, London;
Consultant Surgeon, King Edward VII Hospital for Officers, London

Preoperative

The patient's general condition and fitness for major surgery should be assessed, and the presence of conditions such as cardiovascular disease, bronchitis and diabetes determined by appropriate tests. Some degree of anaemia is common among patients with carcinoma of the colon, particularly those with right-sided growths. All such conditions should be corrected as far as possible before operation.

Preparation of bowel

This subject is dealt with in detail in the chapter on 'Sepsis prevention in colorectal surgery', pp. 21–23. The author's own practice at present in patients without severe obstruction is to give 30 ml of castor oil in the morning 3 days before surgery and a similar second dose the day before surgery. A low-residue diet is given from the start of the preparation and clear fluids only after the second dose of castor oil. No enemas or wash-out need be given.

The author does not at present use preoperative antibiotics as part of the bowel preparation but metronidazole 500 mg is given intravenously at the start of the operation, and the same dose is repeated at 8 hourly intervals for 24 or 48 h.

Blood transfusion

If the haemoglobin level is below 10 G the patient should receive a transfusion at least 48 h before operation; 1000 ml of blood should be available for transfusion during and after operation.

Unless indicated otherwise the cross-references in this chapter refer to *Operative Surgery: Alimentary Tract and Abdominal Wall, Volume 3, 4th Edition*

The operations

Position of patient and incision

For all growths below the splenic flexure it is an advantage to have the patient in the lithotomy-Trendelenburg position (see chapter on 'Abdominoperineal excision of the rectum', pp. 554–569 in this volume) as this allows access to the anus for wash-out of the distal bowel when indicated.

A long right or left paramedian incision is usually the best approach when dealing with colonic tumours. Wide access is always necessary.

Exploration

The tumour should be handled as little as possible. A thorough exploration of the whole abdomen must first be made to determine the resectability of the growth, the presence of metastases or of another neoplasm in the colon, and other associated disease. The condition of the colon proximal to the growth is important, for if the preoperative preparation has been ineffective and the bowel is loaded with faeces, it may be desirable to carry out a preliminary colostomy and perform the resection at a later date (*see* chapter on 'Management of the obstructed bowel', pp. 210–229). In discussing the operation of resection at different sites it will be assumed that the condition and preparation of the bowel are suitable for elective resection.

General principles of colonic surgery

After removal of that part of the bowel containing the growth with its related lymphatic field, the surgeon should aim to restore continuity by end-to-end anastomosis. In order to do this safely the two ends of bowel must have a good arterial supply and must come together without any tension. Therefore, the remaining colon must be mobilized sufficiently to achieve this result. Before carrying out the anastomosis, both of the ends to be joined should be mopped out and cleaned carefully with sterile distilled water or cancericidal solution – this manoeuvre will reduce considerably the risk of implantation recurrence at the suture line.

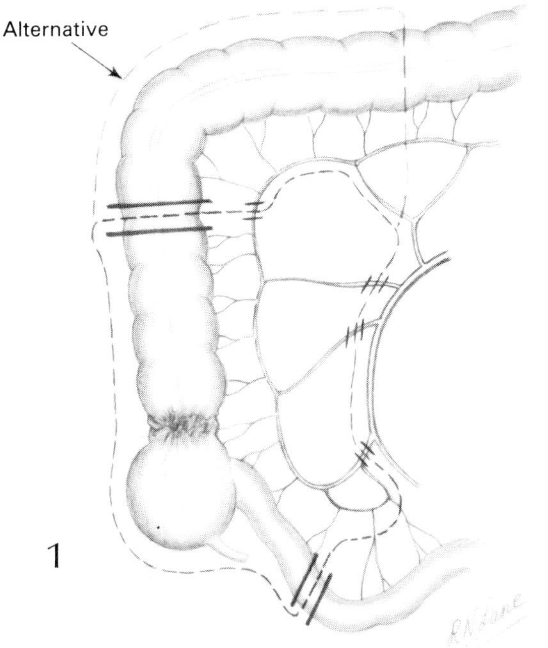

RIGHT HEMICOLECTOMY

1

Parts of ileum and colon removed

In dealing with all malignant growths of the colon it is more important to aim at wide removal of the related lymphatic field than at wide clearance of the bowel itself. Probably 7–10 cm clearance of the bowel suffices and unnecessary removal of terminal ileum and right colon should be avoided. For growths of the caecum, adequate lymphatic removal will usually still allow preservation of the hepatic flexure with plentiful blood supply from the middle colic artery; growths of the ascending colon may need a wider removal of the right colon with ligation of the right branch of the middle colic vessels. There is however considerable individual variation in the 'normal' arrangement of the arterial supply to the colon.

2

Mobilization of growth (I)

It is usually easier to carry out a right hemicolectomy from the opposite side of the patient, i.e. the patient's left side. The operation is best started by entering the lesser sac between the gastroepiploic vessels along the greater curve of the stomach and the omentum attached to the right transverse colon. Small vessels will need ligating and the dissection is continued round the hepatic flexure and down the right paracolic gutter; here there are usually only small vessels which can be touched with the diathermy apparatus.

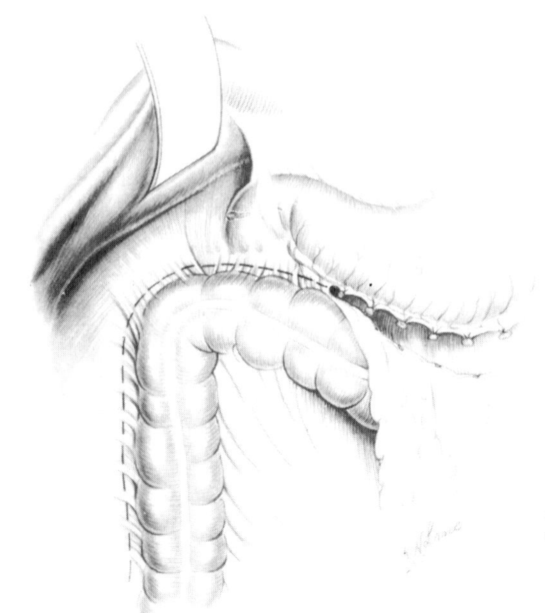

2

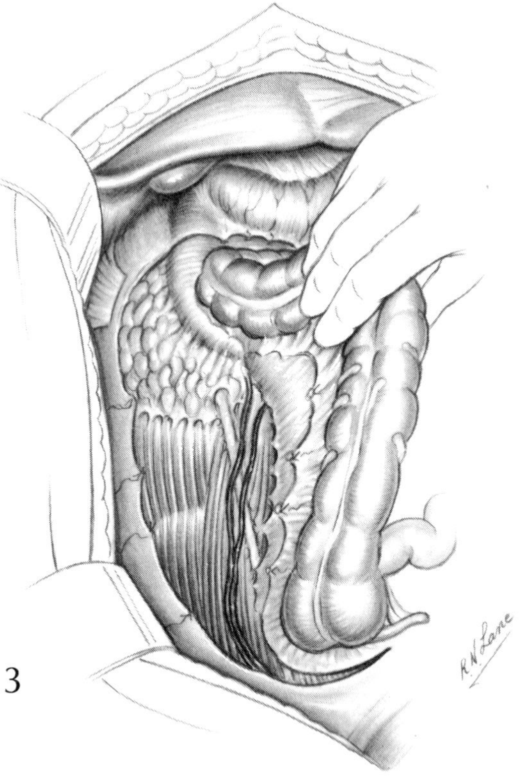

3

3

Mobilization of growth (II)

The colon containing the growth is mobilized medially, exposing the perinephric fat, the right ureter, the second part of the duodenum and the right testicular or ovarian vessels. The last 10 cm of terminal ileum are also freed by division of the posterior peritoneum, so that the whole of the right colon and mesocolon is mobilized.

4

Division of mesentery

After full mobilization, the surgeon should now decide on the exact extent of removal to be carried out. Light forceps of Babcock type are placed on the colon and small bowel at the points of the planned division. With good transillumination the mesentery of the right colon and terminal ileum are divided and the main vessels carefully ligated near the superior mesenteric artery and vein. Near the bowel fine forceps are used to pick up the small vessels and the dissection is taken right up to the bowel at the points previously marked. Clamps are applied across the bowel, slightly obliquely so as to ensure good blood supply on the antimesenteric side. The bowel is then divided and the specimen removed.

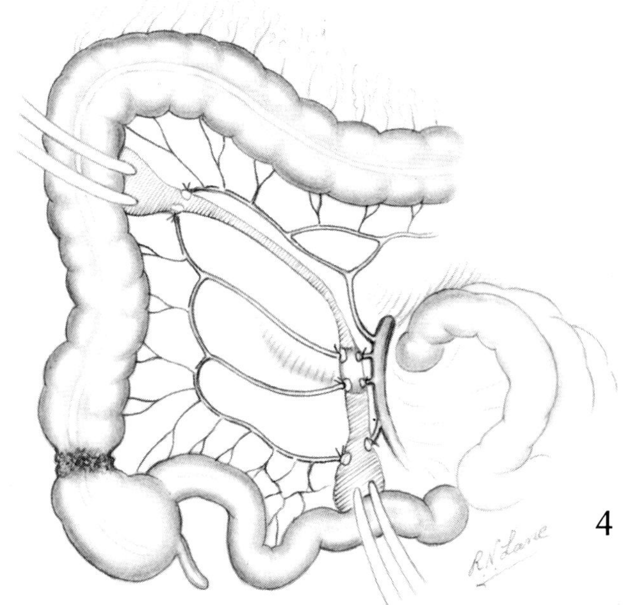

4

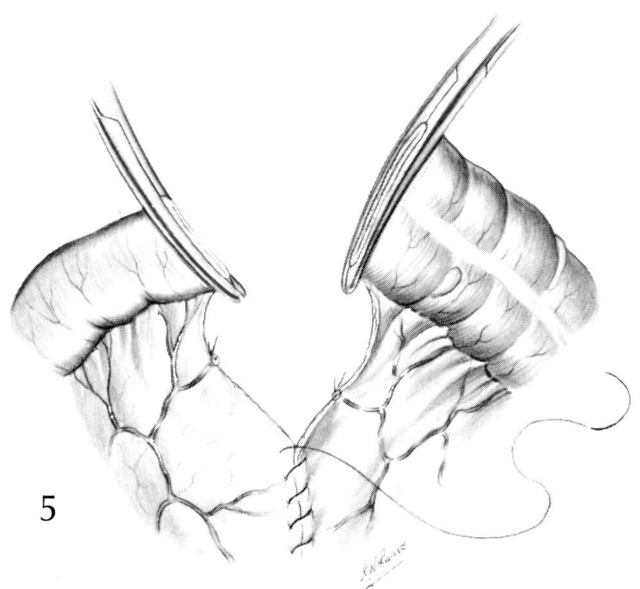

5

5

Closure of mesentery

After ensuring that the mobilization of the two ends of bowel has been adequate to allow them to come together without tension, the next step is to close the mesocolon from its base near the superior mesenteric vessels to within 2.5–5 cm of the bowel ends which remain clamped. A continuous atraumatic catgut stitch is used, taking care not to damage the vessels supplying the two ends of bowel to be joined.

6a, b & c

End-to-end anastomosis

The crushing clamps are then removed and the crushed tissue trimmed away with fine scissors. Light clamps may be placed across the bowel about 3–4 cm from the cut ends if there is likely to be soiling. The two ends of bowel are then mopped out as previously described. A series of interrupted non-absorbable sutures are placed through the seromuscular coats to form the posterior layer of the anastomosis. In this way the disparity of size that often exists between the ends is equalized and the subsequent continuous all-coats catgut suture with an inverting Connell suture on the anterior wall allows a satisfactory and safe anastomosis. A final layer of interrupted non-absorbable sutures completes the anastomosis anteriorly. The mesocolic suture is then completed up to the bowel.

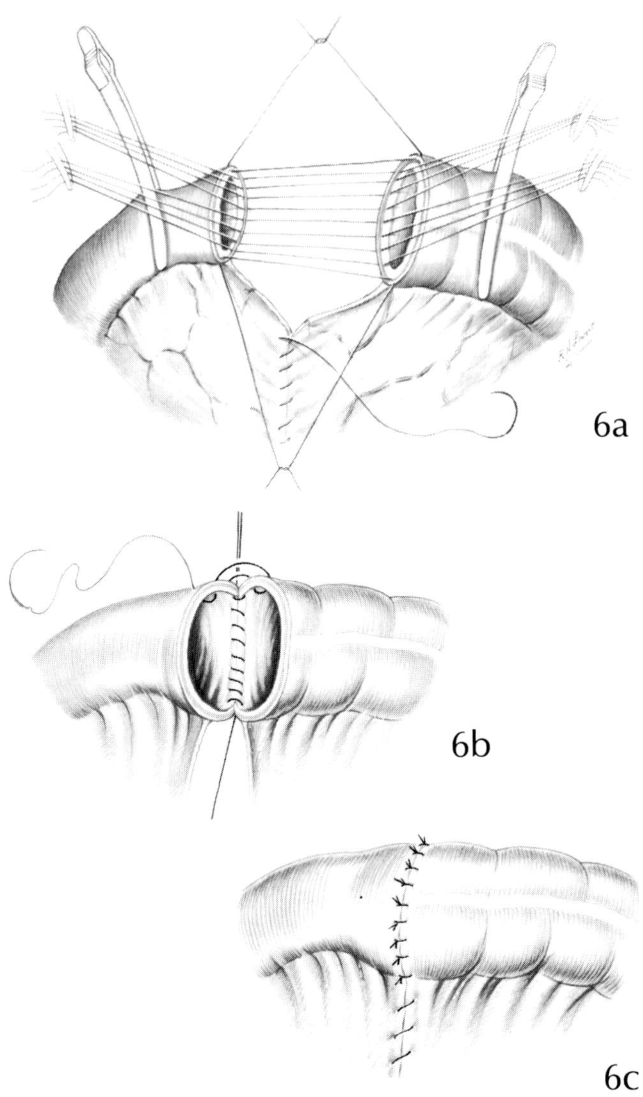

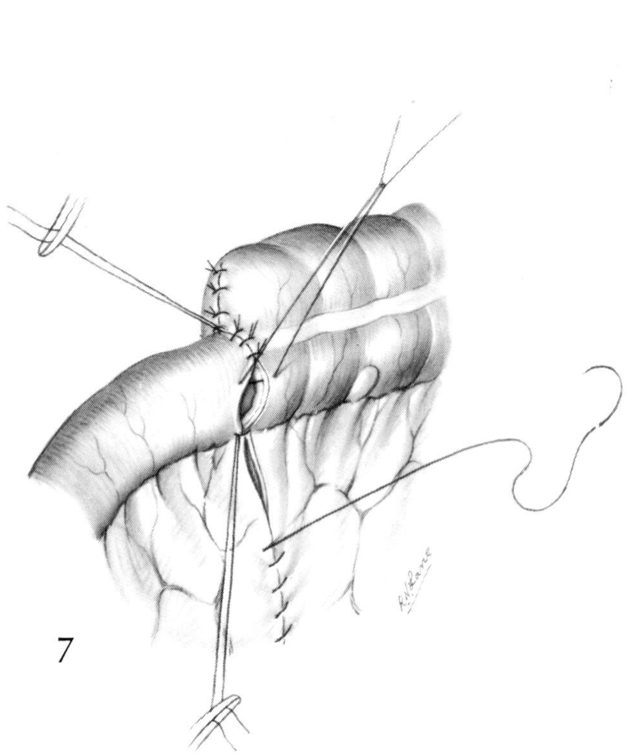

7

Disparity in size

When there is gross disparity in size between the ileum and colon, it may be wiser to close the antimesenteric half of the colon in two layers and then carry out end-to-end anastomosis between the ileum and the remaining open end of colon.

After checking for haemostasis the abdomen is closed. A stab drain may be inserted through the right flank if there has been much oozing or any soiling, but is not always necessary.

CARCINOMA OF TRANSVERSE COLON

Growths arising near the hepatic flexure are resected by right hemicolectomy; those near the splenic flexure are considered later. For growths of the midtransverse colon, resection aims at removal of the greater part of the transverse colon, the attached omentum and the lymphatic field lying in the drainage of the middle colic artery contained in the mesocolon.

8

The first step is the separation of the omentum from the greater curvature of the stomach and from the hepatic and splenic flexures. These flexures are now mobilized by division of each phrenicocolic ligament, though this may occasionally be unnecessary if there is a long transverse colon. The middle colic artery is now divided at its origin and the mesocolon separated from its attachment to the posterior abdominal wall. The sites of resection are selected, and the mesocolon and marginal vessels are divided and ligated up to the bowel.

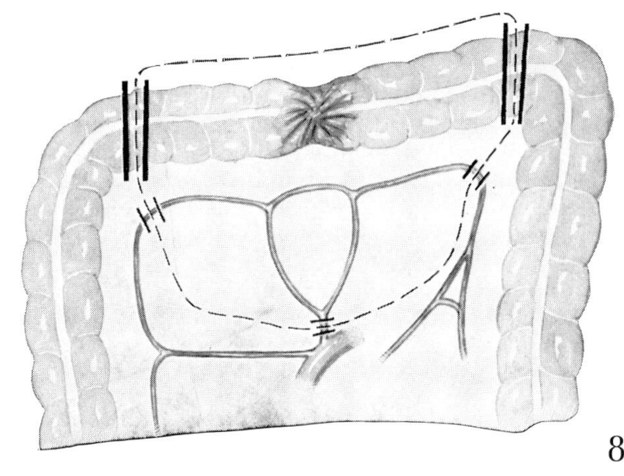

8

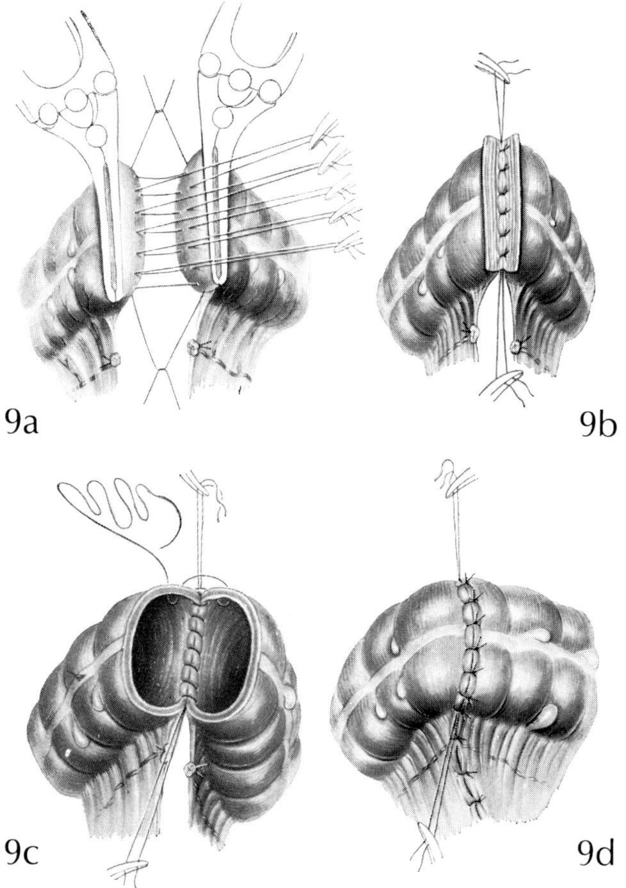

9a 9b 9c 9d

9a–d

End-to-end anastomosis is then carried out in two layers, with outer interrupted non-absorbable sutures and inner continuous absorbable sutures. The posterior interrupted layer may be inserted with the clamps still on as shown here or after their removal as shown in *Illustration 6*. There is seldom much disparity in size between the two ends. The mesocolon must be closed either before the anastomosis (*see Illustration 5*) or following its completion.

CARCINOMA OF SPLENIC FLEXURE AND DESCENDING COLON

Sites of ligation

10

Splenic flexure and upper descending colon

Growths of the splenic flexure and upper descending colon may spread both to glands beside the middle colic artery and to those beside the inferior mesenteric artery. A very radical removal involving ligation of both these vessels at their origin would require removal of most of the transverse and left colon and make restoration of continuity difficult. Such extensive removal is very seldom necessary or justified. It usually suffices to tie the left branch of the middle colic near its origin from the main trunk and the left colic near its origin from the inferior mesenteric artery.

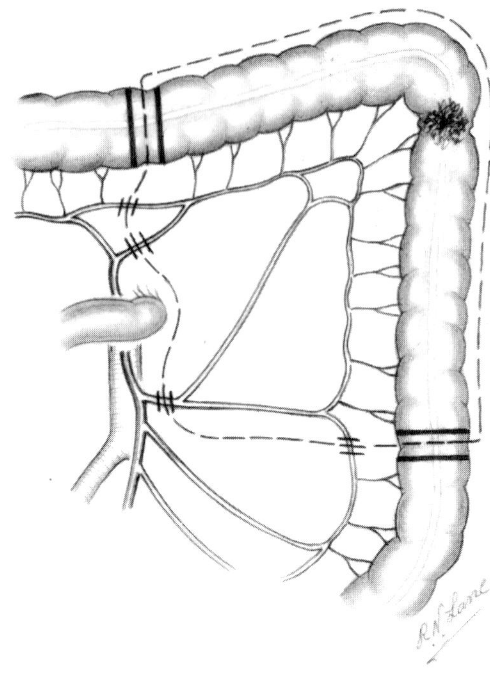

10

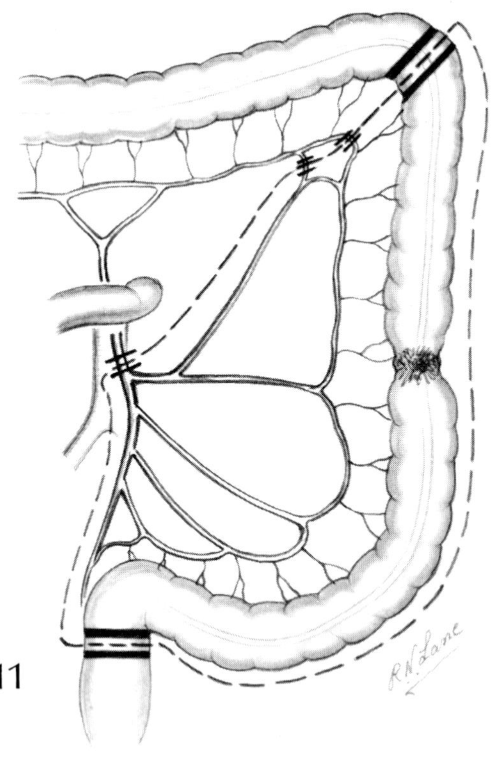

11

11

Tumours of descending colon

When dealing with tumours of the descending colon, ligation of vessels similar to that shown in *Illustration 10* may suffice. If lymph node involvement seems to indicate a more radical clearance then the inferior mesenteric artery should be ligated at its origin and the wider removal of bowel as shown here will probably be needed if good blood supply to both ends of bowel is to be ensured.

12

Mobilization of descending colon (I)

Starting at the outer side of the sigmoid colon, the line of the peritoneal attachment is divided to the splenic flexure and the colon gradually mobilized medially.

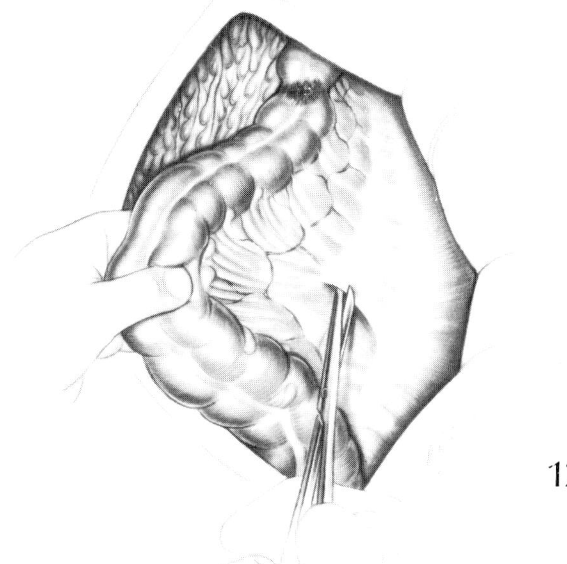

12

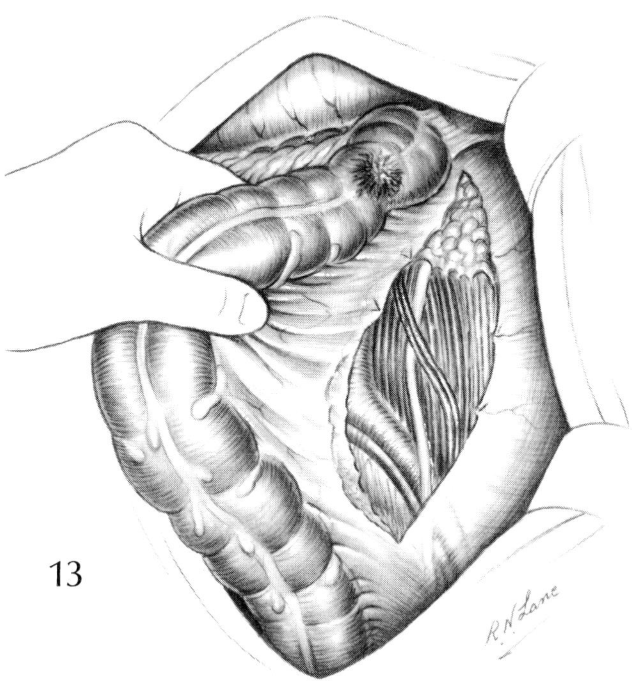

13

13

Mobilization of descending colon (II)

When fully mobilized the perinephric fat, the left ureter, the ovarian or spermatic vessels, the lowest part of the aorta and the left common iliac artery are exposed. Mesocolic vessels can now be clearly seen.

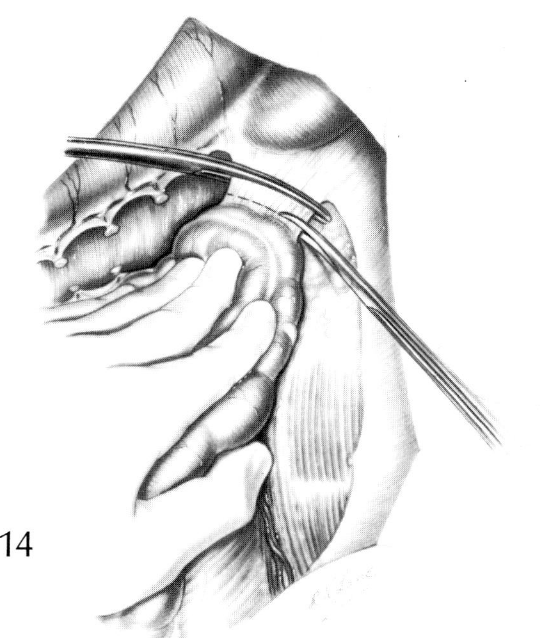

14

14

Freeing of splenic flexure

The lesser sac is entered below the gastroepiploic vessels on the greater curve of the stomach and the dissection continued towards the spleen, ligating and dividing the gastrocolic omentum. The final freeing of the splenic flexure must be done very carefully with good access, lighting and retraction, as the bowel is often in very close relation to the spleen, the capsule of which tears easily. There are often a few small vessels in the adhesions between the spleen and colon and often a 'pedicle' can be gently isolated and then clamped before division. The left colon and splenic flexure are usually then freed enough to allow their delivery outside the abdomen.

The mesocolon can be divided as required, the length of bowel containing the tumour removed and continuity restored by end-to-end anastomosis without any tension.

CARCINOMA OF SIGMOID COLON

15

Sites of ligation (I)

For most cases of carcinoma of the sigmoid colon the superior haemorrhoidal and sigmoid arteries should be tied at their origins from the inferior mesenteric, that is, just below the origin of the left colic artery. This ensures an excellent blood supply to the left colon, which is anastomosed to the upper rectum at the level of the sacral promontory.

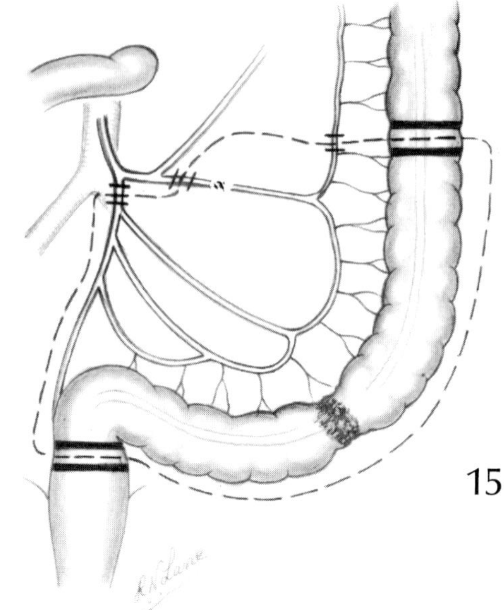

15

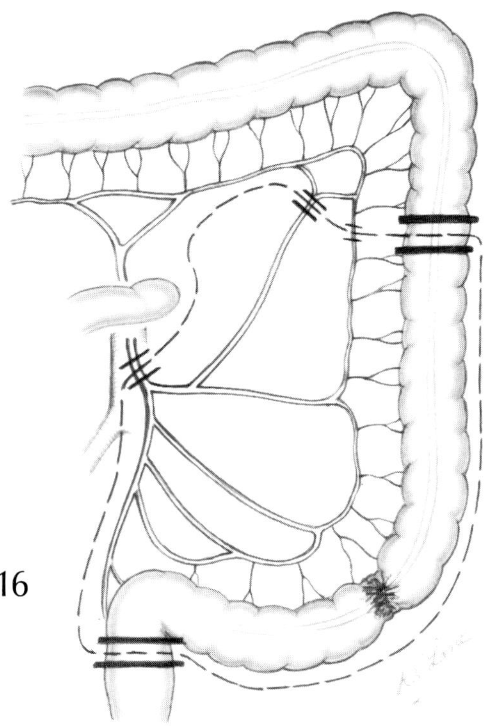

16

16

Sites of ligation (II)

If a more radical lymphatic removal is indicated, the inferior mesenteric artery is ligated at its origin from the aorta. Reliance is then placed on the marginal artery from the middle colic to supply the descending colon and it may be necessary to remove more of the descending colon to ensure that the proximal colon is viable; in that case the splenic flexure may have to be mobilized so that the remaining colon can be brought down to the rectum without tension.

17

Preparation for anastomosis

Following ligation of the main vessels, the mesentery is divided out to the bowel at the level decided. After gentle mobilization of the rectosigmoid from the sacral promontory, the dissection is also taken through the retrorectal tissue, again ligating and dividing the superior haemorrhoidal vessels, which are here running down behind the rectum. When the rectal wall has been bared, a right-angled clamp is applied across the upper rectum, which is then washed out with cytotoxic solution through a proctoscope per anum (*see* chapter on 'Anterior resection', pp. 520–542 in this volume).

The upper end is divided between clamps and a soft occlusion clamp may be applied about 2.5 cm higher to prevent soiling during anastomosis. The upper end should be gently mopped out with water or a mild aqueous antiseptic solution.

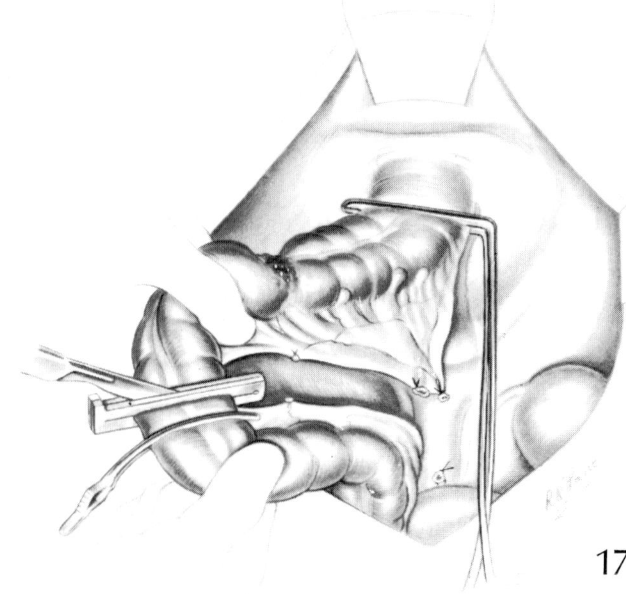

17

18a & b

The anastomosis

For more difficult anastomoses, when both bowel ends cannot be brought up into the wound, it is best to insert all the sutures of the outer posterior layer with the bowel ends separated and then slide the upper end down to the lower before tying them. The continous all-coats suture is then started in the midline posteriorly, brought round on each side and finished anteriorly. Further interrupted seromuscular silk stitches anteriorly complete the anastomosis. The mesentery is sutured to the pelvic peritoneum on the right side with a running catgut stitch. Drainage depends upon the surgeon's preference but is not usually necessary unless there is much oozing. The abdomen is then closed. The anus may be dilated at the end of the operation. This allows an easier escape of flatus which reduces intraluminal tension.

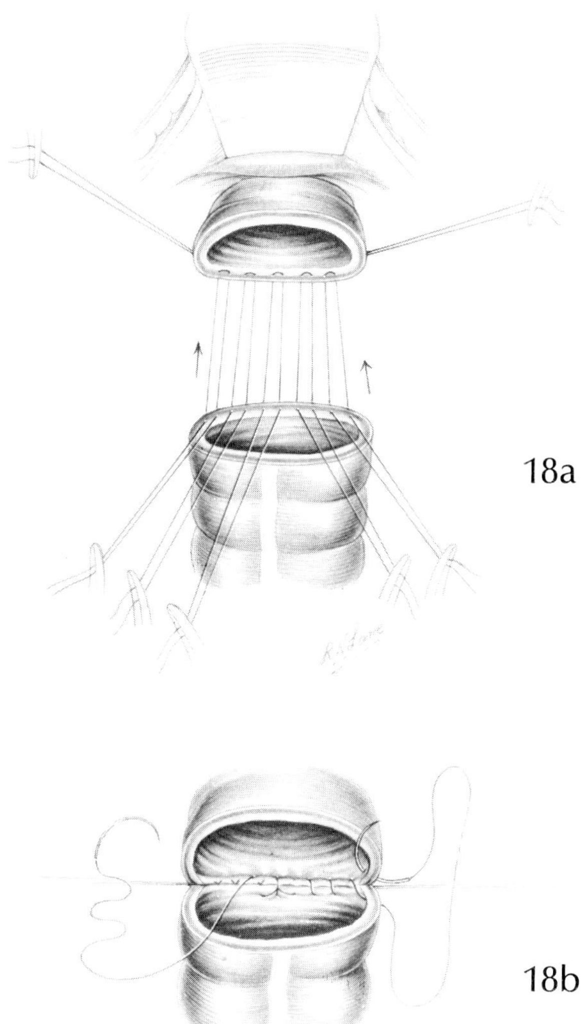

18a

18b

Postoperative care

Postoperative care is essentially the same as that for any major abdominal operation. Blood loss should be made good during and immediately after the operation. Postoperative breathing exercises are commenced as soon as possible. The use of prophylactic antibiotics is a matter of personal decision. Since a period of postoperative intestinal paresis is to be expected, nothing should be given by mouth and the patient is maintained on intravenous fluids until there is positive evidence of the full return of peristalsis by the passage of flatus. Routine postoperative gastric suction is used by many surgeons; others institute this only when it appears desirable.

If a drain has been inserted at the end of the operation, it should usually be shortened by about 2 cm on the third postoperative day and removed on the fourth or fifth day when the bowel has functioned normally.

Anterior resection

J. C. Goligher ChM(Ed.), FRCS(Ed.), FRCS
Consultant in General and Colorectal Surgery, Leeds;
Emeritus Professor of Surgery, University of Leeds;
Consulting Surgeon, St Mark's Hospital, London

L. P. Fielding MB, FRCS
Chief of Surgery, St Mary's Hospital, Waterbury, Connecticut;
Associate Professor of Surgery, Yale New Haven Hospital, Connecticut;
Visiting Clinical Scientist, St Mary's Hospital Medical School, London

Preoperative

Indications

When 'anterior resection' was first introduced for the treatment of carcinoma of the rectosigmoid and upper rectum in the early 1940s, there was considerable controversy about its safety and efficacy for this purpose. But its use has been in large measure vindicated in more recent years by many large-scale studies of the early and late results in comparison with those of abdominoperineal excision[1–7]. Although nearly all these enquiries are open to some criticism of the validity of their comparative data[8, 9], their findings have convinced most surgeons that anterior resection can offer as good a chance of cure as does abdominoperineal excision for many patients with growths in the rectosigmoid or upper half or even upper two-thirds of the rectum. It may thus now be regarded as an established surgical procedure for the treatment of suitable carcinomas in these situations; but, if disappointments are to be avoided, great care must be exercised in the choice of patients for this operation. The main criteria of selection are the following.

Unless indicated otherwise the cross-references in this chapter refer to *Operative Surgery: Alimentary Tract and Abdominal Wall, Volume 3, 4th Edition*

Height of growth, physical characteristics of patient and technique of anastomosis (by hand-placed sutures or by the automatic circular stapler)

These are by far the most important considerations in deciding on the suitability of a case for anterior resection – or other form of sphincter-saving resection. Obviously anterior resection is particularly well suited for growths of the rectosigmoid or upper third of the rectum. But it can also often be applied to carcinomas of the middle third or even the upper part of the lower third – and this applies even more so to large villous adenomas – for at operation, when the rectum is mobilized down to the anorectal ring with division of the lateral ligaments, it loses its anteroposterior and lateral curvatures, straightens out and lengthens (*see Illustration 5*). As a result a growth situated at say 6–7cm from the anal verge on preoperative sigmoidoscopy may rise at operation to 9–10cm. Consequently, it can be resected with a distal margin of clearance of 4–5cm (as was originally thought advisable[8, 10–12]) or of course much more easily with a margin of only 2–3cm (as is now considered adequate by many surgeons[13–16], including ourselves), yet leaving not only an intact anal canal but usually a small fringe of distal rectum as well.

Whether an anastomosis of the colon to the top of such a low anorectal remnant from above will be possible depends on several factors: the sex and build of the patient, the surgeon's familiarity with this type of operation and, in particular, his willingness to use one of the new automatic circular staplers to accomplish the union. The greater width of the female pelvis considerably facilitates the performance of an anterior resection, and in a thin woman it is possible as a rule to carry out an adequate resection with an *ordinary hand-sutured anastomosis* for a carcinoma lying at preoperative assessment as low as 6cm from the anal verge – possibly even less – before operation. But in an obese woman, or in a male patient, even if slim, this operation is seldom practicable for growths lower than 7–8cm, while in obese males lesions as high as 10–12cm may be found technically extremely difficult for anterior resection with hand suture. Clearly, if conventional anterior resection is the only form of resection with preservation of the sphincters being practised by the surgeon, however skilled he may be in its use, a few of the female patients and a larger proportion of the male patients with carcinomas in the middle third of the rectum, which on pathological grounds would be deemed suitable for sphincter-saving resection, will be denied the opportunity of having this type of operation and condemned to an abdominoperineal excision with a permanent colostomy. Alternatively other forms of sphincter-saving resection, such as *abdominoanal or abdominosacral* resection (see chapter on 'The Kraske, sacral or posterior approach to the rectum', pp. 381–390), may be employed. Yet another alternative for these difficult lower growths is to use *anterior resection with the aid of the circular stapler for the anastomosis*, for there is good evidence[17–22] that the use of the stapler makes it feasible to perform colorectal anastomoses at a lower level than is possible by hand suture. In fact the downward extension of anterior resection that this device permits has enabled us, Hughes (personal communication), Fazio (personal communication) and many others, to dispense almost entirely in the last 3 or 4 years with other forms of sphincter-saving resection. We would say that in general it should now be quite possible to treat at least 70 per cent of all rectal carcinomas by anterior resection.

Despite the foregoing guidelines, based on the preoperative assessment of the sigmoidscopic level of the growth, it must be emphasized that, certainly with lower lesions, a firm decision as to whether a sphincter-saving resection is going to be feasible or not and which technique will be most suitable cannot be reached until the abdomen has been opened and the rectum and the carcinoma have been fully mobilized.

The grade of malignancy of the growth

It is known that unusually extensive spread in the rectal wall – sometimes up to 7–10cm distant from the macroscopic edge of the primary lesion – may occur in connection with anaplastic rectal carcinomas[9]. Clearly, in such cases an anterior resection with anastomosis might result in a troublesome local recurrence, and a sphincter-saving resection is probably better avoided in any patient whose preoperative sigmoidoscopic biopsy shows a highly active growth, unless the tumour lies in the upper rectum allowing an exceptionally long distal margin of clearance to be taken in the resected specimen.

By contrast the lower edge of a villous adenoma which seems to be benign as determined by the complete absence of induration on palpation with the finger may be safely removed by a resection excising as little as 0.5–1cm of normal bowel wall distal to the growth.

The presence of hepatic metastases

Occasionally an hepatic metastasis is apparently solitary and it is feasible to remove it either at the same time as the rectal resection or at a subsequent intervention either by a local wedge excision or by a formal hepatic lobectomy with some prospect of lasting cure[23]. Much more frequently liver deposits are multiple and the condition is obviously incurable. In such a situation considerable palliation may nonetheless accrue from removal of the primary growth, which is usually responsible for most of the patient's symptoms. Obviously the palliative value of such an excision will be greatly enhanced if it can be carried out as a sphincter-saving resection instead of as an operation involving the establishment of a permanent colostomy. Bearing this in mind the surgeon may feel tempted to stretch the indications for resection with conservation of the sphincter in such patients. If he is not careful, however, he may incur for his patient a high incidence of complications which may greatly prolong the period of convalescence and thereby diminish the amount of palliation afforded. Particularly is this so with middle-third growths which require a very low resection and are apt to be followed by much diarrhoea and even some incontinence for 4–6 months. If the liver in these cases is found to contain a large volume of secondary deposit, the period of survival may be as short as 9–12 months and much of this time might therefore be spent in coping with a somewhat distressing state of bowel function. An ordinary abdominoperineal excision with colostomy may in fact provide more effective palliation in such a situation. Another much underused alternative is an extended Hartmann operation which has the advantage of sparing the patient the inconvenience of a perineal wound.

Special preoperative measures

Preliminary or simultaneous transverse colostomy

If, as is relatively uncommon with carcinoma of the rectum, the patient is acutely obstructed, a proximal colostomy alone should be performed in the first instance. This is best sited in the extreme right of the transverse colon, at a small transverse wound in the right subcostal region which leaves the left half of the abdomen unencumbered by a stoma at the subsequent resection 2 or 3 weeks later. In the interval between the establishment of the colostomy and resection, the colon is prepared by daily washes through from the colostomy to the anus or vice-versa – and by insertion of suppositories containing metronidazole and neomycin 24–48 h before operation.

An alternative would be to perform an immediate resection completed not by anastomosis at this stage but by closing the top of the rectal stump by suture and bringing the colon stump out as a left iliac colostomy (Hartmanns' operation). However, the subsequent restoration of continuity may be technically very difficult, certainly after any but very high resections. (This subject is considered in more detail on pp. 570–574 in this volume). In the usual unobstructed case a preliminary colostomy is unnecessary, but if at operation the bowel is found to be more heavily loaded than was anticipated, an 'on table' bowel irrigation[24] may be carried out (*see* chapter on 'Management of the obstructed bowel', pp. 210–229). If the anastomosis was effected only with difficulty, it may be advisable also to establish a temporary defunctioning transverse colostomy at the end of the resection. This does not make much difference to the incidence of anastomotic dehiscence, but it probably lessens the seriousness of this complication if it should occur and facilitates its management. The subsequent closure of the colostomy is a simple matter if an interval of not less than 2 months is allowed to elapse for oedema at the colostomy site to subside[9]. One of us (JCG) has tended to perform a simultaneous transver colostomy almost routinely after any particularly low anterior resection, while others, including LPF, Turnbull (personal communication), and Beahrs (personal communication) find this usually unnecessary.

For the average patient the local and general preparation differs in no essential respect from that employed for abdominoperineal excision (*see* p. 555 in this volume), but *mechanical preparation of the bowel is especialy important* because an empty colon facilitates the conduct of these operations and probably results in a smoother recovery. In the anaesthetic room an indwelling urethral catheter is inserted, the bladder completely emptied by compression and an intravenous infusion started, preferably in the right arm as the surgeon will be standing on the left side.

Anaesthesia

General anaesthesia supplemented by relaxant drugs is the most commonly used routine for these operations. However, spinal and epidural anaesthesia have their advocates, because they provide a very 'dry' operative field due to the reduction of blood pressure; the latter method may also be used for control of postoperative pain.

Position of patient

The general set-up for sphincter-saving resections is identical to that for abdominoperineal excision, for, as has already been emphasized, the feasibility of carrying out a sphincter-conserving type of operation usually emerges clearly only at laparotomy, and indeed often only after a certain amount of dissection. It may well be, therefore, that the intervention will finish up as a combined excision. If the synchronous combined technique is preferred for abdominoperineal excision, the patient is placed in the modified lithotomy-Trendelenburg position (*see* p. 212), which also allows a change in plan of operation should resection with restoration of continuity be contraindicated. This particular position has in addition certain technical advantages for the conduct of some types of sphincter-saving resection, because it affords ready access to the anal region while the abdomen is still open.

The operations

LOW ANTERIOR RESECTION

1

Incision, abdominal exploration, mobilization of sigmoid colon and exposure and ligature of inferior mesenteric vessels

The initial steps of this operation are identical with those of the abdominal phase of abdominoperineal excision (see p. 556–558 in this volume) and consist in: opening and exploring of the abdomen through a long paramedian or median incision extending from the pubis to at least 8–10 cm above the level of the umbilicus; ligation of the bowel with a strong silk tie 8–10 cm above the growth to control upward displacement of free cancer cells in the lumen; mobilization of the sigmoid loop by division of the developmental adhesions on the lateral side of the sigmoid mesocolon; identification of the left ureter and exposure of the inferior mesenteric vessels through incisions in the peritoneum on either side of the base of the mesocolon, extended upwards on the right side in front of the abdominal aorta to the lower border of the third part of the duodenum.

The inferior mesenteric artery (IMA) is then ligated and divided at its origin flush with the front of the aorta, and the vein is tied separately at about the same level. Some surgeons prefer to ligate and divide the inferior mesenteric vessels before carrying out any mobilization of the sigmoid. (It greatly facilitates the display of these structures if, at the beginning of the operation, the loops of small gut are turned out of the abdomen into a plastic Lahey bag which retains them on the front of the upper right abdomen and lower chest out of the way of the abdominal dissection.)

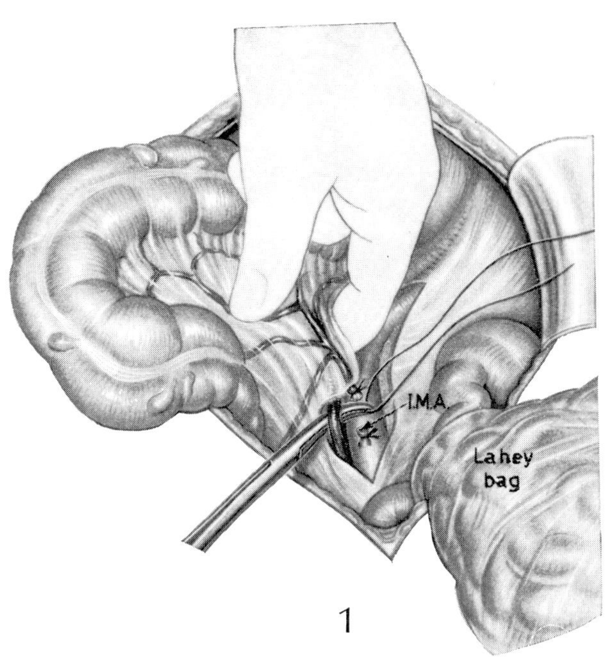

1

2

Preparation of colonic stump

The sigmoid loop is now spread out to display its vessels (aided by transillumination if necessary), preparatory to making an oblique incision with scissors in the mesosigmoid from the site of ligation of the main vessels to a point on the sigmoid colon adjudged capable of extending without any tension – and indeed with *considerable slackness* – to the top of the future rectal stump. Commonly, the cut traverses the ascending and transverse left colic vessels and the marginal arcade between the first and second sigmoid arteries, which must be ligated and divided. Finally the bowel itself is sectioned between two Parker-Kerr clamps applied obliquely from the antimesenteric to the mesenteric border.

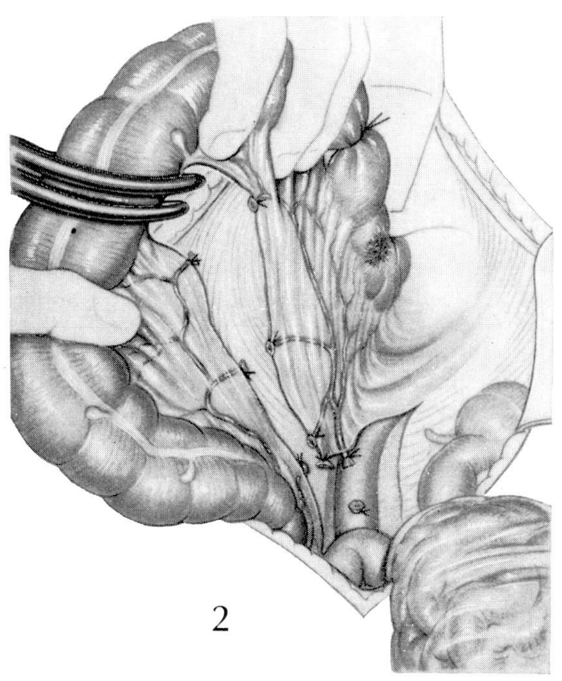

2

3 a–e

Alternative plans of ligation and preparation of colonic stump

The scheme of ligations just outlined leaves the descending colonic and sigmoid stump nourished solely by the middle colic artery through its bifurcation and continuation distally as the marginal artery (*a*). Almost invariably this supply is found to be adequate as shown by the colour of the bowel and the pulsation of the vessels in its wall, or, if there is any dubiety, by free arterial bleeding on snipping one of the small mural arteries. If a longer colonic stump is required, it can often be prepared by retaining more of the sigmoid, supplied by the intersigmoidal marginal arcades (*b*). An alternative plan for securing a longer colon stump is to mobilize the splenic flexure, and this procedure, together with resection to the upper descending or distal transverse colon (c), is also forced upon the surgeon if the blood supply to a sigmoid stump, fashioned as described above, has been found to be inadequate. After a *low* anterior resection it is essential to have enough colon *to lie loosely in the pelvis conforming to the curvature of the sacrum*, rather than stretching straight from the pelvic brim to the top of the rectal stump. It is also a widely held belief that the descending colon has a better blood supply than the sigmoid. Consequently it is an advantage in such low resections to prepare the colonic stump by the method shown in (c) of mobilizing the splenic flexure and resecting up to the descending colon. Naturally if a purely palliative resection is being undertaken a low ligation of the inferior mesenteric vessels suffices from the pathological point of view (*d*), but the preservation of the left colic – and sometimes the first sigmoid – vessels may restrict the mobility of the colonic stump. If so both these sets of vessels can be divided separately, as indicated in (e). preserving the ascending left colic vessels to assist in the blood supply to the long colonic stump

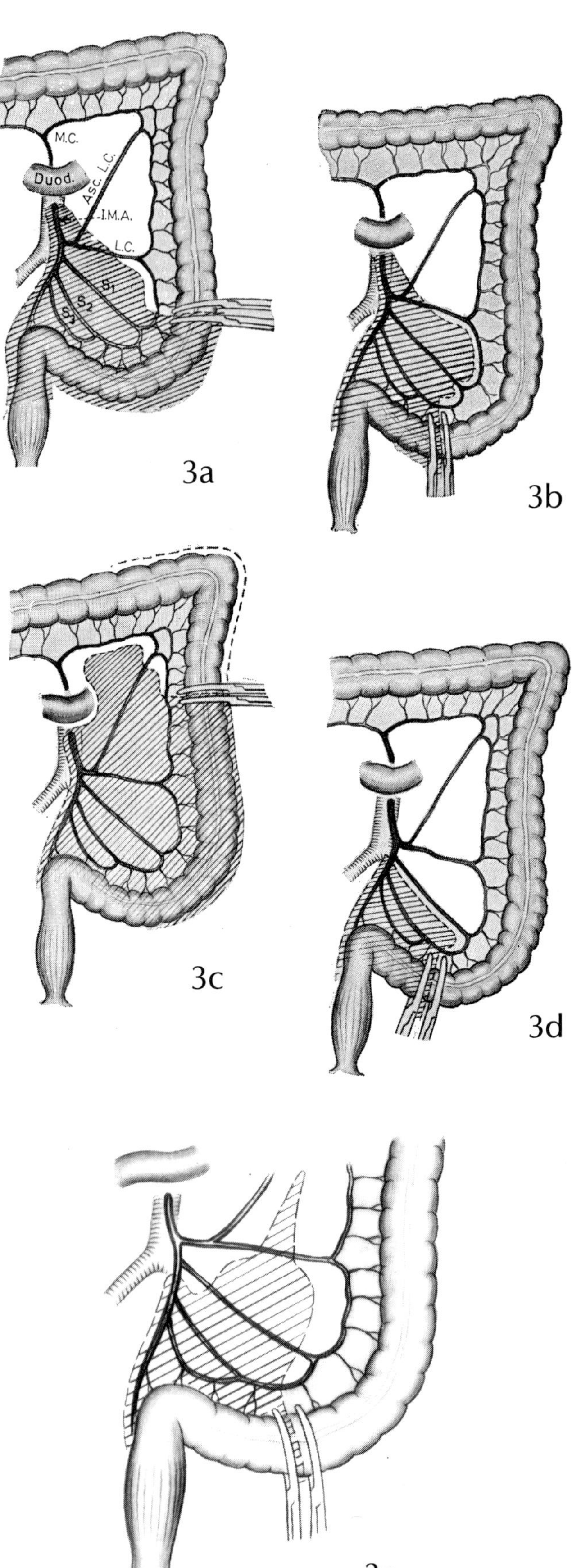

4

Separation of rectum and growth from pelvis

The rectum has now to be dissected free from its surroundings in exactly the same way as in abdominoperineal excision. The lower ends of the incisions in the peritoneum on either side of the sigmoid mesocolon are extended downwards round the brim of the pelvis to meet anteriorly on the back of the bladder. The tongue of tissue including the upper ends of the inferior mesenteric vessels is dissected down off the common iliac vessels and front of sacrum, the separation being completed to beyond the tip of the coccyx by inserting the hand into the presacral space and lifting the rectum forwards. Next, by both scissor and blunt dissection the bladder, vasa deferentia, seminal vesicles and prostate are separated from the front of the rectum and its lateral ligaments. Finally, the lateral ligaments are divided with long heavy scissors either *in toto* or in their upper two-thirds, depending on the height of the growth, any bleeding vessels being fulgurated or ligated.

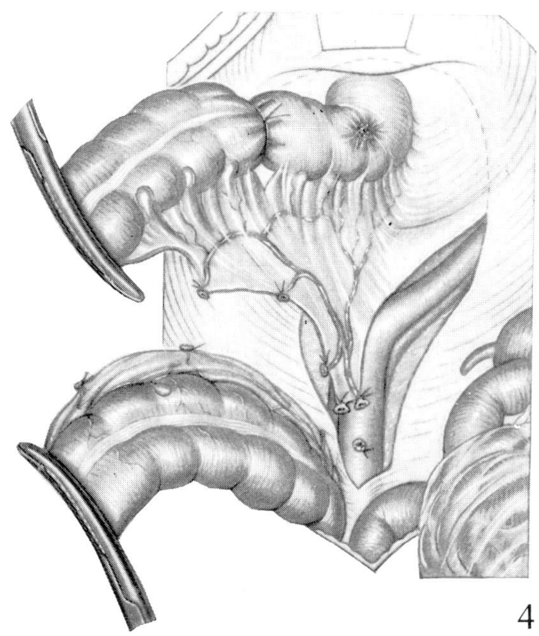

4

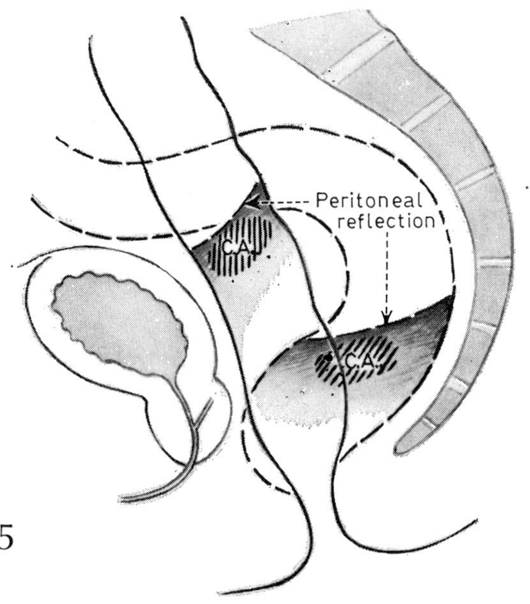

5

5

Final assessment of suitability of growth for anterior resection

The effect of mobilizing the rectum as just described – and particularly of dividing the lateral rectal ligaments – is to allow the bowel to run straight upwards from the anorectal ring without its normal anteroposterior and lateral curves. As a consequence it 'lengthens', and a growth at say 6 or 7 cm from the anal verge on sigmoidoscopy before operation may now lie at 9–10 cm or more from the anus. It is at this stage that the surgeon should make his final decision as to the suitability or not of the lesion for low anterior resection. With the rectum held gently taut he should estimate the top of the anorectal stump which, if an anterior resection is to be performed, must lie 2–3 cm below the lower edge of the growth. If it seems that division at this level will leave a sufficient anorectal remnant to permit construction of a satisfactory anastomosis he will proceed to anterior resection. Otherwise he will contemplate alternative methods of sphincter-saving resection or an abdominoperineal excision with permanent colostomy.

6

Division of mesorectum

The next step is to separate the mesorectum from the back of the rectum at the level selected for division of the bowel below the growth. This is done by scissor dissection aided by gauze dissection. The mesorectum is then clamped with two large curved artery forceps or crushing intestinal clamps and divided between them. These ends are tied off, leaving the rectum bared all round over a segment about 3 cm long, near the lower edge of which the division of the bowel and anastomosis will take place.

The higher up on the rectum the distal line of the resection is to be taken, the easier it is to define and divide the mesorectum in this manner. Lower down, the mesorectum fans out on the back of the rectum and becomes less substantial, so that in very low resections its preparatory isolation and division may not be feasible or necessary.

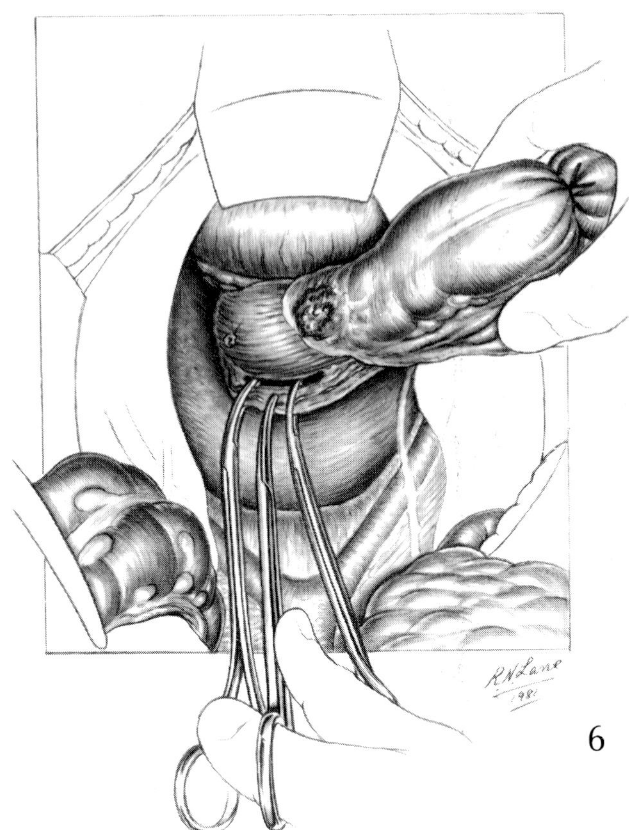

6

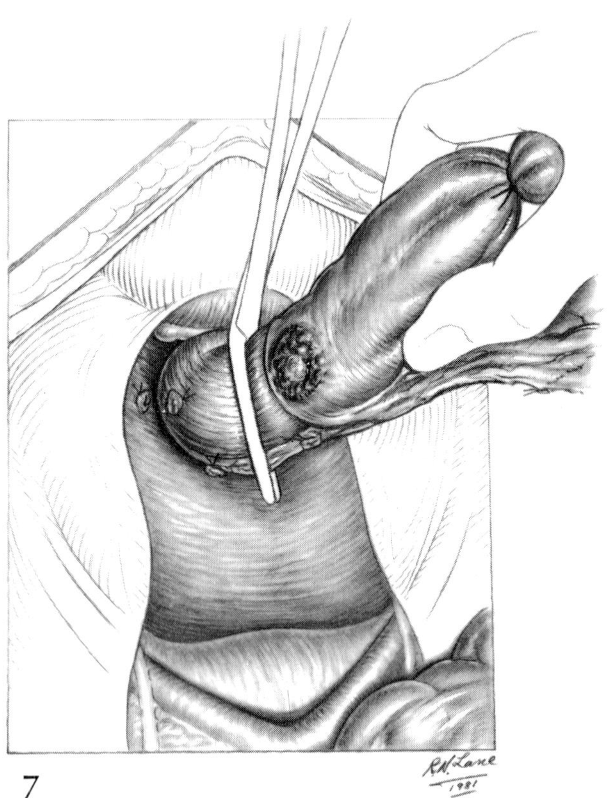

7

7

Clamping of the rectum

As a preliminary to irrigation of the rectal stump a curved Parker-Kerr clamp – or better, a slightly angled clamp – is applied across the rectum exactly in the sagittal or anteroposterior plane to prevent further descent of faeces into the lower segment of bowel. It is placed at least 2 cm below the distal edge of the growth, with its handles just above the pubis.

Irrigation of rectal stump

Before dividing the rectum and proceeding to the anastomosis it is a good plan (when the patient is in the modified lithotomy-Trendelenburg position) to cleanse the distal bowel by irrigation from below. This reduces the amount of faecal contamination when the rectum is eventually divided, for, however quick the surgeon may be with his sucker, there is some leakage of faeces at this stage. It also has the advantage that it washes away – and, if suitable agents are used, may destroy – loose malignant cells mixed with the faeces, and this diminishes the risk of their implantation in the suture line when the anastomosis is done.

8

The irrigation

An assistant now passes a proctoscope per anum and, through a rubber catheter, irrigates the rectum below the clamp, first with cetrimide (500 ml of a 1 per cent solution) as a cleansing agent, and then with nitrogen mustard (500 ml of a 2 per cent solution), which seems to be one of the most suitable cytotoxic agents for this purpose[9, 25].

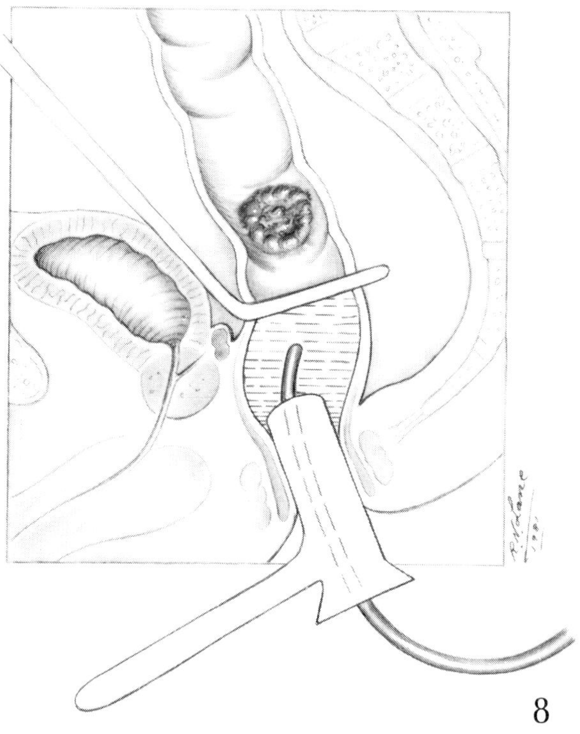

8

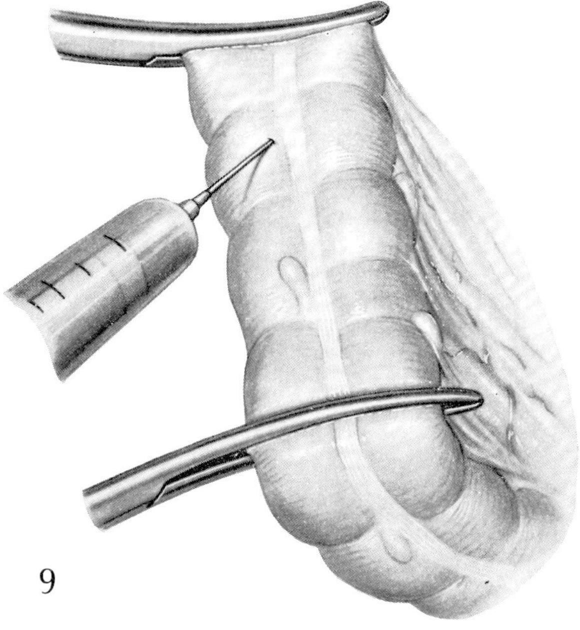

9

9

Injection of cytotoxic agent into colonic stump

If desired a cancericidal agent may be introduced into the colonic stump also. This may be done by clamping the stump 10 cm from its end with a spring clamp and then injecting nitrogen mustard (20 ml of a 2 per cent solution) through a fine needle. This solution is left in place as the anastomosis proceeds and is evacuated by suction when the terminal crushing clamp is eventually removed. An alternative plan for applying a cytotoxic agent to the colon is simply to swab out the open end of the bowel during the construction of the anastomosis, using pledgets soaked in cetrimide and then nitrogen mustard.

The anastomosis: two-layer suture technique

10

Insertion of left lateral row of Lembert sutures

In preparation for the anastomosis, the sigmoid and rectum above the angled crushing clamp are drawn vertically upwards to lift the lower rectum as far as possible out of the pelvis and facilitate the insertion of sutures into it, in the same way as traction exerted on the body of the mobilized stomach is useful during gastrectomy. The Parker-Kerr clamp controlling the end of the colonic stump is rested on the left edge of the abdominal wound, with its mesenteric border directed posteriorly and separated by a distance of 10–12 cm from the rectum. A series of mattress Lembert sutures of 3/0 serum-proof silk is now inserted between the left lateral wall of the rectum and the adjacent surface of the colon, 0.5 mm distant from the controlling clamps in each case, and left untied until all have been placed.

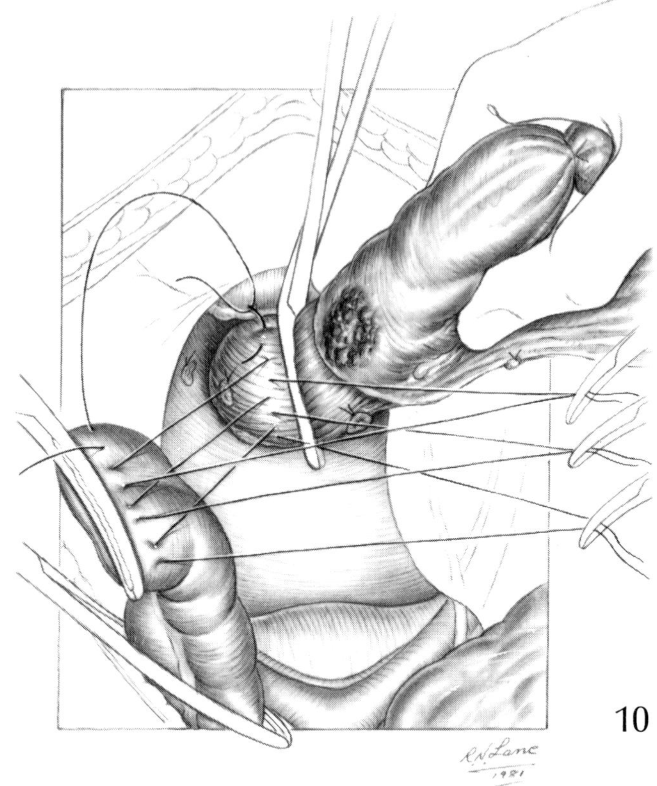

10

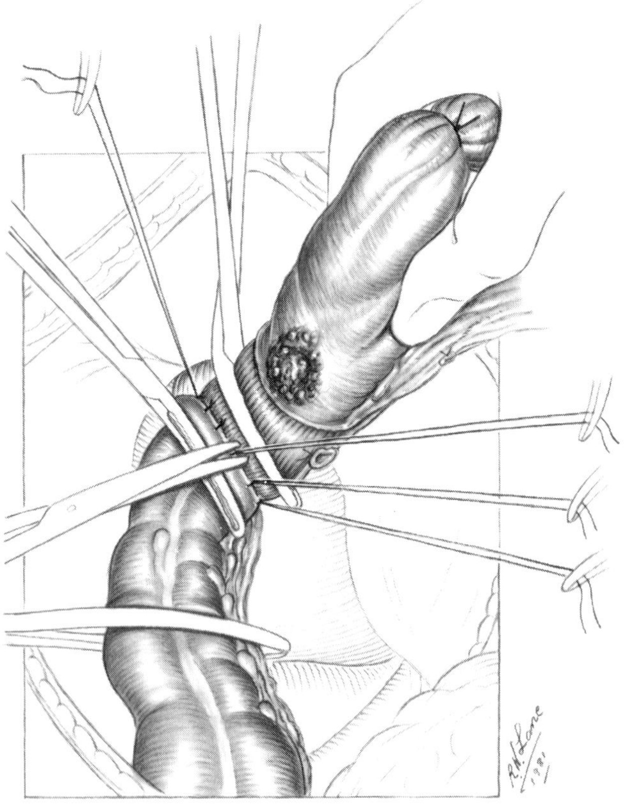

11

11

Apposition of colonic and rectal stumps and tying of left lateral Lembert sutures

The colon is then slid down on these sutures to come into apposition with the rectum, and the stitches are tied so that the tissues are approximated and *just indented but not crushed*. The tails of the first and last are retained for traction, all the others being cut.

12 a–d

Excision of clamps and insertion of continuous through-and-through suture

The crushing clamps, together with the crushed tissue gripped by their blades, are next excised with a scalpel, and in the case of the rectum this means removal of the entire operative specimen also (*a*). If the colonic stump was not previously irrigated with a cytotoxic agent, the cut edges and terminal part of the interior of the colonic stump are now swabbed with cetrimide (1 per cent solution) and then nitrogen mustard (2 per cent solution).

Everything is now ready to continue the colorectal anastomosis, but before doing so a most important step must be taken: *the excised specimen must be checked to make sure that an adequate margin of clearance has in fact been obtained distal to the primary growth, especially if one has aimed only for a 2 cm margin.* It is very easy to misjudge the distance when applying the crushing clamp and to find that there is a distal fringe of only 0.5–1.0 cm in the specimen. At this stage before completing the suture, it is a simple matter to excise more tissue from the top of the rectal stump if necessary.

A continuous 2/0 or 3/0 chromic catgut suture on a fine half-circle atraumatic needle is used to unite the cut edges of the colon and rectum. It is started at the anterior or antimesenteric poles, being inserted from the outer aspect of the rectum to the peritoneal aspect of the colon through the full thickness of bowel lumens. When tied, the knot therefore lies outside the lumen (*b*). The needle is reintroduced through the rectal wall into the lumen for suture of the adjacent halves of the bowel edges, which is done with an ordinary over-and-over stitch. At the mesenteric poles of the lumens, however, the type of suture changes to a Connell or 'loop on the mucosa' stitch (*c*), which is continued along the remote halves of the bowel circumferences (*d*), eventually reaching the antimesenteric angles again. The Connell suture gives good inversion of the cut edges and avoids all mucosal pouting.

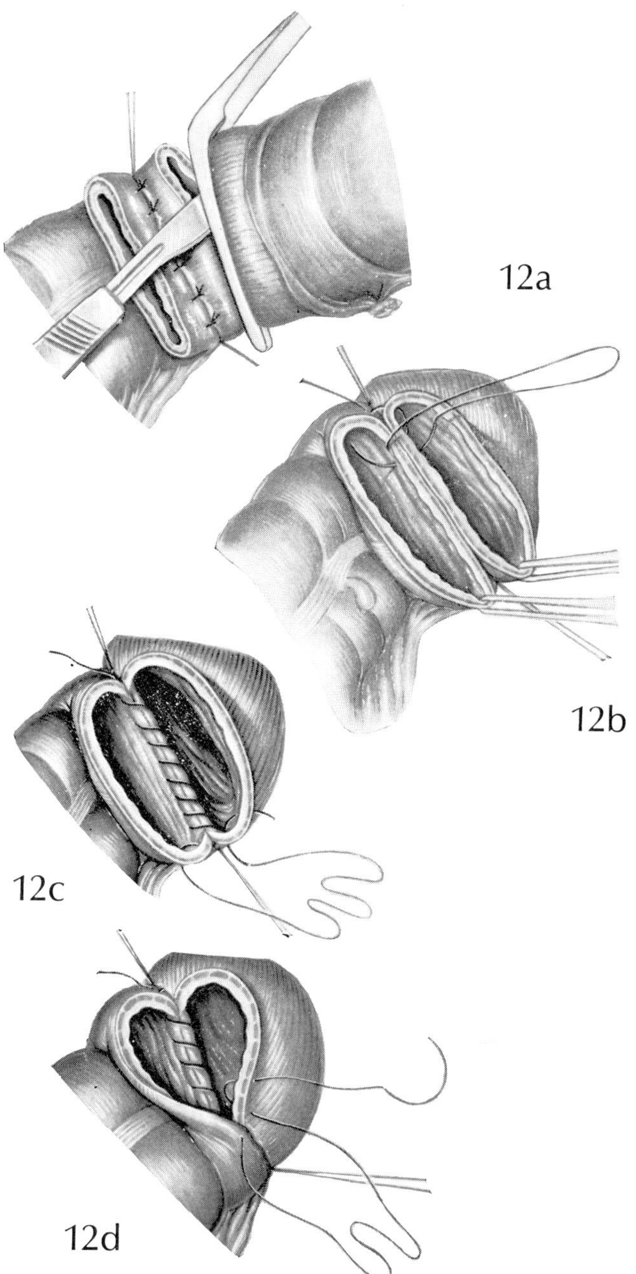

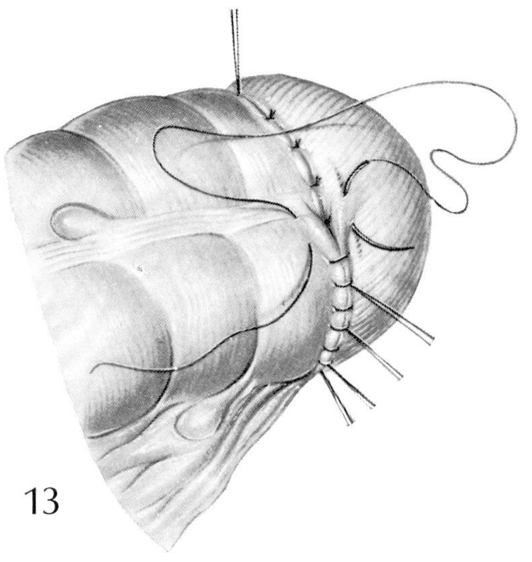

13

Insertion of right lateral Lembert sutures

The anastomosis is completed with a covering row of Lembert stitches of fine silk on the right lateral walls of the colon and rectum. These are inserted in mattress fashion to secure a better grip of the longitudinally running muscle fibres in the rectal wall. The tails of the sutures are left long and held by the assistant, facilitating insertion of the next stitch.

The anastomosis: one-layer suture technique

14

Placement of open colonic and rectal stumps for commencement of suture

Both rectal and colonic stumps having been prepared as shown in *Illustrations 2–8*, the crushing clamps controlling the ends of each stump are excised leaving two open stumps about 15–20 cm apart. The plan is to insert the single layer of interrupted sutures corresponding to the posterior half or preferably two-thirds of the bowel circumference while the colonic and rectal stumps are thus separated and then to slide the colonic stump down into the pelvis on these sutures. Silk (3/0) or corresponding grades of plastic materials, such as Ethiflex or Tevdek, or stainless steel wire mounted on atraumatic needles are satisfactory, but chromic catgut may also possibly be used.

It is convenient to start with a stitch in the midline posteriorly corresponding to the mesenteric border of both stumps. The needle is entered on the mucosal aspect of the colon 6 mm or so from the cut edge and traverses the colonic wall to emerge from the outer surface. It is then inserted through the rectal wall from the outside, again 6 mm from the cut edge, to emerge on the mucosal surface. Next the suture returns from rectum to colon catching the edges of the rectal and colonic mucosae in the process. (The precise relationship of the suture to the layers of the rectal and colonic walls is depicted in *Inset A*.) Finally the needle is cut off the suture material and the two tails of the untied stitch are clipped together with artery forceps.

An alternative way of placing the sutures is to include the muscle coat and submucosa but not the mucosa, so that the stitches do not enter the bowel lumen and are tied from the outside (*Inset B*).

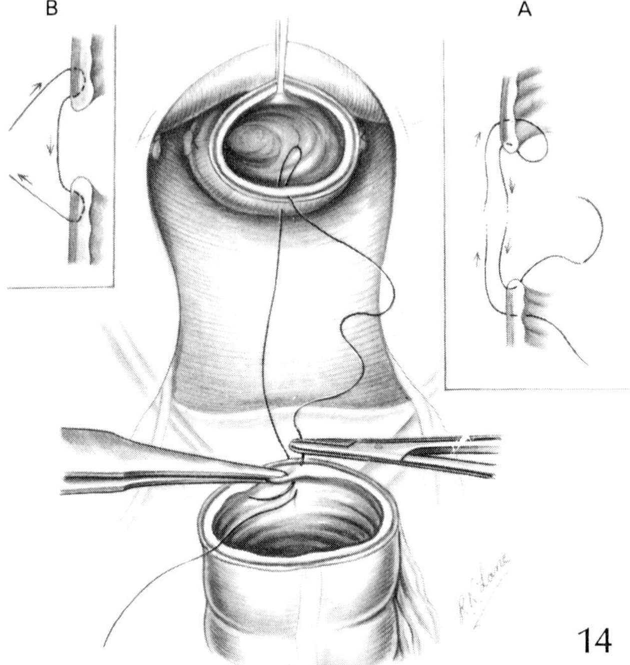

14

15

Insertion of remaining sutures in posterior two-thirds of bowel circumference

It is helpful to mark the anterior limits of the two posterior thirds of the bowel circumference by inserting a vertical mattress stitch on either side in exactly the same way as was used for the median posterior stitch, the ends being left long and clipped untied with artery forceps. Further sutures are then inserted at intervals of 4 or 5 mm between these three main marking stitches, first in the right posterior third and then in the left posterior third.

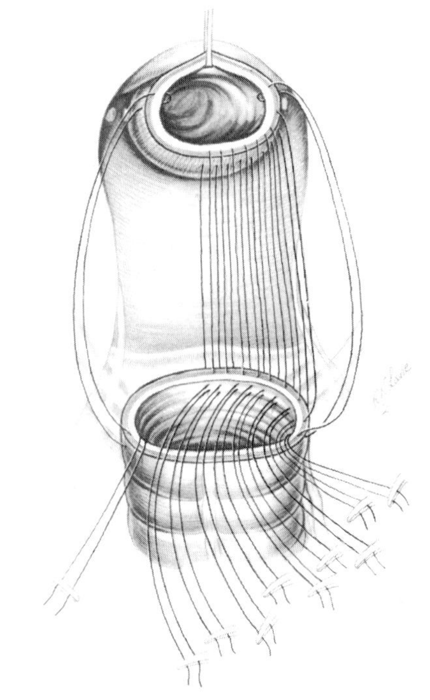

15

16

Sliding colonic stump down on to rectal stump and tying sutures with knots on colonic mucosa

The colonic stump is next slid gently into the pelvis on the tautened strands until the posterior cut edges of the colonic and rectal stumps are in apposition. The sutures are then tied seriatim, commencing near the posterior midline and extending to either side in turn. The knots of these sutures lie on the mucosal aspect of the edge of the colon.

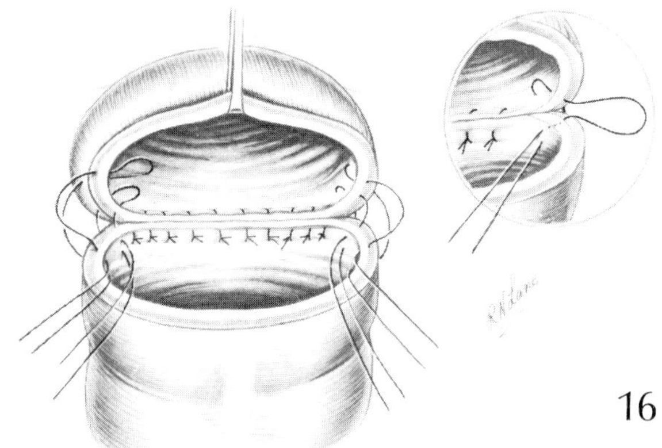

16

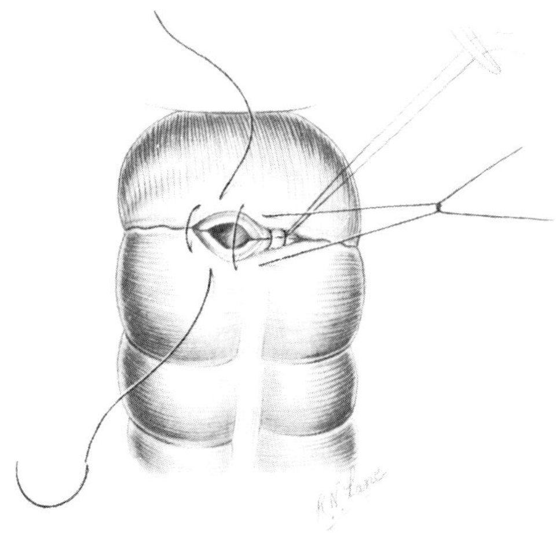

17

17

Closing the gap in the anastomosis corresponding to the anterior third of the bowel circumference

The suture of the anterior third of the bowel circumference must now be completed. Vertical mattress sutures of the Gambee type with the knots on the serosal aspect may be used but are difficult to insert in a bowel situated low in the pelvis. It is easier to use transversely placed mattress sutures, as illustrated, when working at this depth.

The anastomosis: technique with circular stapler

Circular stapling devices available and the principle of use

18

The original instrument of this kind is the Russian SPTU stapling gun, on which the US Surgical Corporation's EEA instrument, here illustrated, is based. The latter has a *disposable end* (head and cartridge), which comes in three sizes preloaded with staples in a sterile package, and is fitted on to the main part of the gun immediately before use. Other *completely disposable* staplers are becoming available from the US Surgical Corporation and Ethicon. Ethicon's ILS stapler is currently being tested and may have certain mechanical advantages over its predecessors.

The essential steps in the use of the stapling guns for anastomosis of the colonic and anorectal stumps after anterior resection are as follows.

1. Insertion of purse-string sutures of 1/0–2/0 monofilament Prolene in the cut ends of the two stumps of bowel.
2. Introduction of stapling gun to the intended site of the anastomosis, preferably from below per anum, but also possibly – though much more traumatically – from above through a side cut in the colonic stump.
3. 'Opening' of end of gun and attachment of rectal and colonic stumps by tying respective purse-string sutures to the central shaft.
4. 'Closing' and 'firing' the gun.
5. 'Opening' the gun slightly and extricating it.
6. Checking on the state of the anastomosis.

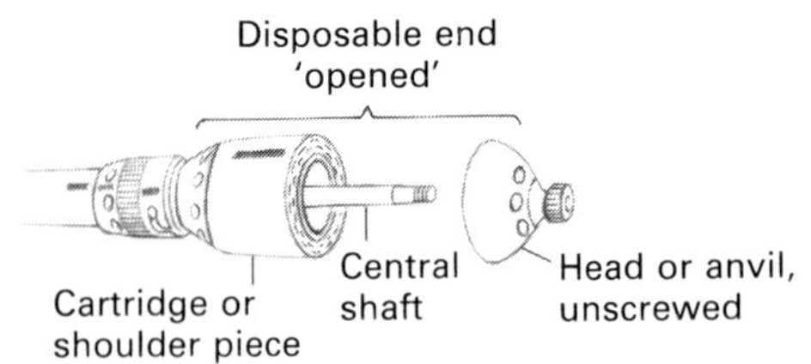

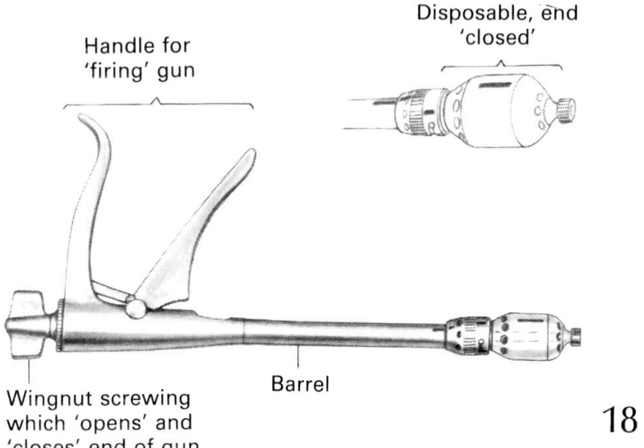

18

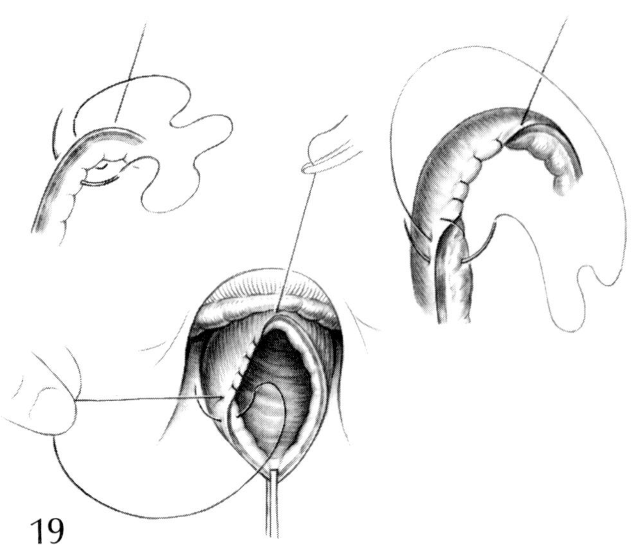

19

Insertion of rectal purse-string suture

This is the *most crucial step in the whole process of constructing a stapled anastomosis*. The reader is referred back to *Illustrations 7* and *8*, in which the rectum is shown as clamped with a sagittally placed Parker-Kerr forceps, 2 cm below the growth. It is important to emphasize that, if a stapled anastomosis is being performed, during the 'firing' of the stapler at least a further 1 cm of bowel wall will be amputated as the 'doughnut' (*see Illustrations 27* and *28*) from the rectal stump and the stapled anastomosis will be that much lower than the top of the stump. Accordingly, in planning the initial extent of the resection, it seems reasonable to allow for this subsequent additional excision and to place the distal Parker-Kerr clamp that much nearer to the lower edge of the tumour – say, within 1 cm instead of 2 cm of it.

19

The rectum is now divided with the scalpel piecemeal from before backwards immediately below the sagitally placed Parker-Kerr clamp, bleeding from the cut edge of bowel being checked by diathermy coagulation as required. The monofilament Prolene suture, which should be 1/0 *in size for the rectal stump* (rarely 2/0 if the wall of the rectum is particularly thin) commences in the midline anteriorly. It is passed from outside to inside 4 mm from the cut edge and then a series of bites are taken at intervals of 4 mm from inside to outside, the effect being to invert the cut margin of the mucosa slightly into the lumen.

20

This whip stitch is continued round the circumference of the bowel until it reaches the starting point anteriorly. The tails are left untied at this stage. There are other ways of placing the rectal purse-string suture, but this technique has proved very reliable in our hands.

Employing a double Furniss clamp and a straight needle as described for the insertion of the colonic purse-string suture (*see Illustrations 23* and *24*) may be applicable to very long rectal stumps after high anterior resection but is quite impracticable for a low stump lying in the depths of the pelvis.

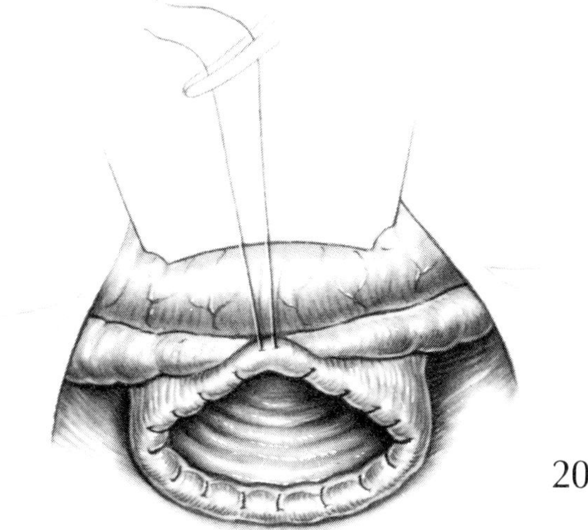

20

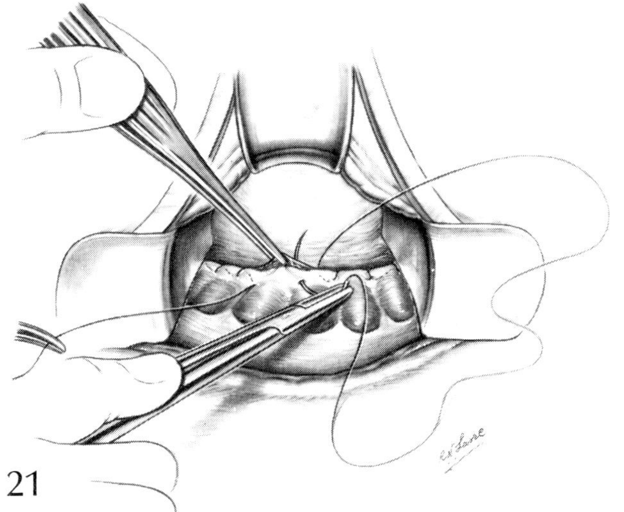

21

21

Very occasionally after extremely low anterior resection in heavily built male patients, it is difficult even to see the rectal stump from above, much less to place a purse-string in it from this aspect. In these circumstances a helpful manoeuvre is to insert this stitch *from below through the anal canal* with the aid of a trivalve anal speculum. The suture begins in the posterior midline and proceeds along the cut edge to the patient's right, the speculum being rotated in a clockwise direction to expose the right lateral, anterior, left lateral and posterior walls of the anorectal stump in turn.

22

The stitch can then either be tied from below on the central shaft of the opened stapling gun (as illustrated), or the untied tails can be passed upwards through the anal canal to the abdominal operator to be tied by him from above in due course.

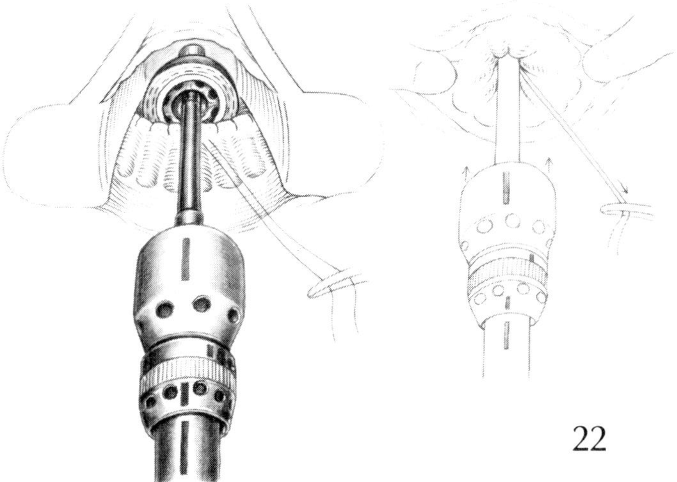

22

23 & 24

Insertion of purse-string suture in colonic stump

For the purse-string suture in the colonic stump 2/0 monofilament Prolene generally suffices. It can be placed as a whip stitch exactly as shown in *Illustrations 19* and *20* for the rectal stump, but the double Furniss clamp provided with the EEA instrument affords a very quick and convenient way of inserting this stitch with a 7.5 cm long straight needle in this accessible part of the bowel.

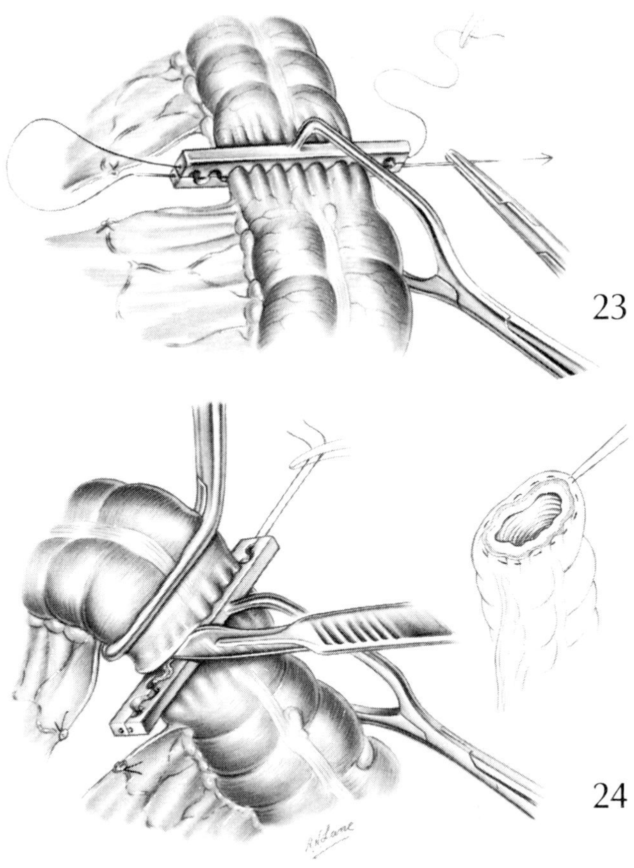

23

24

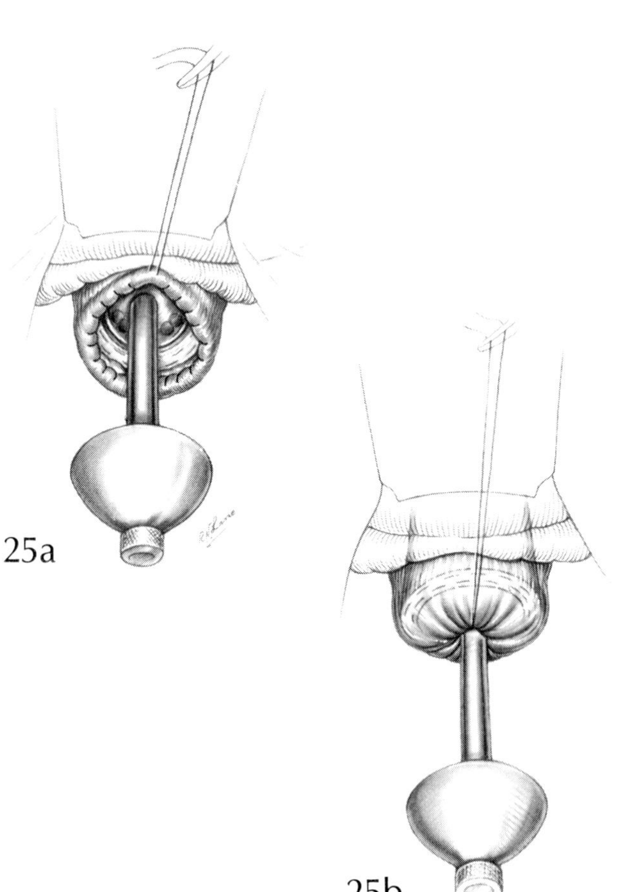

25a

25b

25a & b

Introduction of stapling gun per anum from below and tying of rectal purse-string suture

The size of endpiece to be fitted to the stapler depends essentially on the calibre of the colonic stump, which is generally considerably smaller than that of the rectal stump. The most convenient size as a rule is that with a diameter of 28 mm, but occasionally the 31 mm or 25 mm sizes are appropriate. The endpiece is taken from its sterile package by a scrubbed-up assistant and fitted on to the shaft of the autoclaved gun. It is a wise precaution to 'open' the gun, as in *Illustration 18(top)*, and to advance the staples slightly to show their tips and to check that they are all present. They can subsequently be pushed back into their sockets by gentle patting with the side of a dissecting forceps. The gun is then generously smeared with lubricating jelly both externally and between the head and shoulder piece, 'closed' and introduced through the anus into the anorectal stump.

During this process the surgeon observes the pelvic cavity from above and, as soon as the knob on the top of the head of the instrument emerges through the top of the rectal remnant, he instructs the assistant below to 'open' the endpiece. This advances the head 6 or 7 cm above the cut edge of the stump, *while the upper margin of the cartridge or shoulder piece is still within the stump* (*a*). The rectal purse-string is then tied on the central shaft just above the cartridge (*b*).

26a, b & c

Tying of colonic purse-string suture and approximation of colonic and rectal stumps

The cut edge of the colonic stump is caught with three equidistantly placed Allis forceps which give the distal opening of the colon a triangular shape. The base of this triangle is held with two of the forceps below the basal edge of the head of the gun posteriorly, while its apex is lifted by the third forceps over the top of the head (*a*). The colonic purse-string is then tied to the central shaft (*b*). The next step is to 'close' the gun, but before doing so the instrument is pushed fairly firmly upwards by the assistant into the pelvis to make sure that there is no slack rectal wall or mucosa between the site of contact of the top edge of the shoulder piece and the tied rectal purse-string suture. At the same time the surgeon draws the colonic stump upwards to avoid any slack colonic wall between the purse-string suture and the outer edge of the base of the head. The gun is now 'closed', approximating the head and shoulder piece and firmly apposing the colonic and rectal hoods on these parts between them (*c*). An automatic check incorporated in the instrument prevents the gap between the head and shoulder piece from being reduced to less than 2.5 mm to avoid subjecting to an injurious degree of compression the tissues to be stapled.

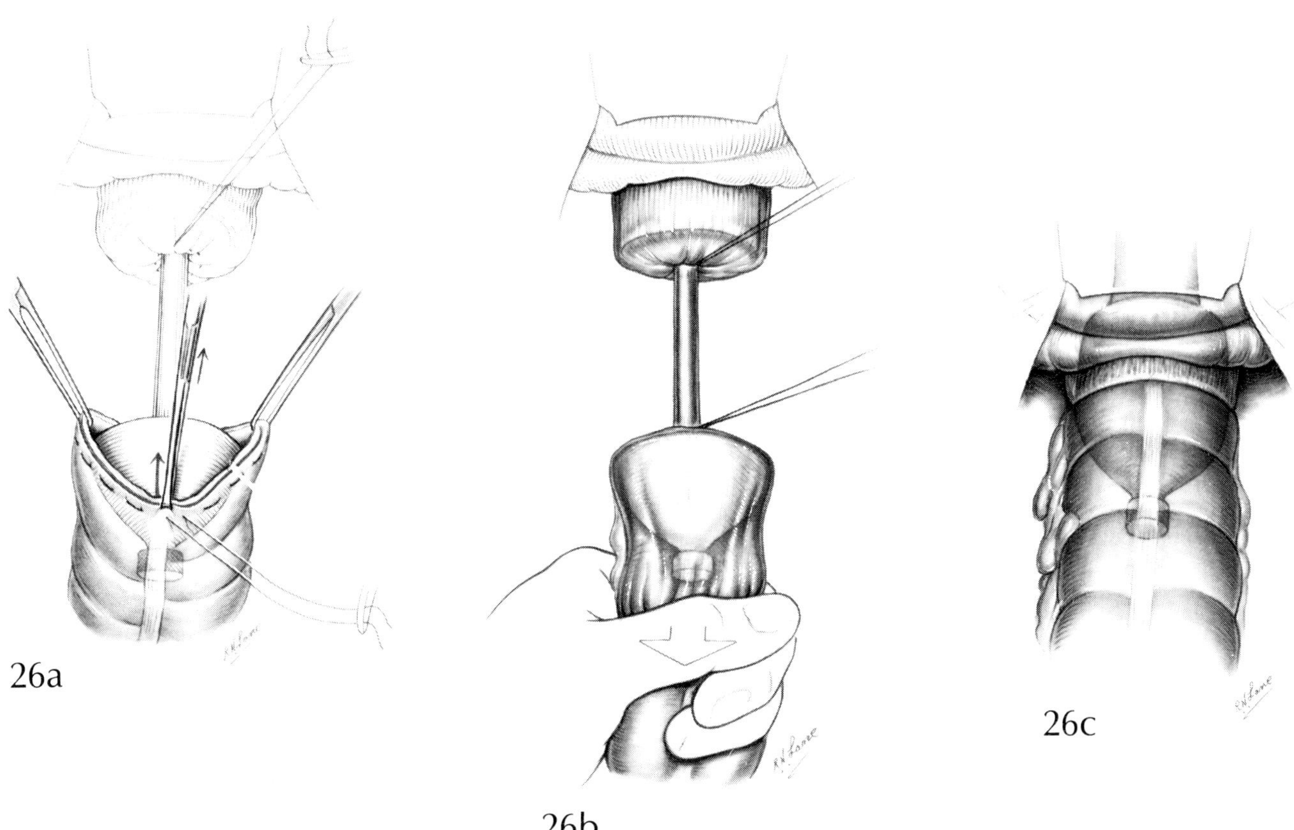

26a

26b

26c

Firing and withdrawing the gun

27

The gun is 'fired' by a sharp forceful approximation of the two limbs of the handle, using the preferred hand, while the other hand grasps the barrel of the gun to stabilize it and avoid jarring movements on the anastomosis during 'firing'. The effect is to project the U-shaped stainless steel staples through the contiguous walls of the rectal and colonic stumps to impinge on corresponding shallow grooves on the peripheral part of the under aspect of the head, which deflect the two limbs of each staple towards one another and then backwards to form a capital B. Simultaneously the 'firing' advances a circular trephine-shaped knife from within the shoulder piece against a plastic washer in the base of the head, which automatically cuts through the inturned parts of the rectal and colonic stumps just internal to the two rings of staples.

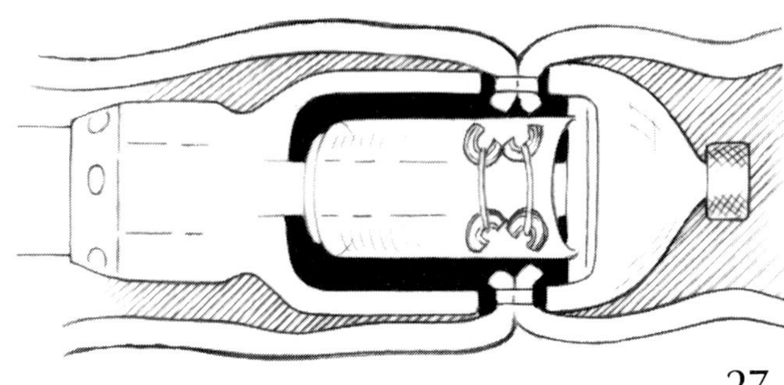

27

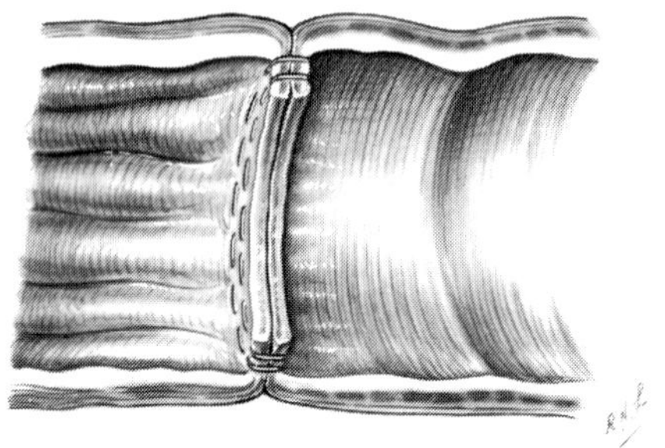

28

28

The gun is now 'opened' 1 cm to allow the stapled flange of colorectal walls to recede outwards from its grasp. Next the gun is rotated to tear any residual strands of mucosa that were not completely divided by the trephine and is then gently extricated leaving a nicely inverted end-to-end stapled anastomosis.

The withdrawal of the gun often seems a very traumatic manoeuvre, likely to damage the recently formed anastomosis. This is especially so when a rather too large end has been used on the instrument. However almost invariably withdrawal is eventually achieved without significant trauma to the anastomosed bowel. Very exceptionally (in one case in 110 in our experience) it proves impossible to extract the gun, probably because of failure to divide all the mucosa. In these circumstances the best plan is to make a 3–4 cm longitudinal cut on the anterior aspect of the colonic stump 2–3 cm above the anastomosis to expose the head of the gun, which can then be unscrewed and removed, allowing the rest of the instrument to be drawn out per anum. The colotomy wound is then closed by one or two layers of interrupted silk sutures.

Examining the so-called 'doughnuts' of rectal and colonic wall excised by the stapler

29

When the gun is inspected after removal two discs of bowel wall will be found skewered on the central shaft. After removal of the head these should be slipped off the shaft and – after extraction of their purse-string sutures – carefully examined, to see whether they are complete discs or not, for this information has considerable bearing on the quality of the anastomosis. An incomplete disc very strongly suggests a defective anastomosis, while complete discs make it highly likely, but not absolutely certain, that a sound anastomosis has been achieved.

The surgeon can of course inspect the outer aspect of the anastomosis from the abdominal aspect. This is easily done when the site is readily accessible, as after a high or only moderately low anterior resection. But with really low resections it can be quite difficult to obtain a good view of all parts of the anastomosis, especially posteriorly, and there is a danger that in the process the staple line may be torn. A helpful and probably safer alternative for low anastomoses is to fill the pelvis with warmed saline to submerge the anastomotic site, while the assistant passes a fine catheter per anum into the lower rectum and inflates a little air into the bowel. If an anastomotic defect is present bubbles of air can be seen rising from the region of the anastomosis to the top of the pelvic saline pool.

Any anastomotic defect should be repaired either by Lembert sutures of silk from the abdominal aspect or, if the anastomosis is very low, by passing a bivalve speculum into the anal canal as shown in *Illustrations 21* and *22* to expose the line of anastomosis from within the bowel lumen and to repair any gap by interrupted inverting through-and-through sutures of silk or Dexon. In any case found to have a defective anastomosis, even though it is subsequently repaired, it is probably a wise precaution to finish the operation by establishing a temporary loop transverse colostomy.

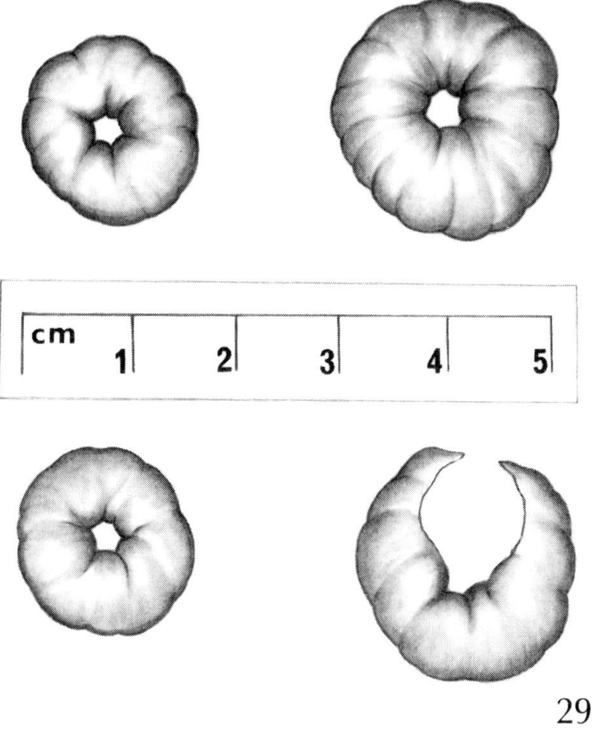

29

30

Irrigation and drainage of pelvic cavity

It is a good plan to irrigate the pelvis at the conclusion of the anastomosis with 2 or 3 litres of normal saline, to which tetracycline 1 g per litre is added[26, 27]. As for drainage, though most surgeons agree that it is important to drain the pelvis after low anterior resection, opinions differ as to the best method of doing so. We prefer to use 2 or 3 suprapubic suction drains extending to the depths of the pelvis (either Shirley sump drains or Redivac type closed drains) one placed anteriorly, the other one or two posteriorly.

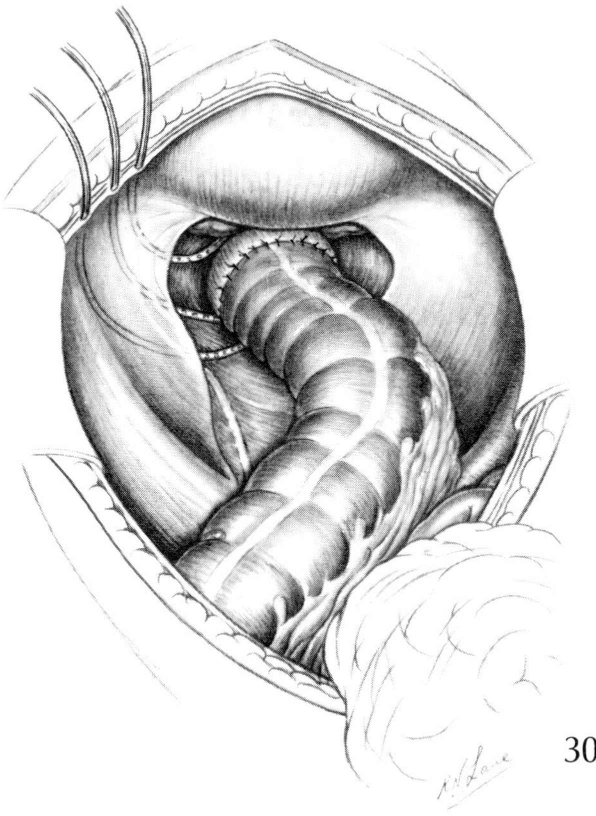

30

HIGH ANTERIOR RESECTION

In resecting carcinomas of the rectosigmoid region the same technique is employed, but the rectum is not completely lifted out of its sacral bed, the anastomosis being between the colon and the intraperitoneal part of the rectum. The preparation of the colonic stump is exactly the same as that described for low anterior resection.

Preparation of rectal stump

31

Incision of right leaf of mesosigmoid and mesorectum

The upper rectum and lower sigmoid are drawn upwards and to the left to render the mesorectum and mesosigmoid taut. Then, starting at the lower end of the incision made in the right leaf of the mesosigmoid for exposure and ligation of the inferior mesenteric vessels, an oblique scissor cut is carried in the peritoneum to reach the back of the bowel 5 cm below the lower margin of the growth. Subsequently the peritoneal cut is deepened through the subjacent fat, especially in its posterior part.

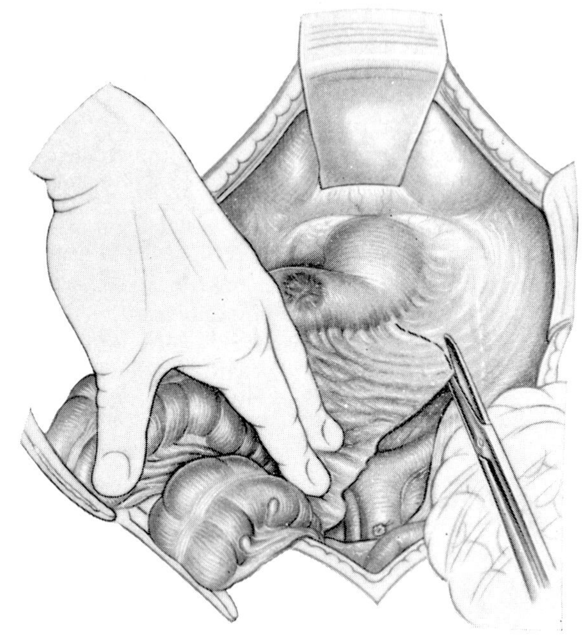

31

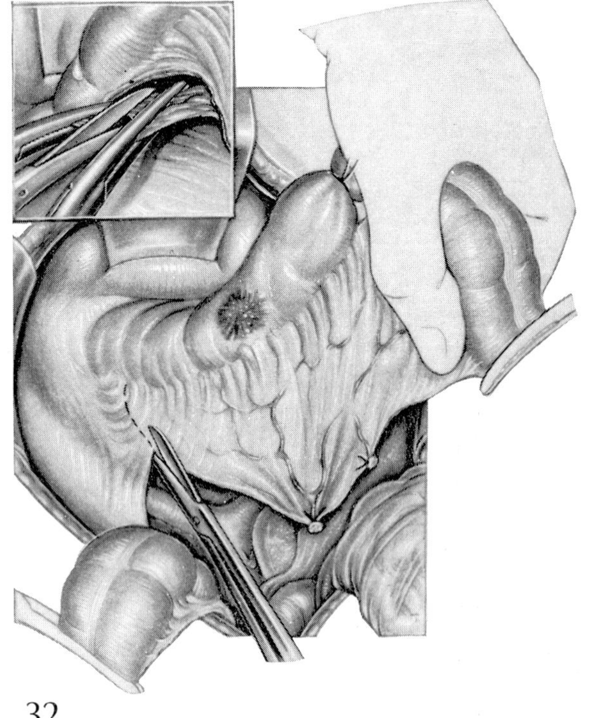

32

32

Incision of left leaf of mesosigmoid and mesorectum, and clamping and division of superior haemorrhoidal vessels

While the rectum is now retracted upwards and to the right, a similar incision is made in the left leaf of the mesosigmoid and mesorectum, care being taken to ensure that its termination at the back of the bowel corresponds accurately with the end of the incision in the right leaf. The underlying fat is also divided with scissors or broken through by blunt dissection in the posterior part of the cut, but just behind the rectum a search is made for the superior haemorrhoidal vessels as they run downwards and forwards close to the back of the bowel. These vessels are isolated, clamped with two large crushing clamps, divided and tied, thus baring the posterior wall of the rectum at this point.

33

Clamping of bowel and colorectal anastomosis

A curved Parker-Kerr or slightly angled clamp is applied across the rectum in the sagittal plane immediately above the level chosen for the lower limit of the resection, and at least 4cm distal to the inferior edge of the growth. Thereafter the anorectum below the clamp is irrigated by an assistant through a proctoscope as in low anterior resection. When this has been completed the end of the colonic stump controlled by a Parker-Kerr clamp is drawn down to the left edge of the abdominal wound. The anastomosis is completed by any of the three methods described for low anterior resection, though there is no special virtue in the use of the stapler at this level – it may in fact be a little difficult to apply because of impingement of the head of the instrument on the front of the sacrum near the promontory.

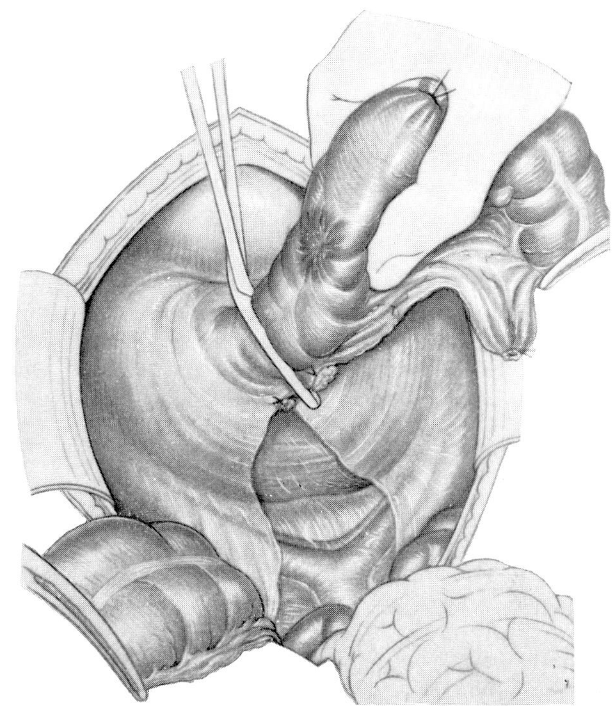

33

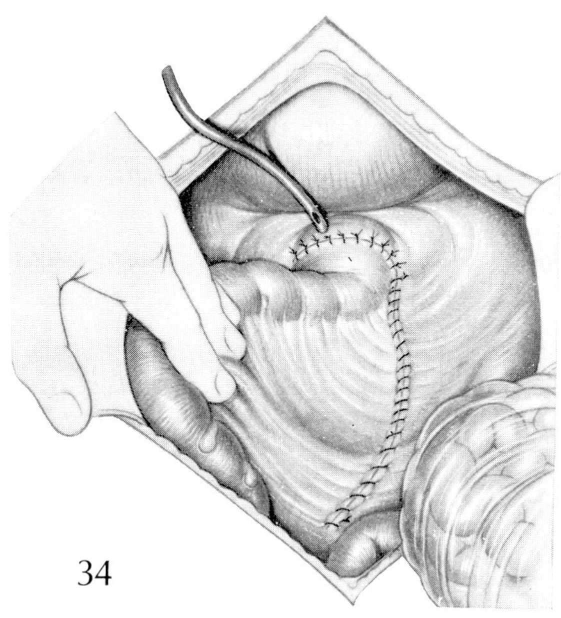

34

34

Completion of operation and drainage

The final result is an entirely intraperitoneal anastomosis between the colon and a very short cuff of intraperitoneal rectum. Peritoneal irrigation is carried out and drainage established by one or two suction drains (*see Illustration 30*). The laparotomy incision is then closed by whatever technique the surgeon favours for abdominal wound closure in general (see pp. 52–56 in *Alimentary Tract and Abdominal Wall, volume 1*).

Special postoperative care and complications

If there has been unusual faecal contamination during the operation it is wise to administer a full course of systemic antibiotic therapy for 4 or 5 days, preferably using two agents one of which should be effective against anaerobic organisms – for example, either gentamicin 80 mg and lincomycin 600 mg intramuscularly 8 hourly or tobramycin 80 mg intramuscularly 8 hourly with metronidazole 500 mg intravenously twice daily. Many surgeons including ourselves favour a short prophylactic course of these drugs, consisting of one dose immediately preoperatively and another 6 or 8 hours later *in all cases*. There is good evidence from controlled studies that this type of regimen lessens the incidence of septic complications[28, 29, 30].

Oral fluids should be withheld initially and an intravenous infusion continued with appropriate solutions, as indicated by daily plasma electrolyte estimations and other considerations, until vigorous peristalsis is heard on auscultation and flatus or faeces is passed per anum or per colostomy; glycerine suppositories on the fourth or fifth postoperative day may help to stimulate bowel function. The suprapubic drain is retained as long as significant quantities of fluid are withdrawn, which is usually for 3 or 4 days. The urethral catheter is removed on the fourth or fifth day.

If a transverse colostomy was established at the time of doing the low anterior resection, it can be closed after 2½ to 3 weeks if the anastomosis heals per primam, but in any event it is probably better to retain it for 2 months, because of the difficulties of colostomy closure sooner due to residual oedema in the everted bowel. It is little hardship to a patient to go home for 6 weeks wearing a modern disposable drainage bag on his temporary colostomy.

Anastomotic dehiscence

Separation of the anastomosis at some part of the bowel circumference, usually the posterior third, is not uncommon after low anterior resection. Everett[31] has provided evidence from a controlled trial that it is less frequent after a one-layer suture technique than after a two-layer technique, but our extensive trial failed to confirm this finding[32]. As for the relative security of stapled and hand-sutured anastomoses after anterior resection, some early uncontrolled experiences suggested that stapled anastomoses might be a little more secure[19, 33], but a recent controlled trial has shown no significant difference in the relative dehiscence rates after stapled and sutured anastomoses[22]. However, it is a surprisingly innocuous complication as a rule, especially if a transverse colostomy was made at the conclusion of the resection. All that need be done in these circumstances is to retain the colostomy until the dehiscence has largely healed, which may require anything from 2 to 4 weeks, depending on the extent of the breakdown. Meanwhile irrigations of the rectum through a proctoscope or washes-through from the colostomy to the anus may help to clear up resulting pelvic infection. If a transverse colostomy was not established at the time of the resection, and there is a *major dehiscence* of the anastomosis with suprapubic leakage of faeces, urgent surgery is required (*see* chapter on 'Surgical management of anastomotic leakage and intra-abdominal sepsis', pp. 185–192).

Though from clinical evidence anastomotic dehiscence is apparently well tolerated by most patients, it does add substantially to the postoperative mortality (threefold difference) and length of stay in hospital when compared to patients without such leakage[34]. The surgeon should therefore make every effort to avoid this complication by good bowel preparation and a delicate and precise operative technique providing accurate apposition of tissues with a well preserved blood supply and without any tension.

Haemorrhage

Reactionary bleeding has been a very rare complication after stapled anastomoses. In fact it is almost surprising that there have not been more instances of this complication because the closed staple is designed not to be completely haemostatic. In our four cases complicated in this way, the bleeding was not severe and stopped spontaneously, a blood transfusion being given in 2 patients. It may be reasonable to place a cotton-wool ball soaked in 1:1000 adrenaline at the anastomosis if bleeding persists.

Stricture

Some degree of narrowing at the anastomosis due to reactionary oedema is a fairly frequent finding in the early weeks after an anterior resection, but this usually corrects itself spontaneously possibly assisted by the dilating effect of passing normal faeces. Only if there has been a major breakdown of the anastomosis involving, say, half the bowel circumference, is a persistent stricture likely to develop, but it is surprising how over a period of 6 to 12 months these strictures may also undergo considerable spontaneous dilatation. Rarely is it necessary to carry out dilatation with Hegar's dilators, at first under a short general anaesthetic and then daily by the patient himself for a time.

Some surgeons have the impression that stricture formation is slightly more common after stapled anastomoses than after hand-sutured ones (Killingback, personal communication), but opinion is divided on this issue.

Local recurrence

Local recurrence of rectal carcinomas is easier to detect after a sphincter-saving resection than after an abdominoperineal excision. Sometimes they may seem to be confined to the region of the anastomosis, but on other occasions they are more widespread in the pelvis and may also be associated with recurrence elsewhere in the abdomen. Rarely in the former group it may be possible to remove the recurrence by an abdominoperineal excision or even a further anterior resection, but this may be technically a very difficult operation. Otherwise supervoltage radiotherapy may be considered.

Anal incontinence

After anterior resection, even of the low variety, the functional result is usually excellent, although, owing to the loss of the greater part of the sigmoid colon and much of the rectum, motions are passed more frequently at first. This applies particularly to patients having the exceptionally low resections now being obtained with the aid of the circular stapler which give anastomoses just above the anal canal (i.e. 3.5–4.5 cm from the anal verge). In such cases severe diarrhoea, often with as many as 8–12 motions per day, and some degree of incontinence are usual for 3–6 months. Most of these patients eventually achieve full control though a few of the more elderly patients continue with partial incontinence indefinitely. Some of these patients would have been better served by an abdominoperineal resection and permanent stoma.

References

1. Waugh, J. M., Block, M. A., Gage, R. P. Three and five-year survivals following combined abdominoperineal resection, abdominoperineal resection with sphincter preservation, and anterior resection for carcinoma of the rectum and lower part of the sigmoid colon. Annals of Surgery 1955; 142: 752–757
2. Mayo, G. W., Fly, O. A., Connelly, M. E. Fate of the remaining rectal segment after subtotal colectomy for ulcerative colitis. Annals of Surgery 1956; 144: 753–757
3. Mayo, C. W., Laberge, M. Y., Hardy, W. M. Five year survival after anterior resection for carcinoma of the rectum and rectosigmoid. Surgery, Gynecology and Obstetrics 1958; 106: 695–698
4. Deddish, M. R., Stearns, M. W. Anterior resection for carcinoma of the rectum and rectosigmoid area. Annals of Surgery 1961; 154: 961–966
5. Cullen, P. K., Mayo, C. W. A further evaluation of the one-stage low-anterior resection. Diseases of the Colon and Rectum 1963; 6: 415–421
6. Morgan, O. N. Carcinoma of the rectum. Annals of the Royal College of Surgeons of England 1965; 36: 73–97
7. Vandertoll, D. J., Beahrs, O. H. Carcinoma of rectum and low sigmoid; evaluation of anterior resection of 1766 favorable lesions. Archives of Surgery 1965; 90: 793–798
8. Goligher, J. C. Preservation of the anal sphincters in the radical treatment of rectal cancer. Annals of Royal College of Surgeons of England 1958; 22: 311–329
9. Goligher, J. C. Surgery of the anus, rectum and colon, 4th ed. London: Baillière Tindall, 1980
10. Quer, E. A. Dahlin, D. C., Mayo, C. W. Retrograde intramural spread of carcinoma of the rectum and rectosigmoid. A microscopic study. Surgery, Gynecology and Obstetrics 1953; 96: 24–30
11. Grinnell, R. S. Distal intramural spread of carcinoma of the rectum and rectosigmoid. Surgery, Gynecology and Obstetrics 954: 99: 421–430
12. Hernerck, P., Gall, F. P. Sicherheitsabstand bei der sphintererhaltenden rectunresektion. Der Chirurgie 1981; 52: 25–29
13. Penfold, J. C. B. A comparison of restorative resection of carcinoma of the middle third of the rectum with abdominoperineal excision. Australia and New Zealand Journal of Surgery 1974; 44: 354–356
14. Localio, S. A., Eng, K. Malignant tumors of the rectum. Current problems in surgery. Sept 1975: 1–48
15. Manson, P. N., Corman, M. L., Coller, J. A., Veidenheimer, M. C. Anastomotic recurrence after anterior resection of carcinoma: Lahey clinic experience. Diseases of the Colon and Rectum 1976; 19: 219–224
16. Killingback, M. Annals of the Royal College of Surgeons of England (in press)
17. Goligher, J. C. Recent trends in the practice of sphincter-saving excision for rectal cancer. Annals of the Royal College of Surgeons of England 1979; 61: 169–176
18. Goligher, J. C. Use of circular stapling gun with peranal insertion of anorectal purse-string suture for construction of very low colorectal or colo-anal anastomoses. British Journal of Surgery 1979; 66: 501–504
19. Goligher, J. C. Faltin lecture. The use of stapling devices for the construction of low rectal anastomoses. Annales Churgiae et Gynaecologiae 1980; 69: 125–131
20. Heald, R. J. A new approach to rectal cancer. British Journal of Hospital Medicine 1979; 22: 277–281
21. Heald, R. J. Leicester, R. J. The low stapled anastomosis. British Journal of Surgery 1981; 68: 333–337
22. Beart, R. W., Kelly, K. A. Randomized prospective evaluation of the EEA stapler for colorectal anastomoses. American Journal of Surgery 1981; 141: 143–147
23. Wilson, S. M., Adson, M. A. Surgical treatment of hepatic metastases from colorectal cancers. Archives of Surgery 1976; 111: 330–334
24. Dudley, H. A. F., Radcliffe, A. F., McGeehan. Intraoperative irrigation of the colon to permit primary anastomosis. British Journal of Surgery 1980; 67: 80–81
25. Goligher, J. C. Further reflections on preservation of the anal sphincters in the radical treatment of rectal cancer. Proceedings of the Royal Society of Medicine 1962; 55: 341–346

26. Stewart, D. J., Matheson, N. A. Peritoneal lavage in appendicular peritonitis. British Journal of Surgery 1978; 65: 54–56

27. Stewart, D. J., Matheson, N. A. Peritoneal lavage in faecal peritonitis in the rat. British Journal of Surgery 1978; 65: 57–59

28. Stokes, E. J., Waterworth, P. M., Franks, V., Watson, B., Clark, C. G. Short term routine antibiotic prophylaxis in surgery. British Journal of Surgery 1974; 61: 739–742

29. Keighley, M. R. B., Arabi, Y., Alexander-Williams, J., Youngs, D., Buidon, D. W. Comparison between systemic and oral antimicrobial prophylaxis in colorectal surgery. Lancet 1979; 1: 894–897

30. Condon, R. E., Bartlett, J. G. Nichols, R. L. Schulte, W. J., Gorbach, S. L., Ochi, S., Preoperative prophylactic cephalothin fails to control septic complications of colorectal operations: result of controlled clinical trial. American Journal of Surgery 1979; 137: 68–74

31. Everett, W. G. A comparison of one- and two-layer techniques for colorectal anastomosis. British Journal of Surgery 1975; 62: 135–140

32. Goligher, J. C., Lee, P. W., Simpkins, K. C., Lintott, D. J. A controlled comparison of one- and two-layer techniques of suture for high and low colorectal anastomoses. British Journal of Surgery 1977; 64: 609–614

33. Goligher, J. C., Lee, P. W. R., McFie, J., Simpkins, K. C., Lintott, D. J. Experience with the Russian model 249 suture gun for anastomosis of the rectum. Surgery, Gynecology and Obstetrics 1979; 148: 517–524

34. Fielding, L. P., Stewart-Brown, S., Blesovskly, L.,Kearney, G. Anastomotic integrity after operations for large-bowel cancer: a multicentre study. British Medical Journal 1980; 281: 411–414

Peranal endorectal operative techniques

The late Sir Alan G. Parks MCh, PRCS, FRCP
Consultant Surgeon, The London Hospital and St Mark's Hospital, London

R. J. Nicholls MChir, FRCS
Consultant Surgeon, St Thomas' Hospital and St Mark's Hospital, London

Introduction

1

The rectum is particularly amenable to the application of endocavity techniques. Excellent exposure of the lower rectum may be obtained by holding the anal canal open with a suitable retractor. The self-retaining retractor illustrated can easily be inserted through the anal sphincter and, owing to their contour, the blades when opened hold the walls of the rectal ampulla apart and maintain the instrument in place. A third insertable blade further improves exposure.

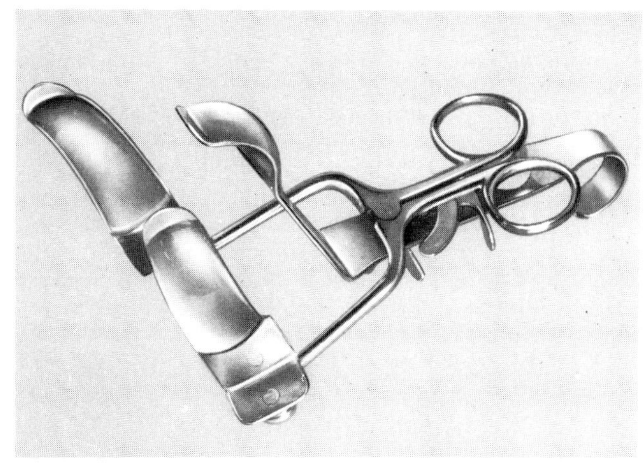

1

Not only is it possible to deal with a lesion directly exposed in the rectum itself but access can often be obtained to more proximal rectal polyps by intussuscepting the rectosigmoid region to the level of the lower rectum or anal canal. An operating sigmoidoscope is not suitable for this as it gives inadequate exposure.

Special angled instruments are available which enable the surgeon to work via this approach without the hands obscuring vision. Illumination may be obtained by a light source attached to the retractor, by a headlamp or by the main theatre light placed behind the operator.

Submucosal excision of sessile adenomas using the peranal route was described in 1966[1]. The same approach has since been used to excise selected carcinomas and to perform an anastomosis between the colon or ileum and the anal canal. The latter can be carried out with precision and is especially useful when an abdominal anastomosis is difficult or impossible.

SUBMUCOSAL EXCISION OF SESSILE ADENOMA OF THE RECTUM

Principle

A sessile adenoma is a benign mucosal lesion and thus only the mucosa needs to be excised for its removal. This is possible owing to the distensibility of the submucosa which only contains blood and lymphatic vessels with loose areolar tissue. In its natural state it is approximately 1 mm thick but by submucosal infiltration of physiological saline, it may be distended to some 2 cm thick. The adenoma is lifted along with the submucosa from the underlying circular muscle and can then be excised by dissecting with scissors in the fluid-filled submucosal plane. This should be carried out as close to the mucosa as possible to avoid blood vessels although the addition of adrenaline 1:300 000 to the solution prevents most bleeding. The tumour can be removed without any damage to the circular muscle.

Preoperative assessment

The entire colonic mucosa of a patient with a sessile adenoma of the rectum should be considered to be unstable. In approximately 10 per cent of cases there is a synchronous tumour at some other site in the large bowel. It is therefore essential to have a barium enema examination or endoscopy before treatment to detect the presence of other neoplastic lesions, benign or malignant.

It is usually possible to identify a sessile adenoma of the rectum by palpation. If the lesion is entirely soft then it is probably benign. Ulceration or indurated areas indicate that malignant change may have occurred and it is important to take a sigmoidoscopic biopsy (*1*) to confirm the diagnosis of adenoma and (*2*) to attempt to diagnose malignant invasion if suspected. Unfortunately the pathological report of a benign lesion does not rule out the possibility of malignancy elsewhere in the tumour and removal of large pieces of tumour for biopsy may interfere with the submucosal excision by obliterating the submucosal space (especially if diathermy is used). Unless malignancy is confirmed on the biopsy it is better to perform a total excision of the tumour and to subject this to pathological examination.

A palpable sessile adenoma can almost always be removed per anum, although extensive tumours of the entire rectum or lower sigmoid may require a combined abdominal approach (*see Illustration 10*). It is not generally recognized, however, that many impalpable tumours located in the upper rectum and lower sigmoid can also be removed per anum, delivering the tumour into the field of operation by intussuscepting the proximal bowel (*see Illustrations 11 and 12*).

Preoperative preparation

It is essential that the rectum is empty of faeces and the patient should receive an enema containing a contact laxative the night before and a few hours before the operation.

Anaesthesia and position of the patient

The operation is performed under general anaesthesia, using muscle-relaxing drugs to allow the anal canal to be readily dilated. It may be done with equal facility with the patient in the lithotomy or the jackknife position, although the latter may give better exposure of anterior tumours.

The operation

2

Insertion of the retractor

The retractor is gently inserted into the anus and when fully in position the blades are slowly opened. A third blade can be inserted and is particularly valuable if the tumour is proliferative and bulky.

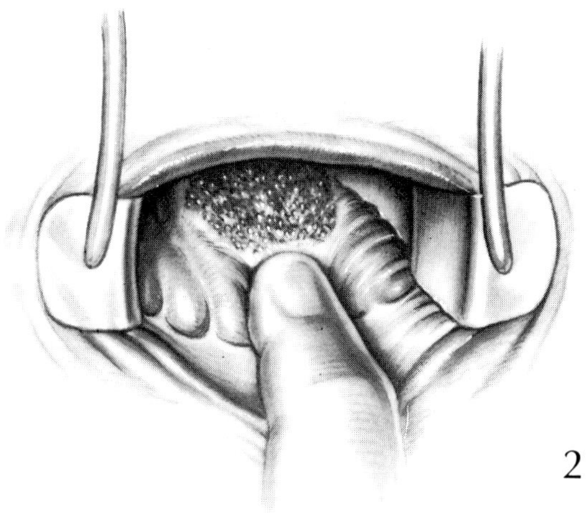

2

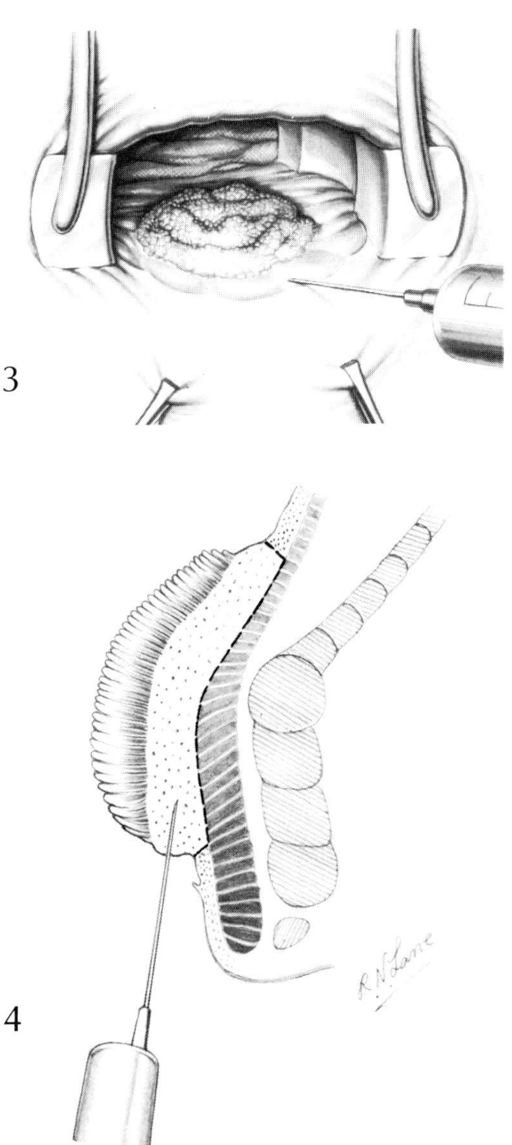

3

4

3 & 4

Injection of the submucosal plane

Several millilitres of isotonic saline containing adrenaline 1:300 000 are injected into the submucosa by placing a needle into this layer 1–2 cm away from the tumour itself. The solution rapidly spreads in all directions and the adenoma is seen to be lifted off the underlying muscle.

5 & 6

Excision of the adenoma

A 1 cm margin of adjacent normal mucosa is excised with the tumour. Injection of the submucosal plane renders the mucosa tense and small extensions of the tumour which would otherwise be overlooked are rendered obvious and can be removed. An incision is made about 1 cm from the edge of the tumour with sharp-pointed scissors. With the same scissors connective tissue within the oedematous submucosa is divided just deep to the mucosa and the tumour. The tumour should be removed in one piece if at all possible. The edge of the specimen, which is fragile and tears easily, should be handled with care. Fine tissue forceps such as Babcock's are suitable. It may be necessary to inject further quantities of saline-adrenaline solution as it tends to diffuse out from the submucosal plane once the mucosa has been incised. Bleeding points are controlled using diathermy coagulation; even a small amount of blood may obscure the correct plane of dissection.

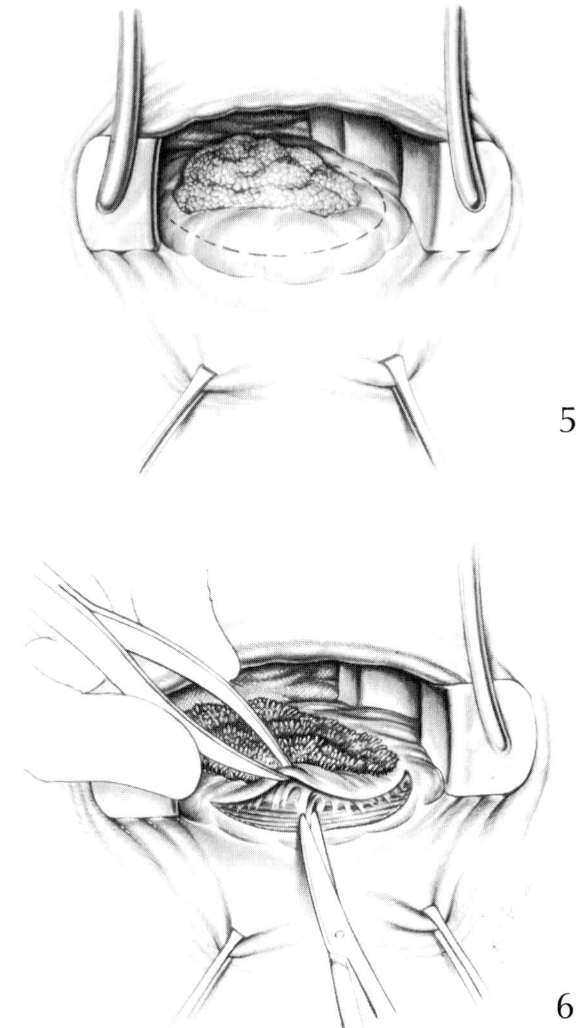

5

6

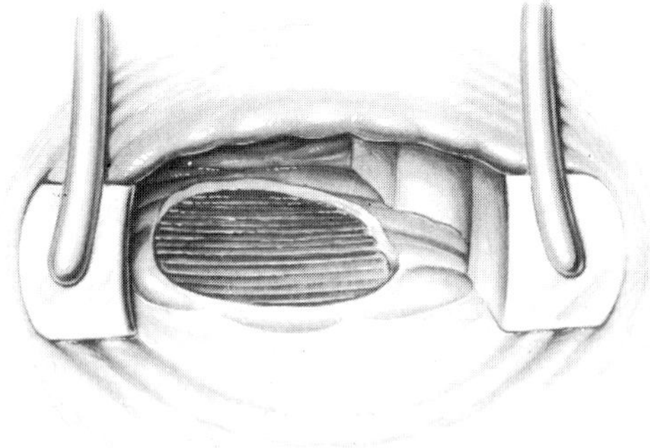

7

7

If the lesion is not circumferential, as is usually the case, the wound may be left open. It will heal without infection or stenosis.

Extensive circumferential lesions

The technique is almost identical to that described above with the obvious difference that the whole tumour cannot be exposed at one time. It is therefore necessary to withdraw the retractor and reinsert it at a different angle in order to excise tumour from an area of rectum not originally seen. Sometimes the tumour can still be removed in one piece but often, especially if proliferative, it may need to be removed in segments.

Should the lesion extend up to 12 or 15 cm it is still possible to excise it by drawing the rectal wall down into the area exposed by the retractors using tissue forceps or stay sutures. Repeated injections of the saline-adrenaline solution are required as new areas of tumour are exposed.

8 & 9

After excision of a circumferential tumour the remaining wound may heal with stricture formation unless the denuded area of muscle is covered with mucosa. Circumferential wounds even 10–12 cm in length can be readily closed by plicating the muscle of the rectal wall with non-absorbable sutures. Commencing at the lower edge of the wound, multiple 'bites' of the circular muscle of the rectum are taken until the upper edge is reached. About 10 such sutures are placed around the rectum and when tied these have a concertina-like effect, drawing the mucosal edges together, which may then be sutured with a layer of catgut stitches.

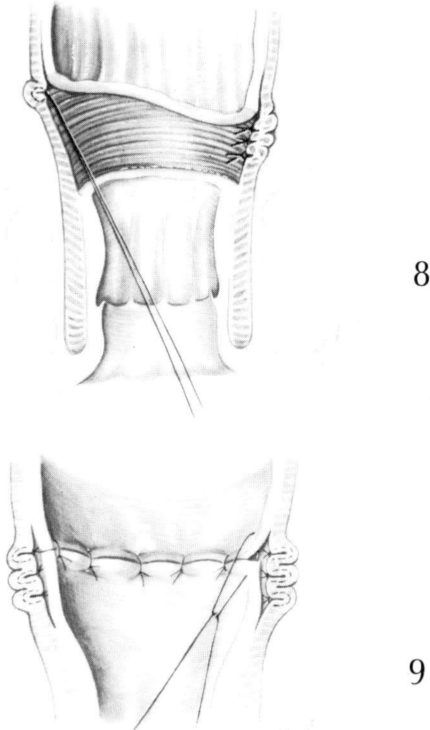

8

9

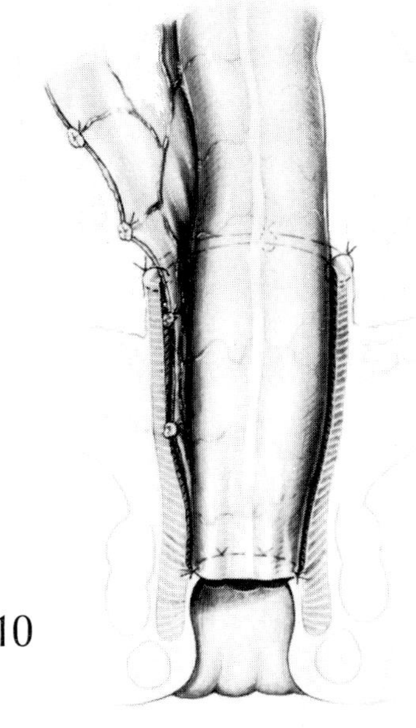

10

10

In a few cases the tumour may extend from the upper anal canal into the lower sigmoid colon when it will not be possible to excise the upper part per anum. As much of the tumour as possible should be removed using the technique described above but the part of the tumour in the upper rectum and sigmoid will require an abdominal approach. An abdominal incision is made, and after mobilization the rectum is transected at a point distal to that reached by the submucosal excision carried out per anum. The remainder of the adenoma is removed by resection of the upper rectum and sigmoid colon and the descending colon is brought through the muscle tube of the rectal stump which has already been denuded of mucosa down to the upper anal canal. Bowel continuity is restored by carrying out a peranal coloanal anastomosis as described on p. 551 in this volume.

Sessile adenomas of the upper rectum and lower sigmoid

It may be possible to deliver tumours at these levels into the lower rectum by intussusception of the rectosigmoid by traction. The direct access to the tumour afforded then permits a submucosal excision as described above.

11

The anal retractor is passed as for excision of a low rectal sessile adenoma. A wide-bore sigmoidoscope is then introduced through the parted blades of the anal retractor and advanced to the level of the lesion. The tumour or neighbouring mucosa is grasped by long 'crocodile' sigmoidoscopy forceps and the sigmoidoscope and forceps are then gently withdrawn together, causing intussusception of the bowel.

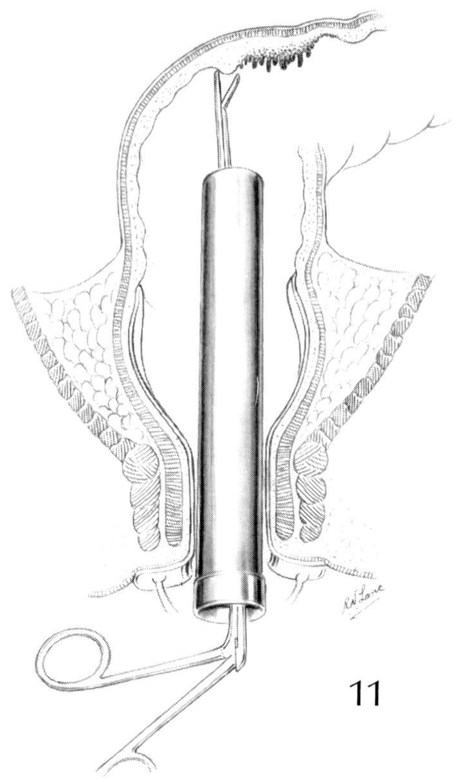

11

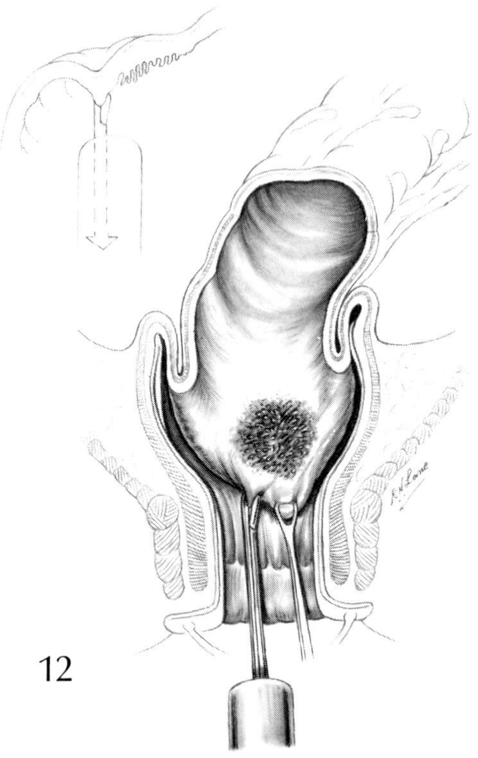

12

12

The sigmoidoscope is removed over the shaft of the forceps enabling tissue forceps of the Babcock pattern or stay sutures to be applied to the edge of the tumour which is now situated at the level of the lower rectum or anal canal.

13

The long forceps are released and submucosal excision carried out.

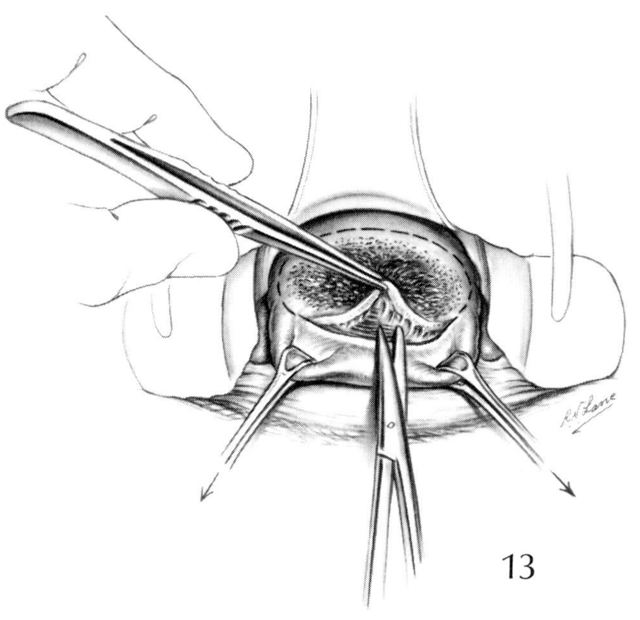

13

Preparation of the specimen for the pathologist

The surgeon should pin out the excised specimen on to a cork board spreading it as widely as possible. It is then fixed in this position by floating the cork upside down in a bath of formaldehyde/saline solution (10 per cent). By this means the histopathologist obtains the specimen in an optimal state for examination which includes a search for possible foci of malignant invasion.

Postoperative care and complications

Patients who have had a purely endorectal excision need no special postoperative care. A normal diet is given immediately and it is wise to administer a hydrophilic laxative to ensure that the initial bowel action is soft.

The commonest complication is haemorrhage from the wound although this is rare if haemostasis has been carefully established. If this occurs it may be necessary to examine the patient under anaesthesia so that the bleeding point can either be under-run with a suture or coagulated with diathermy.

Recurrence

It is well known that villous adenomas have a tendency to recur whatever method of excision is used. This may be a result of either incomplete initial removal or independent growth of another lesion. The patient should therefore be examined by sigmoidoscopy at least every 3 months for the first year and then at 6-monthly intervals indefinitely thereafter. Metachronous lesions elsewhere in the colon may occur after some years and a barium enema examination should be performed at approximately 5-yearly intervals.

LOCAL EXCISION OF RECTAL CARCINOMA

Principle

Avoidance of a permanent colostomy is a laudable aim if cure of the disease is not prejudiced. An elderly patient often finds a colostomy such an indignity both to himself and his family that all possible attempts should be made to avoid it. In recent years local excision has gained an established place in the treatment of selected carcinomas of the lower rectum. A histologically well-differentiated lesion that has not penetrated the full thickness of the rectal wall will have produced lymph node metastases or invasion of extramural veins in about 10 per cent of cases. It is argued therefore that local excision of these tumours is likely to result in the eradication of the disease in 90 per cent of patients. Survival rates obtained indicate the policy of local excision of this selected group of carcinomas is justified.

Preoperative assessment

As with a sessile adenoma, there is an increased chance of a synchronous neoplastic lesion being present and a barium enema examination or endoscopy should be performed. The diagnosis of carcinoma must be obtained by a preoperative sigmoidoscopic biopsy and a well differentiated (low-grade) tumour histology established. Assessment by digital examination is the only means available of determining depth of penetration and involvement of lymph nodes. Only a small tumour or a pedunculated one is suitable for local excision and its size and height above the anal canal must be assessed. Depth of penetration should be limited to the rectal wall as judged by full mobility of the tumour and the absence of any palpable extrarectal spread. Careful palpation of the retrorectal tissues is carried out in an endeavour to detect enlargement of mesorectal lymph nodes, which is a contraindication to local excision.

Once a tumour has been removed in this limited way, the pathologist may report that the excision is inadequate or that the tumour is of a higher grade of malignancy than had been suspected. In this case the procedure must be regarded as an excision biopsy and further, more radical treatment planned. A similar argument, or course, applies to a sessile adenoma found on histopathological examination to contain infiltrating malignancy.

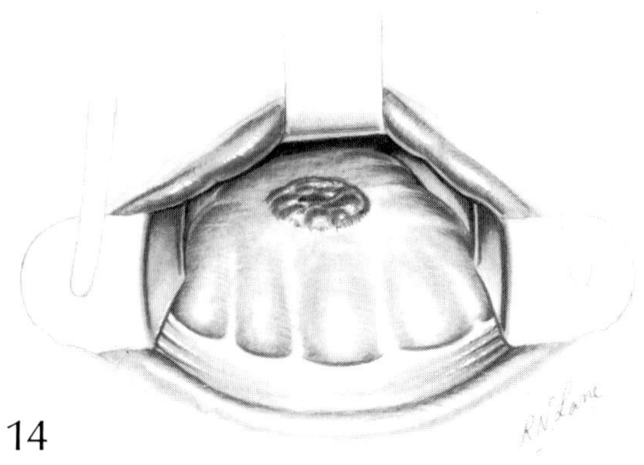

14

The operation

14

Insertion of the retractor

This is done in a similar way to that previously described.

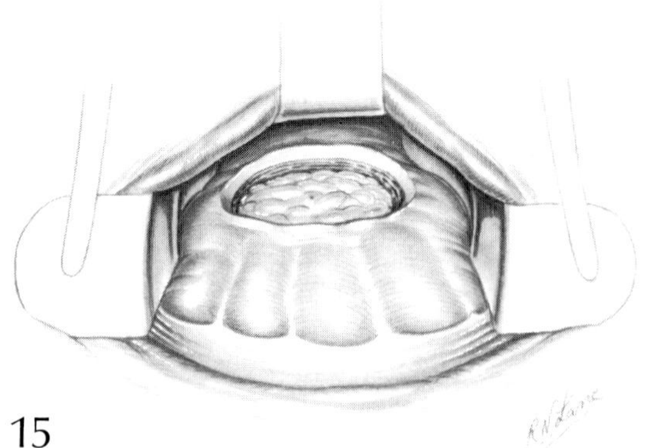

15

15

Excision of the tumour

An incision is made in the normal mucosa about 2 cm away from the edge of the neoplasm. It is necessary to incise the full thickness of the rectal wall and expose the extrarectal fat. Dissection is carried out in the extrarectal fat so that the lesion together with 2 cm of surrounding normal rectum is excised as a disc. Removal is facilitated by infiltrating the extrarectal fat with isotonic saline containing adrenaline 1:300000 which reduces bleeding and therefore improves visibility for the surgeon.

16

Closure of the wound

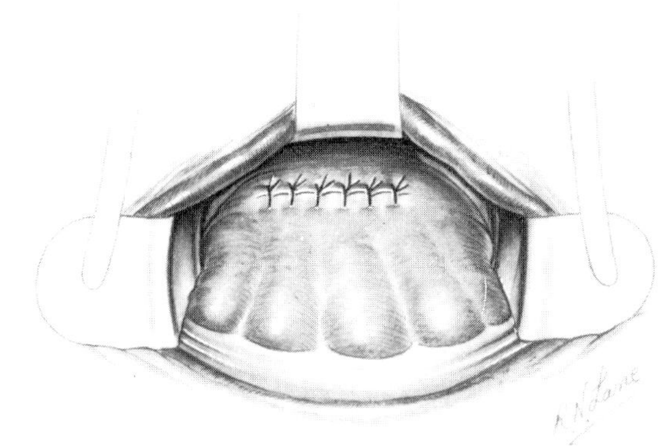

16

Haemostasis must be carefully secured; otherwise, a haematoma will collect in the loose extrarectal tissues causing infection and breakdown of the wound. The wound is closed transversely with one layer of absorbable sutures which should be tied so that the edges of the bowel are just approximated without strangulating tissue.

Sometimes a part of the suture line separates postoperatively leaving a defect which then heals by secondary intention. Spreading infection has so far not been encountered with this technique and if separation occurs this does not usually produce symptoms. There is no special postoperative management other than the avoidance of constipation.

COLOANAL ANASTOMOSIS

Introduction

Major operations for carcinoma of the rectum fall into two groups: total excision of the rectum (with a terminal colostomy) and restorative procedures. Tumours of the lower third usually require excision of the rectum (unless local excision is possible), whereas those of the upper third may be treated by either, depending on the histological grade of the tumour and its local extent. In some patients, particularly men, an abdominal anastomosis may be impossible because the patient's build prevents adequate access to the lower pelvis. In this circumstance the technique of coloanal anastomosis using the peranal route enables the surgeon to restore intestinal continuity.

Principle

The abdominal dissection is identical to that for low anterior resection and after applying a clamp below the tumour and washing out the distal rectum the specimen is removed. The distal ano-rectal stump is then denuded of mucosa down to the dentate line by a perineal operator using the peranal route. In this way a short length of ano-rectal musculature is left proximal to the anal canal. The distal colon is then brought into the upper anal canal and an anastomosis carried out per anum.

Preoperative assessment

In earlier years, patients were carefully selected and the operation confined to those with tumours showing no evidence of extension into the perirectal fat or enlargement of retrorectal lymph nodes. With increasing experience, the operation has been used to treat carcinomas of the middle and occasionally the lower third of Dukes' B and C stages. An anaplastic tumour judged by histological examination of a preoperative biopsy is still considered a contraindication. Full examination of the colon by barium enema is routinely carried out.

Preoperative preparation

This is the same as for any restorative resection. The large bowel must be completely free of faecal material.

Position of patient

The patient should be placed in the lithotomy-Trendelenburg position so that both the abdominal dissection and coloanal anastomosis using the peranal route may be performed without moving the patient.

The operation

Mobilization of left colon

It is advisable to use the descending colon for the anastomosis because the sigmoid colon has a tendency to undergo necrosis in the early postoperative period. The reason for this is not known but it may be that the relatively poor vascularity of the sigmoid is compounded by atheromatous changes in older patients causing the vessels to become readily thrombosed particularly if the blood pressure is temporarily reduced. It is therefore necessary to carry out a mobilization of the distal transverse colon and the splenic flexure and preserve the marginal artery. The inferior mesenteric artery should be divided at its origin from the aorta because, if preserved, these vessels tend to tether the colon when it is brought to the anus.

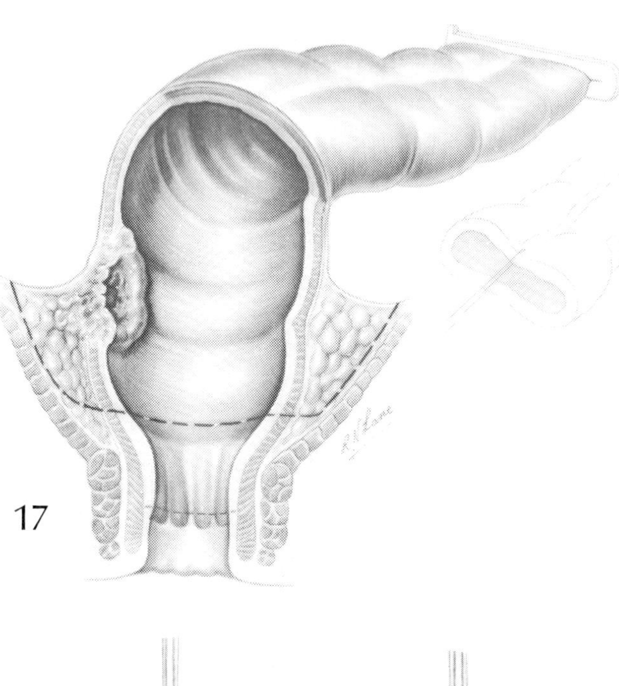

17

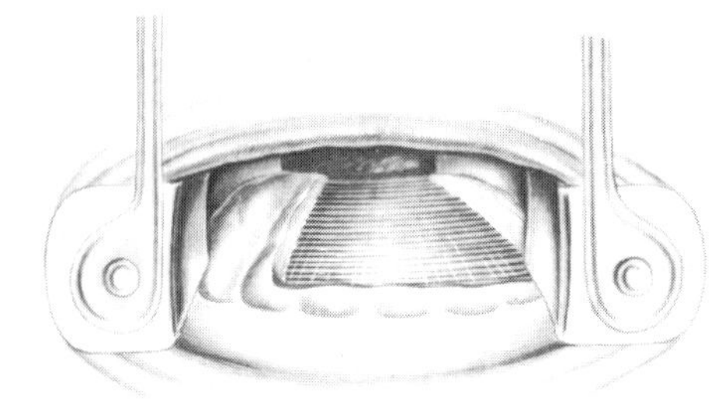

18

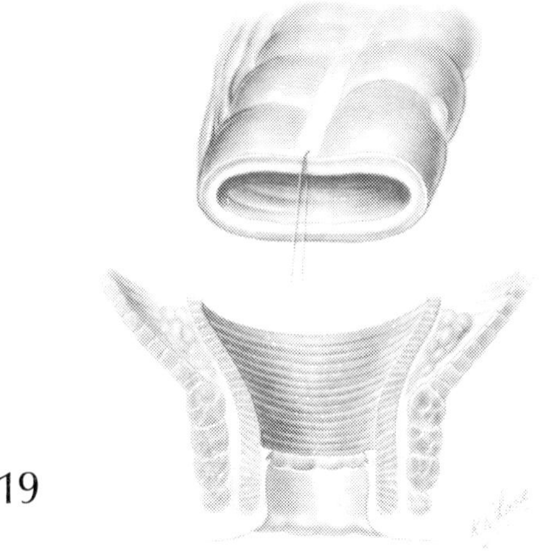

19

17

Rectal dissection

The rectal dissection is performed as for a low anterior resection. It is most important to identify the correct plane anteriorly. In the male an incision is made in the peritoneum behind the bladder just above the peritoneal reflection, and the plane between the seminal vesicles and Denonvilliers' fascia is identified. This plane is pursued by blunt dissection downwards towards the prostate. Blunt dissection laterally sweeps both the vas and the ureter away from the field of operation on each side and exposes the lateral ligaments without risk.

Once the dissection has reached the lower level of the prostate, Denonvilliers' fascia is divided and the dissection continued to the upper part of the anal canal in the perirectal fat to display the levator ani muscle almost entirely. The lateral ligaments are divided and a clamp is placed across the rectum below the tumour, which is often at the level of the anorectal junction. The anorectal stump is irrigated with a cytotoxic agent (e.g. 1:500 mercuric perchloride). In the female the dissection is somewhat easier as the rectovaginal plane can be readily opened down to the anal canal. It is very important to preserve the integrity of the vagina because a rectovaginal fistula may occur if the vaginal mucosa is exposed. The rectum is divided below the clamp and haemostasis is then carefully secured.

18

Removal of mucosa from anorectal stump

The surgeon moves to the perineum to make the anastomosis. The anal retractor is passed and the submucosa from the dentate line to the level of division of the anorectal stump is infiltrated with saline adrenaline solution (1:300 000). The mucosa is excised using sharp-pointed scissors, usually in three or four strips. This dissection is performed as close to the mucosa as possible to avoid submucosal vessels. Complete haemostasis of the denuded anorectum must be secured.

19

Delivery of colon through anorectal stump

Two stay sutures, one on the mesenteric, the other on the antimesenteric border, are placed through the divided end of the colon. These are then passed into the pelvis and through the anal canal to the perineal operator who gently draws the colon into the anorectal stump.

20

The anastomosis

An anal retractor with narrow blades is passed through the anus into the colon. This permits direct exposure of the divided end of the colon above and the proximal limits of the anorectal mucosa below. An anastomosis is then carried out. Interrupted non-absorbable sutures are placed through the anal mucosal edge taking the stitch deep into the internal sphincter and the full thickness of the colon. It is easiest to place a suture in each of four quadrants and then to complete the anastomosis by further sutures between them. About 12–20 sutures are required.

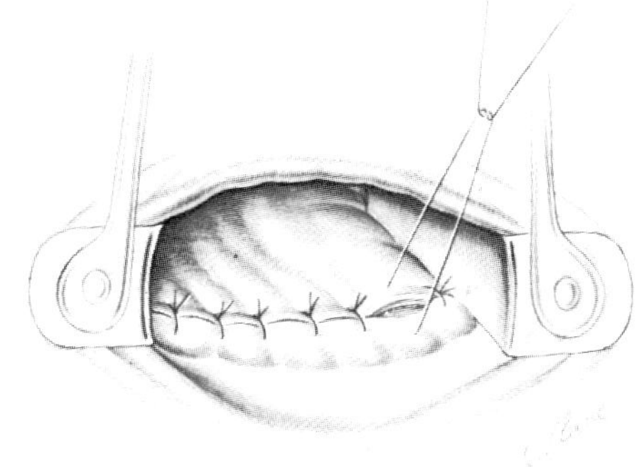

20

21

Final arrangement of colon

To avoid tension it is often convenient to arrange the colon to the right of the small intestine, attaching its mesentery and the mesocolon to the posterior abdominal peritoneum.

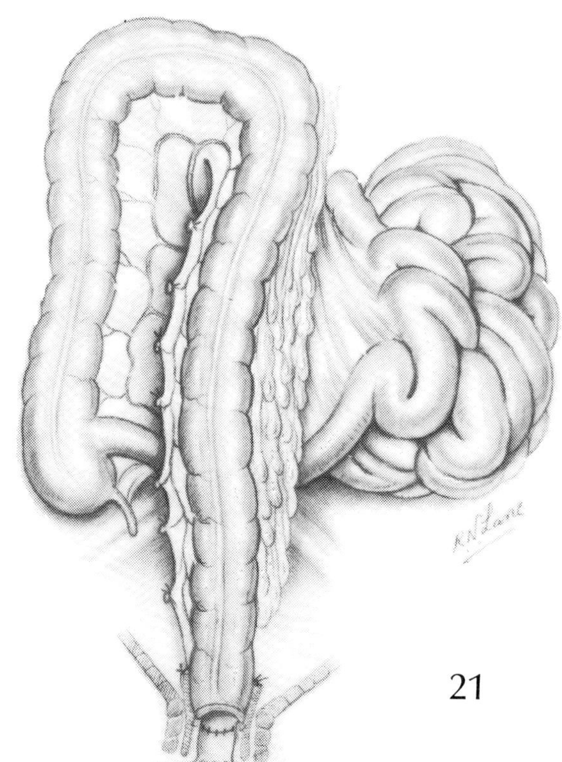

21

Conclusion of the operation

It is essential that good haemostasis is obtained in the pelvis to avoid haematoma formation. Infection leads to a pelvic abscess which may then discharge through the anastomosis. Not only does this increase the morbidity but subsequent fibrosis between the colon and pelvic floor may impair sensation resulting in functional difficulties later. Adequate suction drainage of the pelvis should therefore be established. A temporary loop transverse colostomy or caecostomy is made at the end of the operation.

Postoperative care

This is identical to that following anterior resection. Once the anastomosis has healed satisfactorily, the colostomy may be closed.

Results

There is every indication that rate of survival of patients is similar to that obtained after total rectal excision and anterior resection. There may be some frequency of defaecation with occasional difficulty in controlling loose stool initially after closure of the colostomy; however, after a few weeks to months these problems resolve, frequency being around 2–4 times per 24 h with normal or acceptable continence in 95 per cent of patients.

Reference

1. Parks, A. G. Benign tumours of the rectum. In: Rob, C., Smith, R., Morgan, C. N. Abdomen and rectum and anus. Clinical Surgery, Vol. 10; London: Butterworths, 1966: 541–548

Abdominoperineal excision of the rectum

P. R. Hawley MS, FRCS
Consultant Surgeon, St Mark's Hospital and King Edward VII Hospital for Officers, London

Preoperative

Abdominoperineal excision of the rectum should always be carried out in the lithotomy-Trendelenburg position of Lloyd-Davies as this gives the best exposure and avoids altering the position of the patient during the operation. The procedure can be undertaken by a surgeon and his assistant carrying out the abdominal part of the operation and then proceeding to the perineal excision but it is best carried out synchronously by two surgeons working together.

Indications

Over the last decade the number of abdominoperineal excisions of the rectum undertaken for adenocarcinoma has gradually decreased as more restorative resections have been undertaken. This has been helped by the availability of the circular stapler which has enabled surgeons to carry out lower anterior resections. However, at the present time approximately 30 per cent of rectal carcinomas will require abdominoperineal excision. In most surgeons' hands the operation will also be undertaken for squamous carcinoma of the anal canal and in those carcinomas of the anal verge which cannot be adequately treated by local excision. Occasionally the rectum will be excised for carcinoma when the primary is situated in the vagina or cervix with involvement of the rectum. It should be noted, however, that when the rectum is excised as part of a proctocolectomy for ulcerative colitis and in some patients with Crohn's disease a more conservative method of rectal excision is preferable to avoid damage to the presacral nerves and nervi erigentes with subsequent bladder and sexual dysfunction. Conservative excision of the rectum in inflammatory bowel disease is described on pp. 493–496 in this volume.

Contraindications

The operability rate for rectal cancer however treated should approach 95 per cent of all cases. In a few cases the tumour will be totally inoperable as it will be fixed onto the sacrum or lateral pelvic walls. It is difficult to be certain on clinical examination or even on examination under anaesthesia whether a tumour is really inoperable and a laparotomy and trial dissection are usually justified. A patient with an inoperable tumour will require a palliative defunctioning colostomy. The presence of hepatic metastases is not a contraindication to abdominoperineal excision as this operation usually gives the best local palliation even if the patient has only months to live. Abdominoperineal excision is contraindicated when there is confluent growth in the pelvic peritoneal floor which cannot be removed as this often results in carcinoma growing throughout the perineal wound. It must be remembered that when residual tumour is left within the pelvis with extension of the growth along the lateral ligaments to the pelvic wall, or when the internal iliac nodes are involved, a palliative Hartmann's operation may be a more suitable alternative for the patient.

Unless indicated otherwise the cross-references in this chapter refer to *Operative Surgery: Alimentary Tract and Abdominal Wall, Volume 3, 4th Edition*

Preoperative preparation

The patient is admitted 3 days before the operation for assessment and bowel preparation; the chest is X-rayed and an intravenous pyelogram carried out in advanced tumours. Laboratory tests include a blood count, blood grouping, and estimation of urea and electrolytes. Urine examination is carried out and severe anaemia treated by blood transfusion. It is advisable for the haemoglobin to be at least 11g before an abdominoperineal excision is undertaken. The operation generally requires 4u of blood to be cross-matched. Prostatic obstruction is best dealt with in the postoperative period as all patients require an indwelling Foley catheter during the operation and for the first week postoperatively. Mechanical bowel preparation is carried out in all cases. The author's preference is still to use castor oil 30ml by mouth on the third day before operation together with a low-residue diet. On the second preoperative day the patient is given fluids only by mouth and on the day before the operation the patient receives another 30ml of castor oil and fluids only by mouth. In the majority of cases a rectal wash-out or enema will not be necessary after this preparation. If it is thought necessary a hypophosphate enema (1.5g in 1 litre of water) can be given on the evening preceding surgery. The operation and the immediate postoperative period are covered with broad-spectrum antibiotics such as gentamicin which is given initially with the premedication and intravenous metronidazole commenced during the operation. These are administered intravenously for 48h postoperatively but if the perineal wound is closed by primary suture with suction drainage in a male patient the antibiotics are continued until the suction drainage is discontinued, usually on the fifth postoperative day.

Marking the colostomy

It is important that the site of the colostomy is accurately marked on the day preceding the operation by either the surgeon or a stoma therapist. The author prefers to mark the site of the stoma himself as the satisfactory positioning of the stoma is ultimately the responsibility of the surgeon and many postoperative problems can be avoided by a colostomy which is situated in the optimal position. A suitable colostomy appliance is fixed in the left iliac fossa and at the apex of the infraumbilical fat pad away from the umbilicus and the antero-superior spine. Care is taken to ensure that the colostomy is not situated on a skin crease when the patient is sitting.

Anaesthesia

A suitable general anaesthetic is administered, the particular technique depending upon the preference of the surgeon and anaesthetist. The author has found the technique of intrathecal heroin injection by the anaesthetist after induction to be of great benefit to the patient. The dose of both relaxant and analgesic drugs given during the course of the operation is reduced and the patient is almost pain-free for the first 24h after the operation resulting in considerably more movement and deep breathing with a subsequent reduction in pulmonary complications. Intravenous infusion is essential and is commenced before the start of the operation.

The operation: synchronous method of excision of the rectum

1

Position of patient

The patient is placed in the lithotomy-Trendelenburg position with Lloyd-Davies leg supports and the sacrum is raised on a Vac-Pac positioning pad or a Goligher sacral rest. With the patient in this position two surgeons may work together, one in the abdomen and the other in the perineum, with no hindrance to either.

The position may be used by a surgeon working alone or by two surgeons working synchronously. The distinguishing features between these two methods are the timing of the various procedures and the amount of dissection carried out from either the abdominal or perineal aspect.

A Foley catheter is inserted into the bladder and connected to a Uribag. In males the catheter and scrotum are fixed to the right thigh with adhesive strapping so that the perineum is clear for the surgeon carrying out the perineal resection. The anus is closed by a strong encircling suture of thread or silk (*see Illustration 17*).

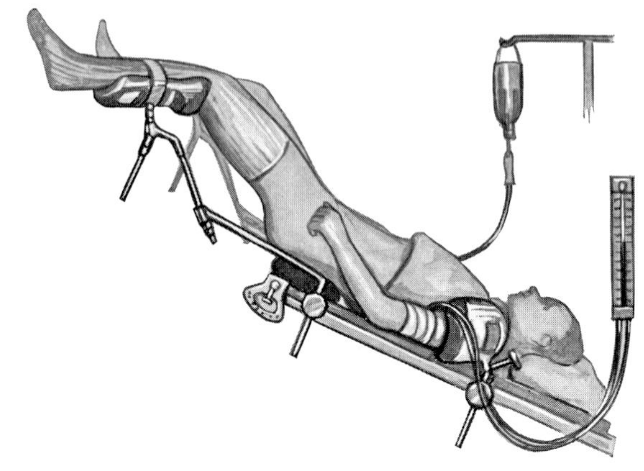

1

ABDOMINAL EXPLORATION AND DISSECTION

2

Colostomy manufacture

If it is certain that an abdominoperineal excision of the rectum will be caried out a colostomy trephine should be made before opening the abdomen. The trephine wound is made through the left rectus muscle at the site previously marked by cutting a disc from the skin 1.5–2.0 cm in diameter, removing a core of subcutaneous fat and cutting a disc from the anterior rectus sheath. In an elderly patient with poor muscles the rectus muscle is not divided. The posterior rectus sheath and peritoneum are then opened with a cruciate incision. Too large a colostomy trephine will result in the common complication of a paracolostomy hernia. The subcutaneous space between the rectus sheath and the superficial fascia is closed with four interrupted catgut sutures.

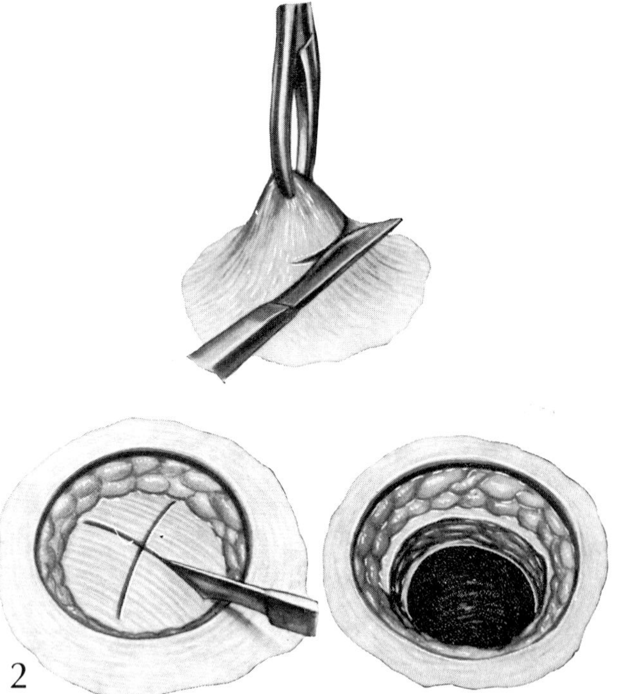

2

3

The incision

The abdomen should then be opened through a long right paramedian incision which extends from the pubis to about 5 cm above the umbilicus, or through a midline incision. The author prefers the right paramedian incision as this keeps the wound as far as possible from the site of the colostomy. Only in those patients in whom a definite decision cannot be reached as to whether continuity can be restored or not should the abdominal incision be made prior to the formation of the colostomy trephine. A midline or left paramedian incision is preferable when an anterior resection is contemplated.

When the abdomen has been opened a thorough systematic examination of all the organs is carried out; the surgeon must look at the liver carefully as small retention cysts can be mistaken for metastases. Definite metastases must be biopsied for histological confirmation. If only one or two small secondary deposits are present close to the liver edge or on its surface and there are no other obvious metastases present in the peritoneal cavity, they may be excised and the defect in the liver closed with a catgut suture using a liver needle. The whole of the peritoneal cavity must be examined carefully, with the mesentery and lateral pelvic walls being inspected for the presence of enlarged lymph nodes. If an abdominoperineal excision is to be undertaken the primary tumour will be situated completely beneath the peritoneal reflexion. The tumour is palpated and its mobility assessed.

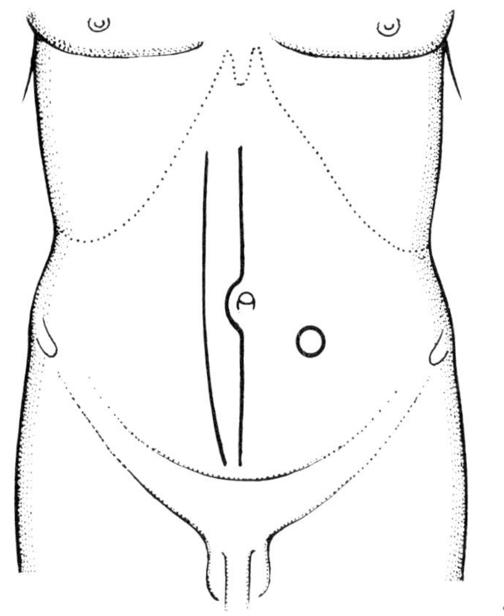

3

4

Extent of bowel removal

This plan of the vascular and lymphatic field which is to be removed shows the usual arrangement of the vessels to be ligated: inferior mesenteric, left colic, transverse colic, middle and inferior rectal.

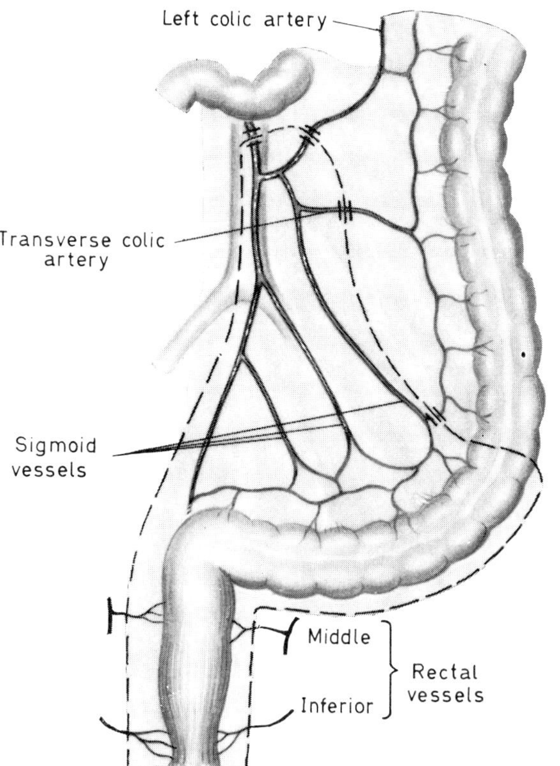

5

Mobilization of the colon

The wound edges are covered with moist packs and a self-retaining retractor of the Comyns–Berkeley type inserted. Small intestine can be packed away in the upper abdomen; or alternatively can be lifted out of the abdomen and placed under a warm pack or in an Aldon bag. The iliac portion of the colon is then mobilized by incising the congenital peritoneal folds attached to the lateral aspect of its mesentery. The left ureter is identified and swept away from the vascular pedicle. The sigmoid colon is retracted to the left and the peritoneum is incised to the right of the midline. The vascular supply of the rectum can now be approached from either side of its mesentery.

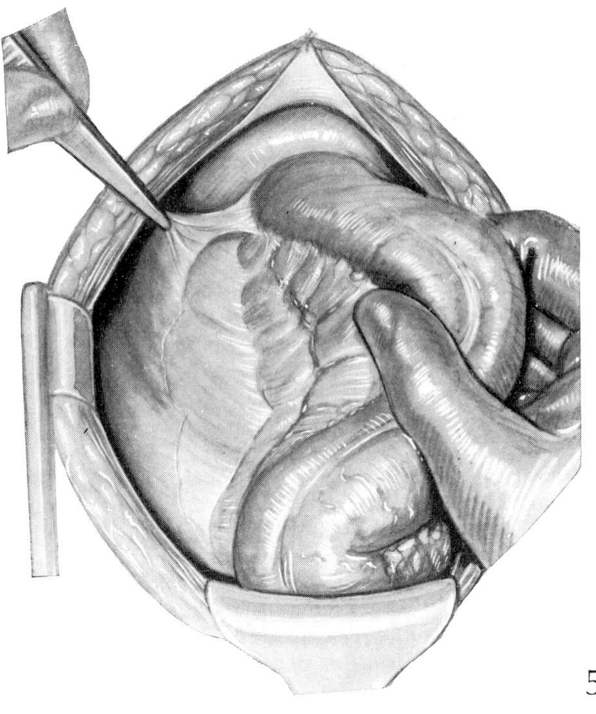

5

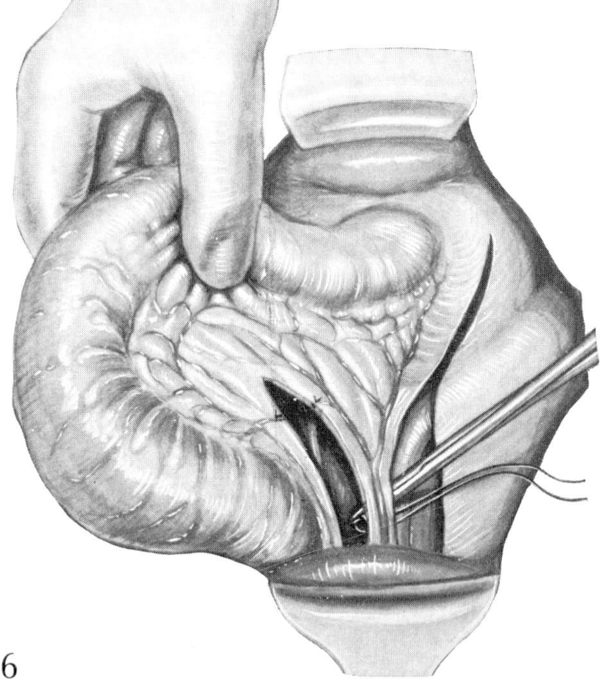

6

6

Ligation of the pedicle

The inferior mesenteric artery and vein are isolated by passing a finger between the mesentery and the anterior surface of the aorta. If lymph nodes are not obviously involved with tumour the presacral sympathetic plexuses should be identified and left intact. In all cases where large nodes are palpable and in tumours of the upper third of the rectum it is advisable to clear all the tissue anterior to the aorta including the sympathetic plexuses. The inferior mesenteric artery should be tied close to its origin from the aorta with thread or silk ligature. The inferior mesenteric vein lying to the left of the artery is then ligated and divided. The colostomy will be supplied by the middle colic vessels often via the bifurcation of the left colic artery (which should be preserved whenever possible) and the marginal artery of the descending colon.

7

Pelvic dissection

No attempt at pelvic dissection should be made until the vessels have been ligated, except in large tumours where an initial trial dissection is carried out to assess if excision is possible. The peritoneal incisions are carried down on each side of the rectum to the level of the vesicles.

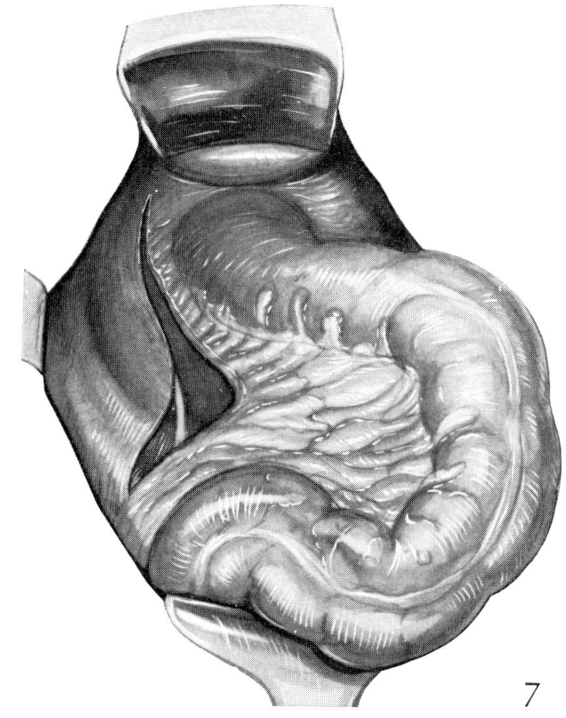

7

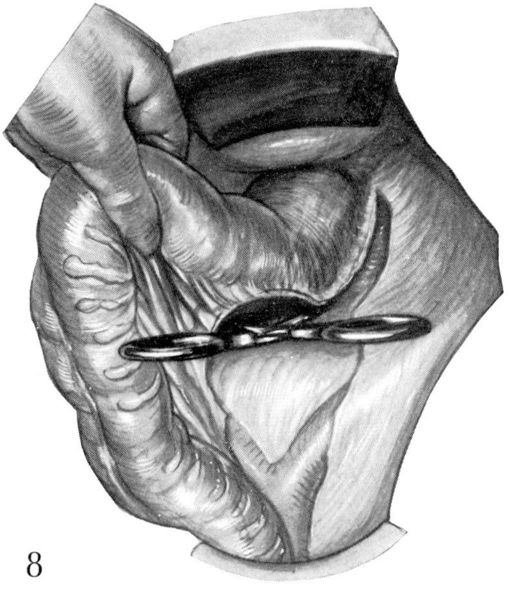

8

8

Production of line of cleavage

The rectosigmoid mesentery is lifted forwards from the promontory of the sacrum and a pair of blunt-ended scissors inserted in the midline downwards and backwards immediately in front of the first piece of the sacrum and behind the mesorectum; a presacral line of cleavage is thus defined.

9

Further mobilization

The fingers and finally the hand are introduced into the presacral space and the mesorectum deliberately pushed forwards from the front of the presacral fascia and the sides of the pelvis as far downwards as the coccyx. Any tough strands of pelvic fascia are divided with scissors. At this stage the abdominal and perineal dissections meet behind the mesorectum, the rectum being completely freed posteriorly (not illustrated).

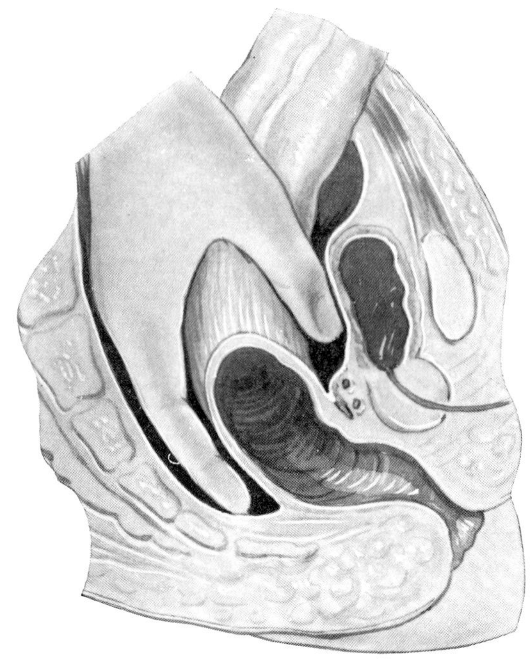

9

10

Peritoneal incisions

The peritoneal and subperitoneal tissues which have been incised on either side of the rectum are now joined anteriorly by dissecting across the peritoneal reflection 1 cm in front of the lowest part of the peritoneal pouch.

The course of both ureters should be carefully noted at this stage and in bulky tumours in the midpelvis both ureters should be exposed throughout their course to the bladder to avoid damage.

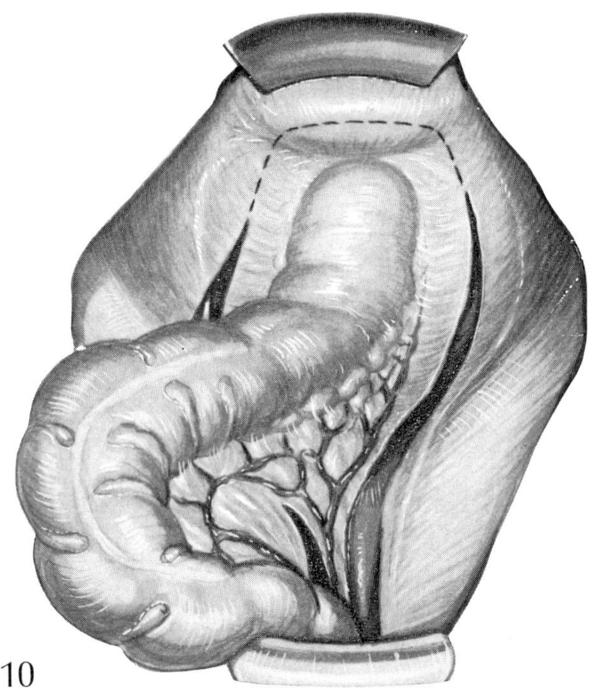

10

11

Incision of the fascia of Denonvilliers

The apex of the incised peritoneum is drawn upwards and the base of the bladder and both vesicles (or vaginal wall in the female) exposed by blunt-nosed scissor dissection. A lipped St Mark's retractor is inserted behind the vesicles which are drawn upwards exposing the fascia of Denonvilliers on the anterior rectal wall. This is incised transversely and a distinct line of cleavage extending downwards as far as the apex of the prostate will be found with the fingers. While in this space the fingers are swept laterally to define the anterior border of the lateral ligaments.

This anterior dissection can be carried out as described before posterior mobilization if the surgeon wishes. This has the advantage that the seminal vesicles and vasa deferentia can be clearly seen and the fascia divided with a completely dry field before commencing the posterior dissection.

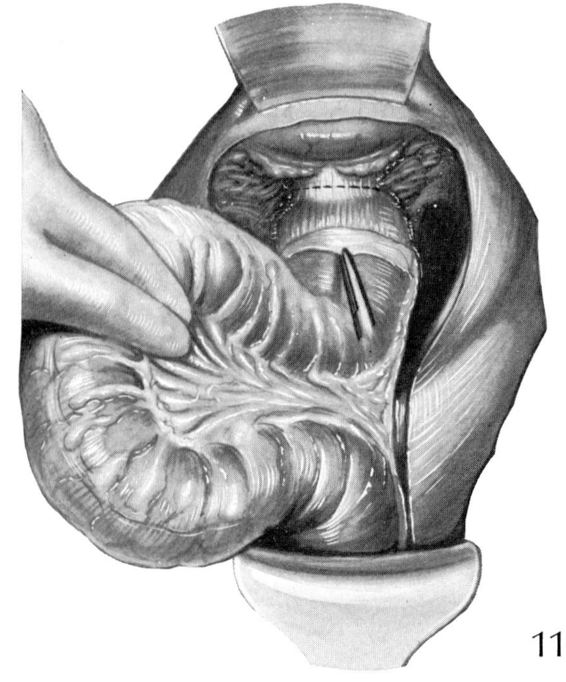

11

12

Division of the lateral ligaments

Each lateral ligament is made taut in turn by displacing the rectum to the opposite side of the pelvis with the left hand and is then divided with scissors well out on the pelvic wall as far downwards as possible. Any remaining inferior portions will be divided by the perineal operator. Middle haemorrhoidal arteries should be picked up and ligated after division. If clamps are placed across the lateral ligament prior to its division incision is usually not so radical as part of the lateral ligament remains protruding from the pelvic wall. Abdominal dissection is now complete and the remaining dissection is left to the perineal operator.

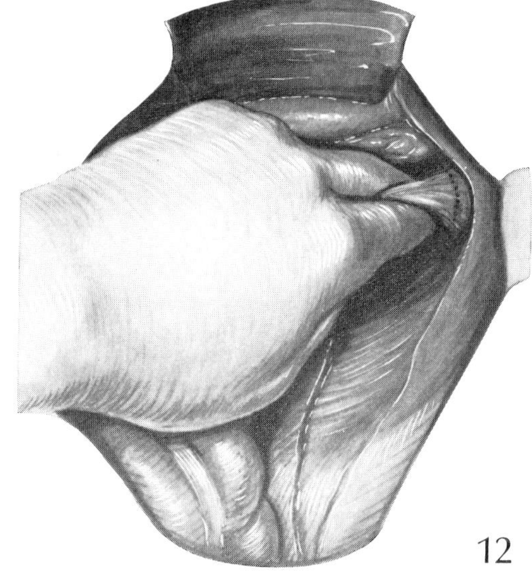

12

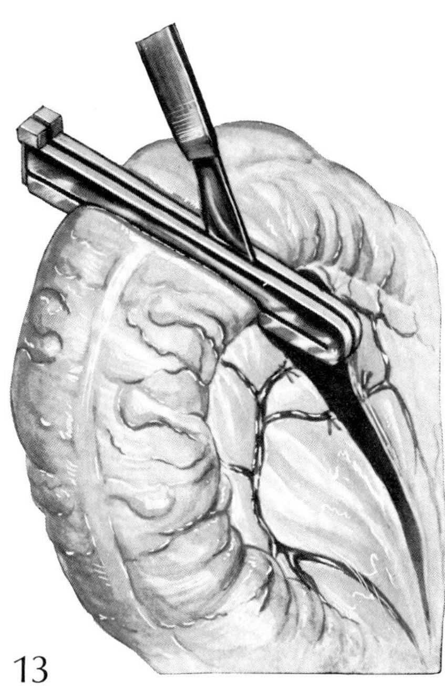

13

13

Division of colon

The colon is prepared for division at a suitable site, the correct length is determined approximately by drawing the descending and sigmoid colon down until it reaches the pubis. This will normally allow a satisfactory length of viable colon and make a colostomy which is raised 0.5 cm from the surrounding skin. If in doubt, particularly in an obese patient, it is much better to have too much colon which can be trimmed before the colostomy is finally constructed, than too little and have the bowel under tension. The mesentery should be divided at right angles to the bowel which is divided between a Zachary-Cope clamp. Perineal dissection having been completed the excised colon and rectum are withdrawn through the perineum.

14

Closure of lateral space and passing the colon through the incision

The left border of the laparotomy wound is now elevated by passing a long forceps through the colostomy incision exposing the paracolic gutter. A non-absorbable thread purse-string suture is inserted from the lateral edge of the colostomy site, including some muscle fibres, and continued under the peritoneum of the paracolic gutter to the mesenteric border of the colon. When the suture is tied the space to the outer side of the colostomy is obliterated preventing small bowel obstruction through what would otherwise be a narrow foramen. The proximal clamped colon is passed through the colostomy incision.

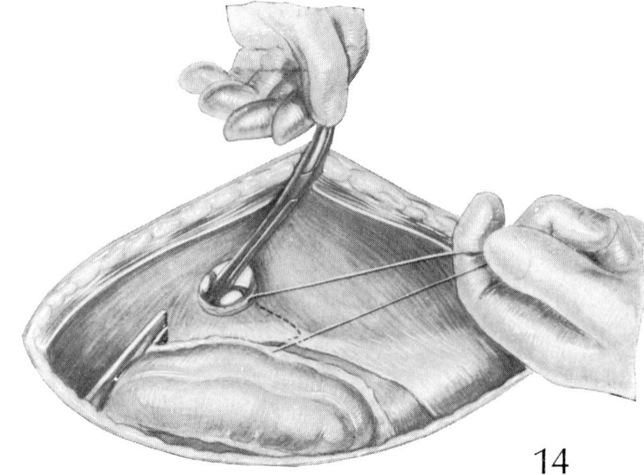

14

15

Closure of the abdomen

Before the pelvic peritoneum can be closed it is important for both the abdominal and perineal operators to obtain complete haemostasis. The pelvis is then irrigated with a suitable chemotherapeutic solution in order to minimize the risk of pelvic recurrence. A solution of 500 ml of 1:500 mercuric perchloride is suitable for this purpose. The peritoneum from the lateral walls of the pelvis and the iliac fossa are gently mobilized with the fingers and the edges sutured together over the empty pelvis by an invaginating continuous Lembert suture to diminish the chance of adhesion formation using 2/0 chromic atraumatic catgut.

The main pedicle ligature is covered during this process and the suture continued laterally between the free edge of the mesocolon and the peritoneum of the left iliac fossa to the point of exit of the colon. The abdomen is closed without drainage and the wound sealed with Whitehead's varnish and a waterproof top dressing.

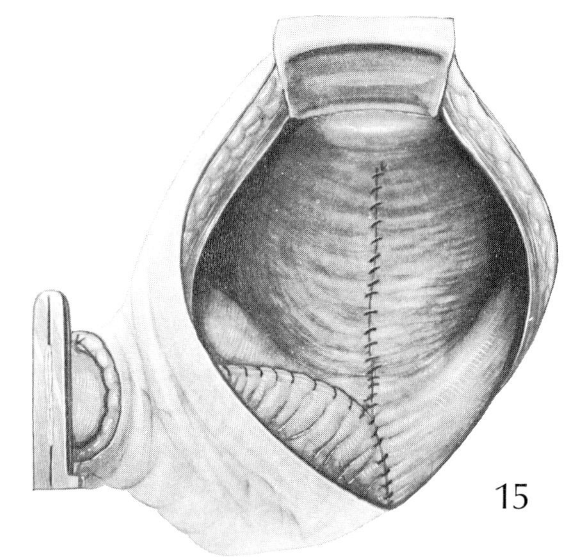

15

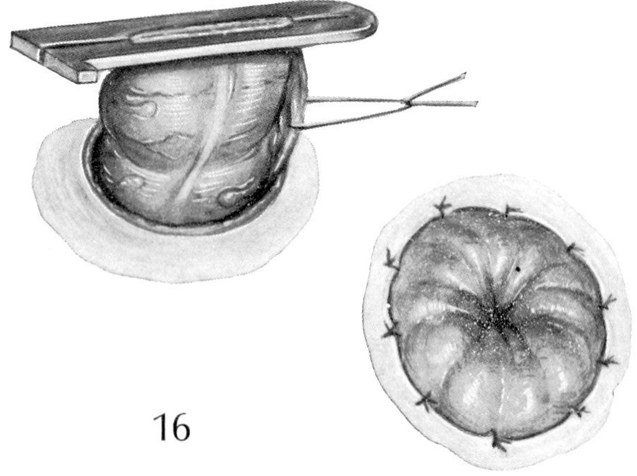

16

16

Formation of the colostomy stoma

The Zachary-Cope clamp is now removed and the colon trimmed to leave 0.5–1 cm projecting above the skin surface. The edges of all coats of the colon are carefully sutured to the surrounding skin with interrupted 2/0 chromic catgut sutures on a cutting needle. This produces a very satisfactory stoma with no tendency to skin stenosis.

PERINEAL DISSECTION IN THE MALE

17

The incision

A swab soaked in 1:500 mercuric perchloride solution is inserted into the anal canal and the anus is then closed with a strong subcutaneous purse-string suture to prevent soiling. No dissection is commenced until the abdominal surgeon has completed the exploration and decided that a combined excision is the correct procedure.

An elliptical incision is made round the anal canal from a point midway between the anus and the bulb of the urethra anteriorly and extending backwards to the sacrococcygeal articulation. This incision is deepened until the lobulated fat of the ischiorectal fossae is seen and the coccyx exposed. Tissue forceps on the lateral margins of the incision and on the anus, pulled appropriately, facilitate dissection of the ischiorectal fossae up to the plane of the pelvic floor muscles.

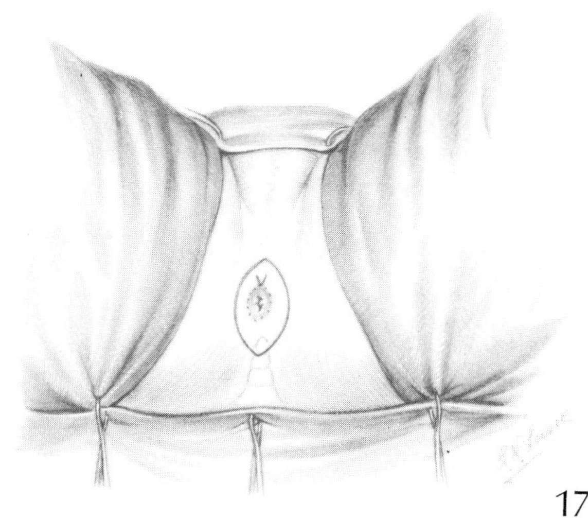

17

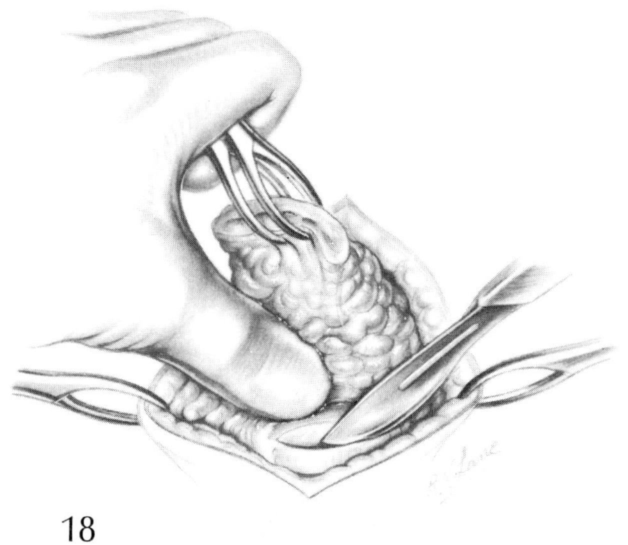

18

18

Removal of part of coccyx

The coccyx is not routinely removed but in males with a narrow pelvis and in patients with a large posterior tumour situated in the lower third of the rectum, removal facilitates the dissection and extends the clearance of the tumour.

The coccyx is flexed with the thumb to open up the sacrococcygeal joint and the point of a scalpel is inserted. The distal portion of the coccyx is separated, care being taken to keep the knife close to the superior surface of the bone to avoid damaging the rectum. The middle sacral vessels may require diathermy coagulation or ligation at this stage.

19

Isolation and division of iliococcygeal muscles

Small lateral incisions are made with a scalpel on either side of the coccyx through the fibrous attachment of the coccygeal muscles and a finger is inserted on each side in a forward and outward direction to separate the levator muscles from the underlying rectal fascia of Waldeyer. The overlying ischiorectal fossa fat and the iliococcygeus muscles are now divided well out on the lateral walls of the pelvis. The inferior haemorrhoidal vessels require diathermy coagulation or ligation.

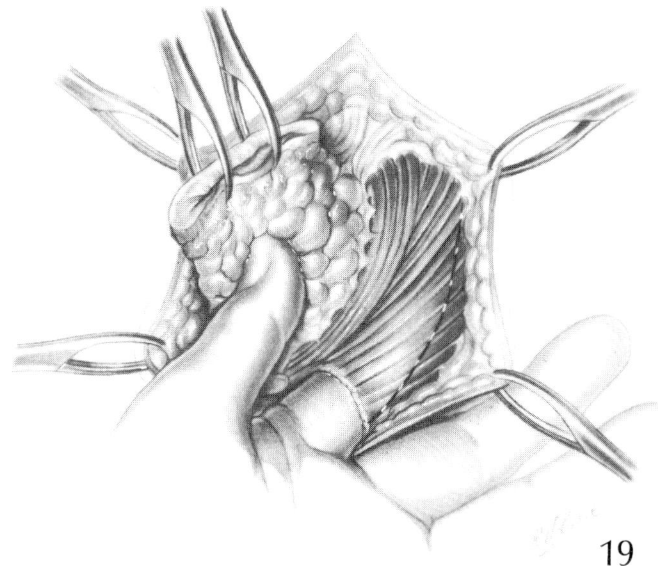

19

20

Exposure of mesorectum

A St Mark's pattern self-retaining perineal retractor is then placed in position and the fascia of Waldeyer, which can be clearly seen, incised just in front of the divided coccyx. If this fascia is not divided the presacral fascia will be stripped from the sacrum producing nerve damage and severe haemorrhage from the presacral venous plexus. This incision is continued laterally at the outlet of the bony pelvis to expose the mesorectum.

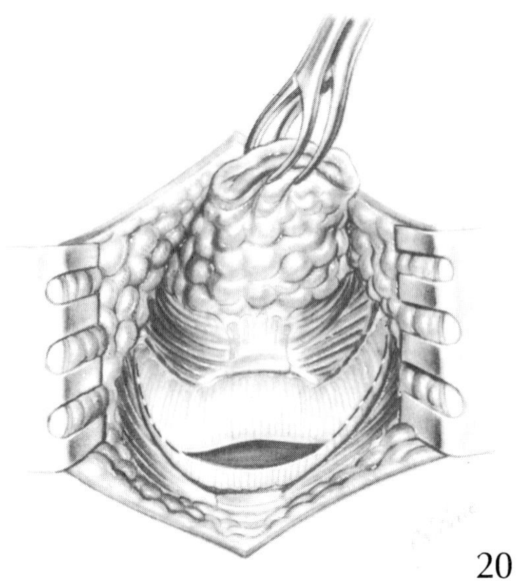

20

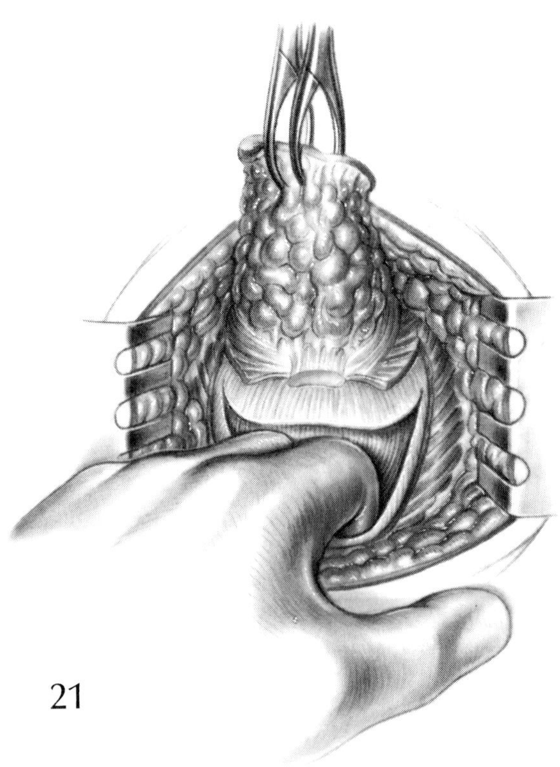

21

21

Separation of mesorectum

The fingers are inserted in front of the cut edge of the fascia and the mesorectum can be separated from the front of the presacral fascia and the lateral pelvic walls to the level of the sacral promontory.

Perineal and abdominal operators meet in this plane at this stage in the operation (*see Illustration 9*), the rectum being completely freed posteriorly.

22

Anterior dissection

The rectum is then retracted posteriorly and transverse incisions are made from either side of the wound to expose the superficial and then the deep transverse perineal muscles. The plane of the dissection must be behind these muscles to avoid injury to the urethra, and when the deep transverse perineal muscles are completely exposed by dividing the decussating fibres of the external sphincter muscle, whitish longitudinal fibres of the anterior rectal wall will be seen.

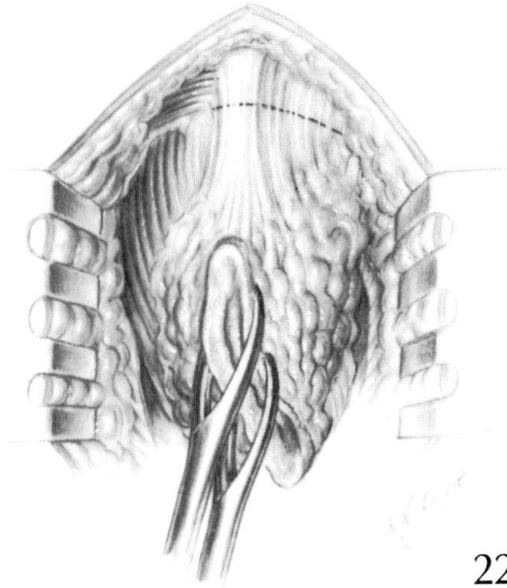

22

23

Separation and division of pubococcygeus muscles

The broad strap-like pubococcygeus muscles now become evident on either side of the rectum and prostate or vagina. A finger is inserted between the superior borders of these muscles, separating them from the underlying pelvic fascia while they are being divided almost completely from their origins as far lateral as possible on each side.

The underlying fascia, which is the lateral continuation of the fascia of Denonvillier and Waldeyer, is divided to expose the rectal wall. The prostate will then be clearly felt anteriorly and the plane between the rectum and prostate defined. If the surgeon does not cut this fascial layer he will not enter the plane between the rectum and prostate and his dissection will be carried forward lateral to the prostate, producing a deep fossa anterior and lateral to the prostate and causing an unnecessary large wound and increased bleeding which can be difficult to control.

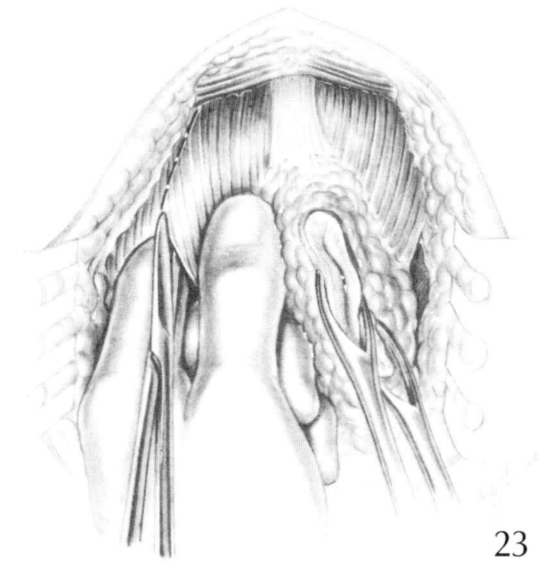

23

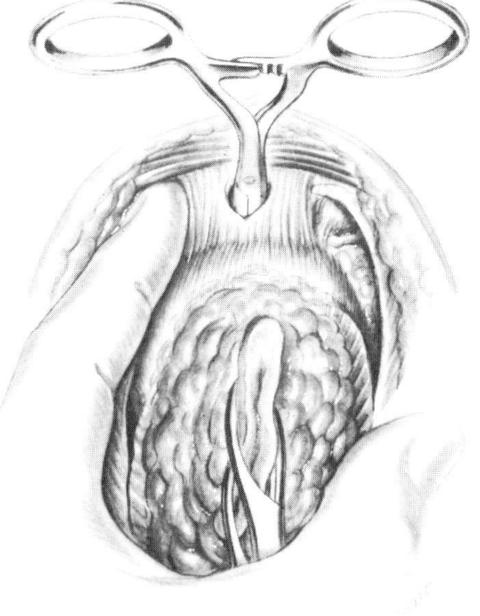

24

24

Separation and division of fibromuscular bundle

The thick anteroinferior borders of the puborectalis muscles, together with longitudinal muscle fibres passing from the anterior rectal wall to the apex of the prostate and membranous urethra (rectourethralis muscle), still hold the anorectal junction forwards in the middle line.

This barrier is separated into two bundles by blunt dissection with an artery forceps. The forceps are directed towards the apex of the prostate which is located with the index finger of the left hand and must lie parallel with the posterior aspect of the gland to avoid injury to the urethra. The separated fibromuscular bundles are divided in turn and the capsule of the prostate exposed.

Occasionally a few readily recognized longitudinal fibres obscure the capsule and require separate division to avoid injury to the rectum and expose the true plane of cleavage which will already have been found by the abdominal operator.

25

Division of pelvic fascia

The visceral pelvic fascia, which is condensed anteriorly and passes forward to the lateral aspects of the prostate, is divided, exposing the whole of the posterior aspect of the prostate and then the seminal vesicles above. At this stage the abominal and perineal operators meet anteriorly.

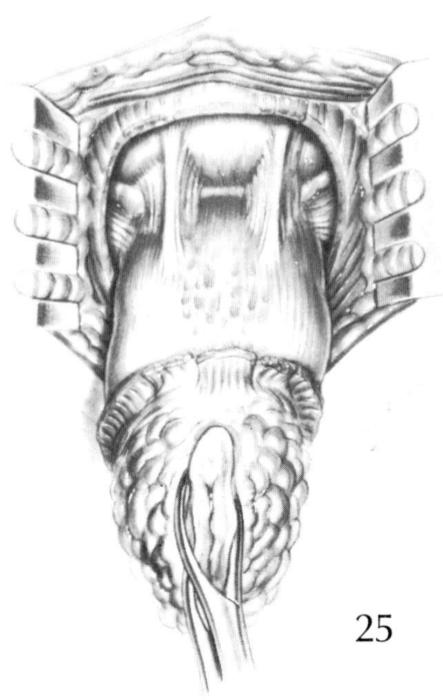

25

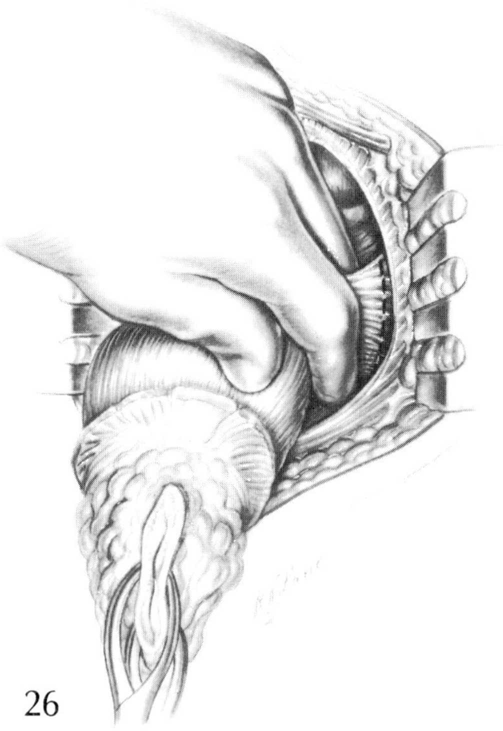

26

26

Removal of rectum

The anterior and posterior aspects of the rectum are now completely isolated and only the remaining lower portions of the lateral ligaments require division. The bowel is alternatively displaced to the opposite side and the stretched ligament divided close to the pelvic wall. The excised rectum and sigmoid colon is then passed down from the abdomen and removed through the perineum. Haemostasis is secured and to avoid the risk of reactionary haemorrhage the patient's blood pressure at this stage of the operation should not be much lower than normal. Open veins may be located by levelling the table.

Closure of perineal wound

27

In the majority of cases the perineal wound in males can be completely closed. No attempt is made to suture the levator muscles which cannot be approximated if a wide excision has been carried out. Really good haemostasis must be obtained. A large suction drainage tube of the sump type, such as the Shirley or the Fuller-Elliott drain, is inserted into the pelvis through a lateral stab wound and positioned to lie in the sacral hollow. The wound is closed with interrupted subcutaneous sutures of 3/0 Dexon or Vicryl and the skin closed with small vertical mattress sutures of a similar material. Continuous suction is started immediately and continued for 5 days. The wound is sealed with gauze dressing using Whitehead's varnish and adhesive tape and left undisturbed. Sutures may be left or removed on the tenth postoperative day but in a heavy and obese patient they should be left undisturbed.

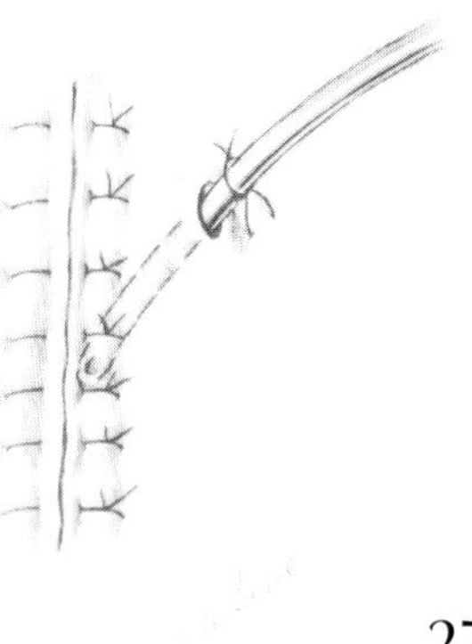

27

28

In a few patients where good haemostasis has not been achieved or there has been pre-existing sepsis or soiling due to perforation of the rectum, the wound can be closed as shown. Skin anteriorly and posteriorly is closed with vertical mattress sutures of Dexon or Vicryl leaving a space in the middle of the wound through which three fingers can be inserted. A corrugated drain is placed into the pelvic cavity through this open aspect of the wound and sutured to the skin. It is only necessary to pack the perineal cavity firmly with dry gauze in the rare case where severe haemorrhage persists and cannot otherwise be controlled; this is removed 3 days later.

When the pelvic floor cannot be closed in any way a thin plastic bag lightly packed with gauze is inserted into the pelvic cavity to prevent downward prolapse of the small intestine, and is left in place for 3–5 days.

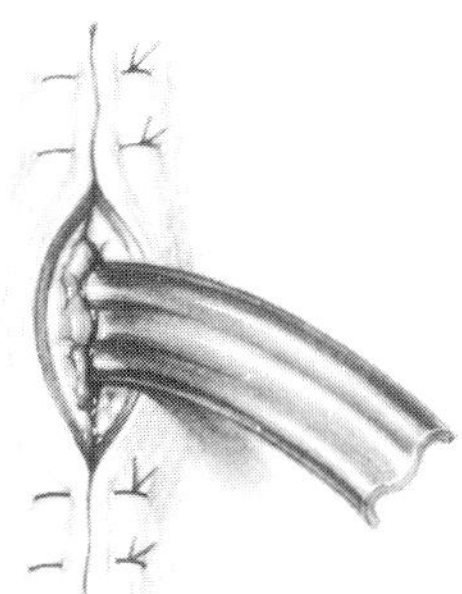

28

PERINEAL WOUND DISSECTION IN THE FEMALE

29

The incision

In excision of the rectum for malignant disease, unless the tumour is small and situated in the midline posteriorly, the posterior vaginal wall should always be excised in continuity with the rectum. Attempts to preserve the vagina result in inadequate clearance of the tumour and an increased pelvic recurrence rate with metastases in association with the lateral or posterior vaginal walls. The incision therefore extends from the posterolateral aspects of the labia around the anus to the coccyx.

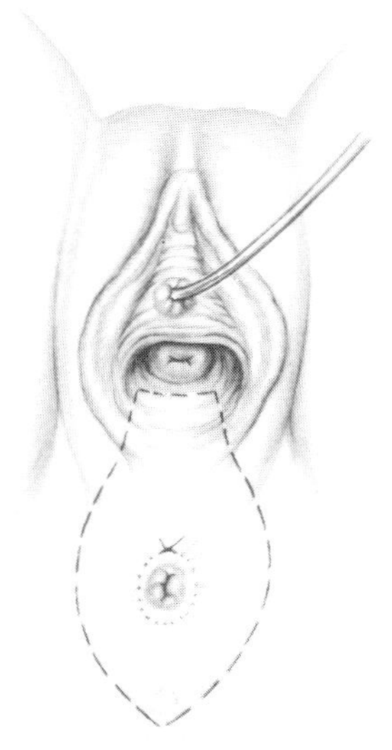

29

30

The extent of the anterior dissection

Excision of the rectum proceeds as in the male until the anterior part of the dissection is reached. The anterior incisions are then carried upwards through the lateral aspects of the vagina as far as the posterior fornix. A transverse incision is then made through the posterior fornix to join the two lateral incisions. This is deepened to expose the rectal wall, at which point the abdominal and perineal operators meet anteriorly. The lateral ligaments are divided and the specimen removed.

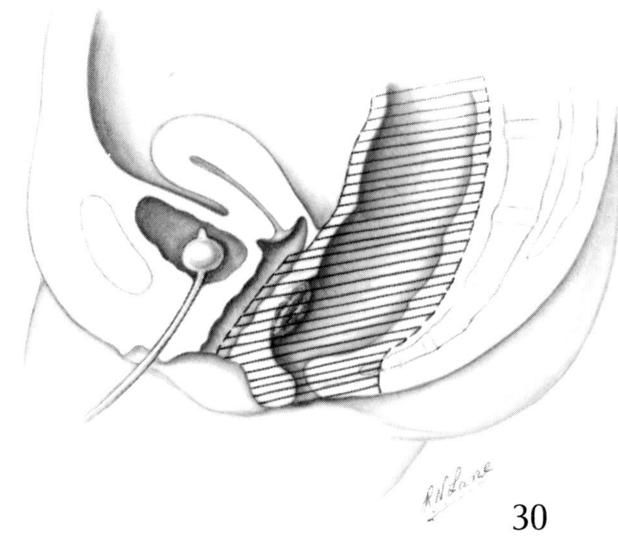

30

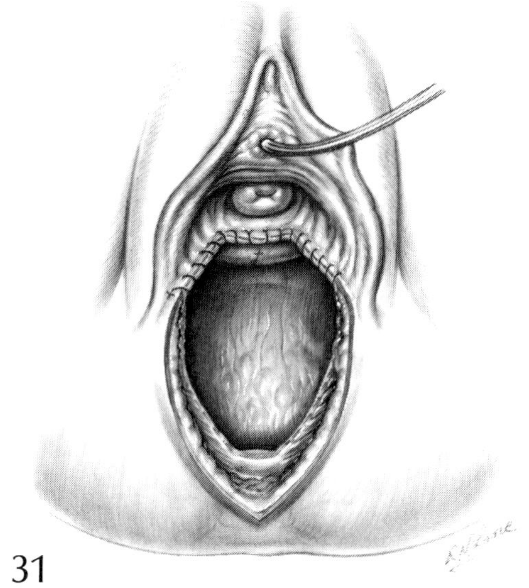

31

31

Haemostasis

No attempt at reconstructing the vagina is necessary. Haemostasis is attained by oversewing each half of the cut edge of the vagina with a continuous 2/0 chromic catgut suture.

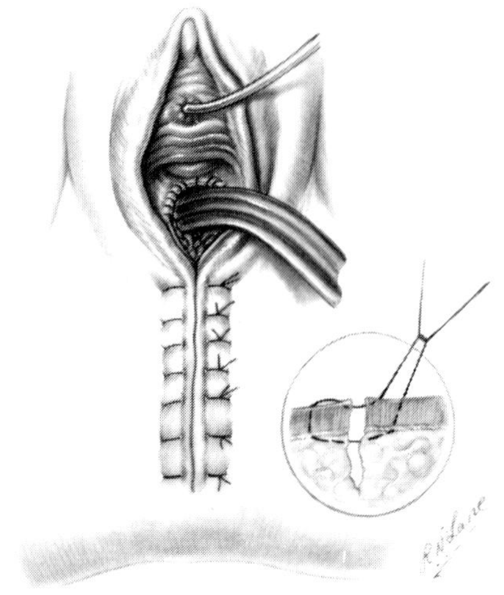

32

32

Perineal closure

As in the male no attempt is made to approximate the cut edges of the levator muscle. The incision is closed by suturing the subcutaneous tissue with interrupted 3/0 Dexon or Vicryl sutures and the skin is closed with interrupted vertical mattress sutures of the same material. The wound is sutured as far forward as the cut edges of the labia which are approximated to leave an orifice that will take three fingers. A corrugated drain with a suction catheter of the Shirley type sutured to it is placed into the pelvic cavity through the reformed vaginal orifice and sutured to the edge of the labia to keep it in place. The suction catheter has the great advantage of obviating the need for repeated dressings.

Postoperative care and complications

These are of particular importance after operations which have included removal of the rectum because not only may the patient suffer from any of the complications of a major abdominal operation but, in addition, the colostomy, urinary tract and perineal wound require special attention.

Intravenous infusion

The infusion of whole blood given during the operation may be continued afterwards. It is followed by intravenous dextrose and electrolyte solutions until normal peristalsis returns and flatus is passed through the colostomy which usually occurs between the third and fifth postoperative days.

Gastric complications

Gastric aspiration through a nasogastric tube is unnecessary in the majority of patients. Small quantities of water by mouth are commenced as the postoperative ileus is relieved.

The perineal wound

The perineal wound is closed with suction drainage in most male patients. The dead space between the skin and the pelvic peritoneum will be obliterated more rapidly if the patient is encouraged to sit up or if the head of the bed is raised as soon as the general condition of the patient permits. Continuous suction is maintained until drainage is minimal usually after a period of 5 days. The suction catheter is then removed. The Dexon sutures in the skin, though soluble, become uncomfortable and may be removed on the tenth postoperative day or later when sound healing has occurred. If the wound has been closed by only partial suture with a corrugated drain this is removed after 3 days, the Dexon sutures remaining until the wound is soundly healed. If it has been found necessary to pack the wound to keep the small intestine from prolapsing the gauze is gradually removed from the plastic bag during the first 3–5 days after which the bag itself is removed. This can be done in the ward without pain. If the wound has been packed with gauze directly to stop severe haemorrhage it can usually be removed on the third postoperative day. This should be done in the operating theatre under a general anaesthetic so that the wound can be thoroughly examined and any residual bleeding points secured. Secondary suture of the wound may be worthwhile.

Retention of urine

In any radical operation some temporary or permanent damage to the nerves of the bladder is inevitable. All patients have an indwelling catheter of the Foley type connected to a sterile plastic bag on open drainage. The catheter is usually removed on the fifth to seventh day and a trial made to establish normal micturition. This may be helped by distigmine bromide or similar drug by injection. Those who fail are given open drainage as before for another 24–48 h when a further trial is made. The process may be repeated several times and even when micturition appears to be established it is important to ensure that there is little or no residual urine. If normal micturition cannot be established cystoscopy and a transurethral resection of the prostate will normally be required. Those with complete bladder paresis may also be assisted by a small transurethral resection. Bladder emptying is then accomplished at regular intervals by suprapubic pressure. The need for this, however, is uncommon.

The colostomy

The action of the colostomy is usually spontaneous and it will be found that on the fourth or fifth day after the operation flatus will be passed. Should delay occur a glycerin suppository may be inserted into the colon, but in the absence of distension it is usually wise to leave the bowel alone until it begins to function normally. Only occasionally will an enema be required. A transparent adhesive colostomy appliance will have been placed over the colostomy at the end of the operative procedure. No other dressings are required, though the colostomy stitches should be removed in 10 days if they have not resorbed.

Hartmann's operation

J. D. Griffiths MS, FRCS
Consultant Surgeon, St. Bartholomew's Hospital and The Royal Marsden Hospital, London

Preoperative

Introduction

The principle of Hartmann's operation is the excision of the upper two-thirds of the rectum and sigmoid colon with the construction of a left iliac colostomy and closure of the lower third of the rectum which is left *in situ*, along with the pelvic floor. This operation was first described by Hartmann[1] and was the operation of choice for carcinoma of the upper and middle thirds of the rectum before anterior resection became a safe procedure. Hartmann's operation need rarely be performed in modern practice – now being the operation of choice only where anterior resection or abdominoperineal resection are contraindicated.

Advantages

The advantage of Hartmann's operation in diverticulitis is that it enables removal of the diseased area of bowel which allows inflammation to settle before performing an end-to-end anastomosis. It has advantages over the staged operation in which the transverse diversionary colostomy leaves the affected bowel *in situ*. This procedure is often followed by attacks of infection which delay excision of the area and subsequent anastomosis.

This operation may also be performed with safety when the bowel has not been prepared. (see chapter on 'Management of the obstructed bowel', pp. 210–229)

Indications

Hartmann's operation is indicated in two main groups of patients.

1. Those patients with carcinoma of the upper two-thirds of the rectum who are either: (*a*) bad risk patients in whom excision of the pelvic floor would add to the mortality or morbidity of the operative procedure without subsequent benefit to the patient; (*b*) patients in whom carcinoma of the upper two-thirds of the rectum has perforated with associated peritonitis or with diffuse metastatic pelvic floor seedlings, in whom anterior resection is unwise.
2. Some patients with diverticulitis. The operation has been used in recent years as the initial stage in cases where there has been perforation and peritonitis or gross pelvic inflammation which make primary anastomosis a hazardous procedure.

Contraindications

This operation should not be performed in the following circumstances.

1. The patient is fit for either an anterior resection or abdominoperineal resection;
2. There is carcinoma of the lower third of the rectum. Removal of the pelvic floor is a necessary part of curative excision of this lesion;
3. There has been perforation with peritonitis in a case of diverticulitis and the toxaemic state of the patient indicates that a transverse colostomy, as a quick, safe procedure, is the method of choice. (*Editors' comment*: This is a controversial subject and some surgeons would advocate, even in this situation, excisional surgery.)

Unless indicated otherwise the cross-references in this chapter refer to *Operative Surgery: Alimentary Tract and Abdominal Wall, Volume 3, 4th Edition*

The operation

Position of the patient

The patient should be in an extended lithotomy-Trendelenburg position (Lloyd-Davies). It is often necessary, especially in cases of carcinoma of the rectum for a rectal wash-out to be performed, using a cancericidal agent, before closure of the rectal stump.

Incision

A long left paramedian incision, as for anterior resection or abdominoperineal resection, should be made.

PROCEDURE

1

Mobilization

The sigmoid colon and rectum should be mobilized as described for anterior resection. The inferior mesenteric artery pedicle should be ligated appropriately. Care should be taken to identify the left ureter.

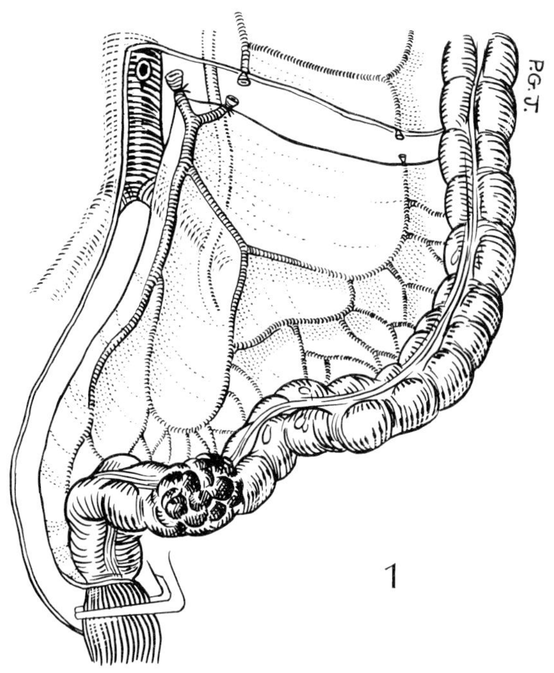

1

Ligation of superior rectal artery

The superior rectal artery should be ligated on the rectal stump.

Clamping

A clamp should be placed between the upper two-thirds and lower third of the rectum. A rectal washout below the clamp is advised using a cancericidal agent or antiseptic solution as required.

2

Division of the rectum

The rectum is divided and the rectal stump oversewn with chromic catgut as the division is made. It is better to avoid non-absorbable suture material. If possible the stump is covered with peritoneum.

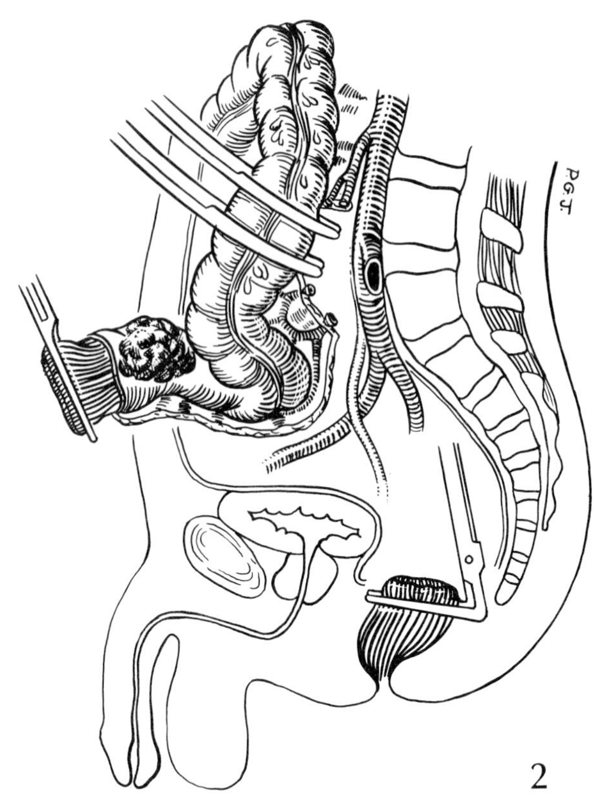

2

Division of the sigmoid colon

The sigmoid colon should be divided at an elected site – in cases of diverticulitis above the affected area and in cases of carcinoma at a convenient site, allowing a colostomy to be constructed without tension.

Construction of left iliac colostomy

A separate incision should be made in the left iliac fossa at a point equidistant from the anterior iliac spine, the umbilicus and the pubic tubercle, as in the case of abdominoperineal excision of the rectum. The bowel should be brought through this incision, and the lateral space between the peritoneum and mesentery closed with a continuous thread stitch to prevent herniation of bowel on the lateral side of the colostomy (*see* chapter on 'Abdominoperineal excision of the rectum', p. 562 in this volume).

The colostomy should remain clamped until the abdominal wound is closed.

Suturing the abdominal wound

The abdominal wound should be closed in layers. The pelvis is drained through a stab incision using a Redivac or corrugated drain. The incision should be sealed.

Fixation of the colostomy

The colostomy should now be unclamped and the wall of the colon stitched to the skin using interrupted chromic catgut sutures around its circumference.

Anal sphincter

It is important at the end of the operation to dilate the anal sphincter or to insert a large soft rubber tube drain to prevent retention of secretions and blood in the rectal stump.

Postoperative care

Patients should be managed as for an anterior resection or abdominoperineal excision (*see* P. 569 in this volume).

Drains

The pelvic drain should be shortened after the first 24h then shortened each day before removal after 4 days. The rectal tube should be removed after 48h.

Complications

Pelvic abscess A pelvic abcess may develop and may discharge spontaneously through the rectal stump. In such cases gentle irrigation of the stump with physiological saline is indicated.

Small bowel obstruction Small intestine can enter the pelvis and become attached to the rectal stump by adhesions. This may produce intestinal obstruction postoperatively or at any time subsequently. It is one of the main disadvantages of this operation.

RESTORATION OF CONTINUITY OF THE BOWEL FOLLOWING A HARTMANNS PROCEDURE

In situations where the patient's general and local conditions permit, continuity of the bowel can be restored by a two-layer anastomosis (as in anterior resection) or by using a stapling gun, which has made this procedure easier in low anastomosis. It is wise in cases of severe pelvic sepsis, as in the case of diverticulitis, to defer the restorative operation for at least 3 months to allow the sepsis and inflammatory reaction to subside completely.

Preoperative preparation

Bowel preparation is similar to that for anterior resection; that is pre- or peroperative antibiotics, colostomy wash-outs and a low residue or fluid diet for 48 h prior to the operation. Preoperative wash-outs of the rectal stump with physiological saline should be carried out twice during the 24 h before the operation or until clean.

The operation

The patient should be in the lithotomy-Trendelenburg position. Following the skin preparation the colostomy is dissected from the abdominal wall and mobilized from the skin surface down to the peritoneal cavity. A sterile glove is placed over the mobilized colostomy and secured with a tape tie. The colostomy is then returned into the abdomen, the resulting abdominal wound being left open. The towel and instruments for the procedure are discarded and the operator changes gown and gloves. Skin preparation is again carried out. The previous left paramedian incision is reopened. Intraperitoneal adhesions are divided and the small intestine packed away from the operation site.

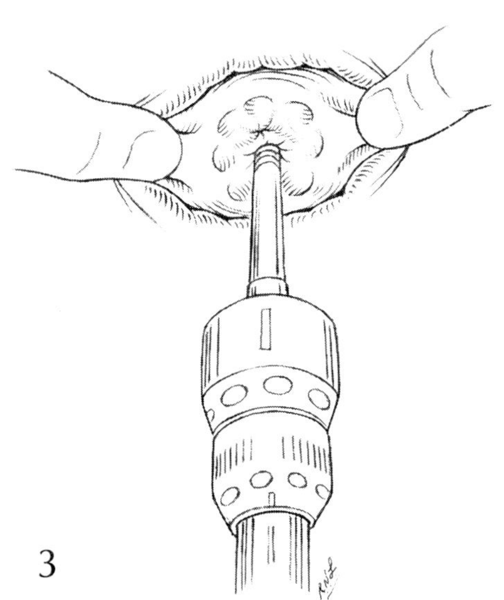

3

3

A difficulty often experienced in this operation is the localizing of the rectal stump caused by inflammatory and fibrous reactions, and the rectum may be contracted. To facilitate dissection of the rectal stump, an assistant passes an obturator of a small sigmoidoscope through the anus. This enables the abdominal operator to identify the rectal stump and to mobilize it sufficiently so that anastomosis may be performed by either the hand-sewn technique or use of the stapling instrument.

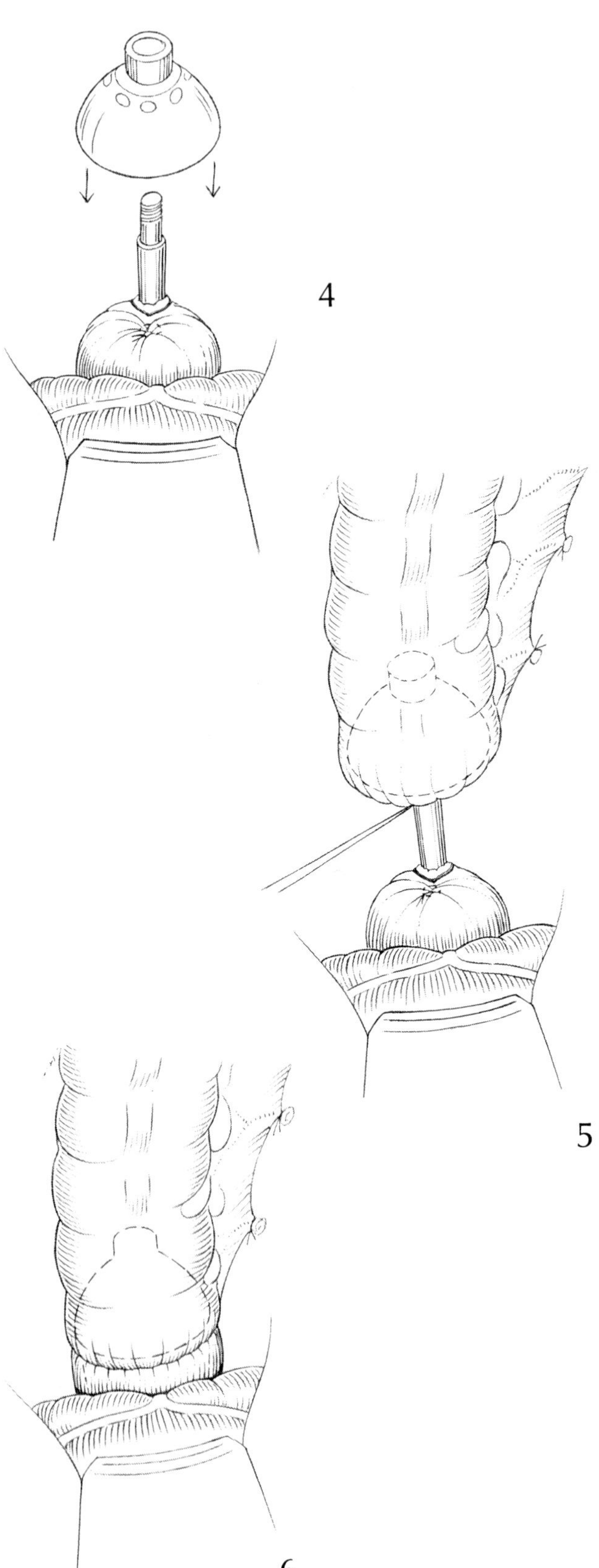

4, 5 & 6

If a stapling instrument is used, the anastomosis is most simply performed by introducing it through the anus (after dilatation). The central stem alone is passed through the top of the closed rectum via a tiny incision in its anterior wall, the anvil is then replaced and the proximal colon is passed over it. The purse-string suture is then firmly tied and the anvil approximated to the rectal stump (see chapter on 'Anterior resection', pp. 520–542 in this volume). Once the necessary technical precautions have been taken the anastomosis is completed by 'firing' the gun.

Drains are placed in the pelvis, the wound of the previous colostomy is closed and the abdominal wound secured.

The anus may be mildly stenotic owing to the lack of function of the anal canal and in such cases it should be stretched before the termination of the anaesthetic.

Further reading

Hartmann, H. Nouveav procédé d'ablation des cancers de la partie terminale du Pelvier. Congrès Français de Chirurgie 1921; 30: 411–418

Complete rectal prolapse: anterior wrap (Ripstein operation)

Robert Britten-Jones MB, BS, FRCS, FRACS
Senior Visiting Surgeon, Royal Adelaide Hospital, South Australia

Preoperative

A simple procedure to treat rectal prolapse, in which the rectum is retained in the hollow of the sacrum by a plastic mesh sling, has been described by Ripstein[1]. It is based on the fact that, in this disease, the rectum is unusually mobile and easily displaced forward from the sacral concavity to form a straight tube. In this position, when the patient strains, all the intra-abdominal forces act in the long axis of the tube, favouring prolapse. By means of this operation the sacral curve of the rectum is restored and maintained when straining, so that the intra-abdominal forces tend to push the rectum backwards against the hollow of the sacrum rather than vertically downwards. The sling can be made of Mersilene, Teflon or polypropylene (Marlex) mesh. The latter is now favoured because it excites less tissue reaction and is a little more rigid than the other materials (Ripstein, 1976, personal communication).

Personal experience with this operation has proved it to be safe, simple and effective. The Lahey Clinic figures reported by Jurgeleit *et al.*[2] confirm this view, with no deaths in 55 patients undergoing Teflon sling repair over 10 years and 7 per cent recurrence rate. Morgan[3], in a similar number of operations, reports one postoperative death and no cases of recurrent complete prolapse. Ripstein is quoted by Morgan as having only two cases of recurrence after 500 sling operations.

Indications

All patients with complete rectal prolapse who are fit to undergo laparotomy are suitable for the procedure. The frail and aged, in whom prolapse is relatively common, withstand it well.

An advantage of the operation is that only minimal mobilization of the rectum is necessary. The lateral ligaments are not divided and no dissection is required anteriorly; thus blood loss is slight and there is no risk of postoperative impotence in the occasional male patient.

Contraindications

It is most important to exclude partial or 'mucosal' prolapse, which is better treated by ligature and excision of the prolapsing mucosa. When concomitant symptomatic diverticular disease exists, anterior resection of the rectum and sigmoid is preferred as this treats both conditions adequately.

Investigations and preparation

Sigmoidoscopy is essential to exclude the occasional case of associated carcinoma, villous tumour or polyp which, by inducing constant straining, may precipitate prolapse. A barium enema to exclude colonic lesions is advisable.

The most important preoperative measure is to empty the large bowel completely. This is achieved by admitting the patient to hospital 3 clear days before operation. On Day 1 the patient has a low residue diet and Agarol 15 ml is given orally. On Day 2, nourishing fluids only are given by mouth along with Agarol 15 ml morning and evening and a tap water enema. On Day 3, clear fluids only are given by mouth, colonic lavage is performed and oral metronidazole 400 mg is given at 8-hourly intervals. On the day of operation a further bowel washout is given. Anaemia, if present, is corrected and the patient in whom incontinence is a problem should be warned that, although the bowel will no longer protrude after the operation, incontinence may not be cured completely.

Anaesthesia

A general anaesthetic with muscular relaxation is essential. An intravenous infusion is set up and gentamicin 80 mg intravenously is given at the beginning of the operation.

The operation

1

Incision and laparotomy

The patient is placed supine, the bladder catheterized and any residual urine expressed. Fifteen to twenty degrees of head-down tilt facilitates exposure of the rectum. A left paramedian incision is made extending from the pubis to the level of the umbilicus with the operator, if right-handed, standing on the left side of the patient. Laparotomy is carried out; the intraperitoneal organs are carefully palpated and any co-existent large bowel disease is particularly looked for. A self-retaining retractor is placed in the wound; the colon and small bowel are pushed into the upper part of the abdomen and held out of the pelvis by packs. In the female, the uterus is held forward by stay sutures passed through the broad ligaments and anchored to the rectus sheath where it is inserted into the pubis.

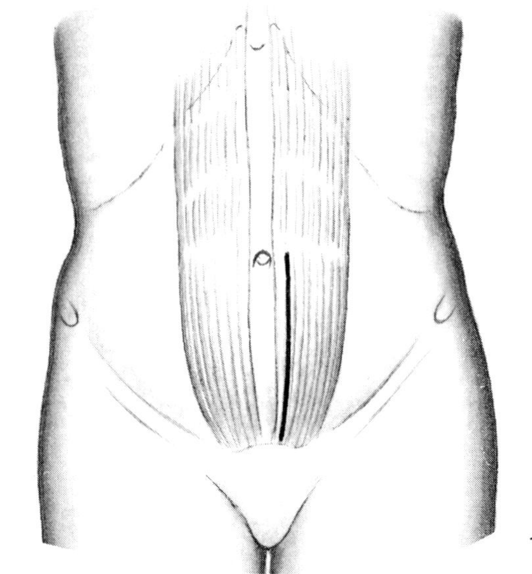

1

2

Left lateral peritoneal incision

After the congenital adhesions between the sigmoid mesocolon and the parietes have been freed, with the assistant holding the apex of the sigmoid loop forwards and to the right, the peritoneum and subperitoneal tissue immediately to the left of the base of the mesorectum are incised with dissecting scissors from the level of the pelvic brim as far down as the peritoneal reflection. Diathermy is used to coagulate any small vessels that have been divided. It is essential to recognize and avoid the ureter where it crosses the pelvic brim at the level of the common iliac artery bifurcation.

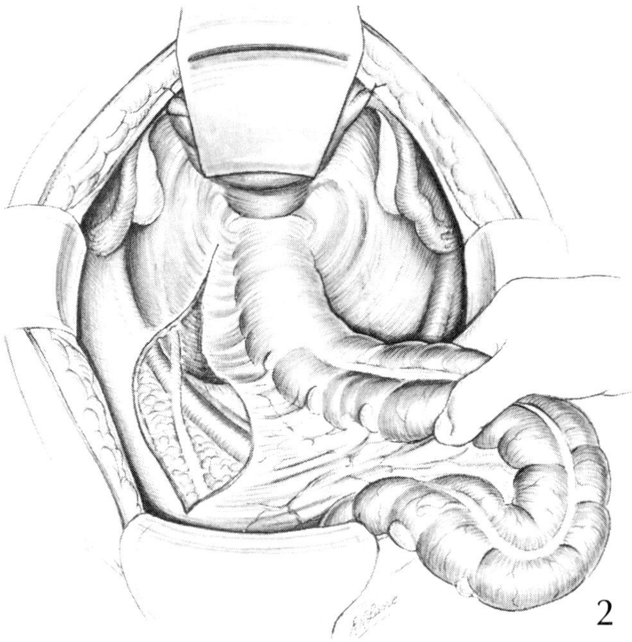

2

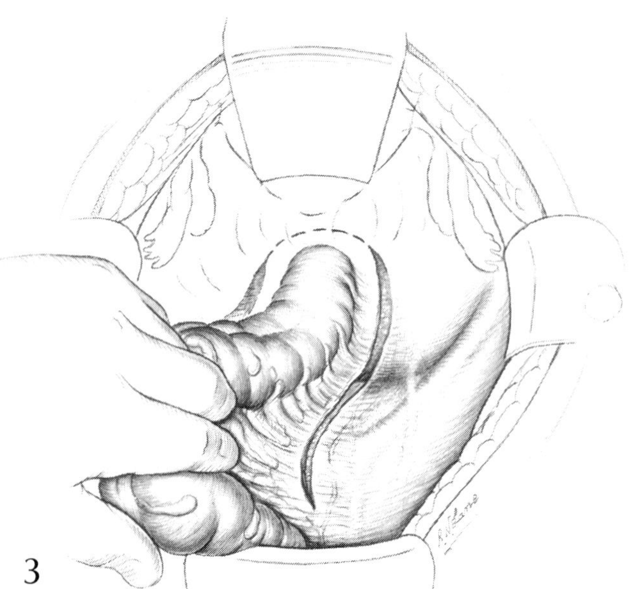

3

3

Right lateral peritoneal incision

A similar incision is made in the peritoneum on the right side of the base of the mesorectum. The peritoneum on the anterior surface of the rectovesical pouch, about 3 cm above its deepest point, is divided transversely to join the lower ends of the two lateral incisions.

4, 5 & 6

Opening of the areolar plane

With the left hand holding the rectosigmoid junction forward, the operator's right index finger is introduced into the loose areolar plane between the rectum and the sacral promontory, behind the inferior mesenteric artery at the upper end of the right lateral peritoneal incision. The left index finger is then substituted, holding the mesorectum with the inferior mesenteric vessels forward and allowing the right hand to introduce dissecting scissors to open the areolar plane until the four fingers of the right hand can be gently inserted between the presacral fascia and the upper half of the rectum. This must be carried out with care to avoid rupturing small presacral veins. The rectum is not mobilized further and the lateral ligaments are left undivided. Anterior to the rectum, below the peritoneal reflection, only sufficient dissection is done to take up the slack of the lower rectum. In many cases this can be carried out without dissecting at all in this plane.

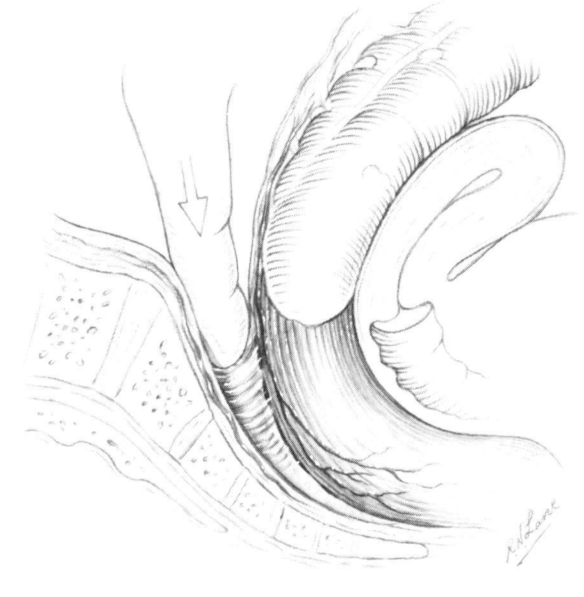

4

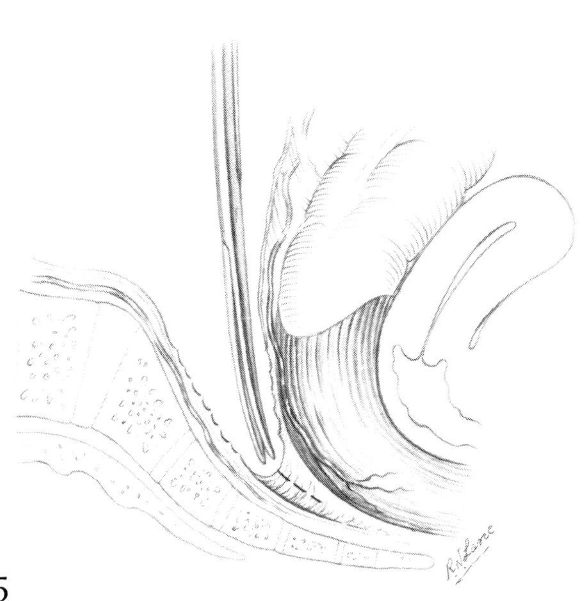

5

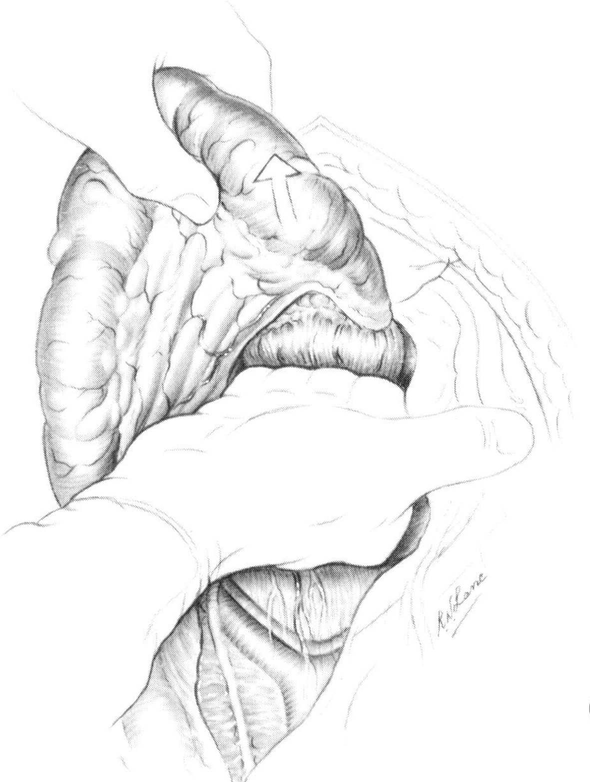

6

7

Fixation of sling to sacrum

A piece of presterilized Teflon or Marlex mesh is cut to form a rectangle, measuring 12 cm × 5 cm. The rectum is held forward by an assistant to expose the anterior surface of the sacrum. One of the two narrower edges of the rectangular plastic mesh is then sutured to the sacrum just to the right of the midline so that its centre lies approximately 5 cm below the promontory, using four interrupted non-absorbable sutures in a vertical line. Each suture is threaded on a No. 14 round-bodied Mayo needle held on a strong needle holder. Initially, the lowest suture is placed with the needle and thread piercing the mesh close to its edge and then taking a wide, deep bite of the presacral fascia and underlying periosteum. This is the most difficult part of the operation. Care must be taken to avoid any visible presacral blood vessels in this region and if one is inadvertently pierced, the suture should be removed and firm pressure applied to the bleeding point either digitally or with a swab on a holder. Pressure should be maintained for 4 min. If bleeding persists, the bleeding vessel should be under-run with 00 catgut on an atraumatic curved needle. (On one occasion the author was forced to pack the pelvis with gauze rolls to control bleeding. The operation was terminated and the packs were removed uneventfully 48 h later.)

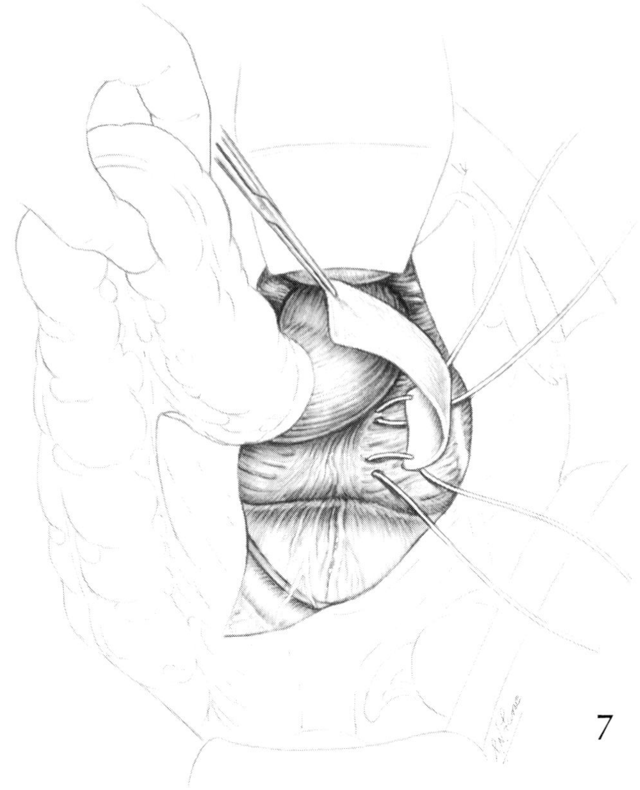

7

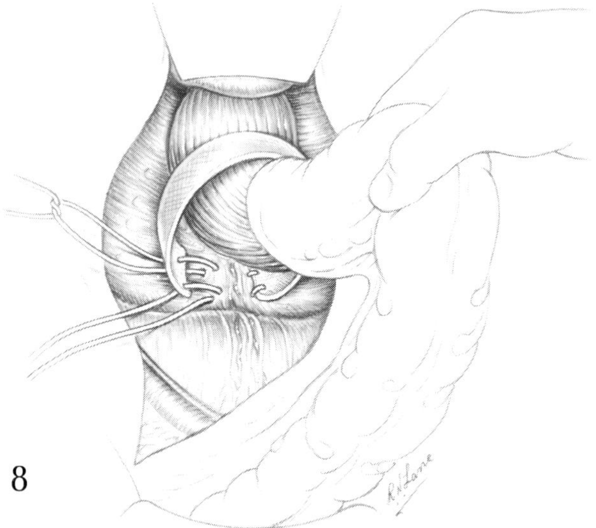

8

8

Encircling of rectum with sling

The opposite short edge of the plastic mesh sling is then carried around the rectum anteriorly and similarly sutured to the sacrum just to the left of the midline. Before tying these sutures the surgeon must ensure that the sling is sufficiently lax. This is checked by pulling both ends of the sutures taut after tying one throw of the knot. With the sling thus held temporarily in position, it should be possible to insert the index and middle fingers easily behind the rectum. If the sling is too tight, faecal impaction may result.

9

Fixation of sling to rectum

The rectum is pulled upwards and rendered taut. The upper and lower borders of the sling are then attached by fine non-absorbable sutures to the seromuscular layer of the rectum at about the level of the peritoneal reflection. Wrinkling of the sling is avoided by spreading the plastic mesh in the vertical plane over the anterior surface of the rectum before inserting the sutures in the anterior and lateral rectal wall. Angulation of the rectum by the sling occurs in most cases and to avoid this, a 'hitch' suture of non-absorbable material is placed between the fascia covering the anterior surface of the lumbosacral disc and the mesosigmoid close to the bowel wall at the rectosigmoid junction. A second 'hitch' suture may be necessary between the left lateral surface of the mesosigmoid close to the bowel and the parietes so that the lower sigmoid forms a gentle curve rather than a sharp angle with the rectum. The author has never had to resect a redundant sigmoid but can envisage that it may be necessary in the rare case where volvulus appears to be a danger.

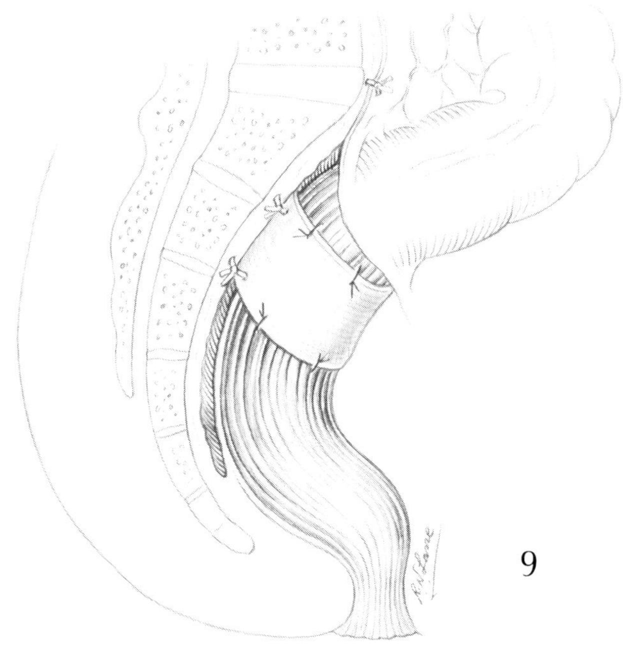

9

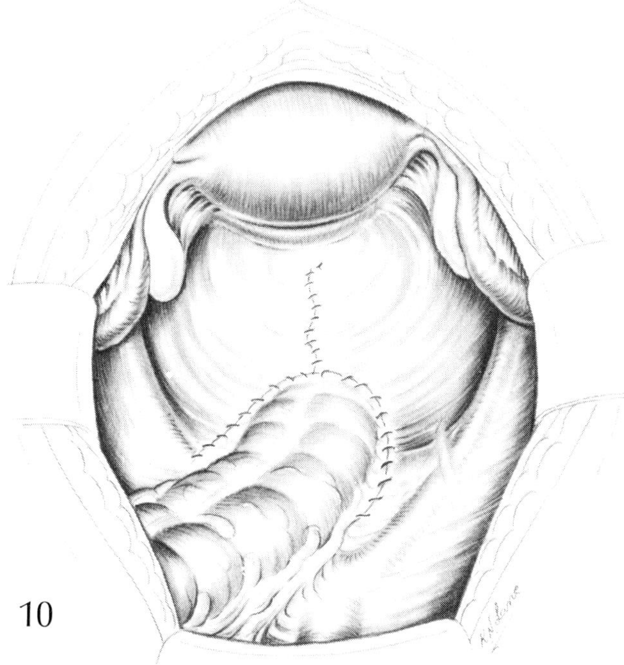

10

10

Closure

If Teflon is used, the sling should be buried beneath the pelvic peritoneum to avoid the possibility of small bowel adhering to it, by a running suture of chromic catgut closing the anterior and lateral peritoneal defects. However, using Marlex with its minimal tissue reaction, adherence to small intestine is most unlikely and the peritoneal defects may be left open. If they are closed, it is most important that a sump drain be placed in the presacral space and brought out through a stab incision in the anterior abdominal wall. The abdominal wound is then closed in layers.

Postoperative care and complications

Oral feeding may commence early and nasogastric suction is unnecessary. It is wise to continue the prophylactic antiobiotic given preoperatively for 24 h (gentamicin 80 mg 8 hourly intravenously) as the plastic mesh is a foreign body and, as such, predisposes to infection, particularly if the bowel is inadvertently punctured by a suture. A soft-formed daily bowel action should be induced by administering lubricant aperients from the second day after operation and if no bowel action has occurred by the third day, a tap water enema is given. Thereafter, to ensure that faecal impaction does not occur, daily rectal examination is performed until normal bowel actions are established. If faecal impaction occurs, the scybalous mass must be broken up and removed manually. The patient whose bowel habit hitherto has been faulty is encouraged to develop a satisfactory bowel action with increased roughage in the diet and added daily bran or bulk-forming laxatives.

Persistent incontinence, especially for flatus, occurs in a number of patients but they should not feel discouraged as improvement is often gradual and may take many months. If the patient's bowel can be managed adequately after the operation so that the stool is normally soft-formed, continence is considerably improved[4].

Residual mucosal prolapse is best treated by ligature and excision.

Faecal impaction should not occur if care is taken to make the sling around the rectum sufficiently loose, if angulation is avoided and soft faecal consistency maintained.

Abscess formation is rare, but if it occurs a faecal fistula inevitably results. Drainage of the area with removal of the mesh and a defunctioning transverse colostomy are essential.

References

1. Ripstein, C. B. Surgical care of massive rectal prolapse. Diseases of the Colon and Rectum 1965; 8: 34–38

2. Jurgeleit, H. C., Corman, M. L., Coller, J. A., Veidenheimer, M. C. Procidentia of the rectum: Teflon sling repair of rectal prolapse, Lahey Clinic experience. Diseases of the Colon and Rectum 1975; 18: 464–467

3. Morgan, B. P. Procidentia of the rectum: the Ripstein operation. Diseases of the Colon and Rectum 1975; 18: 468–469

4. Hawley, P. R. Procidentia of the rectum: Ivalon-sponge repair. Diseases of the Colon and Rectum 1975; 18: 461–463

Postanal pelvic floor repair for anorectal incontinence

The late Sir Alan G. Parks MCh, PRCS, FRCP
Consultant Surgeon, The London Hospital and St Mark's Hospital, London

John Percy FRACS, FACS
Consultant Surgeon, North Shore Medical Centre, St Leonard's, New South Wales

Introduction

Anorectal incontinence, although not common, is such a distressing condition that every attempt must be made to relieve it. Careful examination of the incontinent patient is important to determine the cause of the condition. In particular, evidence of division of the sphincter muscles during childbirth, at fistula and other perineal operations, or as a result of external trauma should be sought. These patients should be treated by direct muscle suture, as described on pp. 439–442. Cauda equina lesions, either congenital or acquired, will also be disclosed by the history and physical examination. However, some patients have anorectal incontinence which occurs without evidence of direct muscle damage or overt neurological disease; this is termed idiopathic anorectal incontinence and, although found in all age groups, is most commonly seen in the middle years. Women are affected 10 times more commonly than men.

Patients with this condition can be divided into two main groups, those with a coincidental large rectal prolapse and those in whom any prolapse is minimal. In those with a complete rectal prolapse, the usual first step in treatment is the performance of some form of abdominal repair, which will relieve the incontinence in about half the patients. The remainder and those without significant prolapse have a profound weakness of the pelvic floor. Recent evidence indicates that this weakness is caused by damage to the innervation of the muscles but the nature of this nerve damage remains obscure. In a number of patients, usually the younger ones, the incontinence follows difficult childbirth but many are either nulliparous or give no history of obstetric difficulty.

Anal canal manometry and electromyography of the anal sphincter muscles, particularly single fibre EMG studies, may prove helpful in the assessment of these patients and may be useful in predicting which patients require more than a rectopexy to relieve the incontinence associated with rectal prolapse. Simple digital examination, however, will usually provide as much information about muscle function as is necessary. The superficial part of the external sphincter is seldom functioning at all in this condition and, as a result, the anal reflex is absent. However, the puborectalis and pubococcygeus muscles may still be active and it is important that an assessment of the power of contraction of these be made. A good contraction in response to voluntary effort and to coughing are the most helpful prognostic signs.

The cross-reference in this chapter refers to *Operative Surgery: Alimentary Tract and Abdominal Wall, Volume 3, 4th Edition*

1

In planning an operation designed to relieve incontinence account must be taken of the fact that the muscles are already partially degenerate; the repair must be aimed at making residual function maximally effective. One of the most important features in the maintenance of continence is the valve effect caused by the double right-angle which normally exists between the anal canal, the lowermost rectum and the midrectum.

The force of abdominal pressure acts upon the anterior rectal wall, thrusting it on to the closed anal canal and so effectively blocking it. This angulation is maintained by the sling of functioning puborectalis muscle and on defaecation straining the muscle relaxes, making the angulation less acute. As a result the flap valve effect is lost and defaecation can take place. Patients with incontinence due to weakened pelvic floor muscles lose both the angulation and the valve so that any increase in intrarectal pressure is likely to lead to involuntary defaecation.

The essential part of an operation for this condition is therefore the reconstruction of the anorectal angulation with the restoration of a reliable flap valve mechanism which does not give way under stress. This is accomplished by approximation of the pelvic floor and sphincter muscles behind the anorectal junction, displacing them anteriorly and increasing the angulation at this point.

Although the main effect of the operation is geometric, namely an increase in the anorectal angulation, the shortening of the effective length of the puborectalis muscle allows those muscle fibres which remain innervated to function more efficiently. In addition, the repair incorporates ileococcygeus and pubococcygeus muscles, which are usually considerably less degenerate than the lower muscles.

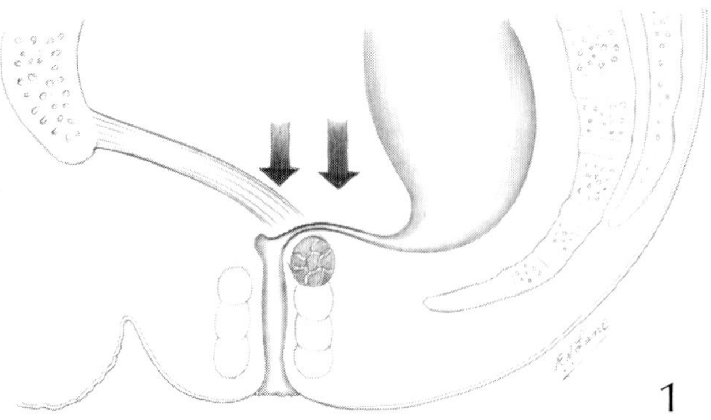

1

The repair is best performed by approaching the muscles from their inner surface so that sutures can be placed from the limb of one side of each muscle across to the equivalent part of the other side. The anatomical approach is interesting and not difficult. All that is required is to displace the termination of intestinal viscus forwards to obtain access to the posterior and lateral inner surfaces of the external anal sphincter, puborectalis and levator ani muscles. The approach is made behind the anorectal viscus, because it is here that muscles must be approximated to narrow their field of action and to restore the normal anorectal angulation.

Preoperative preparation

The colon and rectum must be completely evacuated during the 48 h before operation.

The operation

2

The patient is placed in the lithotomy position (although the jack-knife would be equally suitable). After routine skin preparation, a solution of saline containing adrenaline 1:300 000 is injected into the fat and subcutaneous tissue around the posterior part of the anal canal. This reduces capillary bleeding and enables the operator to differentiate between the internal and external anal sphincters, a vital first stage in the dissection.

A V-shaped incision is made in the perineum about 6 cm behind the anal canal. The wound is placed so far behind the anus because in the course of the repair the skin of the anal region is drawn into the canal itself; if the wound were put too close, it would be pulled into the anal canal and infection would result. The skin anterior to the incision is then raised with scissor dissection until the anal verge is reached.

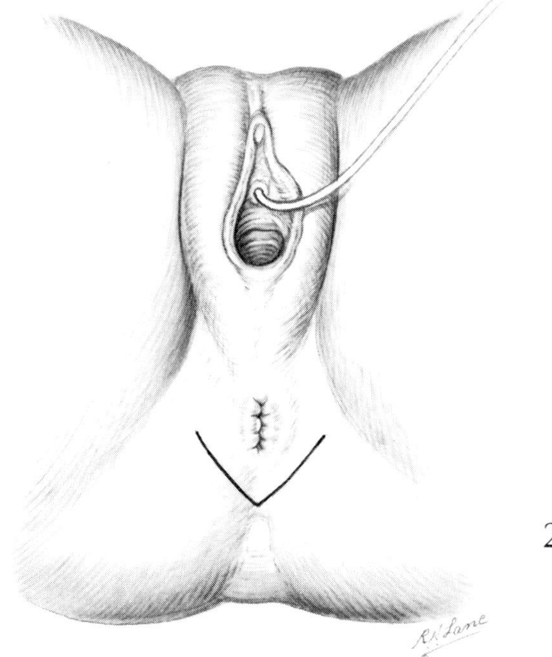

2

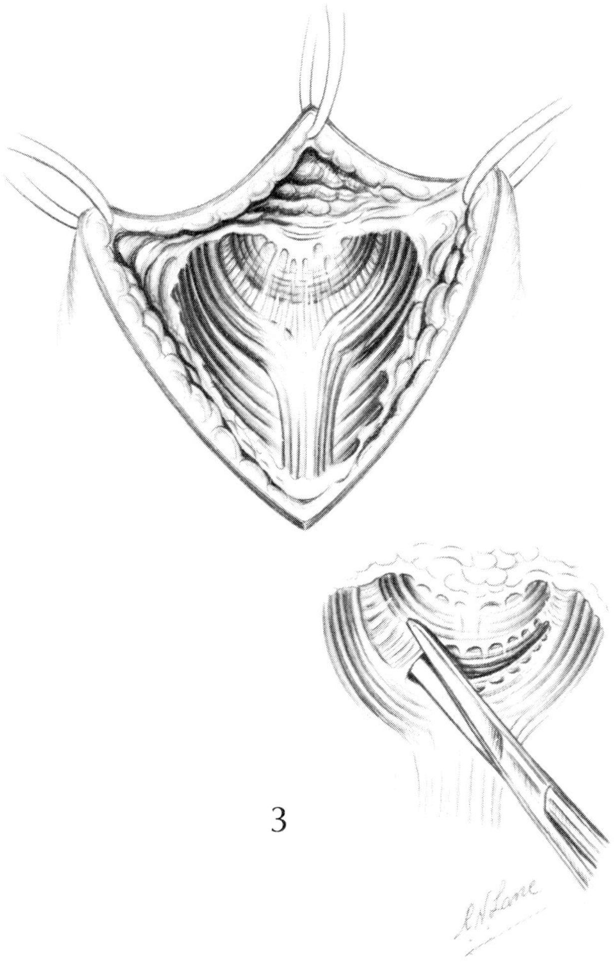

3

3

The lower borders of the internal and external anal sphincters are exposed. The plane between the two is relatively bloodless and can be identified anatomically; the longitudinal fibres help to guide the operator to the correct site. The external sphincter is usually red and easily identified, whereas the internal sphincter is white. However, when the external sphincter is degenerate, the distinction between the two muscles becomes blurred. Stimulation of the tissue with the diathermy or an electrical nerve stimulator will usually cause contraction of the external sphincter. The internal sphincter, being smooth muscle, does not contract with electrical stimulation. By gentle scissor dissection the internal sphincter is displaced from the lower part of the external sphincter through about half its circumference.

4

As the dissection progresses, the viscus is lifted off the upper part of the external sphincter, progressively onward and upward until the sling of puborectalis muscle at the anorectal junction is reached. It is important to avoid straying from this plane as it is not difficult to enter the rectum and somewhat easier to dissect through the external sphincters into the ischiorectal fat. Throughout the dissection the separation between the two layers is carried as far forward on each side of the anal canal as possible. At the anorectal junction the condensation of Waldeyer's fascia and the levator fascia is encountered where it is attached both to the rectal wall and to the puborectalis muscle. It is incised near the muscle to enable the rectum to be separated from the pelvic floor, providing direct access to the superior aspect of the pelvic floor muscles.

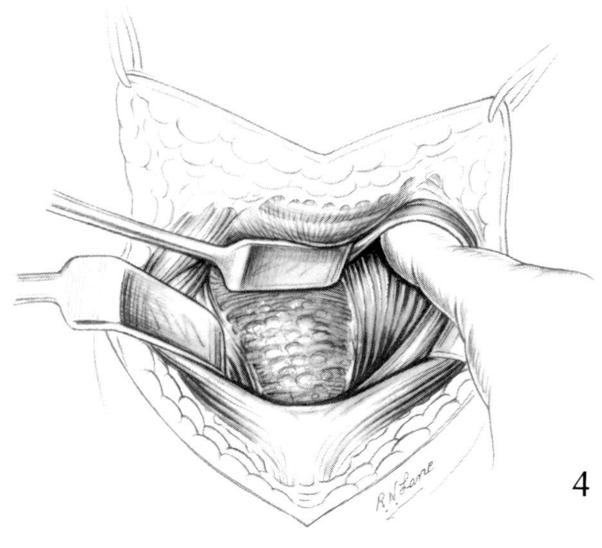

4

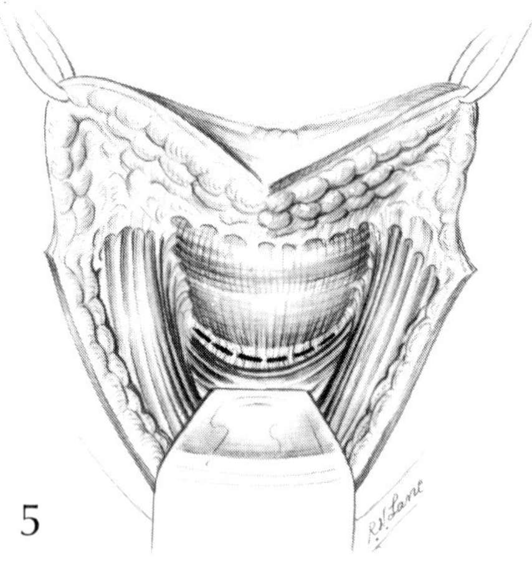

5

5

Retractors are then placed into the pelvis to hold the rectum forwards so that the origin of the levator ani muscles on both sides can be seen.

6

Sutures of atraumatic polypropylene are placed across the two limbs of the ileococcygeus muscle in the following manner. The highest and most lateral point of the levator group is identified with blunt dissection, close to the spine of the ischium, which is readily palpable. A small curved atraumatic needle is then passed under a fairly large bundle of the levator on one side. The retractor is then moved to expose the exactly equivalent site of the muscle on the other side and the needle containing polypropylene picks up a similar bundle of muscle on that side. About three layers are placed at this topmost level and are tied only lightly, without tension, to form a lattice across the pelvis.

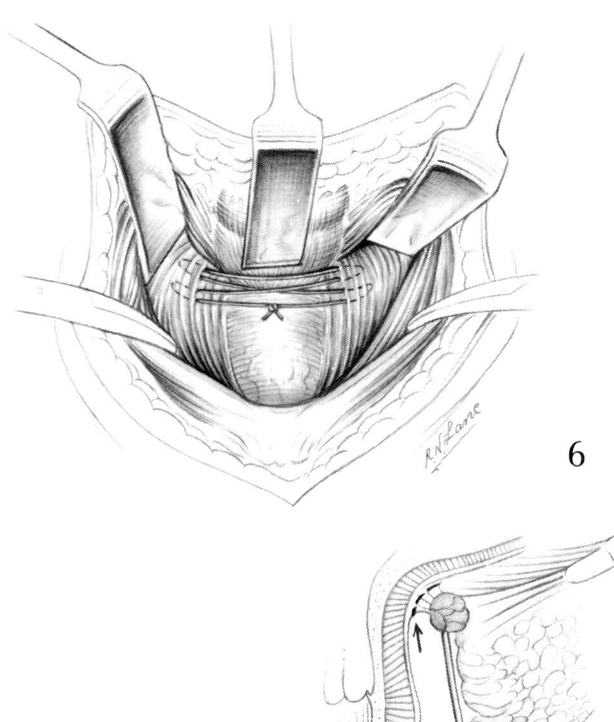

6

7

The next layer of sutures is placed in the upper part of the pubococcygeus muscle and again each is tied only lightly with the formation of a lattice. The lower part of the pubococcygeus, however, is a stronger bar of muscle and its origin is much nearer the midline on the pubic arch. Sutures are placed as close to its origin on each side as possible and again about three layers are used.

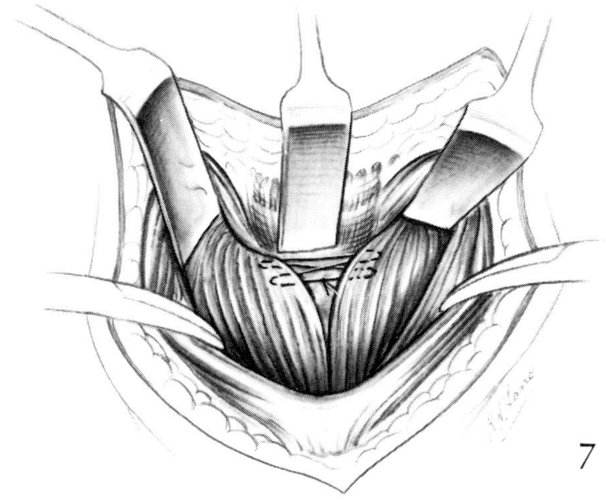

7

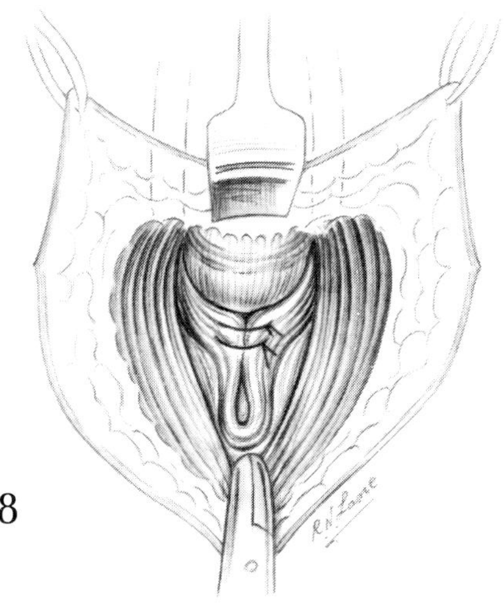

8

8

The most important layer of all is that put into the puborectalis. The muscle is the strongest and thickest of all those encountered and can be seen with ease. Once more the suture is placed as near to the pubis as possible. It is tied so that the muscle is approximated but a small gap is left to take into account swelling which may occur in the tissues postoperatively.

9

Another layer of sutures is placed in the external sphincter below the puborectalis and, finally, at the anal margin a layer of catgut sutures is used to avoid putting a non-absorbable suture near the skin. A Redivac drain is placed in the pelvis.

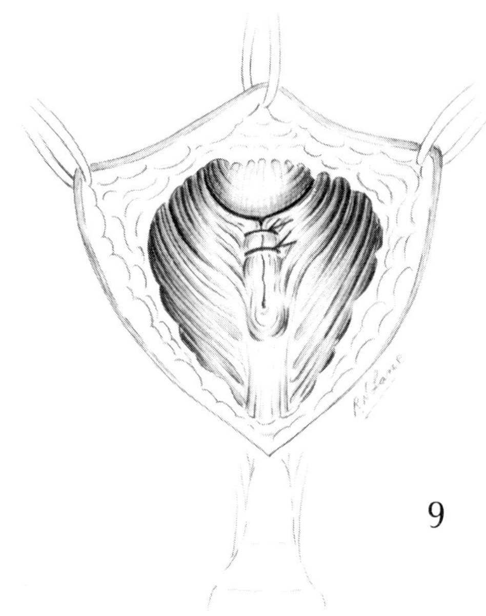

9

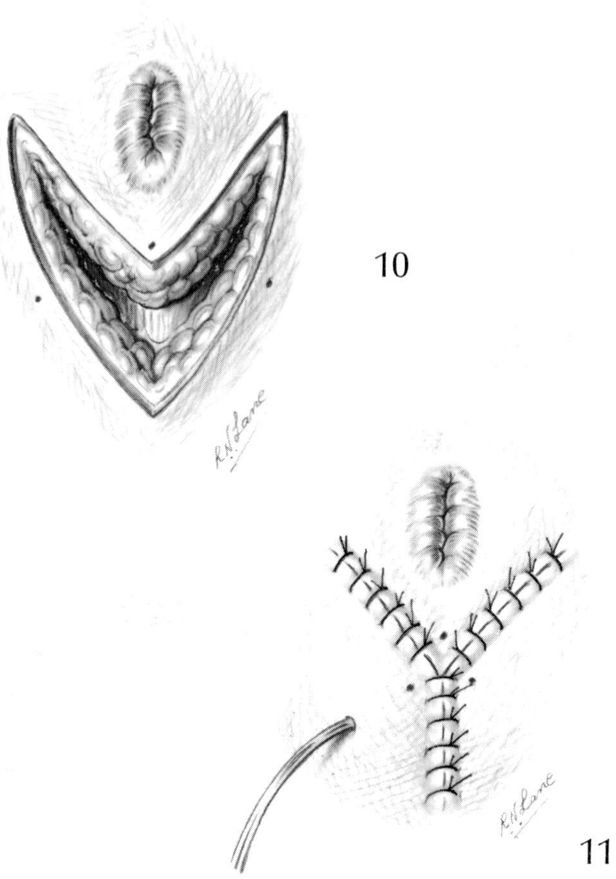

10 & 11

As a result of the repair, the anterior skin flap is drawn forwards and cannot be resutured to the posterior skin edge without undue tension. The wound is therefore reconstituted in the shape of a Y. It is not uncommon for local necrosis to occur at the apex of the anterior flap but this always heals uneventfully.

Postoperative care

A catheter is placed into the bladder for 2–3 days. Were the patient to strain in the immediate postoperative period and pass a large stool through the anal canal, it might disrupt the whole repair. The two ways of avoiding this are either to fashion a temporary colostomy or to create a state of permanent diarrhoea for 10–12 days. Neither alternative is pleasant but the diarrhoea regimen is preferable and, to this end, magnesium sulphate is prescribed in sufficient doses to maintain about three semiformed stools a day. Once this period has passed, the chance of damaging the muscles by defaecation straining is over. However, it is essential that straining habits are not resumed because the repair will gradually weaken, or more likely the muscle itself will weaken over months and symptoms recur. The patient must therefore steer a course between hard stool which cannot be expelled easily and diarrhoea which may only be controllable with difficulty. To accomplish this, one of the bulk-forming laxatives may be given by mouth if required, and each morning one or two glycerine suppositories are routinely inserted. The latter induce rectal contraction, so that the stool is expelled by the 'vis a tergo' of the rectal wall rather than by abdominal straining. This regimen is continued indefinitely and it is necessary to reiterate this to the patient on several occasions. Only too frequently they feel that there is now no longer a problem and that they can give up using the suppositories. The result may be either intermittent impaction of faeces or gradual resumption of straining efforts.

Results

In general, the best results are obtained in younger patients who still have good powers of voluntary contraction and in whom the muscle degeneration seen on histological appearances is minimal. In patients who have a complete rectal prolapse, the first step is to perform an abdominal repair. This will relieve the incontinence in about half the patients, while the remainder will require a postanal repair as a second procedure. It should be noted that even the patients without a complete rectal prolapse will usually have a degree of prolapse of the lower rectal mucosa in association with lax sphincter muscles. A rectopexy, however, is not required in these cases, as the mucosal prolapse is usually controlled by the postanal repair.

Intelligent cooperation in the postoperative regimen is essential and the operation should be avoided in a patient who is unlikely to follow instructions conscientiously. Partly for this reason, and also because they generally have more muscle degeneration, patients above the age of 70 years also tend to do less well. If the patient is cooperative, however, age alone should not prevent an attempt to restore continence.

The operation does not return the degenerate muscle to normal. It restores the anatomical situation of acute angulation at the anorectal junction and allows the remaining functioning muscle to act more efficiently. More than 80 per cent of patients are improved sufficiently by this operation, together with the postoperative regimen, to enable continence to be maintained under normal circumstances. Follow-up studies have shown that, once a good result has been obtained, functional deterioration seldom occurs.

Management of patients with symptomatic haemorrhoids – an introduction

L. P. Fielding MB, FRCS
Chief of Surgery, St Mary's Hospital, Waterbury, Connecticut;
Associate Professor of Surgery, Yale New Haven Hospital, Connecticut;
Visiting Clinical Scientist, St Mary's Hospital Medical School, London

In this section of the book no less than eight chapters have been devoted to the treatment of 'piles'. This plethora of treatment methods suggests that patients who complain of 'piles' may have one or more of a number of individual problems; that no single treatment method can be advised for all patients; and that several different methods may achieve equally good results – hence this short introduction.

The haemorrhoidal tissues (piles) are normal structures which are thought to play some part in anal continence. Their size, shape and details of anatomical configuration vary in the population who *do not* complain of any local problems. Thus any classification of clinical 'disease' must be based on patients' symptoms arising from or caused by an ill defined derangement of anal canal function. These symptoms may occur singly or in combination: pain, bleeding, prolapse, mucous discharge, perianal itching, constipation, and incontinence to flatus and/or faeces.

Despite this variety of symptoms two main types of symptom complex appear to exist and are associated with the level of anal tone and the patient's age.

1. *High anal tone.* Occurs most frequently in the young patient complaining of discomfort (pain), constipation and bleeding, Although these symptoms may be 'cured' by a local attack on the bleeding, congested haemorrhoidal plexus by injections with phenol-in-oil*, Barron's bands or cryosurgery, it seems more logical to carry out a manual dilatation of the anus or a lateral internal sphincterotomy after which anal tone returns to within the normal range. However, it must be remembered that manual dilatation of the anus must always be conducted with great care *and slowly* if permanent damage to the anal sphincter mechanism is to be completely avoided. Furthermore, it is essential that the diagnosis be correct. Manual dilatation must *not* be done for an undiagnosed anal pain.
2. *Low anal tone.* Occurs in the older patient with haemorrhoidal prolapse, bleeding and some degree of incontinence or its consequences – mucous discharge and perianal itching (pruritis).

   The combination of low anal tone and excess bulk to the haemorrhoidal cushion results in disruption of anal canal function. Clearly anal dilatation for this type of patient is contraindicated and treatment must be directed to 'fixing' the haemorrhoidal cushion high in the anal canal with either (*a*) injection of phenol-in-oil, Barron's bands or Cryosurgery; or (*b*) excision of the pile by haemorrhoidectomy. The ultimate effect of either of these treatment approaches results in the obliteration of the vascular cushion which stops the bleeding, and the removal of the bulk of the pile from within the anal canal itself allows any secondary incontinence to be relieved.

Thus a 'single' type of treatment method (e.g. injection of phenol-in-oil) may achieve its results by a number of mechanisms: thrombosing a bleeding area; reduction in the bulk of an oversized pile cusion; and fixation of the lax submucosal tissues to hold the pile above the anal canal, preventing its descent. Although these 'mechanisms' are put forward as statements they are, of course, merely rationalizations based on clinical observations.

When attempting to choose a treatment for an individual patient the methods described in this section of the book can be considered in three groups of increasing complexity.

1. Haemorrhoidal cushion size reduction and fixation: injection of phenol-in-oil; Barron's bands; cryosurgery.

* The oil used is usually almond or arachis (ground nut) oil. It must never be a mineral oil

2. Anal sphincter tone reduction: manual dilatation of the anus; lateral internal sphinterotomy.
3. Haemorrhoidal cushion obliteration: 'open' or 'closed' haemorrhoidectomy.

It seems reasonable to proceed from group 1 (the simple method requiring no anaesthetic) to group 2 (the non-excisional treatments) and then to group 3 (a last resort and if other treatments fail).

With such an approach most patients will be well treated in an out-patient – office setting and approximately 10 per cent of patients will require hospitalization for haemorrhoidectomy.

Irrespective of treatment method it is worthwhile emphasizing the benefits of stool bulking agents prescribed as an adjunct because they probably help prevent recurrent problems and, if taken early in the development of 'troublesome piles', may result in normal function and the disappearance of all symptoms before more invasive treatments are required.

There is no doubt that this collection of chapter will not be the 'last words' on the subject – already infrared photocoagulation is gaining some popularity but we have chosen to await its formal evaluation before adding to the multiplicity of treatments described in this text.

Barron band ligation of haemorrhoids

C. V. Mann MCh, FRCS
Consultant Surgeon, The London Hospital and St Mark's Hospital, London

Preoperative

Indications

Many internal haemorrhoids are too large to respond satisfactorily to injections but do not give rise to such severe symptoms that the patient is willing to have an operation. This is the situation in larger second degree haemorrhoids and some smaller third degree piles. In some cases, haemorrhoids recur after excision and the patient is reluctant to have further surgical treatment.

The ideal case for treatment by this method is a patient with one or two large isolated prolapsing haemorrhoids.

Contraindications

For small haemorrhoids injection treatment is preferred, and for third degree haemorrhoids surgical excision is more certain to produce a good result. Banding treatment should not be attempted if an anal fissure or fistula is present.

Previous injection treatment makes the technique more difficult to apply because submucosal fibrosis prevents the pile being drawn into the applicator.

As with all other anal procedures banding should not be done in the presence of active colitis, Crohn's disease of the anorectum or other inflammatory lesions such as dysentery. Preliminary diagnostic sigmoidoscopy is required to exclude a rectal neoplasm, proctocolitis, etc. A general and abdominal examination should be carried out to exclude conditions such as heart failure or portal hypertension requiring a different approach for treatment.

Unless indicated otherwise the cross-references in this chapter refer to *Operative Surgery: Alimentary Tract and Abdominal Wall, Volume 3, 4th Edition*

Preparation

No special preparation is necessary. The rectum should not be loaded and constipation should be corrected before banding is carried out. If necessary the rectum can be emptied by preliminary treatment with two Dulcolax (bisacodyl) suppositories or by giving a Fleet's (disodium hydrogen phosphate) enema.

An operative assistant is required.

Anaesthesia and position of patient

If expertly performed, banding treatment is painless apart from a mild ache afterwards. No local or general anaesthesia is required but if the patient is uncooperative through apprehension or shyness a light general anaesthetic can be given. Pain at the time of banding suggests that it should be removed immediately because it has been applied to the sensitive anoderm.

The left lateral (Sims) position with the pelvis raised on a sandbag (see p. 490) is a good position for the procedure, which can also be carried out in the knee-elbow or jack-knife positions.

The lithotomy position is not a good posture in which to carry out banding because the anterior haemorrhoid is difficult to visualize and manipulate.

The operation

1

Instruments

The banding instrument consists of a double drum carrying elastic bands 1/16 inch (1.5 mm) in diameter when unexpanded ('O' rings). The doubly overlapping drum is mounted on a long shaft, at the base of which is a trigger-mechanism which can release the elastic 'O' rings as required by forward movement of an outer drum over an inner one which is loaded with the elastic bands. The 'O' rings are loaded by a separate conical device which slots into the end of the barrel of the drum and enables the bands to be stretched and slipped up and over onto the inner drum, ready to be squeezed off by the trigger mechanism. The third essential piece of equipment is a pair of special toothed grasping forceps which are passed through the hollow centre of the drum to grasp the base of the pile in order to pull the base of the haemorrhoid into the barrel.

The drum is loaded with *two* bands before each application.

Banding is carried out through a standard tubular proctoscope illuminated proximally. The proctoscope is passed and adjusted by the operator to obtain an optimal view of each haemorrhoidal mass in turn. Once the haemorrhoid for treatment has been identified and its neck clearly seen, the assistant steadies the proctoscope in position.

Self-operated instruments which do away with the need for an assistant by combining the functions of the proctoscope and the banding instrument are also available.

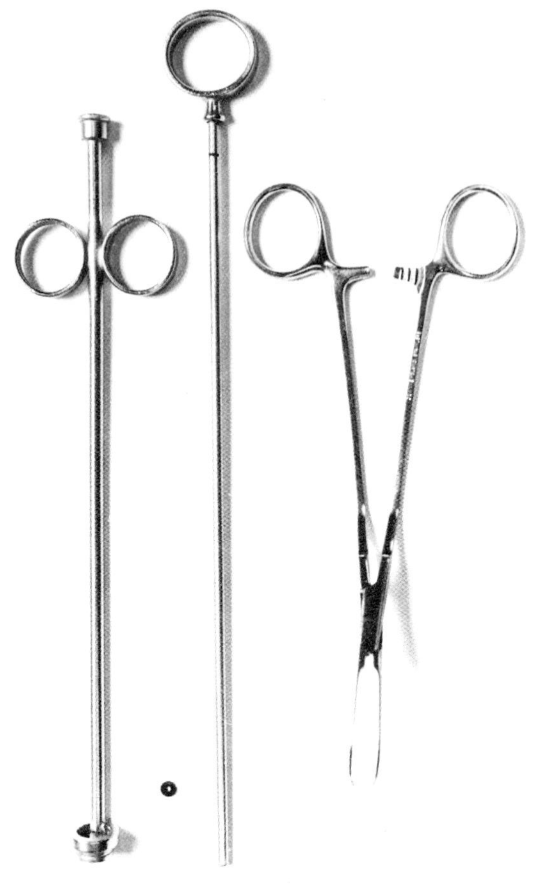

1

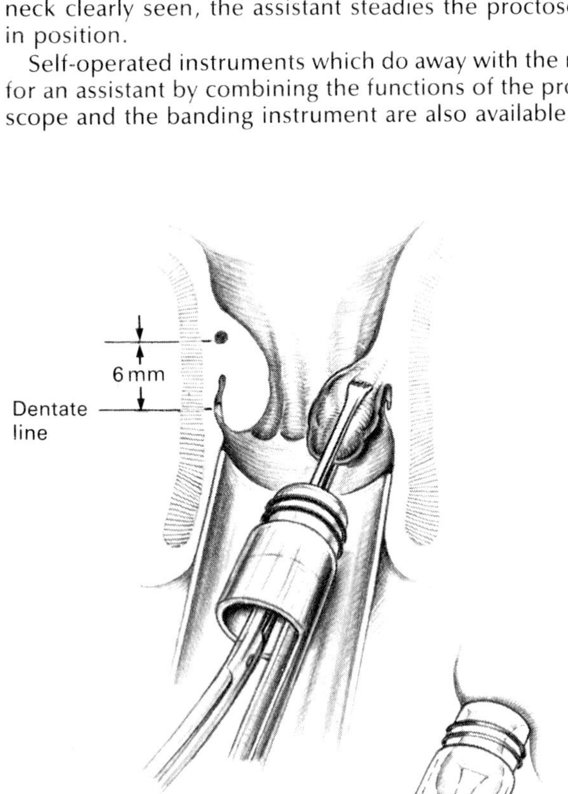

2

2

The banding procedure

Once the proctoscope has been positioned each haemorrhoid is grasped at its neck by the forceps. It is important that the point selected for application of the forceps is at least 6 mm above the dentate line, and that the patient does not experience *any* pain when the forceps are closed.

Gentle sustained traction is then applied through the forceps to draw the pile mass by its neck into the barrel of the drum, while at the same time the banding instrument is pressed firmly forwards into the anal wall: this combination of traction and pulsion pulls the bulk of the haemorrhoid into the drum, the distal edge of which comes up to the edge of the neck of the haemorrhoid.

The trigger mechanism is now 'fired' and the 'O' bands are squeezed off, snapping them onto the neck of the haemorrhoid.

3

The end-point

After the bands are in position and the instruments have been withdrawn a ball of tissue (which is usually cherry-sized) is left with its base tightly constricted.

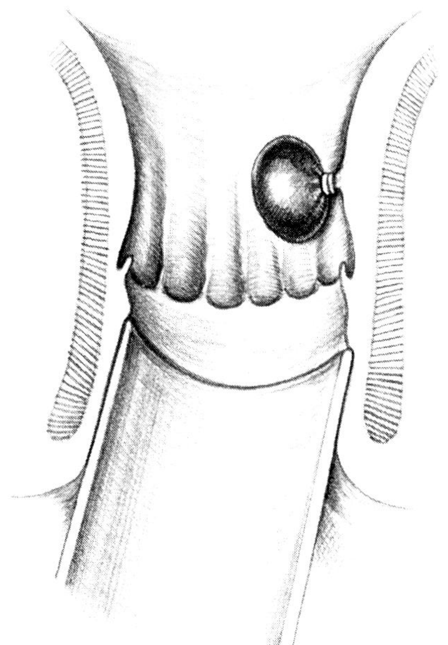

3

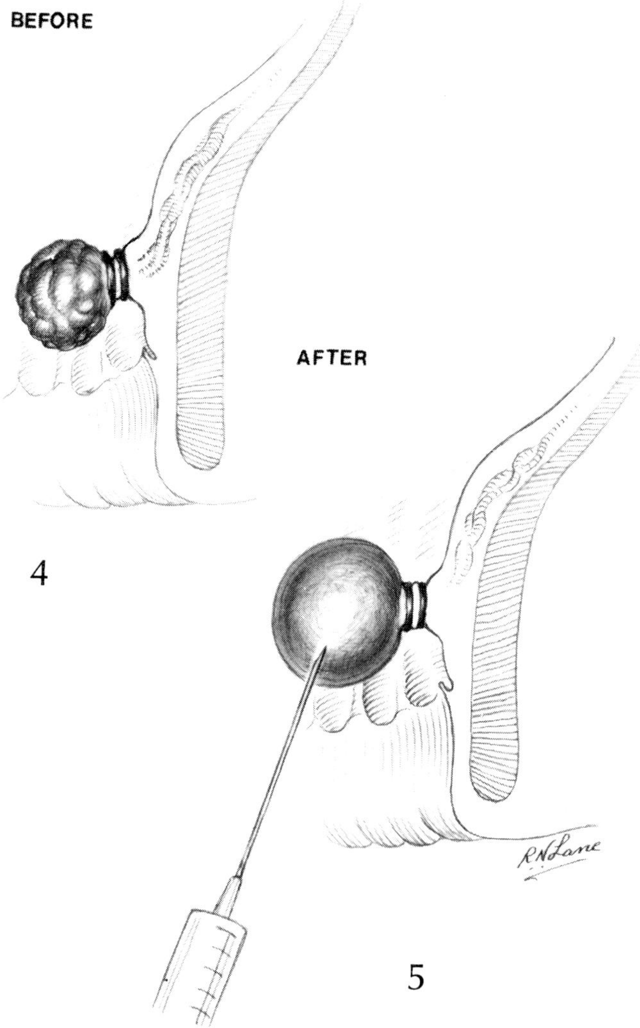

4

5

4 & 5

The procedure is now complete, but many surgeons perform an additional measure which consists of injecting the strangled mass with 1 or 2 ml of 5 per cent phenol in arachis oil (author's preference) to sterilize the ischaemic process and reduce the risk of secondary haemorrhage. Others prefer local anaesthetic solutions because this reduces the post-treatment discomfort.

Furthermore the fluid 'blows up' the banded tissue and makes it more difficult for the bands to become dislodged.

It is recommended that no more than two haemorrhoids be banded at any one occasion to reduce the amount of post-treatment oedema and pain, and at least 3 weeks should elapse between treatments.

Postoperative care and complications

Provided the bands have been put on correctly, the patient will not experience pain during or after treatment. A mild ache is usual for up to 48 h, but it can be controlled by a few paracetamol or Distalgesic tablets. Opiates are not usually necessary and should be avoided if possible because they increase sphincter spasm and cause constipation.

Constipation should be prevented by giving 15 ml Milpar every evening and the patient is directed to avoid straining.

The piles necrose and separate between the fourth and tenth days when the patient may notice slight bleeding. He should be warned that the 'O' rings may be seen after separation. A shallow mucosal ulcer is left behind after the pile has sloughed away and this may take up to 2 weeks to heal.

Severe pain

If too many haemorrhoids have been banded at one treatment, or if the 'O' rings have been applied too low, i.e. too near the dentate line (thereby including sensitive squamous epithelium in the constricted zone) severe pain can result. The pain is usually too intense to be treated by analgesics (even Pethidine 100 mg every 6 h may be insufficient to give adequate relief) and the elastic bands must be removed. This is difficult and may be associated with troublesome bleeding: therefore it may have to be carried out under a general anaesthetic, the rings being divided by a small straight-pointed tenotomy knife or pointed scissors.

Oedema and thrombosed external haemorrhoids

Occasionally after a banding treatment the tissues at the anal verge become slightly swollen. This subsides after a few days and does not require treatment, but hot baths (Sitz) are soothing and may hasten resolution of the oedema.

Very rarely, secondary thrombosis of an external haemorrhoid may occur. This should be treated conservatively with frequent hot baths and the application of hygroscopic ointments (ung. magnesium sulphate). It can also be treated surgically (*see* pp. 464–466).

Prolapse

Provided straining is prevented this complication can be avoided. However, if the patient *does* strain within a few days of banding, a general prolapse and thrombosis of the whole haemorrhoidal complex can occur. This is usually treated conservatively, but the patient may require admission to hospital for a few days. Alternatively a maximal anal dilatation may be employed (*see* pp. 593–598 in this volume) to effect a quicker cure.

'Ulcer' and secondary haemorrhage

In 1–2 per cent of cases, separation of the dead slough is associated with a deeper than usual ulcer crater and a haemorrhoidal vessel may be eroded. This can cause a severe secondary haemorrhage requiring the patient to be admitted urgently to hospital for a blood transfusion. The bleeding may need to be controlled by packing and/or suture/ligation (*see* p. 606 in this volume).

Further reading

Barron, J. Office ligation of internal haemorrhoids. American Journal of Surgery 1963; 105: 563–570

Goligher, J. C. Surgery of the anus, rectum and colon. 3rd ed. London: Ballière Tindall, 1975: 137

Maximal anal dilatation

Peter H. Lord MChir, FRCS
Consultant Surgeon, Wycombe General Hospital, High Wycombe, Buckinghamshire

Introduction

Haemorrhoids consist of normal tissue which is present in the form of vascular cushions or pads situated in the submucosa at the lower extremity of the rectum and upper anus. These pads are in the well recognized positions – left lateral, right posterior and right anterior. The vascular pads are present at birth, become larger at puberty and persist throughout life[1]. They can give rise to symptoms if they become overfilled with blood and are then called haemorrhoids. They may bleed, thrombose or prolapse. Overfilling is always associated with defaecation and is presumably due to obstruction of venous return by increased intrarectal pressure. This in turn is believed to be caused, certainly in the vast majority of sufferers, by a constricted outlet which will not dilate sufficiently to allow the faecal bolus to pass easily. The congested haemorrhoids further restrict the outlet, and it is the aim of the dilatation procedure and regimen to break this vicious circle.

All degrees of haemorrhoids respond to the dilatation procedure and regimen. Minor degrees should respond to diet, bran and bowel regulation without dilatation, and where there are very large haemorrhoids with much prolapse, dilatation alone may be insufficient. The method can then be combined with cryotherapy, Barron band ligation or clamp excision.

Preoperative

Assessment

The assessment of haemorrhoids relies mostly on the history given by the patient. Their presence can be seen on inspection and proctoscopy, but only the patient can tell if they bleed or prolapse on defaecation and whether they retract spontaneously or have to be replaced.

Preoperative preparation

As dilatation requires an anaesthetic there is no need to subject the patient to painful procedures preoperatively. If the anus is tender, particularly in the presence of a fissure, sigmoidoscopy, etc. can be carried out with the patient anaesthetized and without any preoperative bowel preparation. Dilatation as described below is an excellent treatment for fissure-in-ano.

If the anus is not tender and the rectal mucosa has been visualized preoperatively and proctitis and colitis excluded, it is advantageous to prepare the bowel preoperatively with a disposable enema or Dulcolax (bisacodyl) suppository. If the rectal mucosa has not been seen, this form of preparation makes it difficult to assess whether the mucosa is normal or inflamed.

Anaesthetic

The procedure is usually carried out in the anaesthetic room. The patient is asked to lie on the left side before the anaesthetist starts. Intravenous Epontol (propanidid) is used for induction, supplemented by halothane inhalation anaesthetic if necessary. Normally the procedure takes only a few minutes, including the sigmoidoscopy.

The operation

1

Identifying the constriction

The surgeon must first identify the constrictions involving the lower end of the rectum and the anal canal. These are not apparent in the non-anaesthetized patient, nor can they be felt with the fingers of one hand. The surgeon stands at the patient's back, inserts two fingers of the left hand and pulls upwards. Then the index finger of the right hand is inserted, pressing downwards, and the constriction can be felt. This is often at the level of the pecten, and in most patients consists of the lowermost fibres of the internal sphincter, which have undergone a change and are no longer able to relax. There is a thickening of the muscle, abnormal motor activity and some fibrosis similar to the changes seen in the sigmoid colon in diverticular disease[2].

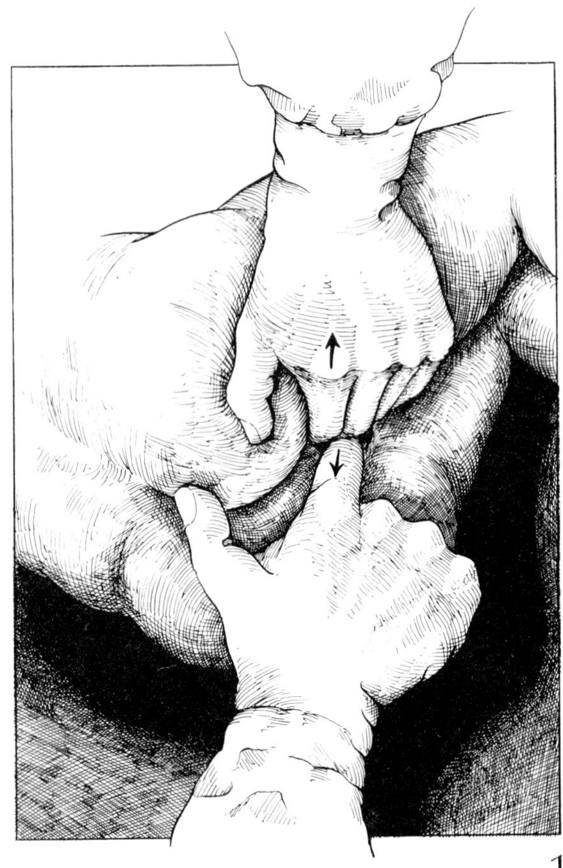

1

2

The dilatation

The dilatation procedure should be gentle and controlled. It starts using the index finger of each hand, the surgeon gradually inserting more fingers as the constriction is overcome. By careful manipulation it is possible to throw the strain of the dilatation on to the constricting bands in the left lateral and right lateral positions, i.e. 3 and 9 o'clock, and to avoid damaging the sphincter at 12 o'clock and particularly at 6 o'clock where it is relatively weak. The degree of dilatation varies, and it is clearly better to do too little than to risk damage to the sphincter; usually six to eight fingers can be inserted, and often constrictions can be felt in the lower rectum as high as the fingers can reach. These also should be made to give way laterally.

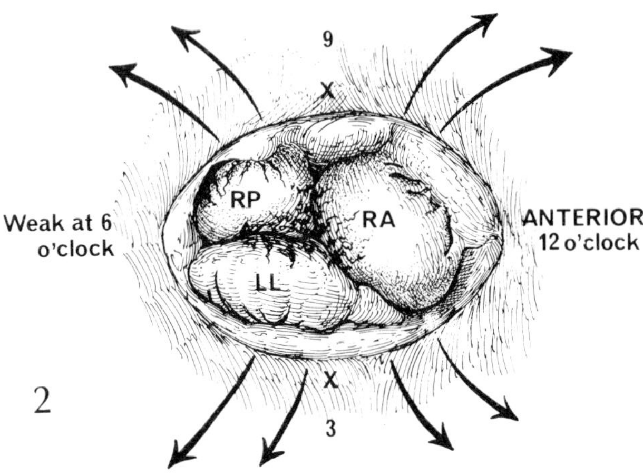

2

The sponge

At the end of the dilatation procedure it should be clear that there is no constriction between the upper rectum and the exterior, and that defaecation is able to take place without any significant rise in intrarectal pressure.

3, 4, & 5

At this point, without removing his fingers, the surgeon stands to the side, and the theatre nurse inserts the sponge using a sponge-holding forceps. This is easier if the specially designed forceps are employed, though these are not essential. The sponge should be inserted gently and goes in more easily if it is well soaked in a soapy solution such as Hibitane, 1:200 000. The surgeon's fingers guide the sponge into position, and if the special introducer is used, the nurse can then spring open the sponge-holding forceps and remove the blades one at a time. With an ordinary forceps there is a tendency for the sponge to be pulled down again as the forceps are removed. The sponge exerts gentle pressure on the walls of the lower rectum and anal canal where the dilatation has been carried out, thereby reducing the risk of haematoma formation.

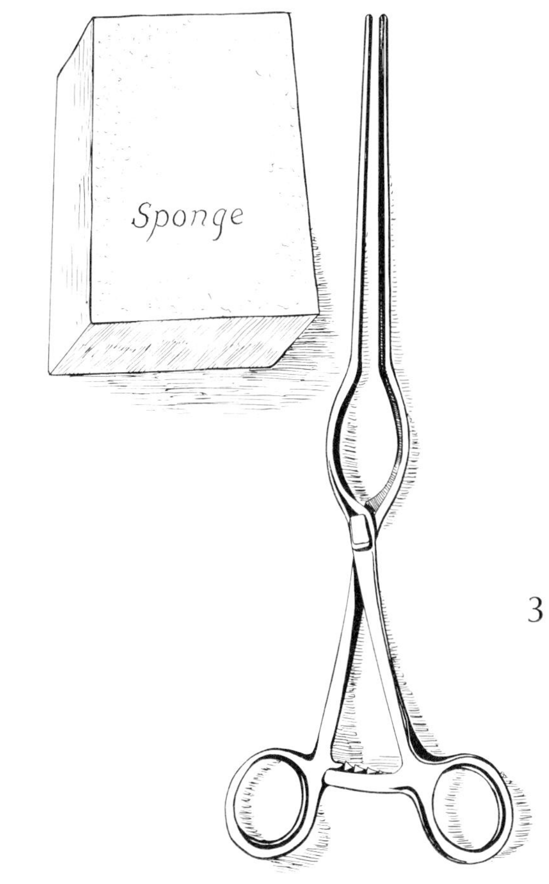

3

Important note

It is important to stress that all these manoeuvres are carried out with great gentleness and that the surgeon must feel what he is doing – there should be no tearing of mucosa or damage to the delicate anorectal sphincter mechanism. It is worth repeating that it is far better to do too little than to do too much and thus cause damage.

The sponge stays in place for at least 1 h and can then be removed. This part of the procedure may cause pain to the patient, so intramuscular pethidine 100 mg can be given half an hour before removing the sponge.

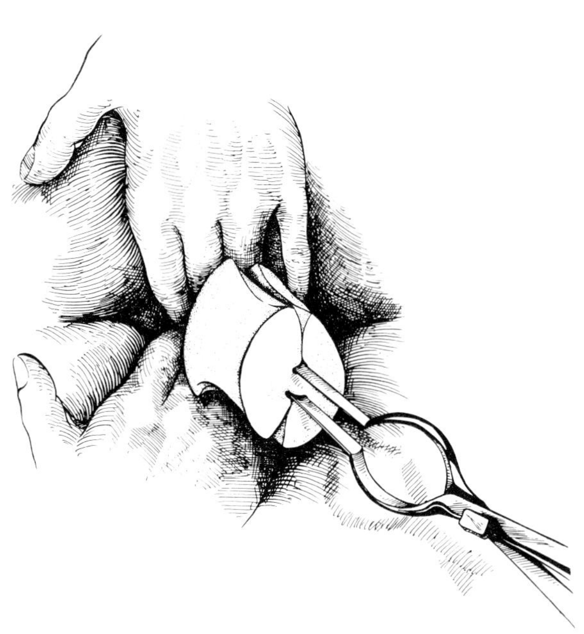

4

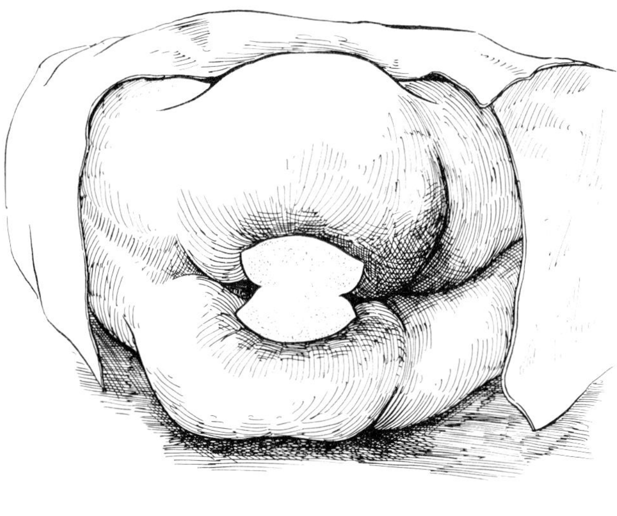

5

Postoperative regimen

6

The anorectal region might narrow down again during the healing period, and the aim of the postoperative regimen is to prevent this possibility. A special dilator has been designed for this purpose, and the patient is trained to insert this when well relaxed after a hot bath in the evening before retiring. If the dilator goes in easily then it can be used less often, but once a day for 2 weeks, then twice a week, once a week, etc., has usually been the pattern among the author's patients.

A bulk evacuant, Normacol, is used as a routine postoperatively so that the patient passes a soft bulky stool. Once a good bowel habit is established, it is usually a wise precaution for the patient to supplement the normal diet with natural bran.

The patient is seen 2 weeks after the procedure to make sure that all is well and 2 months afterwards for a final check and discharge.

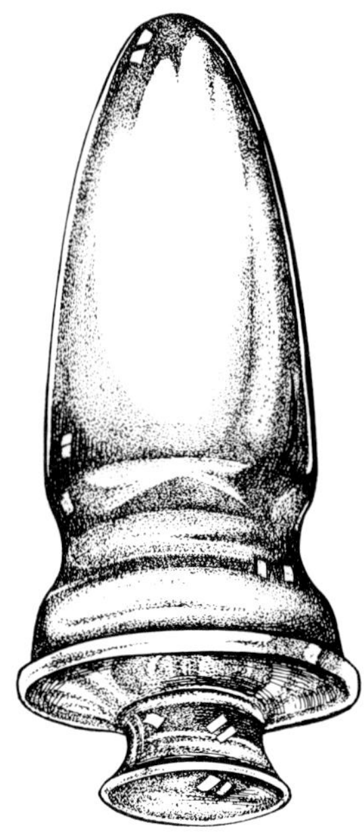

6

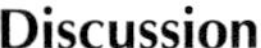

Discussion

Although the author carries out the procedure and regimen in much the same way as originally described[3] the method has been modified by others who claim satisfactory results. Some surgeons have stopped using the sponge and say it has made no difference to their haematoma rate.

It is difficult to know if the dilator is vital to the success of the method. Some surgeons claim that they get good results without its use. On the other hand, many of the author's patients have volunteered that they find the dilator very helpful in the early postoperative phase and that they feel more comfortable after using it.

The dilator

The dilator is left with the patient who is instructed that if at any future date any anal symptom occurs, the dilator should be used a few times to make quite sure that the constriction has not recurred.

Complications

Incontinence

This is the complication most feared by the patient and by the surgeon not familiar with the method. It is a fair statement that this complication does not occur, and that if it did, the method would be unacceptable, but this statement needs to be qualified as follows.

1. Incontinence of flatus for a few days after dilatation is usual, and this may persist for a few weeks.
2. If the patient previously had a particularly tight outlet, the situation is very different after dilatation, and the patient may take a little time to get used to the new condition. There may be a feeling of unsureness of the sphincter mechanism and encouragement and sphincter exercises are needed for a few weeks.
3. A number of cases have now been reported where the sphincter mechanism has been damaged at 6 o'clock, producing the so-called keyhole deformity of the anus. Faecal-stained mucus can escape down the groove leading to soiling and soreness. This complication is avoided by good technique and particularly by ensuring that the strain of the dilatation is thrown on to the lateral aspect of the anus.

Bruising

Modest perianal bruising is normal after this procedure and is of no significance. A large amount of bruising can lead to pain and may require several days' treatment with analgesics, but fortunately this does not adversely affect the end result.

Excessive haematoma formation may occur in a patient with a bleeding diathesis, e.g. haemophilia. The method is not contraindicated in these patients but should be carried out with great gentleness – in stages if necessary – and with full haematological cover.

Mucosal prolapse

Some degree of postoperative prolapse is commonly seen after the dilatation in those patients who had appreciable haemorrhoidal prolapse preoperatively. This will gradually improve with the postoperative regimen and sphincter exercises and the majority resolve, but if still persistent at 2 months, a further procedure is necessary.

A prolapse is abolished by: (*1*) Barron band ligation; (*2*) cryodestruction; or (*3*) clamp excision using the author's perianal clamp.

7a

7a–d

Use of the clamp

Persistent mucosal prolapse is usually in the right anterior position (*a*). Under general anaesthetic and with the patient in the left lateral position, as already described, this is grasped in Duval forceps, pulled down, a Lord pattern perianal clamp (*b*) applied across the base (*c*) and the excess mucosa removed (*d*). The clamp, which is curved to fit the buttocks, is strapped in position and left on for 1 h (*c*). The jaws are of a crushing haemostatic design so that when the clamp is removed, there should be no bleeding and the patient is allowed home when recovered from the brief anaesthetic. This clamp can also be used for removing skin tags and anal polyps.

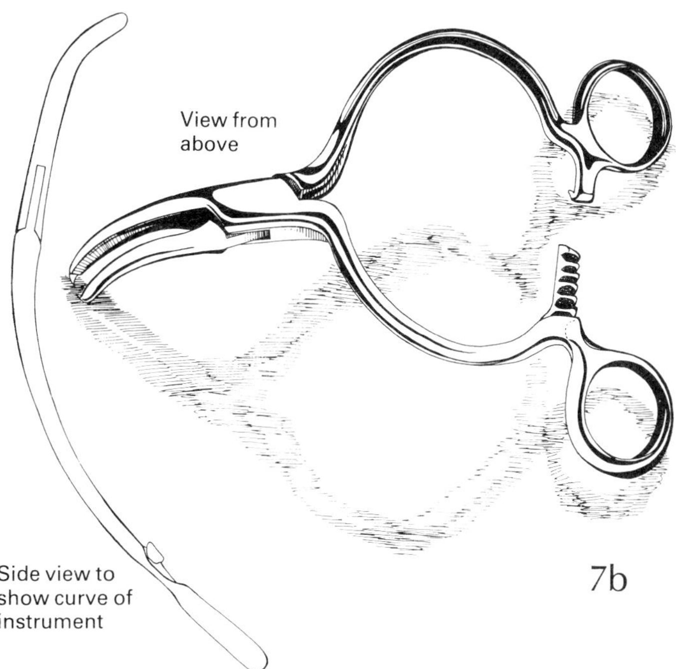

7b

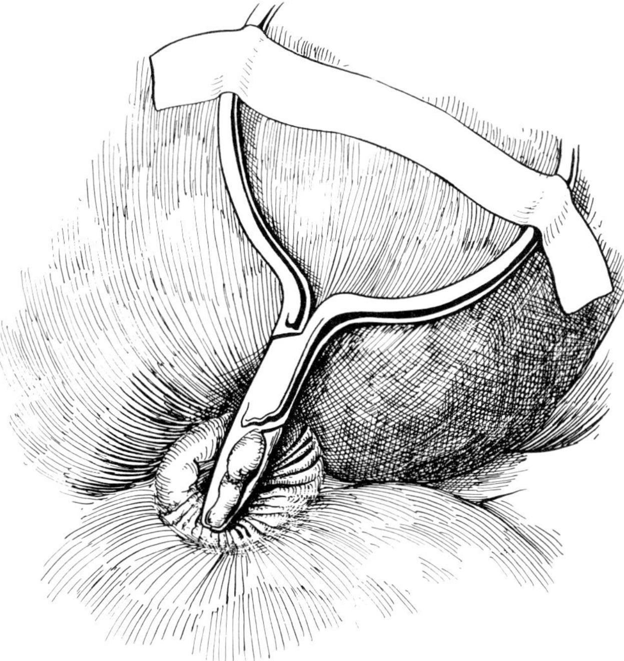

7c

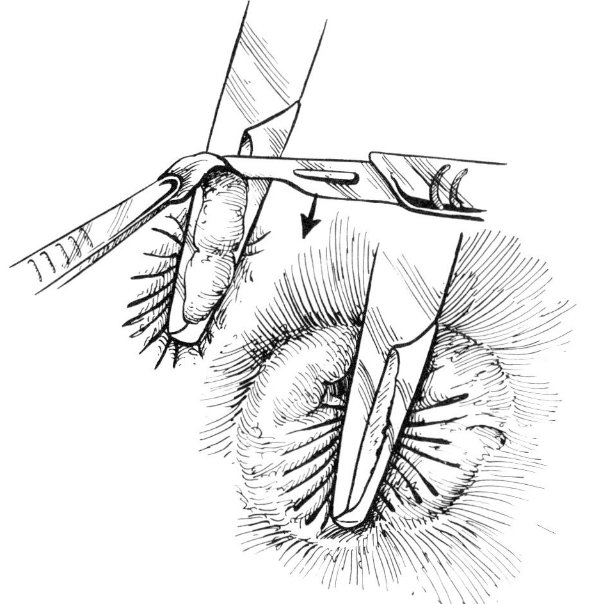

7d

Acute thrombosis of the haemorrhoidal tissue

This complication is fortunately rare – it is not clear why it occurs in these few patients nor what can be done to prevent it. It is an embarrassment as there is a considerable swelling with some soreness, though usually not severe pain. This settles gradually and usually leads to an excellent end result, but the patient requires much reassurance.

Complications not seen

Urinary retention; faecal impaction; deep vein thrombosis; pulmonary embolus.

References

1. Thomson, W. H. F. The nature of haemorrhoids. British Journal of Surgery 1975; 62: 542–552

2. Hancock, B. D. Internal sphincter and the nature of haemorrhoids. Gut 1977; 18: 651–655

3. Lord, P. H. A day-case procedure for the cure of third-degree haemorrhoids. British Journal of Surgery 1969; 56: 747–749

4. Lord, P. H. A new approach to haemorrhoids. Progress in Surgery 1972; 10: 109–124

Open haemorrhoidectomy (St Mark's ligation/excision method)

C. V. Mann MCh, FRCS
Consultant Surgeon, The London Hospital and St Mark's Hospital, London

Preoperative

Indications

Surgical treatment offers the best chance of permanent cure of haemorrhoids. For large *third-degree* haemorrhoids with prominent skin tags no other method approaches the precision and certainty of an expertly performed operation. If other treatments, such as banding or maximal anal dilatation, have failed, an operation can still cure the patient.

Associated anal pathology (e.g. chronic fissure, large skin tags or a fistula) are reasons for removal of any coexistent haemorrhoids.

Rarely, severe anaemia can be caused by persistent bleeding from haemorrhoids.

The open method combines removal of the haemorrhoidal cushions with excellent drainage of what is theoretically a septic wound. Complications are rare and the successes high.

Contraindications

Although symptomatic recurrent haemorrhoids are rare after a properly performed haemorrhoidectomy, the younger the patient the greater the risk of recurrence. It is the author's preference not to operate on patients with haemorrhoids below the age of 35 years when a suitable alternative method exists to relieve symptoms until the patient is older, particularly when there is a strong family history of the condition or an occupation (e.g. publican) that predisposes to piles.

All operations on the anal area are best avoided if a dysenteric infection, active Crohn's disease or colitis are present: not only are the wounds likely to be indolent and slow to heal, but complications (e.g. fistula) may occur.

Gross obesity should be reduced before surgery, and any skin sepsis (e.g. fungus infection) eradicated.

During pregnancy palliative treatment is best and the piles usually improve after delivery. If they do not, then an elective operation can be recommended, although future pregnancies may cause new piles to appear.

Acute prolapse/thrombosis of haemorrhoids ('strangulated piles') can be operated on if the patient comes to the hospital within a day or two of the complication, but once there is obvious cellulitis of the anal margin, or if there is so much oedema that adequate skin bridges cannot be preserved, it is safer not to operate. Piles, however painful or disabling, are harmless in themselves, and treatment should never introduce a significant element of risk.

Providing a safe anaesthetic (even by a caudal method) can be given, old age is not a contraindication to surgical treatment, but irregular bowel habit, especially constipation, should be corrected before surgery. If the patient fails to pass a regular formed stool after operation, or uses purgatives to liquefy the motions, anal stenosis may result.

Patients who have active pulmonary or intestinal tuberculosis should not be operated on as tuberculous infection of the anal wounds can occur.

Preparation

Sigmoidoscopy to above the rectosigmoid junction (>20 cm) is necessary to confirm the absence of rectal disease and in particular to exclude a carcinoma. When suspicious symptoms are present a barium enema should be performed. If a rectal polyp is found, this should be removed totally before haemorrhoidectomy for histological examination: if it is an adenomatous lesion colonoscopy should be performed before operative treatment of the piles.

The usual preparation to ensure a fit patient and a safe anaesthetic should be performed; the programme should include haematological tests for sickle-cell disease, thalassaemia and Australia-antigen in appropriate cases.

The patient is admitted to hospital the day before surgery and a simple soap and water enema should be given soon after admission.

The perianal region should be carefully shaved and the patient should bathe.

A laxative should be given (2 Senokot tablets) the night before, and a disposable Fleet's (sodium dihydrogen phosphate) enema 2 h before the operation. If this does not work, a rectal wash-out is administered 1 h before surgery, but care must be taken to ensure that *all* the enema fluid is retrieved before the patient leaves for the operating suite.

Anaesthesia

Most patients remain very nervous at the prospect of a haemorrhoidectomy and premedication is an important preparation for the anaesthetic.

General anaesthesia supplemented by local anaesthesia is the best method; the local anaesthetic infiltration enables a much smaller dose of general agents to be administered because painful anal stimuli during the operation are reduced or even abolished. In particular, the risk of laryngeal spasm or cardiac arrhythmias from anal sphincter dilatation is avoided. The addition of adrenaline (1:200 000) added to lignocaine (1 per cent solution) produces an insensitive and bloodless operation field.

In elderly or unfit patients a caudal block can be used and some surgeons employ the caudal or epidural method routinely to supplement the general anaesthetic because they produce excellent relaxation of the anal sphincters and reduce peroperative oozing from the anal wounds. They also improve analgesia during the postoperative period. Epidural or low spinal blocks can be used as alternatives to general anaesthesia but both carry a greater risk than caudal block.

Position of patient

The patient is placed in the full lithotomy position with the buttocks lifted well down over the edge of the table, the lower flap of which should be removed. This can be an embarrassing and uncomfortable position if the operation is being carried out under local anaesthesia. In these circumstances the left lateral Sims position with the buttocks raised on a sandbag (see p. 490) offers reasonable exposure, especially if the upper buttock is retracted by strapping. If the patient has cardiac or respiratory problems this position is tolerated better than full lithotomy because there is no embarrassment of diaphragmatic action and no gross posturally related change in venous return to the heart so that cardiac output remains stable.

The operation

1

Injection of local anaesthesia

With the patient anaesthetized and in the lithotomy position, the perianal skin is carefully cleaned with a mild antiseptic solution (cetrimide 1 per cent or aqueous Hibitane 1:2000). The anal canal is carefully swabbed with cotton-wool pledgets soaked in cetrimide until all faecal particles have been removed.

Local anaesthetic solution (1 per cent lignocaine) containing adrenaline 1:200 000 is injected subcutaneously into each haemorrhoidal mass to be removed: 2–3 ml at each site is enough to ensure a dry field. The infiltration should extend beneath the mucocutaneous junction and the lining of the lower part of the anal canal, but need not include the upper half of the anal cushion.

Further amounts of local anaesthetic solution (3–5 ml) are placed in each ischiorectal fossa just to the medial side of the ischial tuberosity to block the inferior haemorrhoidal branches of the pudendal nerves. Using a No. 20, 5 cm needle with a finger in the anal canal as a guide, the needle is passed from a central puncture forwards and laterally until it is felt to strike the periosteum of the ischial tuberosity 2.5 cm above its lowest point. The needle is then withdrawn 1–2 mm and the infiltration carried out having ensured by aspiration that a vein has not been entered. This partial pudendal nerve block relaxes the sphincter ani externus and provides a helpful period of analgesia postoperatively.

It is advisable to wait 3–5 min after the local infiltration to allow the full haemostatic and anaesthetic effects.

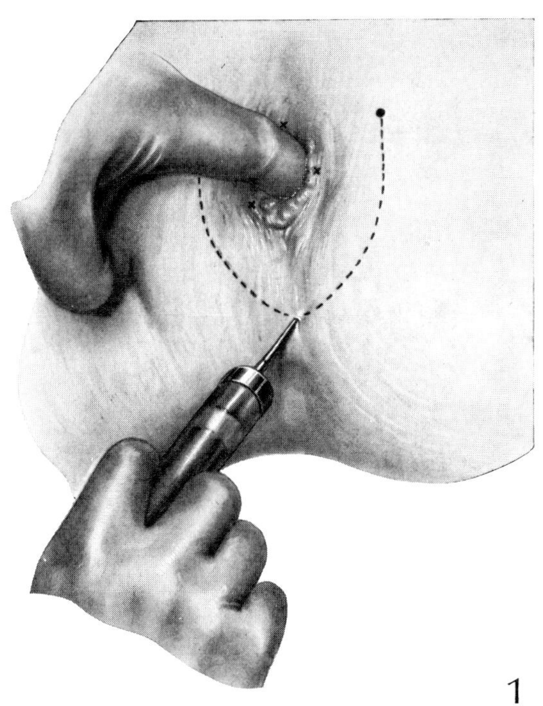

1

2

Display of operation field

A gentle two-finger dilation of the anal sphincters is performed to allow the anal canal to be opened. If the sphincter is very atonic, either naturally or as a result of the nerve block, this step is unnecessary and may be dangerous.

Dunhill forceps are placed on the perianal skin just outside the mucocutaneous junction opposite each primary haemorrhoidal cushion (left lateral, right anterior and right posterior – 3, 7 and 11 o'clock). Skin tags should be included in the area of perianal skin removed. Gentle traction on the forceps brings each haemorrhoidal mass into view.

At this stage careful note is made of the selected areas of skin and mucosa ('skin bridges') that will be left between each area of dissection and from which healing of the wounds will originate. If too few (less than 3) or too narrow (less than 1 cm) skin bridges are left there is a risk of postoperative anal stenosis.

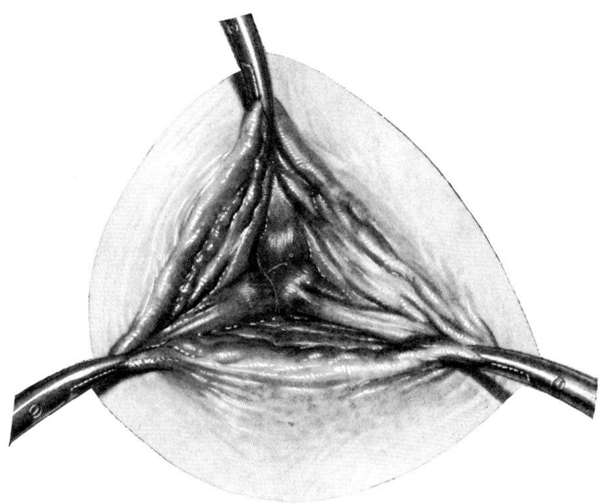

2

3

Triangle of exposure

As the internal haemorrhoids are pulled down, a second Dunhill forceps is put onto the main bulk of each haemorrhoidal mass; further traction exposes the pedicles of the haemorrhoids, and produces the so-called 'triangle of exposure': this is caused by the stretching of pink columnar-cell mucosa between the apices of each taut pedicle. When the second pair of Dunhill forceps are clipped to each haemorrhoid, care must be taken not to include the internal sphincter muscle by too deep a bite. Intervening small secondary haemorrhoids are taken with separate forceps, and approximated to the nearest primary forceps, so as to be included with the main haemorrhoid in the subsequent dissection.

Once the triangle of exposure has been achieved, the haemorrhoids are ready to be dissected and removed. It is a mistake to carry the pedicle dissection higher than this exposure allows because troublesome arterial bleeding will be encountered in the upper anal canal and there is a risk of narrowing the anal canal if too much mucosa is gathered in at the anorectal junction.

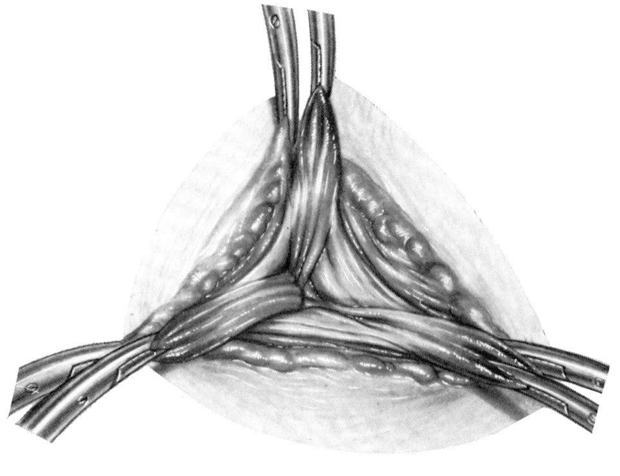

3

4

Start of the dissection

The haemorrhoids are dissected in turn. For a right-handed surgeon, it is convenient to start with the left lateral, the others being temporarily held out of the way with slight traction by the assistant. The two forceps are held in linear fashion in the palm of the left hand with the left forefinger in the anal canal on the pedicle of the haemorrhoid and pressing lightly outwards to stretch the pedicle gently over the pulp of the finger. The blades of a pair of blunt-nosed scissors (or knife) are placed alternately at each edge of the base, as seen from its cutaneous aspect, and the tissues divided towards the median plane until the incisions meet. The subcutaneous space superficial to the lowest ('white') fibres of the sphincter ani internus muscle and deep to the superficial sphincter ani externus ('red') muscle is now exposed and can be opened up.

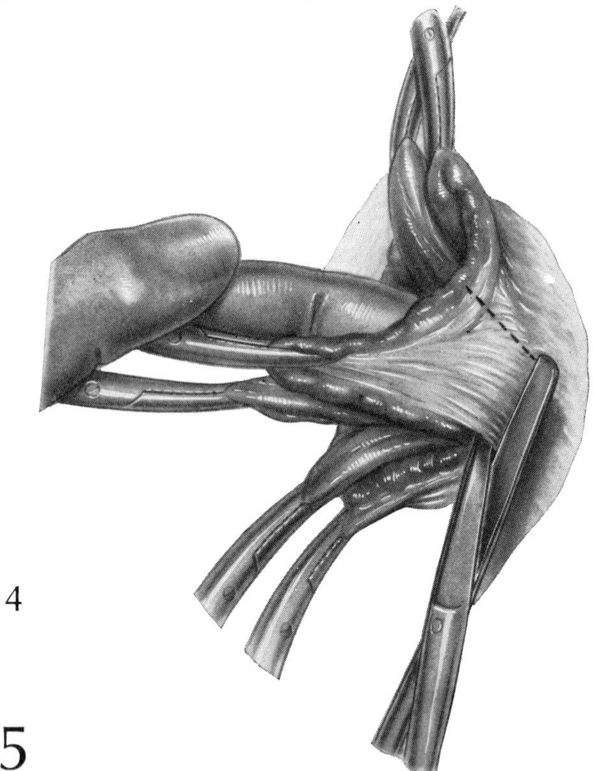

4

5

Further dissection

Dissection is continued in a coronal plane superficially at first but almost at once medial to the sphincter ani internus muscle and directed towards the pedicle of the haemorrhoids in the submucosal plane. The borders of the dissection taper towards the base of the pile and upward mobilization is not continued more than is necessary to allow easy control of the pedicle as previously defined by the 'triangle of exposure'.

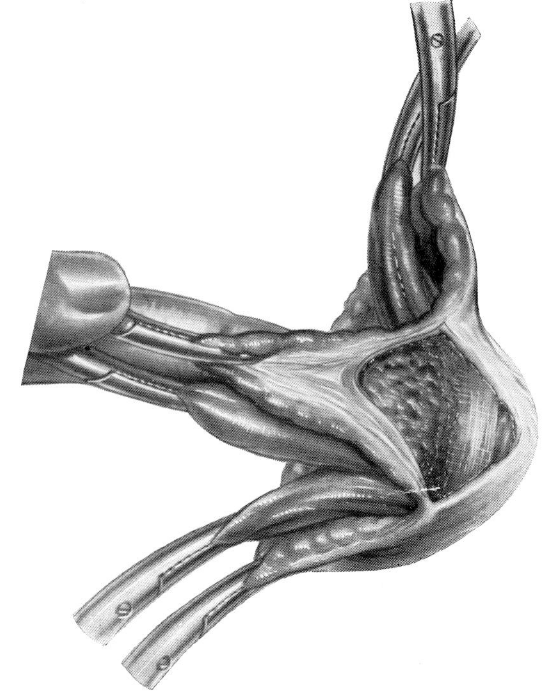

5

6

Ligation of pedicle

As the pedicle is exposed by dissection, traction on the haemorrhoid should be eased. Once it has been defined, the pedicle is transfixed with silk or catgut, with the knots tied on the lumen aspect. It is not necessary to use very strong material for the pedicle ligation, and too large a knot of unabsorbable material can excite a foreign-body reaction and even cause a fistula.

If the pedicle is large a second ligature can be applied, and double ligation with 00 chromic catgut is safer than single ligation with No. 1 catgut or braided silk.

Once the pedicle has been secured, and traction released to check that the vessels have been safely controlled, the pedicle can be cut through allowing a good cuff of tissue distal to the ligature so that it is not displaced by the first act of defaecation. The ends of the ligatures are left long, and the pedicles are allowed to retract to their normal position in the upper one half of the anal canal.

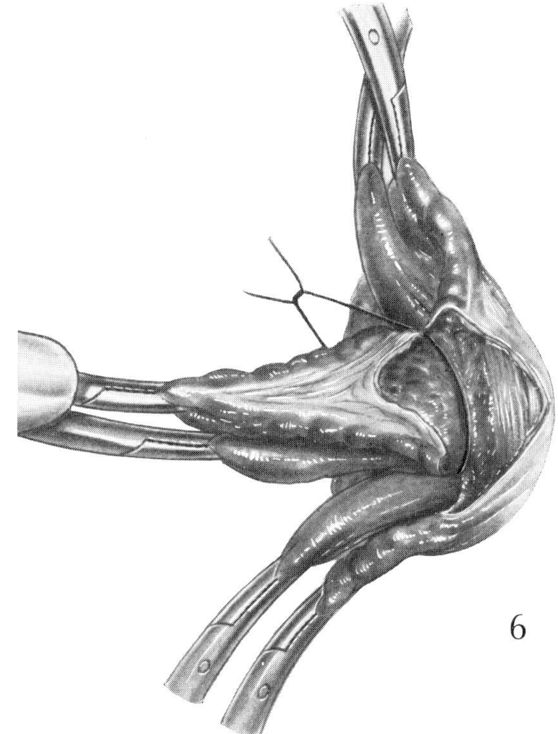

6

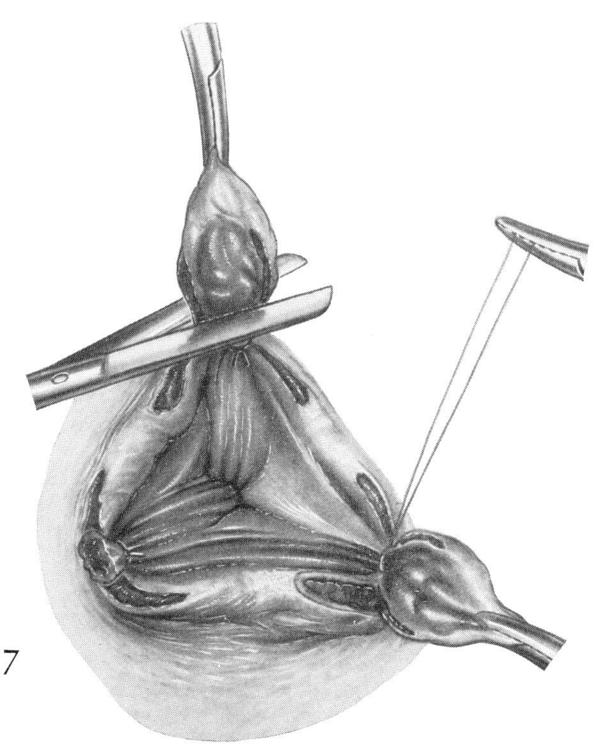

7

7

Procedure for the remaining haemorrhoids

The other haemorrhoids are dealt with each in turn by an identical process. The right anterior haemorrhoid is usually the smallest and easiest to eliminate and is frequently left to the last, especially as any bleeding from the front of the anal canal may obscure any subsequent dissection posteriorly. Intact 'bridges' of skin and mucosa (which should not be less than 1 cm in width) are preserved between all dissection sites.

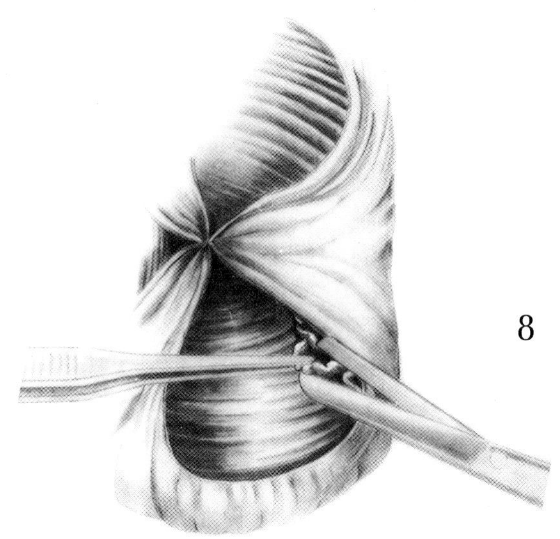

8

8 & 9

'Filleting' of skin bridges

If large external veins are seen beneath the residual bridges, these can be removed by dissection beneath the margins of the bridges from each side ('filleting') or by dividing across the bridges, removing the underlying veins, and then sewing the bridges back in place ('bridge division') with fine catgut.

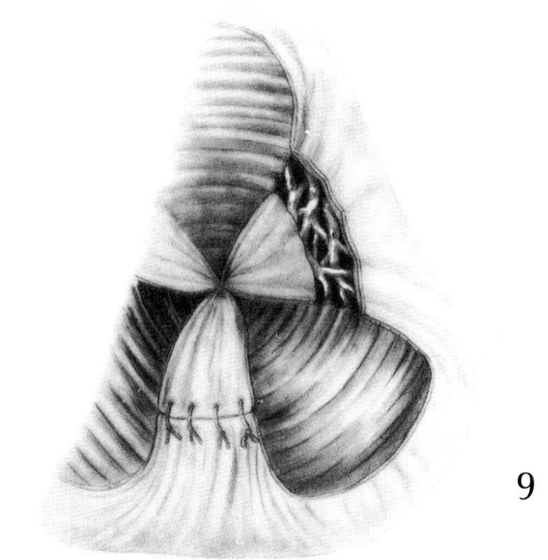

9

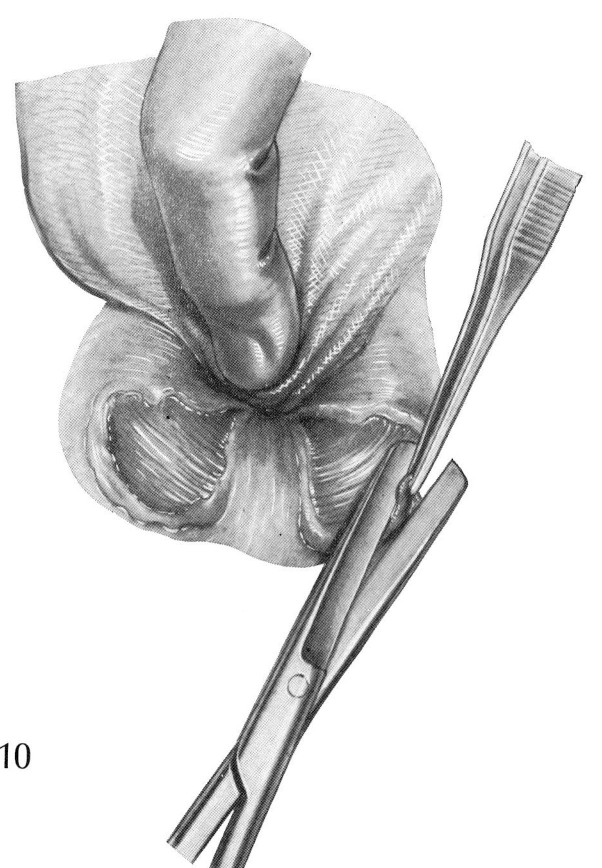

10

10

Trimming of wounds

The pedicles having retracted into the upper anal canal, the wounds are critically inspected for neatness and drainage, as well as haemostasis. Any redundant tags of skin are removed, and any puckering of the skin bridges is reduced by anchoring sutures of fine 000 chromic catgut. Haemostasis of any small bleeding points either from the mucosal edges or from the raw area of the wounds is controlled by light application of diathermy or by ligation with 000 catgut. Occasionally, in the presence of diffuse bleeding, the application of a swab soaked in adrenaline solution 1:1000 is preferred to excessive electrocoagulation.

11

Final appearance and dressing

The final appearance of the operated area should resemble a three-leafed clover, and the wounds should be absolutely dry before a dressing is applied.

Dressings are a matter of choice, except that oily substances and greasy materials should be avoided as they tend to clog the wounds and prevent proper drainage of serosanguinous exudate.

An excellent dressing is gauze lightly soaked in Milton (sodium hypochlorite 1:40 solution), or aqueous Hibitane (1:2000 solution). Whatever solution is used, it should not be painful or harmful to the healing process, and the gauze should lie flat without wrinkling or puckering. Finally, a thick pad of cotton-wool or Gamgee is laid over the perineum and held in place by a T-bandage or Netelast. Large endoanal plugs or tubes are unnecessary and painful and should not be used.

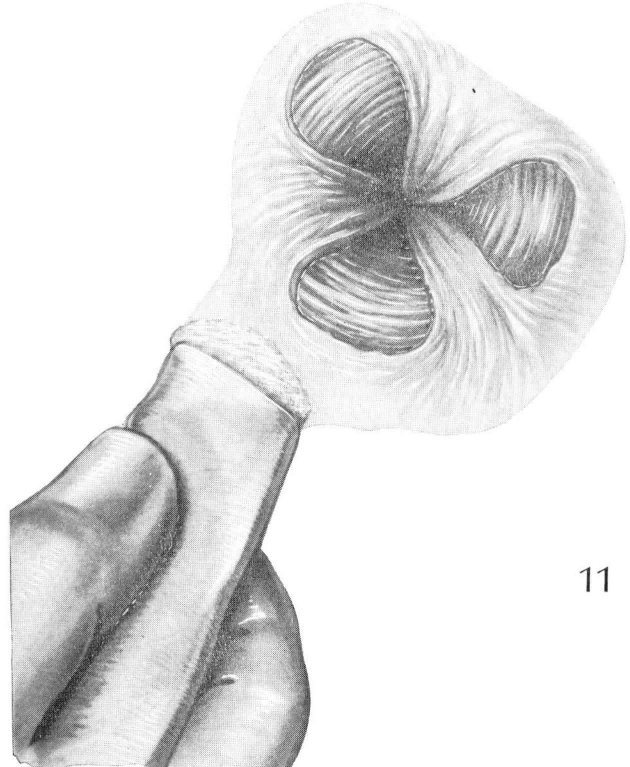

11

Postoperative care and complications

The dressings are left undisturbed for 24 h, after which they are changed twice daily. Before each dressing the patient should have a warm bath and on returning to bed the wounds are thoroughly irrigated with hydrogen peroxide followed by aqueous Hibitane (1:2000 solution). Finally gauze dressings lightly soaked in Milton solution (1 per cent sodium hypochlorite) are applied and adjusted to lie flat.

The patient should have a bath and his dressings reapplied after each bowel action, and in order to make the first evacuation easier Milpar (magnesium hydroxide and liquid paraffin – 15 ml 8 hourly) is started the day after operation. Once defaecation commences Milpar is stopped and Normacol, 1 tablespoon once or twice daily, is given instead. If the patient has not achieved defaecation by the third postoperative day, a disposable (sodium dihydrogen phosphate) enema is administered.

On the fifth postoperative day, a finger should be passed to check that healing is proceeding satisfactorily. If there is any stenosis (there should *not* be if the operation has been properly performed) or if there is any undue spasm or pain, the patient should be taught to use an anal dilator twice daily (St Mark's pattern anal dilator – size No. 2 is generally the most suitable for this purpose). If there is difficulty in establishing a regular daily bowel action with the passage of a properly formed stool, the use of an anal dilator may assist in obtaining regular healing without narrowing of the anal canal.

The patient can be permitted to leave hospital between the sixth and the tenth postoperative days, but final healing of the internal wounds will not occur for 6 weeks.

Before discharge from hospital the patient is recommended a high roughage diet with a bran supplement. If this does not ensure regular passage of a formed stool of reasonable size and soft consistency, Normacol-Special, 1 tablespoon (10 ml) night and morning, should be prescribed, although other hydrophylic colloids can also be given (Isogel, Celevac granules, Cologel) according to the patient's preferences.

The patient should return for examination 3 weeks after the operation. A finger should be passed to check that stenosis has not developed, but a proctoscope should not be employed as it is liable to break down the healing wounds and precipitate the development of an acute fissure.

Retention of urine

This can occur unexpectedly even in stoical patients, but is more common in nervous subjects or those who have a lot of immediate postoperative pain. The incidence is reduced by fluid restriction, the use of sedatives pre- and postoperatively, the employment of adjuvant local or epidural anaesthesia over the operation itself, and by generous use of analgesics. The condition usually responds to simple conservative measures and reassurance, but catheterization is occasionally required.

Immediate (reactionary) haemorrhage

Haemorrhage from a properly ligated pedicle is very rare in the immediate period after operation. However, brisk bleeding may occur from small arteries in the mucosal edge or raw surface of the wound. They can be stopped in most cases by application of a gauze swab soaked in adrenaline (1:1000 solution). If this fails, the application of a haemostat or diathermy coagulation may be required. An alternative would be the application of an infrared coagulation probe. In most cases it is not necessary to take the patient back to the operating theatre for these bleeding episodes.

If a ligature on a main pedicle slips, profuse blood loss may occur and blood transfusion is often necessary. The patient must be reanaesthetized when the blood pressure is stable, and either the rectum is packed for 24 h or the bleeding point located and underrun. The latter is the better procedure. It may be necessary to wash out the blood clot before the bleeding site can be seen.

Delayed (secondary) haemorrhage

This occurs unpredictably between the sixth and twentieth days postoperatively in 1–2 per cent of cases. The haemorrhage is often severe, requiring blood transfusion as well as local measures to arrest the bleeding.

Occasionally a single bleeding point can be identified after washing the blood clots out of the rectum, in which case an underrunning suture will arrest the haemorrhage. More frequently the bleeding must be stopped by applying firm pressure on the wall of the anal canal and lower rectum. This is done by packing the rectum with dry gauze through a large proctoscope. An anaesthetic is unnecessary but the patient needs to be sedated and helped with pain relief: an intravenous injection of opiate is ideal (Omnopon 10–20 mg). The patient must be instructed not to strain down while the packing is in progress. The gauze can be partially removed after 24 h, and completely removed after 48 h. The bowels are confined for several days by giving codeine phosphate (30 mg tablets 6 hourly). A Foley catheter in the rectum blown up to 30 ml can be tried as an alternative to packing: after the balloon is distended, traction is applied to the stem of the catheter, which is then strapped under moderate tension to the thigh and left *in situ* for 24–48 h. As a general rule, sepsis follows most cases of secondary haemorrhage and, in the author's view, broad-spectrum antibiotics should be given (intramuscular ampicillin 250 mg every 6 h for 5 days).

Fissure and fistula

Occasionally the anal wounds narrow but do not heal, and a fissure develops. This can be prevented by good postoperative care and the use of an anal dilator when necessary during the early healing period. If an anal dilator can not be used because of pain, gentle anal dilatation under a general anaesthetic may be required.

In some cases, the superficial margins of the wound fall together and heal over, leaving a fistulous track below the surface. If this happens, the wound must be laid open to allow secondary healing to occur from the depths of the wound towards the surface.

Anal stenosis and cross-healing

If the anus is not regularly expanded postoperatively (by a formed stool, or a dilator) the anal orifice can contract, leading to stenosis. If this occurs, the anus must be dilated under a general anaesthetic. An anal dilator should be used after dilatation to prevent recurrence.

If the patient is not encouraged to pass a regular stool of reasonable size after surgery and digital examination is neglected, adhesion between opposite wounds can occur. Such cross-healing requires breaking-down under a general anaesthetic if it is not detected early in the recovery period. It is extremely rare.

Further reading

Goligher, J. C., Leacock, A. G., Brossy, J. J. The surgical anatomy of the anal canal. British Journal of Surgery 1955; 43: 51–61

Milligan, E. T. C., Morgan, C. N. Surgical anatomy of the anal canal. Lancet 1934; 2: 1150–1157; 1213–1217

Milligan, E. T. C., Morgan, C. N., Jones, L. E., Officer, R. Surgical anatomy of the anal canal and the operative treatment of haemorrhoids. Lancet 1937; 2: 1119–1124

Lateral subcutaneous internal anal sphincterotomy for fissure-in-ano

M. J. Notaras FRCS, FRCS(Ed.)
Consultant Surgeon, Barnet General Hospital;
Honorary Senior Lecturer and Consultant Surgeon,
University College Hospital, London

Introduction

Examination of the lower half of the anal canal by separation of the buttocks to open up the perianal region will reveal the presence of any simple anal fissure as it is located below the dentate line and is always confined to the anoderm in the midposterior position (90 per cent) or the midanterior position (10 per cent). The anoderm is that part of the anal skin which lies between the dentate line and the anal verge and is the squamous lining of the anal canal. The acute fissure is a superficial splitting of the anoderm and may heal with conservative management. Once the fissure is recurrent or chronic, operation is required for a permanent cure. The chronic fissure is recognized by the presence of transverse fibres of the internal sphincter in its floor. A late stage in the development of the chronic fissure is the formation of a large fibrous polyp from the anal papilla on the dentate line at the upper end of the fissure. Infection of the sentinel pile which develops at the lower end of the fissure at the anal verge may lead to the formation of a superficial fistula.

Fissures which are multiple or extend above the dentate line should be viewed with suspicion as the simple fissure-in-ano never extends above the dentate line. These complex fissures are usually signs of more serious diseases such as ulcerative colitis, Crohn's disease, tuberculosis or syphilis. When associated with large rubbery inguinal lymph nodes they may indicate a primary syphilitic infection and smears from the anal canal should be taken for dark ground illumination before digital or endoscopic examination contaminates the field with lubricant.

A biopsy should always be taken from any suspicious fissure or ulcer.

An intersphincteric sinus or abscess may be mistaken for a chronic anal fissure unless excluded by careful examination. A subcutaneous fistula may also be present in a sentinel pile (*see* illustration on stages of fissure-in-ano).

Treatment of fissure-in-ano

Lateral subcutaneous internal anal sphincterotomy has been shown to have many advantages over other forms of treatment such as anal dilatation and the midposterior internal sphincterotomy performed through the floor of the fissure. It has rapidly gained acceptance as it may be performed as an outpatient procedure under local or general anaesthesia. Its main advantages are that it avoids an open intra-anal wound, the divided internal sphincter is bridged by skin, there is minimal anal wound care, postoperative anal dilatation is unnecessary and relief from symptoms is almost immediate with the fissure becoming painless and healing within 3 weeks.

The cross-reference in this chapter refers to *Operative Surgery: Alimentary Tract and Abdominal Wall, Volume 3, 4th Edition*

Stages of fissure-in-ano

(Illustrated below)

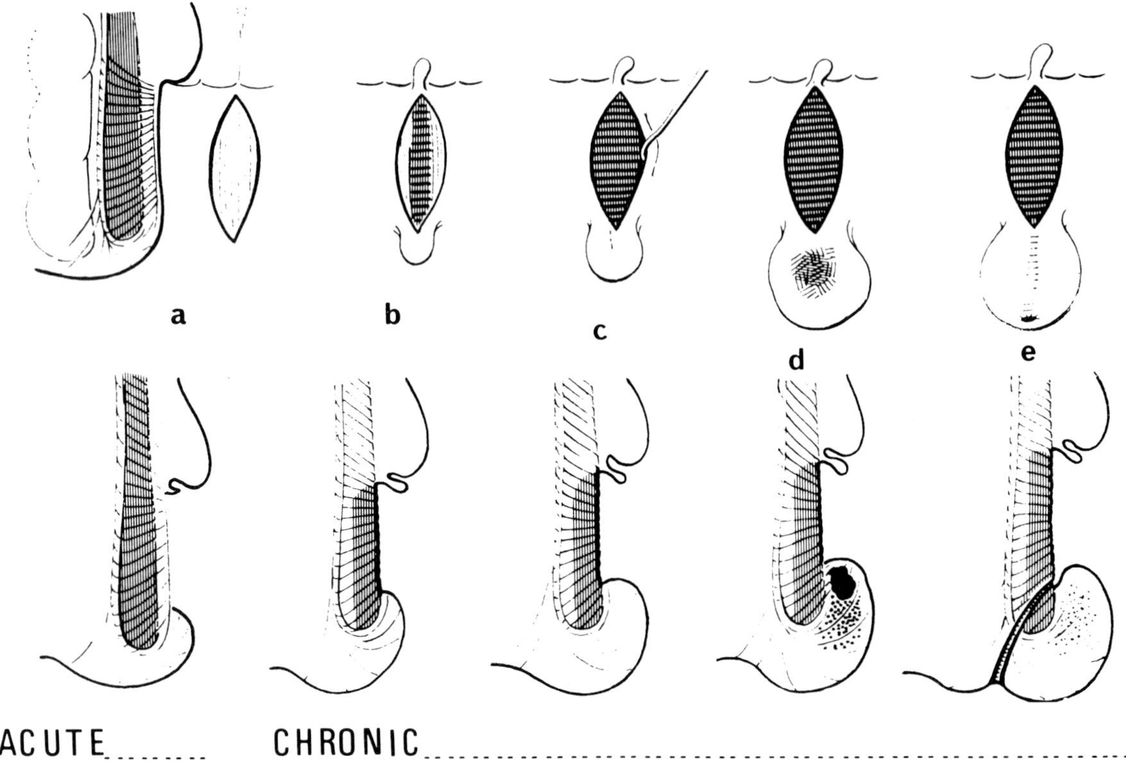

Preoperative

Preoperative preparation

The author prefers no bowel preparation so that the urge to defaecate after the operation is not delayed. The patient may be placed in the lithotomy, lateral or 'jack-knife' positions according to the preference of the surgeon. Sigmoidoscopy should be performed on all patients.

Anaesthesia

The procedure may be performed under general or local anaesthesia or a combination of methods. The author supplements a general anaesthetic with local anaesthesia which permits a lighter general anaesthetic to be used and local dilute adrenaline solution helps to reduce bleeding and immediate postoperative pain.

Approximately 10 ml of local anaesthetic agent (0.5 per cent lignocaine with 1:200 000 adrenaline) is infiltrated subcutaneously into the perianal area on each side of the anus. The inferior haemorrhoidal nerves are blocked on each side by injection of 5–7 ml into each ischiorectal space along the medial aspect of each ischial tuberosity. A further 5 ml is injected directly into the external sphincter muscle on each side of the anus.

When local anaesthesia is used alone it should be supplemented by diazepam 10–20 mg intravenously (according to age and weight), and sometimes also pethidine 50–100 mg intravenously. This technique sedates patients adequately and although conscious throughout the procedure they usually have no memory of the event. After the operation patients will need to rest for 1–2 h until the effects of local anaesthesia have subsided and the sphincters have recovered.

The operations

CLOSED TECHNIQUE (lithotomy position)

1 & 2

A bivalved anal speculum (Parks, Eisenhammer or Goligher) is introduced into the anal canal and opened sufficiently to place the anus on a slight stretch. The internal sphincter is then felt as a tight band around the blades of the speculum. Its lower border is easily palpated and can be demonstrated by gently pressing a pair of forceps into the intersphincteric groove. The floor of the fissure should be probed for a sinus or fistula.

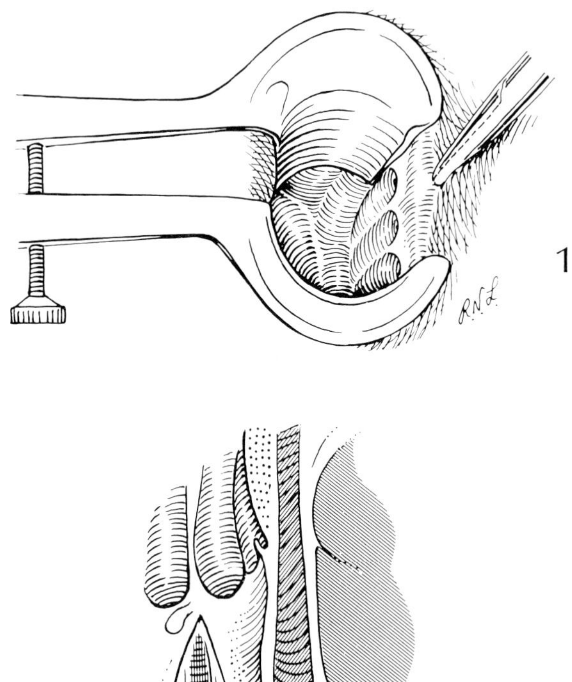

1

2

3

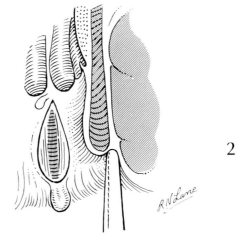

Two or three millilitres of the local anaesthetic agent is then introduced under the mucosa and anoderm. The illustration shows how the anal lining is lifted away from the internal sphincter, thus reducing bleeding and the risk of perforation by the scalpel blade in the closed technique. It also facilitates dissection if the open technique is used.

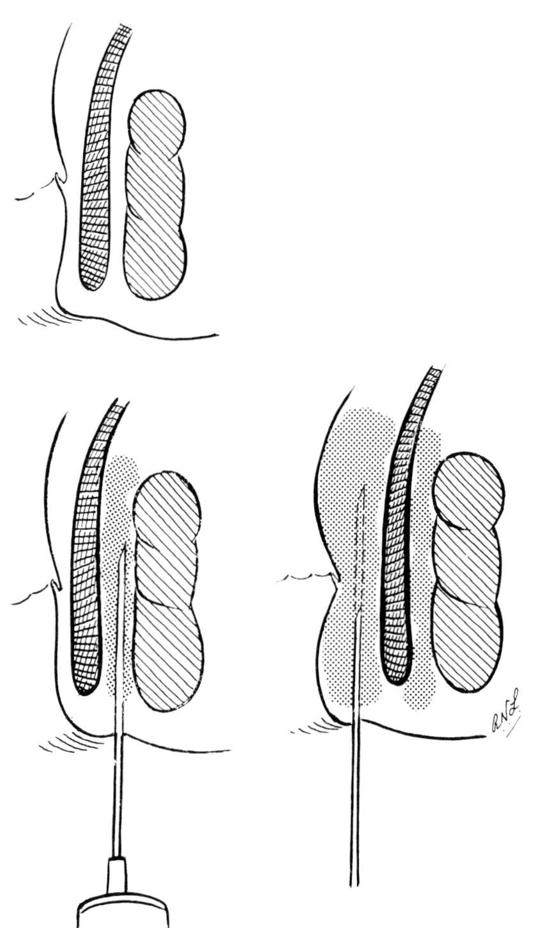

3

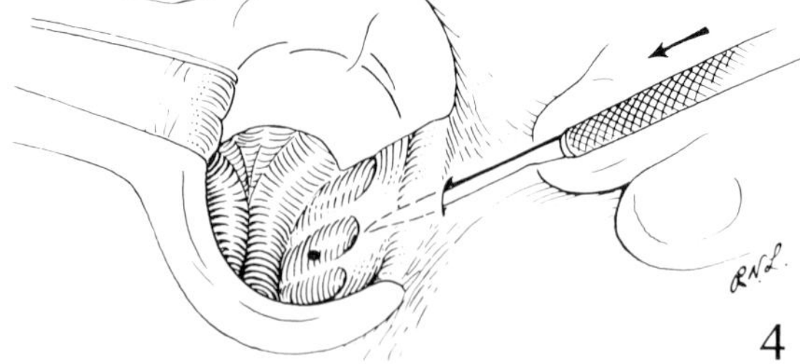
4

4 & 5

After the internal sphincter has been identified a narrow-bladed scalpel (52L 'Beaver' cataract knife) is introduced through the perianal skin at the midlateral aspect of the anus (3 o'clock). It is pushed cephalad with the flat of the blade sandwiched between the internal sphincter and anoderm until its point is just above the dentate line.

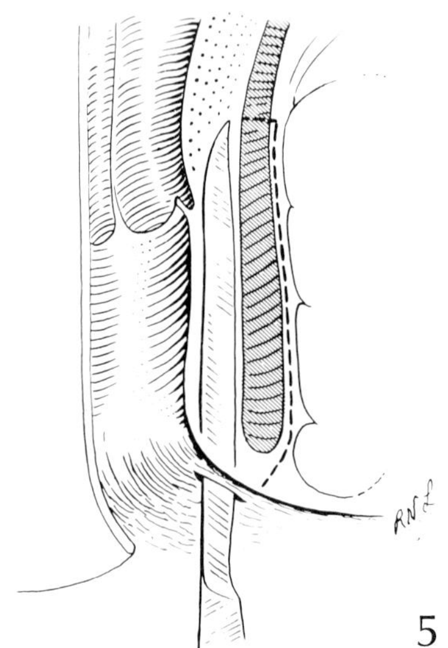
5

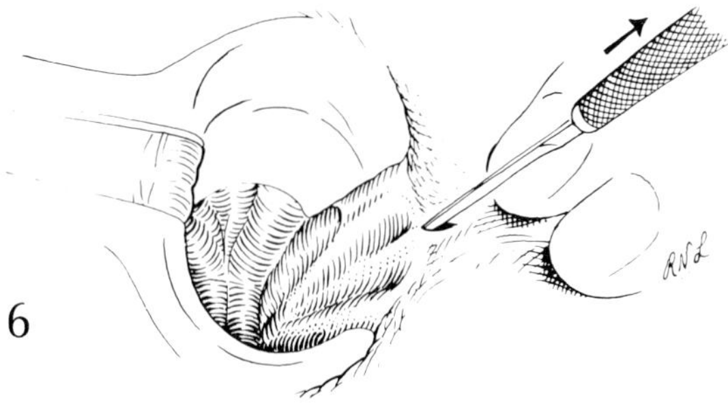
6

6 & 7

The sharp edge of the blade is then turned towards the internal sphincter and by incising outwards and laterally the internal sphincterotomy is performed. As the scalpel blade cuts through the internal sphincter there is a characteristic 'gritty' sensation and with completion of the division there is a sudden 'give', indicating that the blade has reached the outer surrounding ring of external sphincter muscles.

Another variation of the technique is to introduce the blade between the external and internal sphincter muscles via the intersphincteric groove and then to perform the sphincterotomy by cutting inwards towards the mucocutaneous lining.

Whichever technique is used, the aim is to preserve a skin bridge over the divided internal sphincter.

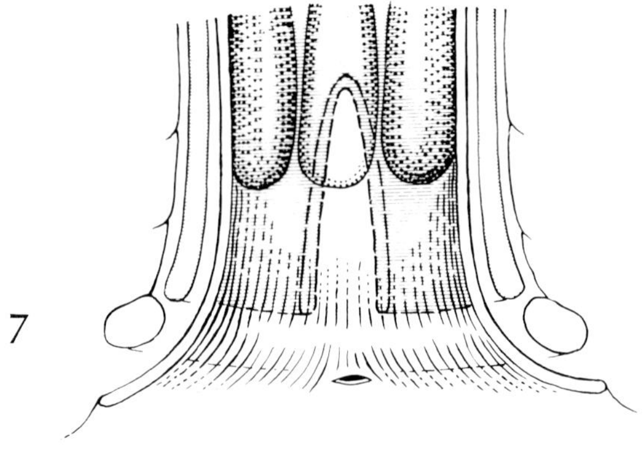
7

8

Following division of the internal sphincter the completeness of the sphincterotomy may be assessed after withdrawal of the knife by pressure of the finger tip over the site. This will rupture any residual internal sphincter fibres.

Usually there is a slight ooze of blood from the small external wound but this is soon arrested by tamponade as the external sphincters recover and contract around the internal sphincter. The external wound is left open to allow drainage of this blood. A local anaesthetic combined with adrenaline injected into the area prior to performance of the sphincterotomy will help to minimize blood loss.

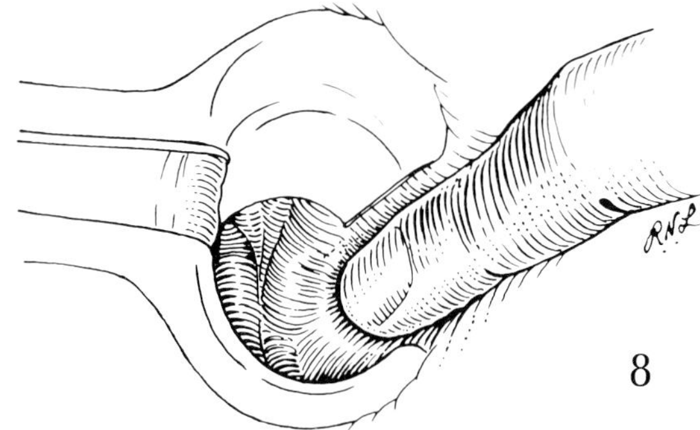

8

9

If there is a large sentinel pile, it is removed with sharp-pointed scissors without damaging the sphincters and with minimal excision of the perianal skin. All overhang is removed. Fibrous polyps are excised if present.

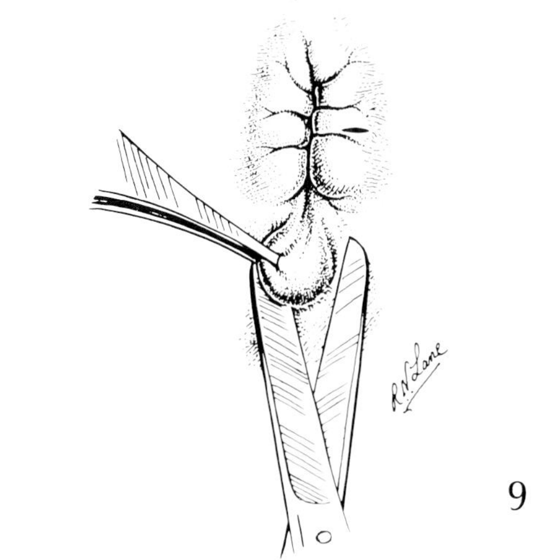

9

10

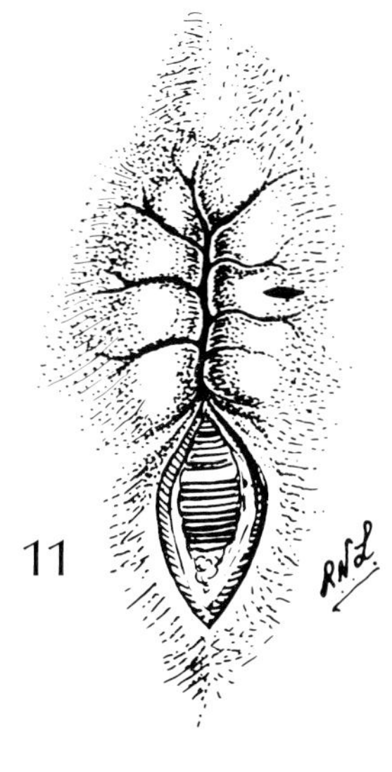

11

10 & 11

A fistula in a sentinel pile when present should be laid open. The track passes through some of the superficial fibres of the lower border of the internal sphincter. It is tempting to perform also a complete internal anal sphincterotomy through the fissure and the rest of the sphincter above the sentinel pile but results are better if the surgeon confines himself to merely laying open the fistula and then performing a lateral subcutaneous sphincterotomy. This avoids the development of a 'key-hole' deformity in the midposterior position which may lead to perianal soiling (*see* chapter on 'Anoplasty', pp. 586–592).

A dressing is laid on the anal area. Intra-anal dressings are contraindicated as they cause postoperative pain. Once bleeding has ceased no dressings are required. The patient is encouraged to have a bowel action as soon as the inclination develops.

OPEN TECHNIQUE

If the surgeon is not happy with the closed technique because of fear of damage to the external sphincter muscle the open method is equally applicable. The author originally practised this technique but with experience found the closed technique simpler and more expeditious.

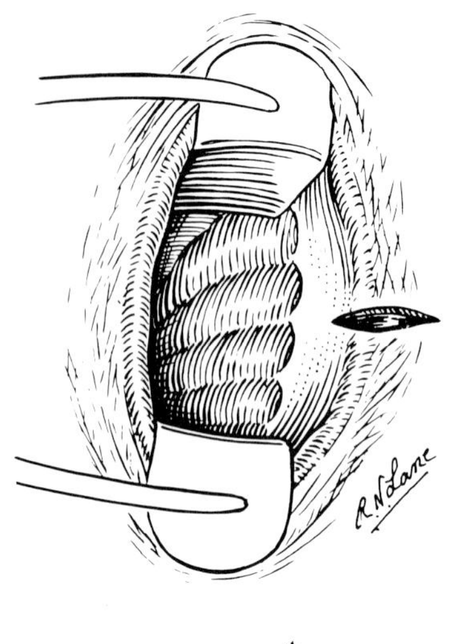

12

12 & 13

A bivalved anal speculum is inserted into the anus to place the internal sphincter on a slight stretch to assist its identification as described in the closed method.

A local anaesthetic with adrenaline is injected into the subcutaneous area selected for the procedure. A radial incision is made into the perianal skin just below the inferior border of the internal sphincter. This incision is preferred to the circumferential type as the wound is left unsutured and open for the egress of blood and the edges of the wound will approximate naturally.

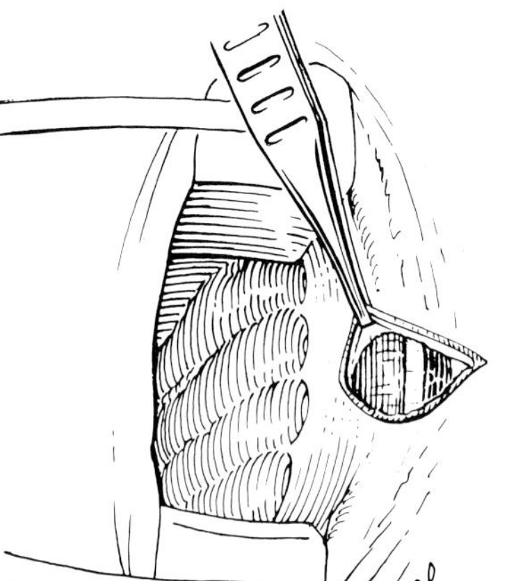

13

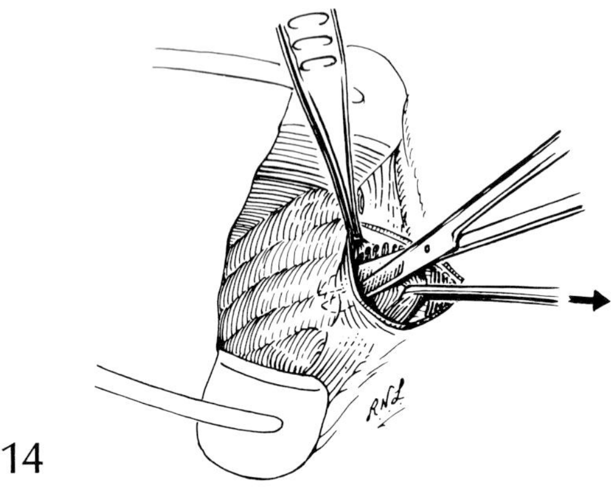

14

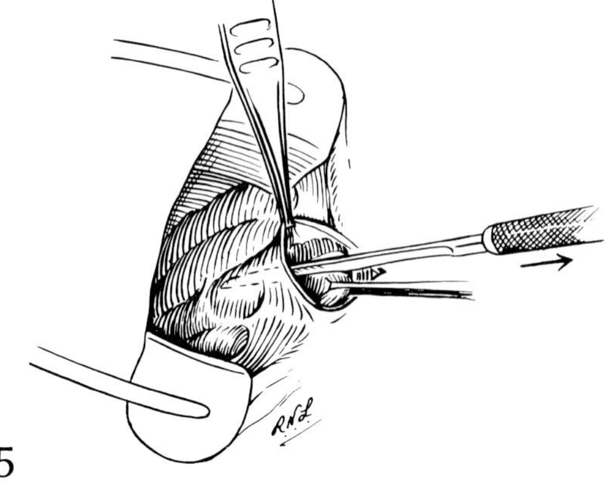

15

14 & 15

The upper end of the incision is grasped with forceps and dissection with narrow-bladed scissors is carried out so as to separate the anoderm from the internal sphincter. The latter is recognized by its white fibres. To facilitate dissection and the sphincterotomy its lower border may be grasped with forceps.

The exposed internal sphincter is then divided by a narrow scalpel blade or scissors.

16

The wound is left open to allow free drainage. A 'lay-on' dressing of gauze is placed over the anus. Intra-anal dressings should not be used as they cause postoperative pain.

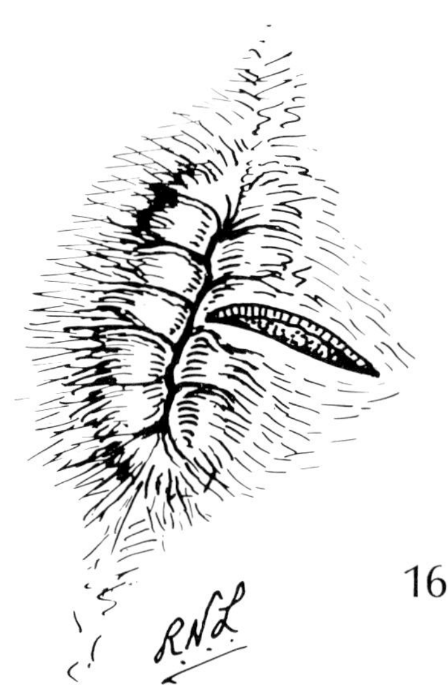

16

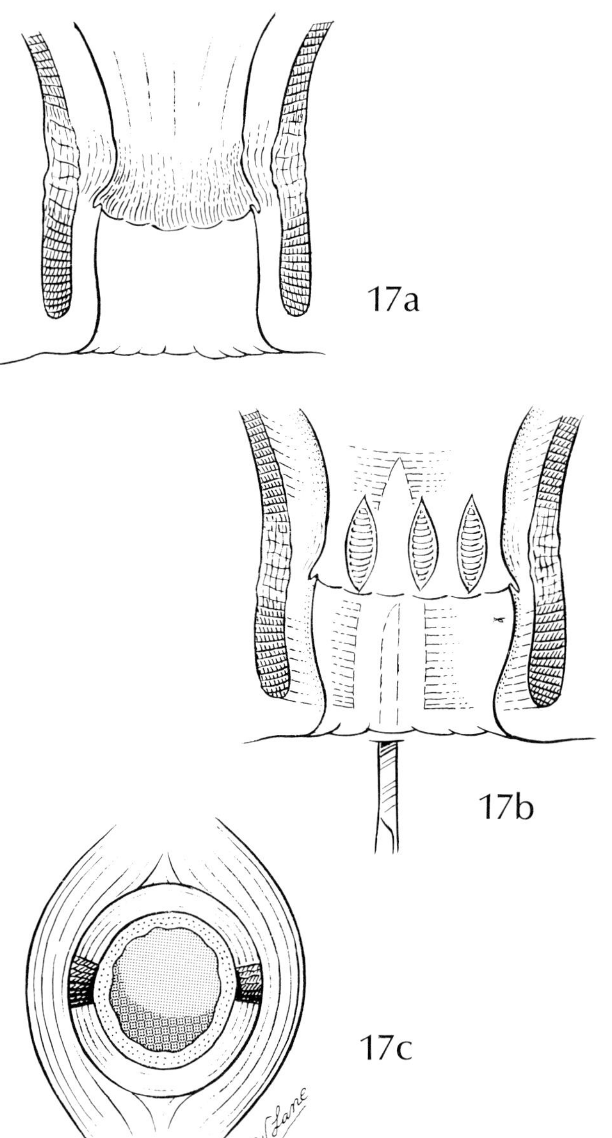

17a

17b

17c

17a, b & c

ANAL STENOSIS

Patients may have a marked anal stenosis caused by chronic and repeated ulceration. It may also follow a previous haemorrhoidectomy or the prolonged use of mineral oils ('paraffin anus').

In those cases where there has been no previous anal surgery a bilateral subcutaneous lateral sphincterotomy may be of value. The sphincterotomy is performed on one lateral side and if considerable tension remains in the internal sphincter on the opposite side then a second lateral subcutaneous sphincterotomy is indicated.

When there has been a previous haemorrhoidectomy it is usual for scarring of the anoderm to extend beyond the dentate line to the rectal mucosa. There is usually fibrosis in the internal sphincter deep to these areas. In such cases the author selects a site for the sphincterotomy in the healthiest tissue between the areas of scarring. It may also be necessary to make release incisions in the scarred mucosal areas (as illustrated) but these are made superficially. The patients are advised to use an anal dilator for up to 2 months after the procedure.

Anorectal sepsis

Roger Grace FRCS
Consultant Surgeon, The Royal Hospital, Wolverhampton

Introduction

The diagnosis of anorectal sepsis is usually obvious. The patient complains of a painful lump by the anal canal and the severity of pain is such that the history is short. Examination reveals the swelling and there is usually associated erythema of the overlying skin with local tenderness to palpation. There is, however, a small group of patients in whom the diagnosis may be delayed. This group complains of pain but there is no obvious swelling and no erythema; rectal examination is very tender and a diagnosis of fissure is supposed. The true diagnosis of sepsis is made only at an examination under anaesthetic; any patient who complains of persistent anal pain of short duration in whom no fissure is visible should undergo an examination under anaesthetic as an emergency.

Surgical management

1

The correct management of anorectal sepsis must relate to the aetiology of the abscess. It has been accepted that anorectal abscesses begin as an intermuscular abscess secondary to infection of an anal gland[1–5]; extension of this intermuscular abscess downwards between internal and external sphincter muscles or through the lower fibres of the external sphincter produces a perianal abscess; extension through the external sphincter complex into the ischiorectal fossa produces an ischiorectal abscess; extension upwards or medially into the submucosal plane produces a high intermuscular or a submucous abscess. Anorectal sepsis should therefore be associated with a fistula-in-ano. However, recent microbiological studies have shown that, whereas abscesses from which a bowel organism has been cultured are likely to be associated with a fistula, those abscesses from which a skin organism is cultured (mainly *Staphylococcus aureus*) will not be associated with a fistula[6].

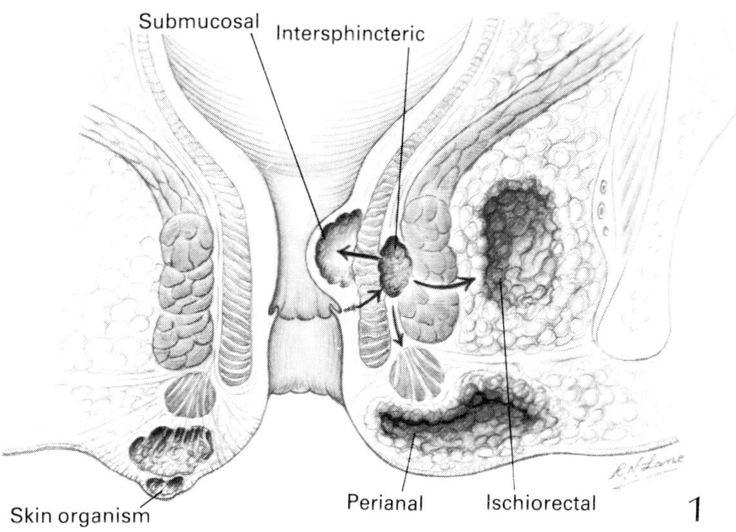

1

Any rationale for the initial treatment of anorectal sepsis must assume that a fistula is present because microbiology is not immediately available; a past history of sepsis at the same site is further strong evidence that a fistula is present.

Surgical management should be designed to:

1. relieve the immediate symptoms;
2. prevent recurrent sepsis; and
3. minimize healing time and thereby time lost from work.

Three drainage procedures have been described.

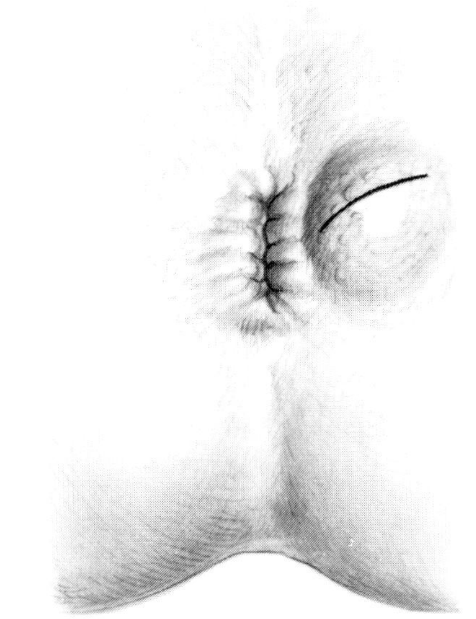

2a

2a & b

Incision and drainage

Linear incision over the point of maximal tenderness/induration releases the pus; a small drain may be left *in situ*. This technique will relieve the immediate symptoms and minimize healing time but will do nothing to prevent recurrent sepsis if a fistula is present.

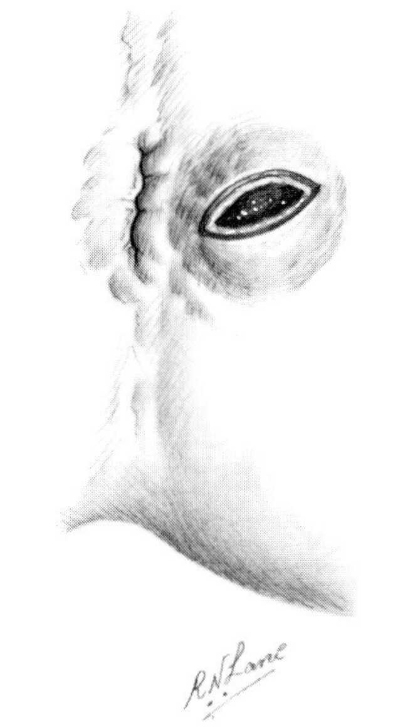

2b

3

Saucerization

A cruciate excision is made over the point of maximal tenderness/induration followed by excision of the triangles of skin to allow 'good drainage'. If a fistula is present this technique will relieve the immediate symptoms but does nothing to prevent recurrent sepsis and, with a large wound, healing time is prolonged.

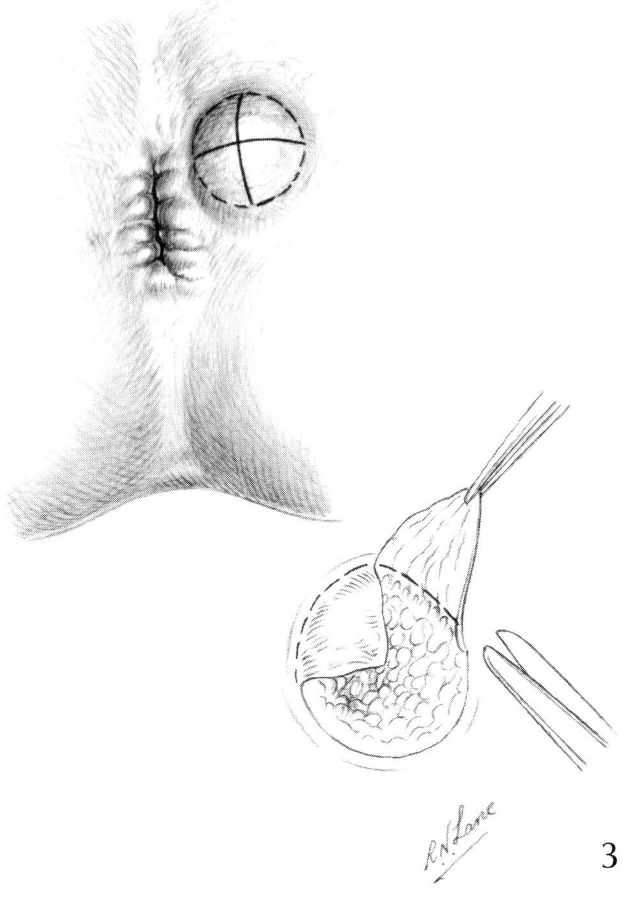

3

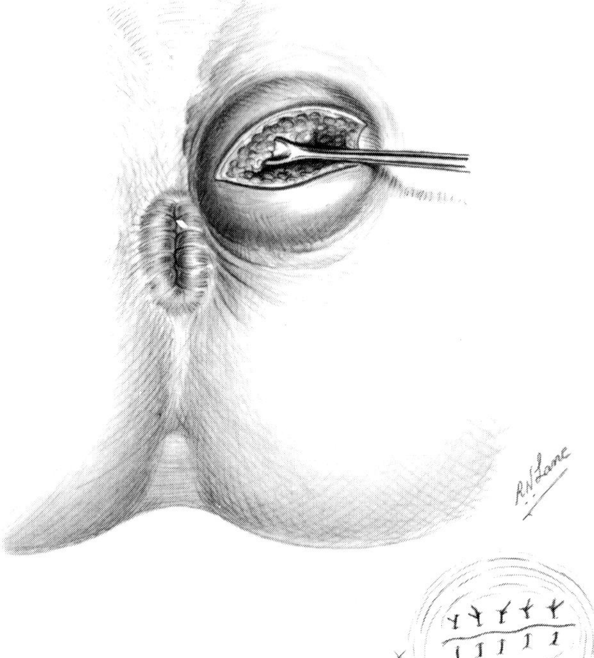

4

4

Incision and primary suture

A linear incision is performed over the point of maximal tenderness/induration; the abscess cavity is curretted and the wound is sutured, under antibiotic cover, to obliterate this cavity. This technique will relieve the immediate symptoms and minimize healing time but it does nothing to prevent recurrent sepsis should there be an underlying fistula.

Taken in isolation, these three techniques all ignore the possible aetiology of the sepsis, i.e. the presence of a fistula-in-ano. Logical management requires the search for a fistula-in-ano and, if one is found, laying it open, as well as drainage of the abscess. This management relieves the immediate symptoms, prevents recurrent sepsis if a fistula is found and is associated with minimal healing time if no fistula is found.

Operative technique

Examination under anaesthetic

5

The patient is examined under general anaesthetic in the lithotomy position. Visual examination and then careful palpation defines the extent of induration and determines whether the abscess is perianal or ischiorectal; a large area of cellulitis does not necessarily indicate ischiorectal sepsis.

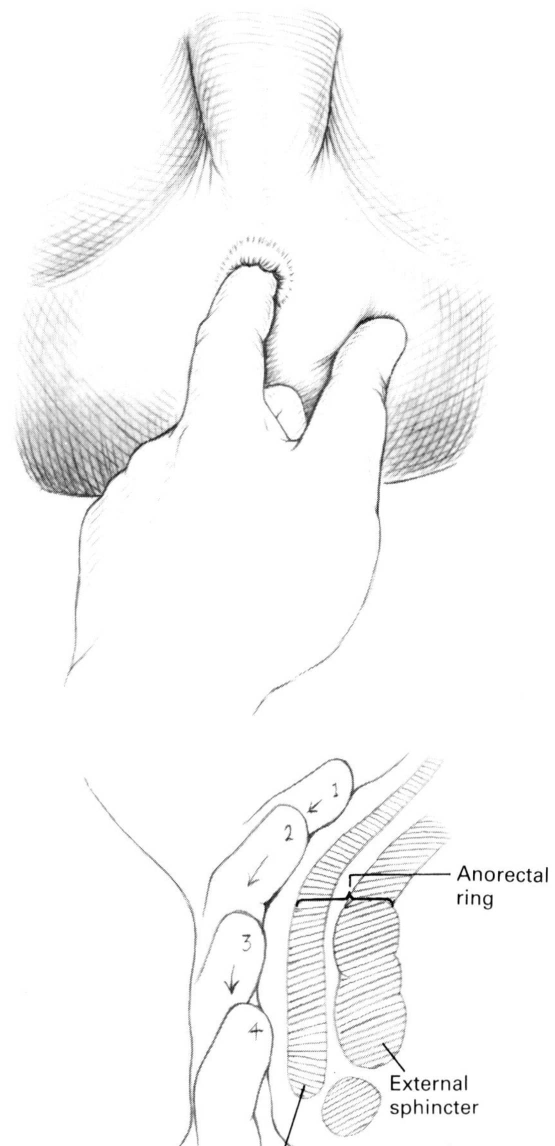

5

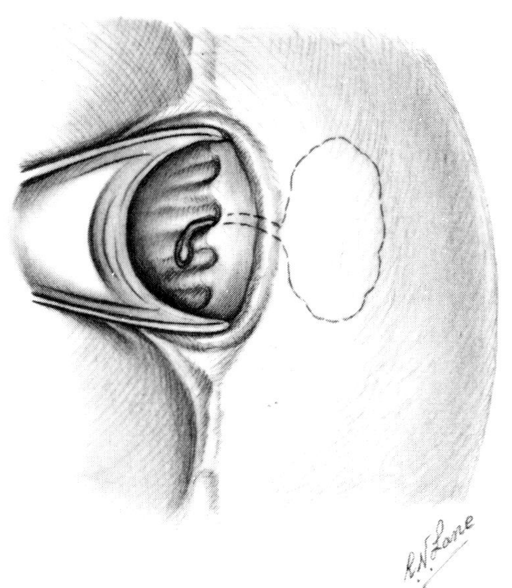

6

6

The anal canal is inspected using a Sims speculum; the surgeon is looking for pus draining into the canal through an internal opening at the dentate line. Gentle pressure on the abscess from outside may help to identify the internal opening by the appearance of pus at the dentate line.

Incision and drainage

7a & b

The abscess is drained through a linear incision, the cavity curretted and pus sent for culture. The incision may be radial (*a*) or circumanal (*b*); a theoretical danger of the radial incision is damage to the underlying sphincter musculature. It is suggested that the line of incision should reflect the direction of any potential associated fistula. A perianal abscess will probably be associated with a low fistula track running directly towards the anal canal, and a radial incision is indicated. An ischiorectal abscess may be associated with a 'high' fistula running posteriorly, or sometimes anteriorly, and a circumanal incision is preferred.

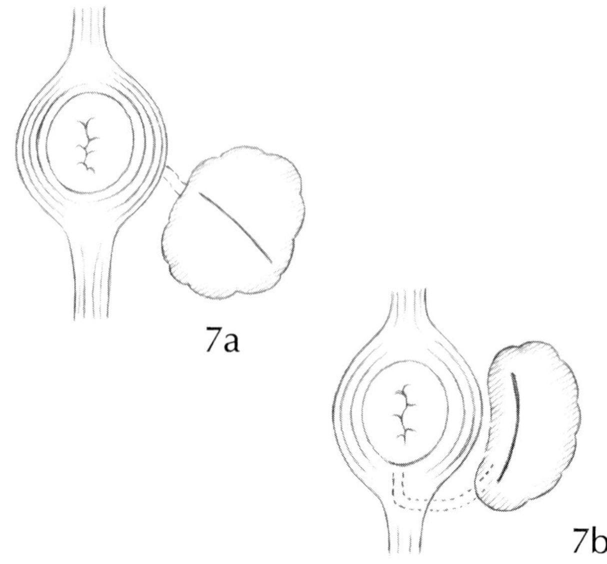

7a

7b

8

Anorectal sepsis sometimes presents with bilateral abscesses. These abscess cavities connect in the midline posteriorly and are associated with a fistula but drainage of the abscess cavities will certainly require at least one incision on either side and, depending on the anterior extent of the sepsis, may require further incisions anteriorly.

If an internal opening has been defined, a hooked Lockhart-Mummery probe is passed through the internal opening in an attempt to define the fistula track; a forefinger in the abscess cavity will help to identify the tip of the probe. A probe may also be passed from the abscess cavity towards the internal opening. These manoeuvres should be done with extreme care as the area is oedematous and friable and too much pressure will produce a false track; with the probe *in situ* the relationship between the fistula track and the sphincter is defined by careful palpation. This is easier with a posterior fistula than an anterior one where the sphincter is more difficult to define. Inexperienced surgeons should take particular care while looking for a fistula.

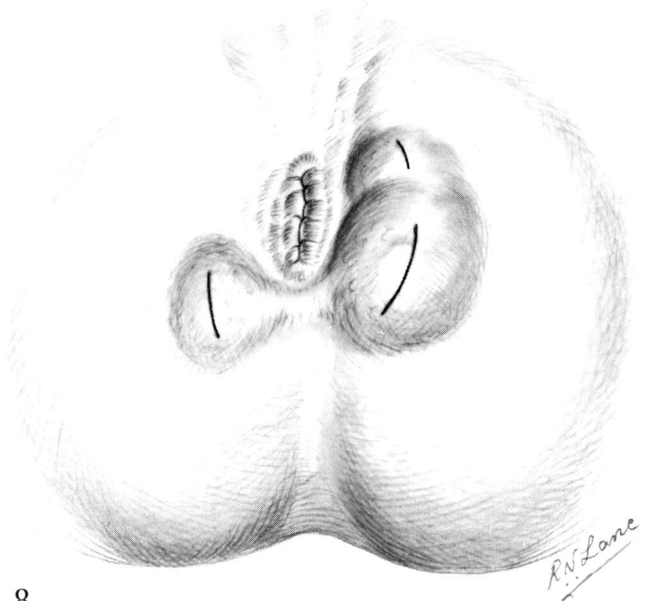

8

9

Laying open

The fistula track is laid open by incision through the sphincter down onto the groove of the Lockhart-Mummery probe (*see* chapter on 'Fistula-in-ano', pp. 622–635 in this volume). The wound edges are trimmed to produce a wound with sloping edges, i.e. with no overhanging edges which might harbour infection and delay healing. If there is any doubt as to where the fistula track lies in relation to the external sphincter (oedema may make definition difficult), the fistula may be marked with a Seton suture or, if preferred, left unmarked until a second examination under anaesthetic.

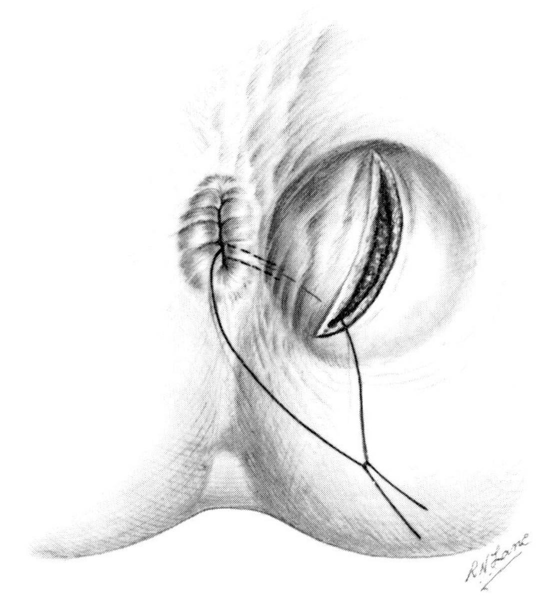

9

Microbiology

If no fistula is found, further management depends upon microbiology. Culture of a bowel organism requires a second examination under anaesthetic 7–10 days later whereas the growth of a skin organism means that a second examination under anaesthetic is not required[6].

Second examination under anaesthetic

If a fistula was found but not laid open at the initial examination under anaesthetic, this is now laid open (*see* chapter on 'Fistula-in-ano', pp. 622–635 in this volume).

If no fistula was found at the first examination, the incision is extended to give a good view of the abscess cavity which is then curretted. The fistula track will be marked by granulation tissue projecting from the fistula track orifice; this will remain even after the area has been curretted. The Lockhart-Mummery probe is passed into the track which is laid open. If no fistula track can be found, nothing further is done.

Postoperative management

Drainage of abscess alone

First examination under anaesthetic

If no fistula has been found, the abscess cavity should be packed as necessary for haemostasis with a Milton dressing which will be removed on the following day. The patient should be discharged home with instructions to bathe twice daily and apply a flat dressing to, but not into, the incision. The dressing will be held in place with elastic pants.

Second examination under anaesthetic

If no fistula is found, management is as above with a dressing being worn until the wound has healed.

Drainage of abscess and laying open of fistula

Analgesia

Analgesia will be required but the patient with a fistula wound will rarely experience as much pain as a patient who has undergone haemorrhoidectomy.

Bowel habit

The patient should be encouraged to have a normal bowel action by the third or fourth postoperative day. A high fibre diet along with a mild laxative will ensure that there is little problem.

Management of the wound

The patient bathes at least twice a day and again after the bowels have been opened. The wound is irrigated with a dilute Milton (1:40) solution and dressed with a flat dressing soaked in dilute Milton which is tucked into the wound; the wound should not be packed and ribbon gauze should never be used. The anal dressing should be held in place with a pair of close-fitting elastic pants which are best for all anal and perineal wounds.

Anal dilator

The passage of an anal dilator twice a day from the third postoperative day ensures that the smaller, low fistula-in-ano wounds heal without bridging; the patient will normally manage this without any trouble. The larger, high fistula wounds do not require an anal dilator but a further examination under anaesthetic may be required 2 weeks later to ensure that no bridging has taken place and the wound is healing satisfactorily. If pus is present there is often an unresolved problem.

Antibiotics

With adequate surgical drainage of the abscess there is no place for antibiotics in the postoperative management of these patients. There are however two exceptions to this rule: fulminating gangrene and tuberculosis. There may also be a place in patients with Crohn's disease or diabetes mellitus requiring insulin.

SPECIAL SITUATIONS

In three special situations management may need to be modified.

Crohn's disease

The management of anorectal sepsis in Crohn's disease is part of the overall management of the disease and certain principles should be understood.

1. Sepsis is always associated with a fistula.
2. Large anal wounds do not heal well.
3. Management should be aimed primarily at relieving symptoms with prevention of recurrent sepsis depending upon the nature of the fistula.
4. There is a high incidence of recurrent sepsis if treatment does not include surgery to the fistula.

Surgical management

Abscess plus low fistula Management may include the laying open of a fistula as the wound will be small but simple drainage may be preferred.

Abscess with high fistula The fistula should only be laid open with extreme caution as the resulting large wound may be very slow to, or may never, heal.

Abscess with multiple fistulae The management almost certainly consists of drainage of the abscess; continuing sepsis, however, may eventually become an indication for excision of the rectum.

Tuberculous infections

This possibility should be considered in populations in whom tuberculosis is endogenous. However, surgical management of the acute abscess should be on the principles already discussed as results of culture will not be available for at least 6 weeks. When tuberculous infection is suspected, pus should be sent with a special request for a suitable culture and if positive the patient will require standard antituberculous therapy. The patient usually has evidence of tuberculosis elsewhere.

Fulminating anorectal sepsis

Under this heading may be grouped those patients with gas-forming infection and acute dermal gangrene which may or may not be clostridial in origin[8,9]. These infections are rare but are associated with a definite mortality and considerable morbidity. Surgery must aim to excise all the necrotic tissue and further procedures should be carried out if the first operation is not sufficiently radical. These patients are the only ones with anorectal sepsis who require broad-spectrum antibiotics taking account of microbiology when it becomes available. There may be a place for hyperbaric oxygen if there are gas-forming organisms but the need for this has not been well defined. Diabetic control in those patients with diabetes mellitus is not usually a difficult problem.

References

1. Nesselrod, J. P. In: Christopher, F., ed. A textbook of surgery, 5th ed. Philadelphia and London: Saunders, 1949: 1092

2. Eisenhammer, S. The internal anal sphincter and the ano-rectal abscess. Surgery, Gynecology and Obstetrics 1956; 103: 501–506

3. Eisenhammer, S. A new approach to the ano-rectal fistulous abscess based on the high intermuscular lesion. Surgery, Gynecology and Obstetrics 1958; 106: 595–599

4. Eisenhammer, S. The ano-rectal and ano-vulval fistulous abscess. Surgery, Gynecology and Obstetrics 1961; 113: 519–520

5. Parks, A. G. Pathogenesis and treatment of fistula-in-ano. British Medical Journal 1961; 1: 463–469

6. Grace, R. H., Harper, I. A., Thompson, R. G. Ano-rectal sepsis: microbiology in relation to fistula-in-ano. British Journal of Surgery 1982; 69: 401–403

7. Hobbiss, J. H., Schofield, P. F. Management of perianal Crohn's Disease. Journal of the Royal Society of Medicine 1982; 75: 414–417

8. Ledingham, I. McA., Tehrani, M. A. Diagnosis, clinical course and treatment of acute dermal gangrene. British Journal of Surgery 1975; 62: 364–372

9. Brightmore, T. Perianal gas-producing infection of non-clostridial origin. British Journal of Surgery 1972; 59: 109–116

Fistula-in-ano

Ian P. Todd MS, MD(Tor), FRCS, DCH
Consulting Surgeon, St Bartholomew's Hospital, London;
Consultant Surgeon, St Mark's Hospital and King Edward VII Hospital for Officers, London

Sir Hugh Lockhart-Mummery KCVO, MD, MChir, FRCS
Consulting Surgeon, St Thomas' Hospital and St Mark's Hospital, London;
Consultant Surgeon, King Edward VII Hospital for Officers, London

Introduction

A fistula is an abnormal communication between any two epithelial-lined organs. An anal fistula is one in which there is an opening between the anal canal and perineal skin. Commonly a fistula is preceded by an abscess and if an abscess in this region of the body is recurrent, it is almost certain that a fistula exists, even if its track cannot be identified. Spontaneous healing of an anal fistula is very rare. A neglected fistula may flare up, causing repeated abscesses and considerable ill health. An abscess treated at an early stage by drainage, without antibiotics, may heal completely without fistula formation.

Most fistulae are due to infection arising in the anal glands which open into the crypts in the anal canal at the level of the dentate line. The glands, some six to eight in number, are mucus secreting, branching and tend to penetrate through the internal sphincter into the intersphincteric plane. Infection arising in them is probably related to obstruction leading to abscess formation. If the abscess is drained early, its cavity is not lined by granulation tissue and will heal and the tip of the gland will fibrose. If the abscess becomes chronic, or is undrained or partly sterilized by antibiotics, it becomes lined by granulation tissue and when it ruptures a fistula results. This is a common fistula. The abscess undrained may enlarge and spread in any direction: downwards, upwards, laterally and medially, but above all circumferentially. In this lies the difficulty in understanding and treating fistulae surgically.

There are various other aetiological factors: tuberculosis, inflammatory bowel disease, foreign bodies, lymphoma etc. If a fistula persists for many years, malignant change may occur. Malignancy can also arise primarily in an anal gland or be implanted in a fistulous track from a primary tumour elsewhere in the bowel. A biopsy should always be taken when operating upon any fistula.

Preoperative

Indications

A discharging sinus in the perineum, particularly if recurrent, indicates that a fistula is probable. In view of the recurrent ill-health related to this condition, surgical cure is advised.

The patient should be fully investigated before curative surgery is undertaken. Gastrointestinal and abdominal symptoms should be investigated and sigmoidoscopy is mandatory in all cases. A chest X-ray should be carried out.

Contraindications

Active pulmonary tuberculosis may be associated with an anal fistula. In this case the fistulous opening may show the typical appearance of a tuberculous ulcer, the tracks may not be indurated and treatment of it should not be instituted until the pulmonary disease is controlled when it should be treated in a normal manner.

The appearance of the fistulous opening may make one suspect Crohn's disease, there being a cyanotic discoloration of the skin, oedema, lack of induration and an indolent sinus. It is usually wise to avoid extensive surgery in this fistulous condition.

Preoperative preparation

The lower bowel should be emptied by an enema the night before operation and a rectal wash-out given on the morning of operation. The anal region should be widely shaved.

Anaesthesia

General anaesthesia is necessary for all except the most superficial fistulae. Full relaxation should be avoided, as there should be sufficient tone in the muscles to enable the operator to palpate the main parts of the anal sphincters, particularly the anorectal ring.

Position of patient

The patient should be in the lithotomy position with the buttocks well down over the end of the table.

Preoperative examination

Before starting the operation, the whole anal area should be carefully palpated. The index finger should feel around the anus externally, feel the intersphincteric groove between internal and external sphincter and identify any induration, whether radial or circumferential. Now with the index finger within the anus, induration should be identified, in which quadrants, whether above, at or below the anorectal ring and whether any tiny pit or dimple can be felt which might indicate an internal opening. The area is then felt with the index finger within and the thumb outside to gauge the extent of induration. Most tracks can be felt as indurated ridges except when they are parallel to the anorectum. A proctoscope should then be passed to note any anal canal abnormality when pus or an internal opening may be seen. Only then should a malleable probe be passed.

Pathological examination

As stated before, a portion of the granulation tissue and fibrous tissue of the fistulous track should always be submitted for microscopic examination.

Anatomy and classification of fistulae

1

Anatomy

The essential anatomy of the anal region is shown in the diagram. Note that the ischiorectal fossa is a pyramidal space, the apex of which is above the anorectal ring. The anorectal ring marks the junction of rectum and anal canal and is formed by the puborectalis fibres of levator ani passing round the bowel and blending with the external sphincter. Complete incontinence results if all the anal sphincters, including the anorectal ring, are divided; section of muscle below this level may lead to some impairment of control or mucous leakage, depending on the amount of muscle divided. The illustration shows (A) anorectal ring; (B) levator ani; (C) ischiorectal fossa; (D) internal sphincter; (E) subcutaneous external sphincter (F) other parts of external sphincter; (G) perianal space; (H) circular muscle of bowel.

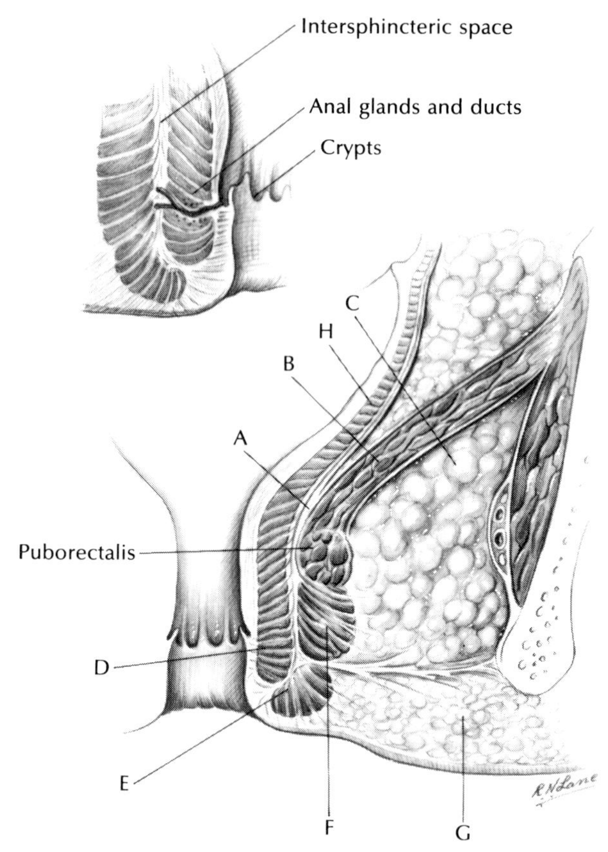

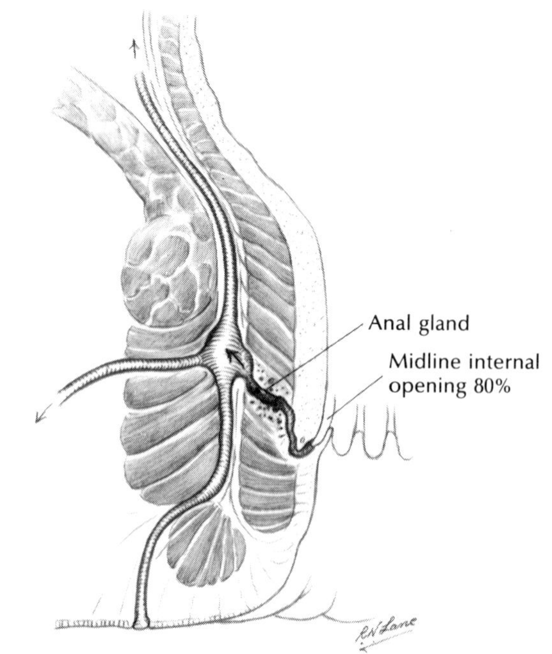

Classification of fistulae

2

The majority of anal fistulae result from infection of the anal glands, which arise from the anal crypts and penetrate into and often through the internal sphincter muscle. The infected gland is commonly in the midline and in 80 per cent of anal fistulae the internal opening will be found in the midline posteriorly.

Infection in the deeper part of the anal gland leads to an abscess cavity in the potential space between the internal and external sphincter muscles, i.e. the intersphincteric space. From this focus infection may track laterally, medially, upwards or downwards, before or after tracking circumferentially. These diagrams can only present the fistula in two dimensions, but it must be remembered that in reality they are three dimensional.

3

If the infection tracks from the tip of the gland in the intersphincteric plane directly downwards to the perianal skin it forms a perianal abscess, and when it has discharged a fistula results. This is the commonest type of fistula. It is commonly radial and is classified as intersphincteric. It may be laid open simply (*see Illustration* 15).

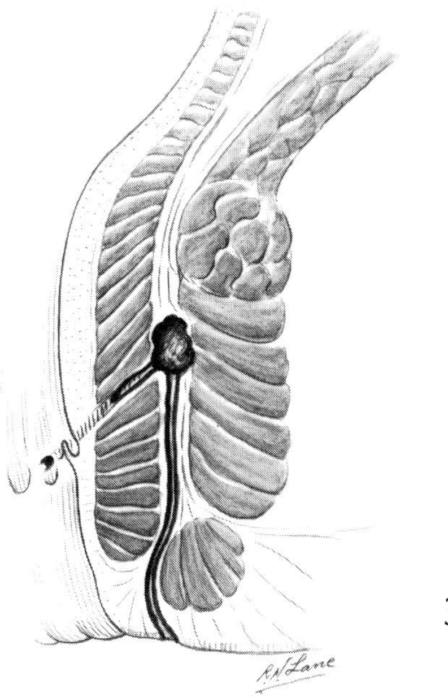

3

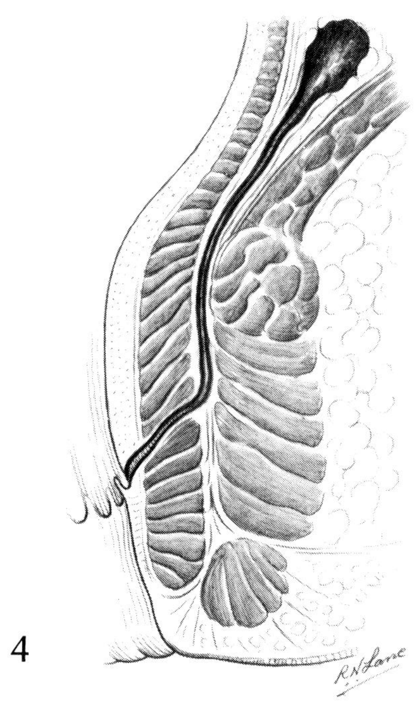

4

4

The pus may track upwards from the primary abscess site, remaining in the intersphincteric plane but pushing its way above the anorectal ring, bulging the overlying rectal mucosa. This type of abscess often extends circumferentially which accounts for induration surrounding part of the circumference of the anorectal ring and sometimes above it. It can be drained by opening up the intersphincteric plane adequately. The primary opening must however always be laid open adequately.

5

The abscess may break back into the anal canal by tracking medially. This gives rise to a secondary opening, usually at a higher level than the primary opening which is normally at the level of the crypts at the dentate line. The secondary opening may well heal spontaneously or if lightly sutured once the primary opening has been adequately dealt with.

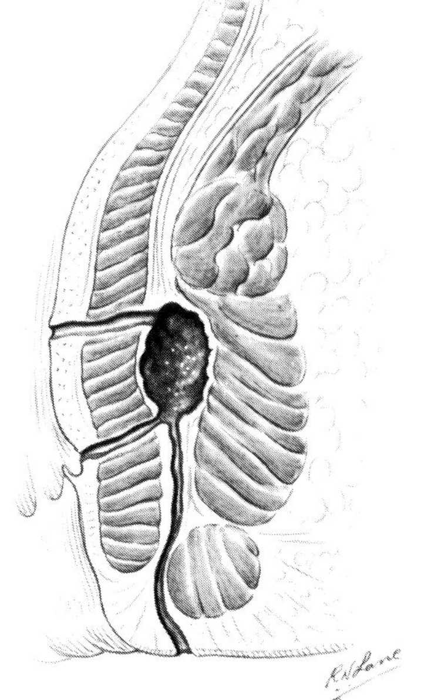

5

6

The intersphincteric abscess may spread laterally through the external sphincter muscle to infect the ischiorectal fossa. It is then said to be a trans-sphincteric fistula. Most of these fistulae can be dealt with by simple laying open provided the anorectal ring is left intact (see chapter on 'Anorectal sepsis', pp. 614–621 in this volume).

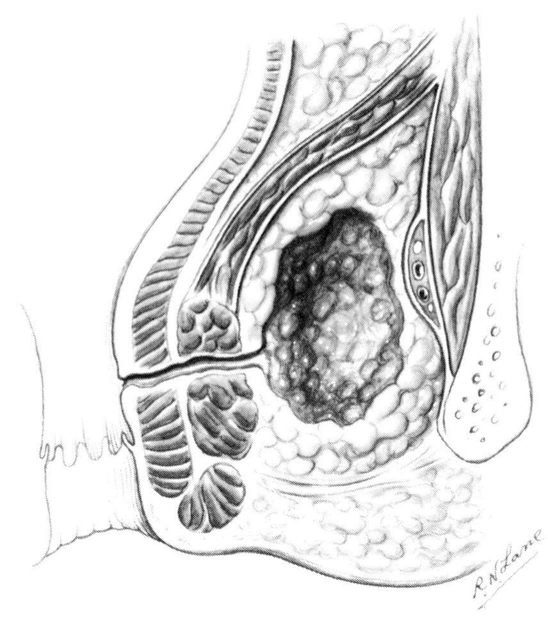

6

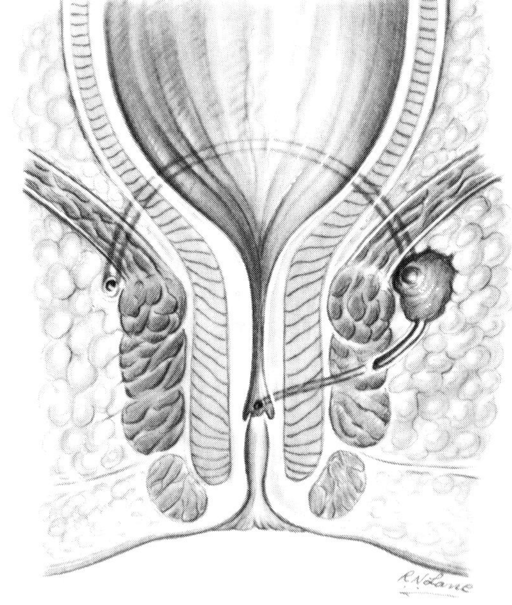

7

7

The infection in the ischiorectal fossa may track round circumferentially. However the difficulty here is that the site of penetration of the infection through the external and internal sphincter may not overlie one another: i.e. the anal gland in the midline posteriorly may be the origin and penetrate the internal sphincter in this plane; the intersphincteric abscess then spreads circumferentially and penetrates the external sphincter at (say) 3 and 9 o'clock in the lithotomy position, causing bilateral ischiorectal abscesses, which may of themselves track around circumferentially. Ischiorectal abscesses usually open at least 2.5 cm from the anus, are felt between finger and thumb as a swelling and indicate a trans-sphincteric fistula. They are normally limited above by the levator muscles but may bulge them upwards suggesting a supra-levator origin.

8

Rarely the track may truly spread through the levator muscle plate, or even more rarely into the rectum above the anorectal ring. It is possible that these two varieties are both iatrogenic, that is, due to surgical interference with excessive enthusiasm in opening an ischiorectal abscess, 'breaking down loculi' and insertion of a rigid drain. They do however occur with foreign bodies.

The supralevator abscess associated with ischiorectal involvement must be adequately drained over a prolonged period with adequate antibiotic therapy, or else it will recur because of closing off of the cavity by the muscle fibres pulling together.

A supralevator hole in the rectum will need to be closed, probably by an intersphincteric approach, possibly with a covering colostomy, but the primary cause must be dealt with first.

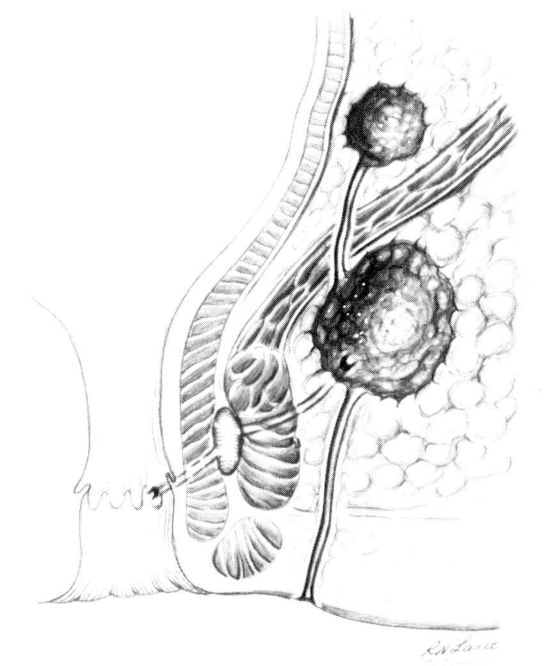

8

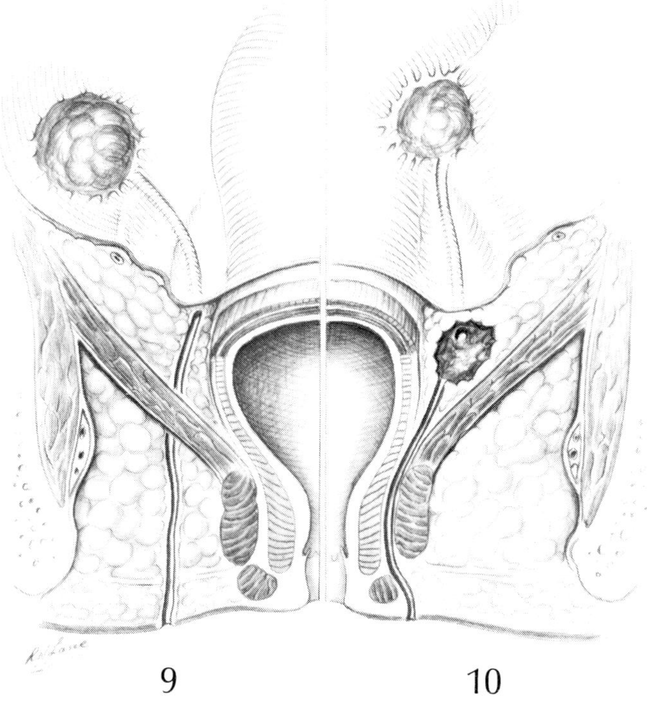

9 10

9 & 10

Very rarely a fistula arises from a supralevator origin, passes directly through the pelvic floor either intersphincterically or through the levator to open on to the perineal skin. This is not a fistula-in-ano but a supralevator or extrasphincteric fistula. It usually arises from bowel or gynaecological disease, e.g. diverticular disease, Crohn's disease, appendix abscess, pelvic abscess or pyosalpinx. It may arise from a pelvic fracture penetrating the intestine. In these circumstances the primary cause is dealt with and the fistulous track curetted when it will usually heal without any problem. These tracks usually run directly parallel with the anorectum but some distance from the bowel. No induration may therefore be apparent.

Operative treatment

THE SIMPLE LOW RADIAL FISTULA

11, 12 & 13

Insertion of probe-pointed director

The indurated radial track is felt. A malleable probe-pointed director is passed from the external opening along the track until its tip emerges into the anal canal through the internal opening. It is helpful to have a finger palpating on to the point of the director, thus steadying the anus, but the director must be worked gently along the track and should never be forced through the tissues.

A finger passed into the anus checks the level of the internal opening in relation to the dentate line and anorectal ring, to ensure that division of the muscle superficial to the director will not lead to incontinence.

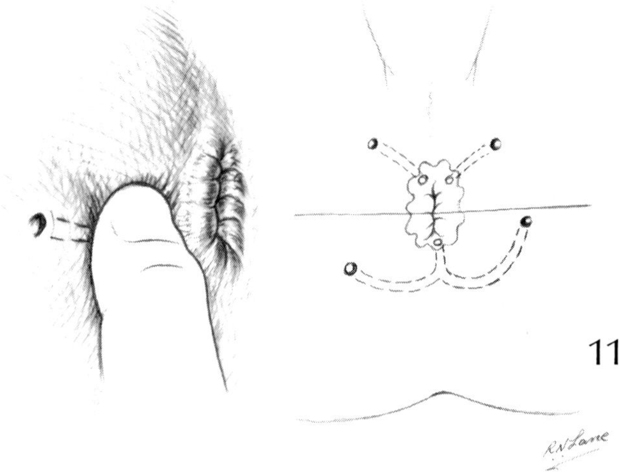

Goodsall's Law: anterior tracks are often radial; posterior tracks may be horseshoed

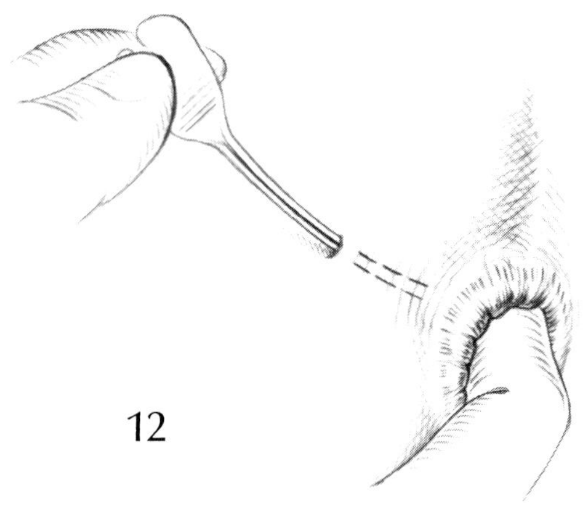

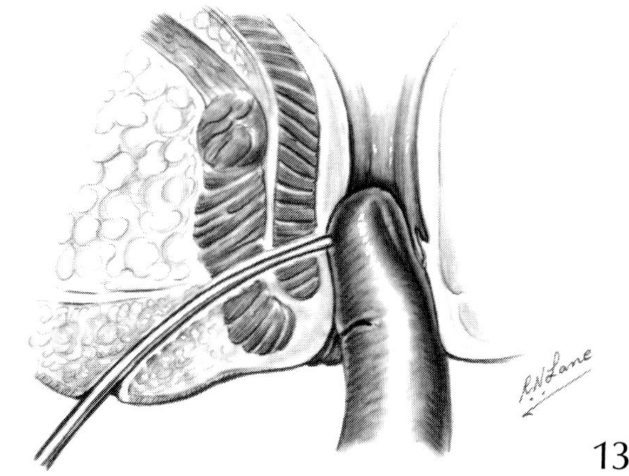

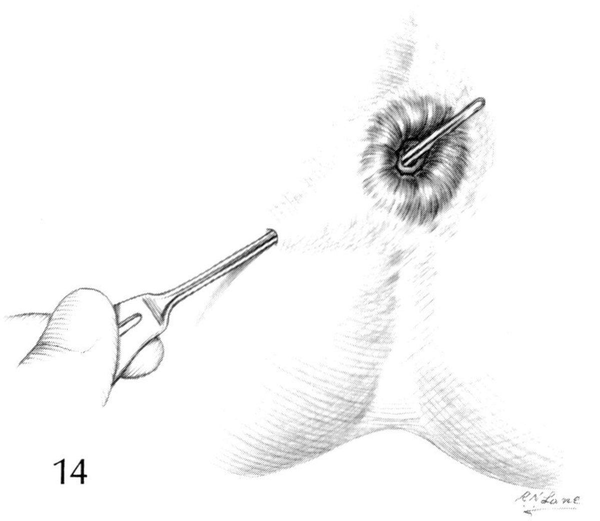

14

Exit of director through the anus

Once right through the track the tip of the director is angled towards the operator and is then pushed on to the outside of the anus. A curved director (*see illustrations 12* and *13*) may be particularly useful when dealing with less direct tracks.

15

Incision over the director and curettage of granulation tissue

The track is laid open by cutting onto the groove in the director which is then removed. The edges of the wound are held apart with Allis' forceps and the granulation tissue curetted away. Search is made by looking, feeling and probing for any other track opening out of the main one, and if such a track is found, it is also laid open

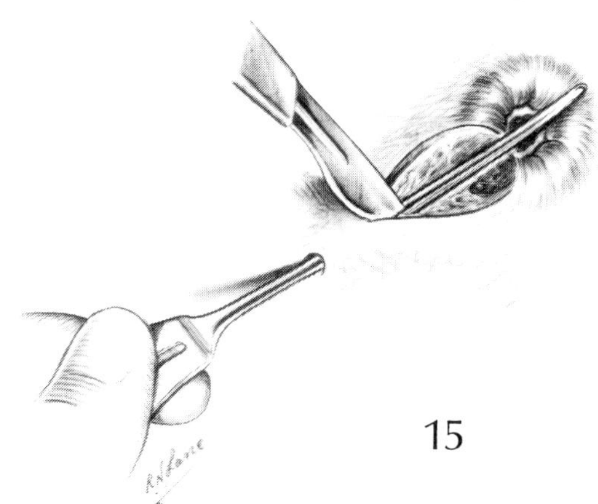

15

16

Extension of the wound

The wound is extended outwards for a short distance so that the external opening is removed and mobilized (Salmon's back cut). The edges are then trimmed to make a shallow wound without overhang. A portion of the track is sent for histology.

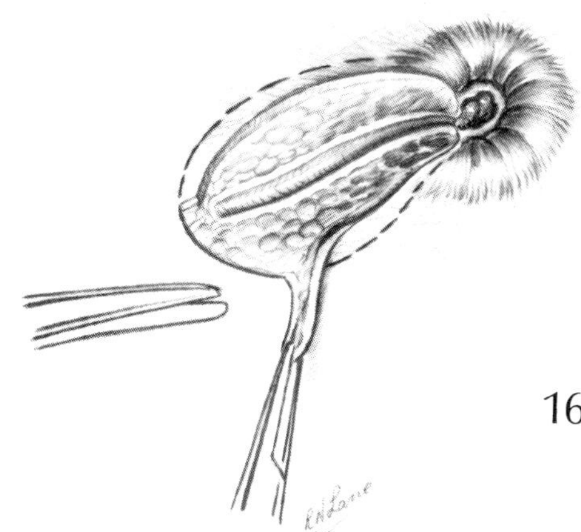

16

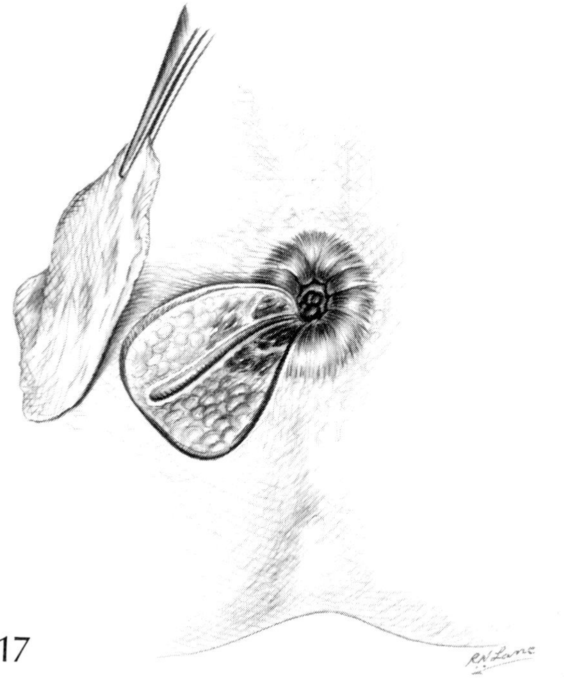

17

17

Healing of the wound

Such a wound may appear unnecessarily large, but experience has shown that the healing of anal wounds is better and free from complications when there is good external drainage. The outer edge of the wound should be larger than the inner portion with a tendency to a triangular shape.

A flat gauze dressing moistened with Eusol (1:8) or Hibitane (1:2000) is placed into the wound, covered with a cotton-wool pad and held in place with a T-bandage or Netelast. Adhesive plaster should be avoided as it may cause hair follicle infection.

Subcutaneous fistulae and those fistulae with an intermuscular extension are laid open in a similar way. The size and shape of the external wound varies according to the length and direction of the track and the depth of the internal opening, the surgeon always attempting to get a shallow shelving wound.

HIGH INTERSPHINCTERIC FISTULA

18

Insertion of speculum; probing the fistula

A Sims speculum is passed into the anal canal and held by an assistant. It is probable that the operator has already laid open the lower part of this fistula which opened into a crypt at the dentate line. It may then become apparent that a higher intersphincteric track is present (this was probably suspected because of induration in the region of the anorectal ring) as the cavity can not be curetted clean and a further sinus track is seen. The director is then passed into the sinus opening, up along the track and sometimes back into the lumen as a secondary opening.

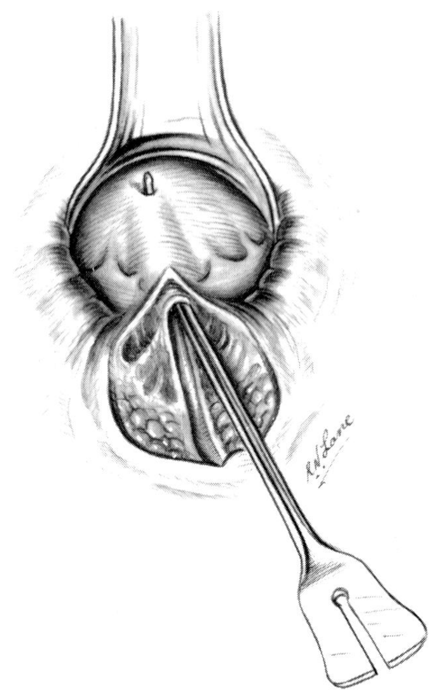

18

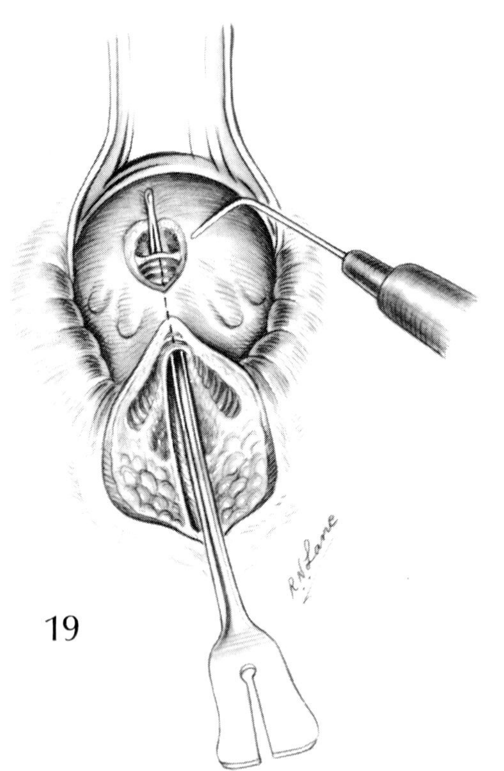

19

19

Laying-open on to probe

The mucosa and internal sphincter muscle on the director are then slowly divided with a diathermy needle in order to minimize bleeding. In this way the whole length of the fistula is laid open into the upper anal canal. The only muscle divided in this phase of the procedure is the internal sphincter.

FISTULA INVOLVING THE ISCHIORECTAL FOSSA (TRANS-SPHINCTERIC FISTULA)

20

Course of the main track

The main track of this type of fistula follows the roof of the ischiorectal fossa, that is, it lies on the undersurface of the puborectalis and pubococcygeus muscles. The track is horseshoe shaped if both sides are involved, with the anterior extension on each side passing deep to the transverse perineal muscle. The communication with the anal canal is most frequently in the midline posteriorly but not invariably so. The track leading to the external opening on the skin is not shown in the diagram but is usually vertical and may descend from any part of the main circumferential track. The communication with the lumen is usually angled as in *Illustrations 3, 4, 8,* and *21* and is frequently not found for this reason.

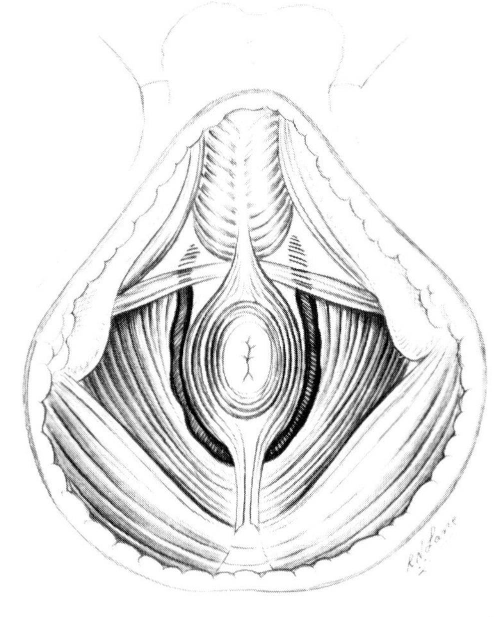

20

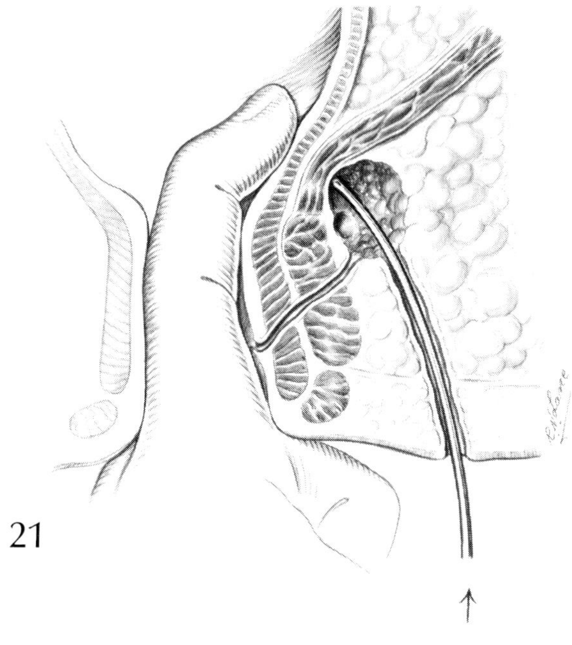

21

21

Insertion of probe to apex

If a probe is passed into the external opening it will enter deeply, *parallel* to the anal canal, and its tip can often be palpated through the rectal wall at a level apparently above the anorectal ring. It must never be forced through here, as the real internal opening is nearly always below the anorectal ring, still following the undersurface of the puborectalis.

22

First incision

The director is passed up the vertical track and is held with the groove posteriorly by an assistant. The left index finger steadies and protects the rectum. A scalpel is slid up the groove in the director and cuts out backwards towards the coccyx, thus laying open the posterior part of the track on that side. This track may prove to be either intersphincteric or outside the external sphincter but, being essentially circumferential, it does not cut muscle.

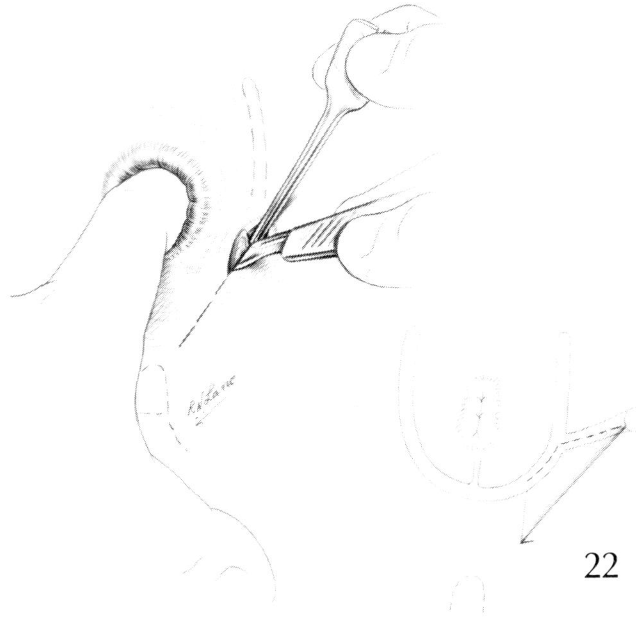

22

23

Exposure of anterior extension

The edges of the wound are held apart with Allis' forceps and the main bleeding points secured. They should not be fulgurated at this stage as the eschar may later suggest a further track. The anterior extension is sought in the depths of the wound. The director is passed along the track, which is then laid open by dividing the overlying tissues. The posterior part of the perineal membrane and contained muscles may very rarely need to be divided in laying open this part. A finger passed into the laid-open track will often confirm adequate drainage and that the top of the fistula has been reached.

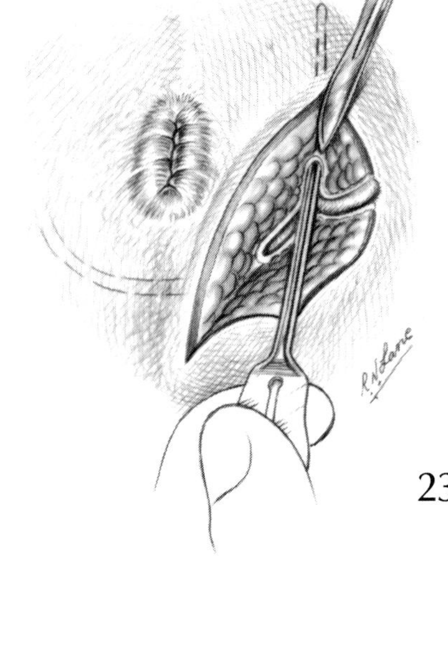

23

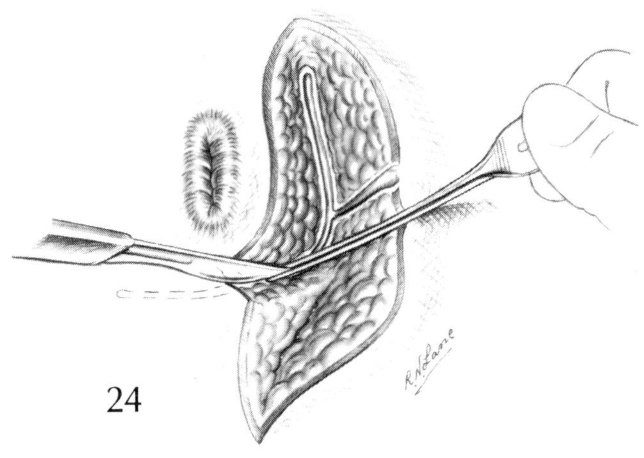

24

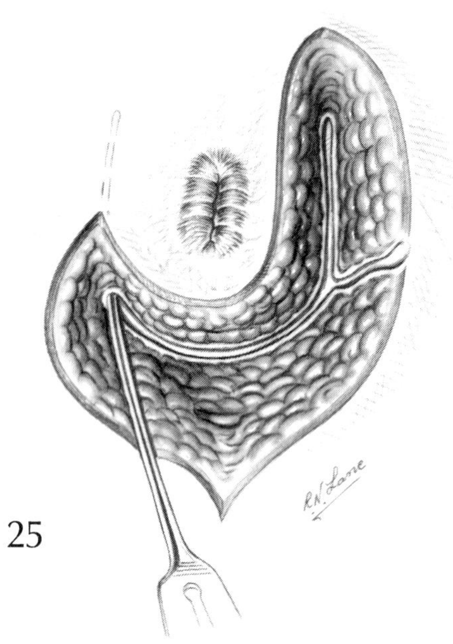

25

24 & 25

Extension of track to opposite ischiorectal fossa

Attention is now turned to the posterior end of the wound, where an extension to the opposite ischiorectal fossa is sought in the depths of the wound. Probing must be gentle but must seek particularly where there are visible granulations that will not curette away or where there is palpable induration.

26

Exposure of extension to opposite ischiorectal fossa

If an extension of the track to the opposite fossa is found, it is laid open for its full length by the division of overlying tissues, as on the other side. The laying open of these deep tracks must be carried out carefully and thoroughly, and many vessels in the fat may require controlling. Once again no muscle need be divided at this stage. The track may be either intersphincteric or outside the external sphincter, that is trans-sphincteric.

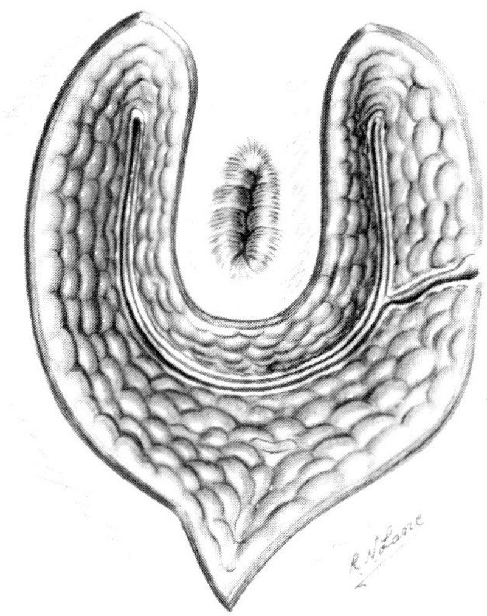

26

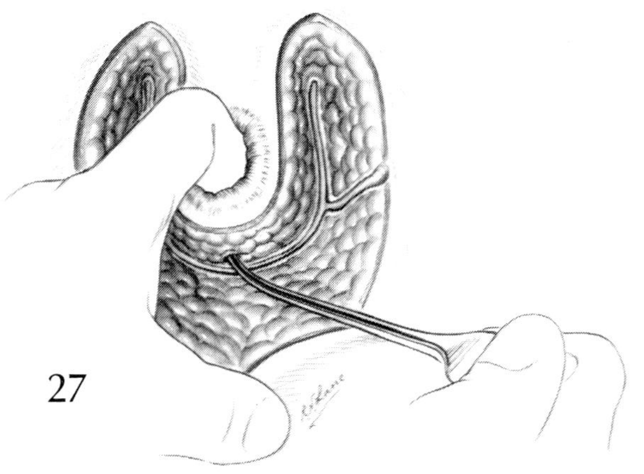

27

27

Search for internal opening

The internal opening should now be sought. The area nearest the midline posteriorly should be searched first, as this is the most frequent site. The communicating track is often very oblique (*see Illustrations 3, 4, 8* and *21*) and a hook or angled director may be necessary to find it. When found, one must first ensure by careful palpation and inspection through a proctoscope that the internal opening is below the anorectal ring. Occasionally it is necessary to search for the internal opening from within, using a Sims speculum and probing the crypt area gently. Often two probes, one within the anal canal and one in the wound, can be made to touch in this way.

28 & 29

Division of sphincter muscles

If it is certain that the internal opening is below the anorectal ring, the contained muscles are divided by cutting on the probe. If there is doubt, the superficial muscles only are divided and a nylon suture (seton) is passed round the deeper part and knotted loosely. Later examination when the patient is conscious and can actively contract the sphincter muscle will allow better assessment of the height of this opening. If findings are favourable, the contained muscles can be divided a few days later or the seton may be left in place for a while. Muscles should always be divided at right angles to their fibres if possible and not divided obliquely. The probe can be angled in such a way as to achieve this.

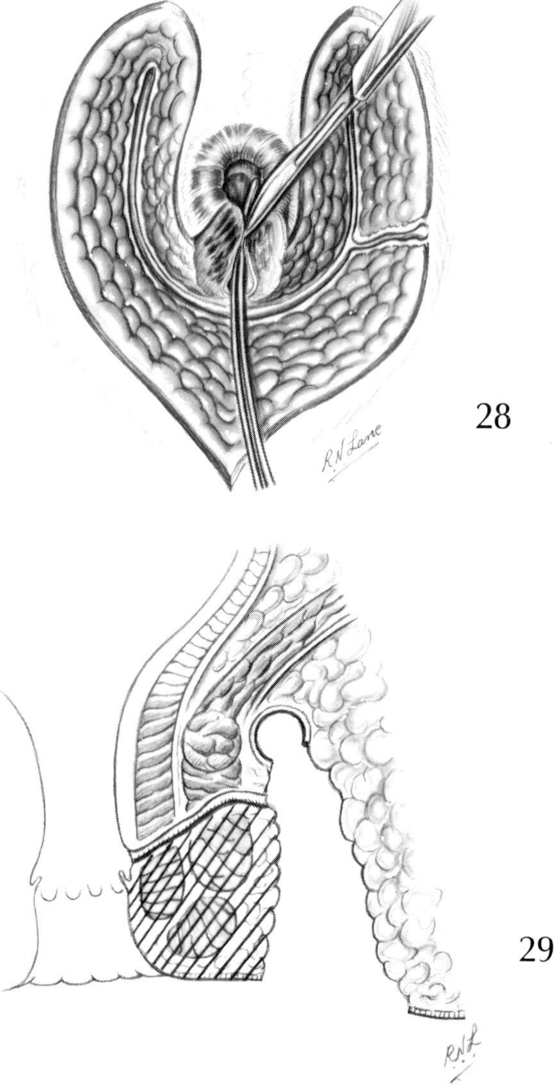

28

29

30

Extension and trimming of the wound

The wound is trimmed and enlarged by excising some skin edges and redundant fat, and the whole wound fashioned so as to shelve as shallowly as possible. All granulation tissue is meticulously curetted away and a careful search should ensure that no section of track has been overlooked.

Flat gauze dressings moistened with Eusol (1:8) or Hibitane (1:2000) are applied lightly to keep the edges of the wound apart, covered with a large cottonwool pad and held in place by T-bandage or Netelast.

Skin excision should be kept minimal and scars should be fashioned circumferentially away from the ischial tuberosities.

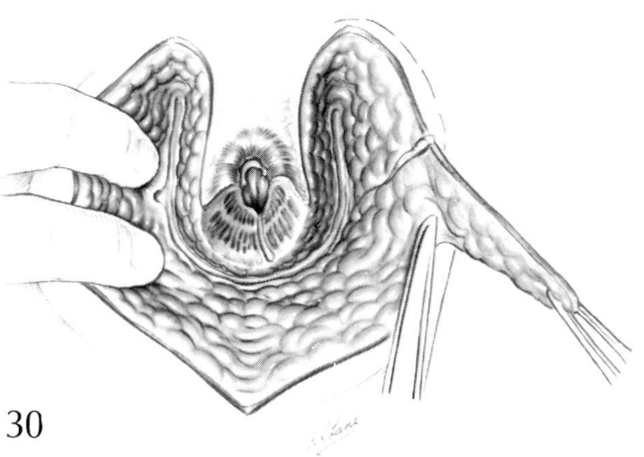

30

31

Healed appearance and sphincteric function

The wound heals slowly, the final scar being much smaller than the initial wound, and the anal appearance may not be grossly altered. Sphincteric function is usually adequate. If necessary the wound should be reviewed under anaesthesia, particularly if there is a persistent discharge of true pus.

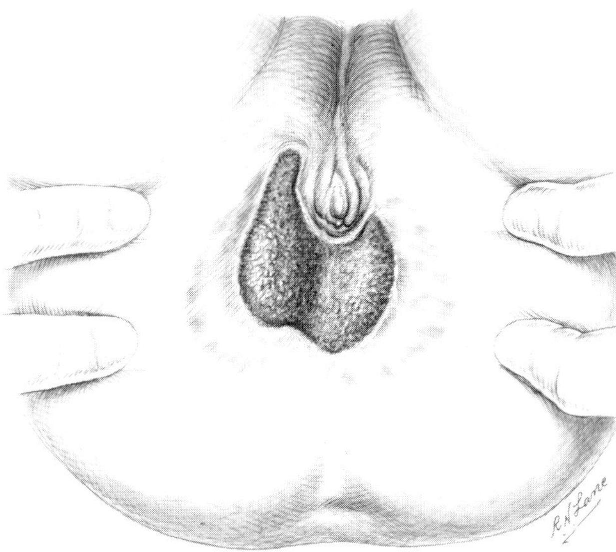

31

Uncommon fistula-in-ano

In a very few of the more complicated fistulae, particularly when there is a secondary opening into the rectum above the anorectal ring, a temporary diverting sigmoid colostomy may be advisable. Then the track into the rectum may be dissected out and the wall closed by suturing with fine monofilament steel wire or fine Dexon, with a very high chance of success and firm healing. The lower part of such a fistula, including the original anal opening, is dealt with as already described.

The use of a seton

As stated above a seton may occasionally be useful. If it is apparent postoperatively with the patient conscious that adequate muscle for continence exists above, the muscle may be divided at once. If however there is doubt, the seton should be left *in situ* for at least 3 months when it will probably have migrated downwards towards the anus with healing above. It may then be possible to divide the remaining muscle surrounded by it.

It is unnecessary for a seton to be tight initially nor need it be tightened later.

The precoccygeal space

Infection may occur in this space where it can spread upwards close to the bone and to the left and right but not apparently involving the ischiorectal fossae and fat as such. It often becomes a very rigid, ill drained cavity which may rarely extend through Waldeyer's fascia. Should this space become infected, adequate and prolonged drainage with frequent checking is necessary. It is important not to allow an overhanging undrained sump at its lowest extremity and adequate division of muscle must be undertaken to avoid this. Curetting and irrigation will slowly heal it.

Special postoperative care and complications

The postoperative care of anal wounds and the attention needed to regulate the bowel action has been fully described in the chapter on 'Open haemorrhoidectomy (St Mark's ligation/excision method)', pp. 599–606 in this volume. The same regimen should be followed in the care of the small and superficial wounds following an operation for fistula.

Larger wounds, and particularly those following operation on complicated fistulae, require rather more detailed attention. The first few dressings may be painful, and a light general anaesthetic may be necessary to allow them to be properly applied, or alternatively an analgesic drug may be given. The bowels should be encouraged to move on the third or fourth postoperative day and thereafter kept regular and the motions soft with suitable medicines and a full diet.

After the first few days, a bath, irrigation and dressing should follow each bowel action and a similar sequence should be adopted each evening. Two experienced nurses may be needed for the dressings and good lighting is essential. After a thorough irrigation, the moist flat gauze is placed gently into the depths of the wound by one nurse while the other holds the wound edges apart.

There is a tendency for large deep wounds to form pockets which delay healing; it is therefore advisable to examine them carefully once weekly throughout the period of healing, with the patient in the lithotomy position in the operating theatre. The first few such examinations should be carried out under anaesthesia. In this way the wound can be trimmed as necessary during the healing process and any pockets or tracks that have been overlooked can be laid open. Final healing may take 6–12 weeks and patience on the part of both surgeon and patient is necessary.

In those cases in which division of the greater part of the anal sphincter has been necessary, the power and function of the remaining portion may be improved by active sphincter exercises throughout the period of healing, and the patient should be instructed to carry them out.

Packing with ribbon gauze should be strenuously avoided at all stages.

Further reading

Hawley, P. R. Anorectal fistula. Clinics in Gastroenterology 1975; 4: 635–649

Milligan, E. T. C., Morgan, C. N., Lloyd-Davies, O. V., Thompson, H. R. Fistula in ano. British Surgical Practice, Vol. 4. London: Butterworths 1948; 102–130

Parks, A. G., Gordon, P. H., Hardcastle, J. D. A classification of fistula-in-ano. British Journal of Surgery 1976; 63: 1–12

Procedures for pilonidal disease

Douglas M. Millar FRCS, FRCS(Ed.)
Consultant Surgeon, Essex County Hospital, Colchester

Introduction

Although the aetiology of pilonidal sinus is a subject of debate the pathology of the established lesion is well recognized: there are one or more midline pits in the natal cleft and deep to these pits is a cavity lined with granulation tissue which usually contains hair. Running cephalad, either in the midline or laterally into the buttock from this midline cavity, there may be one or more tracks which are also lined with granulation tissue and which discharge on the surface often some distance from the midline.

General assessment

Numerous surgical treatments are employed for postanal pilonidal sinus disease. The procedures vary in their effectiveness but all are reported to carry a significant failure rate.

In the author's opinion the exact procedure for an individual patient will depend on the surgeon's preference, the size and complexity of the lesion, and the type of medical facilities which are available.

Simple non-operative measures

Removal of hair from sinus

For small central sinuses without lateral tracks simple measures may be used. Removal of hair from the sinus with forceps, followed by meticulous shaving of the surrounding skin and then good local hygiene can give good results. The sinus tract lined by granulation tissue will heal provided the foreign material is removed and observation continues until sound healing is achieved. Repeated local shaving at weekly intervals is necessary to keep the hair short until the scar has matured. To achieve depilation using irradiation seems unjustifiable.

1

Phenolic injection therapy

An area of skin approximately 15 cm in radius around the sinus is generously smeared with petroleum jelly to protect it from Phenol overflow. A wedge of cotton wool is placed in the natal cleft to cover the anus.

The main sinus and its side tracks are gently probed.

A blunt hypodermic needle is inserted into the orifice of the main tract and pure Phenol is injected slowly without pressure until it is seen to issue from all the side openings. Excess Phenol is immediately wiped away from the surrounding skin. The Phenol is left *in situ* for about 1 min and then expressed by pressure. The procedure is repeated until the total period of Phenol contact is approximately 3 min, after which it is finally expressed.

A light dressing of petroleum jelly gauze is applied.

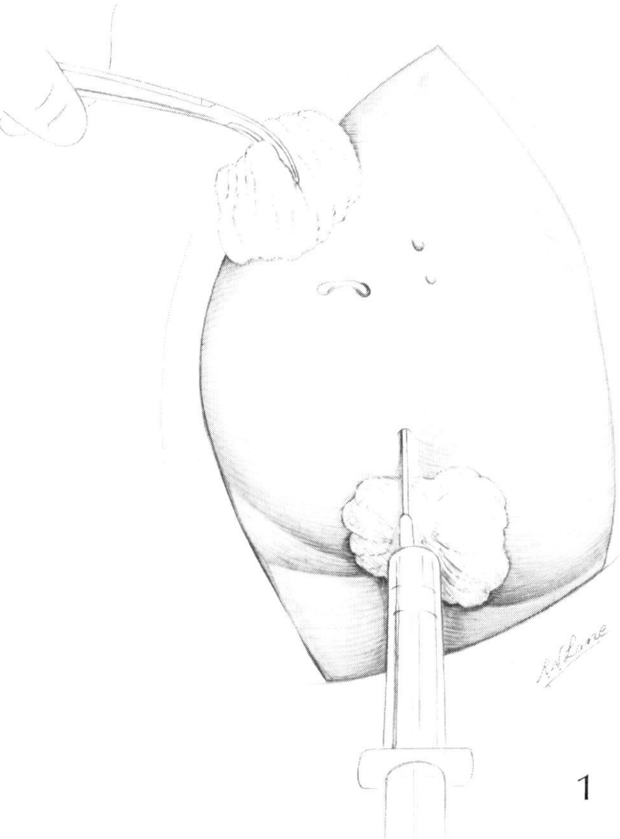

1

Preoperative

Position of patient and anaesthesia

For simple debridement type operations and the treatment of acute pilonidal abscess the left lateral position is suitable. The patient lies on his left side turned slightly face downwards. The right buttock is retracted by an assistant or by adhesive tape to open up the natal cleft. Local anaesthesia may be used (1 per cent lidocaine with 1:200 000 adrenaline).

For excisional procedures with primary suture or flap closures, the prone jackknife position is recommended but endotracheal intubation is necessary for the general anaesthetic.

Preoperative preparation

The areas immediately around the midline pits and the lateral sinuses are meticulously shaved for a distance not less than 5 cm. A wider area is required for operations involving primary suture or flap procedures.

Residual hair long enough to enter the operation wound will interfere with healing. After shaving more midline epithelial pits may sometimes show up.

The operations

EXCISION OF SINUS PITS AND CURETTAGE

2

Surgical excision is limited to an area immediately surrounding the midline pits and the lateral sinus openings with removal of not more than 0.5 cm of skin on either side.

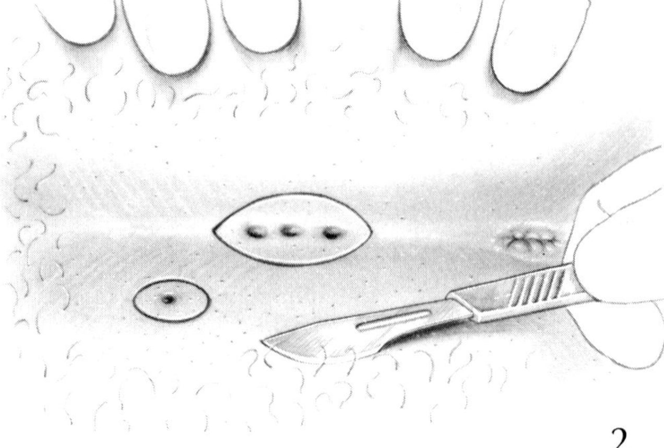

2

3

This excision is carried down to the underlying cavity from which all hair is carefully removed and debris cleaned out. No attempt is made to excise the cavity completely.

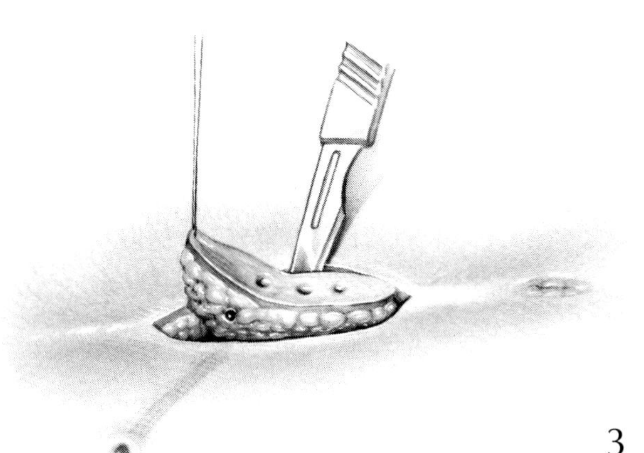

3

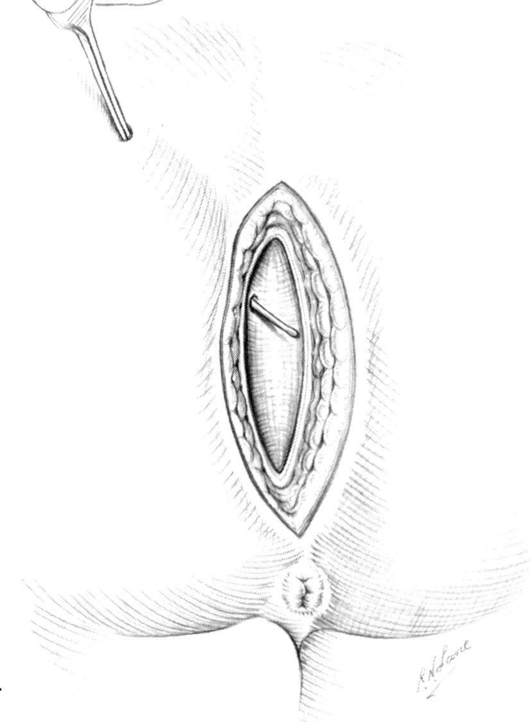

4

4

The lateral sinus track is probed to demonstrate its connection with the main central cavity. The track can then be enlarged with sinus forceps.

5

The opening of the lateral sinus is excised with a circular incision to gain good access to the connecting track. If there is a lateral abscess this must be unroofed by a similar circular incision to obtain full drainage.

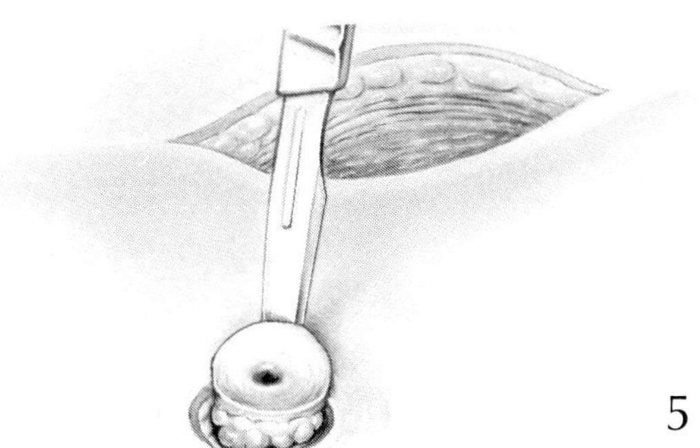

5

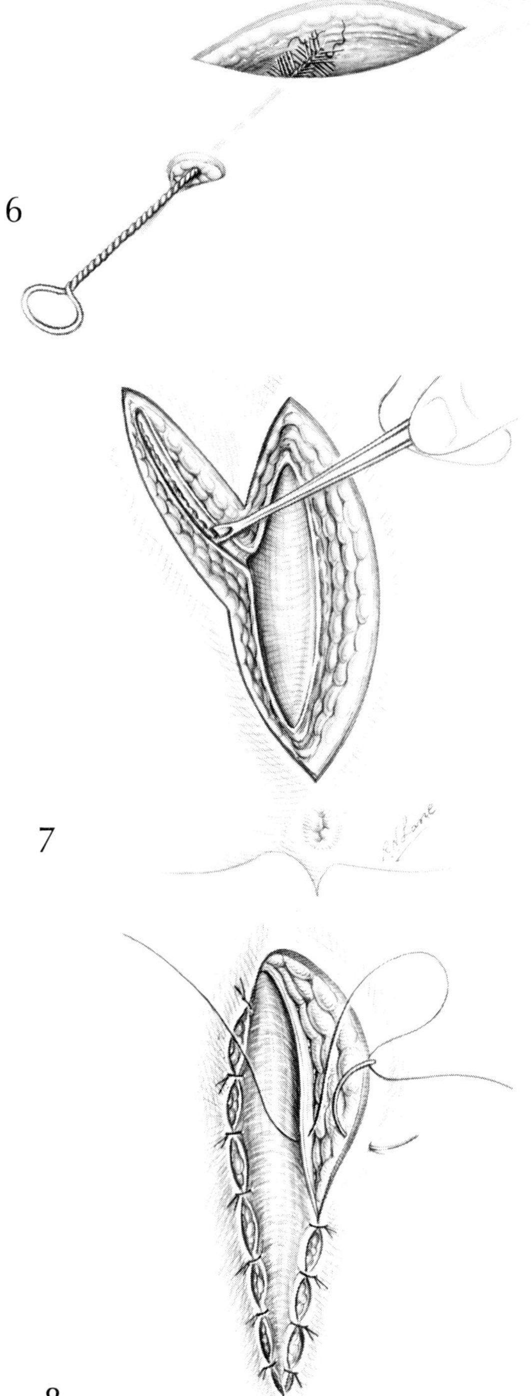

6

7

8

6

All hair and foreign material must be removed by thorough cleaning and the cavity curetted. Hair in the lateral sinus and foreign material can be removed by inserting successively several small bottle brushes and a spoon curette. These are rotated and moved backwards and forwards to clean out the track.

7

Alternatively a lateral track can be incised throughout its full length and the granulation tissue and hair curetted and cleaned out.

8

In obese patients or cases in which the exposed sinus cavity appears to be overlapped by the skin edges with a danger of bridging over then marsupialization may be employed.

After excision of the sinus pits, interrupted chromic catgut sutures are placed between the raw skin edge and the margin of the opened sinus. The objective is to turn the skin edge down to prevent a skin bridge over the site re-establishing a sinus tract.

EXCISION AND PRIMARY SUTURE

9 & 10

A wide excision of the sinus is performed to expose healthy fat on either side and the glistening sacral fascia in the depths of the wound. Deep sutures of nylon are placed at 2.5 cm intervals across the wound, picking up the sacral fascia, and left untied. The skin edges are then sutured.

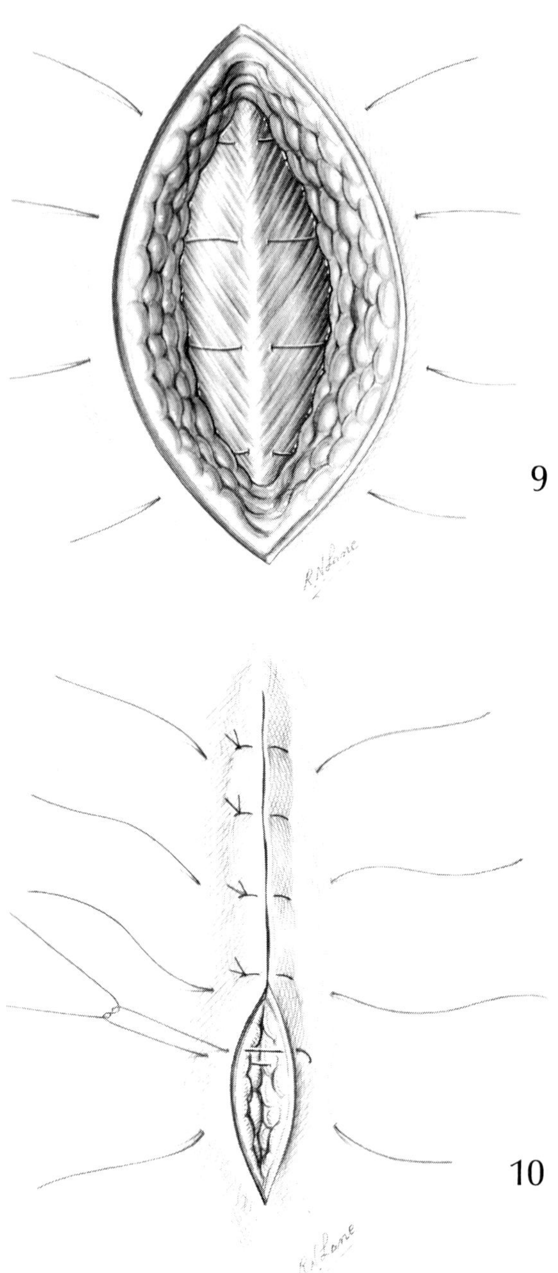

9

10

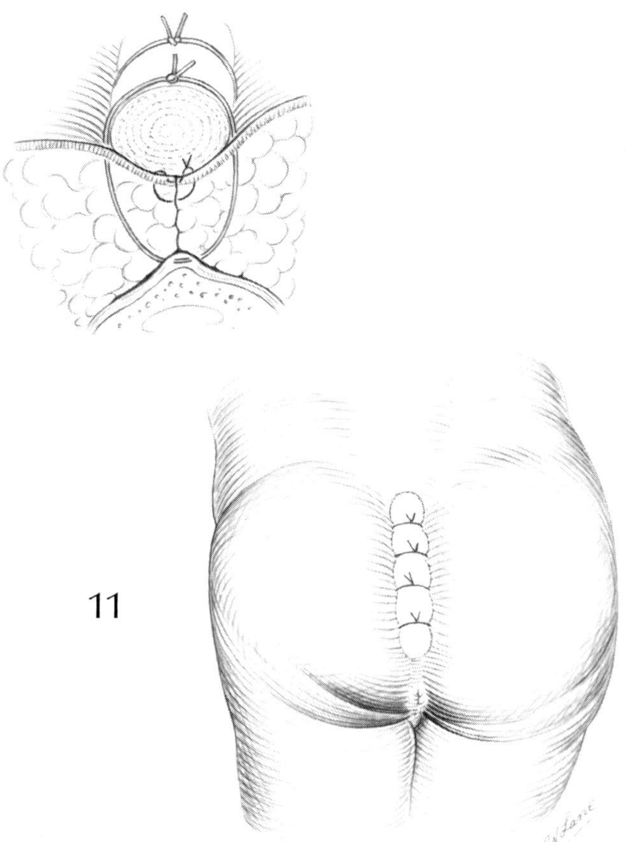

11

11

A roll of gauze dressing is placed along the wound and the deep sutures tied over it.

EXCISION AND LATERAL FLAP

This is an alternative method of primary closure and is designed to flatten the natal cleft and eliminate a midline scar. A short lateral track can be included in the excision.

12 & 13

The excision of the cavity is 'semilateral'. It closely follows the midline pits and median cleft on one side but is wider on the contralateral side and should excise any short lateral track.

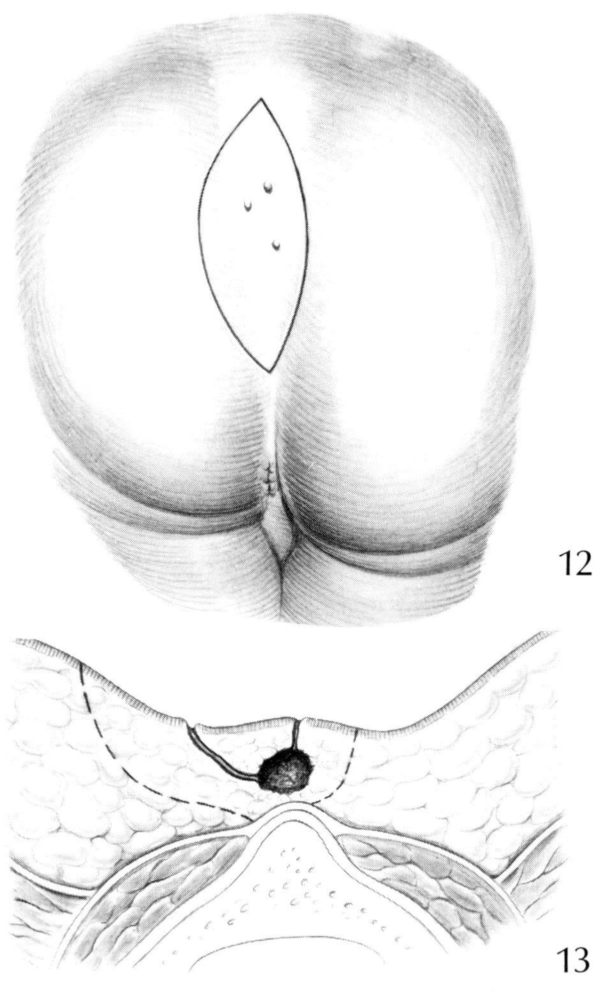

12

13

14 & 15

At the depth of the sacral fascia a lateral flap is undermined.

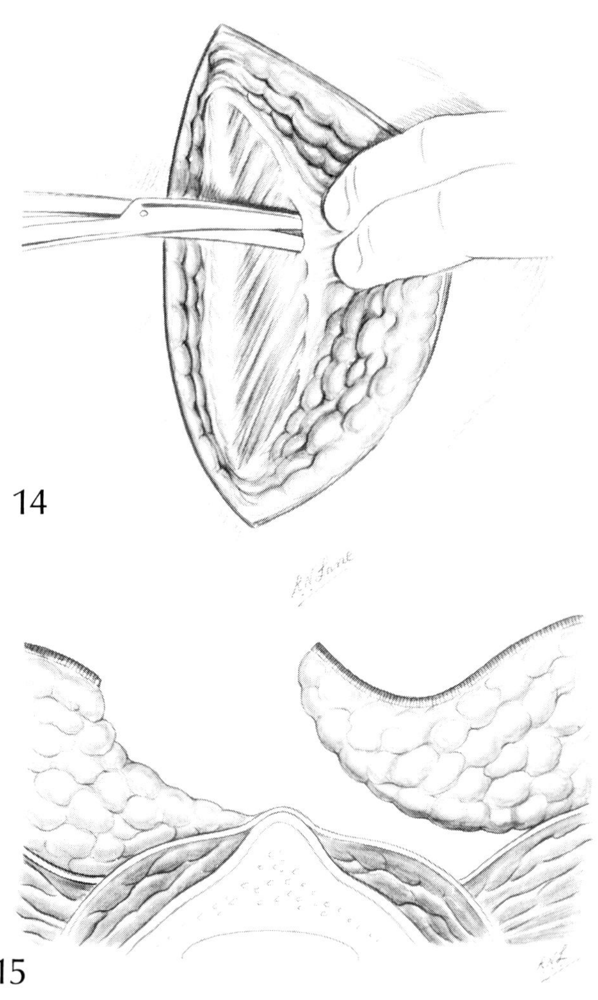

14

15

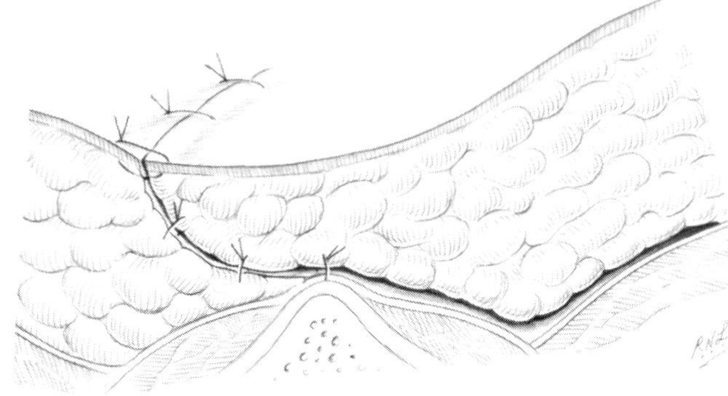

16

16 & 17

It is essential that the underside of the flap is sutured with catgut to the sacral fascia. The skin sutures will be to one side of the original natal cleft.

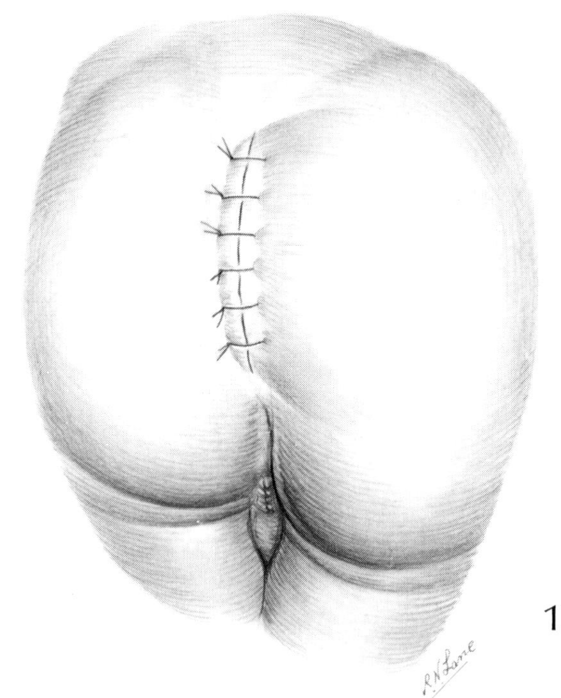

17

EXCISION AND Z-PLASTY FLAP

Primary suture and lateral flap suture is not suitable for bilateral or long lateral tracks.

18

Following total excision of the midline sinus and its lateral tracks incisions are made at 45° to the midline.

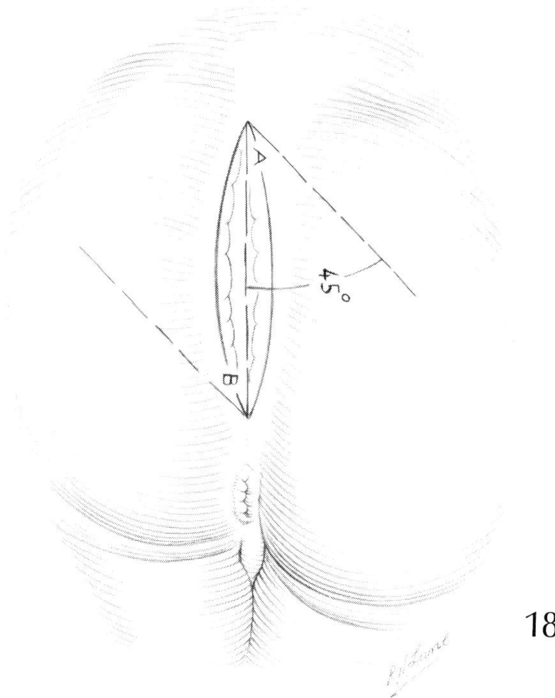

18

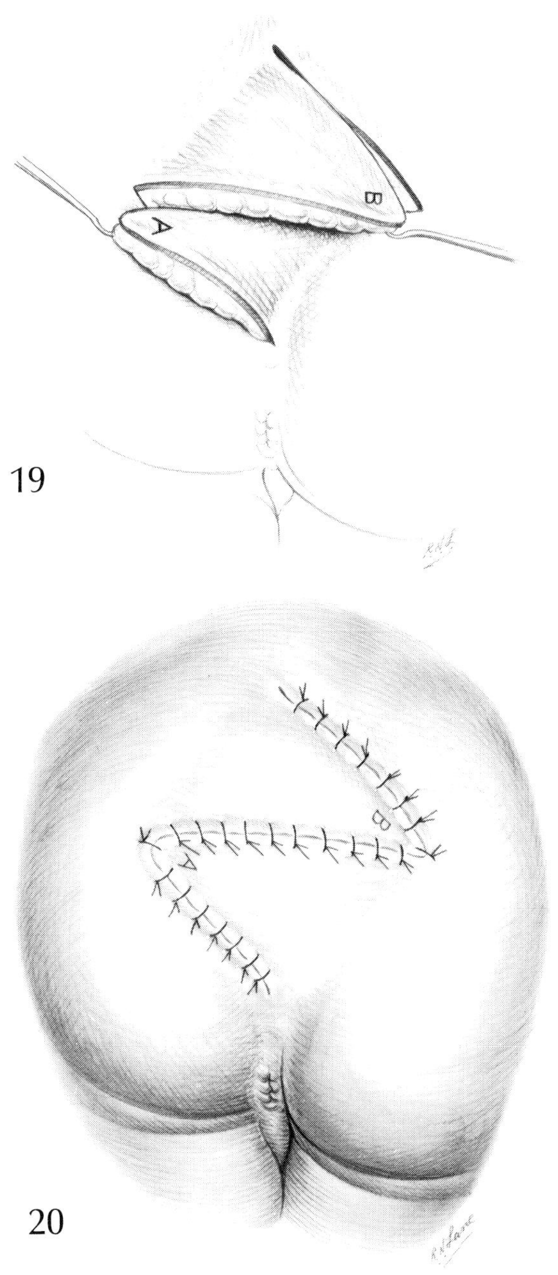

19

20

19 & 20

The two triangular flaps with their apices at A and B are mobilized to include skin and fat down to the level of the sacral fascia. Further mobilization of the other tissues may be required at the same level.

The triangular flaps are transposed and the skin sutured. Suction drainage may be employed through small stab incisions.

Postoperative care

After the simple procedures all that is required is a dry gauze pad for dressing. On the first day after the procedure a bath is taken and the dressing removed. After careful drying of the area the gauze pad is replaced. This routine is repeated daily and can be carried out at home. Leisure and work activities may be resumed immediately and only restricted by local discomfort.

Primary suture and flap repair methods generally require 7–10 days' bed rest. Deep sutures are removed on the seventh day after operation but the superficial ones are retained until the tenth day. A low residue diet is given and the bowels should be confined for a few days.

For open methods it is essential that the patient attends an outpatient clinic at least at 2 weekly intervals, when any skin bridging across the deeper cavity can be broken down so that healing takes place from the base towards the surface. Any accumulated debris is cleaned out. Hair must be shaved on the surrounding skin for a margin of 5 cm. After complete healing the patient is advised on careful personal hygiene and the use of a simple astringent lotion which allows the scars to become pale and firm.

Suture methods also require good outpatient follow-up particularly to ensure good hygiene and prevention of intertrigo. Shaving around the suture line until the scar is firm prevents inturning of local hairs.

Acute pilonidal abscess

A simple incision over the pointing abscess results in a very high recurrence rate and should therefore be regarded as a temporary expedient before definitive surgery. If, however, the sinus pits are excised and the whole cavity laid open and thoroughly cleansed into the lateral tracts a high percentage of primary cures result which require no further surgery.

Recurrent pilonidal sinus

Simple excision of sinus pits and laying open of the underlying cavity as well as cleansing with or without marsupialization is effective. Sometimes there is considerable scarring in the region which is better treated with an excisional procedure. Simple primary closure must never be used and reconstruction should be achieved by flap advancement or Z-plasty as already described.

Further reading

Simple treatment techniques

Edwards, M. H. Pilonidal sinus: a five year appraisal of the Millar-Lord treatment. British Journal of Surgery 1977; 64: 867–868

Goodall, P. Management of pilonidal sinus. Proceedings of the Royal Society of Medicine 1975; 68: 675

Lord, P. H., Millar, D. M. Pilonidal sinus: a simple treatment. British Journal of Surgery 1965; 52: 298–300

Notaras, M. J. A review of three popular methods of treatment of postanal (pilonidal) sinus disease. British Journal of Surgery 1970; 57: 886–890

Ortiz, H. H., Marti, J., Sitges, A. Pilonidal sinus: a claim for simple track incision. Diseases of the Colon and Rectum 1977; 20: 325–328

Primary suture techniques

Bentivegna, S. S., Procario, P. Primary closure of pilonidal cystectomy. American Surgeon 1977; 43: 214–216

Goligher, J. C. Surgery of the anus and rectum and colon, 3rd Ed. London: Baillière Tindall, 1975

Flap–suture techniques

Fishbeir, R. H., Handelsman, J. C. A method for primary reconstruction following radical excision of sacrococcygeal pilonidal disease. Annals of Surgery 1979; 190: 231–235

Karydakis, G. E. New approach to the problem of pilonidal sinus. Lancet 1973; 2: 1414–1415

Middleton, M. D. Treatment of pilonidal sinus by Z-plasty. British Journal of Surgery 1968; 55: 516–518

Acute pilonidal abscess

Millar, D. M., Lord, P. H. The treatment of acute postanal pilonidal abscess. British Journal of Surgery 1967; 54: 598–599

Hernia: general introduction

In all the abdominal wall hernia operations the main mechanical principle is to repair each layer of the defect discretely and thus restore the patient's anatomy, insofar as is possible, so that it resembles the normal unoperated condition. Only tendinous/aponeurotic/fascial structures can be successfully sutured together: suturing red fleshy muscle to tendon or fascia will not contribute to permanent fibrous union of these structures. Nor will it reconstruct anything resembling the normal anatomy!

The suture material must retain its strength for long enough to maintain tissue apposition and allow sound union of tissues to occur. A non-absorbable or very slowly absorbable suture material must therefore be employed.

The inherent disadvantageous properties of non-absorbable suture materials – proneness to sepsis, adverse tissue reaction and sinus formation – have led surgeons to seek compromises which have often not proved effective when used for hernia repair.

The suture material of choice for the repair is metric 3 polypropylene (Prolene) and this is used for all fascial/aponeurotic layers in adults. Stainless steel wire is a most effective suture material but it is difficult to use; polypropylene is as effective and is much easier to handle.

For haemostasis we ligate the larger vessels, especially the veins in the subcutaneous tissue, using metric 3.5 chromic catgut. Otherwise diathermy is used for haemostasis. Careful haemostasis is most important if haematoma and consequent sepsis is to be avoided.

Sepsis is the great hazard to herniorrhaphy particularly when non-absorbable suture material is used. Scrupulous surgical technique is vital if infection is to be avoided. The skin is routinely covered at the site of operation with sterile adherent film which is not removed until the subcutaneous fat is closed. Sutures are never used to close the skin for by their very nature they have potential for introducing dermal and epidermal bacteria into the subcutaneous tissue along their tracks. Each suture is a linear abscess lined with granulation tissue, and if the 'infection' in these abscesses spreads and involves the buried non-absorbable sutures sinuses may result.

In adults local or general anaesthesia may be used. In British practice general anaesthesia is more frequently used but local anaesthesia with lignocaine or bupivacaine (Marcaine) is effective and this technique may be more appropriate in some environments.

H. Brendan Devlin

Epigastric hernia

H. Brendan Devlin MA, MD, MCh, FRCS, FRCS(I)
Consultant Surgeon, North Tees General Hospital, Stockton on Tees, Cleveland;
Associate Lecturer in Clinical Surgery, University of Newcastle upon Tyne

Introduction

An epigastric hernia is a protrusion of extraperitoneal fat between the decussating fibres of the linea alba. These hernias usually occur in the midline of the epigastrium between the xiphisternum and the umbilicus; but small hernia can occur away from the midline and may protrude into the rectus muscle sheath. If these hernias enlarge considerably they may develop a peritoneal sac, which may be subcutaneous in the midline hernia or interstitial, within the rectus sheath in more lateral hernias.

Preoperative

Indications

Epigastric hernias may cause symptoms quite out of proportion to their size as the very narrow opening in the linea alba predisposes to attacks of strangulation of the peritoneal fat in which the patient may suffer severe abdominal pain when the swelling becomes tense and tender. The occurrence of such attacks is an adequate indication for operative treatment. It is, however, important to investigate the patient fully, as a small innocent epigastric hernia is sometimes blamed for symptoms which are in fact due to some intra-abdominal condition, such as a peptic ulcer. At the same time it is true to say that an epigastric hernia may sometimes produce symptoms which closely resemble those due to a peptic ulcer.

Anaesthesia

A general anaesthetic is usually employed but repair can be quite satisfactorily performed under local infiltration with lignocaine or bupivacaine.

The operation

Position of patient

The patient is placed supine on the operating table.

Suture materials

For repair metric 3 polypropylene sutures are used.

Drapes

Drapes are arranged so that the whole of the epigastric area from the costal margin to just below the umbilicus is exposed for surgery. Not infrequently the hernia is found to be larger than anticipated and placing the drapes widely has the advantage of facilitating an extended incision.

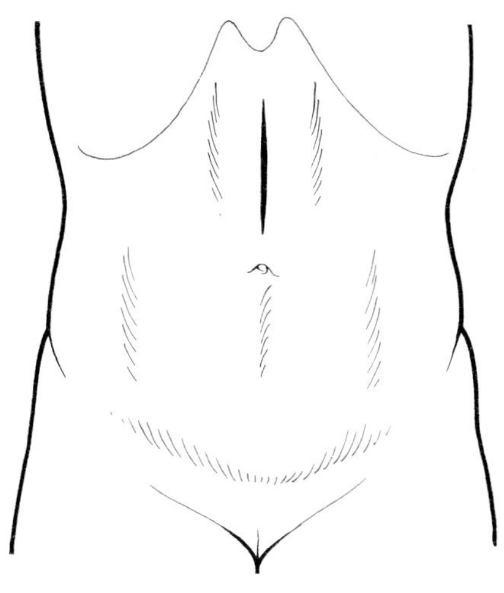

1

1

The incision

A vertical incision has the advantage that the abdomen can easily be opened if this is deemed necessary.

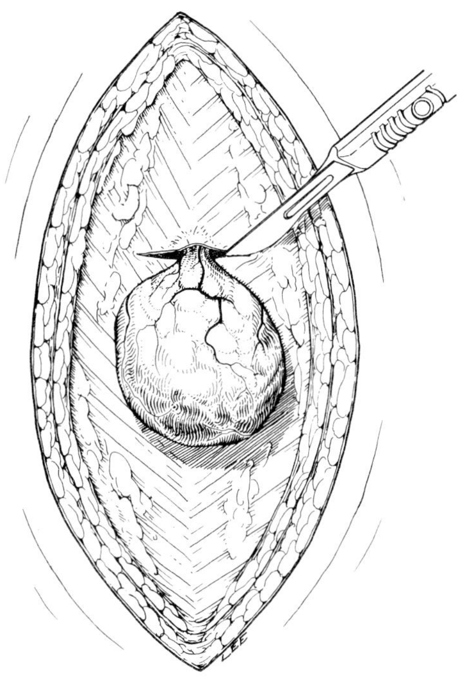

2

2

The fatty hernia which is enclosed within a fine capsule is dissected out from the surrounding abdominal fat. The opening in the linea alba which is usually tiny should be enlarged by incisions from opposite sides running laterally into the linea alba.

3 & 4

The hernia is incised at its neck to determine whether there is a peritoneal sac and to reduce its contents if present into the abdomen.

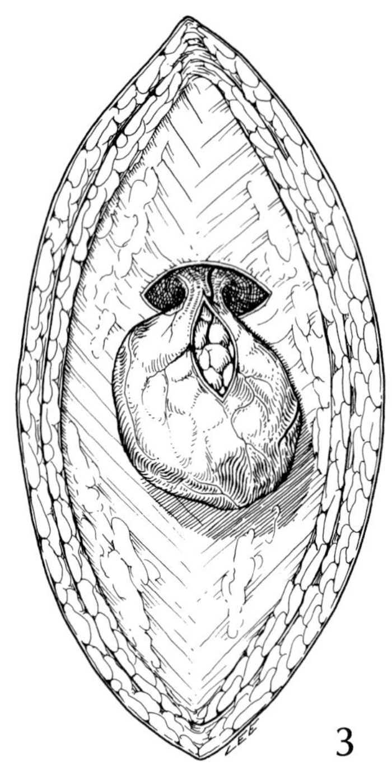

3

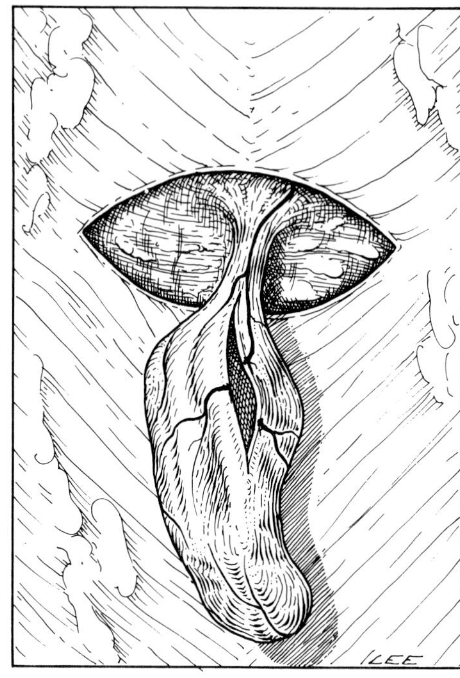

4

5 & 6

The neck of the hernia is then ligated with a transfixion suture of metric 3 chromic catgut and the hernia excised.

The opening in the linea alba is then closed by overlapping its edge as shown with two rows of interrupted polypropylene or nylon sutures, the first row inserted as mattress sutures and the second as simple sutures.

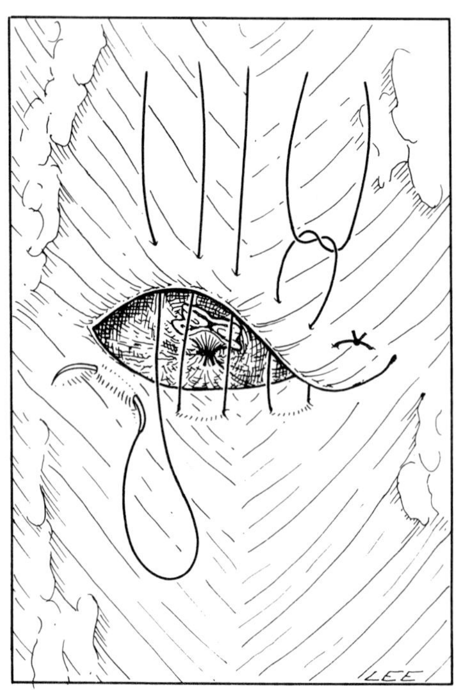

5

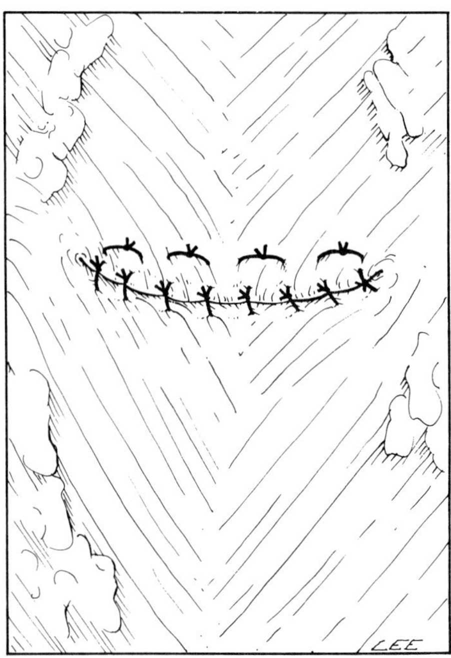

6

7

The subcutaneous fat is closed with interrupted catgut sutures. No 'dead space' should be left and the fat should be closed so that the skin is closely approximated.

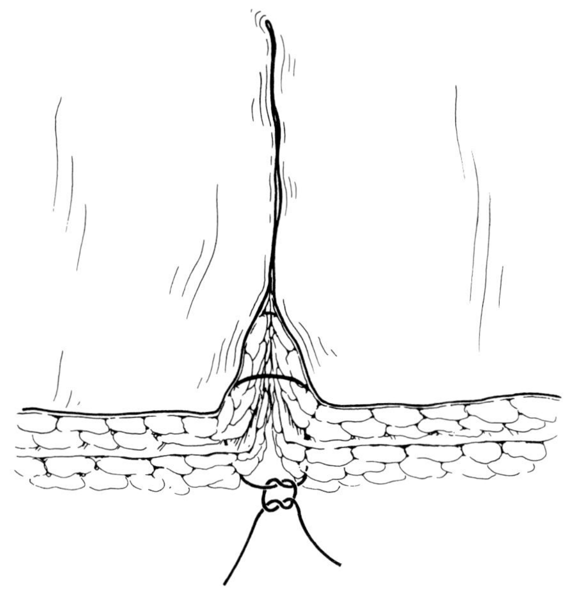

7

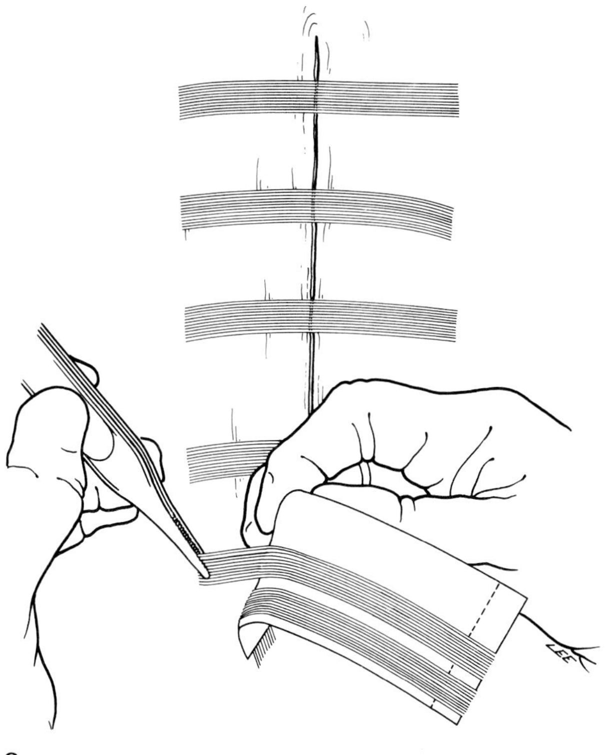

8

8

The skin is closed with microporous adhesive tape or a strip of gauze impregnated with collodion or similar adhesive. Non-penetrating skin clips give an equally good closure but require skilled attention when they are removed. Sutures should not be used.

Postoperative care

No special postoperative care is needed.

Umbilical hernia in babies and children

H. Brendan Devlin MA, MD, MCh, FRCS, FRCS(I)
Consultant Surgeon, North Tees General Hospital, Stockton on Tees, Cleveland;
Associate Lecturer in Clinical Surgery, University of Newcastle upon Tyne

Introduction

Historical note

Umbilical hernias frequently contain omentum and stomach, transverse colon or small intestine; in adults they are prone to obstruction and strangulation. Without surgical intervention strangulation inevitably progresses to abdominal wall suppuration, peritonitis and death except in the rare instance when a fistula or preternatural intestinal stoma develops at the umbilicus. Such a remarkable case of strangulation of the transverse colon was described by Cheselden in 1784[1]; consequently, in surgical hagiography Cheselden is credited with the first colostomy!

Surgical repair of umbilical hernia remained unsatisfactory until Dr William Mayo described his 'vertical method' of repair to the American Academy of Railway Surgeons on October 4th 1898[2]. This operation rapidly improved the results of umbilical hernia closure and was commended by Drs A. J. Oschner and J. B. Murphy to the Fifty-fourth Annual Session of the American Medical Association in 1903. This eponymous operation is the standard method of treatment today.

Incidence

Childhood umbilical hernias requiring surgery are much less frequent than inguinal hernias. In Stockton on Tees there were 15 667 live births in the 6 years 1974–1979. Of these children 36 had umbilical hernias which required surgical correction, an incidence of 2.3 per 1000 live births.

Personal experience

The author's experience of surgery of umbilical hernias in children is primarily drawn from the Stockton on Tees sample already mentioned: in the 9 years from 1970 up to and including 1979, 58 children (34 male and 24 female) with umbilical hernia have been operated on.

Preoperative

Indications

The usual infantile umbilical hernia is a protrusion through the umbilical cicatrix with a small peritoneal sac and a relatively narrow neck. These hernias become very obvious when the infant cries or strains and are often a source of worry to the parents. Almost all infantile umbilical hernias undergo spontaneous regression and cure as the child grows; however, if the hernia is unusually large, with a neck diameter greater than 1.5 cm, or fails to regress by school age it should be operated upon. It is important for psychological reasons to preserve the umbilical cicatrix when undertaking surgery.

Arrangements for surgery and anaesthesia

Children with umbilical hernias can be treated on an outpatient day case basis[3]. The arrangements for this surgery are similar to those described in the chapter on 'Inguinal hernia in babies and children', pp. 675–680 in this volume.

The operation

Principles

A simple excision of the peritoneal sac and closure of the aponeurotic defect by double-breasting in the vertical plane – Mayo's operation – is recommended. The umbilical cicatrix is carefully preserved and its base sutured to the deep fascia to present a cosmetically attractive appearance after surgery.

Haemostasis and suture materials

Careful haemostasis is achieved by ligating all bleeding points with metric 3 chromic catgut. Diathermy may be used safely for the smaller vessels.

The aponeurosis is sutured using metric 3 chromic catgut on a curved, round bodied needle. The subcutaneous fat and skin are closed with metric 3 chromic catgut as described in the chapter on 'Inguinal hernia in babies and children'.

Position of patient

The child is placed on his back (supine) on the operating table. A light cotton blanket is placed over the chest and upper abdomen and a similar blanket over the lower limbs. This precaution prevents undue heat loss during surgery.

Draping

Drapes are applied so that the umbilical area is exposed throughout the operation.

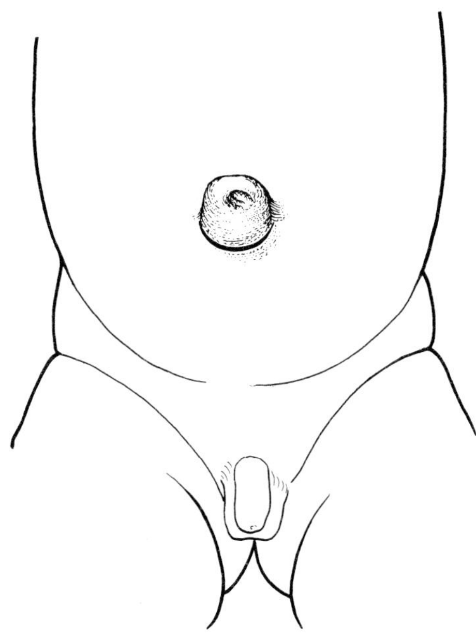

1

1

The incision

A curved transverse incision is made below the umbilicus. There is usually a skin fold skirting the umbilicus and the incision can be placed in it to give the most cosmetically acceptable result.

2

Skin flap and exposure of hernial sac

A skin flap, including the umbilical cicatrix, is dissected back to expose the hernial sac which is dissected free from the surrounding fat. When the neck of the sac is defined the more rigid outline of the linea alba should now be easily identified.

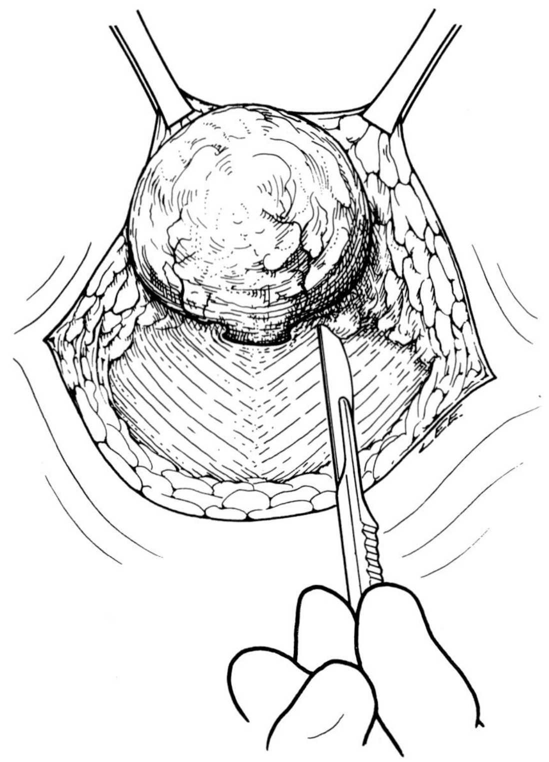

2

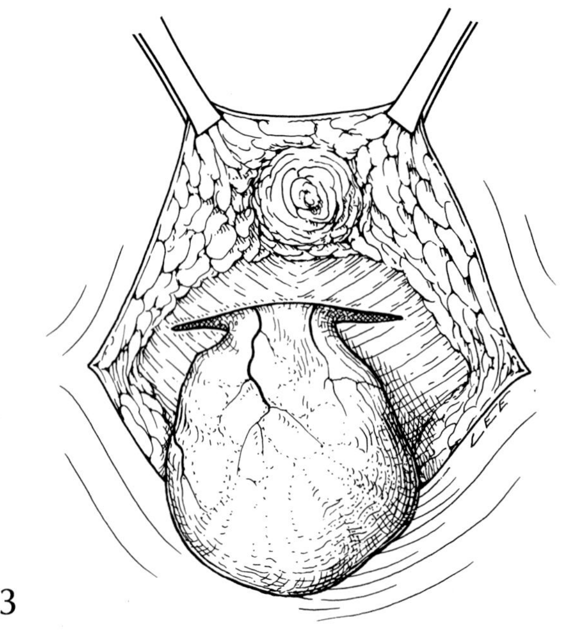

3

3

Enlargement of opening

It is usually possible to reduce the contents of an infantile umbilical hernia without enlarging the opening of the linea alba. However, if the contents cannot be reduced the opening should be enlarged by small horizontal incisions into the rectus sheath on either side.

4

Removal of sac

The sac should be opened and then divided from the parietal peritoneum at its neck. As the sac is divided its edges are picked up and held in small haemostats.

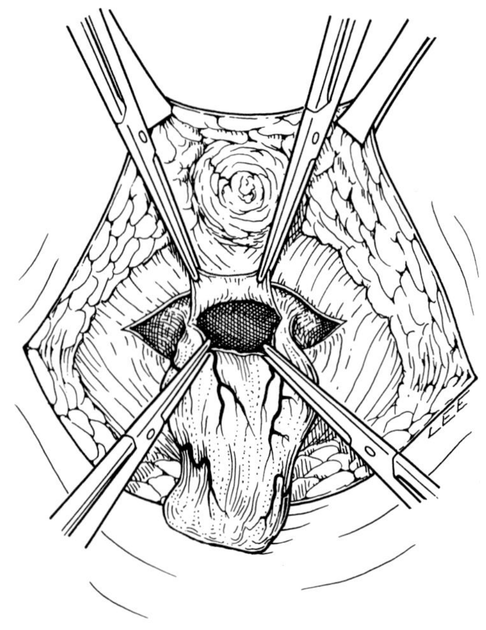

4

Repair of linea alba

The linea alba and the peritoneum are sutured as one layer.

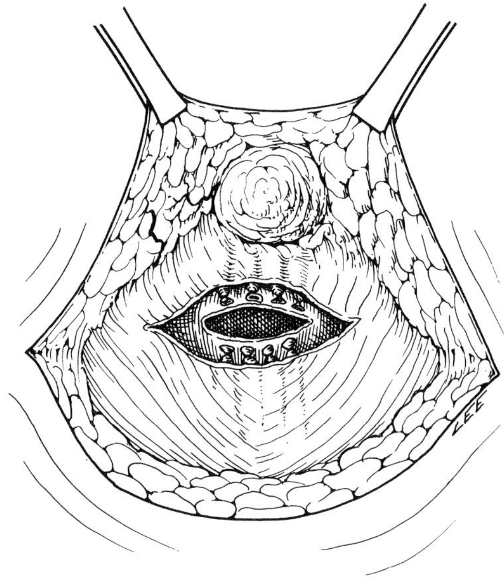

5

5

Haemostasis must first be secured. Often in children there are some substantial vessels running between the peritoneum and the aponeurosis and [illegible] best ligated with catgut.

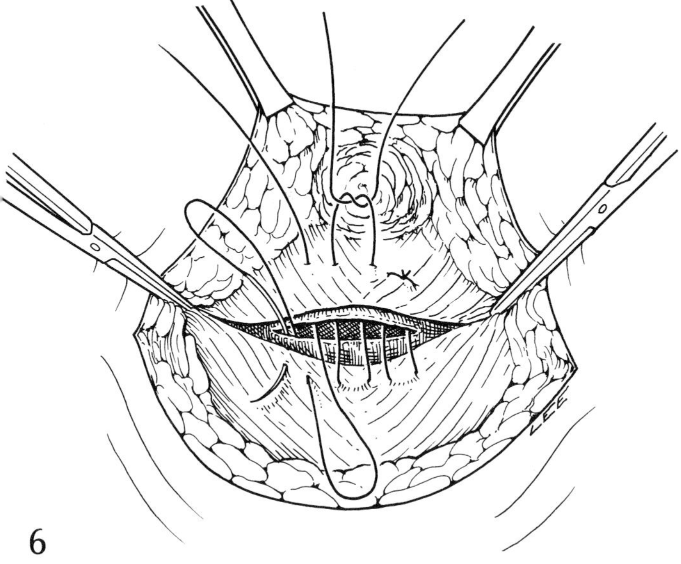

6

6

A double-breasting technique (Mayo) is used. The placement of the sutures is facilitated if the lateral extremities of the cut in the linea alba are held up in small haemostats. Three metric 3 catgut sutures are used; they are introduced through the upper flap, then through the lower flap and back through the upper flap. The sutures should traverse the upper flap about 0.5 cm from its margin (the condensation of the fascia at the linea alba aperture). As each suture is introduced it is held, not tied.

7

When all three sutures have been placed they are gently tightened and tied. Thus the lower aponeurotic flap is sutured to the undersurface of the upper flap.

The repair is now completed by suturing the edge of the upper flap to the anterior surface of the lower flap. Metric 3 chromic catgut is used as a continuous suture.

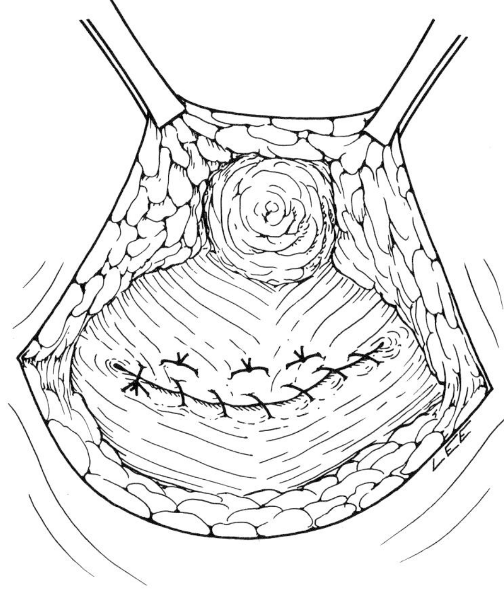

7

Reconstruction of umbilicus and skin closure

8

The deepest part of the delve of the umbilical cicatrix is now sutured to the linea alba with catgut, so preserving the appearance of the umbilicus.

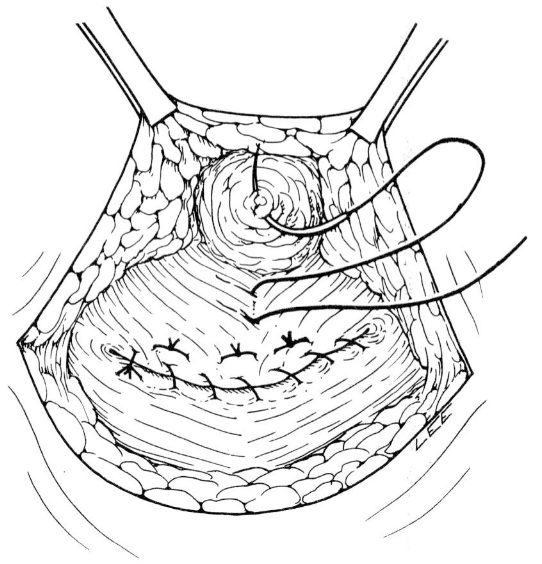

8

9 & 10

The subcutaneous fat and the skin are closed by interrupted subcuticular sutures of fine catgut, the knots being tied deeply.

The final integrity of the skin closure is maintained by a surface dressing of gauze soaked in collodion or with hypoallergenic skin tape.

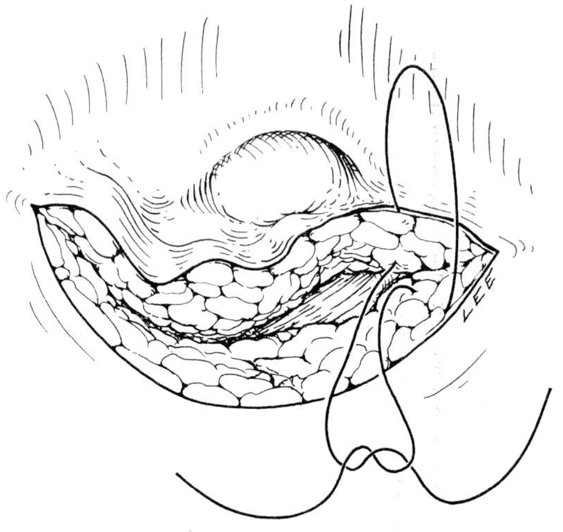

9

Postoperative care

No postoperative care other than normal maternal nursing care is required.

The child can be caressed and fed by his mother as soon as he is recovered from the anaesthetic. He can be allowed to play and bathed as soon as necessary. The adherent dressing generally falls away after 24–48 h. No attempt is made to remove it prematurely.

Personal results

Because umbilical hernias generally regress spontaneously the author's policy is to operate on very few of them. Consequently operations for umbilical hernias are numerically much fewer than operations for inguinal hernia in infancy and childhood.

In the past 9 years the author has operated on 58 children with umbilical hernia, 34 male and 24 female, compared with 346 operations for inguinal hernia in childhood. None has sustained complications or recurrence.

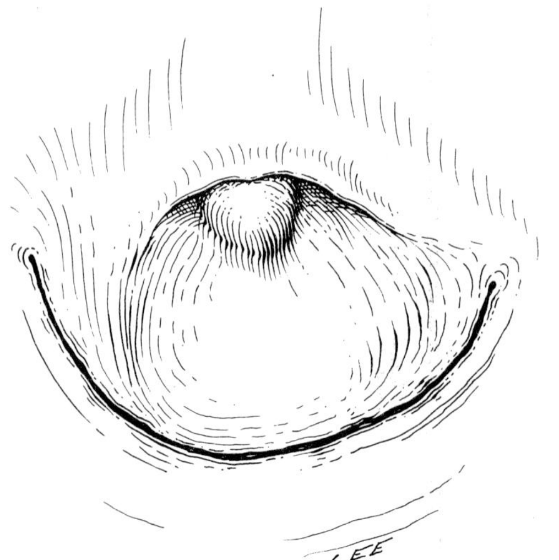

10

References

1. Cheselden, W. Colostomy for strangulated umbilical hernia. In: Cheselden, W. The anatomy of the human body. 12th ed. London: J. E. & C. Rivington, 1784: 324
2. Mayo, W. J. Further experience with the vertical overlapping operation for the radical cure of umbilical hernia. Journal of the American Medical Association 1903; 41: 225–228
3. Atwell, J. D., Burn, J. M. B., Dewar, A. K., Freeman, N. V. Paediatric day case surgery. The Lancet 1973; 2: 895–897

Umbilical hernia in adults

H. Brendan Devlin MA, MD, MCh, FRCS, FRCS(I)
Consultant Surgeon, North Tees General Hospital, Stockton on Tees, Cleveland;
Associate Lecturer in Clinical Surgery, University of Newcastle upon Tyne

Introduction

Umbilical hernias in adults can be a cause of considerable morbidity and if complications supervene they can lead to death. Umbilical hernias are much less frequent in the adult population than inguinal hernias (in the last 9 years the author has operated on 19 cases – 10 male and 9 female – compared with 603 primary inguinal hernias).

Preoperative

Indications for operation

Most patients with umbilical hernias complain of a painful protrusion at the umbilicus and this discomfort may be indication enough for operation. Absolute indications for surgery include obstruction and strangulation. Irreducibility is not an absolute indication for surgery: many long-standing umbilical hernias have many adhesions in a loculated hernia and are thus irreducible. In larger hernias the overlying skin may become damaged and ulcerated. Such hernias are best treated by operation after the skin sepsis has been controlled. In general the author's policy is to advise surgery for all umbilical hernias unless there are strong contraindications which would include obesity, chronic cardiovascular or respiratory disease, or ascites (umbilical hernias can be manifestations of cirrhotic or malignant peritoneal effusions).

Suture materials

For repair of the aponeurosis, metric 4 polypropylene or metric 3.5 nylon is used. The subcutaneous fat is closed with metric 3.5 chromic catgut. The skin is best closed with metal clips.

Anaesthesia

General anaesthesia with full muscle relaxation should be employed.

Patients who require an extensive intraperitoneal dissection often have considerable adynamic ileus after surgery and may require a postoperative regimen of nasogastric suction and fluid and nutritional support.

Position of patient

The patient is laid on his back on the operative table.

Drapes are applied to allow good access to the umbilical area and the abdomen if extended access is required.

Preoperative preparation

Sepsis is the great hazard to herniorrhaphy using non-absorbable suture material. Scrupulous surgical technique is vital if infection is to be avoided. The skin is routinely covered at the site of operation with sterile adherent film which is not removed until the subcutaneous fat is closed. Sutures are never used to close the skin for, by their very nature, sutures have the potential of introducing dermal and epidermal bacteria into the subcutaneous tissue along their tracks. Each suture is a linear abscess lined with granulation tissue and, if the 'infection' in these abscesses spreads and involves the buried sutures, sinuses may result.

For haemostasis both ligation with catgut and diathermy are used. Careful haemostasis is most important if haematoma and consequent sepsis are to be avoided.

The operation

1

The incision

Two semilunar incisions joined at their extremities are used. The ellipse of stretched skin and the enclosed umbilical cicatrix are excised. Care must be taken when deciding the dimensions of the incisions. Though the umbilical cicatrix is best excised, removal of too much skin will place the final wound under tension and jeopardize its healing. It is better to aim on the side of caution and take little skin away at the commencement of the operation; more skin can always be excised later.

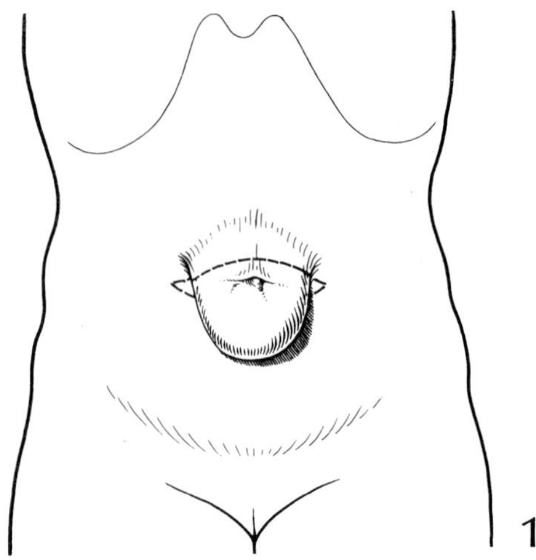

1

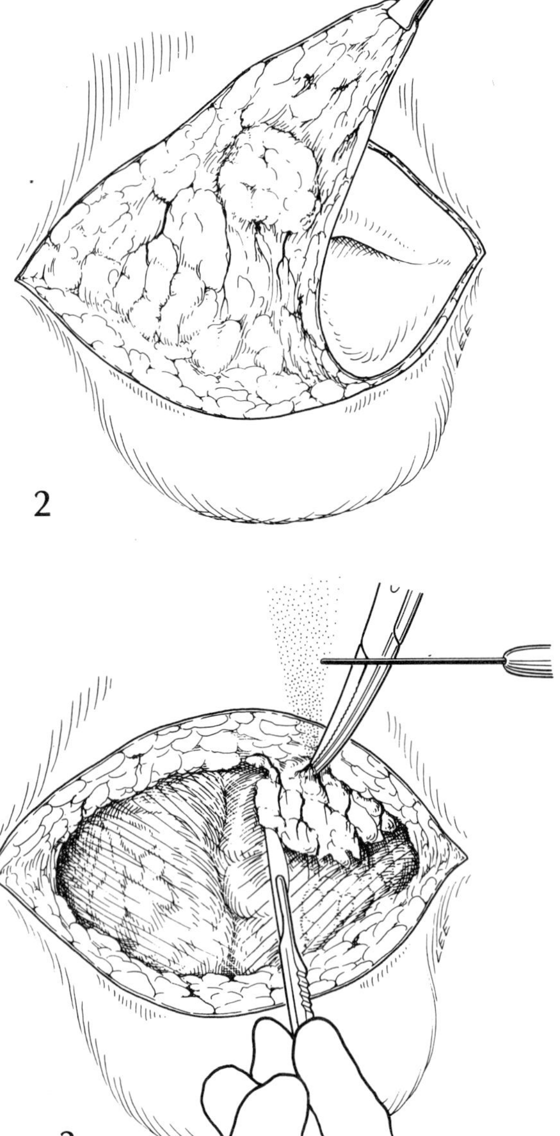

2

3

2 & 3

Removal of redundant skin and fat

The area of skin and subcutaneous fat enclosed by the semilunar incisions is removed. The incisions are deepened down to the muscular aponeuroses, care being taken to ensure that the incisions are vertical and at right angles to the fascia and that the skin is not undermined and its blood supply hazarded. This part of the dissection can be very bloody, and a cautious aproach and careful sequential haemostasis are recommended. The avoidance of blood loss at this stage is very important if blood transfusion and its considerable hazards in an obese and elderly patient is to be avoided.

Identification of neck of the sac

When the incisions have been deepened to the aponeurosis the margins of the aponeurosis about the peritoneal neck of the sac can be sought and dissected.

4, 5 & 6

Management of the Sac I

Having isolated the neck of the sac all the overlying fat and skin can be dissected off leaving the peritoneum of the sac protruding bare through the defect in the abdominal wall. The sac can now be opened and its contents inspected. Often the contents are densely adherent to the lining of the sac particularly at the fundus. Adhesions must be divided and ligated where necessary to control bleeding. Again the admonition about the avoidance of blood loss should be remembered. Densely adherent omentum, particularly if it is partly ischaemic, is best excised. After the contents have been freed from the sac they are ready to be returned to the main peritoneal cavity.

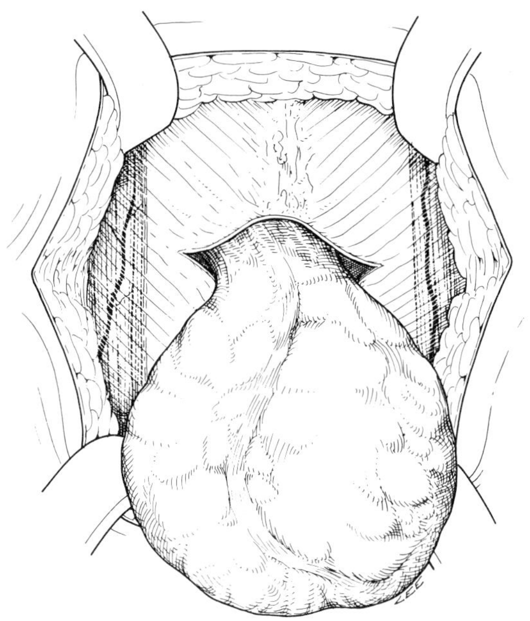

4

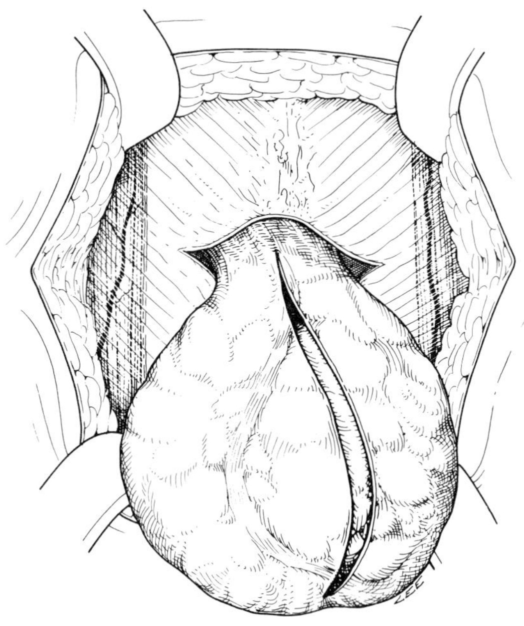

5

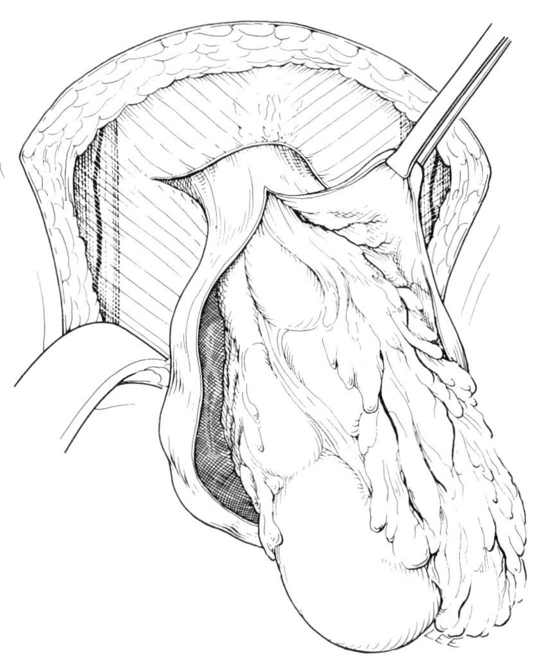

6

Management of the sac II

If the sac is vast and multiloculated an alternative strategy can often usefully be employed.

7

Once the peritoneum of the neck at any one point has been identified it should be opened and a finger inserted.

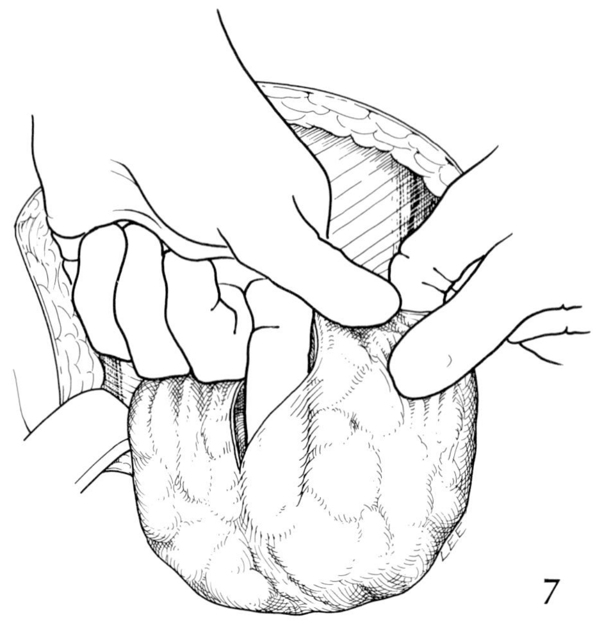

7

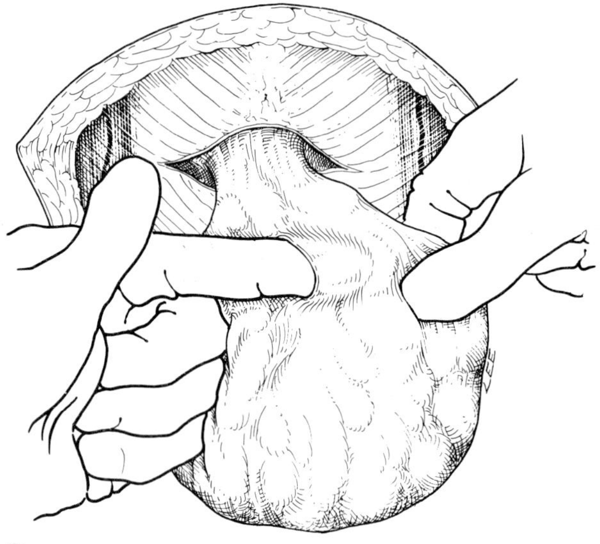

8

8

The whole mass of sac, contents and overlying fat and skin is then held up by assistants while the neck is dissected around using the finger in the sac as a direction finder. This dissection can be tedious if the sac is multiloculated and the contents very adherent. It is well for the operator to change from side to side of the operating table to facilitate this manoeuvre. Once the neck has been divided attention can be turned to the contents of the sac. Adhesions are divided and doubtfully viable omentum excised.

Enlargement of the aponeurotic aperture

9

The opening in the abdominal wall is next enlarged laterally for 3 or 4 cm on either side, the rectus muscle being retracted as the posterior rectus sheath is divided, taking care not to injure the epigastric vessels.

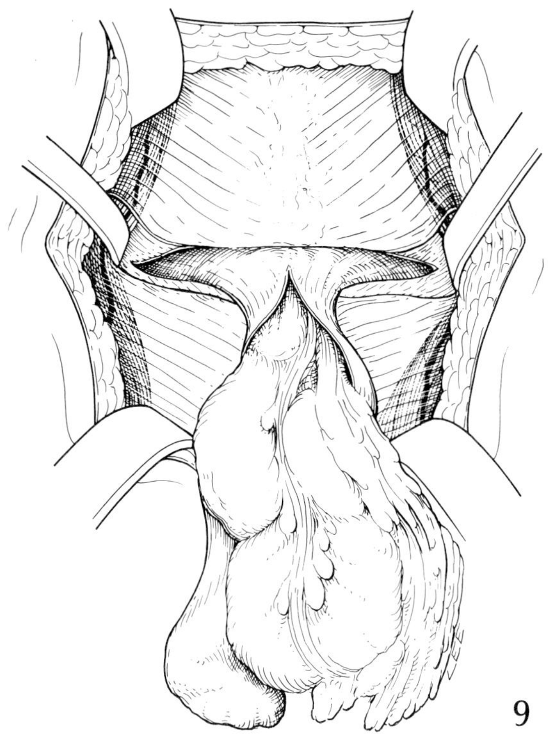

9

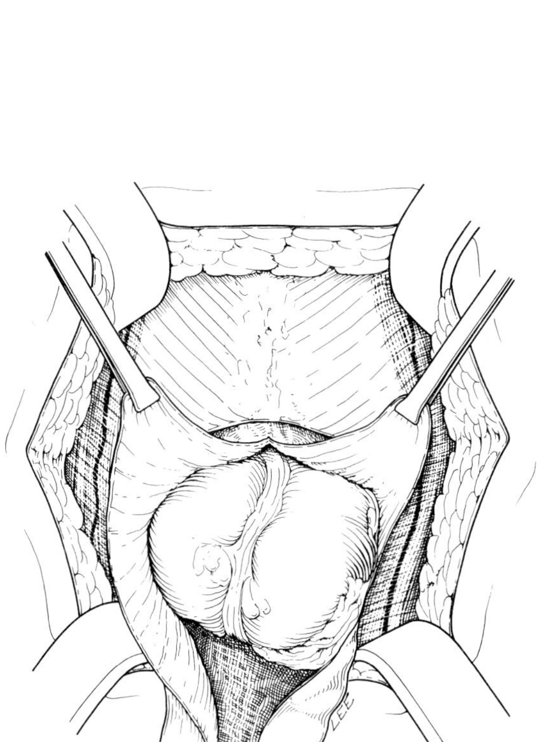

10

10

Once the fibrous ring of the neck has been divided the contents of the sac can be reduced back into the abdomen.

The repair of the defect – Mayo technique[1]

11

The margins of the opening – aponeurosis, posterior rectus sheath and peritoneum – are now grasped in large haemostats and held up by assistants.

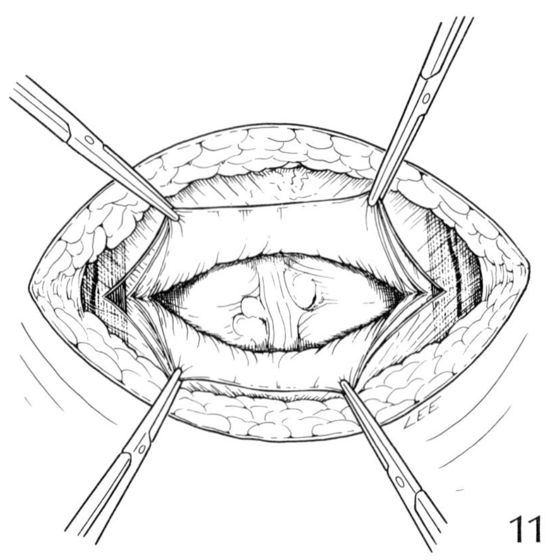

11

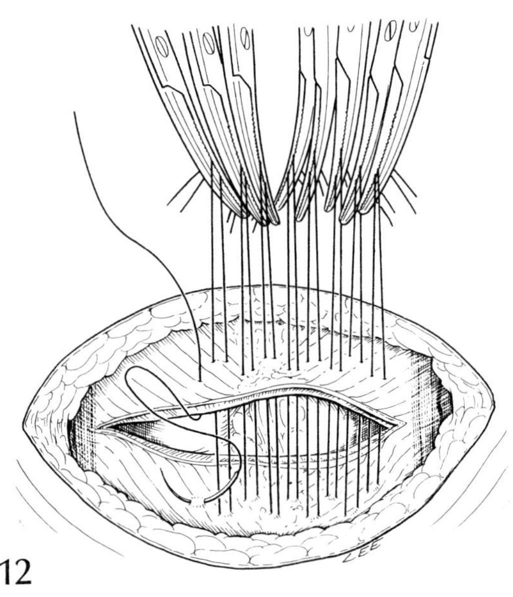

12

12

The deep sutures are next placed. Strong non-absorbable material (metric 4 polypropylene or metric 3.5 nylon) is used on a round-bodied needle.

The suture enters the upper (cephalad) flap from without, between 2 cm and 3 cm from its margin. The needle is then grasped on the deep surface of the upper flap, passed across the defect and then from the outside through the lower flap. Then the needle is pulled back through the lower flap, across the defect and through the deep surface of the upper flap. The suture thus placed is held in a clip. Many more such sutures are now inserted and held untied until all are in place.

There are four useful technical points.

1. In the upper flap the sutures must all be placed further than 2 cm from the margin – up to 4 cm is permissible.
2. In the lower flap the sutures must all be at a distance greater than 1 cm from the margin.
3. It adds to the stability of the suture lines if the sutures are staggered, not all at the same interval from the margins of the defect.
4. The more sutures that are put in the easier they are to close and tie, and the strain is more evenly distributed.

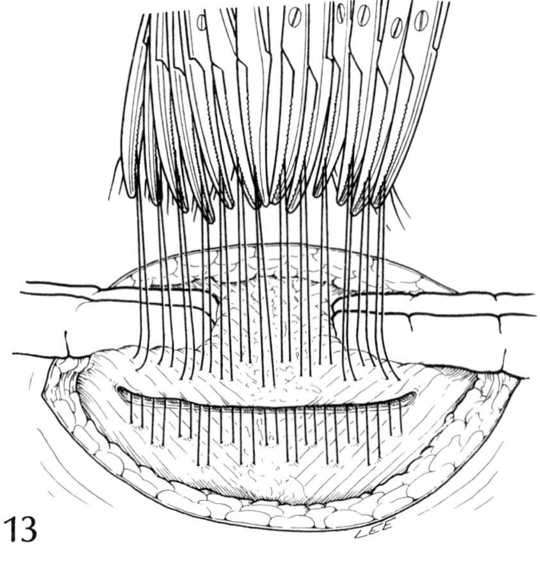

13

13

After the sutures have all been placed the flaps are brought together, the upper being 'railroaded' down the sutures until it lies overlapping the lower flap.

14

The sutures are now tied, fixing the tissues firmly (but not too tightly) together. A triple-layer, double-throw knot is used. When all the knots are complete the ends are cut short.

A fine suction drain is now placed in between the two flaps of the aponeurosis.

The edge of the upper flap is now sutured to the anterior surface of the lower flap using the same non-absorbable suture material as previously. Suture bites of over 1 cm into both upper and lower flaps are used.

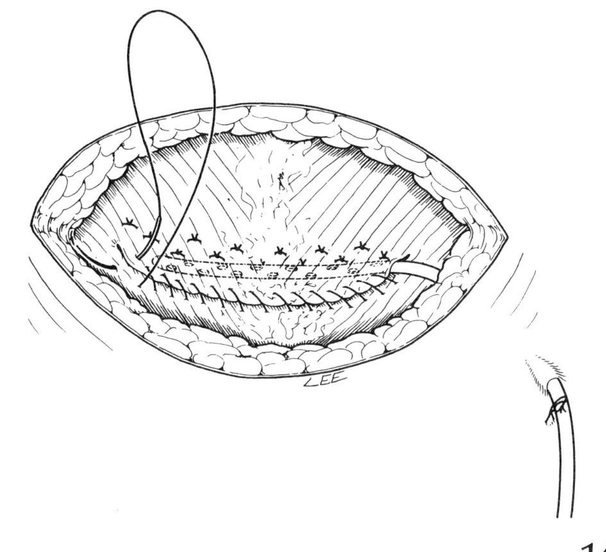

14

Closure

Meticulous haemostasis, suction drainage and obliteration of any dead space are the essential components of this part of the operation.

The subcutaneous fat is closed in terraces using fine (metric 3) chromic catgut. Suction drainage is employed.

15

The skin is closed using skin clips. Suturing of the skin is not recommended: it is often poor and infected in the vicinity of a longstanding umbilical hernia and sutures may carry skin bacteria along their tracks to the deeper parts of the wound or introduce sepsis adjacent to the non-absorbable hernia repair.

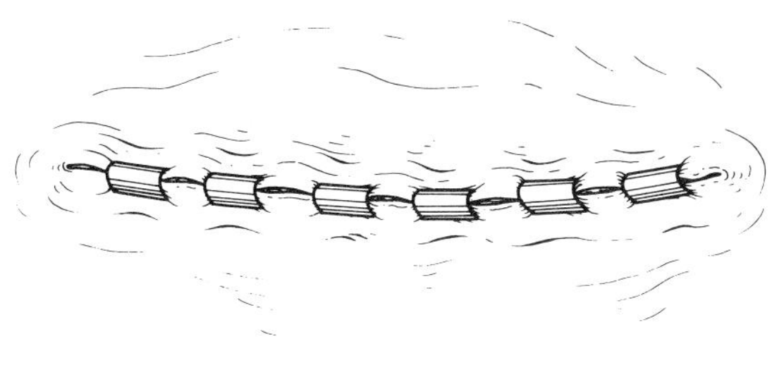

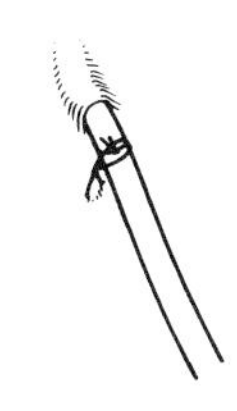

15

Postoperative care

If there has been extensive handling and dissection of the small gut and omentum during the operation, postoperative nasogastric suction and parenteral metabolic support will be needed until normal peristalsis is re-established.

Early ambulation and breathing excercises are essential. The postoperative problem which most frequently arises is respiratory embarrassment caused by the wound pain and the newly raised intra-abdominal pressure.

Reference

1. Mayo, W. J. Further experience with the vertical overlapping operation for the radical cure of umbilical hernia. Journal of the American Medical Association 1903; 41: 225–228

Incisional hernia

(excluding peristomal hernia)

H. Brendan Devlin MA, MD, MCh, FRCS, FRCS(I)
Consultant Surgeon, North Tees General Hospital, Stockton on Tees, Cleveland;
Associate Lecturer in Clinical Surgery, University of Newcastle upon Tyne

Historical note

Incisional hernia is iatrogenic and its incidence has increased with each increment of abdominal surgical intervention. The development of abdominal surgery in the nineteenth century – the excision of an ovarian cyst by McDowell in 1809, partial gastrectomy by Billroth in 1881, cholecystectomy by Langenbuch in 1882 – has been followed by operations to manage the incisional hernias which flowed along as complications. Gerdy is recorded as having repaired an incisional hernia in 1836; Maydl is credited with an incisional hernia repair in 1886; Judd in 1912 and Gibson in 1920 both described repair techniques based on extensive anatomical dissection of the scar and adjacent tissues. Prosthetic materials were introduced early on: autografts of fascia lata were employed by Kirschner in 1910[1], and Gallie and LeMesurier used autologous fascial strips in 1923[2]. Tendons, cutis and whole skin grafts, both homografts and heterografts, have been advocated, and found to have problems[3]. Non-biological prosthetics include stainless steel[4,5], tantalum gauze[6,7], Marlex[8], Mersilene[9] and nylon[10].

Incidence

The overall incidence of incisional hernias is difficult to estimate. Homans in 1887[11] stated that 10 per cent of abdominal operations were followed by incisional hernias, and this figure is consistent with the recent study from Cardiff giving an incidence of 7.9 per cent at 5 years[12]. However, the number of incisional hernias coming to surgical operation is lower than the incidence: in Stockton on Tees over a 9 year period of 1970–1979, 214 cases are recorded (119 males and 95 females), which is 8.4 per cent of the total number of hernias treated surgically.

Aetiological factors

The important causative factors include sepsis (about 60 per cent of patients developing an incisional hernia have had significant wound infection); the placement of drainage tubes through the original incision; a previous operation through the same incision within 6 months; initial closure with catgut alone; steroid and other immunosuppressant therapy; and inflammatory bowel disease. Less significant factors include age and sex, anaemia, malnutrition, hypoproteinaemia, obesity, diabetes, type of incision and postoperative chest infection.

Of particular importance as an aetiological factor is the wound drain. Ponka[13] records that of 126 patients with herniation through a subcostal incision for biliary surgery, all had had drains delivered through the wound at the time of the initial operation.

Lower midline incisions seem to be at greater risk than upper midline incisions. Many of the lower midline incisions are done for gynaecological interventions and the subsequent hernia are often not included in purely 'surgical' follow-up data; hence, there may be under-recording of the true overall incidence of this problem.

Principles of repair

1. Whenever possible the normal anatomy should be reconstituted. In midline hernias this means the linea alba must be firmly reconstructed; in more lateral hernias there should be layer-by-layer closure so far as possible.
2. Only tendinous/aponeurotic/fascial structures should be sutured together.
3. The suture material must retain its strength for long enough to maintain tissue apposition and allow sound union of tissues to occur. A non-absorbable material must therefore be used.
4. The length of suture material is related to the geometry of the wound and to its healing[14, 15]. Using deep bites at not more than 1 cm intervals, the ratio of suture length to wound length must be 4 : 1 or more.
5. Repair of an incisional hernia inevitably involves returning viscera to the confines of the abdominal cavity and a resultant *rise* in intra-abdominal pressure. It is important to minimize this. Every precaution must therefore be taken to prevent abdominal distension due to adynamic ileus which will lead to additional stress on repair suture lines. For this reason handling of the viscera should be minimized.
6. Postoperative coughing can put an additional unwarranted strain on the suture lines. Hence, pulmonary collapse, pulmonary infection and pulmonary oedema must be avoided. Restriction of preoperative smoking, chest exercises, weight reduction and avoidance of excessive blood or fluid replacement (and their haemodynamic effects on the heart) are important components in the successful repair of an incisional hernia.
7. The repair must be performed aseptically: inoculated bacteria, traumatized tissue and haematoma should not be features of these wounds.

Drawing these seven points together I favour three methods of incisional hernia repair which will be described in detail. These three methods are:

1. layer by layer closure;
2. the keel operation[16];
3. prosthetic mesh operation[8, 17].

Preoperative

Suture materials and haemostasis

The suture material of choice is either metric 3.5 polypropylene or 34 gauge monofilament stainless steel wire. Metric 4 monofilament nylon can be used. For preference I use polypropylene but in any patient where there has been sepsis or sinuses since the development of the hernia steel wire is the material of choice.

Very careful haemostasis is achieved using catgut ligatures on larger vessels and diathermy of smaller bleeding vessels. The possibility of haematoma formation is further reduced by using suction drainage in *each layer* of the repair.

dermis and potentially carry infection into the subcuticular fat. Skin sutures are not recommended as they may carry skin bacteria deeply into the wound and lead to infection of the many metres of buried non-absorbable repair material.

Indications

Many incisional hernias produce symptoms of discomfort and pain and often recurrent colic if subacute obstructive episodes occur. Such symptoms are reason enough for operative intervention. Irreducibility and a narrow neck are further indications for surgery. Obstruction and strangulation are absolute indications.

Contraindications

Extreme obesity may be a contraindication to surgery. Obese patients frequently have other problems such as cardiorespiratory decompensation and diabetes, making weight reduction essential prior to surgery. Subcutaneous and intra-abdominal obesity make the repair more difficult and postoperative complications more likely.

Continuing deep sepsis in the wound is a contraindication to repair surgery. Such cases frequently have a history of more than one repair attempt, and the wound may be indurated with many sinuses in it. If the sepsis is longstanding, calcification may be present. Usually wounds with continuing infection contain buried and heavily infected non-absorbable material; it is best to open these wounds, remove all the foreign material, drain all the pockets of pus and saucerize all the sinuses. The wound is then left to granulate over. Only when the wound has been without deep sepsis for some months should repair surgery be undertaken.

Skin infections and *intertrigo* beneath a vast incisional hernia are common, and require vigorous preoperative treatment. If possible, operation should be delayed until the skin is sound.

Choice of operative technique

It is important to make an accurate assessment of the anatomy of the hernia prior to surgery. How big is the defect? Does the size of the defect increase or decrease on movement? Are the contents easily reducible?

The sac and fibrous margins of the sac are examined with the patient supine and at ease and then standing erect.

Finally the patient is laid flat again, and as much of the sac as possible is reduced and held reduced by the examining surgeon. The patient is then asked to sit up while the surgeon continues to hold the hernia reduced. In some hernias, particularly upper midline, the margins of the defect close together on movement and the contraction of the abdominal wall will then hold the sac reduced.

Layer-by-layer repair

If the sac is small, does not protrude and become pendulous in the erect patient, and if the margins can be approximated when the patient is relaxed and draw themselves together when the patient tenses the muscles, there is relatively normal anatomy and a layer-by-layer anatomical repair should be done.

Keel operation

If the margins of the aponeurotic defect can be approximated but the sac is large, diffuse and pendulous – that is, it contains viscera with many adhesions – and the patient has no history of obstruction, a keel repair is advised. The keel operation does not involve opening the large sac. Because it avoids trauma to the gut it also is not associated with postoperative ileus.

Mesh operation

If the aponeurotic margins of the defect cannot be approximated in the conscious patient and do not spontaneously draw together when the patient moves, it is probable that there is a tissue defect (or loss) and that a mesh operation will be required.

Anaesthesia

Full general anaesthesia is necessary. Muscle relaxants will assist in reducing the contents of the sac and drawing together the margins of the defect during the repair.

The operation

Position of patient

The patient is placed on his back on the operating table.

The incision

1

An elliptical incision is made to enclose the cutaneous scar. The incision must generally be extended at either end to give adequate access to all the margins of the defect. The direction of this initial incision will of course depend on the shape of the original scar through which the hernia has come.

Care should be taken not to excise too much skin, and at this stage the minimum excision of cutaneous scar tissue is done.

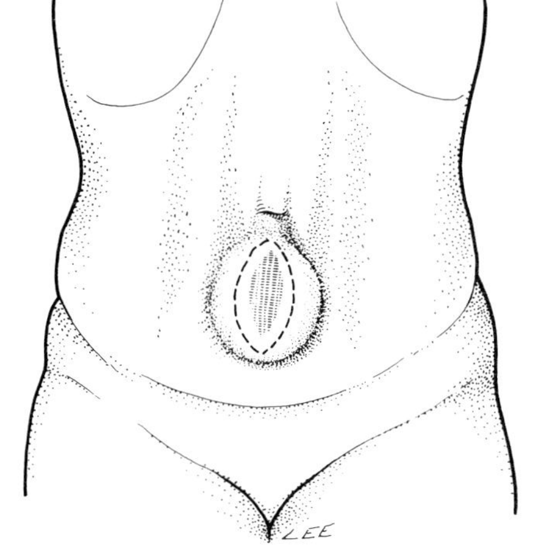

1

Removal of overlying redundant tissue

2

The redundant skin and scar are separated from the underlying hernial sac, which is often just subcutaneous especially near the centre of the hernia, and are removed.

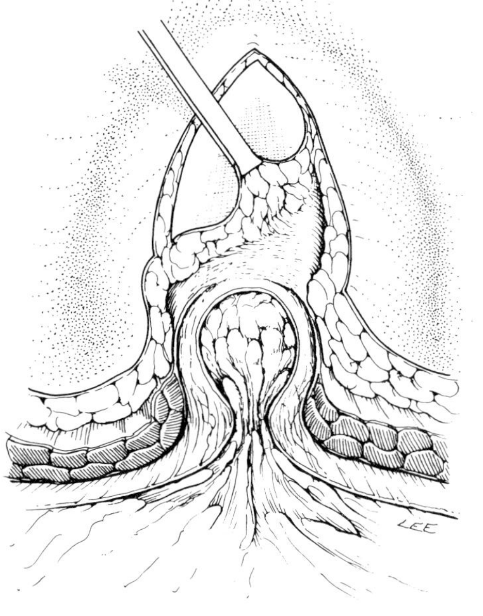

2

3

If the hernia is very large the skin and underlying peritoneal sac may be virtually fused into one layer near the fundus of the hernial protrusion. When removing the redundant skin care is necessary to avoid damage to the hernial contents, which may be adherent over wide areas of the inside of the sac.

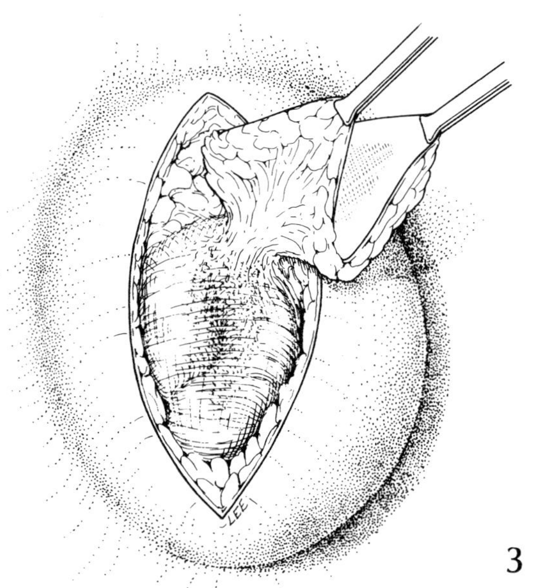

3

Exposure

4

The hernia is dissected from the surrounding subcutaneous fat. Its coverings are stretched scar tissue merging into the stretched abdominal wall aponeurosis at the circumference of the protrusion and a variable amount of extraperitoneal fatty tissue.

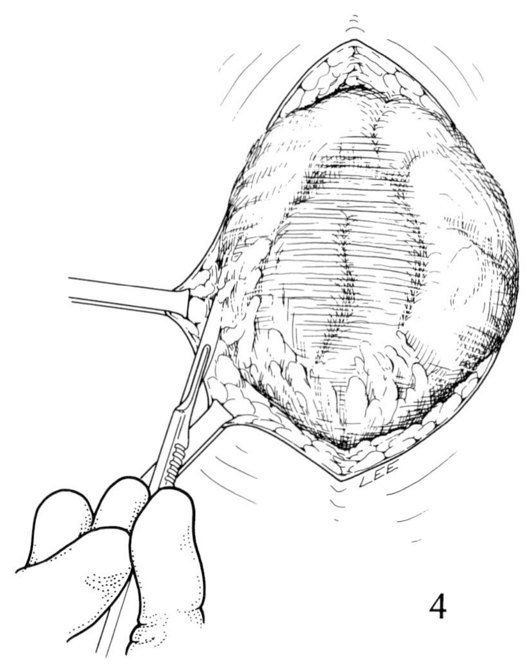

4

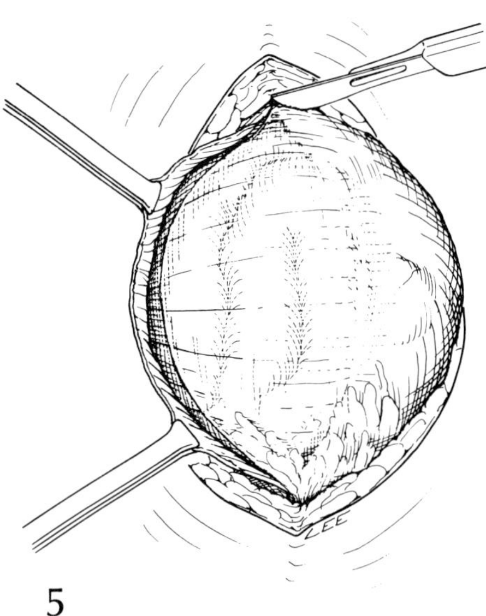

5

5

The scar tissue is incised in an elliptical fashion around the hernial neck where it merges with the stretched aponeurosis. The peritoneal hernial sac is thus defined all around at its attachment to the muscle/aponeurotic layer.

Managing the peritoneal sac

If intestinal obstruction or strangulation is present the sac must be opened and its contents explored, as is the case also if a layer-by-layer or mesh repair is contemplated.

If a keel repair is to be effected the sac must be dissected free but not opened.

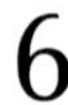

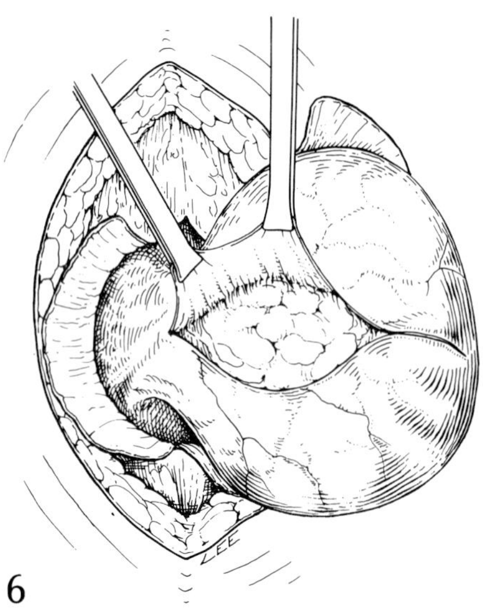

6

6

Opening of the peritoneal sac

The sac should be opened near its neck as shown. The presence of a great deal of extraperitoneal fat may make this difficult as the peritoneal sac is then deeply buried in layers of fat which is often surprisingly vascular.

The peritoneum is often very thin over the fundus of the sac and the cavity is frequently loculated here by adhesions between the sac and its contents. Such adhesions are often less marked at the neck of the sac and the peritoneum is usually less stretched and thin at this point.

The contents of the sac

7

The sac may contain almost any intraperitoneal viscus but usually omentum, small bowel and transverse colon.

Unless the hernia is strangulated and the small bowel non-viable, any adhesions are divided and the small bowel is returned to the abdominal cavity. Strangulated small bowel or omentum can be resected at this stage. The diagnostic decision is now made as to what should be done about very adherent and frequently partially ischaemic omentum. If there is any doubt about omentum it is best excised; to return omentum of doubtful viability to the peritoneal cavity does not serve any useful purpose and invites the formation of adhesions.

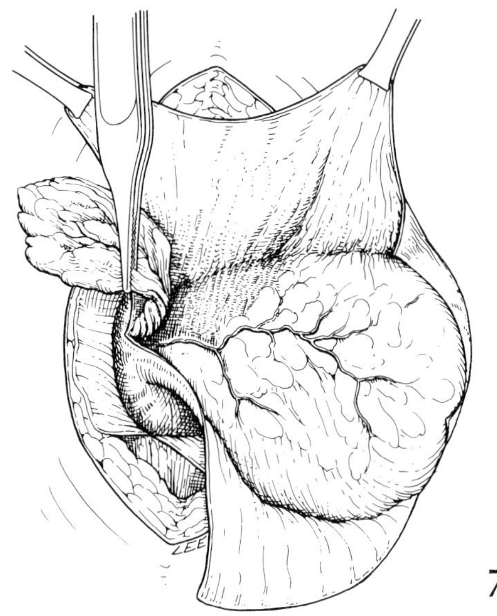

7

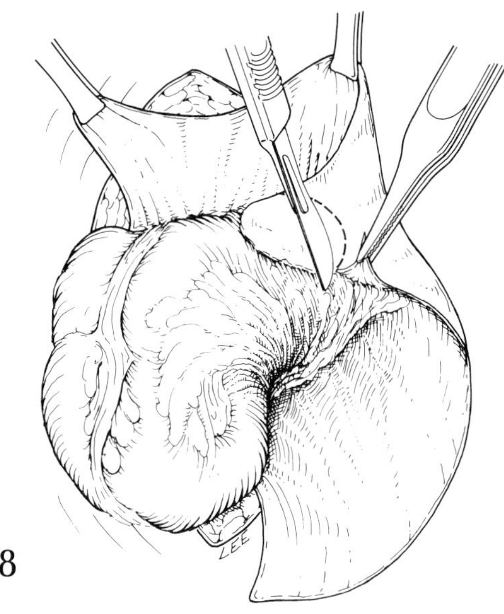

8

8

Particular care must be taken in manipulating and dissecting any colon in the sac. If the colon is strangulated it should be exteriorized with the formation of a colostomy and distal mucus fistula. If it is not strangulated it should be mobilized and returned to the peritoneal cavity, and any densely adherent hernial sac should be trimmed and left adherent to the bowel and returned to the peritoneal sac. The greatest care must be taken to avoid puncturing the colon. If the colon is punctured the safest action is to exteriorize it, conclude the operation and repair the colon at a subsequent date.

9

Excision of sac and suture of the peritoneum

The redundant peritoneum of the sac is now excised and the peritoneal edges are united with a continuous catgut suture. In the upper part of the wound it will be seen that the peritoneal layer is strengthened by the incorporation of the posterior layer of the rectus sheath, which is of course deficient below the semilunar fold of Douglas halfway between the umbilicus and the pubes.

A suction drain is now placed down to this suture line.

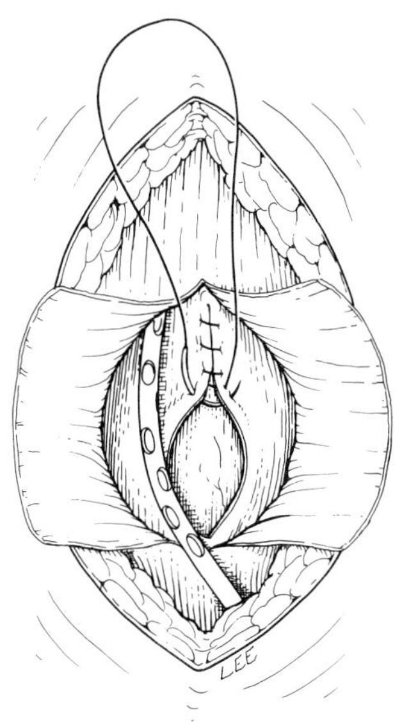

9

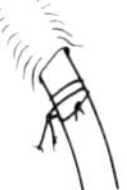

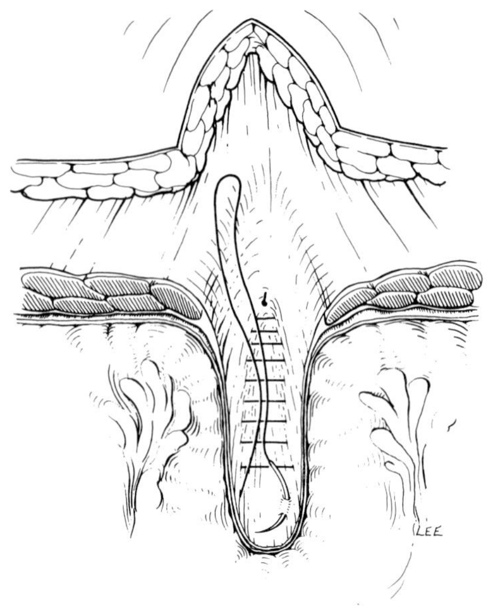

10

Keel operation

10, 11 & 12

In the keel operation the peritoneal sac is not opened. The sac is inverted from above downwards by a series of closely applied 'snaking' sutures of continuous catgut. These sutures are introduced with great care to avoid puncturing any coil of adherent intestine. Each is slowly pulled tight thus pleating and inverting the sac which is gradually obliterated. This process is continued until the fibroaponeurotic margins of the defect become approximated to each other. Viewed in cross-section the appearances of the tissues resemble a ship's keel pointing inwards, hence the name.

A suction drain is then placed along this suture line. The fibroaponeurotic layer is now sutured over the drain using polypropylene as described below.

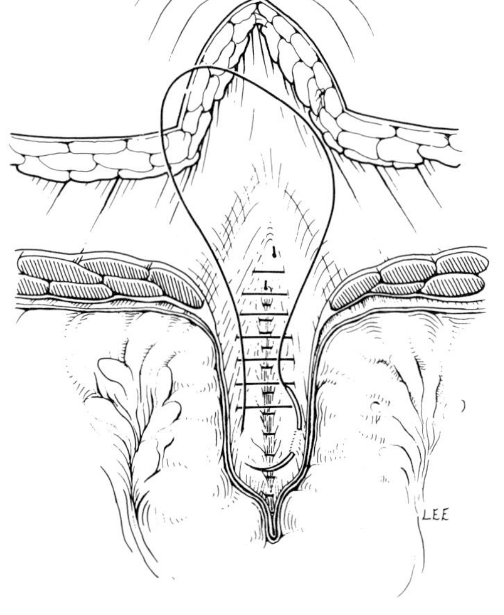

11

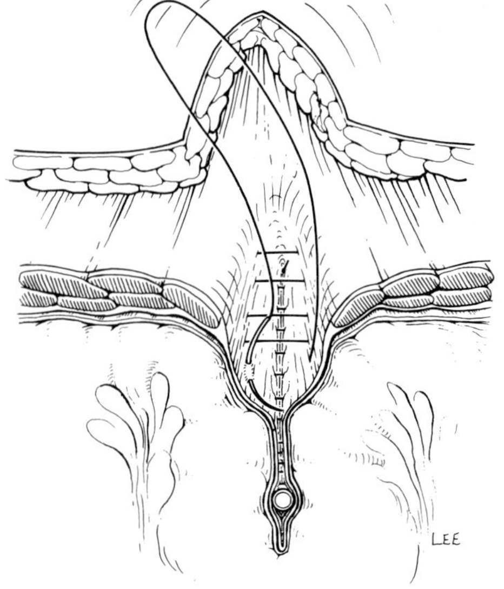

12

Closure of the aponeurotic layer

13

The aponeurosis must be dissected until normal aponeurosis and not scar tissue is identified. Then the full thickness of the margins of all of the aponeurotic layer (that is the abdominal wall in midline and paramedian areas) are approximated and held together by sutures until healing is complete.

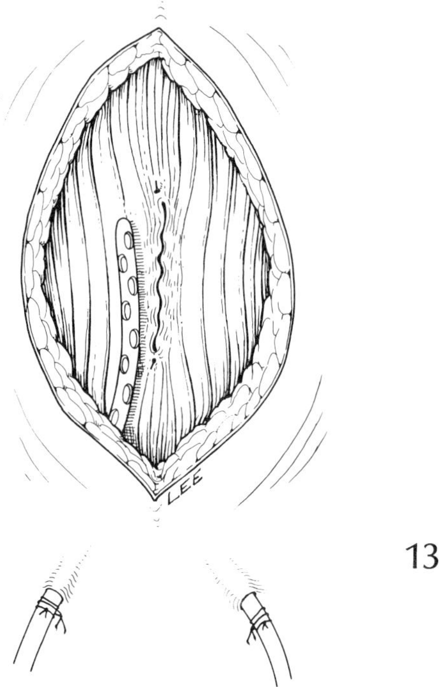

13

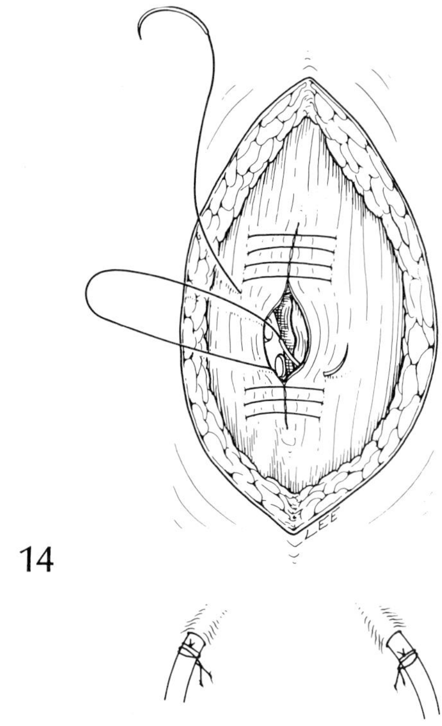

14

14

A polypropylene (or steel) suture is started at each end of the defect. Suturing is continued towards the centre of the defect, one suture alternating with the other and slowly being used to draw together the margins of the defect. Stitch intervals of no more than 0.5 cm are used and bites must be taken more than 2.5 cm from the edges to be sutured.

15

After one layer has been inserted and the margins closed together, at least one further layer of polypropylene (or steel) is inserted, taking bites in between and slightly wider than the first layer. Very large quantities of suture material, up to 44 times the length of the wound, are inserted[15].

When completed, the defect in the aponeurosis should resemble a very closely meshed darn. A suction drain should now be inserted down to this suture line.

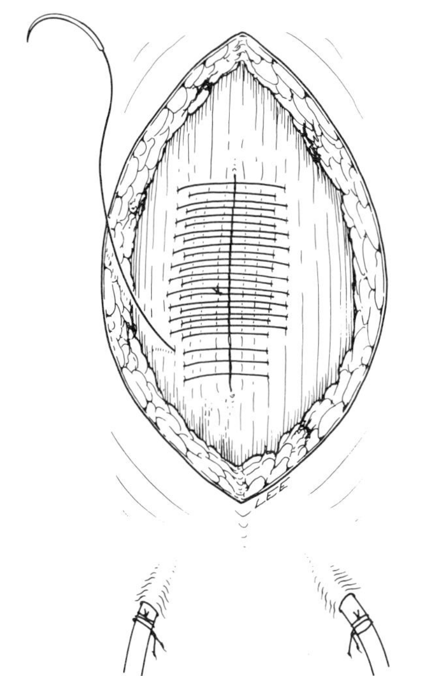

15

16

Haemostasis in the subcutaneous tissue is rigorously checked before further closure of the wound.

17

The subcutaneous fat is now closed in layers with interrupted catgut sutures.

18

The skin margins are now approximated. Skin closure must be effected without any tension but undue redundant skin can be excised at this stage. Many closely placed non-penetrating clips are used and not sutures.

The wound is finally sealed with spray or sealant. A dressing is not applied. The suction drains are fixed with adherent tape or sutures placed well away from the main wound.

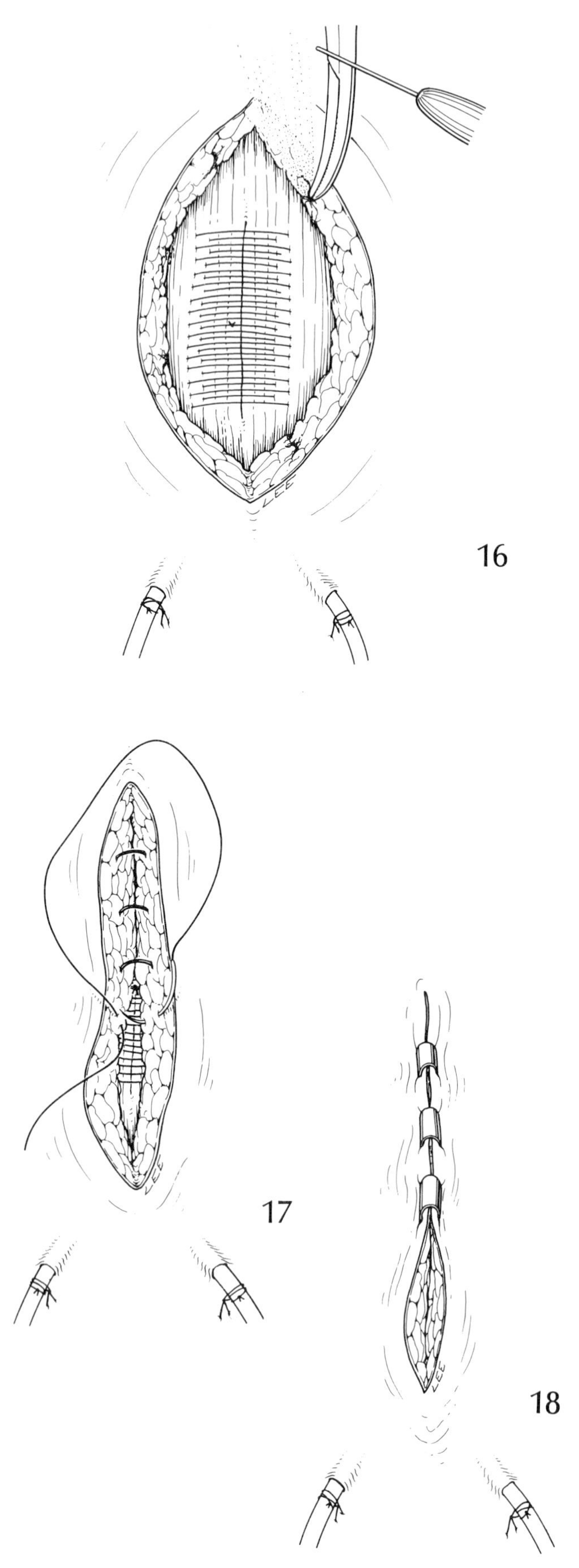

Postoperative care

Immediate active mobilization is the key to rapid convalescence.

In the absence of extensive handling of the intestines (for instance in the keel operation) there is no postoperative adynamic ileus and no need for encumbrances such as nasogastric suction or intravenous drips. The patient is made to take deep breaths; breathing exercises and, where necessary, chest percussion are given. As soon as possible the patient gets up and walks. Fluids are given for the first day then a light diet started. Alternate clips are removed on the second postoperative day and the remainder on the fifth day. Any wound discharge and the contents of the suction drains are cultured and any incipient infection treated vigorously with antibiotics.

Alternative operative technique – mesh repair

Introduction

This technique is applicable to the large diffuse incisional hernia when there is a tissue defect demonstrated preoperatively.

Incision and dissection

The elliptical incision, removing the skin cicatrix, is used as previously described. The dissection is carried down to the neck of the sac. If the sac needs to be opened – because it is irreducible or its contents are compromised – this is done and the peritoneal opening is then closed with chromic catgut. If the sac does not need to be opened, and opening the sac should be avoided if possible, it is imbricated with 'snaking' sutures of chromic catgut as in the keel operation.

If the peritoneum is deficient and cannot be closed over the viscera, an attempt should be made to lay the greater omentum over the intestines. It is best to put the mesh on a 'bed' of omentum rather than in direct contact with the intestine.

After the sac has been dealt with the margins of the defect can be identified and the repair begun. The mesh is inserted as two leaves which are then sutured together. This manoeuvre[18] enables the aponeurotic margins of the defect to be approximated and the mesh to be inserted at the correct tension.

19

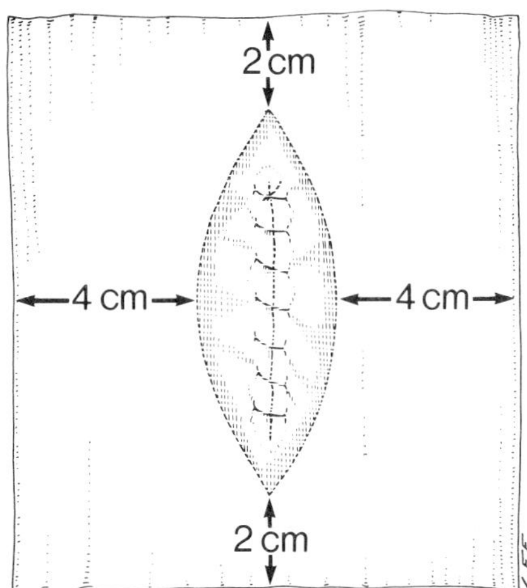

Preparation of the mesh

19

Marlex (polyester) is not currently available on the British market but polypropylene mesh is. The mesh is cut so that it is 4cm longer and some 8cm wider than the defect.

The rectangle of mesh is then divided into two equal halves down its central long axis.

Insertion of the mesh

The mesh is applied as an onlay to the external surface of the aponeurosis and fixed with polypropylene sutures. Generally three lines of continuous suture are placed.

20

The farthest one is placed first, at the margin of the mesh, which should be some 3.5–4cm from the edge of the aponeurotic defect. The sutures should take good bites of the aponeurosis and mesh at intervals of not more than 0.5cm.

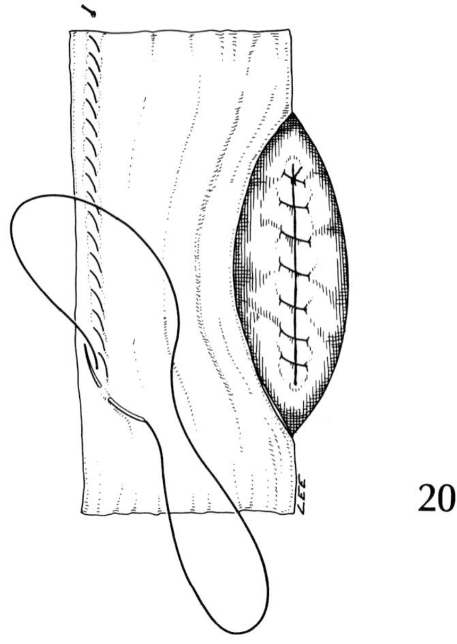

20

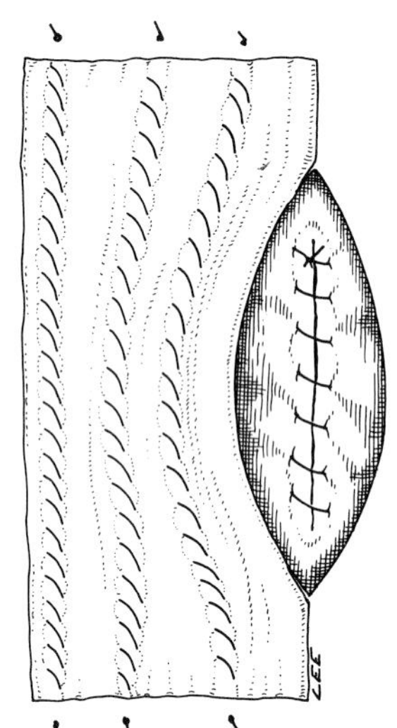

21

21

With the mesh spread taut by traction by an assistant a second line of sutures 1cm closer to the margins of the defect is placed and finally a third line of sutures at the margin of the defect.

22

The mesh is now put into the contralateral side using the same technique. A fine suction drain catheter is now placed to lie along the suture line in the peritoneum deep to the mesh.

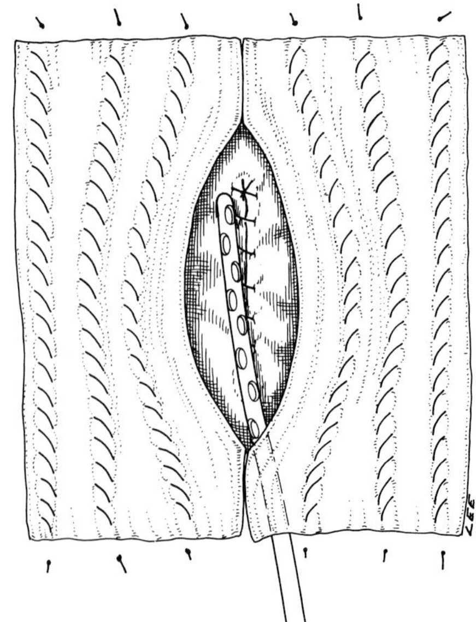

22

Closing the defect

23

The two leaves of mesh are apposed and sutured together with continuous polypropylene, the tension being adjusted according to the size of the defect.

A suction drain is then placed down to the surface of the mesh.

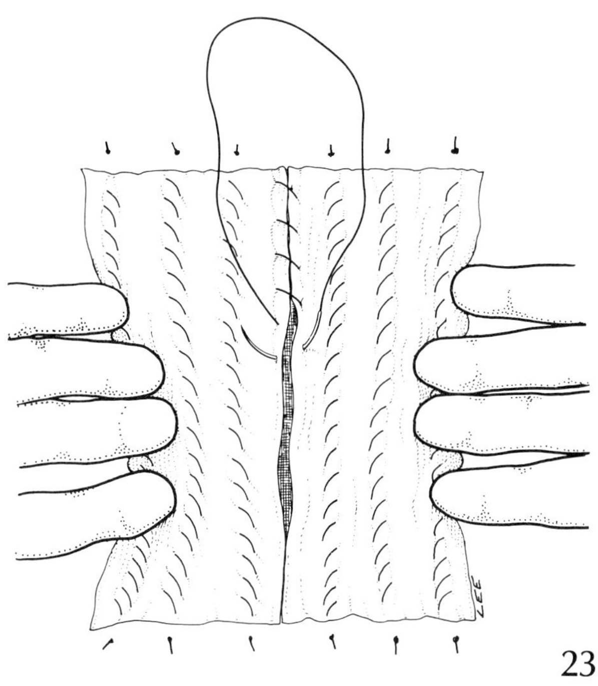

23

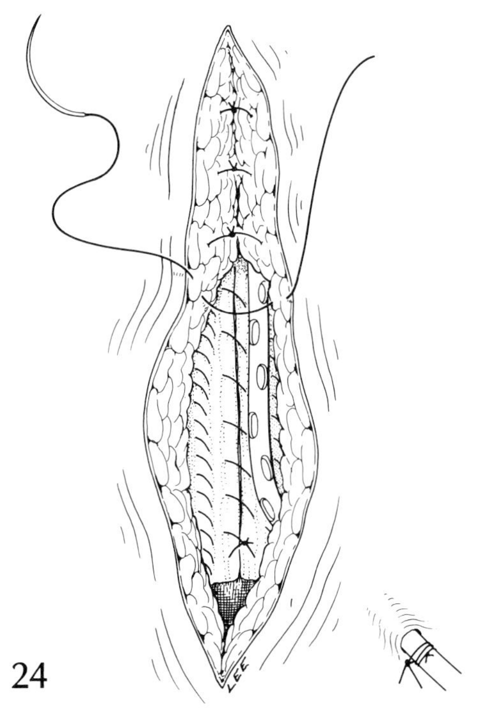

24

24

The subcutaneous fat is tacked down to the underlying aponeurosis to obliterate the 'dead space'. Closure is then completed as described previously with interrupted catgut and clips to the skin.

Postoperative management

This is as described previously for the two other techniques of repair.

References

1. Kirschner, M. Die praktischen Ergebnisse der freien Fascient Transplantation. Archiv für klinische Chirurgie 1910; 92: 888–912

2. Gallie, W. E., LeMesurier, A. B. Living sutures in the treatment of hernia. Canadian Medical Association Journal 1923; 13: 469–480

3. Koontz, A. R. Dead (preserved) fascia grafts for hernia repair. Journal of the American Association 1927; 89: 1230–1235

4. Abel, A. L., Hunt, A. H. Stainless steel wire for closing abdominal incisions and for the repair of herniae. British Medical Journal 1948; 2: 379–382

5. Babcock, W. W. The range of usefulness of commercial stainless steel cloths in general and special forms of surgical practice. Annals of Western Medicine and Surgery 1952; 6: 15–23

6. Throckmorton, T. D. Tantalum gauze in the repair of hernias complicated by tissue deficiency. Surgery 1948; 23: 32–46

7. Koontz, A. R. Tantalum mesh in the repair of ventral and inguinal hernia. Southern Surgeon 1950; 16: 1143–1148

8. Usher, F. C., Ochsner, J., Tuttle, L. L. D., Jr. Use of Marlex mesh in the repair of incisional hernias. American Surgery 1958; 24: 969–974

9. Abul-Husn, S. The use of polyester mesh in hernia repair. Journal Medical Libanais 1974; 27: 437–449

10. Doran, F. S. A., Gibbons, R. E., Whitehead, R. A report on 313 inguinal herniae repaired with nylon nets. British Journal of Surgery 1961; 48: 430–434

11. Homans, J. Three hundred and eighty-four laparotomies for various diseases with tables showing the results of the operations and the subsequent history of the patients. Boston: N. Sawyer, 1887

12. Harding, K. G., Leister, S. J., Mudge, M., Hughes, L. E. Aetiology of incisional hernia – a prospective follow up of 564 patients undergoing major abdominal surgery. Presented to the Surgical Section of the Royal Society of Medicine, London on 10th June, 1981

13. Ponka, J. L. Hernias of the abdominal wall. Philadelphia, London, Toronto: W. B. Saunders

14. Jenkins, T. P. N. The burst abdominal wound: a mechanical approach. British Journal of Surgery 1976; 63: 873–876

15. Jenkins, T. P. N. Incisional hernia repair: a mechanical approach. British Journal of Surgery 1980; 67: 335–336

16. Maingot, R., ed. Abdominal operations. 7th ed. New York: Appleton-Century-Crofts, 1980: 1032–1035

17. Usher, F. C. Further observations on the use of Marlex mesh: a new technique for the repair of inguinal hernias. American Surgeon 1959; 25: 792–795

18. Looijen, S. E. Cited in Kalsbeck, H. L. Experience with the use of Teflon mesh in the repair of incisional hernias. Archivum Chirurgicum Neerlandicum 1974; 26: 71–75

Inguinal hernia in babies and children

H. Brendan Devlin MA, MD, MCh, FRCS, FRCS(I)
Consultant Surgeon, North Tees General Hospital, Stockton on Tees, Cleveland;
Associate Lecturer in Clinical Surgery, University of Newcastle upon Tyne

Incidence

Inguinal hernia is the commonest indication for surgery in early life. The processus vaginalis was found to be open at birth in 94 per cent of infants examined at autopsy by Campers[1]. However, 94 per cent of newborn infants do not have demonstrable inguinal hernias. The most reliable estimate of the incidence of inguinal hernia in England is that of Knox[2], who found among children of Newcastle upon Tyne that operation for primary inguinal hernia was performed on 10.2 per 1000 children surviving at the age of 12 years. The ratio of boys to girls was 12:1 so that the incidence of inguinal hernia in male children, in this community, was 1.9 per cent. Scorer and Farrington[3], in common with most other authors, report that there is a marked preponderance of right-sided hernia in boys – 70 per cent right-sided, 26 per cent left-sided and 4 per cent bilateral – whereas in girls the incidence of right-sided hernia is 50 per cent.

Personal experience

The author's personal experience with these operations is broadly in accord with the reported series. In the past 9 years 346 children with hernia have been operated upon. Of these, 299 (86.4 per cent) were male and 47 (13.6 per cent) female. Of the 299 boys, 184 (61.5 per cent) had right-sided hernia, 97 (32.4 per cent) left-sided hernia, and in 18 (6.0 per cent) the hernia was bilateral. The girls showed an unusual preponderance of right-sided hernia: 32 (68.1 per cent) right-sided, 11 (23.4 per cent) left-sided, and 4 (8.5 per cent) bilateral. No nuclear sex anomalies in the girls were identified in this series (*see below*).

Preoperative

Examination

Most inguinal hernias are apparent within the first 3 months of life. Operation should be recommended for all cases that are clinically apparent. The problem of the inguinal 'bulge', usually associated with screaming, which causes great alarm to the parents, must be mentioned. Sometimes it is impossible to demonstrate a hernia in the clinic, but in many of these cases if a hernia is present, careful palpation will demonstrate a thickened cord. Even if there are no clinical findings but the mother's description of the hernia is convincing and accurate the groin is best explored.

Because inguinal hernias in children are not uncommonly bilateral, should both groins be routinely explored? The chance of the hernia being bilateral is greater if the presenting lump is on the left side and in such instances it is well to question the parents carefully when the child is initially examined: have they seen a lump in the right groin? Making the child cry and then carefully examining both groins is a useful clinic manoeuvre. The author does not routinely explore both groins and only recommends bilateral surgery when there is evidence of bilateral hernia. As anaesthesia is induced the child may strain slightly and if a contralateral hernia is present it will become apparent. In cases of doubt the child should always be re-examined at this stage to ensure that bilateral hernias are not overlooked.

It is important to examine the scrotum in male children in order to ensure that concomitant undescended testicles are not overlooked. If an undescended testicle is overlooked its future prospects may be compromised.

Inguinal hernia in girls should raise the surgeon's suspicions about the child's nuclear sex, particularly if the condition is bilateral. Approximately 1.6 per cent of these children, presenting with inguinal hernia and having apparent female genitalia, prove to be of male nuclear sex with intra-abdominal testes but female anatomy and endocrine function – the 'testicular feminization syndrome'[4]. All female children with inguinal hernia should have their nuclear sex ascertained and skilled paediatric advice should be sought where anomalies are found.

A further note of caution about inguinal hernia in girls should also be introduced. Many of these indirect congenital sacs are in fact sliding hernias containing genital structures, ovaries, fallopian tubes or even the uterus in the walls. Therefore, in female children the sac *must* be opened and its contents examined before it is tied off and excised.

Arrangements for surgery and anaesthesia

Children with inguinal hernias can usually be treated on an outpatient basis. Only for compelling medical or social reasons does the child need to be admitted to hospital. In this case, the mother should be encouraged to accompany the child to hospital and to nurse him or her after recovery from the operation.

To operate on children with inguinal hernia effectively as day cases requires good hospital organization and excellent hospital-to-community communications. It is essential to have printed advice and instructions for the parents and a 'safety net' system which can cope with situations that go wrong[5].

The operation should be performed as soon as possible after the diagnosis has been established. Young, even newborn, children tolerate this surgery well, and parental anxiety and the risk of incarceration of the hernia are minimized by early operation.

Day case surgery in young children should be performed between 10:00 and 15:00. Before 10:00 there may not be time for travel, unhurried preparation and sedation. A screaming child and an anxious mother are not the ideal prelude to elective surgery. Hypoglycaemia and dehydration are of rapid onset when small children are starved unnecessarily. These physiological 'complications' should be prevented by giving the child a normal morning feed and then a preoperative drink of maltose and metoclopramide[6].

Operation, on a day case basis, should always be completed before 15:00 in order to ensure that the effects of anaesthesia are gone before the child is sent home. Children should not be discharged in a sedated or semicomatose state.

The operation

Principles

In babies and young children the inguinal canal has not yet developed its oblique adult anatomy. The superficial ring is directly anterior to the deep ring and the sac is a congenital indirect sac. There is no acquired deformity of the canal. In these cases the fascia transversalis is normal and a simple herniotomy is all that is necessary.

Haemostasis and suture materials

Haemostasis is secured by careful ligating of bleeding points with metric 3 chromic catgut. Diathermy haemostasis is inadvisable because its inexact propagation may thrombose the small vessels in the delicate spermatic cord and cause subsequent testicular damage.

All suturing is carried out using metric 3 chromic catgut on a small, curved round bodied needle.

Position of patient

The child is placed on his back on the operating table. A light cotton blanket lies over the chest and upper abdomen and a similar blanket over the lower limbs. This precaution prevents undue heat loss during surgery.

Draping

Drapes are applied so that the groin area and scrotum are exposed throughout the operation.

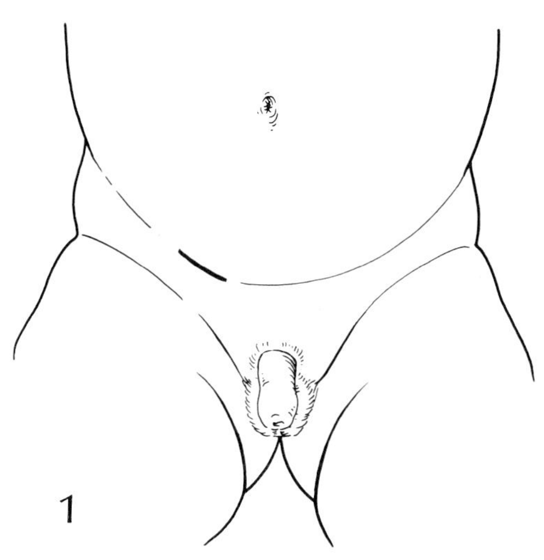

1

1

The incision

A horizontal transverse incision is made in the transverse skin crease just above and medial to the external inguinal ring. The incision should be 1.0–1.5 cm long. The external ring and the emerging spermatic cord can be readily palpated under anaesthesia. The site for incision and the direction of the subsequent dissection are thus confirmed.

Dissection of the external ring

The external ring and cord, which have already been identified by palpation, are approached by gently opening the subcutaneous fat with a blunt haemostat. At this stage the superficial epigastric vessels are encountered and picked up in light haemostats, divided with scissors and ligated.

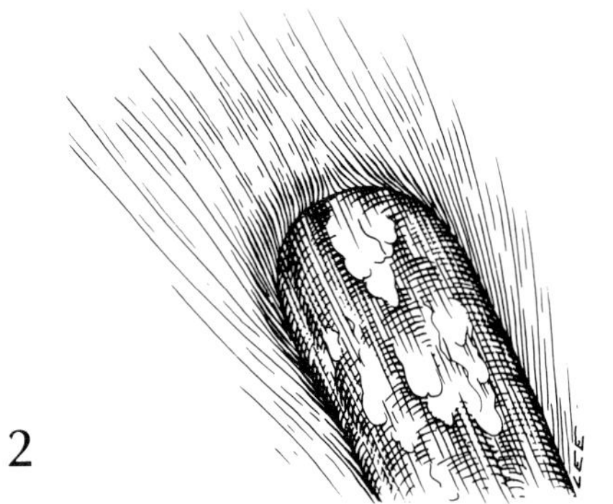

2

2

The external inguinal ring and cord are readily identified when the superficial subcutaneous fat has been opened.

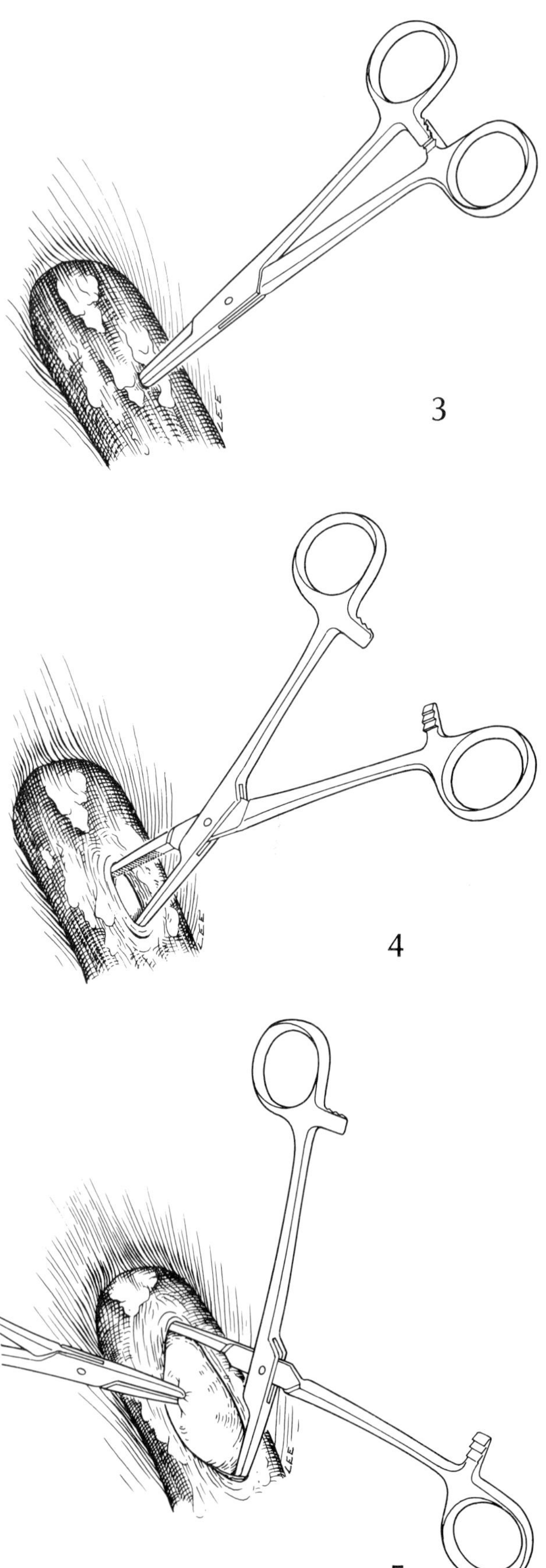

Dissection of the cord coverings

Once the cord has been identified its coverings must be opened to give access to the hernial sac. The sac lies on the anterosuperior aspect of the cord as it emerges from the external inguinal ring. It is covered by the diaphanous external spermatic fascia, the cremasteric fascia, which is readily identified by its neat intertwining pink fascicles of muscle, and by the very delicate internal spermatic fascia. These structures – the three layers of spermatic fascia – are separated from the enclosed contents of the cord by careful blunt dissection with a fine haemostat.

3, 4 & 5

A 'trick of the trade' is most useful here: a *closed* haemostat is pushed through the fascial layers into the cord and then opened slowly so that a rent is made in the long axis. If a hernial sac is present it is immediately apparent in the rent. The rent is held open with the haemostat and the sac grasped with a second haemostat placed between the open blades of the first.

Isolation of the sac

6

The sac can be identified lying on the anterosuperior aspect of the *contents* of the cord. It is pale blue and much thicker than the fascial coverings of the cord. The most difficult manoeuvre in the operation must now be carried out.

The sac is either 'complete', that is, it extends to the scrotum and encompasses the testicles, or 'incomplete', that is, it extends along only part of the length of the cord.

If the sac is 'complete' its posterior wall must be separated from the other cord contents – the vas deferens, the testicular artery and the pampiniform plexus of veins. This must be done very gently and its successful accomplishment is a benchmark by which surgical competence can be measured. A fine haemostat is gently insinuated between each structure and the thin peritoneal sac wall in turn to push them off the sac. When each structure has been pushed off, the proximal sac is held in a haemostat and the sac divided across. The distal sac, testicle and cord can now be manipulated back into place in the scrotum. Gentle traction on the testicle in the scrotum at this time will confirm that it has been returned to its normal site.

The proximal divided sac is now dealt with in the same manner as an incomplete sac.

The fundus of an incomplete sac (or the proximal remnant of a complete sac) is held in a haemostat and the contents of the cord are gently pushed off its posterior wall using a piece of gauze while traction is applied to keep the sac taut. The sac must be stripped of cord contents down to its junction with the parietal peritoneum.

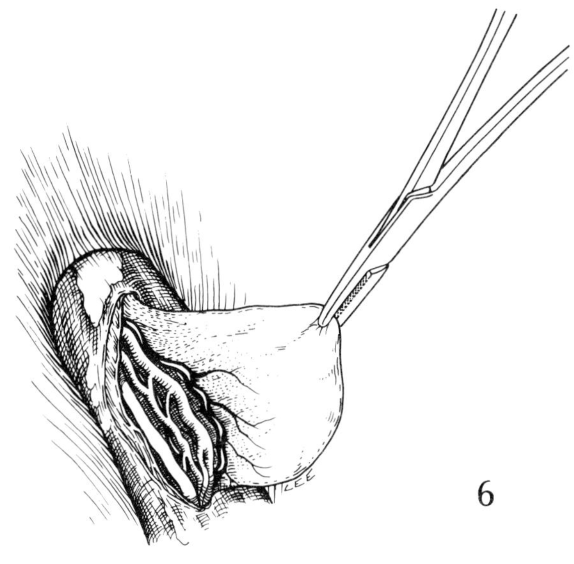

6

Opening the sac

Once the sac has been completely separated from the cord coverings and contents it should be opened. This is most *important in a female child.* If any intra-abdominal contents are in the sac they are pushed back into the greater peritoneal cavity.

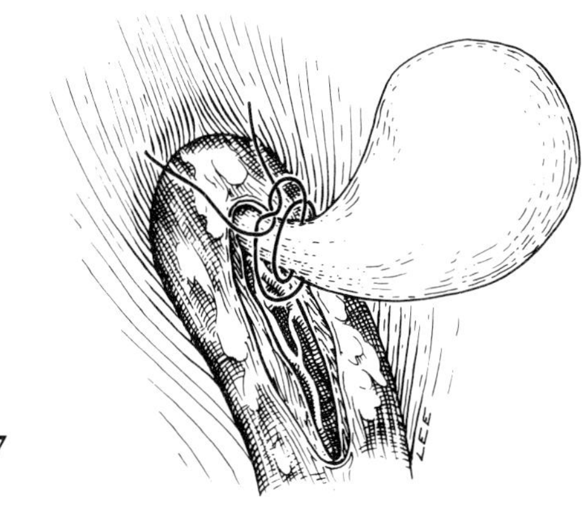

7

Closure

7

The sac is now ligated circumferentially with a transfixion suture of metric 3 chromic catgut. The redundant tissue is excised.

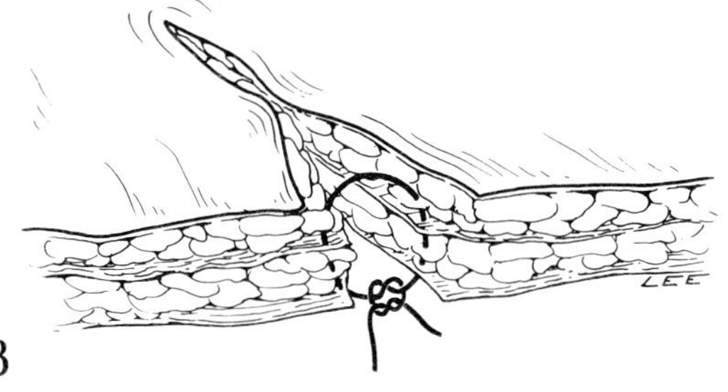

8

8

The subcutaneous tissue

The subcutaneous fat is now closed with two or three metric 3 chromic catgut sutures carefully placed to close the dead space in the depths of the wound and its immediate subdermal layer. The knots are placed deeply.

9

The skin

The skin is closed with porous tapes with a backing of hypoallergic gum or with a strip of gauze impregnated with collodion.

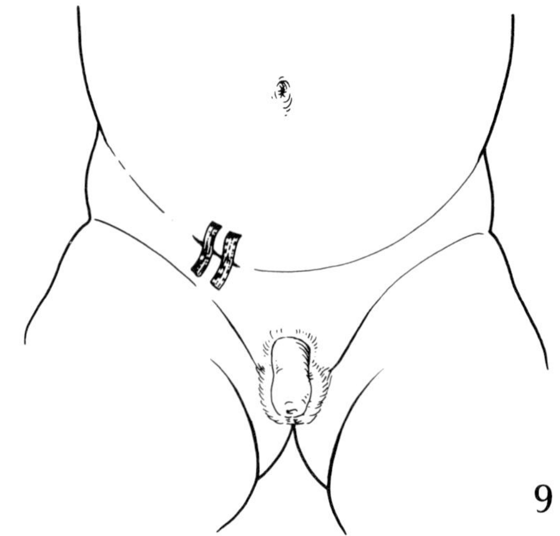

9

Postoperative care

No postoperative care other than normal maternal nursing care is required.

The child can be caressed and fed by his mother as soon as he has recovered from the anaesthetic. He can be allowed to play and be bathed as soon as necessary. The adherent dressing generally falls away after 24–48 h. No attempt should be made to remove it prematurely.

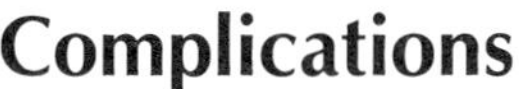

Complications

Some children, perhaps 10 per cent, have bruising adjacent to the wound and in the scrotum, which resolves spontaneously. Wound infections are very rare. In a personal series of 346 cases there was only one wound infection which required community nursing care at home after discharge.

Sometimes the testicle may go 'hard' after surgery. An expectant policy should be adopted with this complication. The 'hard' testicle is in reality suffering from borderline ischaemia and if left alone will recover spontaneously.

Personal results

Over the last 9 years 346 inguinal hernias have been repaired as day cases using this technique. No major complications were encountered and the operation has left a sound cosmetically acceptable scar. The children have been cared for by their mothers with a minimum of psychological trauma to both.

References

1. Camper, P. Sämmtliche kleinere Schriften. Leipzig: Siegfried Lebrecht Crucius 1784–1790
2. Knox, G. The incidence of inguinal hernia in Newcastle children. Archives of Disease in Childhood 1959; 34: 482–486
3. Scorer, C. G., Farrington, G. H. Congenital deformities of the testis and epididymis. London: Butterworths, 1971
4. Kaplan, S. A., Snyder, W. H., Jr, Little, S. Inguinal hernias in females and the testicular feminization syndrome. American Journal of Diseases of Children 1969; 117: 243–251
5. Plant, J. A., Devlin, H. B. Planned early discharge of surgical patients. Nursing Times. Occasional Papers 1978; 74: 25–28
6. Fry, E. N. S. Hypoglycaemia in children undergoing operations. British Medical Journal 1976; 2: 639

Inguinal hernia in adults

H. Brendan Devlin MA, MD,MCh, FRCS, FRCS(I)
Consultant Surgeon, North Tees General Hospital, Stockton on Tees, Cleveland;
Associate Lecturer in Clinical Surgery, University of Newcastle upon Tyne

Historical note

The surgical literature abounds with descriptions of operations for inguinal hernia. However, few of these essays describe new or original principles. The foundations underlying the modern approach to inguinal hernia were laid by Marcy[1] who observed the anatomy and physiology of the deep inguinal ring and correctly inferred the import[2] of the obliquity of the canal. Bassini[3], who built on Marcy's observations, had heard Marcy lecture in 1881, and grasped the significance of the anatomical arrangement, and in particular the role of the transversalis fascia and transversus abdominis tendon. Bassini originally stressed the importance of dividing the transversalis fascia and reconstructing the posterior wall of the canal by suturing the transversalis fascia and transversus muscle to the upturned, deep edge of the inguinal ligament. In his repair, Bassini included the lower arching fibres of the internal oblique muscle where they form the conjoint tendon with the transversus muscle. He called the upper leaf of his repair the 'triple layer', that is, transversalis fascia, transversus abdominis and internal oblique. Bassini's original observations about the fascia transversalis and 'triple layer' have somehow been lost from the later literature. Many of the failures of 'Bassini's operation' occur in cases where the fleshy conjoint tendon only has been sutured to the inguinal ligament.

The three main principles in the operative management of inguinal hernia are as follows.

1. The normal anatomy should be reconstituted as far as possible. The first layer to be defective, in either indirect or direct hernias, is the transversalis fascia; this should therefore be repaired first.
2. Only tendinous/aponeurotic/fascial structures should be sutured together. Suturing red fleshy muscle to tendon or fascia will not contribute to permanent fibrous union of these structures; nor will it result in anything resembling the normal anatomy.
3. The suture material must retain its strength for long enough to maintain tissue apposition and allow sound union of tissues to occur. A non-absorbable or very slowly absorbable suture material must therefore be employed.

Non-absorbable suture materials do have their own inherently disadvantageous properties: proneness to sepsis, adverse tissue reaction and sinus formation. These have led surgeons to seek compromise suture materials which have often not proved effective when used for inguinal hernia repair.

These three principles of repair of the inguinal hernia have been admirably combined in the repair operation outlined by Dr Earl Shouldice of Toronto about 1951[4]. This is the operation described in this chapter.

Dr Shouldice's own results, and the combined results from his clinic, are most impressive. More than 78 000 hernias have been repaired since 1951 with a recurrence rate of 0.8 per cent at 5 years[4]. Myers and Shearburn[5], using the same technique, reported a recurrence rate of 0.1 per cent in 953 consecutive operations for primary inguinal hernia.

Preoperative

Suture materials

The suture material of choice for the repair is metric 3 polypropylene. In the original Shouldice series from Toronto monofilament stainless steel wire was used[4]. Myers and Shearburn[5] and Devlin *et al.*[6] originally used stainless steel wire but have subsequently used polypropylene. Stainless steel wire is a most effective suture material but it is difficult to use; prolypropylene is as effective and is much easier to handle.

Indications and contraindications to surgery

Successful surgical repair is the treatment of choice for inguinal hernias in males. The Shouldice operation is therefore recommended for all male hernia patients from pubescence to retirement. With the elderly male aged over 70 years a less definite policy must be adopted; if the hernia is direct and spontaneously reducible the patient often has few if any symptoms attributable to it and surgery is not advisable. Indeed, the risk of anaesthesia and surgery in this age group are greater than the chances of developing complications necessitating urgent surgery[7].

Administrative and management arrangements for inguinal hernia surgery

A careful administrative policy is necessary if the greatest benefits (for the patients and the community) are to be obtained using the Shouldice technique. At North Tees General Hospital patients are treated on a 'planned early discharge' basis; that is, an assessment of the patient's clinical and social status is made preoperatively and a decision taken about the duration of his hospital stay prior to his admission. In general three regimens are used.

1. Day case – 8 hour stay – applicable to all healthy males who have good home circumstances.
2. Two night – 48 hour stay – applicable to healthy males with less appropriate social status.
3. Five-day stay – most suitable for older patients, patients with contemporaneous medical conditions or patients who are socially disadvantaged.

About one-third of patients fall into each of these categories.

The advantages of this 'planned early discharge' system – apart from the discipline it imposes on the surgical team – are that it keeps the patient mobile and not institutionalized, that there is a challenge to keep complications to a minimum, and finally that it is socially and economically advantageous to the patient and to the community[8,9].

Anaesthesia

Local or general anaesthesia may be employed. General anaesthesia seems more acceptable to British patients, but the clinical and economic advantages of local anaesthesia should not be overlooked. The Shouldice Clinic uses local anaesthesia routinely.

Local anaesthesia

The iliohypogastric and ilioinguinal nerves should be blocked lateral to the inguinal canal, and the skin and subcutaneous tissues in the line of the incision should be infiltrated. The region of the peritoneal neck of the sac will need infiltration during the operation. Traction on the peritoneum is uncomfortable for the patient and the site where the cord comes through the transversalis fascia is infiltrated as soon as the cord is exposed. The anaesthetic agent of choice is 0.5 per cent lignocaine with 1:200 000 adrenaline. About 50–100 ml of this solution are all that is needed for adequate anaesthesia. The maximum dose that can be given to a 70 kg healthy male is 100 ml of the 0.5 per cent lignocaine with adrenaline solution. The infiltration is made easier if a continuously rechargeable syringe is used.

An alternative local anaesthetic is bupivacaine hydrochloride (Marcaine) 0.25 per cent with adrenaline 1:400 000 up to a maximum dosage of 2 mg/kg body weight.

General anaesthesia

General anaesthesia is quicker than local anaesthesia and more comfortable for the patient. No preoperative narcotic drugs are given. Atropine is injected immediately preoperatively and then a short-acting barbiturate and halothane are used, accompanied by muscle relaxants and endotracheal intubation. Light general anaesthesia without any preoperative narcotic agents is safe and allows early discharge after surgery.

The operation

Position of patient

The patient is placed on his back on the operating table. Access is improved if the head of the table is tilted downward by about 15°.

For haemostasis, the larger vessels are ligated, especially the veins in the subcutaneous tissue, using metric 3.5 chromic catgut. Otherwise, diathermy is used for haemostasis. Careful haemostasis is most important if haematoma and consequent sepsis are to be avoided.

Sepsis is the great hazard to herniorrhaphy, particularly when non-absorbable suture material is used. Scrupulous surgical technique is vital if infection is to be avoided. The skin is routinely covered at the site of operation with sterile adherent film which is not removed until the subcutaneous fat is closed. Sutures are never used to close the skin. By their very nature sutures have the potential for introducing dermal and epidermal bacteria into the subcutaneous tissue along their tracks. Each suture is a linear abscess lined with granulation tissue, and if the 'infection' in these abscesses spreads and involves the buried sutures sinuses may result.

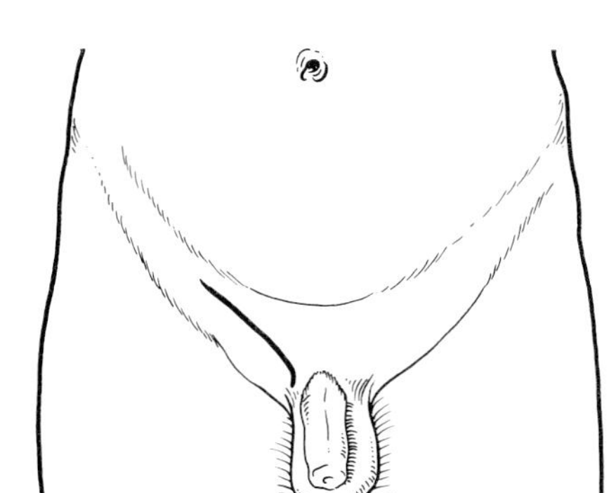

1

1

The incision

The incision is placed 1 cm above and parallel to the inguinal ligament. Laterally the incision begins over the deep inguinal ring, runs to the pubic tubercle, then curves caudally (vertically) and runs down over the pubic tubercle. It is important to keep the knife at right angles to the patient's skin on this corner in the incision in order to avoid undercutting the flap on its lower outer side. More importantly, the extension provides good access to the cord as it emerges from the superficial inguinal ring.

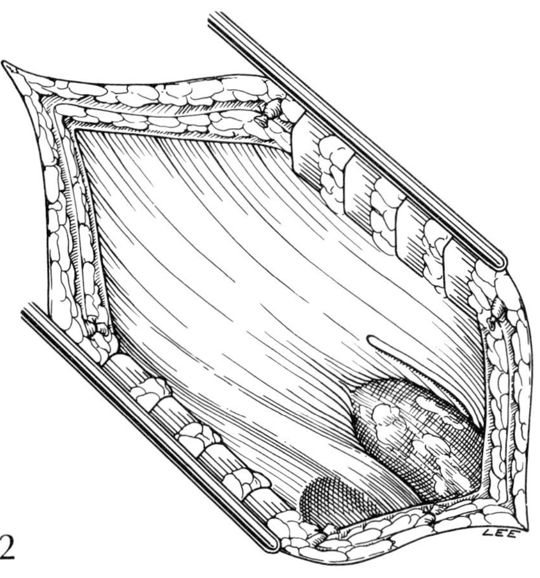

2

2

Exposure

After the skin has been divided the subcutaneous fat is opened in the length of the incision down to the external oblique aponeurosis. Carefully, haemostasis is now attained. The superficial pudendal and superficial epigastric vessels are tied with catgut and the smaller vessels dealt with using diathermy. A self-retaining retractor is now introduced and opened. This retractor serves two purposes: it opens the wound to facilitate access and the slight traction it exerts on the skin ensures haemostasis in the small vessels in the immediate subdermal tissues.

After the subcutaneous fat has been opened down to the external oblique aponeurosis, the deep fascia of the thigh is opened to allow access to the femoral canal. The femoral canal is exposed below the inguinal ligament and checked to make sure it is intact. It is important not to overlook a concomitant femoral hernia which may present in the postoperative period.

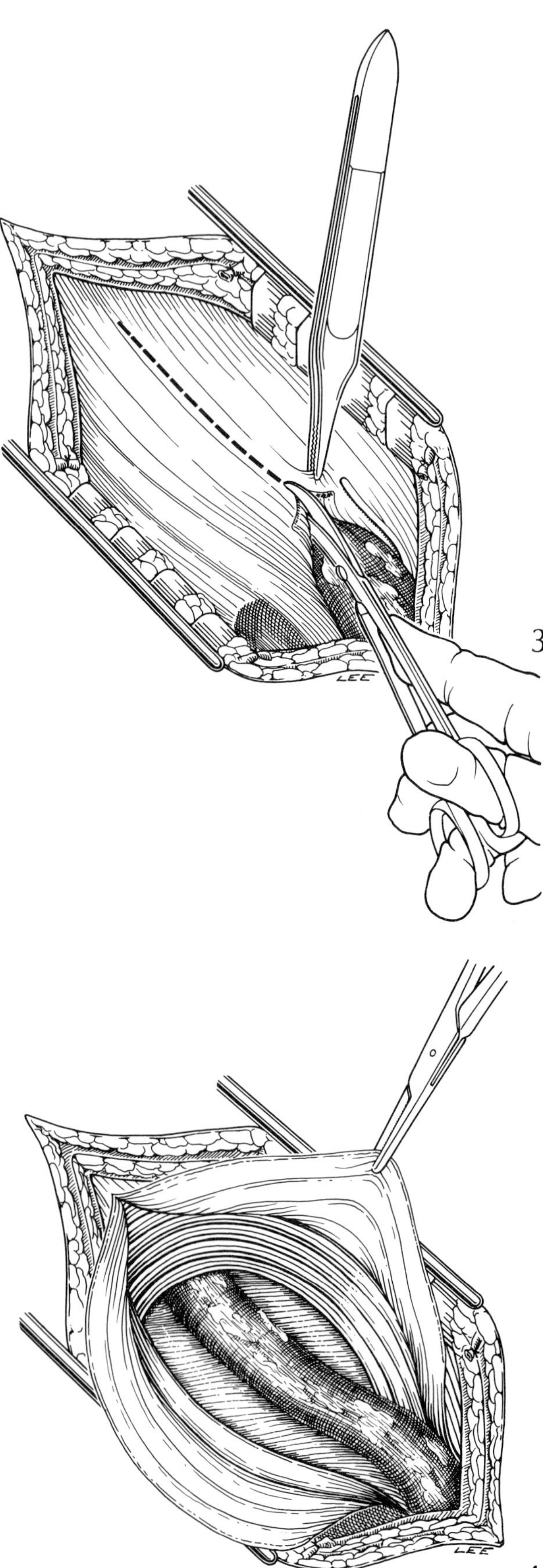

3 & 4

Dissection of the canal

The external oblique aponeurosis is next opened in the long axis of the inguinal canal. This incision extends down to the external inguinal ring, the margin of which is divided. With the ring opened, the upper medial flap of the external oblique is grasped in a haemostat and lifted up off the underlying cremaster fascia. The aponeurosis is gently freed from underlying structures by gauze dissection up to its fusion into the lateral rectus sheath.

Similarly, the lower lateral leaf of the external oblique is mobilized and freed of the underlying cord coverings down to the upturned deep edge of the inguinal ligament, which is exposed.

Thus the whole of the cord is exposed.

Dissection of the cord

5

The cremaster muscle/fascia is now divided in its long axis from its proximal origin down to the level of the pubic tubercle.

The cremaster is made into two flaps, an upper medial and a lower lateral flap. These flaps are raised off the pampiniform plexus of veins, the other contents of the cord and the vas deferens. The flaps of the cremaster are each traced proximally to their origin from the conjoint tendon and distally to the pubic tubercle. The cremaster is clamped, divided and ligated with catgut at its origin from the conjoint tendon and similarly dealt with distally at the level of the pubic tubercle.

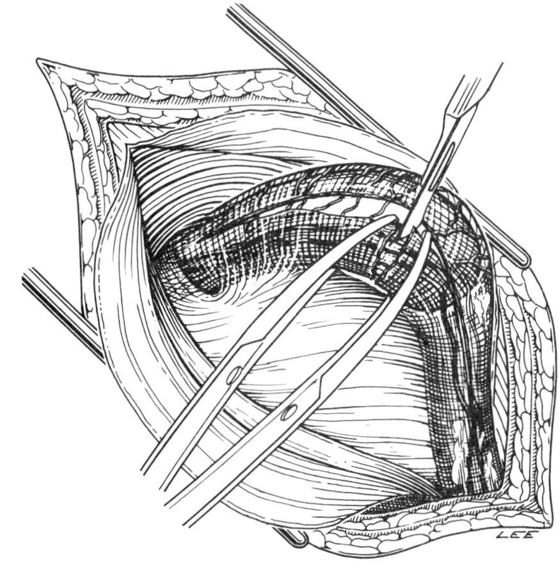

5

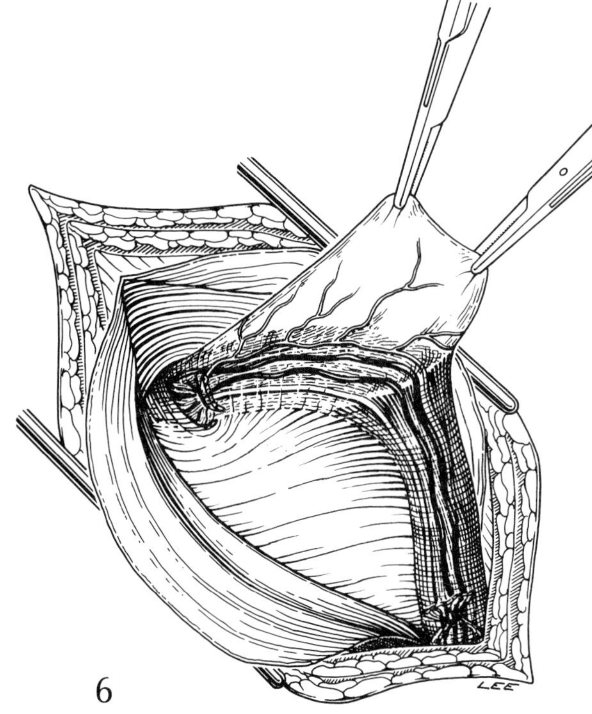

6

6

After the cremaster has been removed the contents of the cord and any hernia contained therein should be visualized. If there is a lipoma in the cord it is excised at this stage, but removal of a lipoma must not be used as an excuse to strip out all the fat and areolar tissue in the cord. If this is done the patient will suffer considerable post-operative testicular oedema and may even develop a hydrocele.

Identification of the transversalis fascia

After the contents of the cord have been adequately visualized they are lifted up and the continuation of the transversalis fascia on to the cord at the deep ring is identified. The condensation of the transversalis fascia about the emerging cord is the deep ring and it must be identified accurately. The correct identification and dissection of the deep ring is crucial to the subsequent repair operation.

Hernial sacs

Indirect

If an indirect hernial sac is present it should be easily found now. It lies on the anterosuperior aspect of the cord structures. Further management depends on the presence and nature of the contents of the indirect hernial sac.

7

No contents If the sac is empty, it is lifted and freed from the adjacent structures by gauze dissection. It is traced back to its junction with the parietal peritoneum, transfixed with a catgut suture which is tied around it securely and the redundant sac excised.

Small bowel and/or omentum, with or without adhesions Unless the hernia is strangulated and the small bowel non-viable, any adhesions are divided and the small bowel is returned to the abdominal cavity. Strangulated omentum or small bowel can be resected at this stage. The diagnostic decision as to what should be done about very adherent and frequently partially ischaemic omentum is a difficult one. If there is any doubt about omentum it is best excised, because to return omentum of doubtful viability to the peritoneal cavity invites the formation of adhesions.

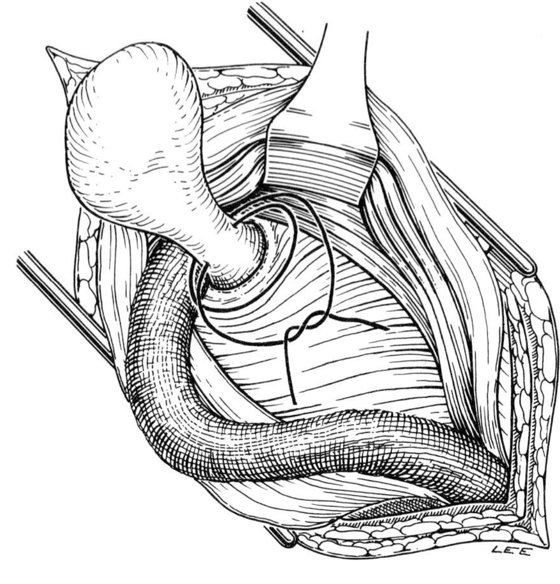

7

8

The sliding hernia Such a hernia may contain the caecum and appendix (on the right side) in its wall, the sigmoid colon (on the left side) or the bladder (in the medial wall on either side). The following guidelines apply in these circumstances.

1. No attempt should be made to separate caecum or sigmoid colon from the sac wall. This may compromise their blood supply and lead to further unnecessary problems.
2. The appendix must not be removed, as this could introduce sepsis.
3. Appendices epiploicae must never be removed from the sigmoid colon – they may harbour small colonic diverticula excision of which will precipitate sepsis.
4. On the medial side of a sac there should be no attempt to dissect the bladder clean. If the bladder is inadvertently opened, a two-layer closure and urethral drainage are required. Recovery will obviously be delayed.

A sliding hernia is dealt with by clearing as much peritoneal hernia sac as possible and then closing it using an 'inside-out' purse-string suture. When it is closed it is pushed back behind the transversalis fascia.

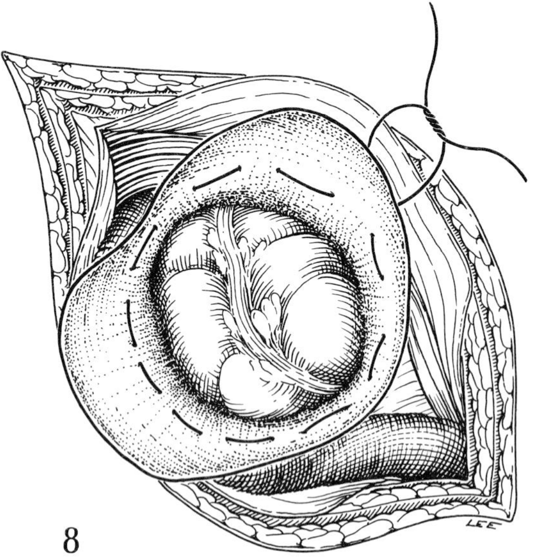

8

9a & b

Direct

The direct sac may be either a broad-based bulge behind and through the transversalis fascia (*a*) or,less commonly, have a narrow neck (*b*). In the first type interference with the peritoneum is not needed – the sac should be pushed back behind the transversalis fascia, which will be subsequently repaired. In the second, which is usually at the medial end of the canal, extraperitoneal fat is removed, the sac carefully cleared, redundant peritoneum excised and the defect closed with a catgut transfixion suture. Care must be taken to avoid the bladder which is often in the wall of such a sac.

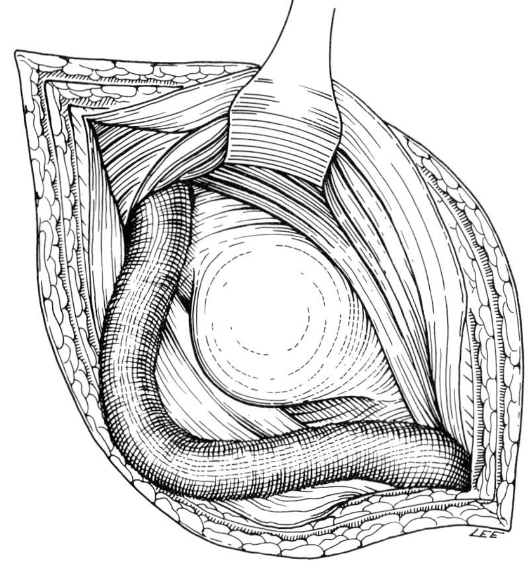

9a

Combined direct and indirect

Lastly a combined direct and indirect 'pantaloon' sac straddling the deep epigastric vessels may be found. In such a case the sac should be delivered to the lateral side of the deep epigastric vessels and dealt with as described for an indirect hernia.

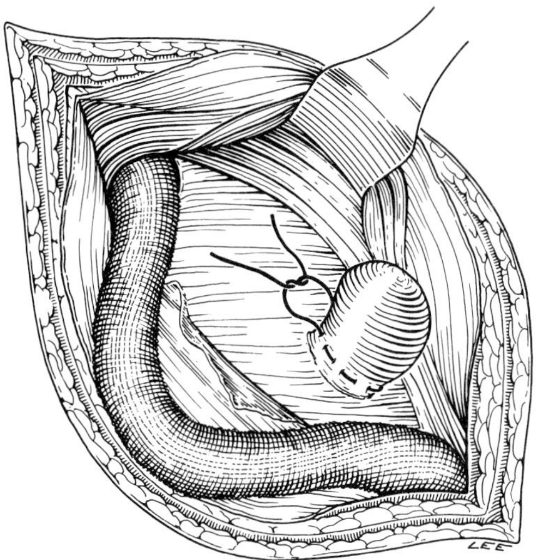

9b

10

Dissection of transversalis fascia

The most essential part of the Shouldice operation is the repair of the transversalis fascia. This structure should already have been identified at its condensation around the cord forming the deep inguinal ring. The condensed deep inguinal ring is freed from the emerging cord by sharp dissection. When this is completed the medial margin of the ring is grasped in a dissecting forceps or a haemostat and lifted up off the underlying extraperitoneal fat. Dissecting scissors are now passed through the ring between the fascia and the underlying fat. By this manoeuvre the fascia is separated from the underlying structures, particularly the deep epigastric vessels. The transversalis fascia is now divided along the length of the canal, beginning at the deep inguinal ring and continuing down to the pubic tubercle. The upper medial flap is lifted up away from the underlying fat.

Attention is now turned to the lower flap. It is penetrated by the cremasteric vessels arising from the deep epigastric vessels; these should now be ligated and divided close to their origin using catgut. If care is not taken with the cremasteric vessels they may be torn off the deep epigastric vessels and troublesome haemorrhage will follow. If a direct hernia is present it will bulge forward at this time and must be pushed back in order to free the lower lateral flap of the transversalis fascia. This flap must be freed down to its fusion to the deep part of the inguinal ligament.

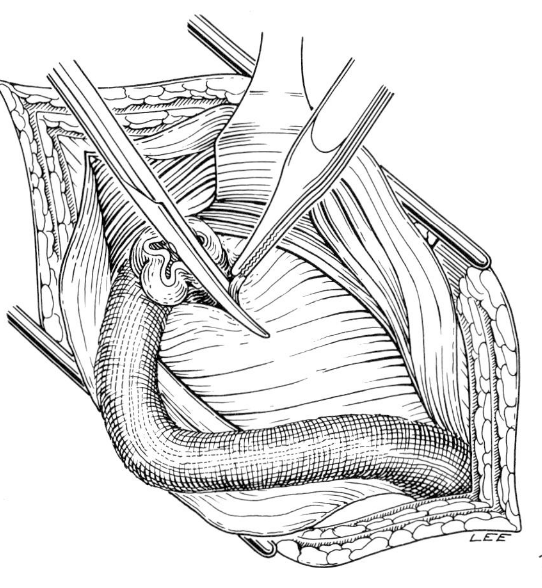

10

Repair of transversalis fascia

11

If the previous dissection has been carried out carefully, and if haemostasis is now complete, the remainder of the operation should be easy. First the transversalis fascia is repaired and the deep ring is carefully reconstituted using a 'double-breasting' technique. The posterior wall of the canal must be reconstituted so that *all* of the peritoneum and the stump of a hernial sac are retained behind it. To do this the lower lateral flap of the transversalis fascia is sutured to the deep surface of the upper medial flap. The repair is begun at the medial end of the canal, the first suture being placed in the transversalis fascia where that structure becomes condensed into the aponeurosis and periosteum on the pubic tubercle. The lower lateral flap of the transversalis fascia is then sutured to the undersurface of the upper flap at the point where the upper flap is just deep to the tendon of the transversus abdominus (conjoint tendon). At this point there is a thickening or condensation of the transversalis fascia which holds sutures easily. The fascia is sutured laterally until the stump of an indirect hernia lies behind it and it has been snugly fitted around the spermatic cord.

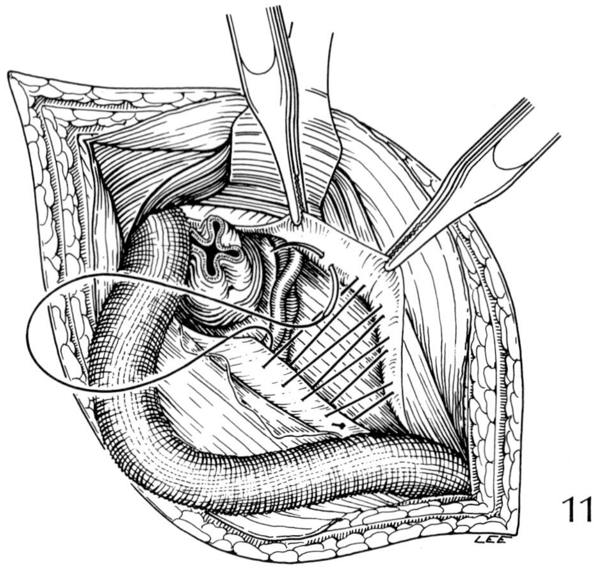

11

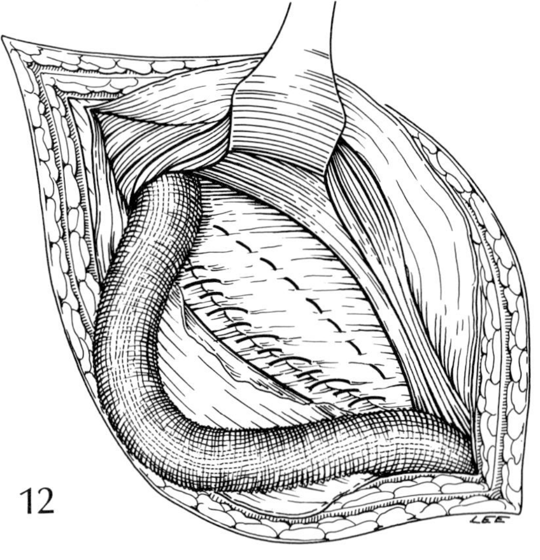

12

12

The direction of suturing is then reversed. The free margin of the upper medial flap is brought down over the lower lateral flap and sutured to the transversalis fascia at its condensation into the upturned deep edge of the inguinal ligament in the floor of the canal. Suturing is continued back to the pubic tubercle, where the suture is tied. By this manoeuvre the transversalis fascia is 'double-breasted' on itself, the 'direct area' of the canal is reinforced and the internal ring carefully reconstituted and tightened.

It is important not to split the fascial fibres. Sutures should be placed about 2–4 mm apart and bites of different depth taken with each so that an irregular 'broken saw-tooth' effect is produced.

The repair of the fascia transversalis is the crucial part of the operation. The fascia must be dissected and handled with care if its structure is to be maintained.

13 & 14

Reinforcement with the conjoint tendon

The conjoint tendon is now used to reinforce the repair of the transversalis fascia. A suture is started laterally through the upturned deep edge of the inguinal ligament at the medial margin of the reconstituted deep inguinal ring and continued to the deep tendinous surface of the conjoint tendon which is directly to the medial side of the deep ring. Sometimes, particularly if the cord is bulky, it is easier to proceed in reverse by passing the needle first through the undersurface of the conjoint tendon and then under the cord and through the upturned edge of the inguinal ligament.

At the point where this suture is inserted, the deep surface of the conjoint tendon is just beginning to become aponeurotic (the tendon of the transversus muscle) and it should hold sutures easily. The suture is continued in a medial direction, picking up the upturned edge of the inguinal ligament and the undersurface – the aponeurotic part – of the conjoint tendon down to the pubic tubercle. The direction is then reversed, suturing the aponeurotic part of the conjoint tendon loosely to the external oblique aponeurosis about 0.5 cm above the inguinal ligament. The 'broken saw-tooth' technique previously mentioned is again used, and as it is done the suture is gently pulled snug, not tight, so that the conjoint tendon and rectus sheath are rolled down on to the deep surface of the external oblique aponeurosis. Suturing is continued laterally until the conjoint tendon is brought up flush with the medial edge of the emergent spermatic cord. The suture is then tied.

The reconstruction of the posterior wall and the floor of the inguinal canal is now complete. The cord is now to be placed back in the canal.

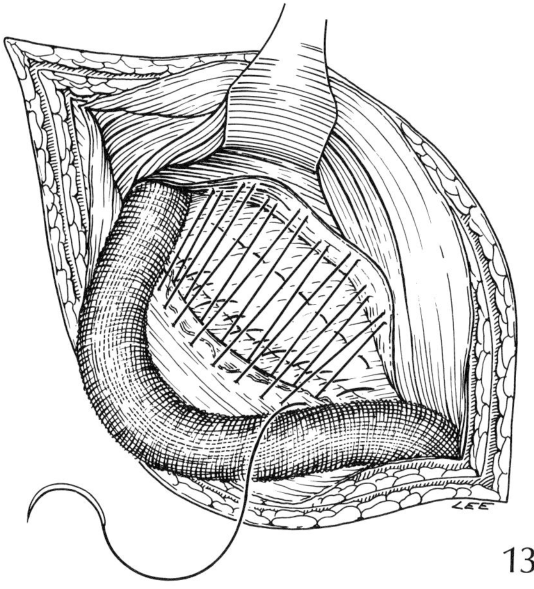

13

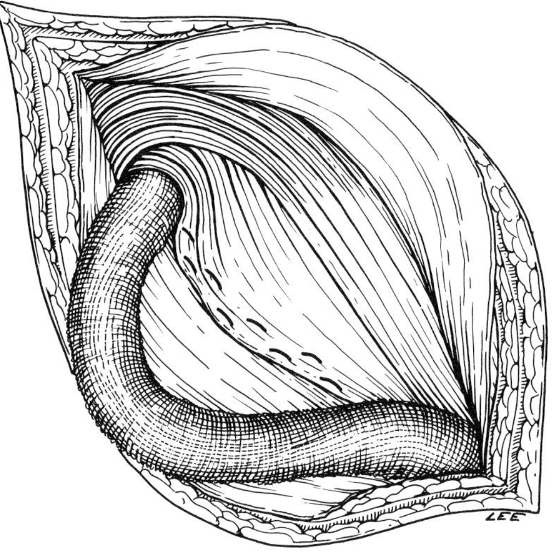

14

Closure

15

The external oblique aponeurosis

Now that the cord has been replaced the external oblique aponeurosis can be closed over it. Again a 'double-breasting' technique is used. The suturing is commenced medially, the lower lateral flap being sutured to the undersurface of the upper medial flap. Suturing is from medial to lateral and back again so that the upper flap is brought down over the lower flap and a new external inguinal ring is constructed at the medial end of the canal.

The repair is now complete and if all the layers have been sutured exactly as described the loads on the suture lines should be well distributed; there should be no undue tension and no splitting of fibre bundles. Indeed the structures should have just 'rolled together'.

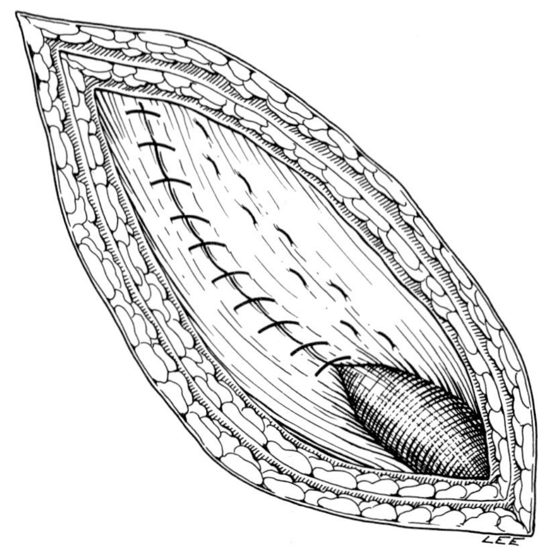

15

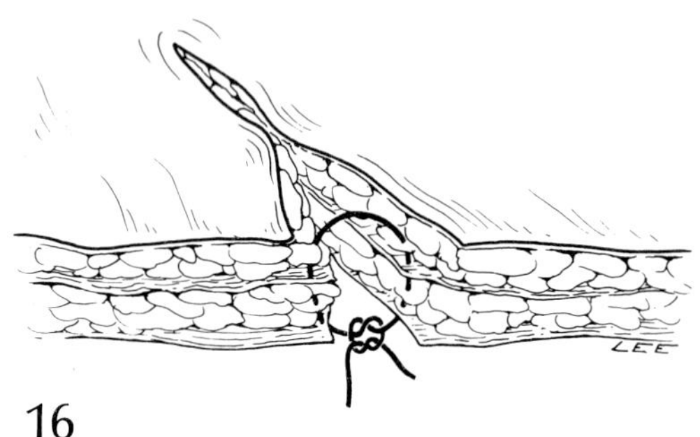

16

16

The subcutaneous tissue

The subcutaneous tissue is carefully closed with interrupted catgut sutures. No 'dead spaces' should be left and the fat should be closed so that the skin is closely approximated.

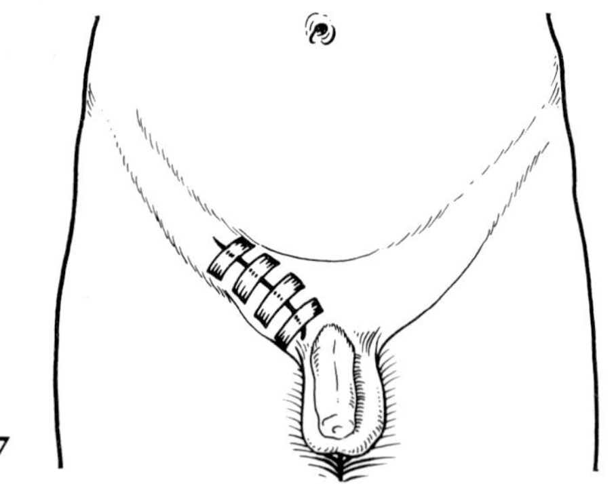

17

17

The skin

The skin is closed with microporous adhesive tape or a strip of gauze impregnated with collodion or similar adhesive. Non-penetrating skin clips give an equally good closure but require skilled attention when they are removed. Sutures should not be used.

18

Suture technique if monofilament stainless steel wire is used.

As an alternative to polypropylene, 34-gauge stainless steel wire can be used. This is the original material used by Dr Shouldice. Stainless steel is an excellent suture material which is strong and causes little tissue reaction. However, special attention must be given to technique if it is not to be broken or kinked in use. It is best to carry the wire as a loop on a long hook between each suture. The assistant must wield the hook carefully while at the same time keeping out of the operating surgeon's way and simultaneously maintaining the tension in the loop constant.

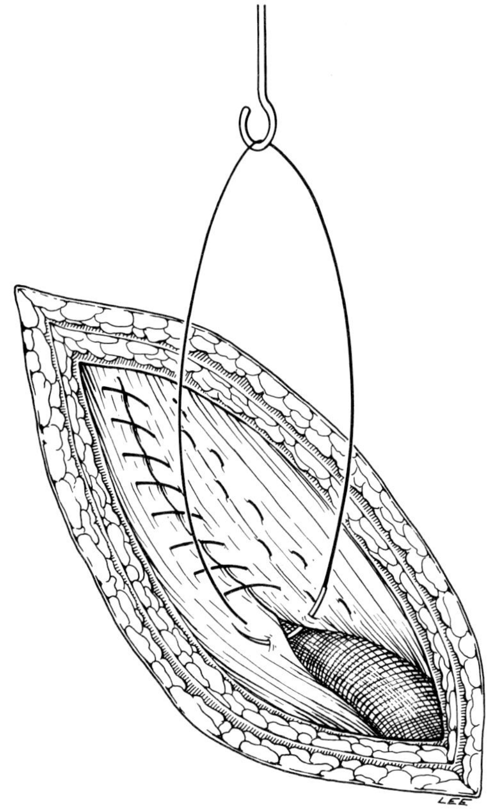

18

BILATERAL HERNIA

Bilateral hernia must never be repaired simultaneously for three reasons.

1. If sepsis occurs it may be bilateral if introduced at the same operation.
2. After simultaneous bilateral herniorrhaphy there is often much oedema and swelling of the penis and scrotum, which can make voiding tiresome and will delay convalescence.
3. There is evidence that simultaneous bilateral herniorrhaphy using the Shouldice technique may stretch the transversalis fascia unduly and predispose the patient to subsequent femoral hernia[4].

It is usual to allow an interval of 3–5 weeks between operations in bilateral hernias.

RECURRENT INGUINAL HERNIA

Recurrent inguinal hernias are always difficult and operation should only be undertaken by an experienced surgeon who is interested in this problem. If there is sepsis or sinus formation, operation should not be undertaken until it has settled. It may be necessary to remove all foreign suture material from the wound at a first operation and then wait some months before attempting the repair. it is always wise to use wire on a recurrent hernia because this material is least likely to cause the sepsis to flare up. The technique is identical to that described above. Generally, tissue planes can be identified if a slow and gentle dissection is made. To date the author has never had to divide the cord in order to repair a recurrent hernia.

THE STRANGULATED HERNIA

The same operative technique can be used to treat a strangulated inguinal hernia. If additional access is required to deal with gangrenous gut the deep ring can be enlarged medially by dividing the deep epigastric vessels between ligatures, taking care to avoid the bladder. It is preferable to perform a standard paramedian incision for access to the main peritoneal cavity rather than to have to do an awkward resection of gangrenous tissue through the groin incision.

Postoperative care

Immediate active mobilization is the key to rapid convalescence. The 'client with a hernia' must not be allowed to become institutionalized into the 'postoperative patient'.

If the operation has been performed under local anaesthesia the patient should be helped to *walk* from the operating table. If general anaesthesia has been used the patient must be made to get up and walk as soon as he is conscious. There may be slight pain after surgery and a suitable mild analgesic should be prescribed. Analgesics with narcotic properties are never needed.

The wound dressing is removed *by the patient* on the fifth postoperative day. After the dressing is removed the patient can shower or bath normally.

Light office or professional work can be resumed after about 7 days and most other heavier jobs after about 8 weeks. Patients are told that they may undertake any work which does not cause pain to their wounds.

Some personal results

Over a period of 9 years 603 primary hernia repairs have been performed using this technique. So far, there have been only 5 recurrences. In 4 of these, multistrand polyester suture material had been used and the wound became septic and formed sinuses. In the remaining recurrence, steel wire had been used; in this case the wound became slightly inflamed some 4 days after the patient had gone home, and the wound was immediately reopened by another surgeon and the wire removed. All 5 primary recurrences were reoperated on and to date these second repairs have been sound[10].

Of 81 patients operated on for recurrent hernia, only one has developed a recurrence.

Conclusion

The Shouldice operation can be recommended for three reasons.

1. It has given uniformly excellent results in Toronto, Philadelphia and Stockton on Tees[4,5,6] and the results are significantly better than those of other techniques reported in the British literature[11,12].
2. It conforms to the principles of good repair surgery, namely, careful and accurate restoration of anatomical planes and their approximation by non-irritative suture material until firm biological union is accomplished.
3. It is, when combined with good management policies, cost effective.

References

1. Marcy, H. O. The cure of hernia. Journal of the American Medical Association 1887; 8: 589–592

2. Zimmerman, L. M., Anson, B. J. Anatomy and surgery of hernia. 2nd ed. Baltimore: Williams and Wilkins, 1967

3. Bassini, E. Ueber die Behandlung des Leistenbruches. Archiv für Klinische Chirurgie 1890; 40; 429–476

4. Glassow, F. The shouldice repair of inguinal hernia. In: Varco, R. I., Delaney, J. P., eds. Controversy in surgery. Philadelphia: W. B. Saunders, 1976

5. Myers, R. N., Shearburn, E. W. The problem of recurrent inguinal hernia. Surgical Clinics of North America 1973; 53: 555–558

6. Devlin, H. B., Russell, I. T., Muller, D., Sahay, A. K., Tiwari, P. N. Short stay surgery for inguinal hernia. Lancet 1977; 1: 847–849

7. Neuhauser, D. Elective inguinal herniorrhaphy versus truss in the elderly. In: Bunker, J. P., Barnes, B. A., Mosteller, F., eds. Costs, risks and benefits of surgery. New York: Oxford University Press, 1977

8. Russell, I. T., Devlin, H. B., Fell, M., Glass, N. J., Newell, J. J. Day-case surgery for hernias and haemorrhoids. Lancet 1977; 1: 844–846

9. Department of Health and Social Security. Administrative arrangements: planned early discharge of patients undergoing surgery. London: HMSO, 1978 (Notes on good practices No. 12)

10. Datta, D., Zaidi, A., Devlin, M. B. Short stay surgery for inguinal hernia. Lancet 1980; 2: 99–100

11. Marsden, A. J. Inguinal hernia: a three year review of one thousand cases. British Journal of Surgery 1958; 46: 234–243

12. Shuttleworth, K. E. D., Davies, W. H. Treatment of inguinal hernia. Lancet 1960; 1: 126–127

Femoral hernia

H. Brendan Devlin MA, MD, MCh, FRCS, FRCS(I)
Consultant Surgeon, North Tees General Hospital, Stockton on Tees, Cleveland;
Associate Lecturer in Clinical Surgery, University of Newcastle upon Tyne

Introduction

A femoral hernia is a protrusion of a peritoneal sac covered with extraperitoneal fat through the femoral canal medial to the femoral vessels as they proceed from the abdomen into the thigh. A femoral hernia sac may contain all or part of an abdominal viscus.

Femoral hernias occur much less frequently than inguinal and, in contradistinction to the latter, are more frequent in females than males. In the author's experience, the ratio of femoral to inguinal hernias is 18:1, and in femoral hernia the ratio of female to male is 3.9:1.

The aetiology of femoral hernia is ill understood. In contrast to inguinal hernia, there is no easy embryological explanation. The fact that femoral hernias are most frequently found in middle-aged and elderly females and the disparity in incidence between parous and nulliparous women suggests that intra-abdominal pressure and the stretching of aponeurotic tissue consequent on pregnancy are important factors. Chronic cough, intestinal obstruction, constipation and excessive physical labour may also contribute to raised intra-abdominal pressure. Weight loss in the elderly female is also associated with femoral hernia.

Operation should always be advised, for two reasons.

1. It is impossible to make and fit an adequate truss to control such a hernia.
2. The incidence of strangulation in these hernias is high – and strangulated hernia in the elderly carries considerable morbidity.

When a patient presents with intestinal obstruction and a femoral hernia, and the hernia is not tender and therefore not strangulated, reduction by taxis may be employed in the short term, but if there is any suggestion that strangulation has occurred taxis should not be employed. Urgent operation is obligatory for all cases of strangulated femoral hernia.

1

Anatomy

Femoral hernia has a sinister reputation because of the unyielding anatomy of the femoral canal. The whole canal (that is, the space between the pubis and the iliopsoas muscle) is bounded anteriorly by the inguinal ligament, posteriorly by the pectineal ligament at its attachment to the pubic bone, medially by the sharp lateral margin of the lacunar ligament and laterally by the iliopsoas muscle with its overlying fascia. The canal is divided into two compartments, the lateral being occupied by the femoral artery and femoral vein, and the smaller medial by areolar tissue, some lymphatics and a lymph node. It is through this small medial compartment that a femoral hernia penetrates into the thigh. In its advancement into the thigh the hernial sac carries with it some extraperitoneal fat about its fundus and it may draw the extraperitoneal anterolateral wall of the bladder down with it on its medial aspect. Once the sac is entrenched in the thigh its medial wall is pressed up against the sharp unyielding margin of the lacunar ligament medially, the unyielding pectineal fascia and pubic bone posteriorly, the inguinal ligament anteriorly and the femoral vein laterally. Compression of the femoral vein and the saphenous vein by a femoral hernia may occur; indeed, visible distension of these veins has been described as a diagnostic sign in the differential diagnosis of a femoral hernia from other groin swellings.

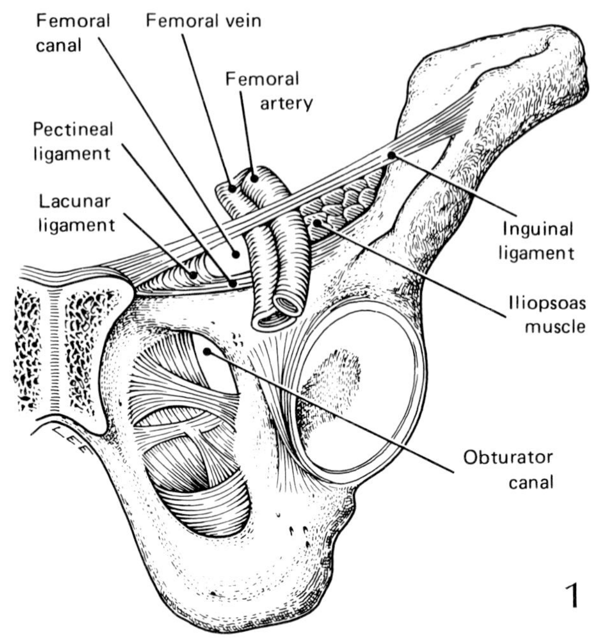

1

Types of operation

Because of its complex anatomical relationships there is no simple access to the femoral canal. Three approaches to femoral herniorrhaphy are described here because no one operation is ideal or uniformly suited to each case.

1. The abdominal, suprapubic or extraperitoneal operation developed by Henry[1]. This is often known as the McEvedy, though Henry used a midline incision and McEvedy a pararectus approach[2].
2. The inguinal or 'high' operation[3,4].
3. The crural or 'low' operation[5].

The extraperitoneal approach gives excellent access to the femoral canal and to the general peritoneal cavity, should that be necessary to deal with a strangulated viscus. However, this approach to the pelvis is unfamiliar to most surgeons and therefore not to be recommended to the inexperienced surgeon operating on his first strangulated femoral hernia at dead of night.

The inguinal approach is familiar but has the twin drawbacks of disrupting the inguinal canal mechanism and not providing adequate access to a strangulated viscus.

The crural approach to the femoral sac is good and bloodless and repair of the hernia is easy by this method. Its very significant disadvantage is that access to a strangulated viscus is often very inadequate.

The crural approach is recommended to the occasional or novice surgeon. If a visceral strangulation is present it is best to perform a standard lower paramedian incision and deal with the crisis through an incision which is familiar to most abdominal operators. With an emergency situation, or for the inexperienced surgeon, there is no place for an anatomical extravaganza. The 'low' operation will be described in detail.

CRURAL OPERATION

Preoperative

Preoperative management

In the uncomplicated case no special preoperative management is required. The lower abdominal and upper thigh area should be shaved and it is best to have the patient catheterized before surgery (the bladder is often involved in the medial wall of the hernial sac and preoperative catheterization will lessen the likelihood of bladder injury).

If the hernia is obstructed or strangulated, preoperative nasogastric aspiration and appropriate fluid replacement will be required.

Anaesthesia

General anaesthesia is preferred, but local anaesthesia can be employed. If it is, the operating surgeon must remember that the parietal peritoneum is very sensitive and manipulation of it can cause the patient much discomfort unless the anaesthesia is adequate. Wide local infiltration with 0.5 per cent lignocaine with adrenaline 1:200 000 is adequate. Up to 500 mg of lignocaine (100 ml of 0.5 per cent solution) can be administered safely to a healthy 70 kg adult but this quantity will need to be reduced in the elderly or in debilitated patients. As an alternative to lignocaine there is bupivacaine hydrochloride 0.25 per cent with adrenaline 1:400 000 which could be used. The dosage should not exceed 2 mg per kg of body weight. Bupivacaine has the advantage that anaesthesia lasts longer than with lignocaine.

Suture materials

The suture material for the repair of the fascia of the femoral canal is metric 3 polypropylene. For haemostasis metric 2 chromic catgut and diathermy are used. The hernial sac and parietal peritoneum are closed with metric 3.5 chromic catgut. The subcutaneous tissue is sutured with metric 3.5 and the skin closed with hypoallergenic microporous adhesive tape.

For the repair of the fascia of the femoral canal a J-shaped 30 mm tapercut needle is best, as it facilitates the deep suturing to the pectineal fascia.

The operation

Position of patient

The patient is placed flat supine on the operating table.

Draping

If the hernia is not strangulated, towels are placed to allow access to the affected groin area only. If strangulation is present or suspected the sterile towels should be placed so that there is easy access to the lower abdomen.

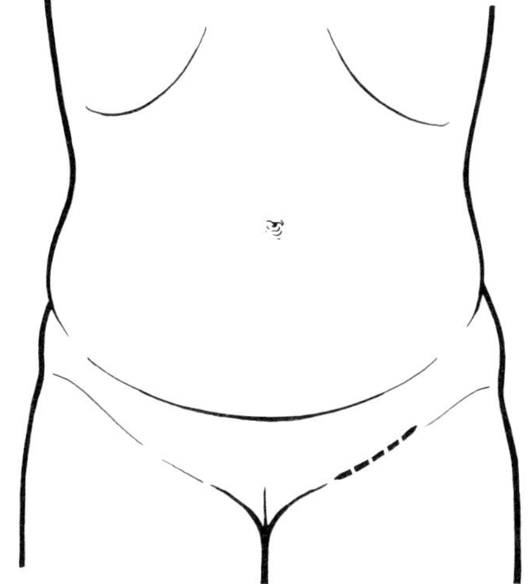
2

2

The incision

A skin incision is made directly over the hernia and about 2.0 cm below the inguinal ligament. The incision should be about 6.0 cm long and oblique so that it is parallel to the inguinal ligament.

After the skin has been divided it is easy to separate the subcutaneous fat down to the coverings of the hernial sac. Secure haemostasis should be attained before the sac is mobilized.

3

Mobilization of the sac

The sac, having emerged from the femoral canal, carries before it transversalis fascia and extraperitoneal fascia in front of which is the attenuated cribriform fascia and femoral vessel fascial layer in the thigh. Because of these fascial layers the sac usually makes a forward and upward turn in its path and its fundus can be found lying over the inguinal ligament. It is important to appreciate this before mobilization is attempted. Once the sac is identified the fascial layers are cleaned from it by blunt dissection, which is best achieved by wiping the fascia off with a gauze swab. These extraperitoneal coverings of the sac are frequently quite thick.

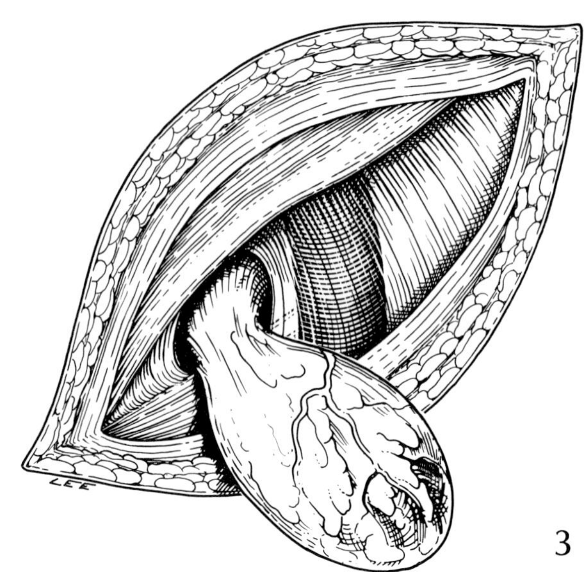

3

Identification of femoral opening

The neck of the sac is now cleared of fat and fascia so that the boundaries of the femoral canal can be identified. It is best to identify the medial and anterior margins of the canal first. The medial margin is the lacunar ligament and is easily seen as it sweeps around from the inguinal ligament to the subjacent pubic bone. Anteriorly, the rolled-over edge of the inguinal ligament can readily be separated from the sac underneath it and the sac should next be lifted up. The fascia on the pectineus muscle is easily recognizable and if this is traced back to the ramus of the pubis, the posterior margin of the canal – the pectineal ligament – can be recognized.

Attention is now turned to the lateral boundary of the canal – the femoral vein. This is the most vulnerable structure in this area and is difficult to identify because it is covered with a quite opaque fascial sheath. One manoeuvre is to identify the femoral artery by touch; the artery lies immediately lateral to the vein so the vein *must* be in any space between the sac and the palpable artery. A careful dissection is made on the lateral side of the sac, preferably using 'curved on the flat' dissecting scissors and keeping close to the sac. The dissection of the sac is only complete when the entire circumference of its neck has been clearly defined.

Inspection of contents of sac

The lateral side of the fundus of the sac should now be opened. The medial side should be avoided, as it may be partly formed by the bladder. There is always much adherent extraperitoneal fat on the fundus which generally contains many distended veins. If these bleed they can confuse the anatomy, so the fat should be gently broken through with a haemostat point and the bleeding carefully controlled.

Inside the extraperitoneal fat the true peritoneal hernial sac will be found. It is grasped in a haemostat and then opened.

Any contents of the sac can now be gently freed, adhesions divided and the contents reduced back into the general peritoneal cavity. If strangulation is present an alternative approach to the remainder of the operation may be necessary (*see* p. 700 in this chapter).

4 & 5

Closure and excision of sac

When it is certain that the neck of the sac is isolated and that the sac is empty it can be closed and excised. Traction is applied to the open sac and, using metric 3.5 catgut on a 40 mm round needle, a transfixion suture should be securely tied around the neck. The redundant sac is cut off, leaving a generous cuff beyond the transfixion suture, and the stump of the sac will now recede through the femoral canal and out of sight.

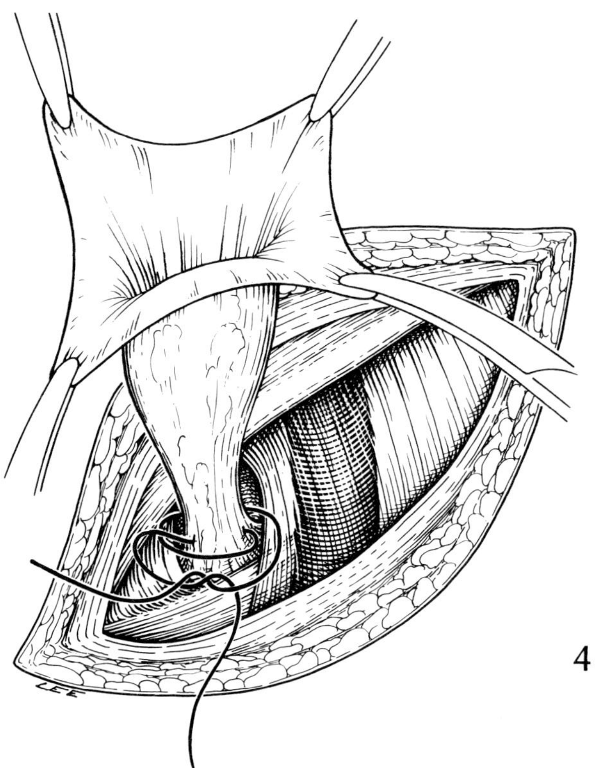

4

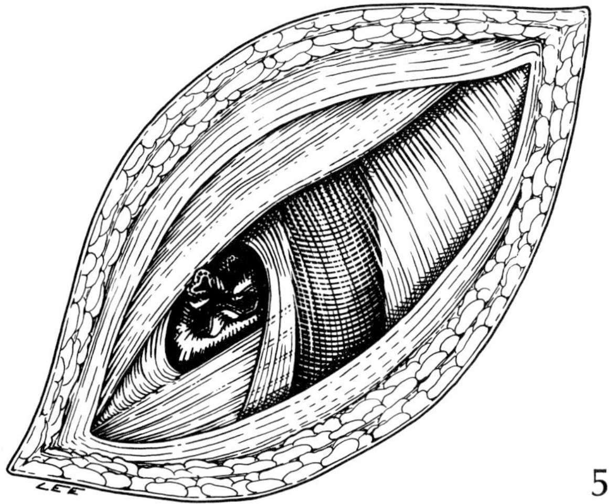

5

Repair of canal

First stage

The canal is repaired using a single figure-of-eight suture of metric 3 polypropylene on a J-shaped needle.

6

The femoral vein is retracted laterally and the pectineal ligament clearly identified on the superior ramus of the pubic bone. The first suture is placed through this ligament from its deep aspect at the point where the medial margin of the femoral vein would lie if it were not retracted. It is necessary to experiment with the retractor and identify this point correctly. If the suture is placed too far laterally the vein will be compromised, and if placed too far medially the repair will be unsound.

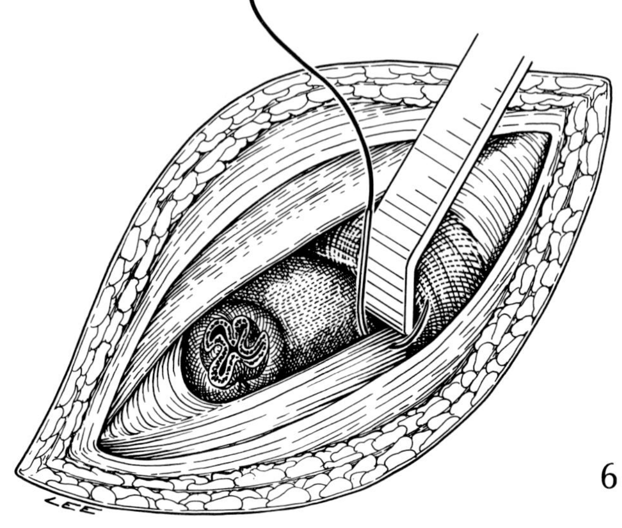

6

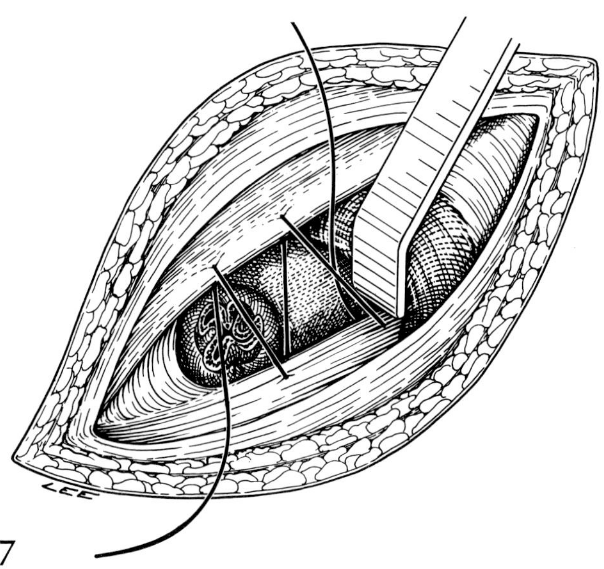

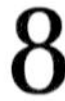

7

7

The next bite must pick up the inguinal ligament at a corresponding distance from its pubic attachment so that the suture forms the base of an isosceles triangle. Next the pectineal ligament is picked up, again from deep to superficial, halfway between the first pectineal suture and the lacunar ligament, and last the inguinal ligament is picked up, again halfway between the first suture and the attachment of the ligament to the pubis.

8

Now the free end of the suture is passed deep to the two loops and the two ends are tied securely. When the suture is pulled tight, the medial 0.75 cm or so of the inguinal ligament will be approximated to the pectineal line and the femoral canal closed. Futhermore, if the knot is placed at the medial side it will be away from the femoral vein which will not be damaged by it.

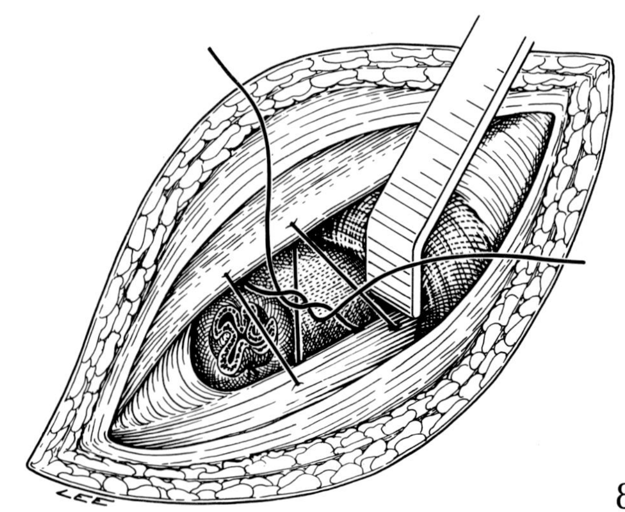

8

9 & 10

Second stage

So far the canal has been closed by the apposition of two tendinous structures under some degree of tension. According to the rules of biological repair tendinous structures drawn together under tension and subject to varying stresses such as respiration and movement do not heal readily. Therefore it is advisable to reinforce the union with a further aponeurotic patch which is not under tension. This is easily achieved by raising a flap of fascia off the surface of the pectineus muscle and suturing it to the external oblique aponeurosis in such a way that it covers the initial repair of the femoral canal. A continuous polypropylene suture is used for this double-breasting manoeuvre.

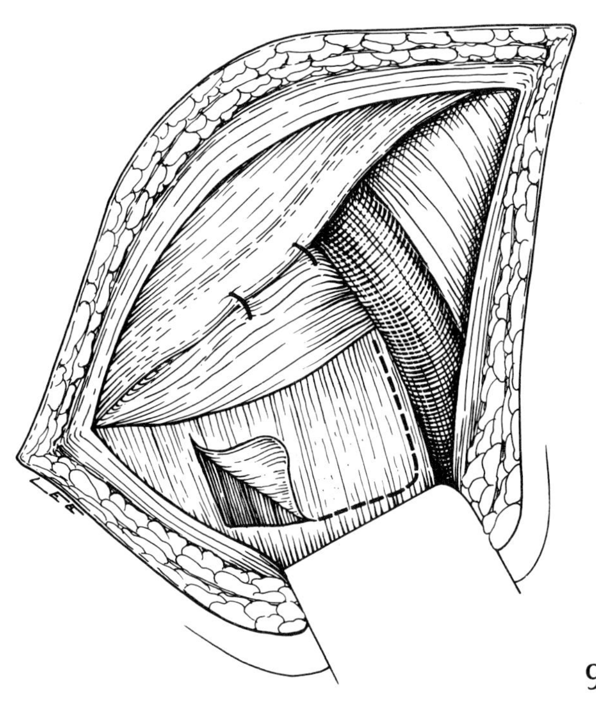

9

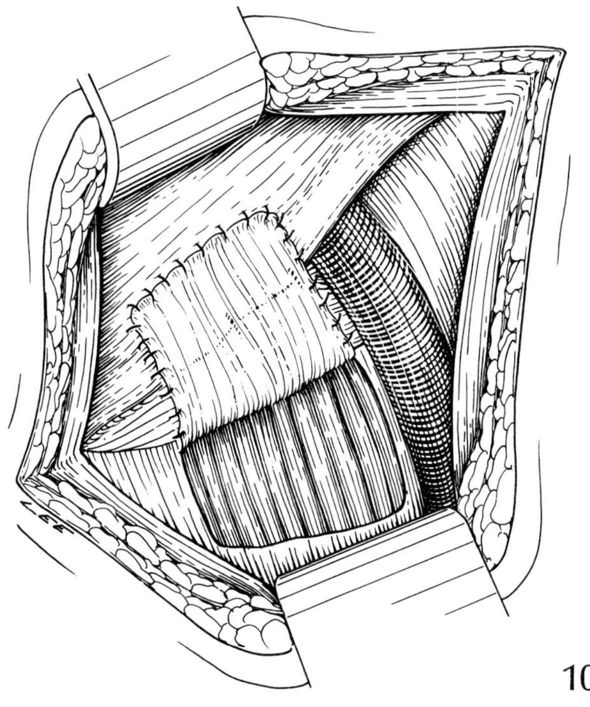

10

Closure

11

The subcutaneous fat is closed meticulously with interrupted metric 3.5 chromic catgut sutures. Haemostasis must be secure and any dead space must be avoided.

The skin is closed with microporous adhesive tape or gauze impregnated with Collodion.

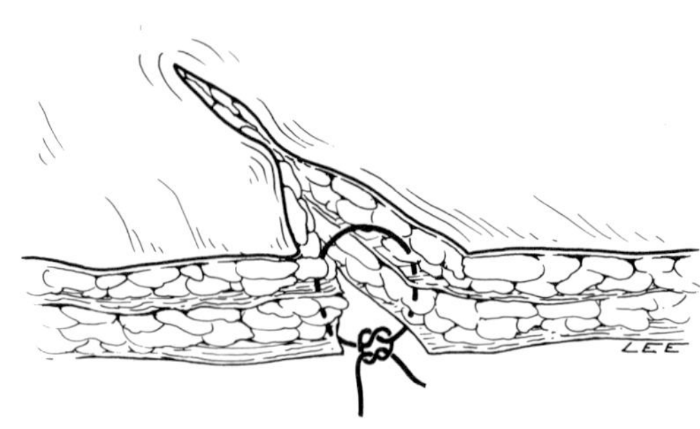

11

Postoperative care

No special postoperative care is required. There should be no postoperative restriction of activity save that imposed in the first few days by postoperative pain which in any case should be minimal.

Strangulation

If strangulation is suspected the sac is approached as described. Once the sac is identified it will be seen to contain blood-stained fluid if strangulation has occurred. The sac should be opened on the lateral aspect of its fundus and the contents inspected. A variety of intra-abdominal viscera may be found in the femoral hernia sac. No viscus should be returned to the peritoneal cavity unless it is definitely viable. Viability of any viscus can only be assessed after its blood supply has been normalized by removing the constriction at the neck of the sac.

Any blood-stained fluid in the sac is sucked out (and some sent for microbiological culture) and the contents of the sac are gently manipulated so that the neck of the sac is revealed clearly. It is very important to be careful with a strangulated loop of gut, as operative perforation can seriously weaken the patient's condition. Quite frequently, careful dissection of the neck of the sac and removal of oedematous extraperitoneal fat about it are all that is required to release the strangulation. The constricting agent is usually the thickened peritoneal neck of the sac and the oedematous extraperitoneal fat about it rather than the ligamentous structures which form the anterior, posterior and medial margins of the sac. The femoral vein is very rarely involved in the strangulation process, which confirms that the neck of the sac itself is most usually the constricting agent.

When the sac has been opened the inguinal ligament can generally be retracted upwards and the femoral vein laterally so that the neck of the sac can be divided.

After the strangulation has been released any contained viscera are wrapped in warm saline packs and left alone for a full 5 min before being inspected. Omentum of doubtful viability is best excised. Small intestine must only be returned to the peritoneal cavity if it has all been inspected and shown to be vital. Often there is a linear necrosis of the bowel where it has been compressed by the neck of the sac and this should be oversewn.

If a considerable segment of gangrenous small bowel needs resection more gut is prolapsed into the wound. Alternatively, if there is technical difficulty, an ipsilateral lower paramedian incision can be made and bowel resected through the groin wound (to avoid contamination of the peritoneal cavity). Anastomosis is then carried out through the main peritoneal cavity. It is worth stressing the importance of not contaminating the main peritoneal cavity and not returning non-viable bowel into it. The use of an ipsilateral lower paramedian incision for all cases of difficulty is strongly recommended.

INGUINAL OPERATION[3,4]

This operation achieves the same objective of fastening the medial portion of the inguinal ligament to the pectineal ligament in order to reduce the size of the femoral canal as has been described above using the crural approach. However, in the inguinal approach the femoral canal is exposed by opening the posterior wall – the transversalis fascia – of the inguinal canal.

The incision and dissection for this operation are exactly the same as those employed in the Shouldice operation for inguinal hernia (*see* pp. 683–686 in this volume). After the transversalis fascia in the posterior wall of the inguinal canal has been opened the extraperitoneal fat on the neck of the femoral hernia can be identified and removed by blunt dissection. The sac can now either be delivered above the inguinal ligament or opened below the ligament and its contents reduced. The neck of the sac is then transfixed and ligated.

The medial extremity of the inguinal ligament is now sutured to the pectineal. Again a figure-of-eight polypropylene suture is used but in this operation it is inserted from above, that is, through the incision in the posterior wall of the inguinal canal. The inguinal canal is then repaired using the Shouldice technique (*see* pp. 688–691 in this volume), care being taken to reinforce the femoral repair with the overlapped transversalis fascia at the medial part of the canal.

The inguinal approach for the repair of femoral hernia is not recommended as the operation of choice because it is technically more difficult and more time-consuming than the crural operation and because it disrupts an otherwise normal inguinal canal.

EXTRAPERITONEAL OPERATION[1]

This operation illustrates the genius of an expert surgical anatomist exploiting fascial plane dissection at its most elegant. Henry's extraperitoneal approach to the anterior pelvis gives an excellent exposure of both femoral canals simultaneously, but it is not an operation for the tyro. In the hands of an expert it is a fine operation enabling bilateral femoral hernia to be dealt with simultaneously through one incision.

The patient is placed on the operating table and the bladder emptied by catheterization. A vertical midline suprapubic incision is made, the aponeurotic layer is opened and the peritoneum exposed. The recti are retracted to either side and the space between the peritoneum and the abdominal wall muscles is opened by gentle blunt dissection in order to approach the femoral canal on either side. Femoral sacs are dealt with by reduction of their contents, transfixion of their necks and resection of redundant sac. If strangulation is present the subjacent peritoneum can easily be opened, the contents of the sac inspected, and so forth. The femoral canal is repaired using a non-absorbable suture as described in the inguinal operation (*see* p. 688 in this volume). The anterior abdominal wall is closed layer by layer.

References

1. Henry, A. K. Extensile exposure. 2nd ed. Edinburgh and London: Livingstone, 1957

2. McEvedy, P. G. Femoral hernia. Annals of the Royal College of Surgeons of England 1950; 7: 484–496

3. Annandale, T. Case in which a reducible oblique and direct inguinal and femoral hernia existed on the same side, and were successfully treated by operation. Edinburgh Medical Journal 1875; 21: 1087–1091

4. Lotheissen, G. Zur Radikaloperation der Schenkelhernien. Zentralblatt für Chirurgie 1898; 21: 548–550

5. Lockwood, C. B. The radical cure of femoral and inguinal hernia. Lancet 1893; 2: 1297–1302

Surgical exposure of the kidney

G. F. Murnaghan MD, ChM, FRCS(Ed.), FRCS, FRACS
Professor of Surgery, University of New South Wales;
Urological Surgeon to The Prince Henry and The Prince of Wales Hospitals;
Consultant Urologist The Royal South Sydney Hospital, Sydney
and The Royal Hospital for Women, Paddington, New South Wales, Australia

Preoperative

Preoperative assessment and preparation

Careful assessment of the patient's respiratory and cardiovascular systems is required before surgical exposure of the kidney is programmed. Retroperitoneal dissection, particularly through the loin, predisposes to respiratory complications and paralytic ileus. Smoking should be discontinued, chest physiotherapy should be used to ensure maximum ventilatory capacity and a control radiograph of the chest should be taken. Regular, adequate bowel action should be assured before operation as part of the routine preparation for general anaesthesia; the level of haemoglobin should be recorded and at least 2 u of compatible blood should be available. The posture and range of lateral flexion in the dorsolumbar spine should be assessed and preoperative skin preparation should extend from the nipple line to the pubis and almost out to the opposite flank on both anterior and posterior aspects of the trunk. Representative and up-to-date radiographs should be chosen from the urological studies and illuminated for easy reference in the operating theatre.

Choice of incision

Choice of incision is influenced by the size, site and mobility of both the lesion and the kidney; by the age and build of the patient with respect to obesity, spinal mobility or curvature; and by the distance between the costal margin and the iliac crest in the midaxillary line where maximum width of the wound is usually obtained.

A standard approach to the kidney through the loin with a subcostal incision will give adequate exposure to a mobile kidney that is not enlarged and when a plain radiograph of the renal region shows that the 12th rib does not project below the midhilar level. The subcostal approach should be carefully considered whenever subsequent re-exposure of the kidney is likely to be required.

Exposure of a high, adherent or enlarged kidney can be significantly improved by resection of the 12th rib or the 11th rib if the 12th is underdeveloped. This transcostal approach is most useful when there has been previous exposure of the kidney by the subcostal route or when reconstructive renal surgery is contemplated.

Easier exposure of a large or fixed kidney with the particular need for access to the upper polar region or pedicle can be obtained without rib resection by a supracostal incision above the 11th rib or, less commonly, the 12th rib to give extrapleural and extraperitoneal exposure. Wide access may also be obtained through a Nagamatsu approach which extends the posterior end of a subcostal incision upwards in a paravertebral line to the 9th intercostal space to allow for resection of 2.5 cm segments of the posterior ends of the lower two or three ribs.

Similar wide exposure may be obtained by a transthoracic approach with a high transcostal or intercostal incision combined with an anterior abdominal extension of the wound to allow for simultaneous transperitoneal exploration and any concurrent lymph node dissection.

An anterior extraperitoneal approach to the kidney may be useful in infants and small children as an alternative to the limited exposure generally obtained through the lumbar incision in young patients. It provides direct but localized access to the lower renal pole, pelviureteric junction and upper ureter in all ages, but is particularly useful for the exposure of one or both kidneys in patients with severe cardiorespiratory limitations or with immobilizing disabilities such as osteoarthritis of the spine, scoliosis or kyphosis. Simultaneous exposure of both kidneys is best obtained through an extensive transverse or curved, muscle-cutting, upper abdominal approach with medial reflection of the organs and peritoneum overlying each kidney.

The operation

All illustrations show access to the right kidney; the posterior aspect of the wound is on the left.

1

Positioning the patient

For any lateral approach the patient lies on the opposite side, somewhat nearer to the operator on the operating table and with any segmented cushions replaced by a continuous sheet of thick sponge and with the kidney bridge just below the costal margin. The patient's back is maintained in the vertical plane by flexion of the lower knee and thigh whilst the upper thigh remains straight and is supported on a pillow. The upper arm is supported horizontally in a rest and is convenient for venous cannulation and monitoring of the blood pressure. The underneath arm is disposed in comfortable flexion with padded support. Rolling of the patient is then prevented by padded fixtures on the table and by a leather strap or broad band of adhesive strapping which crosses between the iliac crest and greater trochanter with firm attachment beneath the table top. Lateral flexion of the spine to open the costo-iliac space is obtained by a convenient combination or choice of sandbag in the opposite loin, elevation of the bridge and breaking of the table. The pelvis should be maintained in the vertical plane and it should be ensured that there is no embarrassment to cardiorespiratory function, that there has been no undue angulation of the spine and that the buttocks remain on the table. Anterior approach to the kidney is facilitated by localized support of the lower posterior chest and loin on one or both sides of the supine patient.

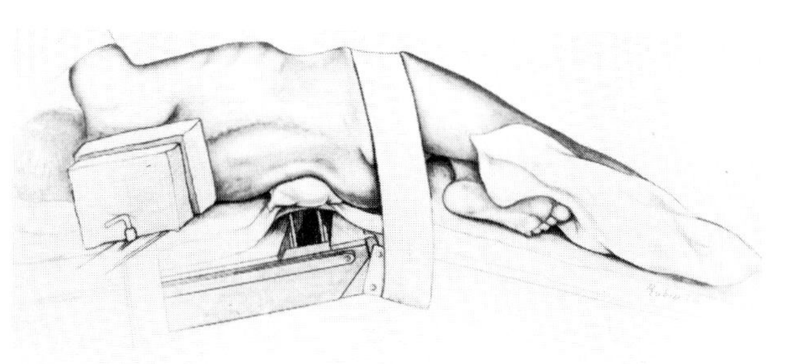

1

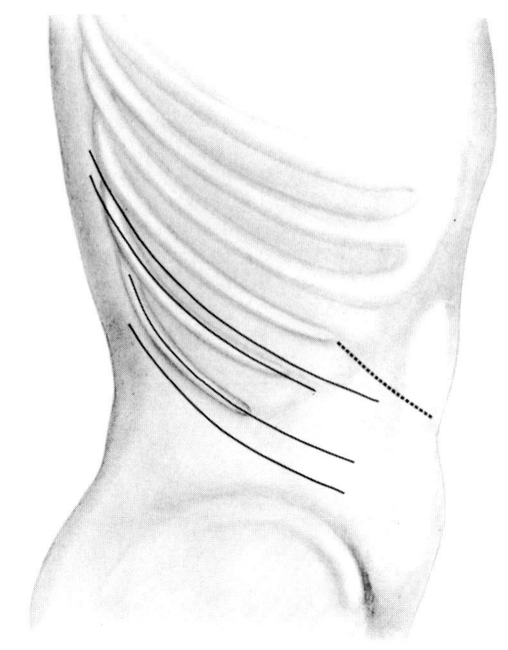

2

2 & 3

The incisions

The lines of skin incision for approach by the subcostal, the transcostal (12th rib), supracostal (11th rib) and thoracoabdominal (10th space) routes of exposure are illustrated. Incisions relating to ribs should curve downwards slightly in their abdominal extension to avoid damage to the neurovascular bundle from the rib above. The foreshortened skin incision for the anterior extraperitoneal exposure of the kidney is shown as a dotted line.

The muscular structures exposed are shown in *Illustration 3*.

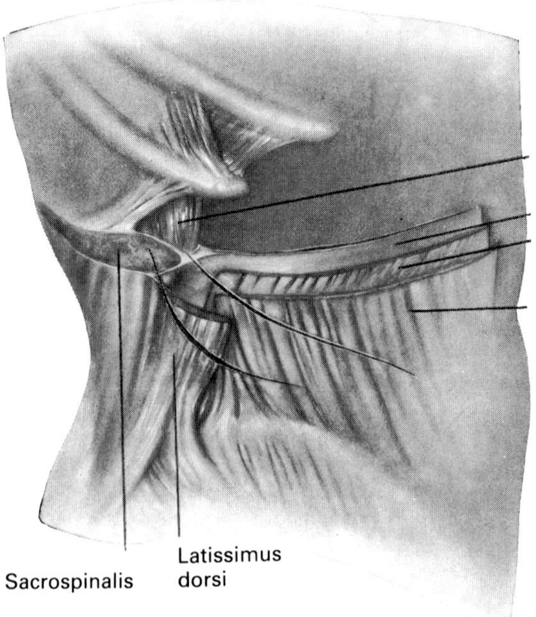

3

SUBCOSTAL APPROACH

4

The skin incision extends from the angle between the 12th rib and the outer border of the erector spinae muscles and passes forwards about 1 cm below and parallel to the rib and then to a point about 2 cm above and anterior to the anterior superior iliac spine. With careful haemostasis the fat and deep fascia are divided to expose the external oblique muscle in the anterior portion of the wound with latissimus dorsi muscle in the posterior portion. The next useful plane is entered by division of latissimus dorsi in the line of the incision to expose the posterior edge of the external oblique muscle and adjacent lumbodorsal fascia.

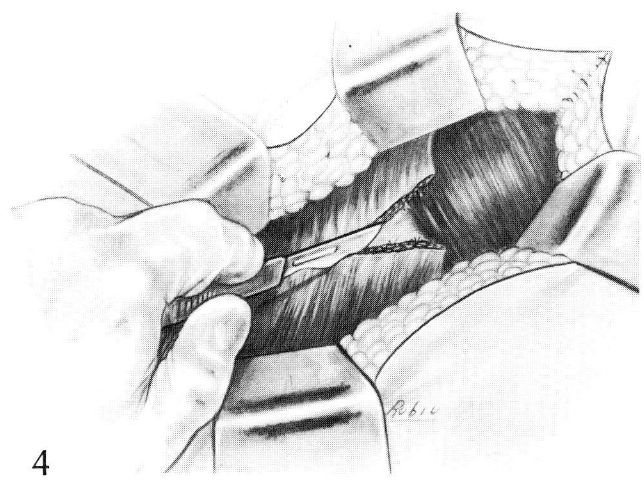

4

5

Division of superficial muscles

Posterior extension of the division of latissimus dorsi exposes the serratus posterior inferior, which is incised to expose the lateral edge of erector spinae beneath the lumbodorsal fascia. Division of the external oblique in the anterior portion of the wound allows for division of the internal oblique muscle from its posterior edge and forwards across the line of its fibres. Care must be taken to avoid the subcostal nerve which in thin patients may be seen crossing the wound beneath the lumbodorsal fascia, having left the 12th rib at about the junction between its middle and distal thirds.

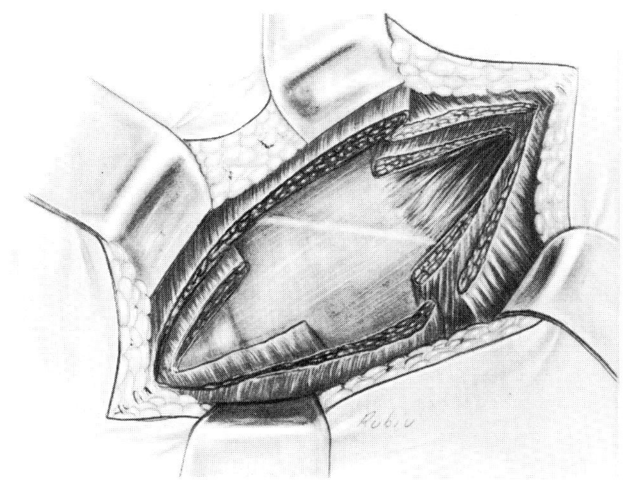

5

6

Division of lumbodorsal fascia

An incision is made into the lumbodorsal fascia in a somewhat more vertical direction than the main line of the incision so that the subcostal nerve is avoided. It can be recognized and dissected clear as the opening in the fascia is extended backwards as far as erector spinae. Blunt dissection forwards beneath the lumbodorsal fascia should proceed carefully to separate the parietal peritoneum from the deep layer of the transversus abdominis muscle, the fibres of which will separate as the fascial incision extends forwards. Careful haemostasis should be obtained and the subcostal neurovascular bundle may be retracted forwards or backwards to obtain the best access.

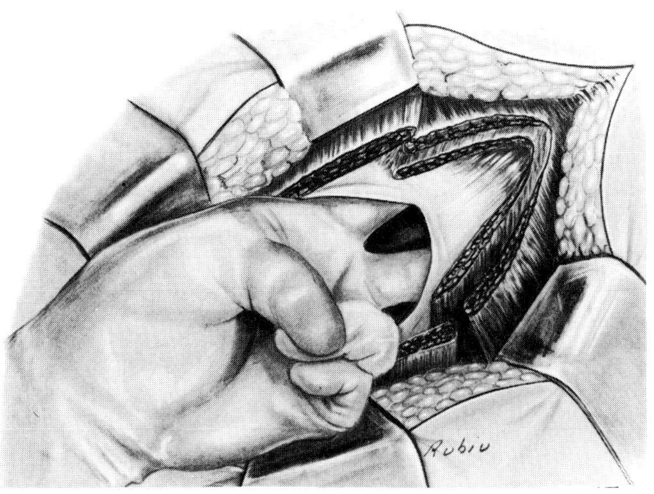

6

7

Exposure of the perinephric space

Retraction of the free edges of the lumbodorsal fascia allows for deep digital exploration of the posterior end of the wound and gentle gauze reflection forwards of the parietal peritoneum and extraperitoneal fatty tissue to expose the perirenal fascia. If the present exposure is considered to be inadequate, further upward retraction of the 12th rib will be facilitated by posterior extension of the incision of the anterior layer of the lumbodorsal fascia to include the external arcuate ligament, but any bleeding from subcostal vessels must be carefully controlled.

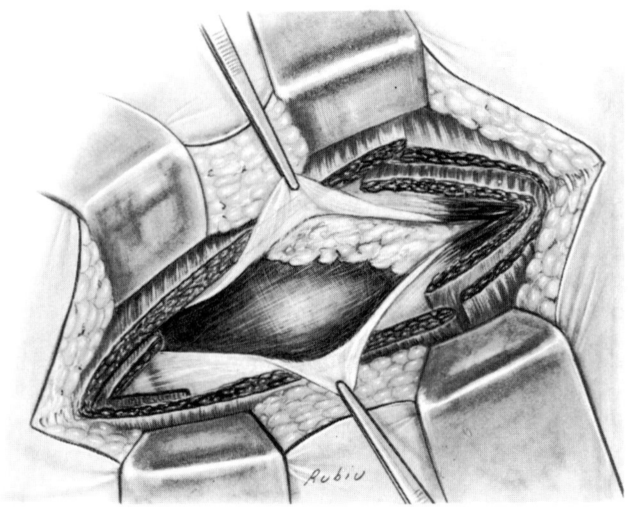

7

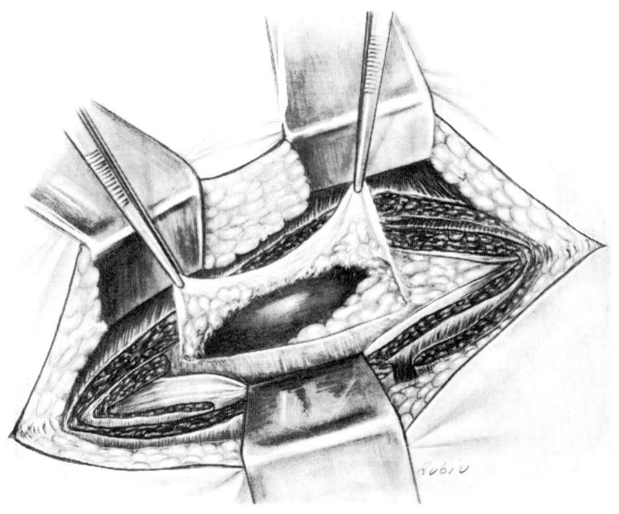

8

8

Incision of the perirenal fascia

A longitudinal cut with knife and then scissors is made through the perirenal fascia a short distance from and parallel to its reflection from the surface of the quadratus lumborum muscle. The anterior edge may be grasped in forceps and elevated to lift the perinephric fat to allow for gentle dissection and exposure of the capsular surface of the kidney.

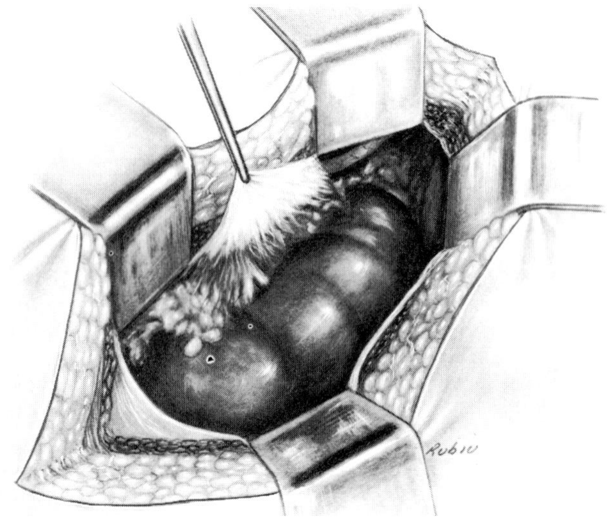

9

9

Exposure of the anterior surface and pedicle

Strong anterior retraction of the peritoneum will allow for continued forward dissection and elevation of the perirenal fascia, with displacement of the overlying abdominal organs. Gentle lateral traction on the kidney aids blunt dissection through the flimsy fascia to expose the pedicle in the hilum. In the presence of adhesions, the plane of the pedicle can more easily be entered after identification of the ureter, medial to the lower pole of the kidney, and by gentle upward dissection in the plane of the ureter and renal pelvis but with care to avoid segmental renal vessels.

10

Exposure of the posterior aspect

Recognition of the ureter near to the lower pole of the kidney is a useful guide into the plane of the renal pelvis. Access is facilitated by delivery of the lower pole of the kidney into the wound whilst the upper pole remains deep. Though the main pedicle usually lies anteriorly, all posterior dissection of the kidney should be careful and blunt in order not to jeopardize segmental renal vessels and ureteric blood supply.

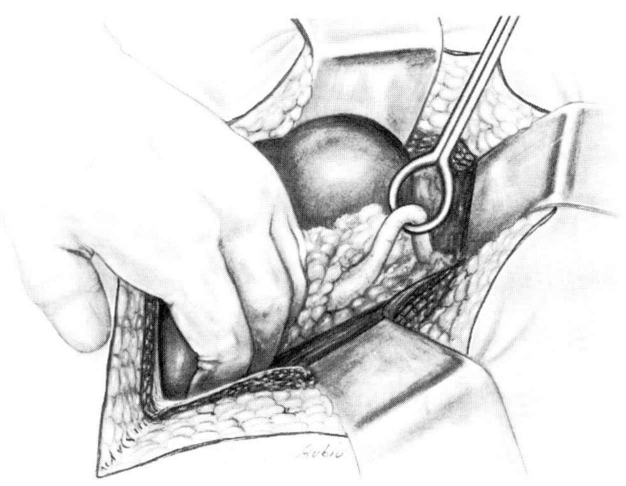

10

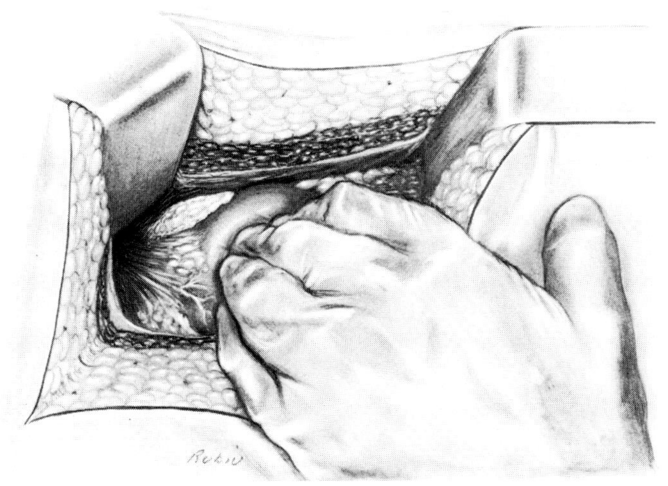

11

11

Exposure of the upper pole

Strong deep retraction of the posterior third of the wound rather than the posterior end of the incision, combined with downward and deep displacement of the kidney, will expose the upper renal pole and suprarenal gland. Strong fibrous brands intermingled with fat may adhere to the renal capsule and may contain quite large blood vessels.

TRANSCOSTAL APPROACH

12

Incision and exposure of rib

Accurate localization of the rib by palpation may be difficult until the skin, fat and superficial fascia have been divided. After subsequent identification a bold incision is made through the latissimus dorsi and serratus posterior inferior muscle onto the rib, which is steadied between fingertips placed in the 11th intercostal space and beneath the 12th rib. Incision should extend into the fascial attachments and periosteum of the outer surface of the rib with clearing of the external oblique muscle from the costal cartilage. Forward extension of the incision with division of the abdominal muscles is postponed until the rib has been resected.

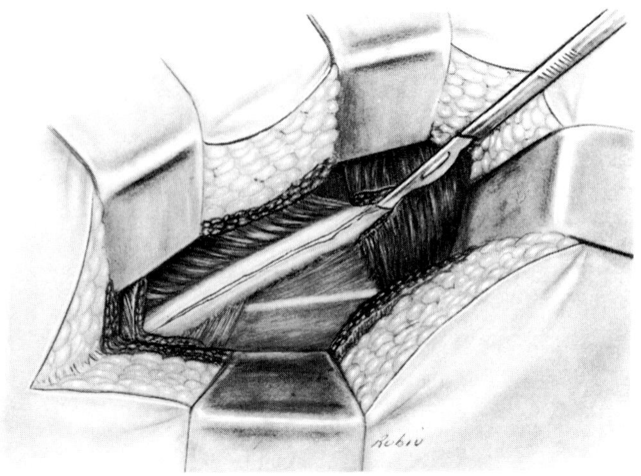

12

13

Excision of rib

The incised periosteum and its attachments on the outer surface of the rib are reflected to the upper and lower borders with a rougine or elevator. Safe and easy entry into the subperiosteal or extrapleural plane on the deep surface of the rib is obtained by careful passage of the rougine along the upper border of the rib from behind forwards and in the reverse direction along the lower rib border. This plane is carefully developed with a raspatory so that the rib is mobilized subperiosteally from the posterior angle to the costal cartilage. The posterior portion is divided with a costotome and the rib is elevated from its bed using a knife to divide the tip and margin of costal cartilage.

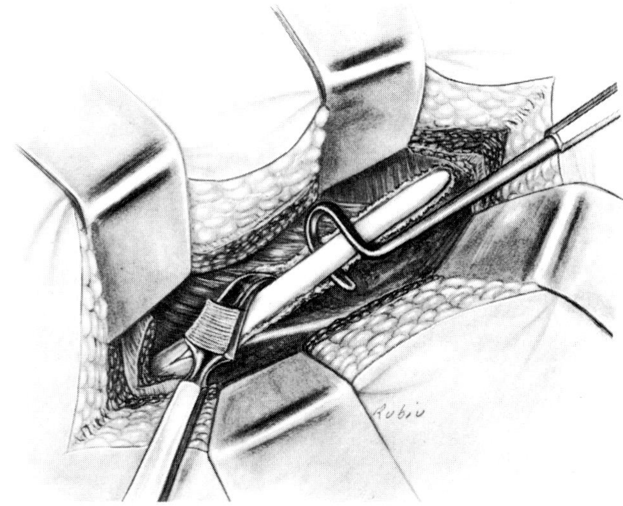

13

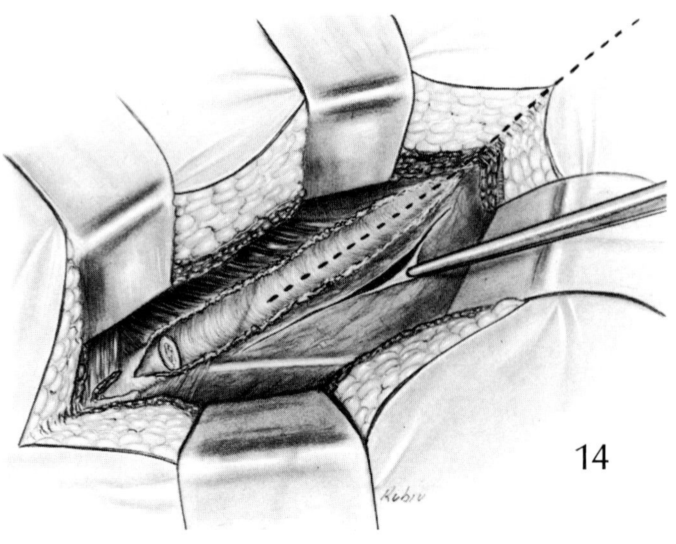

14

14

Division of abdominal muscles

The reflection of the pleura crosses deep to the periosteum of the rib bed. It may be difficult to identify and will restrict safe posterior extension of any incision through the rib bed into the extraperitoneal space. The subcostal neurovascular bundle should be identified as it leaves the lower margin of the rib bed beneath the lumbodorsal fascia. The fascia can be opened safely to avoid both the rib bed and the subcostal vessels and nerve, which can be dissected and displaced posteriorly to allow for easy access to the extraperitoneal space with forward extension of the incision into the abdominal wall muscles. This anterior dissection is similar to the subcostal approach as detailed in *Illustrations 5, 6* and *7*.

SUPRACOSTAL APPROACH

15

Mobilization of the rib

The skin incision extends along the whole length of the 11th rib and is deepened through the overlying muscle to expose but not incise the rib and is carried through the abdominal wall muscles for a short distance beyond the tip of the rib. The intercostal muscle is detached from the upper surface of the rib with a diathermy knife to leave the periosteum bare. A fingertip is inserted into the extrapleural space to protect the deep tissues as the extrapleural plane is developed. The supracostal release must extend posteriorly to allow for division of the posterior supracostal ligament so that the rib is free to rotate downwards at the costovertebral articulation.

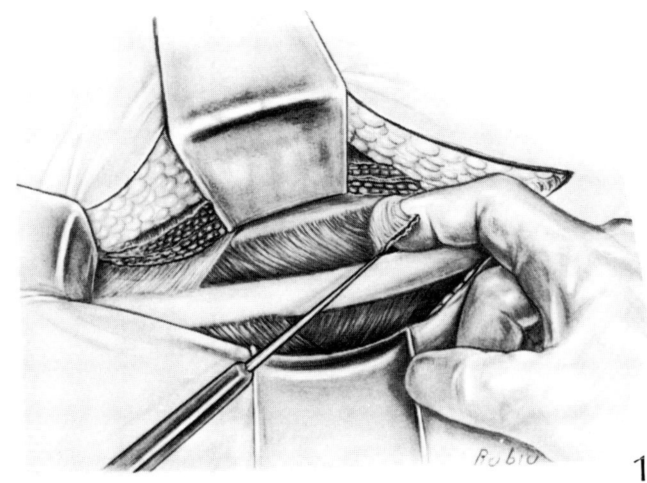

15

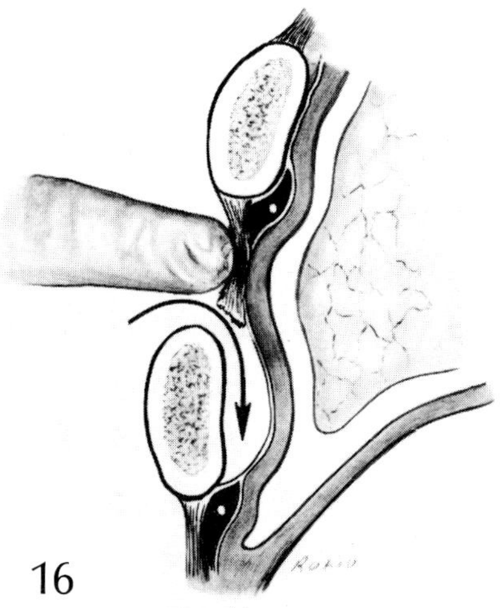

16

16

Release of the intercostal nerve

Incomplete division of the intercostal muscle leaves the innermost fibres intact so that they peel away from the rib with the extrapleural fascia as pressure is applied to the outside surface of the intercostal muscle. The extrapleural fascia splits along the lower border of the rib to enclose the intercostal nerve and the outer layer of fascia must be divided longitudinally with scissors in order to release the nerve and to allow for downward progression of the extrapleural dissection.

17

Division of the diaphragm

The diaphragm is divided as low down as possible to detach it from its origin but with preservation of its full length to facilitate closure. The 11th rib should retract downwards and backwards quite easily to give wide access to the subdiaphragmatic and retroperitoneal space. The peritoneum may be reflected forwards with concomitant fat to expose the perirenal fascia and suprarenal gland.

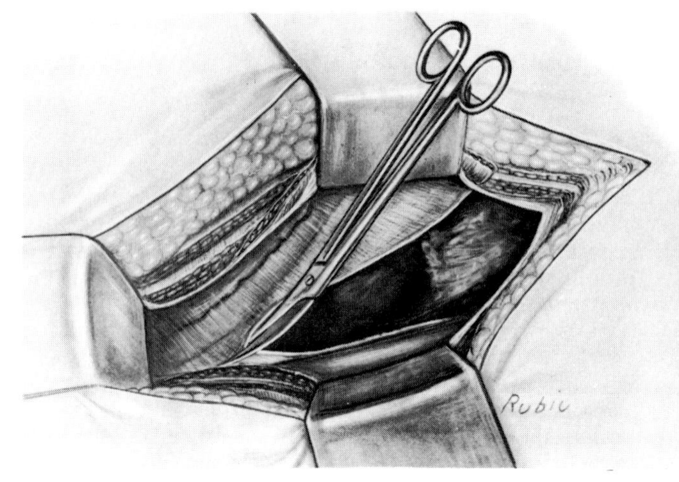

17

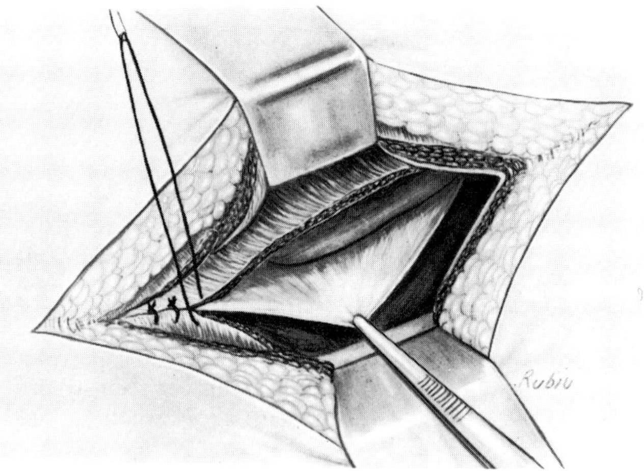

18

18

Closure of supracostal approach

The deeper closure with separation of the thoracic and abdominal compartments is accomplished by pulling the upper margin of the free edge of the incised diaphragm through the intercostal space so that it can be sutured to the intercostal muscles and to the muscles on the outer surface of the rib below, that is serratus posterior inferior posteriorly and latissimus dorsi anteriorly. Any pleural tear can also be approximated in these interrupted sutures after deliberate expansion of the lung by forced ventilation. The superficial muscles are closed in layers and any required drainage is effected through a separate stab incision below the subcostal nerve and 12th rib.

THORACOABDOMINAL APPROACH

19

Thoracotomy

Wide exposure of the kidney with easy access to the pedicle may be obtained by a transpleural approach through the bed of either the 10th or 11th ribs. The chosen rib is resected subperiosteally as described for the transcostal approach, with incision of overlying muscles including the latissimus dorsi, serratus posterior inferior posteriorly and some fibres of the external oblique muscle in the anterior portion of the wound. A similar exposure is afforded more easily by incision through the 9th or 10th intercostal space without rib resection. The superficial layers of muscle must be incised as far back as the lateral edge of the erector spinae.

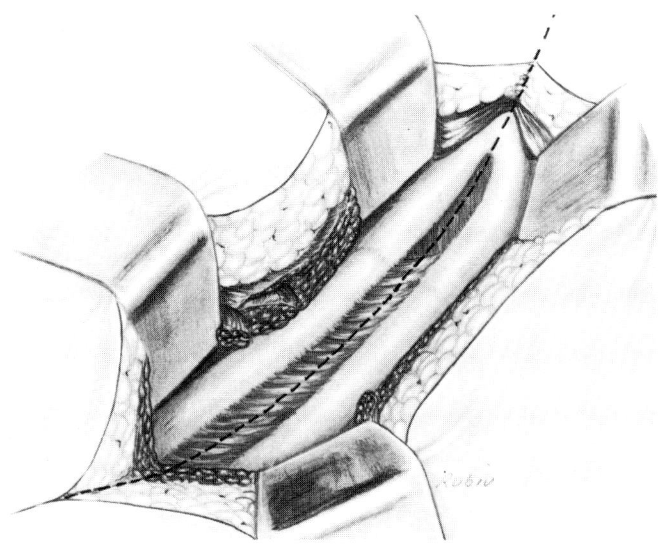

19

20

Exposure and incision of the diaphragm

Incision of the intercostal muscles, intercostal membrane, costal cartilage and underlying pleura exposes the lung, which collapses or is retracted to expose the diaphragm. The retroperitoneal space is then entered by division of the diaphragm and overlying pleura in the midportion of the wound. The diaphragmatic incision is then extended posteriorly towards the angle of the 12th rib so that adherent peritoneum may be dissected free from the undersurface of the diaphragm to allow for forward extension of the incision through diaphragm and the transversus abdominis muscle, which interdigitate. The wound is then extended forwards by incision of the abdominal wall muscles in a manner similar to the description for the anterior extraperitoneal approach (*see Illustrations 21* and *22*). The perinephric fascia is exposed by forward displacement of the subdiaphragmatic peritoneum and fat. The peritoneum may be incised in conjunction with the anterior extension of the thoracoabdominal approach to give extensive access to the abdomen.

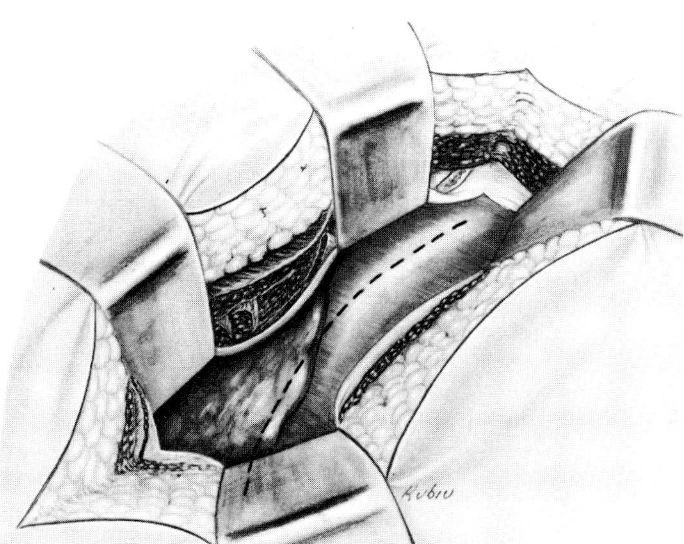

20

ANTERIOR EXTRAPERITONEAL APPROACH

21

Exposure of the peritoneum

The skin incision extends from the tip of the 10th rib to cross the lateral edge of the rectus abdominis muscle in the direction of the umbilicus. The external and internal oblique muscles are divided across the line of their fibres and bundles of the transversus abdominis muscle are gently separated to enter the extraperitoneal plane. Finger or gauze dissection between the peritoneum and the transversalis fascia must be gentle but extensive. The peritoneum becomes more adherent to the posterior rectus sheath in the anterior portion of the wound. Both the anterior and posterior layers of the sheath of rectus abdominis can be incised over a short distance to improve access through this approach, which can also be combined with thoracotomy.

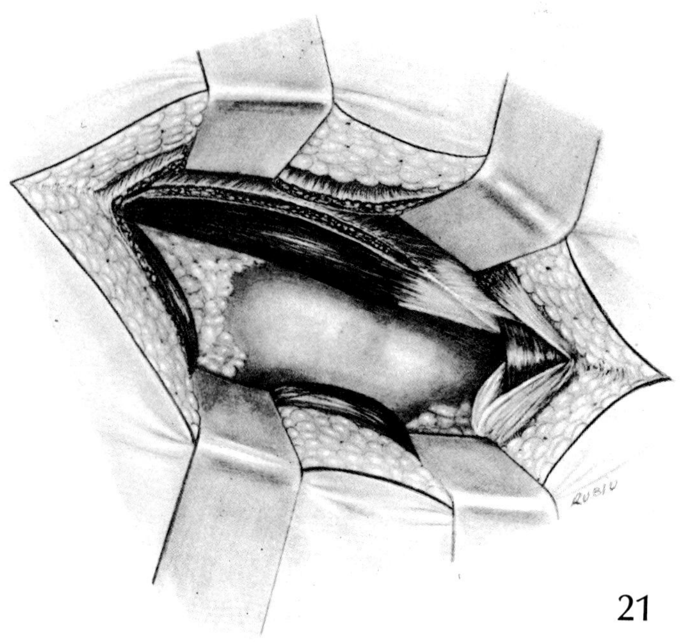

21

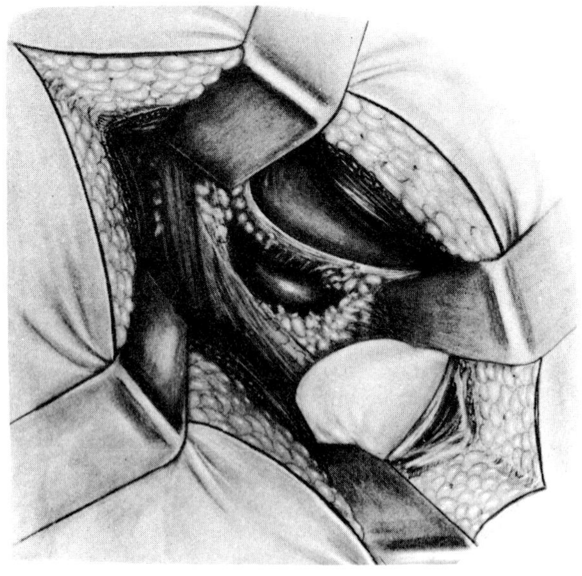

22

22

Retraction of the peritoneum

The extensive and lateral mobilization of the peritoneum allows it to be retracted medially so that the perinephric fascia is exposed on the stretch. The fascia is incised longitudinally, parallel to the renal axis and is mobilized medially with perinephic fat and peritoneum to expose the lower pole of the kidney, the pelviureteric junction and the upper spindle of the ureter.

RE-EXPOSURE OF THE KIDNEY

Most careful review of renal position and mobility and the nature of any previous renal surgery should precede the choice of incision for re-exposure. An alternative to the primary approach is usually desirable and the transcostal route is generally very much easier than direct surgery through the scar of a previous subcostal incision. Re-exploration is cautiously staged. Excessive tension in the parietes from lateral extension of the spine in the 'kidney position' must be avoided in order to prevent sudden splitting of any adherent kidney on the deep surface of the previous muscle closure as the incision is deepened and the wound edges separate. The extraperitoneal plane should be identified at the renal pole away from the major site of previous surgery. The peritoneum may be densely adherent on the lateral as well as the anterior aspects of the kidney and may be included in the scarring of previous drainage sites. Dissection may be started more easily around the upper ureter and a safe plane may be developed proximally to isolate the renal pedicle.

CLOSURE OF WOUNDS AFTER EXPOSURE OF KIDNEY

Despite careful haemostasis during surgery there is a tendency for serosanguinous oozing and there is sometimes risk of urinary leakage. Accordingly it is usually wise to institute drainage of the perinephric space with loose approximation of the perinephric fat and fascia around the drain using a few interrupted absorbable catgut sutures. Drains should be flexible and generally are more effective if corrugated rather than tubular in form. Gross drainage may be collected by surface applicator for measurement and analysis. Drains should be delivered in front of the midaxillary line where they can be included in muscular rather than fascial closure of the wound and will not cause added discomfort to the patient with change in lateral posture. Negligible drainage from the wound would encourage shortening of the drain by 2–3 cm each day and early removal from the retroperitoneal space discourages paralytic ileus.

In wound closure care should be taken to avoid suturing of intercostal or subcostal nerves. The initial deep sutures in the lumbodorsal fascia or rib bed should be placed at the posterior end of any loin wound before the bridge is lowered for the reduction of lateral spinal flexion to aid subsequent wound approximation. Wounds should be closed in separate muscle layers except when this is impracticable after re-exposure. Interrupted sutures of fine non-absorbable material are most dependable for the closure of clean wounds but this technique is time-consuming. Running sutures of 1/0 chromic catgut are a satisfactory alternative provided that independent interrupted sutures are placed on either side of any drain and in each muscle layer separately.

Diaphragmatic incisions must be securely approximated by a reinforced layer of interrupted horizontal mattress sutures of non-absorbable material other than silk. The parietal pleura and any periosteal bed of resected rib are carefully closed with a continuous suture of fine nylon before the parietal muscles are approximated with non-absorbable sutures. It is not necessary to approximate either the parietal pleura or the intercostal muscles in closing a thoracotomy through an intercostal space. The adjacent ribs are brought together and bound with interrupted ties of double 2/0 chromic catgut. The wound becomes airtight with approximation of the superficial muscles by a continuous suture of non-absorbable material. In closing the chest cavity care must be taken to re-expand the underlying lung and a soft intercostal catheter of size 32 Fr is inserted through a stab incision in the 8th intercostal space in the midaxillary line to provide for underwater sealed drainage.

The special technique for closure of the supracostal approach is shown in *Illustration 18*.

Postoperative care

Approaches to the kidney through the loin, lower thorax and retroperitoneal space predispose to pulmonary complications, tympanites and paralytic ileus. If the retroperitoneal dissection has been extensive and particularly in obese patients, oral fluids and food should be withheld and replaced by intravenous fluid and electrolyte therapy until there is evidence of adequate bowel tone. Chest physiotherapy with early mobilization of the patient, supported by analgesics and comfortable wound dressings, promote pulmonary expansion and avoid atelectasis.

Further reading

Nagamatsu, G. Dorsolumbar approach to the kidney and adrenal with osteoplastic flap. Journal of Urology 1950; 63: 569–577

Turner-Warwick, R. T. The supracostal approach to the renal area. British Journal of Urololgy 1965; 37: 671–672

Surgical anatomy and exposure of the ureter

Richard G. Notley MS, FRCS
Senior Consultant Urological Surgeon, Royal Surrey County Hospital, Guildford, Surrey, UK

Surgical anatomy

In the adult the ureter is a thick-walled tube about 24–30 cm in length which can be seen arising within the renal sinus as a funnel-shaped dilatation termed the renal pelvis. Into this open the calyces and the renal pyramids. The renal pelvis funnels down into the narrow ureter which runs caudally on the posterior abdominal wall, plastered to the muscles of the back by the parietal peritoneum. It runs along the surface of the psoas major muscle, across psoas minor if that muscle is present, in the line of the tips of the lumbar transverse processes and crossing the genitofemoral nerve to dip into the pelvic cavity in the region of the bifurcation of the common iliac vessels. During its downward course on psoas the ureter is crossed obliquely by the testicular or ovarian vessels.

On the right side the renal pelvis and upper ureter are usually covered by the second part of the duodenum, and, as it runs caudally, the ureter lies immediately lateral to the inferior vena cava where it is crossed by the right colic and ileocolic vessels. Just before it crosses the pelvic brim the right ureter passes behind the lower part of the small bowel mesentery. On the left the ureter is crossed by the left colic vessels and the pelvic mesocolon.

Having crossed the pelvic brim at the bifurcation of the common iliac vessels over the sacroiliac joint, the ureter continues its extraperitoneal course downwards as far as the spine of the ischium. The internal iliac artery and its branches, together with the obturator nerve, lie on its lateral side. Having reached the ischial spine, the ureter runs forwards and medially to reach the base of the bladder. As it turns forward it is crossed by the vas deferens in the male and the uterine artery in the female.

Throughout its length from the kidney to the bladder the ureter is closely applied to the parietal peritoneum lining the posterior abdominal wall and pelvis so that when the peritoneum is stripped up the ureter is elevated with it. This has the advantage of making surgical access to the ureter relatively simple, but this also means that the ureter is vulnerable to accidental ligature or clamping during the repair of the pelvic peritoneum after surgery. The lowermost part of the ureter may also be damaged during hysterectomy by inaccurate clamping of the nearby uterine artery. This part of the ureter is the most awkward to expose surgically, requiring division of the superior vesical pedicle and the obliterated umbilical artery (and sometimes the inferior vesical pedicle) to demonstrate its union with the base of the bladder.

The blood supply to the ureter is derived from several sources, but, unlike the gut, it receives no regular segmental blood supply. The renal pelvis and the upper ureter are supplied by branches of the renal artery or arteries. The lower ureter receives branches from the inferior and superior vesical arteries, and, in between these extremes, numerous variable vessels reach the ureter from the gonadal arteries and often, too, from the common iliac arteries. All these vessels make longitudinal anastomoses with each other in the adventitia of the ureter. The veins of the ureter drain into the renal, gonadal and internal iliac veins. The lymphatic vessels run back alongside the arteries, from the abdominal portion into the para-aortic lymph nodes and from the pelvic portion into the nodes alongside the internal iliac arteries on the pelvic side wall.

Exposure of the abdominal ureter

Surgical exposure of the ureter is most commonly required for the relief of ureteric obstruction by calculus. It may also be necessary for the relief of extrinsic obstruction, for the repair of injury or for removal of the ureter in combination with the kidney (for transitional cell carcinoma of the ureter or renal pelvis). The surgeon may also wish to expose the ureter in order to affect temporary or permanent diversion of the urine from the bladder.

Lying as it does in intimate relationship to the posterior parietal peritoneum, the ureter may be exposed either by the transperitoneal or extraperitoneal routes. If the object is to open the ureter, the problems of peritoneal contamination and urine drainage make the transperitoneal route less safe than the extraperitoneal, unless the intention is to join the ureter to the bowel intraperitoneally. Bilateral extrinsic obstruction of the ureters due to retroperitoneal fibrosis may be dealt with transperitoneally, but by far the most usual route of exposure is extraperitoneal.

The extraperitoneal approach to the ureter may be carried out either by the lumbar or the abdominal route, each having its own advantages. In general, in dealing with obstructive lesions and injuries, preliminary radiological investigation will permit accurate localization of the site to be exposed. When such accurate localization of the lesion can be achieved the abdominal extraperitoneal route affords good exposure of the required region and has the advantage for the patient of a smaller, anterior skin-crease incision. The exact site of the incision can be matched to the part of the ureter to be exposed, from renal hilum to pelvic brim (*see Illustration* 6). When the lesion is ill defined, or there is a risk that the obstructing calculus may dislocate upwards or downwards, wider exposure of the ureter may be required and the lumbar extraperitoneal approach is then indicated.

The anterior approach to the kidney and the upper ureter has much to commend it in the operation of nephroureterectomy. This approach to the kidney can be combined with the necessary lower abdominal incision without delay and without altering the position of the patient on the table, as will be necessary if the kidney is exposed by the lumbar route.

Position of patient

When the abdominal approach is used the patient is placed in a supine position on the operating table. A small sandbag placed behind the lower ribs on the affected side tilts the trunk sufficiently to facilitate the extraperitoneal approach to the ureter.

Positioning for a lumbar approach is more complex. The patient is placed on his side with the break point of the table level with the waistline. The lower thigh and knee should be flexed and the uppermost leg extended over them to stretch the lateral abdominal muscles, thus increasing exposure when the latter are divided. The table should then be 'broken' to its full extent to create as much lateral flexion of the spine as is feasible for that particular patient. In this way the loin to be operated upon is opened out as the incision proceeds. The patient should be stabilized in this position of full lateral flexion with the upper arm carried forward and secured to an angled arm-rest placed in front of the chest at the level of the shoulder. The pelvis is most conveniently fixed by a length of 3-inch non-stretch adhesive strapping passed across the hips at the level of the greater trochanter and fixed to the operating table on each side. An alternative to 'breaking' the table is to use inflatable pneumatic cushions beneath the loin to achieve the required lateral flexion. Whatever approach is used it is advisable for the surgeon to arrange the position of the patient to his own satisfaction before operating on the kidney or ureter.

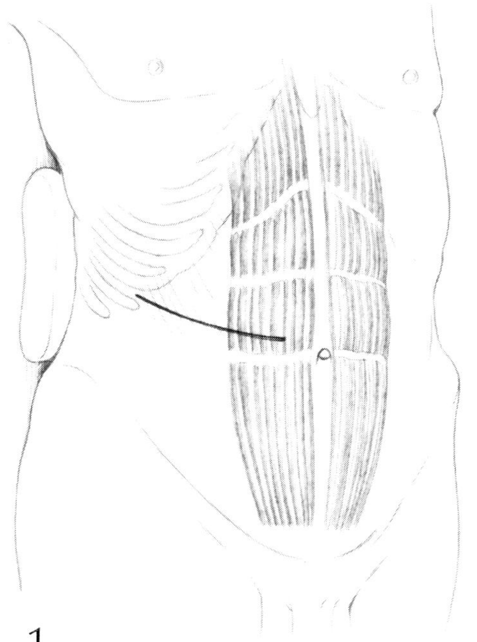

1

THE ANTERIOR APPROACH

1

With the patient supine and a small sandbag beneath the lower ribs on the side of the ureter to be exposed, the incision is planned. Study of the radiographs demonstrating the lesion enables an incision to be made which brings the surgeon accurately to the required part of the ureter. To reach the upper third of the ureter and the pelviureteric segment the incision should commence between the tips of the 10th and 11th ribs, crossing the costal margin laterally by 1 cm or so. The incision runs medially and slightly downwards in the line of the ribs to about midway across the rectus sheath, a total length of 12–15 cm being all that is necessary.

2

After the skin and subcutaneous tissues have been incised, the external oblique muscle fibres are demonstrated laterally, while more medially these fibres give way to aponeurosis which runs medially to form the rectus sheath, exposed at the medial end of the incision. The external oblique muscle fibres and its aponeurosis are divided in the line of the skin incision, the incision being carried on to the rectus sheath to expose the vertical fibres of the rectus muscle.

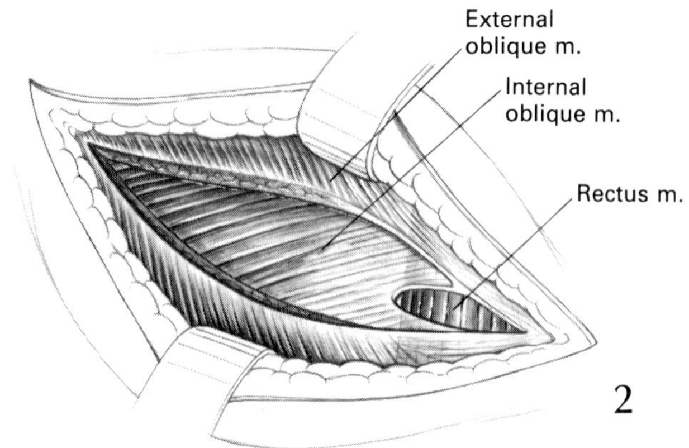

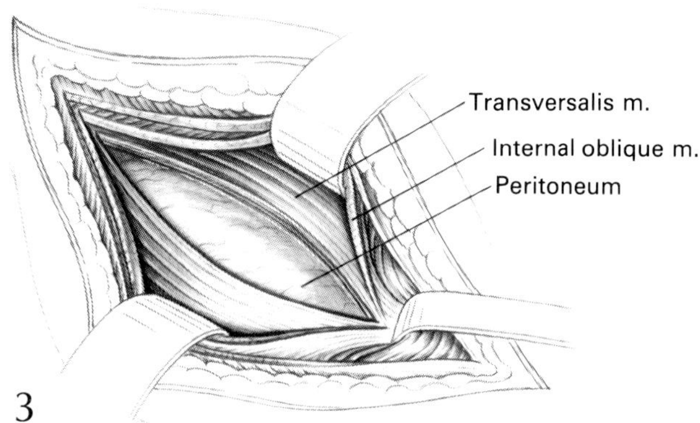

3

The exposed fibres of the internal oblique, running at right angles to those of the external oblique, are now incised to expose the horizontal fibres of the transversalis muscle. This incision is carried medially into the posterior rectus sheath for 1 cm or so, the rectus muscle being retracted medially to permit this. The transversalis muscle is split carefully along its fibres in the depths of the muscle incision to expose the underlying anterior parietal peritoneum.

4

The peritoneum is separated carefully from the anterior abdominal wall muscles. The more medial the incision the more adherent and delicate is the peritoneum and the more care is necessary to separate it from the overlying muscles without breaking its continuity. Gentle blunt dissection with the fingers is usually the most effective method of achieving separation of the intact peritoneum. Once the peritoneum is separated from the muscles for 2–3 cm along both edges of the incision the separation is carried laterally around the flank, down into the gutter lateral to the psoas muscle. The floor of this gutter is the quadratus lumborum muscle. The dissecting fingers must now climb anteriorly, up the steep side of psoas, before continuing the medial lifting of what is now the posterior parietal peritoneum until the great vessels are reached in the midline.

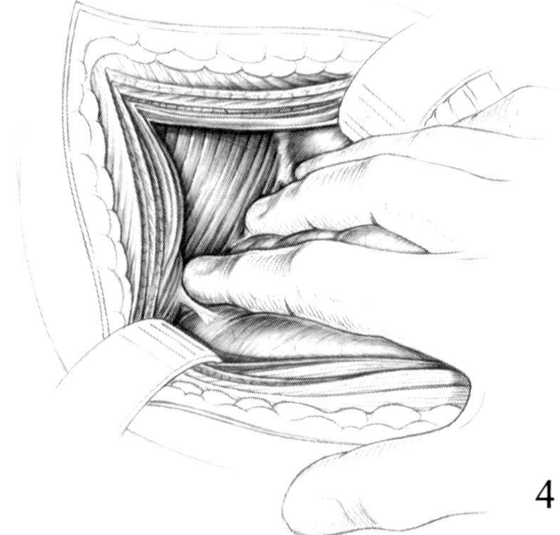

5

A suitable self-retaining retractor is inserted to separate the upper and lower edges of the incision. The peritoneum is retracted medially by an assistant using a wide-bladed, blunt retractor. The ureter is now identified, often lifted off the psoas with the peritoneum to which the ureter tends to adhere. The lower pole of the kidney is exposed and the union of pelvis and ureter can be visualized with a little blunt dissection medial to the kidney. Care must be taken to identify and preserve any lower polar vessels to the kidney during such dissection.

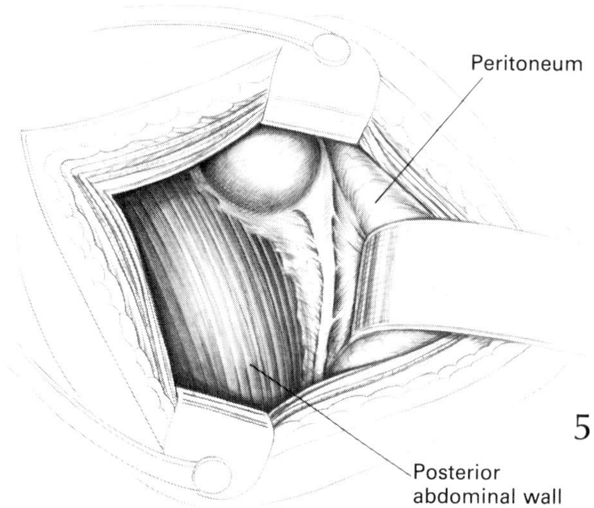

5

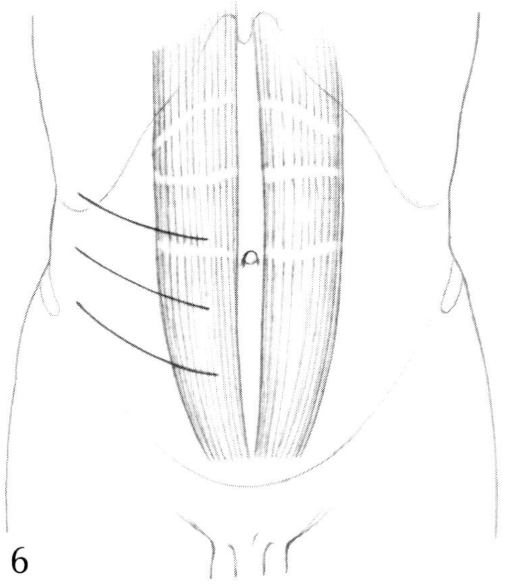

6

6

Access to the lower regions of the abdominal ureter may be obtained by siting the incision lower on the anterior abdominal wall. The precise level may be ascertained by accurate radiological localization of the lesion, but it is important to bear in mind that the lesion always seems to be located more cranially than may appear from the radiographs.

7

A precisely similar method of approach as described above will achieve access to the ureter at the pelvic brim, through the lowermost incision shown (see *Illustration* 6).

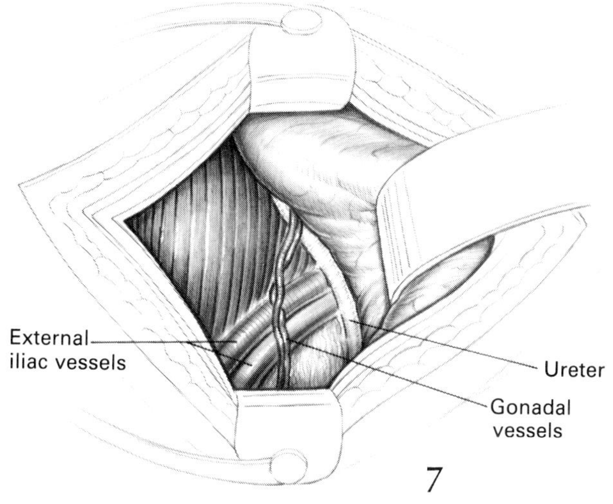

7

THE LUMBAR APPROACH

When localization of the lesion in the ureter is less precise, the lumbar approach to the abdominal ureter has advantages. The disadvantage to the patient of a long incision affecting his back and loin muscles is offset by the surgeon's ability to expose and explore the ureter from the renal hilum to the pelvic brim through a single incision. This approach has particular advantage if it is thought that the risk of upward dislocation of a calculus is high as the whole of the renal pelvis and kidney are accessible through a single incision.

8

With the patient in the lateral position an oblique incision is made in the loin. This incision may be the classical incision excising the anterior end of the 12th rib (see chapter on 'Surgical exposure of the kidney', pp. 702–713 in this volume) or it may be made as an intercostal incision between the 11th and 12th ribs. This incision necessitates careful localization of these ribs so that the knife passes accurately between them. After incision of the skin the anterior fibres of latissimus dorsi and the posterior part of the external and then the internal oblique muscles are divided in the same line. The aponeurotic fibres of transversalis may be pierced just above the tip of the 12th rib to enter the perinephric space and thus achieve early localization of the region to be explored. The fibres of transversalis then separate easily in the line of the incision in front of the surgeon's finger. The peritoneum pushes easily away.

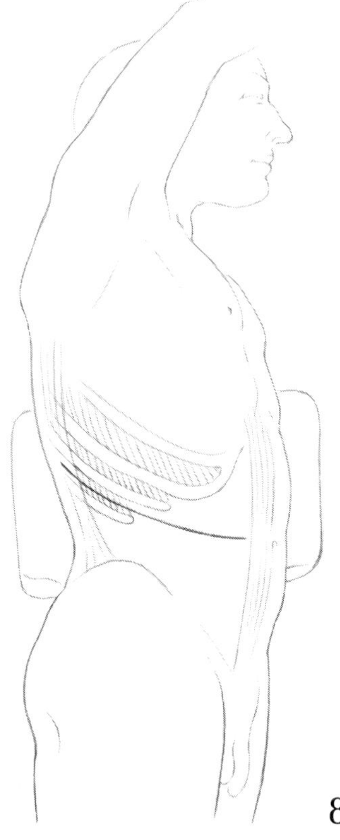

8

The intercostal neurovascular bundles will remain unseen in the layers of this incision if it is kept at the correct oblique angle, but it is wise to keep a sharp lookout for them as it is very easy to be a few degrees off course. By keeping fairly close to the upper edge of the 12th rib, damage to the 11th intercostal bundle can be avoided. As the incision in between the ribs is extended backwards it is necessary to watch out for the lower extent of the pleura which must be identified and preserved. This part of the incision can be deepened conveniently with scissors so that the pleura can be preserved, if necessary dividing some slips of diaphragm which come down to the 12th rib. If the pleura is inadvertently opened it is best left until the wound is being sutured at the end of the operation to effect proper closure. Under such circumstances it is usually not necessary to do more than ensure that the lung is fully inflated before closing the pleura with a continuous catgut suture. Underwater seal drainage to the pleural cavity is not usually necessary.

9

To complete the exposure the incision should be carried posteriorly into the paravertebral muscle mass until the articulation of the 12th rib can be freed from the transverse process. The 12th rib can be swung down and the incision held wide open with a suitable self-retaining retractor. Blunt dissection then enables the posterior peritoneum to be lifted forward to expose the ureter from renal hilum to pelvic brim after opening the perinephric space. The kidney and upper ureter may also be exposed from behind by way of the lumbotomy incision. The exposure of this region through a vertical posterior lumbotomy incision is slightly more difficult. However, it permits a smoother and shorter postoperative course with minimal morbidity. The approach has great advantages where exposure of the kidney is concerned, but for the upper ureter it has little or no advantage over the anterior approach outlined above.

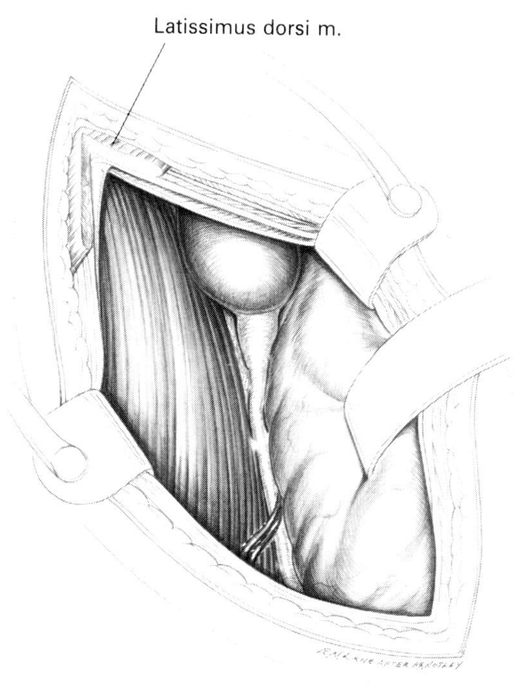

9

Wound closure

Both the anterior and lumbar approach incisions to the ureter require accurate, layer-by-layer closure of the separated muscles. It is a matter of personal choice whether absorbable or non-absorbable sutures are used or whether the sutures are continuous or interrupted as long as the stitches do not strangulate the closed muscles. Drainage of the ureter after incision of its wall is essential; a tube drain placed adjacent to the site is brought out below the main incision and connected to a drainage bag. This drain may be removed as soon as it ceases to drain significant amounts and in all cases should be removed by the 4th or 5th day after operation. The temptation to leave it in position any longer should be resisted even if large amounts of urine are still draining. A drain of this kind offers the line of least resistance for the escape of urine and may perpetuate a urinary fistula which would close spontaneously within a day or two after removal of the drain as long as no distal ureteric obstruction remains.

Exposure of the lower ureter and ureterolithotomy

R. E. Williams MD, ChM, FRCS(Ed), FRCS
Consultant Urologist, The General Infirmary and
St James's University Hospital, Leeds, UK

Principles

Ureterolithotomy is probably the commonest indication for exposure of the lower ureter. Other indications include nephroureterectomy; the repair of injuries, usually following pelvic surgery; urinary diversion by ileal conduit, ureterosigmoidostomy or cutaneous ureterostomy; the relief of ureteric obstruction from extrinsic causes such as retroperitoneal fibrosis or tumour.

Methods of approach

The ureter runs retroperitoneally throughout its course, has a close relationship to the posterior parietal peritoneum and is usually approached extraperitoneally. While it can be approached by the transperitoneal route, this may lead to extravasation of urine into the peritoneal cavity with the risk of infection, and this approach is used only when ureterointestinal anastomosis is intended or when fibrosis or disease has obliterated the extraperitoneal plane. Extraperitoneal exposure may also be difficult when there is severe spinal deformity.

Preliminary investigation with intravenous urography, retrograde ureterography or micturating cystography will have provided the diagnosis, an indication of the site of the ureter to be exposed and the functional activity of both kidneys.

Position of patient

The patient is placed on the operating table in the supine position and dissection deep in the pelvis is made easier if the head end of the table is tilted downwards and if the bladder is empty.

Anaesthesia

The operation is usually done under a general anaesthetic using an endotracheal tube and a suitable muscle relaxant drug.

The cross-reference in this chapter refers to *Operative Surgery: Urology, 4th Edition*

Exposure of the lower ureter

1

The incisions

The ureter follows the curve of the cavity of the pelvis from the brim downwards and is deeply placed in the pelvis as it approaches the bladder. A modified *Gibson oblique incision* (A) may be used; this begins near the anterosuperior iliac spine and curves inwards and medially to a point above the symphysis pubis. If disease is suspected in the bladder also, a lateral extension of the *Pfannenstiel transverse suprapubic incision* (B) will give satisfactory exposure of bladder and lower ureter. The most popular incisions are by an extraperitoneal approach through a *midline incision* (C), extending from the umbilicus to the symphysis pubis, or through a *paramedian incision* (D), especially if transperitoneal exposure is intended for urinary diversion.

In female patients a catheter is passed to ensure an empty bladder, and in male patients the external genitalia are prepared and draped as well as the lower abdominal wall so that a urethral catheter can be passed at any time during the operation. If preliminary cystoscopy has been done, one should make sure the bladder is empty at the end of that procedure.

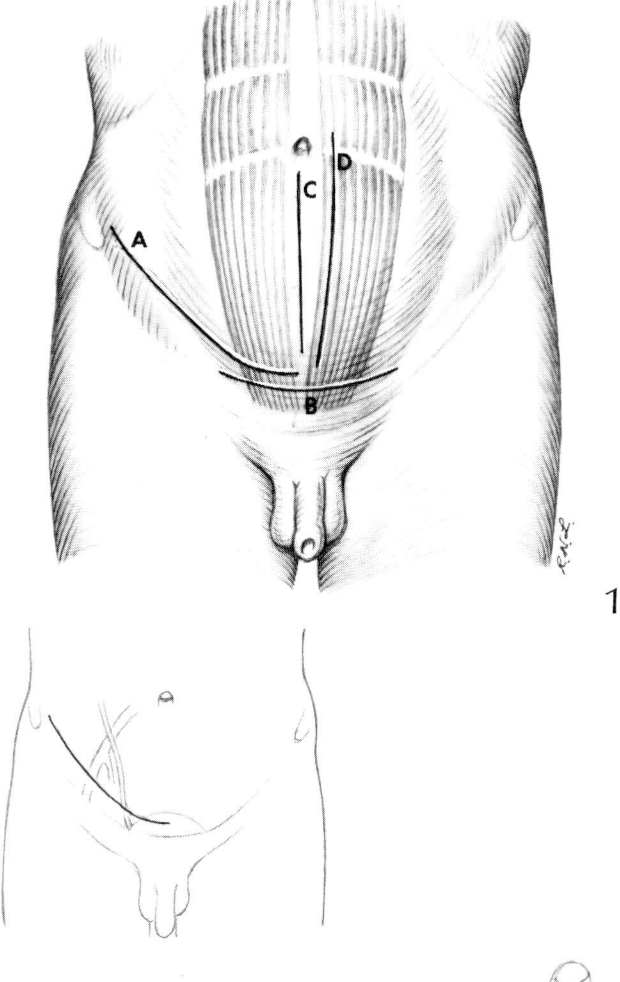

1

2

Modified Gibson incision

This hockey stick incision runs parallel to the inguinal fold and 2.5 cm above it. It starts 2.5 cm medial to the anterosuperior iliac spine and curves inwards and medially to a point one finger's breadth above the symphysis pubis; it may be extended to the opposite side. The skin, superficial fascia and external oblique aponeurosis are divided in this line, as are the external oblique muscle fibres. Medially, the rectus fascia can be divided to the midline and the belly of the rectus muscle retracted medially without being incised. The external and internal oblique muscle fibres may be split bluntly with the scalpel handle or divided with the scalpel blade. The transversalis fascia should be divided carefully by lifting it with forceps, making a nick in it and then separating off the underlying peritoneum by blunt dissection. This is continued until the peritoneum can be retracted medially to expose the ureter in the retroperitoneum where it may remain adherent to the posterior surface of the peritoneum. It may be necessary to divide the deep epigastric vessels and also sometimes the uterine artery overlying the ureter in the female. The ureter is identified high in the incision, encircled by loops and traced downwards.

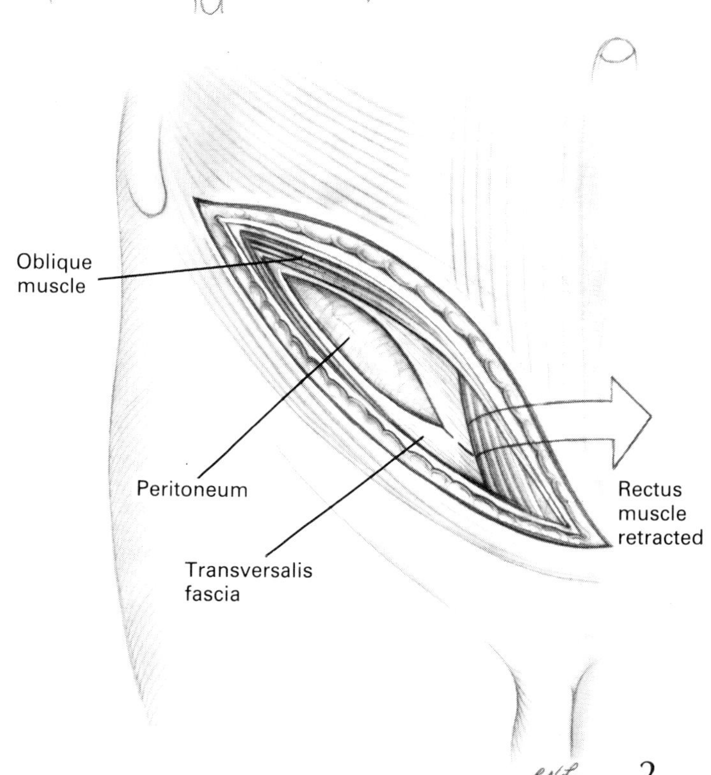

2

The Pfannenstiel approach

This incision may be satisfactory if there is no need to expose the ureter at a higher level than the true pelvis, if there are other lesions affecting the bladder which have to be dealt with simultaneously or if a bilateral approach to the lower ureters is indicated. It heals well with a minimum of scarring but identification of the ureter in the depth of the pelvis may prove to be rather more difficult than when this structure has been identified previously at a higher level as in the other incisions. A slightly curved transverse suprapubic incision is carried through skin, subcutaneous fascia and rectus sheath, after which the rectus bellies may be spread laterally.

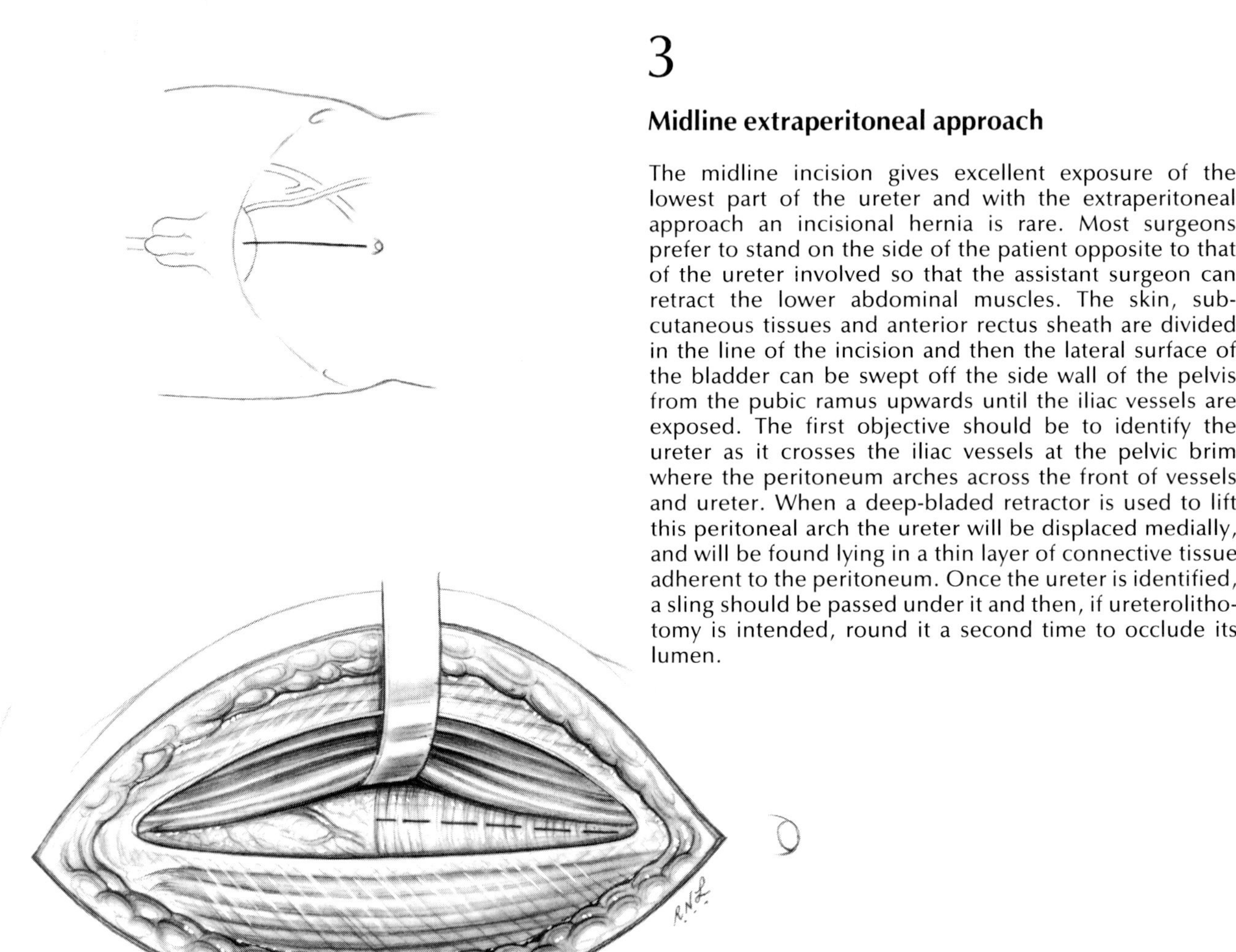

3

3

Midline extraperitoneal approach

The midline incision gives excellent exposure of the lowest part of the ureter and with the extraperitoneal approach an incisional hernia is rare. Most surgeons prefer to stand on the side of the patient opposite to that of the ureter involved so that the assistant surgeon can retract the lower abdominal muscles. The skin, subcutaneous tissues and anterior rectus sheath are divided in the line of the incision and then the lateral surface of the bladder can be swept off the side wall of the pelvis from the pubic ramus upwards until the iliac vessels are exposed. The first objective should be to identify the ureter as it crosses the iliac vessels at the pelvic brim where the peritoneum arches across the front of vessels and ureter. When a deep-bladed retractor is used to lift this peritoneal arch the ureter will be displaced medially, and will be found lying in a thin layer of connective tissue adherent to the peritoneum. Once the ureter is identified, a sling should be passed under it and then, if ureterolithotomy is intended, round it a second time to occlude its lumen.

Paramedian extraperitoneal approach

In the paramedian approach the rectus sheath is incised longitudinally, the muscle is retracted laterally and the posterior rectus sheath is divided in the upper third of the wound to expose the peritoneum throughout the length of the incision. The peritoneum may be separated from the parietal pelvic wall for the extraperitoneal approach or opened for the transperitoneal approach.

Ureterolithotomy

Preoperative

Indications

A round or oval ureteric stone less than 5 mm wide which has a smooth surface is likely to pass spontaneously. A stone larger than 5 mm wide which has a spiculated surface and has not descended in the ureter after 1 week's observation is less likely to pass. Other factors that would indicate surgical removal of the stone are urinary infection and evidence of persistent ureteric obstruction as shown by ureteric dilatation on X-ray or by impaired renal function. Recurrent attacks of severe colic without progression of the stone are also an indication for operative relief. Sometimes a stone may lie symptomless in the ureter for many months and there may be gradual onset of renal damage. In the author's opinion, a stone that has not moved after 1 year should be removed, even though it is not producing symptoms.

Preoperative procedure

Usually an intravenous urogram will have been performed to establish the diagnosis. If the patient is in pain a dense nephrogram will develop with delayed excretion of contrast medium on the affected side and the appearance of a dilated collecting system. Follow-up films may be required at 12 hour intervals before function is sufficient to outline the ureter down to the site of the stone. A stone in the lower ureter may be obscured by the dye in the bladder unless a satisfactory postmicturition film is obtained. If the patient is not in pain, the ureter will fill quickly with dye. When more than one suspicious opacity is present, an oblique film will demonstrate which opacity is within the ureter. It is essential that a plain X-ray of the renal tract be taken on the way to the operating theatre to confirm the position of the stone before surgical exposure is begun.

If urinary infection is present preoperative antibiotics should be given but it is unlikely that the infection will be cleared completely until the obstructing stone is removed.

Preliminary cystoscopy and ureteric catheterization should not be done unless there is some doubt about the diagnosis of a ureteric stone. If a ureteric catheter is passed up to or beyond the suspicious opacity, X-rays with anteroposterior and oblique views will confirm whether or not it is in the ureter. The ureteric catheter may be left in place to help identify the ureter at operation. Care must be taken to ensure that the stone is not pushed into a dilated upper ureter. If no opaque stone can be seen on plain X-ray, retrograde ureterography may demonstrate the presence of a uric acid stone, a ureteric tumour or a sloughed renal papilla. The bladder should be emptied before removing the cystoscope.

Initial stages

When ureterolithotomy has been decided upon, the ureter should be exposed by any of the methods described previously. The author's preference is for a lower abdominal midline incision.

The operation

4a & b

Identification of stone

Often a large stone can be palpated easily and this may help in the identification of the ureter. More often it will be too small to feel or will be surrounded by periureteric fibrosis, and in all cases it is better to identify the ureter at the pelvic brim and dissect downwards from there. The ureter is secured with a controlling tape passed round it twice and then is followed under the arcades of blood vessels crossing from the internal iliac vessels to the bladder.

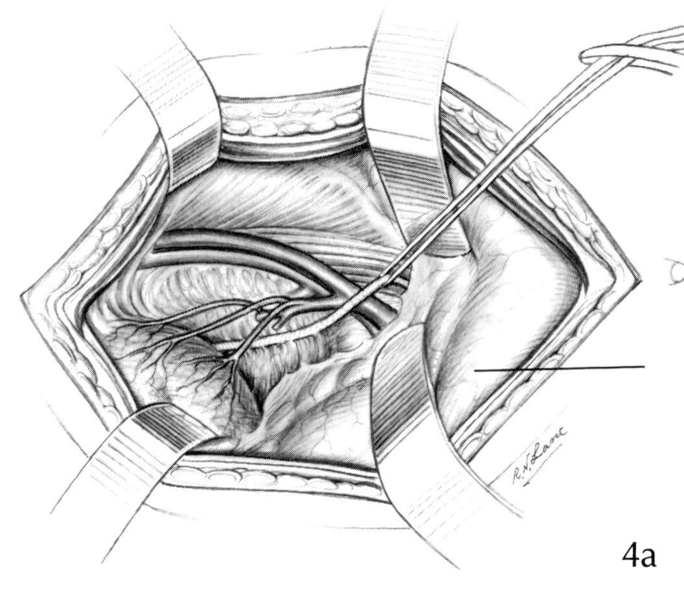

4a

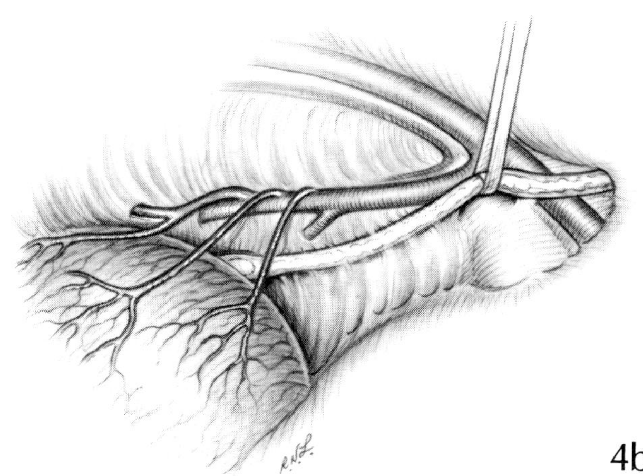

4b

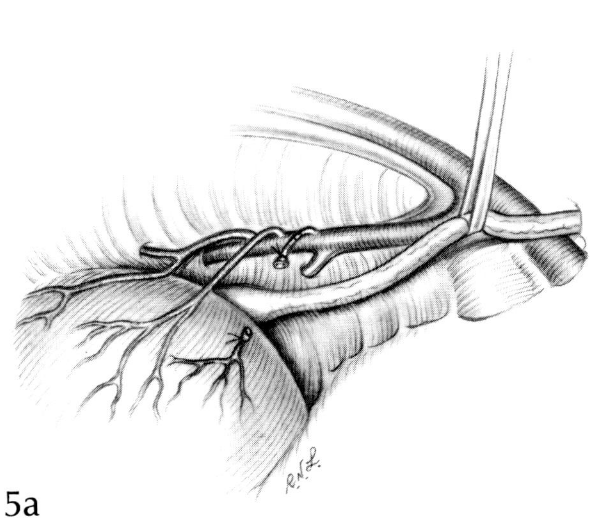

5a

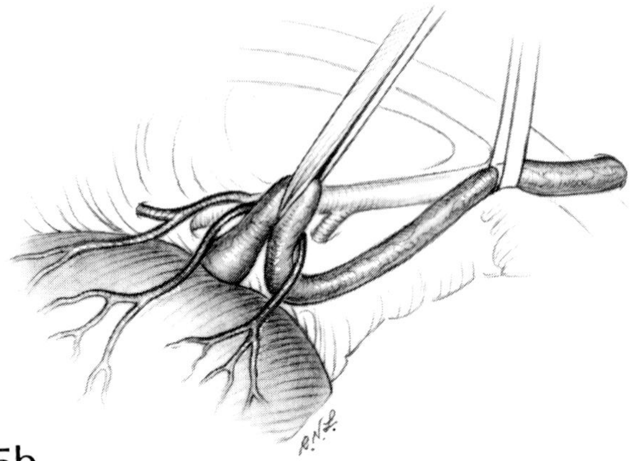

5b

5a & b

Sometimes it is advantageous to divide these arcades (*a*) while on other occasions the ureter can be pulled out through an opening in the arcades and another tape placed round it there (*b*). Care should be taken to avoid injuring the ureteric vessels which run parallel to the ureter. The dissection is continued downwards until the stone can be felt through the wall of the ureter. If the stone is very low in position it may be necessary to dissect the intramural portion of the ureter. The final arcade of vessels covering the stone may be ligated and divided if this makes exposure of the terminal ureter easier. At this stage another sling may be passed round the ureter below the stone.

6

Incision

A longitudinal incision can then be made into the ureteric wall on to the stone and the stone can be removed. The ureter must never be opened unless it is certain the stone is present there.

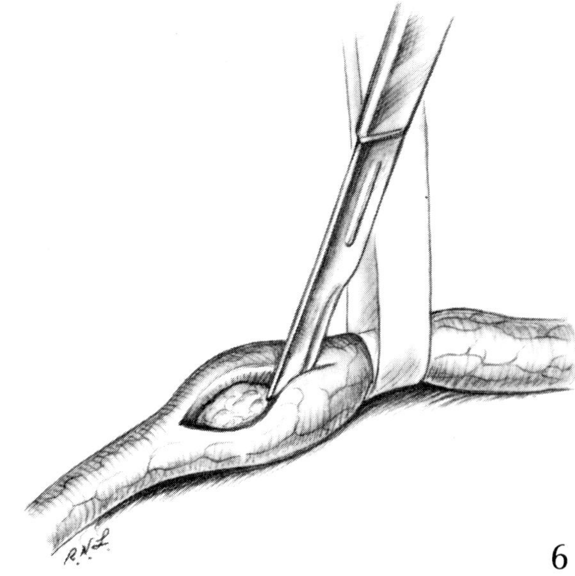

6

7, 8 & 9

Removal of stone

The stone may be removed by using gentle leverage with a blunt dissector and then grasping it with a pair of stone forceps. It is important to make sure that removal is complete and that no fragments have been left behind. If the proximal tape is loosened a flow of urine will appear and some of this can be sent for bacteriological culture.

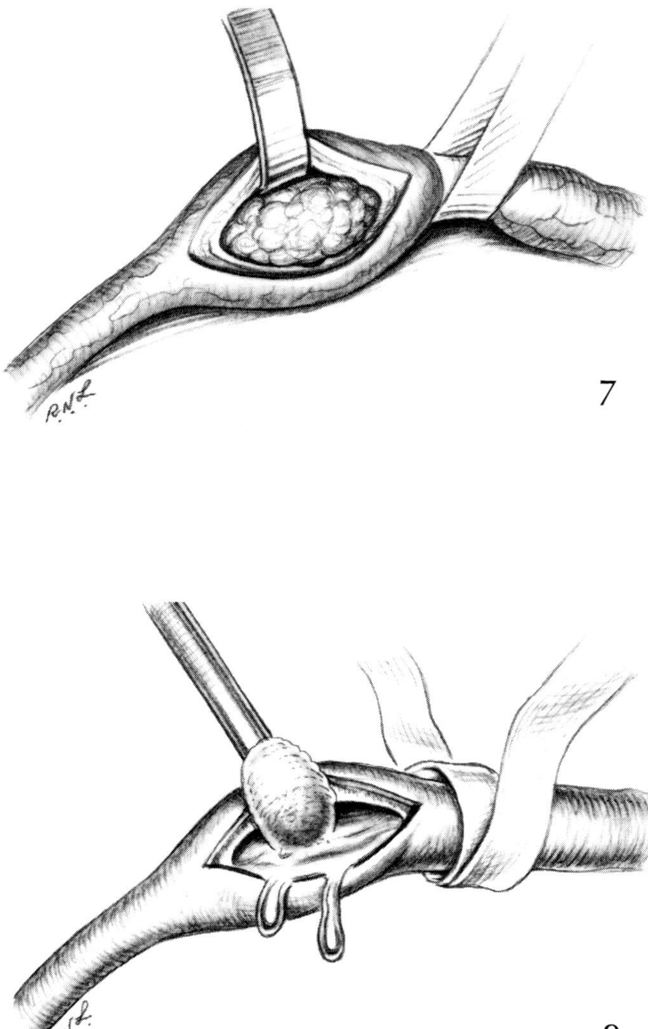

7

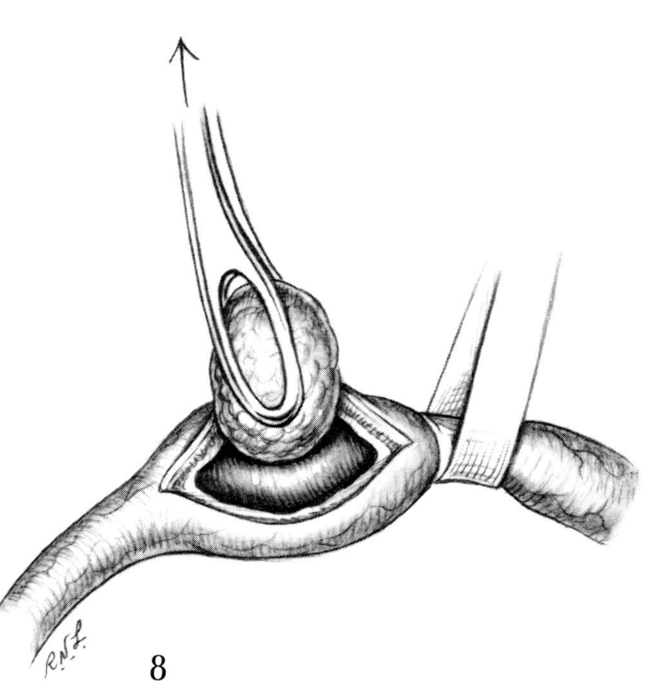

8

9

10

Patency of distal ureter

Once the stone is removed it is essential to ensure that the ureter below that level is not obstructed by a further calculus which might lead to a urinary fistula. A large catheter, preferably of the Braasch bulb type, should be passed down into the bladder.

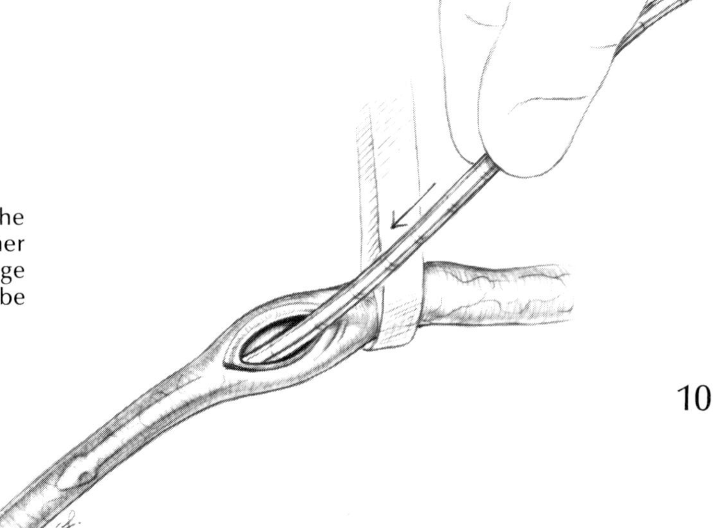

10

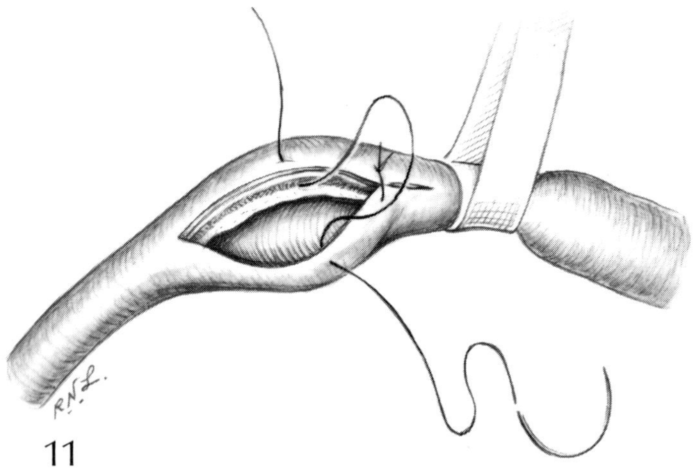

11

11

Closure of incision in ureter

A few interrupted sutures of plain catgut may be placed in the ureteric wall to include the fibrous and muscular coats only. There is no evidence that these sutures help ureteric healing and many surgeons believe that suturing of this incision may be omitted.

Drainage and closure of the wound

A drain is passed through a separate stab incision down to the opening in the ureter. The main wound may now be closed in layers. The drain should be shortened on the third or fourth postoperative day and removed on about the fifth or sixth day depending on the volume of leaking urine.

The removed stone should be sent for analysis.

SPECIAL PROBLEMS

No stone can be found

In these circumstances either the ureter has not yet been dissected far enough down into the pelvis, the stone may have slipped down into the bladder or the suspected opacity may never have been a stone at all! The ureter should be followed into its intramural portion and palpated carefully. If necessary, an X-ray is taken of the patient's abdomen on the operating table to see if the opacity is still present. If the position is still the same, the bladder is opened and a metal probe passed up the ureter until it can be felt to grate on the stone; if necessary further X-rays are taken with oblique and anteroposterior views. If all these attempts fail, the bladder and the wound are closed. The ureter must never be opened unless the stone can be identified with certainty.

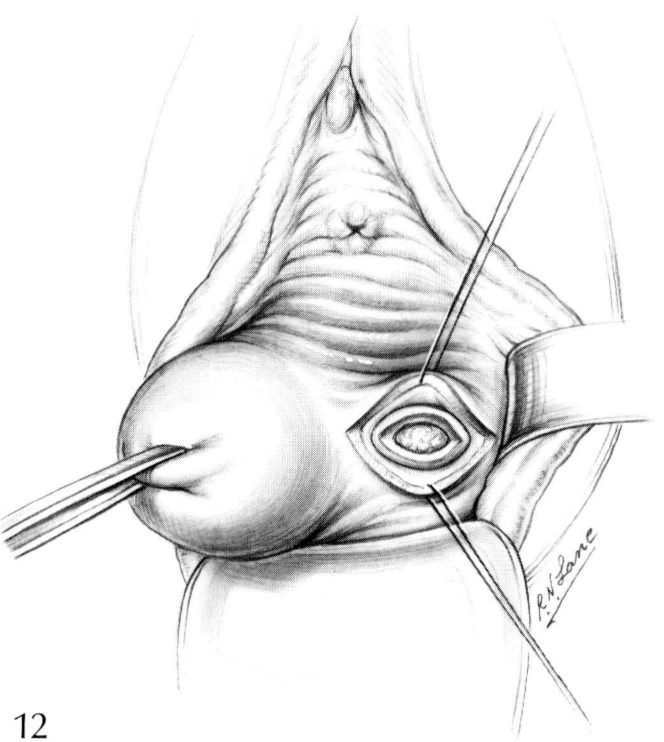

12

Repeat ureterolithotomy

When a previous ureterolithotomy has been done and now a new stone has formed and lodged at the same site in the ureter, further surgery there may prove difficult. Often, dense adhesions around the ureter will prevent extraperitoneal dissection and it may be necessary to open the peritoneal cavity, mobilize the caecum on the right or the sigmoid colon on the left and remove the stone intraperitoneally. In these circumstances urinary leakage may be lessened if a stent is left in the ureter, if the peritoneum is closed over the ureter and if an extraperitoneal drain can be left down to the site of the incision.

Persistent urinary leakage

If urine continues to leak from the drainage site after the 12th postoperative day, an X-ray of the abdomen should be taken to make certain that no further calculi are present and then a ureteric catheter should be passed at cystoscopy under anaesthesia. This ureteric catheter may be kept in place by attaching it to a Foley catheter in the bladder and left for several days until the leakage stops.

12

VAGINAL URETEROLITHOTOMY

This method has limited usefulness but may be used when an easily palpable stone can be felt in the vaginal fornix. With a vaginal speculum holding back the posterior wall, the cervix is grasped with forceps and pulled downwards and towards the contralateral side. An incision is made through the vaginal wall at the lateral margin of the cervix and extended outwards. The vaginal mucosa is dissected to expose the ureter and care must be taken to avoid the uterine vessels. Babcock clamps placed on either side of the stone may prevent it from being dislodged. A longitudinal ureteric incision allows the stone to be removed and the distal ureter to be probed. The ureteric wall should be carefully sutured and the vaginal mucosa closed over it except where a small soft rubber drain has been placed (*see* chapter on 'Vaginal ureterolithotomy', pp. 240–242).

Nephrostomy

W. Scott McDougal MD
Professor and Chairman, Department of Urology,
Vanderbilt University Medical Center, Nashville, Tennessee, USA

Introduction

Percutaneous nephrostomy performed under radiological control and internal ureteral stenting with the double J catheter have markedly reduced the frequency with which open nephrostomy must be performed. The latter provides an internal drainage route and is generally preferred when technically possible over nephrostomies which require an external appliance. There are situations, however, in which open nephrostomy is indicated, either as an adjunctive or as a primary procedure. Such circumstances might include drainage of the pelvis following ureteral pelvic junction repair, following renal stone surgery in which fragments cannot be completely removed, during exploration for trauma when associated duodenal, pancreatic or great vessel injuries occur concomitantly with significant ureteral or pelvic disruptions, following partial nephrectomy and following drainage of perinephric and intranephric abscesses. It may also be used as a primary procedure in rare circumstances where drainage of the kidney cannot be conveniently established by internal means.

There are two types of nephrostomy: single tube and loop nephrostomy. The latter has the advantage of two ports – an irrigation and drainage port. This is particularly useful for continuous irrigation for retained calculi.

Complications

Complications of the procedure include haemorrhage from the nephrotomy site, injury to the renal and/or great vessels, disruption of the ureteral-pelvic junction, calculus formation, pyelonephritis, perinephric abscess, sepsis, and duodenal, splenic and pancreatic injury.

The operations

Position of patient

The patient is placed in the lateral decubitus position with the table flexed as for a standard flank approach to the kidney.

SINGLE TUBE NEPHROSTOMY

The kidney is exposed and a small transverse pyelotomy made in the renal pelvis. The nephrostomy should be placed in the lower pole calyx and exit directly, in a straight line to the skin.

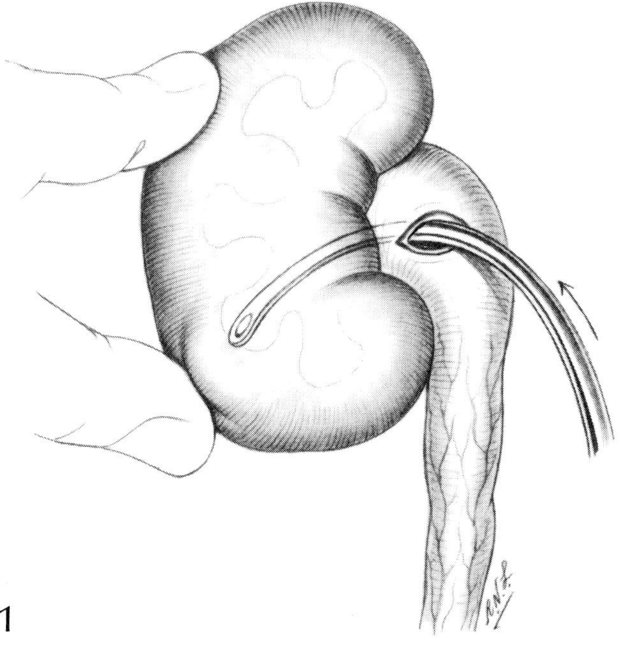

1

1

A transverse pyelotomy is made and a curved Randall stone forceps is gently passed into the inferior pole calyx.

2

A small incision is made in the parenchyma immediately over the stone forceps and it is pushed through the incision. A suture is looped through the Randall stone forceps and tied to a 16 Fr or 18 Fr Foley, Malecot or de Pezzer catheter. The catheter should be larger in size than the nephrotomy site in order to provide parenchymal tamponade.

The catheter is pulled into the renal pelvis, the loop suture cut and removed, and the balloon inflated if a Foley is used. If a Malecot or de Pezzer catheter is used, flanges must be maintained on stretch as they penetrate the renal parenchyma. The disadvantage of the latter catheters is that they cause considerable trauma upon their removal in the postoperative period.

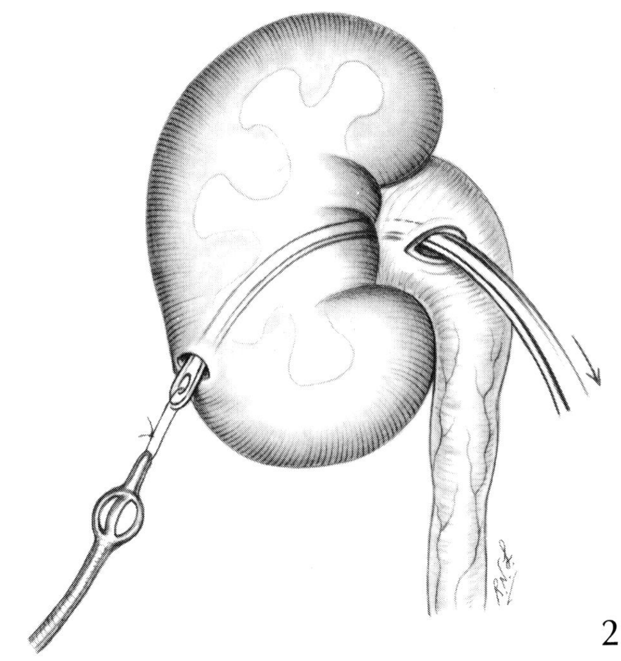

2

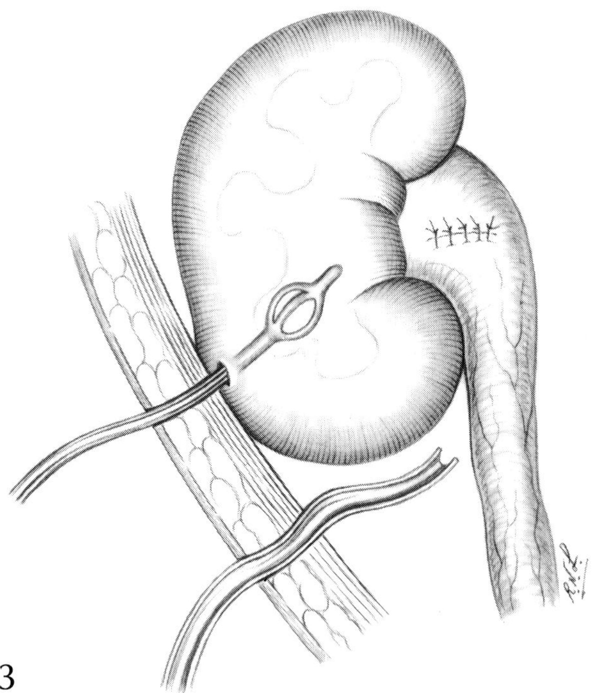

3

3

The pyelotomy is closed, the area drained, Gerota's fascia reapproximated and the nephrostomy tube brought out in a straight line to the skin.

The nephrostomy tube should be situated, if possible, in the anterior aspect of the flank so that the patient can change the catheter with some ease if necessary. The tube should also be secured to the skin with a non-resorbable suture. It should not be brought out through the incision, but rather through a separate stab wound. A straight course into the pelvis facilitates replacement of the catheter.

LOOP NEPHROSTOMY

4

In this instance the catheter is passed through the lower pole calyx and brought out through the pyelotomy incision. Randall stone forceps locate the midpole or upper pole calyx and a nephrotomy is performed immediately overlying the forceps. A suture is drawn back into the renal pelvis and tied to the end of the catheter issuing from the pyelotomy. By gentle traction on the suture the catheter is drawn into the pelvis and out of the middle pole calyx. It is important to note that multiple holes placed in the catheter must be positioned so that they lie within the confines of the renal pelvis. Perinephric extravasation of urine can occur when the holes in the side walls are dislodged and position themselves outside the pelvis.

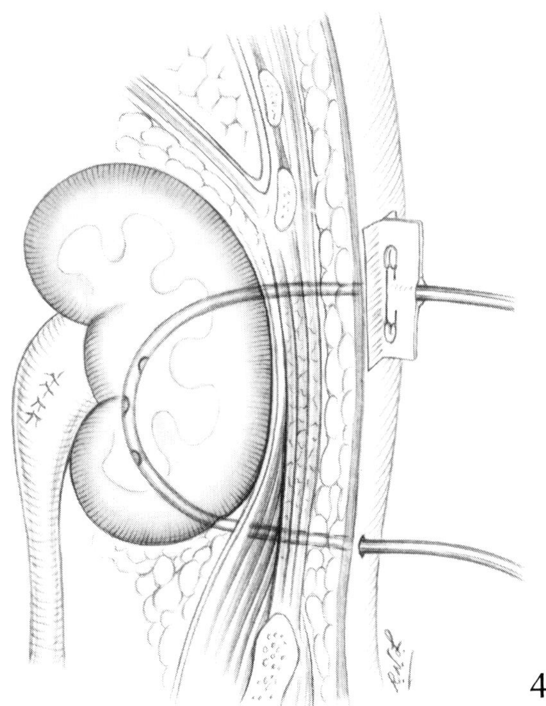

4

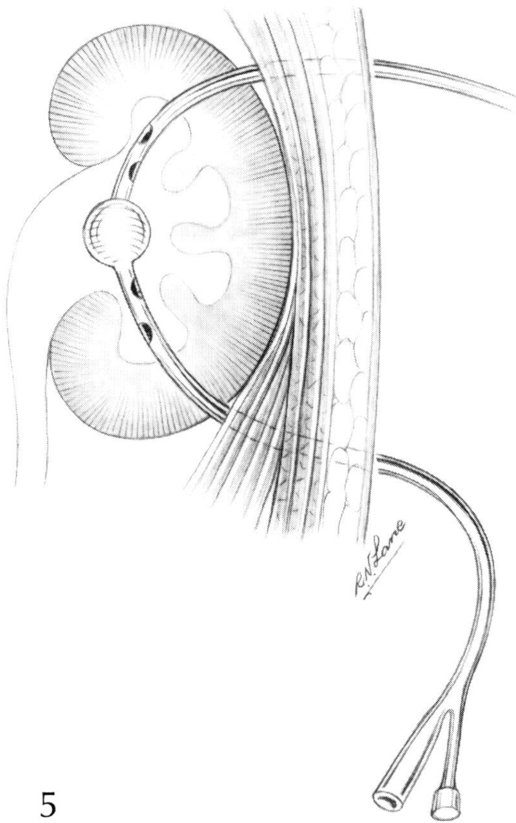

5

5

A loop nephrostomy tube with a balloon in the middle prevents inadvertent dislodgement of the catheter holes outside the confines of the renal pelvis. Some advocate suturing the kidney in a fixed position to the lateral flank side wall so that this distance is constantly maintained.

Penrose drains are placed in the base of the wound and the wound is closed in a standard manner.

Further reading

Brantley, R. G., Shirley, S. W. U-tube nephrostomy: an aid in the postoperative removal of retained stones. Journal of Urology 1974; 111: 7–8

Finney, R. P., Sharpe, J. R. Self-retaining loop nephrostomy. Journal of Urology 1977; 117: 638–640

Gillenwater, J. Y. Loop nephrostomy with the Cummings catheter. Journal of Urology 1977; 117: 641–642

Perinetti, E., Catalona, W. J., Manley, C. B., Geise, G., Fair, W. R. Percutaneous nephrostomy: indications, complications and clinical usefulness. Journal of Urology 1978; 120: 156–158

Operative management of renal calculi

J. E. A. Wickham MS, FRCS
Director of the Academic Unit, Institute of Urology, University of London;
Senior Consultant Urological Surgeon, St Bartholomew's Hospital, London;
Consultant Surgeon, St Peter's Hospital Group, London, UK

Preoperative

Indications

Most renal stones with a diameter of less than 0.5 cm do not require operative removal from the kidney and, if mobile, will pass down the ureter spontaneously. Non-mobile stones lodged in a peripheral calyx may remain silently for many years and do not require operative removal, particularly in the older age groups.

Larger individual or multiple stones, including the staghorn or cast calculi, should, in general, be removed by operation. The principle reasons for removing these stones are:

1. to relieve recurrent renal pain – usually associated with the mobile stone;
2. to prevent recurrent urinary tract infection, seen particularly with phosphatic cast calculi;
3. to prevent loss of renal function produced by chronic intermittent calculous obstruction or sustained infection.

The cross-references in this chapter refers to *Operative Surgery: Urology, 4th Edition*

Preoperative preparation

Radiography

Intravenous urogram (IVU) An adequate and recent IVU should be available to show the precise position of the stone or stones and to demonstrate the functional anatomy of the kidney.

Retrograde studies If an excretion urogram does not demonstrate the intrarenal collecting system and ureter adequately, then retrograde ureteric pyelography should be performed. Most importantly, this is to exclude partial ureteric obstruction by further calculi below the kidney. Removal of renal calculi above an obstructed ureter will result in a persistent urinary fistula.

Plain abdominal X-ray Immediately before operation this is mandatory with all stones, but particularly with the mobile calculus.

Tests of renal function

With severe bilateral stone disease or in the case of the solitary kidney, it is important to estimate renal functional capability with a 24-hour creatinine clearance test. Serum tests of renal function are inadequate. When severe depression of renal function is found, preoperative dialysis may be required to render the patient fit for surgery. Postoperative dialysis may be required to support the patient in the immediate postoperative period.

Renography

Differential isotope renography is often of value in assessing the comparative contribution of a particular kidney to overall renal function, for example a poorly functioning calculus-containing kidney with a normal contralateral organ might be better treated by nephrectomy than by nephrolithotomy. Conversely, when both kidneys show poor function, a conservative operative approach is indicated to preserve maximum overall function.

Metabolic screen

It is now totally inadequate to remove a renal stone without attempting to determine the aetiological cause of its formation. All stone patients should have:

1. duplicate serum calcium, phosphate, oxalate and protein estimates;
2. duplicate 24 hour urinary estimates of calcium, phosphate and oxalate;
3. serum uric acid;
4. spot test for cystine.

Any metabolic abnormality revealed from the tests should be vigorously treated to reduce stone recurrence rates after surgery to more acceptable levels.

Preoperative urinary culture

This should always be performed to identify any infecting organisms. If present, treatment of the infection should be started 24 hours before the operation with an appropriate antibiotic, usually ampicillin or gentamicin. This is particularly important for the avoidance of Gram-negative septicaemia which may be induced by the operative manipulation of an infected kidney.

Crossmatched blood

Crossmatched blood should always be available for any renal surgery. Two units are usually sufficient.

Hydration

Preoperative hydration of the patient is useful in maintaining a good urine flow, especially if ischaemic surgery is to be undertaken. One litre of intravenous dextrose saline given in the hour or two before operation is the best method.

Intraoperative radiology

When any renal stone surgery is performed, facilities should be available for taking contact X-ray films during the operation. It is most unwise to embark on this type of surgery without this ancillary aid.

Anaesthesia

General anaesthesia is required with endotracheal intubation and mechanical ventilation. Obese patients, when placed in the renal operative position, quite often become anoxic and hypercapnic with marked fall in blood pressure if not adequately ventilated.

There is no place for hypotensive anaesthesia in this type of surgery.

The operation

Exposure of the kidney using the lumbotomy incision

The kidney may be approached most easily through the classical loin incision, excising the anterior end of the twelfth rib (*see* chapter on 'Nephrolithotomy', pp. 84–93).

Alternatively, the kidney may be exposed, though with slightly more difficulty, through a posterior lumbotomy incision. This route, although requiring more operative care, undoubtedly results in a much smoother postoperative course with minimal morbidity.

1

Position of patient for the classical loin incision

The patient is placed on the operating table in the lateral position with the lumbar spine across the break. The upper arm is supported horizontally on a rest. The lower leg is flexed at the hip and knee to 90° and the upper leg is kept straight. Three small 'T'-piece rests are attached to blocks at the side of the table which is then tilted laterally so that the patient leans comfortably back on these rests. The table is broken until the lumbar spine just starts to flex laterally. Excessive lateral flexion can cause severe postoperative back pain in old people with osteoarthritis and should be avoided. It is quite often a good idea to insert a urethral catheter so that the anaesthetist may monitor urinary output during the operation.

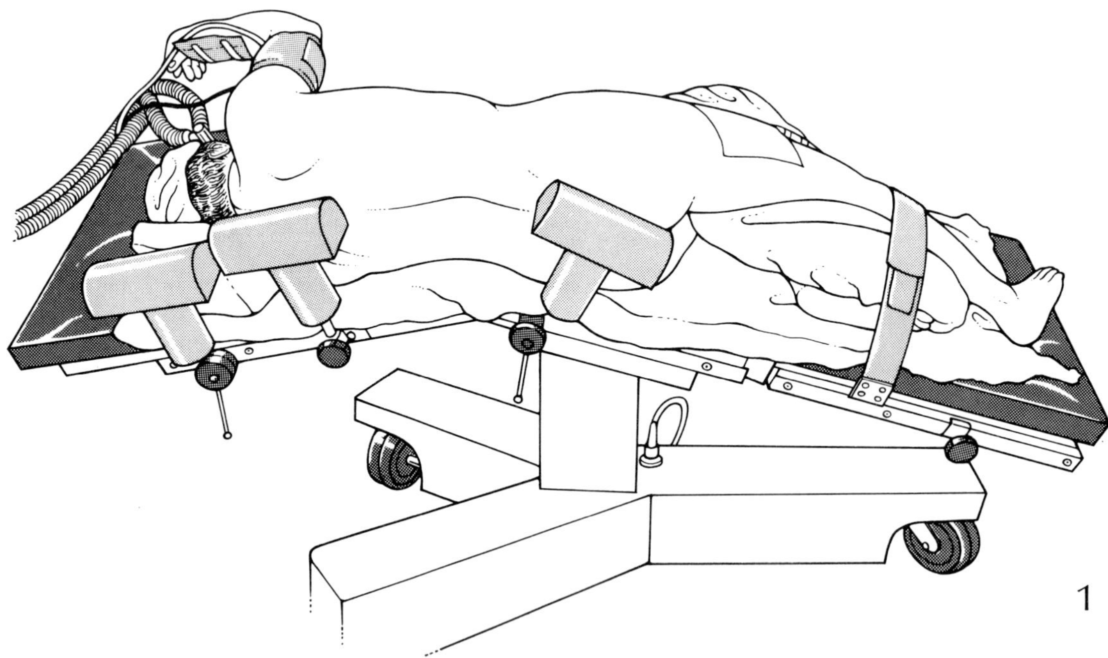

1

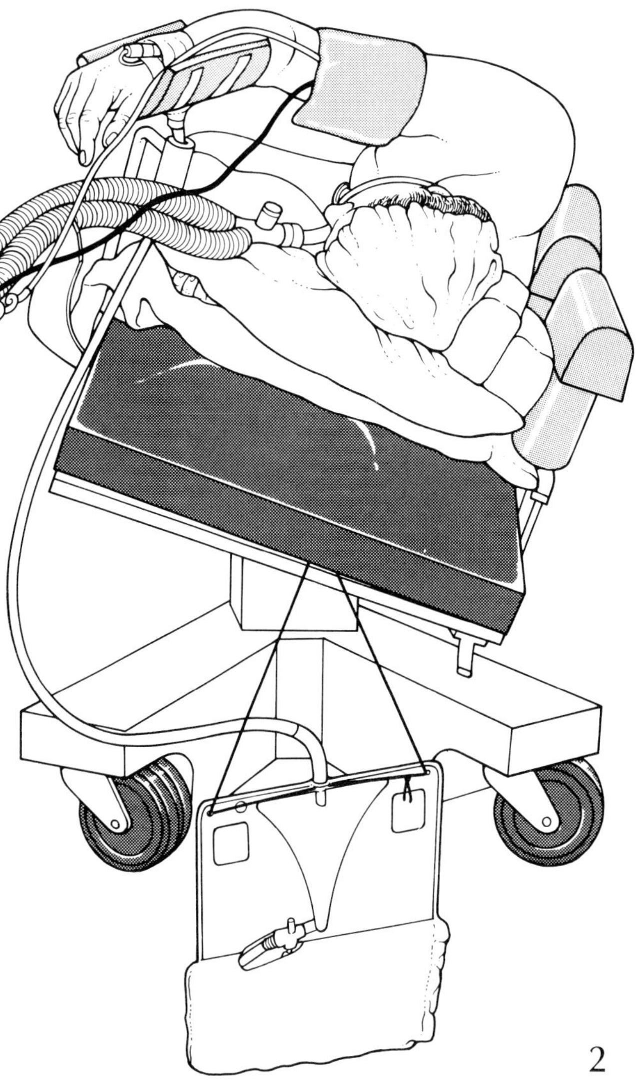

2

2

Position of patient for the lumbotomy incision

Here the patient is placed on the table in the classical prone oblique first-aid position for positioning of the unconscious patient. The lumbar spine is placed over the break and the table broken until spinal flexion just commences. The patient may be stabilized with the 'T' pieces or a length of 7.5 cm Elastoplast across the pelvis and buttocks.

3

The skin incision is made vertically parallel and 2.5 cm lateral to the erector spinae muscle mass. It extends downwards and forwards for approximately 8 cm from the level of the twelfth rib almost to the iliac crest. The incision may be angled forward to parallel Langer's lines rather than the classical vertical lumbotomy which tends to lead to scar formation at the lower end on closure. The underlying subcutaneous fat is incised in the line of the incision to expose the fibres of the latissimus dorsi muscle. This muscle is incised in the line of its fibres to expose the underlying lumbar fascia and the twelfth rib covered by a small portion of serratus posterior.

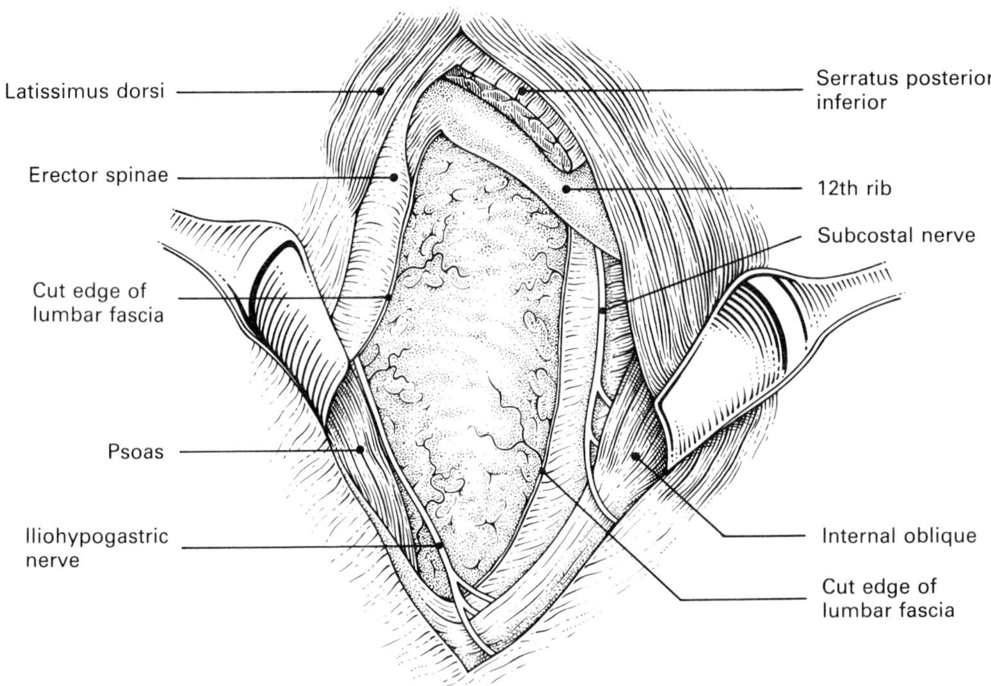

3

4

A 2.5 cm segment of the posterior end of the twelfth rib is removed with bone shears and the lumbar fascia arising from the lower border of the rib is divided in the line of the incision to expose the underlying perirenal fat. Care should be taken to preserve the subcostal nerve at the upper anterior end of the incision and the iliohypogastric nerve running just beneath the lumbar fascia posteriorly. The perirenal fat and fascia are then incised in the line of the incision to expose the kidney. The kidney is gently mobilized from the renal fossa and delivered into the wound.

Should greater exposure be desired, the incision may be enlarged upwards by excising a similar 2.5 cm segment from the posterior end of the eleventh or tenth rib if necessary, the pleura being gently mobilized away from the inner surface of the rib. The intercostal nerve should be retracted.

Very little muscle is transected in this incision and the patient can be mobilized early on the first postoperative day and can leave hospital within a week.

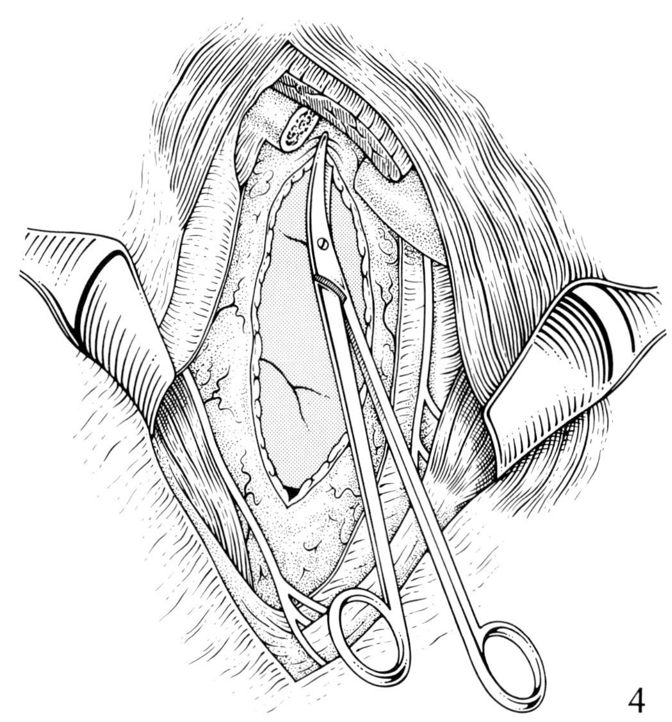

4

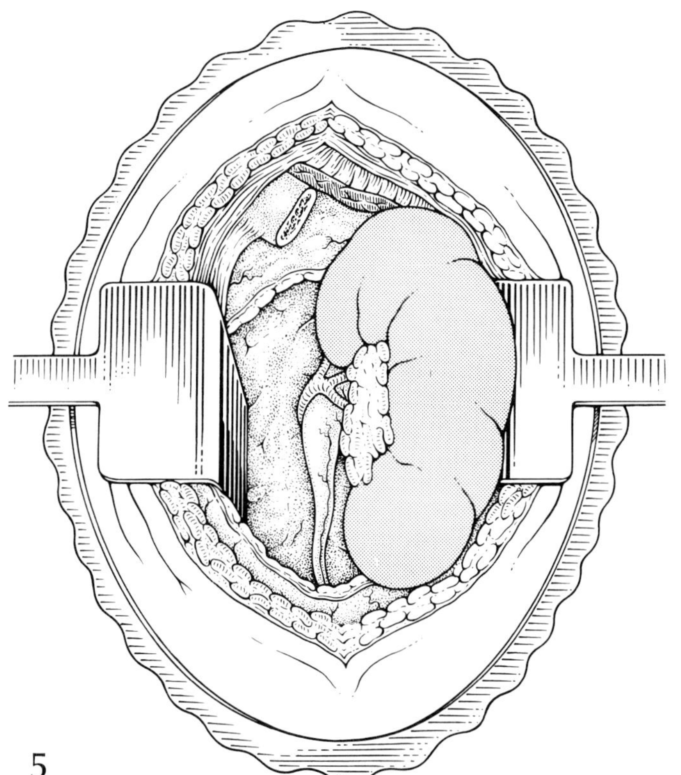

5

5

Retraction

With either the twelfth rib or the lumbotomy incision, exposure of the kidney is considerably facilitated by the use of a self-retaining ring retractor. The author's ring retractor with malleable adjustable blades is most useful (Leibinger, West Germany). A self-retaining twin-bladed retractor of the Finochietto or Pozzi bivalve type is satisfactory.

OPERATIONS AVAILABLE FOR THE REMOVAL OF RENAL STONES

1. Nephrectomy.
2. Pyelolithotomy: (*a*) simple; (*b*) extended.
3. Nephrolithotomy with vascular occlusion: (*a*) with short warm ischaemia or (*b*) with prolonged ischaemia utilizing hypothermic preservation (see pp. 84–93).
4. Percutaneous nephrolithotomy. It should be mandatory that all stones or stone fragments be removed during the definitive operation. This is particularly true of the infective phosphatic stone when residual fragments containing bacteria will perpetuate infection and lead to recurrent stone formation (see p. 93).

Nephrectomy

Nephrectomy is indicated when the renal substance has been so destroyed that significant function is unlikely to return after removal of stones. Obviously it must be established before operation that the contralateral kidney is able to support life.

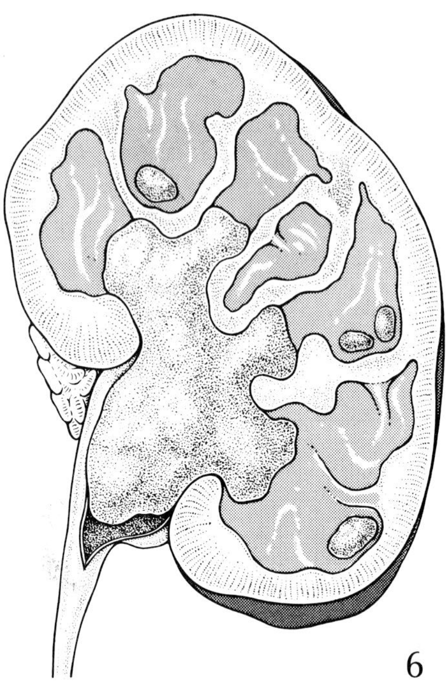

6

Pyelolithotomy

7

Simple pyelolithotomy

When a calculus lies within the renal pelvis the kidney may be rotated forward after exposure and the stone extracted directly through a small posterior vertical incision in the renal pelvis. If the pelvis is intrarenal, the renal substance must be elevated from the pelvis with a small retractor until sufficient exposure has been obtained to permit incision of the pelvis and removal of the stone. The incision in the pelvis is closed with interrupted 4/0 chromic catgut sutures. The wound is closed with 0 chromic catgut to the muscle layers and 3/0 nylon to the skin. A corrugated drain is placed down to the renal fossa.

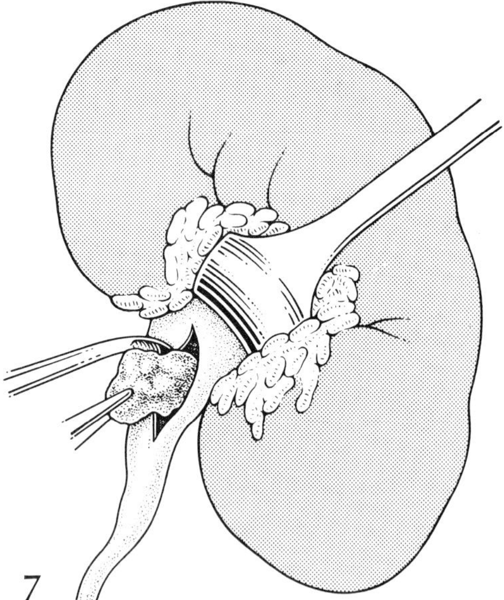

7

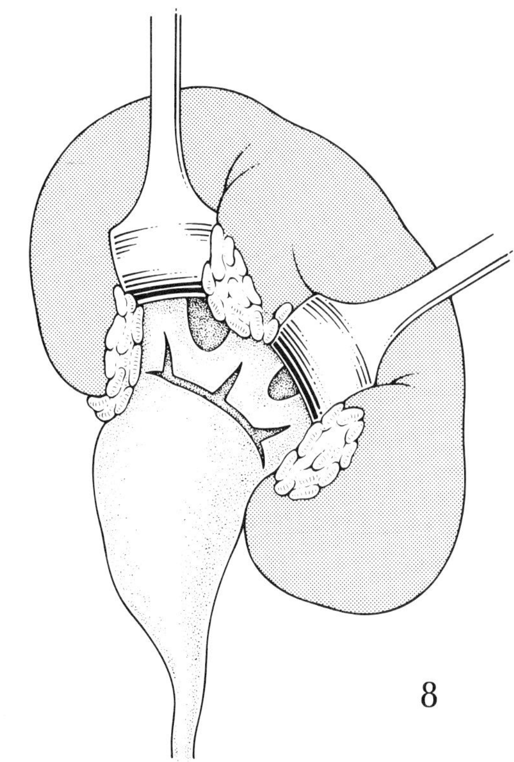

8

8 & 9

Extended pyelolithotomy

When stones lie within the pelvis and also within the major calyces it is often possible, particularly if there is hydronephrotic dilatation of the kidney, to use the technique described by Professor Gil-Vernet (*see* pp. 62–83). Here the relatively avascular plane between the wall of the collecting system and the renal parenchyma is exploited. By blunt dissection the parenchyma is gradually elevated from the pelvis and calyceal necks with small sinus retractors until both can be exposed sufficiently to permit incision and allow extraction of the contained calculus.

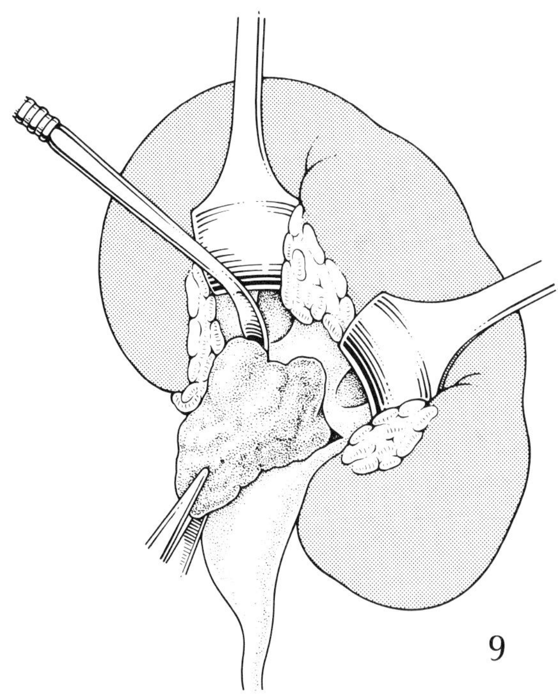

9

Percutaneous renal pelvic and ureteral surgery

W. Scott McDougal MD
Professor and Chairman Department of Urology; Vanderbilt University School of Medicine, Nashville, Tennessee

Introduction

With the advent of extracorporeal shock wave lithotripsy the role that percutaneous endoscopic pelvic stone manipulation will play in the future management of renal stone disease is uncertain. In any event it seems clear that in selected cases it will continue to be a useful procedure. The advantage of this technique over open surgery is that it can be performed through a smaller incision with less morbidity. The disadvantages are that direct control of bleeding may be difficult and access to some stones or lesions, particularly those located in a middle pole calyx, can be difficult. The procedure should not be performed in patients with an active infection of the urinary tract or with a bleeding diathesis.

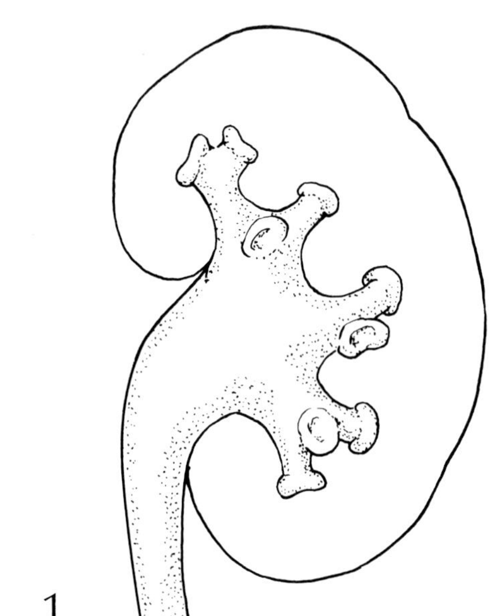

1

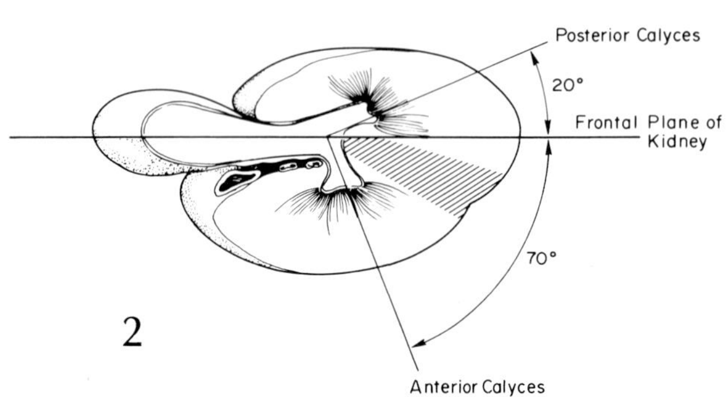

2

The procedure

1 & 2

Renal calyceal anatomy

There are four to twelve calyces in each kidney. Those located in the upper and lower poles are often compound and project directly to their respective poles. The remainder are arranged in an anterior and a posterior row (*see illustration 1*). Those in the anterior row form an angle of 70° to the frontal plane and are the calyces which are seen laterally on the anteroposterior view of an intravenous urogram (*see illustration 2*). The posterior calyces form an angle of 20° with the frontal plane and are those seen medially on the urogram. It is important to locate accurately the calyx in which the calculus or lesion resides for proper placement of the percutaneous nephrostomy and subsequent location of the calculus endoscopically.

Percutaneous nephrostomy

The nephrostomy can be made at the time of stone manipulation or the day before, depending on the preference of the surgeon. Placement and immediate dilatation with stone manipulation can be performed under one anaesthetic and is less likely to result in an infected urinary tract before surgery. To perform percutaneous nephrostomy the renal pelvis must be located. This may be accomplished by four methods: (*1*) by the use of ultrasound, (*2*) with the aid of an intravenous contrast, (*3*) by placement of a ureteral catheter with retrograde injection of contrast and (*4*) by direct injection of contrast through a thin needle inserted into the renal pelvis under fluoroscopic guidance.

3

The kidney is usually punctured through the infundibulum of the lower or middle calyx of the posterior row, provided the stone can be reached through this route. This area is preferred since it can be approached from beneath the 12th rib and most parts of the collecting system can be visualized when the endoscope enters from this area. To perform the puncture the patient is placed in the prone position and tilted up 30° on the side of the kidney to be entered. The posterior calyces thus project vertically, allowing direct access to them. The opacified system is punctured, a guide wire placed down the ureter and the tract dilated. A second guide wire or safety wire is inserted and dilatation continued over the first wire with coaxial dilators or a balloon dilator. The tract is dilated to 24–26 Fr.

It is most important to emphasize the need for two guide wires. Following dilatation placement of the sheath through which the endoscope will enter the renal pelvis requires removal of one of the guide wires. Thereafter, should the sheath become dislodged, one still has a means of finding the renal pelvis using the second guide wire.

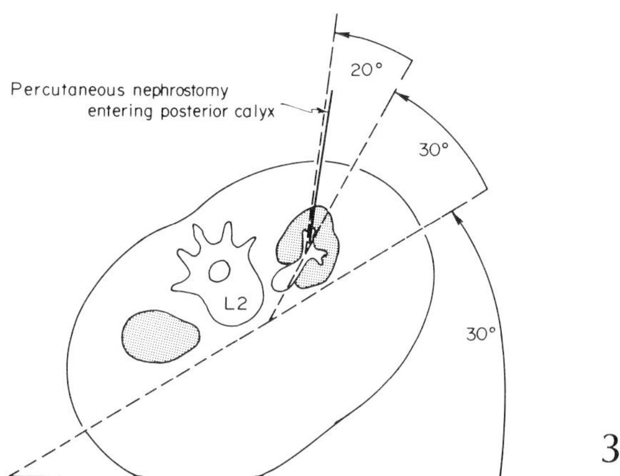

3

Endoscopic manipulation

With the tract dilated a sheath is passed through it into the renal pelvis and the endoscopic instrument is introduced. A craniotomy drape or one which will catch the irrigant is placed about the wound so that the excess irrigant can be collected without draining over the patient, the table and the floor. Stones are grasped and removed or, if too large, they may be broken mechanically with ultrasound or electrohydraulically with shock waves. The irrigant used is usually normal (physiological) saline, but this may need to be modified if electrohydraulic shock wave lithotripsy is preferred. When stones are fragmented care must be taken not to lose fragments down the ureter. This may be prevented by placing a Fogerty balloon catheter up the ureter to occlude the ureteropelvic junction before breaking the stones. Renal pelvic and upper ureteral stones may be approached with this technique. At the termination of the procedure a 14 Fr Malecot nephrostomy is left in place for 4–5 days. Before its removal a nephrostogram is performed to ensure that all fragments have been removed and that fluid can move freely from renal pelvis to bladder.

Chemolysis of calculi

Should retained fragments be discovered on the nephrostogram the renal pelvis may be irrigated with a solution formulated to dissolve the stone. Continuous irrigation may be obtained by placing a second percutaneous nephrostomy tube in the renal pelvis or by passing a ureteral catheter cystoscopically into the renal pelvis. Uric acid stones are treated with sodium bicarbonate or tromethamine solution, cystine stones with sodium bicarbonate, tromethamine or acetylcysteine, struvite stones with Suby's solution G, appatite stones with hemiacidrin and calcium oxalate stones with ethylenediaminetetracetic acid (EDTA).

Complications

Complications of this procedure include bleeding, renal pelvic and ureteral disruption, sepsis, fluid overload from excessive irrigant absorption, loss of the kidney, perirenal fibrosis and injury to the lung, colon, spleen and liver. In most series significant complications resulting in serious mobidity occur in less than 5% of cases.

Further reading

Marberger, M. Disintegration of renal and ureteral calculi with ultrasound. Urologic Clinics of North America 1983; 10: 729–242

Smith, A. D., Lee, W. L. Introduction to endourology: percutaneous nephrostomy and ureteral stents. AUA Update Series 1984; 3: 5

Simple nephrectomy

Thomas J. Rohner, Jr MD
Professor of Surgery (Urology), Chief, Division of Urology, Pennsylvania State University College of Medicine and The Milton S. Hershey Medical Center, Hershey, Pennsylvania, USA

Introduction

The first deliberate nephrectomy was carried out by Professor Gustav Simon of Heidelberg, Germany, in 1869. Simon's patient had a complicated left ureterocutaneous fistula caused by ureteral avulsion during resection of an ovarian tumour 18 months earlier. After four unsuccessful attempts at closing the fistula, Simon considered removal of the kidney. At that time it had not been shown that a kidney could be surgically removed and the opposite kidney provide adequate renal function. After carrying out successful unilateral nephrectomies in several dogs, Simon removed the patient's kidney using an extraperitoneal approach with a good eventual result. An interesting account of Simon's experience is provided by Thorwald[1].

General considerations

Simple nephrectomy involves removal of the kidney and upper ureter without removing the perinephric fat or Gerota's fascia. It is generally performed through a subcostal or anterior 12th rib extraperitoneal flank incision. The choice of incision depends on the position of the kidney.

Preoperative indications

Simple nephrectomy is often done for poorly or nonfunctioning kidneys due to ureteropelvic junction or ureteral obstruction, calculus disease, chronic pyelonephritis, infection, ureteral fistula, vascular disease or late trauma. The decision to carry out nephrectomy indicates that reconstructive efforts to preserve the kidney have been considered and deemed either unreasonable or inappropriate or that the function of the kidney is so poor that further reconstructive procedures are not justified. Simple nephrectomy using an extraperitoneal approach is particularly applicable when it is considered likely that infection is present and one wants to avoid contamination of the peritoneal cavity.

In the past, simple nephrectomy using an extraperitoneal flank approach was used for resection of renal adenocarcinomas. It has been shown that 13–30 per cent of renal adenocarcinomas will extend through the renal capsule into the perinephric fat, and for this reason radical nephrectomy, involving removal of the kidney with surrounding perinephric fat and Gerota's fascia, should provide superior local tumour control[2]. The preferred transabdominal approach to renal tumours provides easier and earlier access to the vascular pedicle. A transperitoneal approach is also recommended for acute trauma and renal injuries within the first 72 hours so that early control of the renal vessels can be gained and associated intra-abdominal injuries can be ruled out.

Preoperative preparation

One unit of blood should be typed and crossed. The procedure is best carried out under general endotracheal anaesthesia in the full flank position. The patient's pulmonary status should be assessed. A specific antibiotic for positive urine cultures should be given 2 hours before surgery. Proper patient informed consent should include discussion of the general hazards related to major surgical procedures and those possible complications peculiar to nephrectomy, including haemorrhage, colon or duodenum injury, and pleural injury with pneumothorax.

The operation

1

After induction of general endotracheal anaesthesia in the supine position, the patient is placed in the lateral decubitus position with kidney bar raised and the operating table flexed so that the upward exposed flank is nearly parallel to the floor. The bottom leg is flexed, with a pillow placed between the knees. Depending on the position of the kidney, either a subcostal or anterior 12th rib incision with resection of the distal portion of the 12th rib is made.

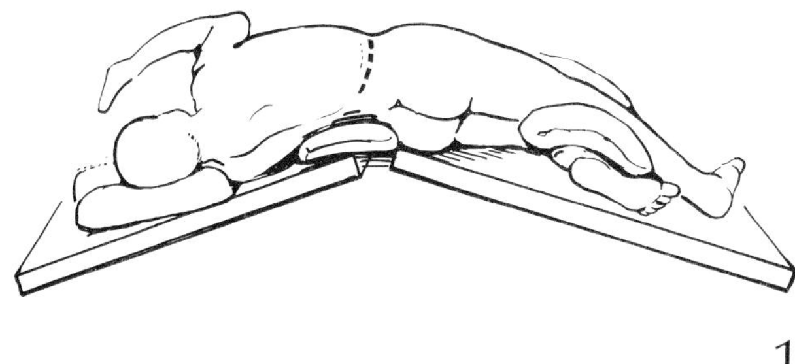

1

2

After the external and internal oblique muscles are sharply incised, the transversus muscle and lumbodorsal fascia at the posterior extent of the incision is bluntly opened with a Kelly clamp and the retroperitoneal space entered. Blunt finger dissection is carried anteriorly to split the transversus muscle in the direction of its fibres.

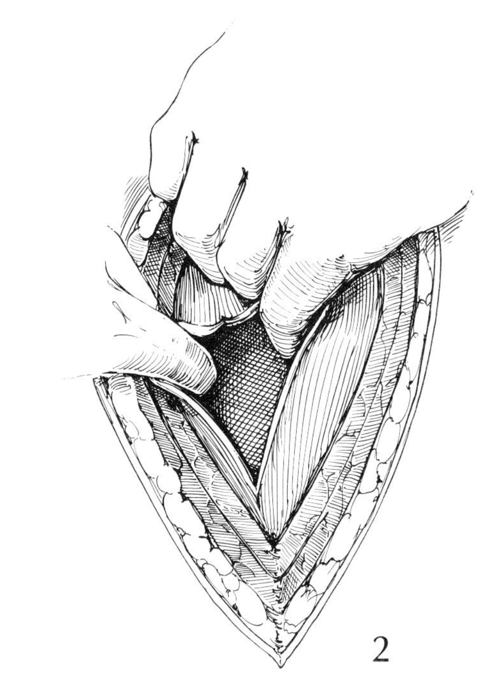

2

Particular attention should be paid to the 12th thoracic intercostal nerve, which lies between the transversus and internal oblique muscles. This nerve should be identified and retracted posteriorly, but not divided, to avoid postoperative abdominal muscle relaxation. The peritoneum is bluntly pushed forward to avoid entering it. Gerota's fascia is identified and the lateral aspect is grasped with smooth forceps and incised, exposing the pale yellow perinephric fat.

Mobilization of the kidney is best done using blunt finger dissection. Dense fibrous bands or fat adherent to the renal capsule is sharply divided, using scissor dissection. The lower pole is mobilized first, followed by the anterior and posterior kidney surfaces. If the kidney has been obstructed and is hydronephrotic, trocar suction can be used to empty the collecting system. This will result in a smaller kidney and will greatly improve surgical exposure.

The upper ureter is identified, divided between clamps and ligated. This manoeuvre permits easier retraction of the kidney and the ureter can be followed to the hilum.

The significant event during nephrectomy is the identification and secure ligation of the renal artery and vein. More than a single renal artery occurs in 25 per cent of individuals and, accompanied by a vein, often supplies the lower or upper pole of the kidney. While freeing the lower pole of the kidney, the possibility of accessory vessels should be kept in mind so that inadvertent avulsion with haemorrhage does not occur. Resistance encountered during blunt finger dissection should be considered a vascular structure and divided between ligatures or clips before division.

The main renal artery and vein in the hilum can be approached either anteriorly or posteriorly. The artery should always be ligated first to minimize vascular congestion and bleeding. It should be remembered that the renal vein lies anterior to the artery, and for this reason the posterior approach has the advantage of providing access to the artery without having to retract the overlying vein. Individual ligation of the artery and vein is more secure and preferable to mass ligation of the pedicle. Arteriovenous fistula is uncommon but has been noted as a complication following mass pedicle ligation.

3

A right-angled clamp is useful in freeing up and passing ties around the artery, following which it is triply ligated in continuity and divided between the distal two ties.

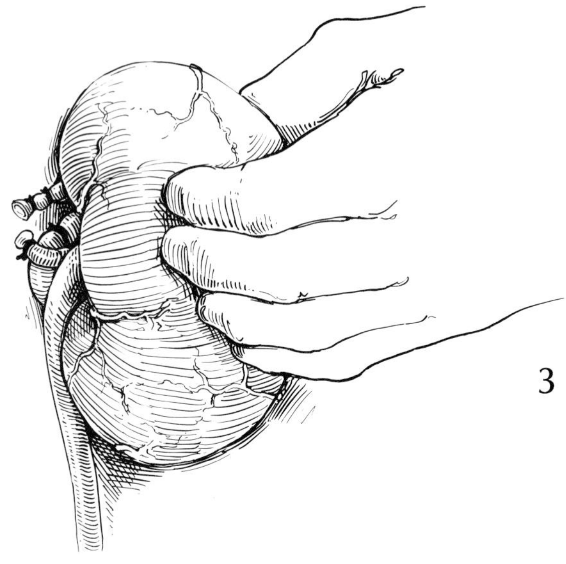

3

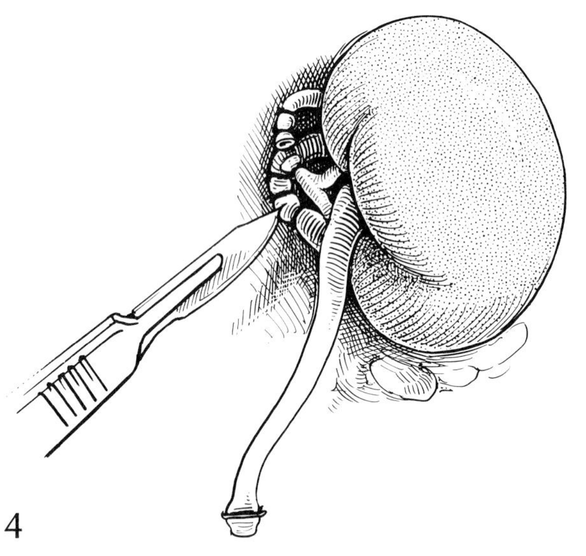

4

4

The vein is then similarly triply ligated and divided.

If extensive perinephric inflammatory disease has been present or several previous kidney operations have been done, the hilum and renal vessels may be encased in thick fibrous tissue, making individual vessel identification and ligation very difficult. In this situation the use of mass pedicle ligation can be considered[3].

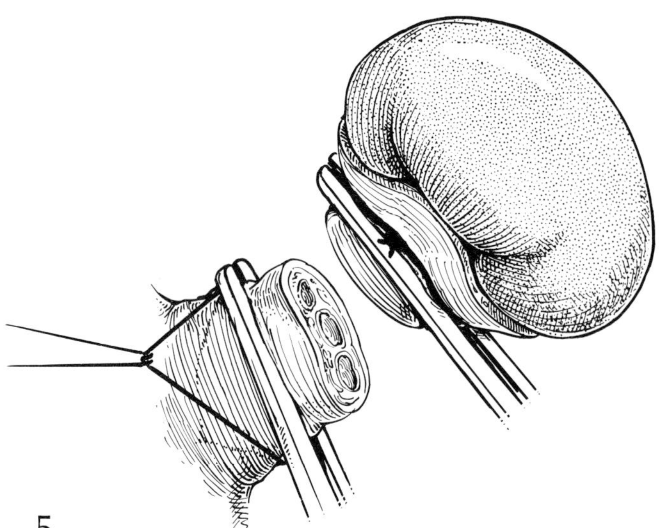

5

5

The renal pedicle, including the artery and vein, is thinned as much as possible and ideally three pedicle clamps are placed across the renal vesels and the pedicle divided between the two distal clamps. Most often only enough pedicle can be mobilized to accommodate two clamps. The pedicle is then ligated proximally using 0 silk ties, loosening the clamps, and then reapplying them after the ties are snugged down.

6

It is important to maintain control of the pedicle and one should be able to reapply the clamps immediately should bleeding occur. A suture ligature between the two proximal ties can be used for added security.

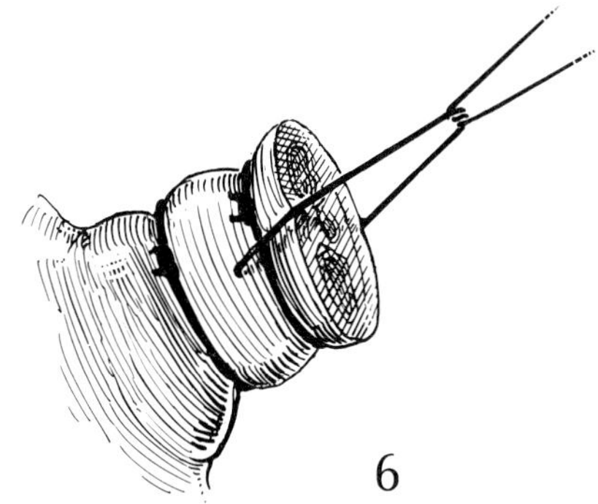

6

In the presence of gross infection No. 1 chromic catgut should be used to ligate all vessels. The use of non-absorbable suture material in this situation may result in a persistent draining fistula or sinus tract.

Sudden haemorrhage during the course of gaining control or tying the renal vessels should be dealt with by direct finger or surgical sponge compression while efforts are organized to deal with the bleeding. These efforts include setting up a second suction line and being certain 5/0 vascular suture material and non-crushing vascular clamps are available. It is also appropriate to inform the anaesthetist of the presence of uncontrolled bleeding and make certain either that blood is available for transfusion or arrange for further blood to be typed and crossed. Blind clamping is to be condemned, since further vascular injury can occur or injury to other structures close to the renal vessels, especially the duodenum, vena cava or colon.

If, during the course of nephrectomy, dense adhesions are encountered binding the renal capsule to the perinephric fat, the surgeon may find an easier plane of dissection between the renal parenchyma and capsule than between the capsule and perinephric fat. In that event, one may continue using the subscapsular technique of nephrectomy (*see* chapter on 'Subcapsular nephrectomy', pp. 116–118).

Another technique to be remembered when one encounters dense adhesions and fibrosis involving the peritoneum and renal pedicle is to extend the incision medially, open the peritoneum and either reflect the colon medially to gain control of the renal artery and vein lateral to the colon, or incise the peritoneum medial to the colon and identify and isolate the renal vessels even more proximally[4]. This area has usually not been exposed during previous urological procedures.

In the distant past, opening the peritoneal cavity during the course of nephrectomy in the presence of gross infection was a serious problem, with fatal peritonitis often resulting. With appropriate antibiotic therapy and reapproximation of the peritoneum, this is now very uncommon, although an extraperitoneal approach is still preferred for simple nephrectomy.

Mobilization of the upper pole is generally done after dividing the renal vessels. This is best done using blunt finger dissection and staying close to the upper renal pole to avoid removing or injuring the adrenal. If the adrenal is torn, haemostasis can usually be achieved either by suture ligation of the torn edge using a running locking 4/0 chromic suture or large haemostatic clips placed along the avulsed edge.

After the kidney is removed, the renal fossa is fully exposed and can be inspected carefully for bleeding. Either suture ligatures or haemostatic clips can be used to achieve haemostasis. We always drain the renal fossa for 24 hours, using a Penrose drain led out from the posterior extent of the wound. Any hypotensive episode or unexplained tachycardia in the immediate postoperative period can then be evaluated, with significant bleeding from the renal fossa unlikely if the drain is dry.

After haemostasis has been achieved, the pleura at the posterior extent of the wound should be inspected for injury. It may be helpful to fill the incision with saline to detect any bubbling as a result of a small pleural tear. If a pleural opening is seen, it should be sutured with a running locking 2/0 chromic suture with the lung expanded as the final suture is tied down. It is important to obtain an upright chest X-ray in the recovery room, with the patient in the sitting position, to detect pneumothorax. If significant pneumothorax is present, an anterior chest tube should be inserted and placed on waterseal suction until the lung has re-expanded.

The wound is closed using a running locking 0 chromic suture to close the transversus layer. Interrupted 0 chromic sutures are used to approximate the internal and external oblique layers individually. The subcutaneous tissue is approximated using interrupted 3/0 plain catgut sutures and either skin sutures or clips used for skin closure. In the paediatric patient we generally use a subcuticular 4/0 chromic suture to minimize scar formation.

References

1. Thorwald, J. Century of the surgeon. New York: Pantheon Books, 1957: 180–199

2. Skinner, D. G., Vermillion, C. D., Colvin, R. B. The surgical management of renal cell carcinoma. Journal of Urology 1972; 107: 705–710

3. Hinman, F. Nephrectomy. Surgery, Gynecology and Obstetrics 1927; 45: 347–358

4. Scott, R. F., Jr, Selzman, H. M. Complications of nephrectomy: review of 450 patients and a description of a modification of the transperitoneal approach. Journal of Urology 1966; 95: 307–312

Traumatic injuries of the kidney

W. Scott McDougal MD
Professor and Chairman, Department of Urology;
Vanderbilt University Medical Center, Nashville, Tennessee, USA

Introduction

Renal injury occurs with a frequency of approximately 2 per 100 000 of the population and is most commonly encountered in men in their 20s and 30s. Blunt trauma is responsible for two-thirds of the cases, while penetrating trauma accounts for the remainder. Only about 7 per cent of patients with penetrating abdominal wounds, however, have injuries involving the kidneys.

The protection afforded the kidney by the ribcage, vertebral column and investing fascia accounts for the relatively low incidence of injury in the adult. However, despite this protection, the kidney is the organ most frequently injured in children as a result of blunt abdominal trauma. The lack of perinephric fat in children (which serves to buffer the kidney from blunt injury) probably accounts for the difference in incidence between children and adults. In addition, pre-existing renal disease may also contribute to the higher incidence of renal injury in children since one-fifth of children with renal trauma have pre-existing renal abnormalities. Renal injuries, blunt or penetrating, are commonly associated with other injuries. Indeed, renal trauma is often unsuspected, since the associated injury is usually recognized initially and may obscure the signs and symptoms of renal injury. Associated injuries are more commonly found in penetrating trauma than in blunt injury. The organs most often injured in descending order of frequency are the liver, lungs, spleen, small bowel, stomach, pancreas, duodenum and diaphragm.

Signs and symptoms

Signs and symptoms of renal injury may be protean. However, those most commonly encountered include haematuria, tenderness or ecchymosis over the flank, a flank mass, and entrance or exit wounds on the skin overlying the renal fossa. Although 80–90 per cent of patients with renal injury present with haematuria, many patients are found to have urine free from blood cells. Indeed, patients with renal pedicle injuries invariably have a normal urine analysis. Because many of the signs and symptoms are not specific for renal injury, a high index of suspicion must be maintained when evaluating the trauma patient if these injuries are not to be missed.

The cross-references in this chapter refers to *Operative Surgery: Urology, 4th Edition*

Diagnosis

Roentgenography is generally the first aid employed in confirming a diagnosis of suspected renal injury. The studies are obtained in a logical progression beginning with the plain film or KUB. Unfortunately, in only about 15 per cent of cases does the KUB suggest the diagnosis. Renal injury is suggested by fractures of overlying ribs or vertebral bodies, obliteration of the psoas outline, blurring of the kidney outline and displacement of loops of bowel away from the renal fossa.

1

Nephrotomogram of a fractured left kidney. Notice the poor concentration of the dye and the lack of clarity of the renal border

1

Nephrotomography

Following the KUB, an infusion or high-dose intravenous pyelogram with nephrotomography is obtained. This investigation has a diagnostic accuracy of about 95 per cent. An injury is suggested by a lack of or delay in visualization, extravasation of contrast, lack of continuous renal outline, an enlarged renal shadow, or radiolucent areas within the confines of the kidney.

Infusion pyelography provides the patient with a large osmotic load and may contribute to haemodynamic instability if it is administered to an inadequately resuscitated patient. Seizures and further aggravation of the shocked state due to loss of fluid, because of the osmotic diuresis, can occur. Moreover, the dye may precipitate acute renal failure if administered to the unstable trauma patient. Therefore, it is necessary to resuscitate the trauma victim properly prior to performing an infusion pyelogram.

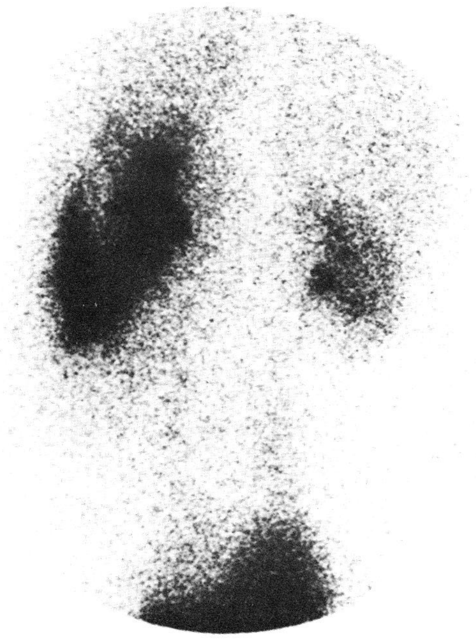

2

Renal scan of a patient with traumatic disruption of the right lower pole and renal pelvis. Notice the extravasation of the radionuclide

2

Renal scans

Renal scans have also been successfully employed in the initial diagnosis of renal injury and have the advantage of neither exacerbating haemodynamic instability nor causing acute renal failure in the inadequately resuscitated patient. Technetium 99m glucoheptonate is the radionuclide usually employed. Pedicle injuries or segmental arterial injuries may be diagnosed by a lack of tracer flow to the kidney or to a part of it. Parenchymal fractures may also be demonstrated provided the defect is large and the parenchymal tissue is separated by more than 1 cm. Unfortunately, the inability to obtain scans in most hospitals on an emergency basis limits their usefulness in the initial evaluation. However, they are of considerable help in following the renal injury over the long term.

3a & b

Ultrasonography

Ultrasonography is perhaps the most significant recent advance in the diagnosis and management of renal injury. With its use, the frequency with which renal angiograms must be obtained has been considerably reduced. This modality is particularly useful in the diagnosis of subcapsular haematomas, confirming the integrity of renal parenchyma when the entire renal outline cannot be visualized by pyelography and confirming the location of a kidney which does not visualize on infusion pyelography.

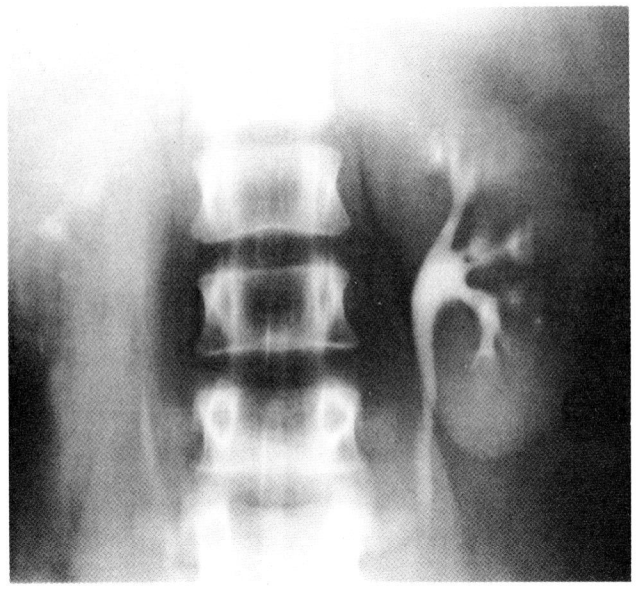

3a

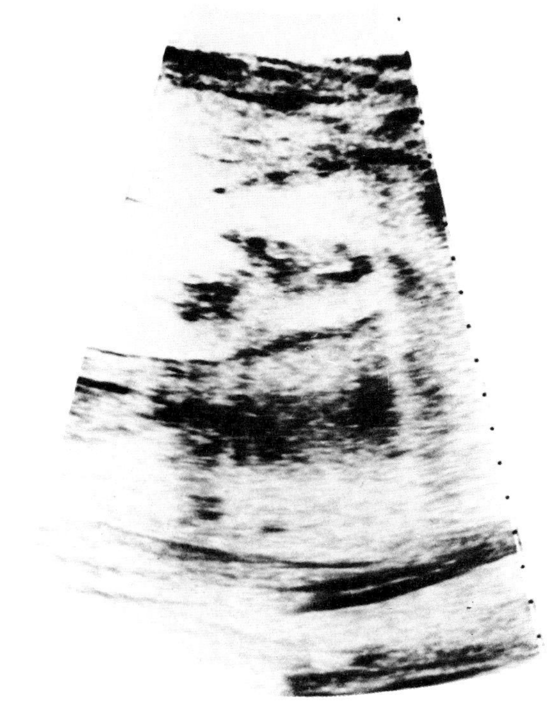

3b

(a) Nephrotomogram of a patient who sustained a traumatic injury to the right kidney. Notice the obscured inferior pole of the right kidney. (b) Ultrasonogram demonstrating a subcapsular haematoma of the inferior pole of the right kidney

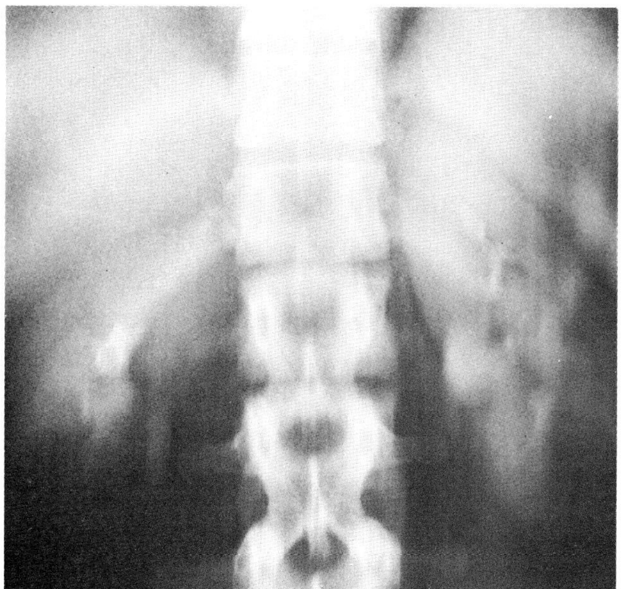

4a

(a) Nephrotomogram of a patient who sustained blunt trauma to the right flank. Notice the poor filling of the inferior calyces. (b) Computerized axial tomograph. Notice the extensive haematoma formation on the lateral border of the right kidney

4a & b

Computerized axial tomography

Computerized axial tomography, obtained routinely in patients suspected of having substantial abdominal trauma, has recently been advocated. Initial reports suggest that this is an excellent modality for determining the presence and extent of renal injury. With the intravenous injection of a radiocontrast agent, parenchymal injuries as well as collecting system injuries can be diagnosed with a high degree of accuracy.

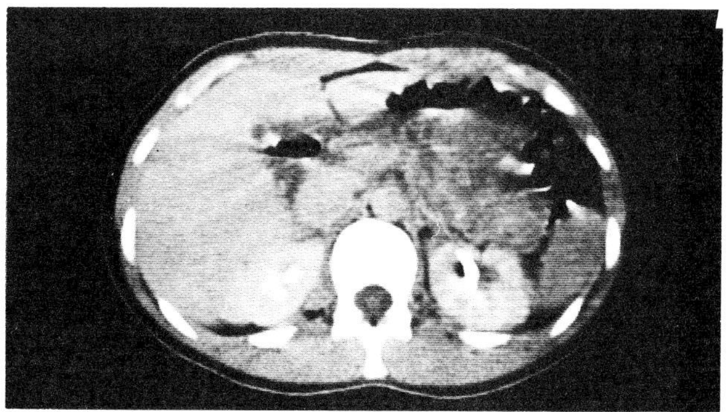

4b

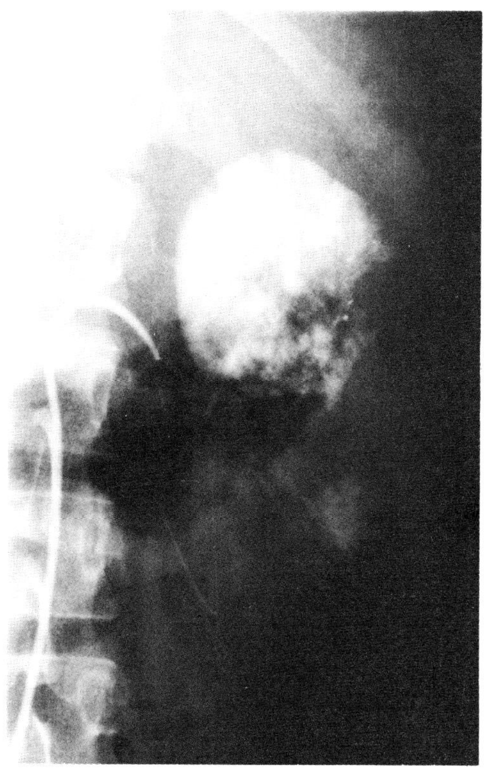

5

Renal angiogram demonstrating extensive fracture of the left kidney (same case as Illustration 1)

5

Angiography

The above diagnostic procedures select a group of patients who are candidates for angiography. Those who should have an angiogram are: those suspected of having a renal pedicle injury; individuals in whom major fractures or separation of renal fragments are suspected and in whom, if confirmed, an operation will be performed; and those who have persistent haematuria or in whom continued bleeding occurs. It is also helpful, usually later in the patient's post-traumatic course, for documenting an arteriovenous fistula.

When extravasation of contrast is extensive, documentation of the size and location of the collecting system injury is best obtained by retrograde pyelography. Indeed, children who sustain acute hyperextension injuries in whom a renal injury is suspected may have disruptions of the ureteropelvic junction and should have a retrograde pyelogram if the intravenous pyelogram does not indicate continuity between the renal pelvis and the proximal ureter.

Classification of injuries

6a–e

Renal injuries are classified into one of five groups depending on their severity and location: (*a*) contusions; (*b*) lacerations; (*c*) fractures; (*d*) pedicle injuries; and (*e*) pelvic injuries.

Contusions

Renal contusions account for approximately 85 per cent of kidney injuries. They are usually due to blunt trauma and include subcapsular haematomas and minor cortical lacerations. Patients commonly present with flank pain and microscopic haematuria. The latter may persist for a week or more. The intravenous pyelogram is often suggestive when a portion of the renal outline cannot be clearly defined (*see Illustration 3a*). However, frequently the intravenous pyelogram is normal and a diagnosis can only be made by ultrasonography (*see Illustration 3b*) or angiography. Clearly, the latter is not indicated in these patients and the non-invasive ultrasonogram is the diagnostic procedure of choice. These patients are treated conservatively with bedrest until the gross haematuria clears; their activity is limited until the microscopic haematuria abates.

Lacerations

Lacerations which extend deep within the parenchyma of the kidney account for somewhat less than 10 per cent of all renal injuries. The treatment of this group remains controversial since there are advocates of both conservative and operative treatment. Those suggesting conservative treatment note that the incidence of nephrectomy in this group is less when non-operative treatment is employed initially than if there is immediate surgical intervention. Moreover, delayed complications in a conservatively treated group are reportedly minimal. They include: delayed rupture of the kidney, persistent haematuria, perinephric abscess, renin-mediated hypertension and arteriovenous fistulae.

Those arguing for immediate exploration, debridement and suture of the laceration with drainage of the wounds suggest that the complications of conservative management are for the most part eliminated and that better preservation of renal function is achieved. A prospective study is required to settle this issue.

Diagnosis of lacerations is generally made by infusion pyelography with the aid of ultrasonography. If these two modalities do not clearly indicate the extent of the lesion, angiography is indicated.

Fractures

Fractures involve multiple portions of the kidney in which segments of the parenchyma are not in continuity with the remaining kidney as a whole. The diagnosis of this injury is made by intravenous pyelography, ultrasonography and, finally, angiography.

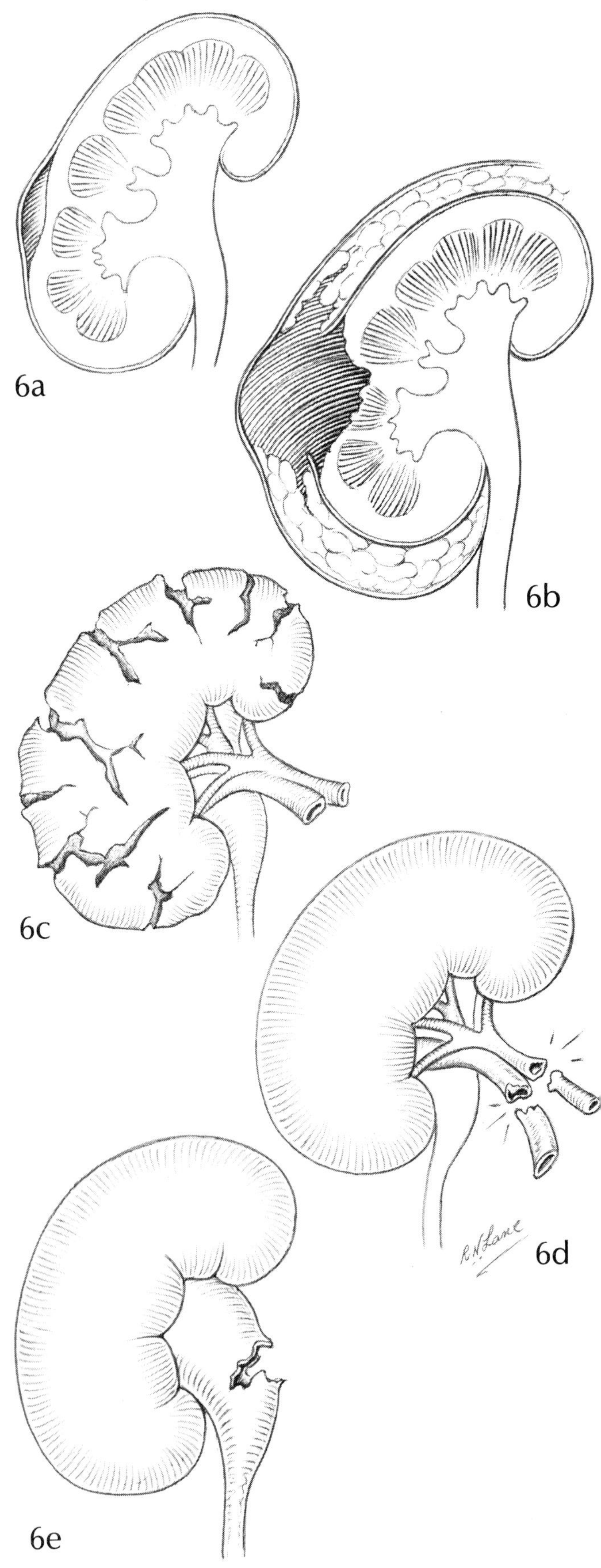

Pedicle injuries

Vascular injuries of the pedicle occur as a result of deceleration-type injury and less frequently as a consequence of blunt or penetrating injuries. When they are due to the latter, associated intra-abdominal injuries involving either the duodenum and/or pancreas often make *in situ* repair difficult. In these circumstances, the kidney should be removed, and, if the patient's stability permits, autotransplanted to the pelvis (see chapter on 'Renal transplantation', pp. 201–212).

An arterial repair adjacent to a major injury of the pancreas or duodenum is fraught with postoperative complications and a very high mortality rate. Less commonly, pedicle injuries are unassociated with multiple injuries and the patient's stability allows for *in situ* repair. These injuries are usually of a deceleration type and involve intimal tears which occur approximately 1 cm from the origin of the renal artery from the aorta. The diagnosis is suspected on intravenous pyelography in which there is marked delay or non-visualization of the kidney. Renal scans may also indicate lack of perfusion of the kidney and angiography is diagnostic. Initial vascular control is absolutely mandatory and therefore these lesions are approached through the abdomen, gaining vessel control before exposing the kidney.

Renal pelvic injuries

Injuries of the collecting system of the kidney are diagnosed by noting extravasated dye on the intravenous pyelogram; their extent is confirmed by retrograde pyelography. If the extravasation is minimal, retrograde pyelography is generally not indicated and the patient may be treated expectantly. On the other hand, if a major laceration is suspected, retrograde pyelography confirms the extent. If there are no other associated injuries, a ureteral catheter may be left in place and this may be all that is necessary. On the other hand, if there is extensive loss of pelvic tissue, then immediate exploration, drainage and repair of the devitalized pelvis is necessary (see *Illustrations 8a–d*). It is important to remember that acute hyperextension injury in a child may result in disruption of the ureteral pelvic junction. Retrograde pyelography is diagnostic in these patients.

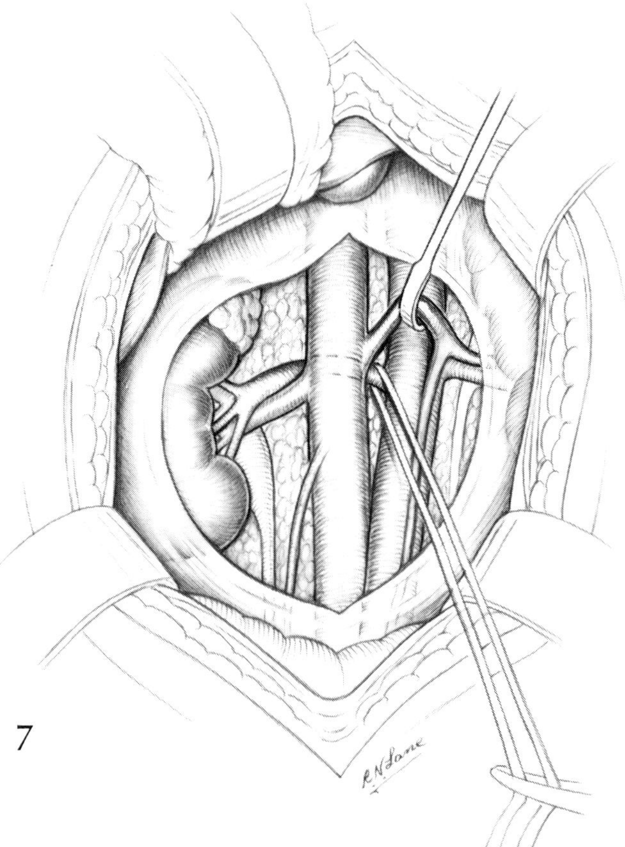

7

Major renal parenchymal injuries which are to be explored must be approached through the abdomen so that vascular control can be obtained before Gerota's fascia is opened. Small bowel contents are swept to the right and placed in a Lahey bag. The retroperitoneum is opened immediately adjacent to the ligament of Treitz, thus exposing the vessels as depicted.

Surgical technique

7

Patients who require immediate exploration of the kidney for trauma should be approached transabdominally so that vascular control can be obtained before Gerota's fascia is opened. The kidney is reached by incising the retroperitoneum from the level of the ligament of Treitz to the caecum. The small bowel mesentery is placed on the abdomen in the right upper quadrant in a Lahey bag. The ligament of Treitz is incised and the retroperitoneum entered thus exposing the vessels as depicted. A large haematoma is often encountered, making identification of the retroperitoneal structures exceedingly difficult. Usually, by careful dissection immediately beneath the ligament of Treitz, the left renal vein can be identified.

Once this structure is identified, the aorta is easily approached, and the right renal artery is identified between the vena cava and aorta. The left renal artery may be a bit more difficult to identify, but again is often found immediately beneath the left renal vein. It should be noted that the origin of the superior mesenteric artery is within 1 cm of the origin of the renal artery. The superior mesenteric artery can often be confused with the renal artery and it is mandatory to confirm the nature and course of the vessel suspected of being the renal artery prior to severing it. The right renal vein is identified generally with a fair degree of ease as it is the first major vessel cephalad to the origin of the right gonadal vein.

Once these vessels are encircled with vascular loops, Gerota's fascia may be opened and the kidney approached. If there is obvious separation of the parenchymal tissue, that which is separated is removed, the borders of the kidney are debrided and full-thickness sutures bring the margins together.

8a–d

A collecting system injury associated with a parenchymal fracture requires debridement of the parenchyma and a watertight closure of the collecting system. Non-viable renal parenchyma is excised (*a*) and bleeding vessels suture-ligated with fine chromic suture (*b*). The collecting system is closed with fine chromic suture (*c*). The capsule is closed (*d*). If the capsule is not sufficient for closure, a piece of peritoneum or fascia may be used in its place (*see Illustration 9d*). Major lacerations, if explored, are brought together with chromic sutures over buttresses of fat or Gelfoam.

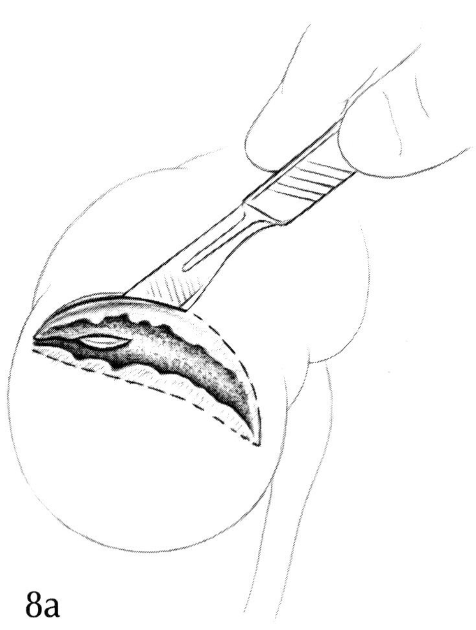

8a

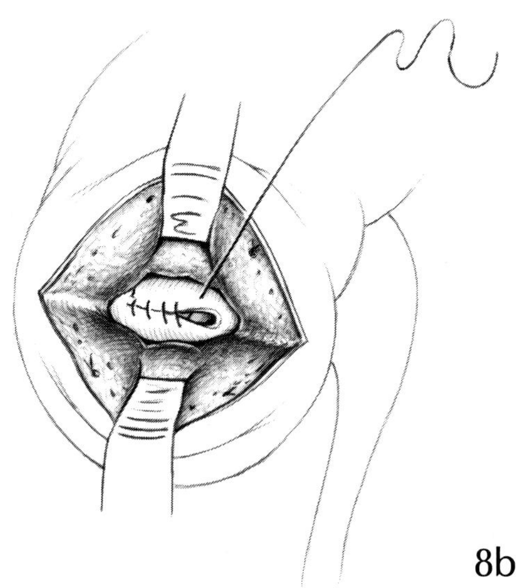

8b

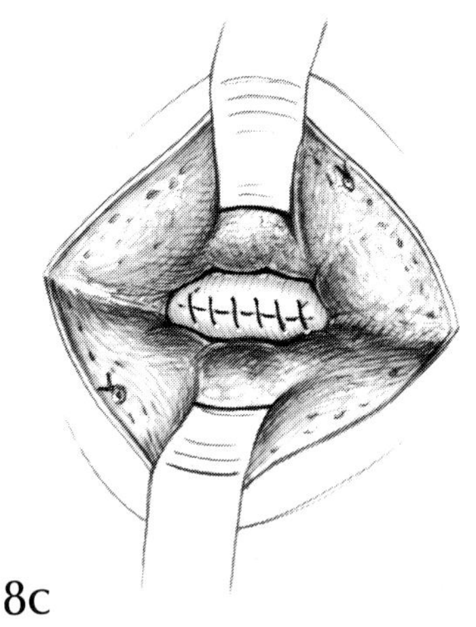

8c

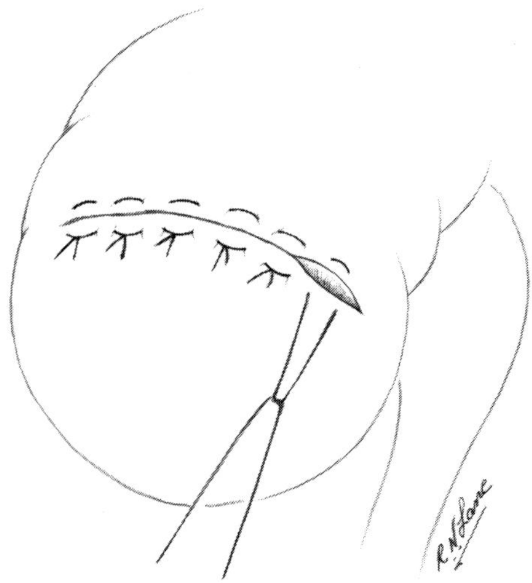

8d

9a–d

On occasion a heminephrectomy is required if the injured parenchyma is extensively fractured and localized to one pole of the kidney. The devitalized tissue is excised, preserving as much capsule as possible(*a*). The collecting system is closed in a watertight fashion with fine chromic suture (*b*). The capsule is closed (*c*), or if it is insufficient, a piece of peritoneum is sutured over the parenchyma (*d*).

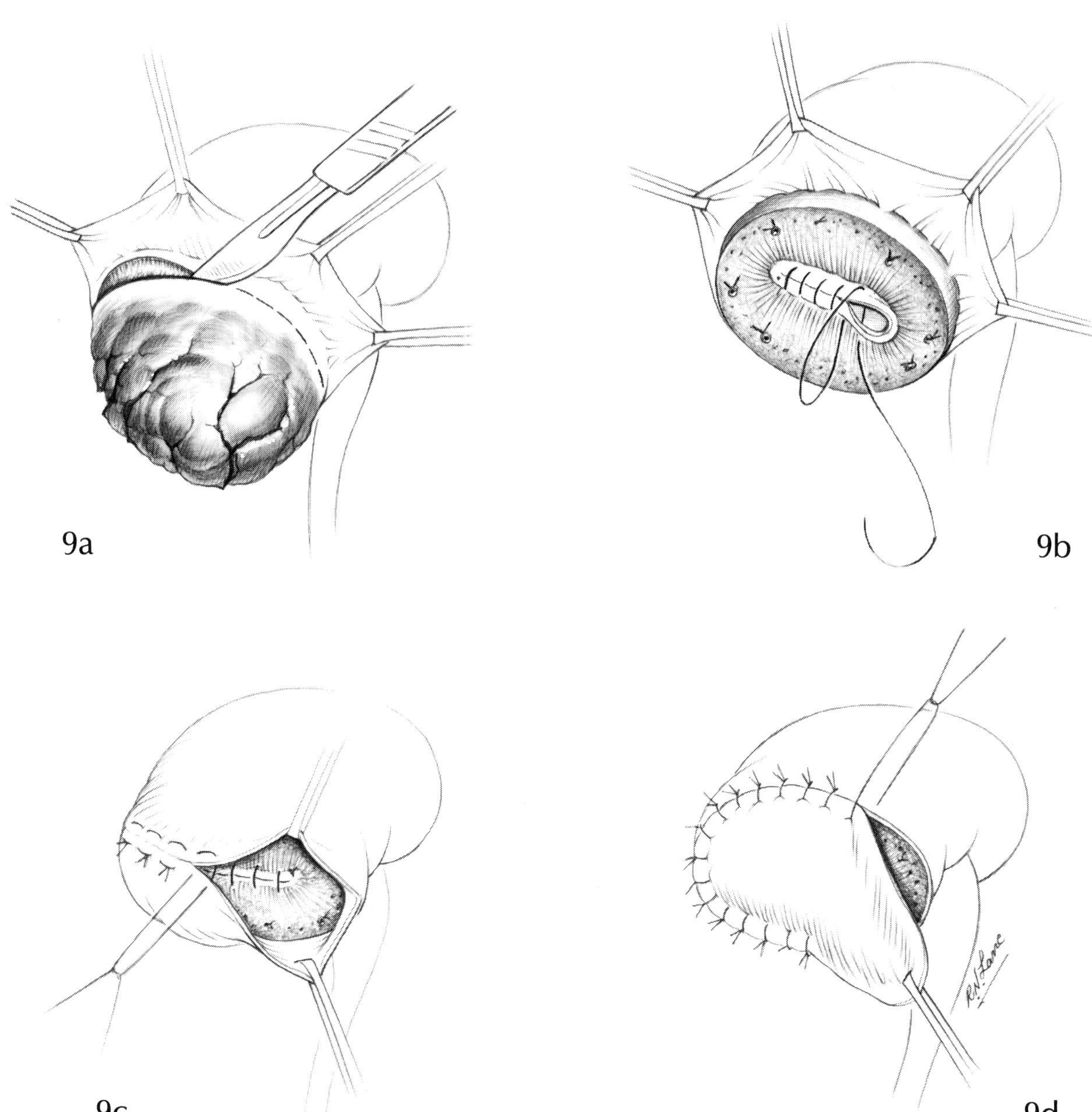

10a–d

Finally, vascular injuries are repaired with 6/0 Prolene sutures. If an intimal tear is present, the segment involved is excised and the ends primarily reanastomosed (*a*). Alternatively, the origin of the renal artery is ligated at the aorta (*b*) and the renal artery itself or a graft is sutured directly into the aorta (*c*). Patch grafts may be necessary in some instances in order to prevent compromise of the small vessel lumen (*d*). If necessary, either Gore-Tex or saphenous vein may be used as an interposed segment. The anastomosis is best made with the aid of magnification, since accuracy is absolutely mandatory for a successful outcome. Prior to occluding the renal artery, an infusion of mannitol is helpful in protecting the kidney from ischaemia and promoting diureses following restoration of renal bloodflow.

When the kidney is injured and there is a major duodenal, pancreatic or vascular injury, the kidney must be separated from these structures. If this cannot be accomplished by reapproximating Gerota's fascia and draining the area away from the above-named structures, then the kidney should either be removed or autotransplanted (*see* chapter on 'Renal transplantation', pp. 201–212, for the technique of autotransplantation). A nephrostomy should be performed if the kidney is left *in situ* in such instances, since if urine bathes wounds of the pancreas, duodenum or great vessels complications and a high mortality rate are inevitable.

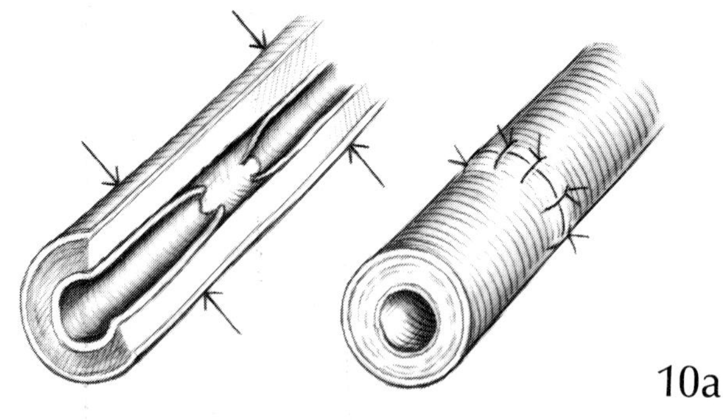

10a

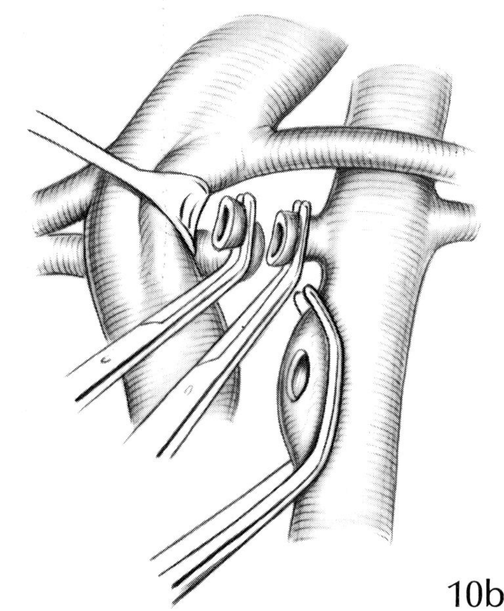

10b

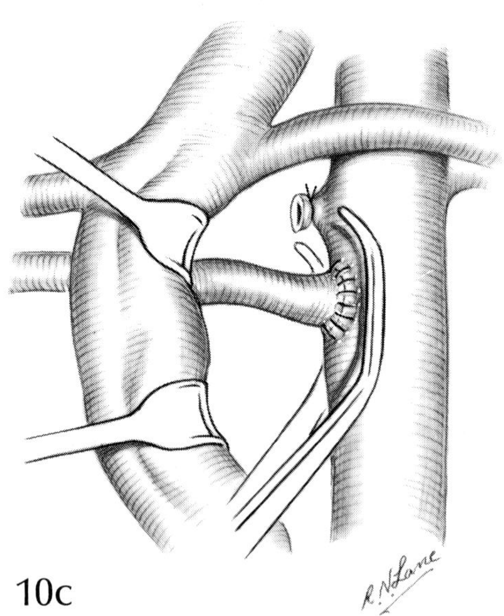

10c

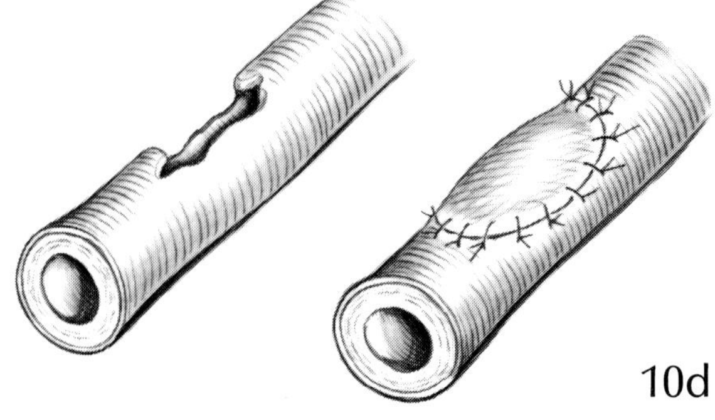

10d

Complications of renal trauma

There are numerous complications of renal trauma which may occur within the first few weeks or as late sequelae. Early complications include haemorrhage, sepsis, urinary extravasation, perinephric abscess, fistula formation, vascular suture line disruption, pancreatic fistula, duodenal fistula, and acute renal failure.

Late complications include hypertension, generally as a result of a compromised vessel or constriction of the kidney (Page kidney), hydronephrosis, chronic renal failure, calculus disease, arteriovenous fistulae, haematocele and non-functioning kidney.

Renal injury in children

Children's kidneys are much more vulnerable to injury than adults' because the retroperitoneal area is not as well protected by fat as it is in adults'. Most children with renal injuries, save for those of the pedicle and complete fracture of the kidney with separation of parts, should be observed initially. They may be explored after being stabilized between the second and the fifth post-injury day if there is urinoma formation, continued haemorrhage, or the extent of the original injury was underestimated. Immediate exploration, of course, should be performed in patients with expanding flank masses or pedicle injury, or in whom major segments of parenchyma are disrupted and disassociated from the remaining kidney with continued bleeding.

Further reading

Bergquvist, D., Hedelin, H., Lindblad, B. Blunt renal trauma, Scandinavian Journal of Urology and Nephrology 1980; 14: 177–180

Cass, A. S. Immediate radiological evaluation and early surgical management of genitourinary injuries from external trauma. Journal of Urology 1979; 122: 772–774

Emanuel, B., Weiss, H., Gollin, P. Renal trauma in children. Journal of Trauma 1977; 17: 275–278

McAninch, J. W., Carroll, P. R. Renal trauma: Kidney preservation through improved vascular control – a refined approach. Journal of Trauma 1982; 22: 285–290

McDougal, W. S., Persky, L. Traumatic injuries of the genitourinary system. Baltimore: Williams and Wilkins, 1981

Wein, A. J., Murphy, J. J., Mulholland, S. G., Chait, A. W., Arger, P. H. A conservative approach to the management of blunt renal trauma. Journal of Urology 1977; 117: 425–427

Williams, J. E. Renal trauma; the place of arteriography. British Journal of Radiology 1976; 49: 743–744

Simple and radical cystectomy

John R. Richardson, Jr MD
Clinical Associate Professor of Urology,
Dartmouth-Hitchcock Medical School, Hanover, New Hampshire, USA

Introduction

In the first half of the 20th century, the development of satisfactory techniques of urinary diversion made the operation of cystectomy increasingly attractive to surgeons as a means of treating patients with invasive bladder cancer. The Bricker ileal conduit, described in 1950, has been the standard diversionary procedure[1]. Recently, colon conduits have enjoyed increasing use, although their superiority over the ileal operation has been disputed[2]. The addition of lymph node dissection and various doses of radiation therapy to this operation seems to increase patient survival in certain circumstances, but routine use of these modalities remains controversial[3,4,5].

1

In our hands, simple cystectomy in the male means removal of the bladder with a portion of overlying pelvic peritoneum, ureteral stumps, prostate, seminal vesicles and a portion of the membranous urethra.

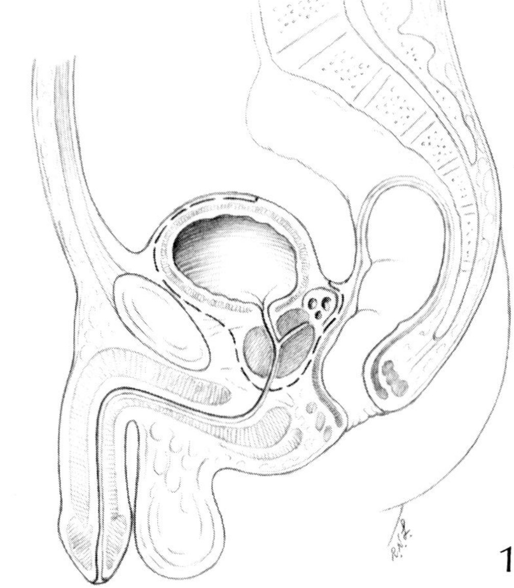

2

In the female patient, the uterus, ovaries, Fallopian tubes and a portion of the vaginal vault and urethra are included in the surgical specimen.

Radical cystectomy denotes the addition of bilateral pelvic lymphadenectomy of the iliac and obturator regions to simple cystectomy. This operation is designed to remove the entire bladder, adjacent organs and the immediate lymphatic drainage areas in one surgical specimen[6]. Indications include localized invading cancers, rapidly recurring superficial cancers and endoscopically unresectable lesions[3,4]. Sexual and voiding functions are sacrificed.

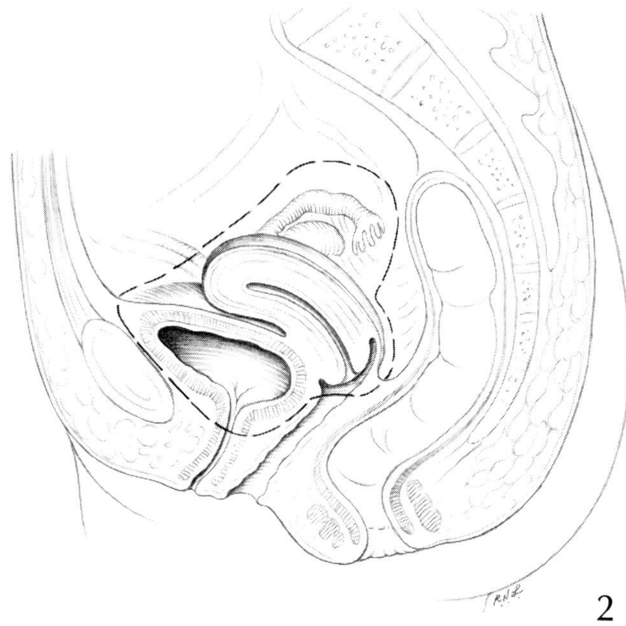

Preoperative

The patient must be an acceptable medical risk for major surgery. Preoperative studies include intravenous pyelography, cystoscopy with biopsy, pelvic examination under anaesthesia and studies to rule out the presence of metastatic disease. Computed tomography of the pelvis has yet to be proved an adequate tool for staging bladder cancer[7]. In patients with normal history, physical examination, liver function tests and alkaline phosphatase levels, liver and bone scans have ordinarily not been helpful in preoperative staging[8].

Any of the standard mechanical bowel preparation routines is satisfactory. This is begun 3 days prior to surgery. We have not used routine digitalization and anticoagulation preoperatively. It is important to instruct the patient in the use of the incentive spirometer preoperatively.

Plans for location of the urinary stoma are begun a few days prior to the operation in order to familiarize the patient with the concept and appliances and to locate a satisfactory site. We try to select a flat area in the right or left lower quadrant below the belt line. The patient is asked to wear a smooth non-adherent face plate with a belt and ordinary clothes for a day – standing, sitting and lying down – in order to locate the most suitable stomal area. This is then marked with a skin pencil and inscribed with a needle in the operating room prior to skin preparation.

In cases of nutritional deficiency, hyperalimentation seems to be indicated preoperatively. Intravenous fluids are begun the night prior to surgery to avoid the hypovolaemia sometimes associated with bowel preparation.

Ordinarily the operation is performed with a single team, although a two-team approach may be useful in some situations. Concurrent urethrectomy is performed in some patients. A general anaesthetic technique is employed. Without excellent anaesthetic support and the presence of an intensive care unit, the surgeon operates at his and the patient's peril.

The operation

The patient is placed on the table in the supine head-down position, so that the intestines gravitate to the upper abdomen. The penis in the male and the vagina in the female are prepared and draped into the operative field. A 20 Fr foley catheter is inserted *per urethram* into the bladder. A midline abdominal incision is made from the upper abdomen to the pubis, skirting the umbilicus and at least 4–5 cm away from the medial aspect of the preselected stomal site. The peritoneal cavity is entered and a careful abdominal and pelvic exploration is carried out. Specific attention is paid to the iliac and obturator node-bearing areas. Frozen section specimens of any suspicious tissues are obtained, and the operation is usually terminated if there is gross evidence of metastic disease. If not, the cystectomy is begun.

A large self-retaining Balfour retractor is placed in the lower portion of the wound. Intestines are packed superiorly using three laparotomy pads and a rolled cloth towel in an inverted U-position. Next the peritoneum overlying the distal ureters is incised. On the left, one must be lateral to the sigmoid colon. The ureters are bluntly freed posteriorly, with finger dissection, from the kidney to the deep pelvis. Care is taken to preserve as much blood supply as possible. The ureters are then divided deep in the pelvis and the distal stumps are ligated with 0 chromic catgut. Sections of the proximal ureter are sent for frozen section diagnosis. If these ends are found to be healthy, they are then ligated with 4/0 chromic catgut ligatures. We believe the resulting dilatation that occurs prior to construction of the conduit facilitates the anastomosis of the ureters to the bowel; it is not associated with an increased incidence of leakage or stricture at the ureteral intestinal sites.

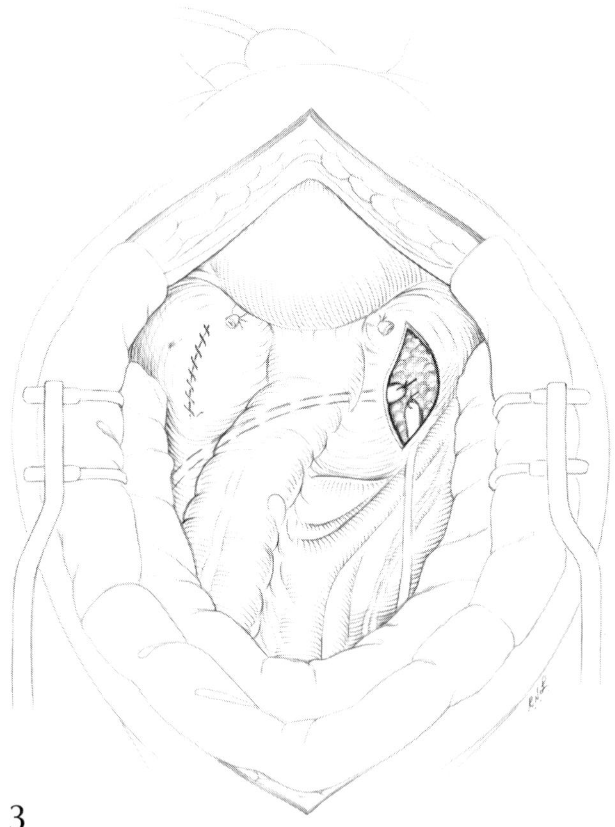

3

3

Next, using two fingers, a tunnel is made beneath the mesentery of the sigmoid colon connecting the two incisions in the posterior peritoneum. Care is taken to avoid mesenteric vessels. The left ureter is then drawn through the tunnel in a gentle arc to the peritoneal incision on the right side. One must take care to avoid excessive angulation of the left ureter which could lead to obstruction. The left peritoneal incision is closed with a running suture of 3/0 chromic catgut. The ureters remain in the right posterior peritoneal incision during the cystectomy.

4a, b & c

Using blunt dissection, the space of Retzius is developed and the bladder is separated from the lateral pelvic walls, the peritoneum being swept superiorly (*a*). The dissection is carried as far distally as the urethral catheter. The presence of the sigmoid colon makes the left side dissection somewhat more difficult. These manoeuvres are easier if the bladder has been partially filled with sterile water. At the completion of the dissection, the bladder is allowed to drain.

In the male, a generous area of pelvic peritoneum overlying the dome and posterior wall of the bladder is incised using the scalpel (*b*). The midpoint should be 2–3 cm above the peritoneal reflection in the pouch of Douglas. On both sides the vas deferens and any surrounding vessels are ligated and divided. Any remaining tissues in this area are bluntly swept towards the bladder until the lateral vesical pedicles are approached. The deep pelvic peritoneum is then sharply dissected in the midline inferiorly from the bladder for a distance of 4–5 cm (*c*). This provides a layer between the bladder wall and the rectum.

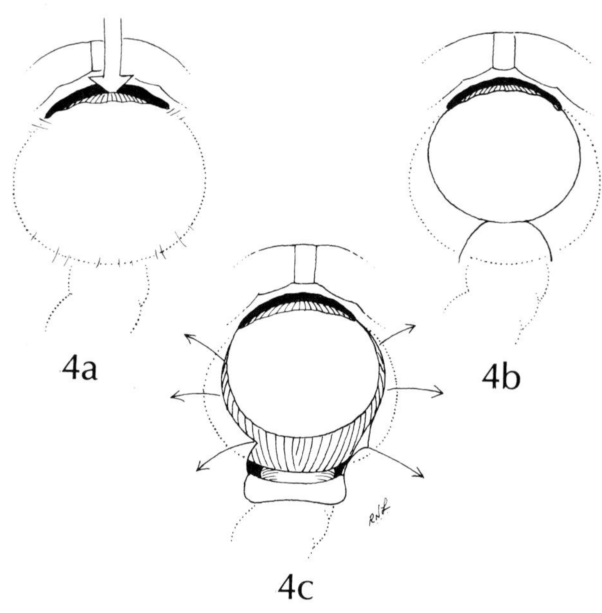

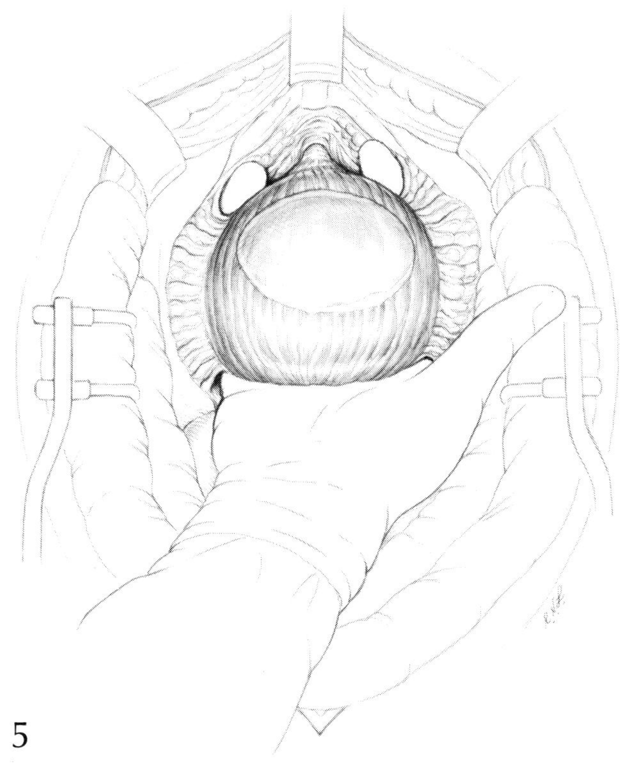

5

5

The upturned fingers and hand are worked bluntly beneath the bladder superficial to the rectum as far distally as the prostate and the urethra. With this manoeuvre two lateral wings of tissue are created containing the blood supply and lymphatic drainage of the bladder. This dissection must be done gently to avoid rectal damage, entry into the bladder and bleeding from torn veins in the area.

6

In the female, the pelvic peritoneal incisions encompass the ovaries and tubes laterally and the uterus and vaginal vault posteriorly. The bladder is freed laterally as in the male, taking care to divide and ligate the ovarian and uterine arteries and the round ligaments. Instead of creating the inferior rectovesical plane as in the male, the upper vagina and cervix are located by palpation and the vaginal vault is entered. A sponge soaked in iodine solution and inserted into the vagina preoperatively renders this manoeuvre easier and safer. The vaginal cuff is incised and whip-stitched to control bleeding. The anterior wall of the vagina is then sharply dissected from the bladder base and upper urethra containing the catheter, which can be located by palpation. When this has been done, two lateral wings of tissue containing the bladder blood supply and lymphatic drainage are created.

If pelvic lymphadenectomy is planned, it is carried out at this time. The left side is approached first as the presence of the sigmoid colon makes this dissection somewhat more difficult. The left external iliac artery is palpated on the lateral pelvic wall, and is approached with sharp dissection as far distally as the area of the inferior epigastric artery and circumflex iliac vein. Here the distal margin is marked with a silver clip. The use of these ligating clips makes the node dissection faster, easier and safer than the use of clamps and ligatures.

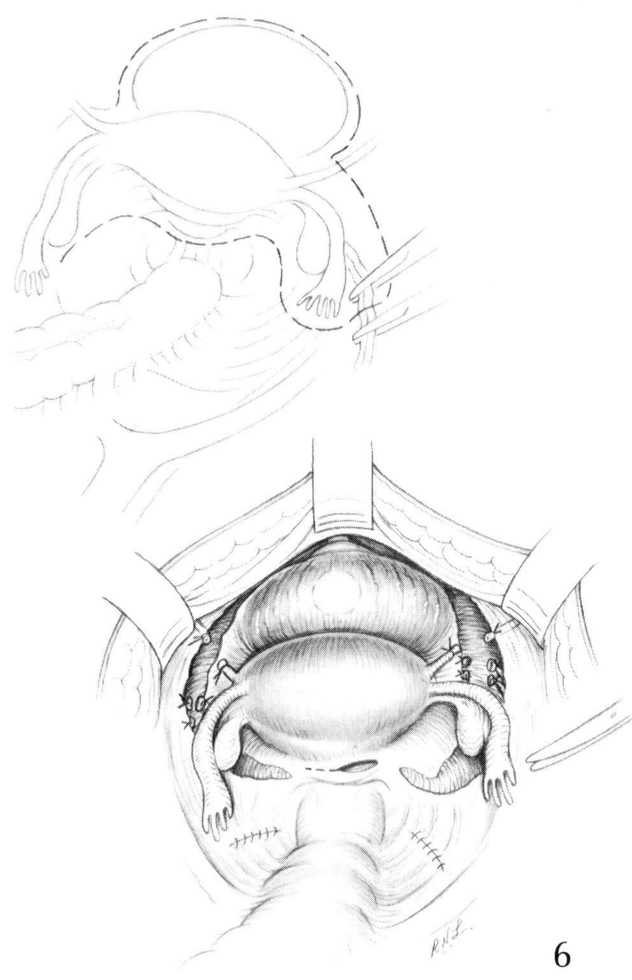

6

7

Metzenbaum scissors are then directed proximally along the wall of the artery and the overlying tissue is incised to an area just above the bifurcation of the common iliac artery. The proper plane is as close to the arterial wall as possible.

The medial and lateral tissue masses thus created are drawn inferiorly along the vessel. Vein retractors and peanut dissectors are helpful in this manoeuvre. An identical procedure is performed on the iliac vein, which lies just below the artery. Now the mass of tissue which lies below the external iliac vein is excised distally after clipping and is drawn inferomedially towards the bladder. At the bifurcation of the common iliac artery, nodal tissue is teased from the crotch. The dissection is carried down the internal iliac artery sweeping lymph-bearing tissue medially. The first two anterior branches of this artery, the superior and inferior vesical arteries, are then ligated with 2/0 silk. This deprives the bladder of its major blood supply. The tissues from the anterior portion of the internal iliac vein are likewise swept medially. Below the external iliac vein, the obturator nerve is located first by palpation and then by dissection. This is the lateral boundary of the deep node dissection. Fat- and lymph-bearing tissue is then teased from the obturator fossa with forceps and pushed medially together with the external and internal iliac specimens.

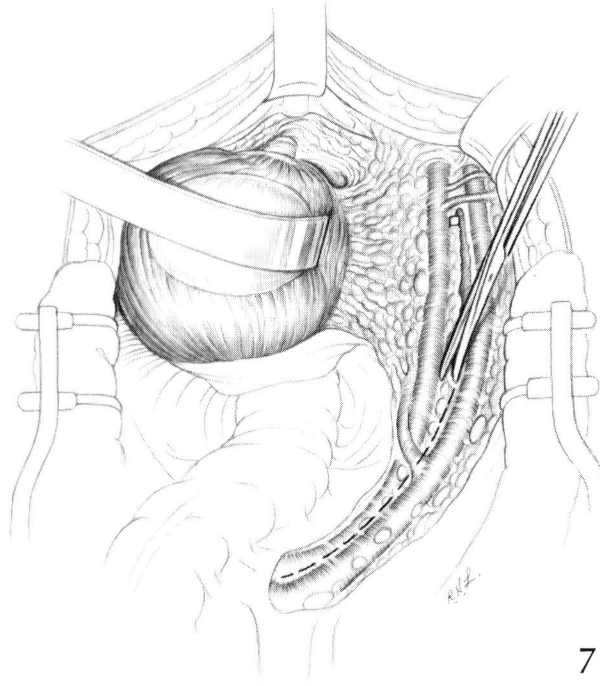

7

8

When this dissection is completed, the lateral pelvic walls and vessels should be clear of lymph-bearing tissue from just proximal to the inguinal ligament to an area just proximal to the common iliac artery bifurcation. All tissues, having been pushed medially, are removed with the bladder specimen. The same dissection is carried out on the right side.

Next the cystectomy proper is begun. If a pelvic node dissection has not been done, the internal iliac artery is exposed and the first two anterior branches are divided. Then the urethral Foley is palpated and a right-angle clamp is driven through the avascular endopelvic fascia lateral to the urethra in the female and lateral to the puboprostatic ligaments in the male. This marks the distal extent of the lateral pelvic wings of tissue on each side.

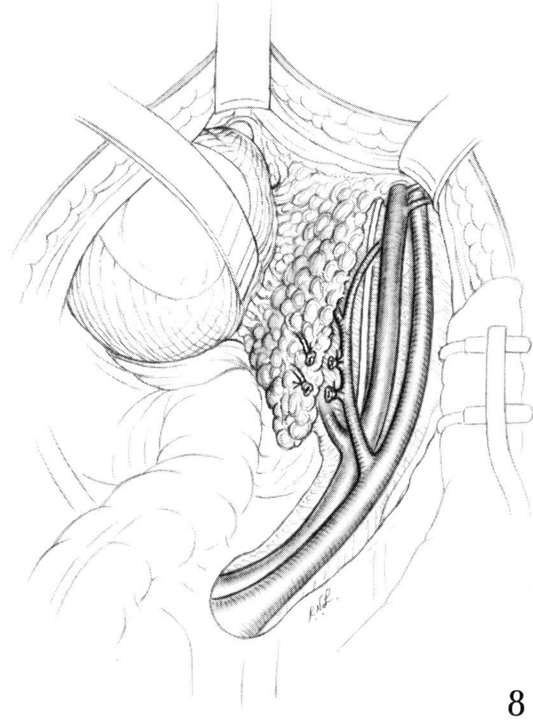

8

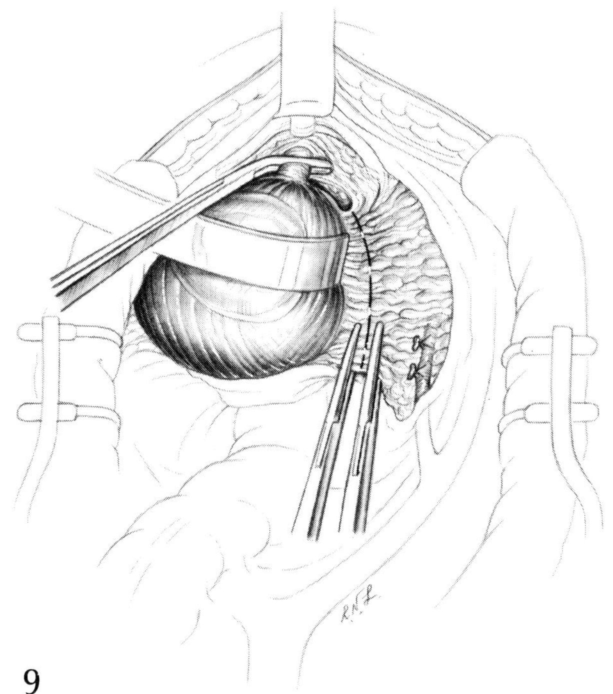

9

9

These wings are divided and suture-ligated with 0 chromic catgut between Kocher clamps. The area to be clamped is carefully palpated prior to placement of the clamps in order to avoid entering either the bladder or the rectum. When this has been accomplished, the specimen is free except for the urethra and periurethral attachments.

In the male, the puboprostatic ligaments are then sharply divided. The resultant bleeding is controlled with pressure. We have had little success in trying to suture-ligate these ligaments and the veins beneath. The urethra is then grasped with a large right-angle clamp, distal to the prostate in the male, taking care to avoid the rectum. In the female, the urethra is grasped distal to the bladder neck. The urethra is then sharply divided distal to the clamp along with the indwelling Foley catheter. This manoeuvre is not carried out if total urethrectomy is indicated.

10

The surgical specimen is removed and a 24 Fr Foley catheter with a 30 ml bag is inserted into the pelvis via the urethral remnant. The bag is inflated with 50 ml of saline and drawn down against the pelvic floor with traction, being held in place by a ring forceps applied to the catheter at the external urethral meatus. This manoeuvre successfully controls bleeding from the periurethral tissues deep in the pelvis.

The rectosigmoid is carefully inspected to make sure it is intact and a diligent search is made to locate any bleeding points in the pelvis. These are controlled with ligatures and electrocautery. Two moist laparotomy pads are then placed in the pelvis to remain there for the rest of the procedure. Appendicectomy is undertaken at this time in the standard fashion.

After the conduit has been constructed the pelvic packs are removed and a final search is made to discover any significant bleeding. Tension on the urethral Foley is removed and the periurethral area is checked to make sure there is no significant ooze. When the surgeon is satisfied, closure is begun. A nasogastric tube is placed in the stomach by the anaesthetist, the location being checked by the surgeon. Infrequently we have used gastrostomy tubes. The wound is closed with No. 2 stay sutures placed 2 cm apart through all layers of the abdominal wall, taking care not to injure the conduit or its blood supply. We place these retention sutures close together in order to provide uniform wound support and to avoid evisceration should wound infection and dehiscence occur. The peritoneal remnants, rectus fascia and subcutaneous tissues are closed in layers with absorbable sutures. A visceral retainer protects the intestines from becoming lodged between the retention sutures during the closure. The skin is closed with staples and the retention sutures are tied over two fingers of the assistant using segments of rubber catheter as bolsters. A minimal dressing is applied.

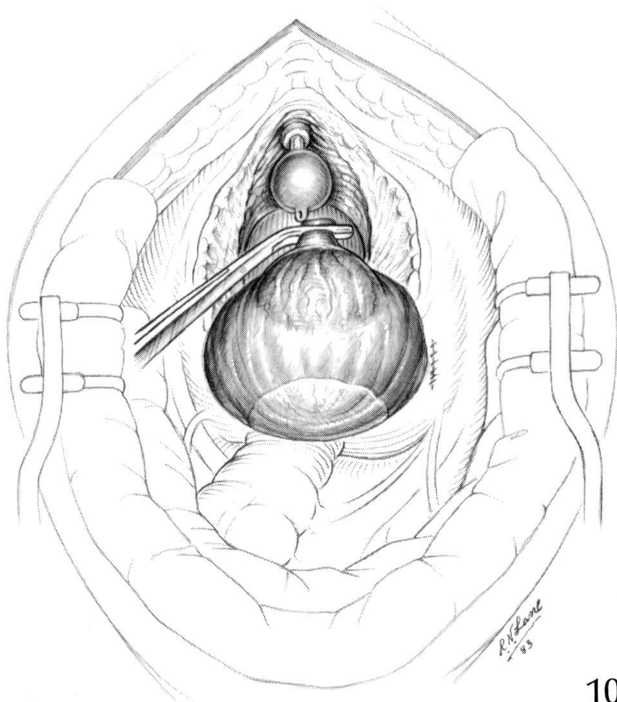

10

Postoperative care

Appropriate antibiotics are administered for 7–10 days. Early ambulation is essential, as is vigorous pulmonary support. The nasogastric tube is removed when the patient has passed gas or had a bowel movement. The average hospital stay is 14–18 days.

Complications have occurred in about a third of our patients. Common early problems are wound infection, prolonged ileus and ureteral intestinal leaks. Common late problems are small bowel and ureteral obstruction and stomal difficulties. The use of radiation therapy seems to increase the surgical complication rate.

In our hands, this is usually a long, difficult, tedious and bloody operation. Aggressive surgical techniques and excellent anaesthetic, medical and nursing support are essential if a good result is to be obtained. These patients require more frequent follow-up than most. About half survive for 5 years, most dying of distant metastatic disease. Further increases in survival rates will probably be achieved only with the development of effective systemic anticancer therapy. Nevertheless, we feel that this surgical procedure, with or without presently available adjuvant therapy, offers most patients with aggressive and invasive bladder cancer the best chance for prolonged survival with an acceptable quality of life.

References

1. Bricker, E. M. Bladder substitution after pelvic evisceration. Surgical Clinics of North America 1950; 30: 1511–1521

2. Sullivan, J. W., Grabstald, H., Whitmore, W. F., Jr. Complications of ureteroileal conduit with radical cystectomy. Review of 336 cases. Journal of Urology 1980; 124: 797–801

3. Mathur, V. K., Krahn, H. P., Ramsey, E. W. Total cystectomy for bladder cancer. Journal of Urology 1981; 125: 784–786

4. Radwin, H. M. Invasive transitional cell carcinoma of the bladder: is there a place for preoperative radiotherapy? Urologic Clinics of North America October 1980; 7: 551–557

5. Heney, N, M., Prout, G. R., Jr. Preoperative irradiation as an adjuvant in the surgical management of patients with invasive bladder cancer. Urologic Clinics of North America 1980; 7: 543–549

6. Prout, G. R. The surgical management of bladder cancer. Urologic Clinics of North America 1976; 3: 149–175

7. Koss, J. C., Arger, P. H., Coleman, B. G., Mulhern, C. B., Pollack, H. M., Wein, A. J. CT staging of bladder carcinoma. American Journal of Roentgeneology 1981; 137. 359–362

8. Berger, G. L., Sadlowski, R. W., Sharpe, J. R., Finney, R. P. Lack of value of routine preoperative bone and liver scans in cystectomy candidates. Journal or Urology 1981; 125: 637–639

Transvesical prostatectomy

Warwick Macky OBE, MS, FRCS, FRACS
Urologist, Auckland Hospital, New Zealand

Introduction

The technique of transvesical prostatectomy was first described and refined by McGill[1], Fuller[2] and Freyer[3]. Significant modifications were made by Thompson-Walker[4], Harris[5], Hryntschak[6,7], Malament[8] and others with the object of improving control of postoperative bleeding to allow primary closure of the bladder with a much lower incidence of sepsis and suprapubic fistula.

Basic considerations

The operation of transvesical prostatectomy is based on the following principles:

1. A small abdominal incision and a limited high cystotomy are used to give adequate surgical access with minimal disturbance of tissue planes.
2. Transvesical enucleation of all adenomatous tissue is effected within the concentric layers of the false or surgical capsule, avoiding interference with the highly vascular, true prostatic capsule. Coincident bladder neck obstruction is relieved.
3. Postoperative bleeding is controlled by ligature of the urethral branches of the prostatic arteries and other vessels at the bladder neck, together with reduction and tamponade of the prostatic fossa.
4. The bladder is closed either by primary purse-string or alternatively by two-layer suture with urethral catheter drainage.

In this chapter, a modified Harris prostatectomy is described with comments on the Hryntschak and Malament operations.

Preoperative

Indications

Transvesical prostatectomy is suitable for all types of intraurethral and intravesical benign enlargement of the prostate, with or without coincident bladder neck obstruction. The operation may be used to advantage when the enlargement of the prostate is associated with such conditions as calculus in the bladder or lower ureter, bladder diverticulum, ureterocele and certain bladder tumours.

A pre-existing suprapubic cystotomy may be extended for the prostatectomy. Inguinal or abdominal hernias may be repaired at the same time as prostatectomy is performed. Those patients who will not tolerate transurethral resection by reason of urethral stricture or unfavourable reactions to the passage of instruments *per urethram*, or those unable to be placed in a lithotomy position because of orthopaedic deformities, are best treated by transvesical prostatectomy.

When retropubic prostatectomy is made difficult by deformity in the bone structure of the symphysis pubis obliterating the retropubic space or by extensive vascular malformations in the anterior prostatic capsule, the transvesical approach is preferable.

Contraindications

Transvesical prostatectomy is not ideal for small fibrous glands, bladder neck obstruction due to fibrous bar, or carcinoma of the prostate. These lesions are best treated by transurethral resection. However, when transurethral resection is not feasible, transvesical resection of bladder neck obstruction gives good results.

Preoperative preparation

As transvesical prostatectomy is an elective procedure, every effort must be made to ensure that the patient is in the best possible condition for surgery. Cardiorespiratory and metabolic diseases are treated adequately and anaemia is corrected. Fluid and acid-base balance is restored.

Adequate time should be allowed for the adverse effects of such drugs as anticoagulants and antihypertensives to be corrected.

Acute retention of urine is relieved by an indwelling, self-retaining urethral catheter, 16 or 18 Fr, inserted under full aseptic precautions and connected to closed-system dependent drainage. Smaller-sized catheters are less likely to give rise to urethritis or pressure necrosis of the urethral mucosa with secondary epididymo-orchitis and late urethral stricture. If urethral drainage is impracticable, a stab suprapubic cystotomy or formal cystotomy may be needed.

When the patient is uraemic, prolonged bladder drainage should be maintained until the optimal level of renal function is established. However, surgery may be considered when renal function is seriously impaired if facilities for dialysis are available.

Urinary tract infection is treated by free drainage of the bladder urine and minimal chemotherapy. Provision is made for prompt treatment of Gram-negative septicaemia. When there is chronic retention with a vesical residue in excess of 1 litre, without uraemia, preoperative catheter drainage may be instituted in some cases, but in general urethral manipulations are avoided as haemorrhage and infection may ensue.

An intravenous pyelogram and micturating cystourethrogram may be requested when associated disease is suspected in the urinary tract, but routine pyelography is seldom warranted. Preliminary cystoscopy may be performed to exclude associated tumour, calculus or other lesions in the bladder or urethra. Provision is made for blood replacement.

Time should be taken to allay the patient's fear of the operation, and to discuss the likely effects on potency and fertility in the younger age group.

The operation

Anaesthesia

General anaesthesia with relaxation is used routinely, although a spinal or epidural anaesthetic may be preferred. Induced hypotension has been advocated by some but has not found general acceptance. Dextrose-saline solution is given intravenously during the operation and significant blood loss is replaced.

Operation time should be as short as possible to reduce the incidence of anaesthetic and cardiovascular complications.

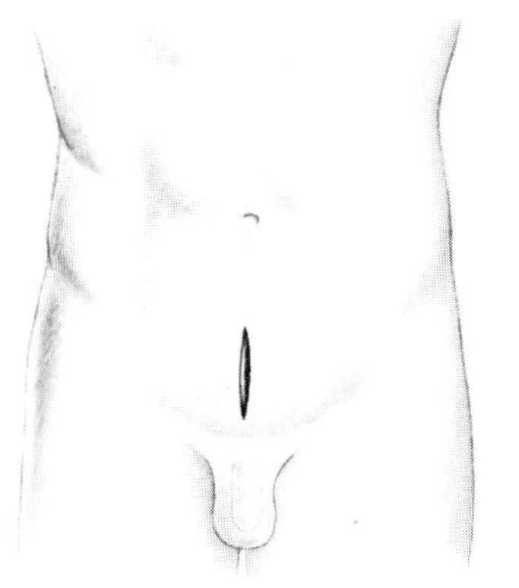

1

2

Position of patient

The patient is placed supine on the table in the head down position to allow abdominal wall fat to drop away from the suprapubic region. Supports are placed under the tendoachillis to relieve pressure on the calf muscles. The diathermy plate is checked after final positioning.

After shaving, the abdomen, genitalia and upper thighs are painted with antiseptic solution and, if desired, adhesive drapes and an O'Connor shield are applied to the lower abdomen and perineum.

Vas ligation is not advised routinely but may be done via small scrotal incisions at this stage in selected cases.

The external urinary meatus and the anterior penile urethra are calibrated. If there is a stricture, Otis urethrotomy, meatotomy or meatoplasty with accurate 4/0 chromic catgut approximation of the penile skin and exposed urethral mucosa is effected. If this is not done, pressure necrosis of the mucosa due to the postoperative, indwelling retention urethral catheter will almost certainly aggravate the stricture.

1 & 2

The incisions

A 5–6 cm vertical midline incision is made through skin, subcutaneous tissue and rectus fascia immediately above the level of the symphysis pubis. This short incision causes minimal disruption of tissue planes and allows adequate rapid exposure of the bladder with the Harris bladder retractor in position. It heals well without undue risk of postoperative incisional hernia. Alternatively, a transverse suprapubic creaseline skin incision 2 cm above the symphysis may be used.

The rectus and pyramidialis muscles are separated in the midline to expose the fascia transversalis and the fibrofatty tissue in the prevesical space.

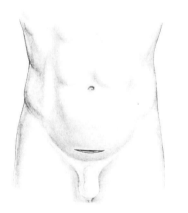

3

Mobilization of bladder

The extravesical fascia is incised in the midline to expose the oyster-coloured bladder muscle with a few veins coursing over the superficial aspect of the vault. If this plane is correctly exposed deep to the extravesical fascia, the peritoneum can be dissected superiorly off the vault in the midline until the dome of the bladder can be brought up to the level of the skin between Allis tissue forceps. There is no need to overdistend the bladder to facilitate this manoeuvre, which is essential to allow a high cystotomy with sufficient mobilization of the vault to ensure subsequent watertight closure.

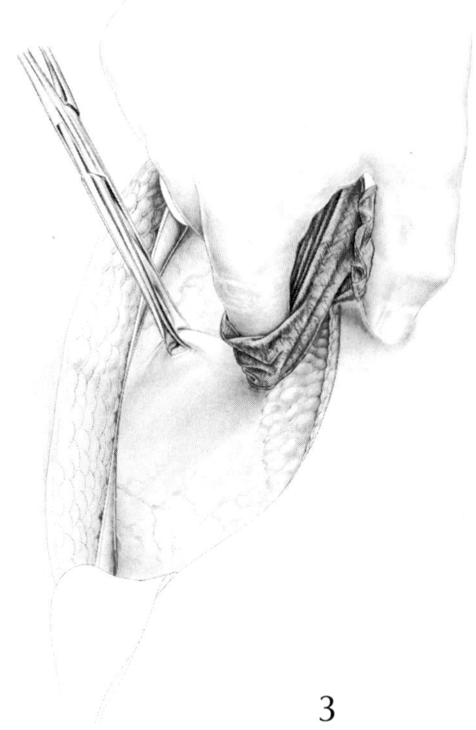

3

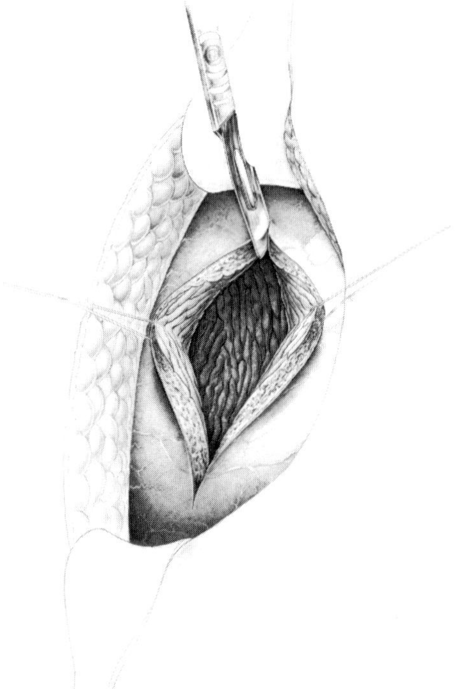

4

4

Opening the bladder

A high 3–4 cm transverse incision is made in the hypertrophied bladder muscle between Allis forceps. The bladder mucosa is seen as a 'pearly bead', which is incised, and the bladder contents are aspirated in such a way as to cause minimal trauma to the bladder mucosa. Two plain catgut stay sutures are inserted in the superior and inferior edges of the cystotomy.

The bladder and prostatic urethra are now explored digitally and any calculi removed. Associated lesions such as bladder diverticulum are best dealt with at this stage.

5

Enucleation of the adenoma

Having assessed the size, type and extent of the enlargement of the prostate bimanually, with one or two fingers of the left hand inserted *per rectum*, the enucleation is started in the urethra, at the apex of the prostate.

The correct plane for enucleation within the concentric layers of the surgical capsule is found by rupturing through the prostatic urethra with firm pressure exerted by the index finger in the anterolateral plane near the midline on either side against the resistance of the peripheral prostatic tissue supported in turn by the bony symphysis. The separation of the apical masses is carried out circumferentially, one side at a time, until the mucosa of the prostatic urethra is separated as far as possible from that of the membranous urethra. Any residual attachments in this plane may be divided by further careful finger dissection, or with scissors, to minimize damage to the membranous urethra, a cuff of which is in danger of being avulsed by traction. This could result in incontinence, although this is rarely a problem.

If enucleation proves difficult due to fibrous tissue or unsuspected infiltrating carcinoma, it is better to stop forthwith and complete the separation of the lateral lobes by sharp dissection under vision when the retractor has been inserted. Ill-advised attempts at enucleation may result in splits of the true prostatic capsule and even rupture of the bladder with severe bleeding and extravasation of urine. When there is gross enlargement, the lateral lobes may be removed separately; on occasion, fenestrated ovum forceps may help to deliver the freed adenomatous tissue from the prostatic fossa.

Due to lack of counter-resistance, it may be difficult to enucleate well-developed subtrigonal or middle-lobe tissue without damaging or avulsing the trigone and bladder base. In such cases the mucosa over the base of the enlarged middle lobe is incised and the dissection completed after the bladder retractor is in position.

Finally, the prostatic fossa is carefully palpated bimanually for residual adenomata which may prolapse into the fossa after enucleation of the main adenomatous mass. These should be removed and any tags of capsule excised.

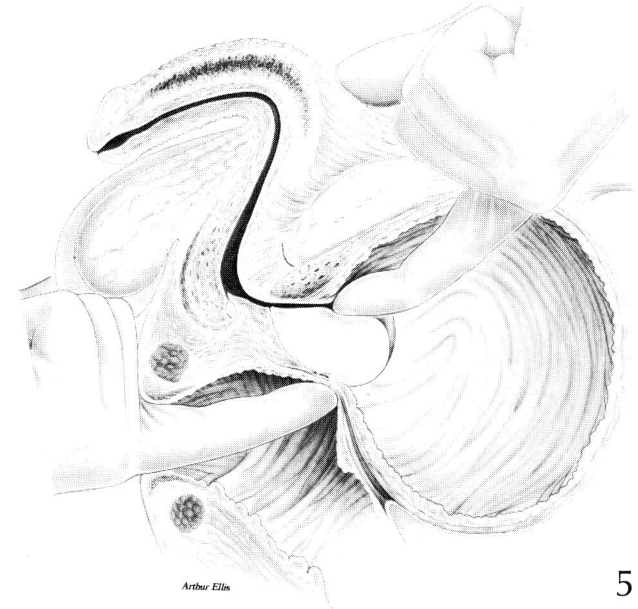

5

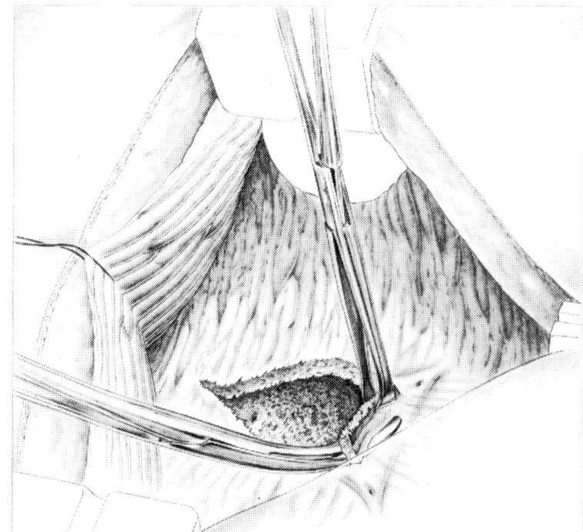

6

6

Excision of bladder neck

The Harris bladder retractor is now inserted in such a way that the vault of the bladder is supported at skin level to ensure an adequate view of the operative field. A pack placed behind the posterior blade may improve the view of the bladder neck and trigone.

The ureteric ridge and trigone are identified, and prominent fibrous bar tissue is excised *en bloc* posteriorly so that the trigonal 'shelf' is reduced in extent. Any further capsular tags, residual adenomata and mucosal remnants are excised under vision, using the curved Harris suction for additional retraction and to maintain a dry field.

7 & 8

Suture haemostasis

To secure the ureteral branches of the prostatic artery, 1/0 plain cross-mattress sutures are inserted in the plane of the bladder neck posterolaterally on each side, parallel and distal to the ureteric ridge. Harris boomerang needles facilitate this manoeuvre. Any obvious bleeding vessels in the lateral aspect of the bladder neck are similarly dealt with. One or two occluding stitches are then placed across the full thickness of the bladder neck anteriorly to reduce the prostatic fossa and support the bladder neck to prevent further extracapsular splits if traction on a bag catheter is subsequently used to tamponade the fossa. The reformed bladder neck should freely admit the tip of the index finger.

Diathermy in the prostatic fossa is not advised as the depth of tissue necrosis cannot be controlled. It is not possible to reconstitute the mucosa of the prostatic urethra by pinning down the trigone prosteriorly, as suggested by Harris.

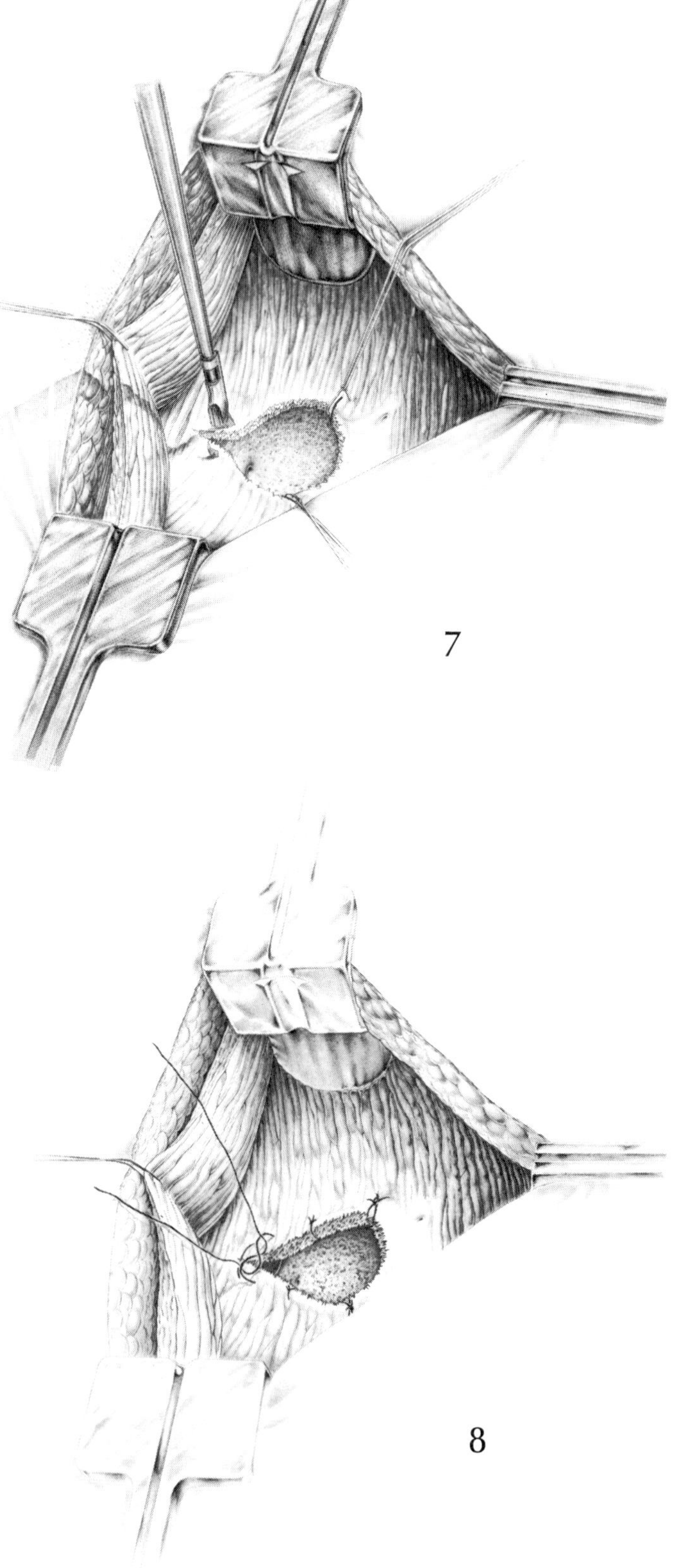
7

8

Insertion of urethral catheter

A 22 or 24 Fr three-way irrigating Foley retention catheter is passed *per urethram* and, after inflation, the bag is seated down on the bladder neck. If excessive bleeding persists, the fossa may be tamponaded by firm, gentle traction on the catheter for up to 6 hours postoperatively. When difficulty is encountered in passing the catheter through the posterior urethra, a flexible curved introducer may be used to guide the tip over any persisting trigonal shelf. The retention bag should not be inflated until the tip of the catheter is properly placed within the bladder, as overdistention of the membranous urethra may cause incontinence. The routine use of the inflated bag, positioned within the prostatic fossa for haemostasis, is not recommended. The catheter is connected to a non-return drainage bag and continuous irrigation started with normal saline at 37°C. Occasional irrigations with a sterile syringe are advisable to ensure that drainage is in fact satisfactory.

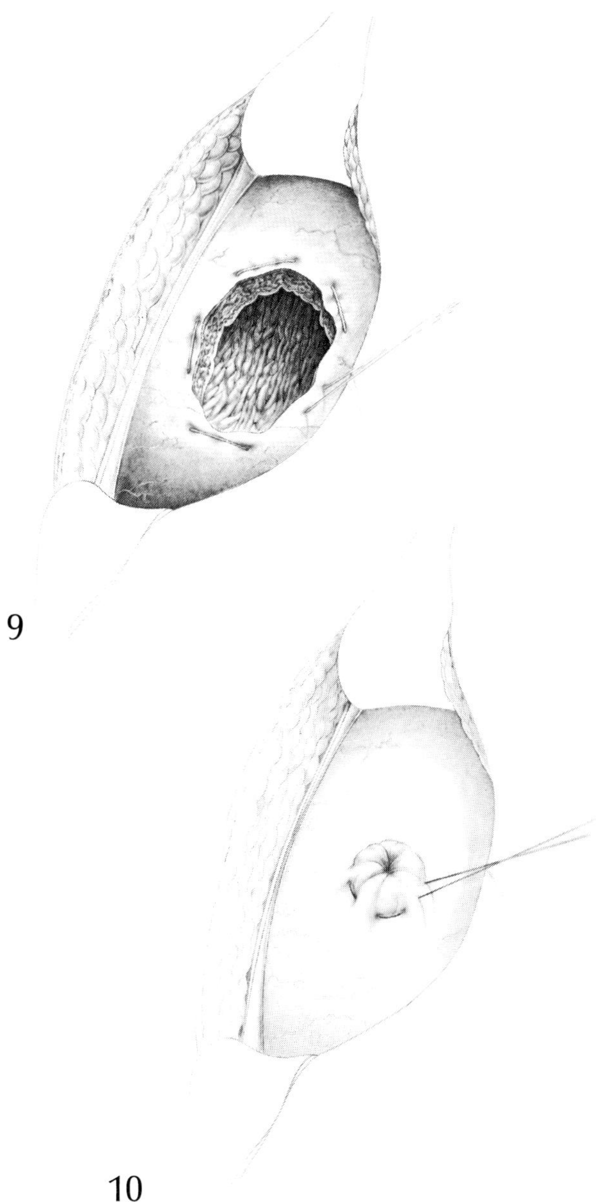

9 & 10

Bladder closure and drainage

After removal of the retractor and aspiration of any residual clots, the bladder is closed by a 2/0 plain purse-string stitch inserted deeply into the muscle so as to produce adequate inversion of the edges of the incision and to ensure watertight closure.

Alternatively, when the bladder wall is greatly thickened, two-layer closure with a deep continuous and superficial interrupted 2/0 plain catgut stitch may be used. The purse-string stitch is most effective but may be less haemostatic than two-layer closure.

A suction drain is placed in the extravesical space and the abdominal wound is closed in layers using 1/0 chromic catgut in the rectus sheath, 2/0 chromic in the subcutaneous tissue and interrupted unabsorbable stitches in the skin.

11 & 12

Hryntschak modification

In addition to the Harris stitches placed posterolaterally, Hryntschak[6,7] advocated the use of deep transverse stitches at the bladder neck, so placed as to incorporate the urethral catheter when tied. These stitches were designed to tamponade the prostatic fossa by occluding the bladder neck completely. When the catheter is removed, tension on the stitches is relieved, allowing the bladder neck to assume its normal contour.

In practice, the use of these occluding stitches has resulted in an unacceptably high incidence of bladder neck stenosis and while the method may serve to control excessive haemorrhage, its routine use is not advocated. Hryntschak also recommended purse-string closure of the bladder and he designed a useful bladder retractor.

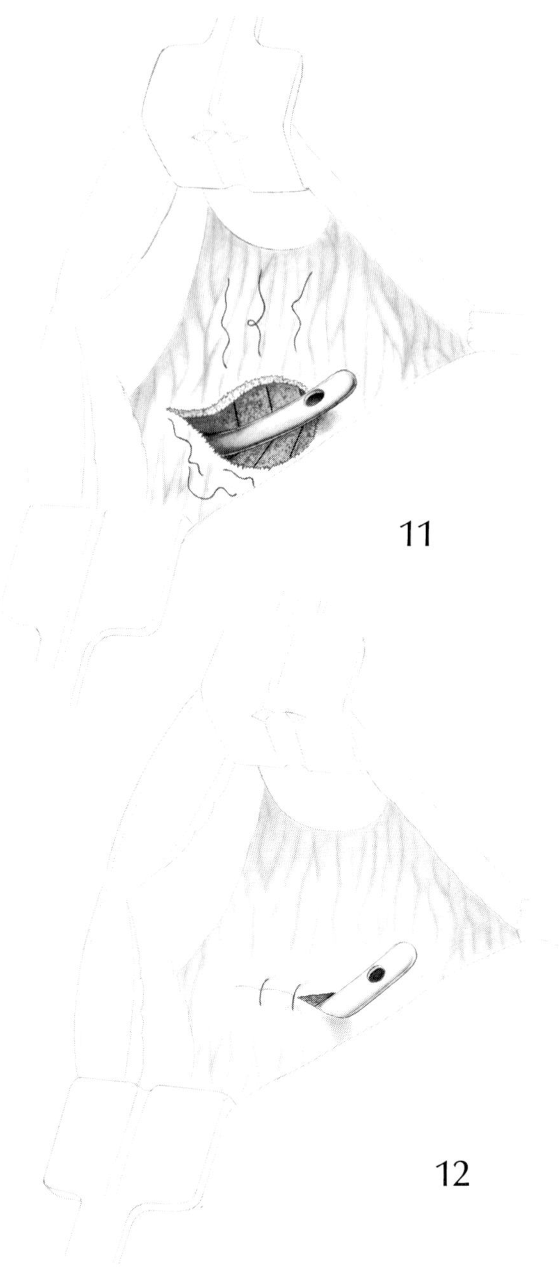

11

12

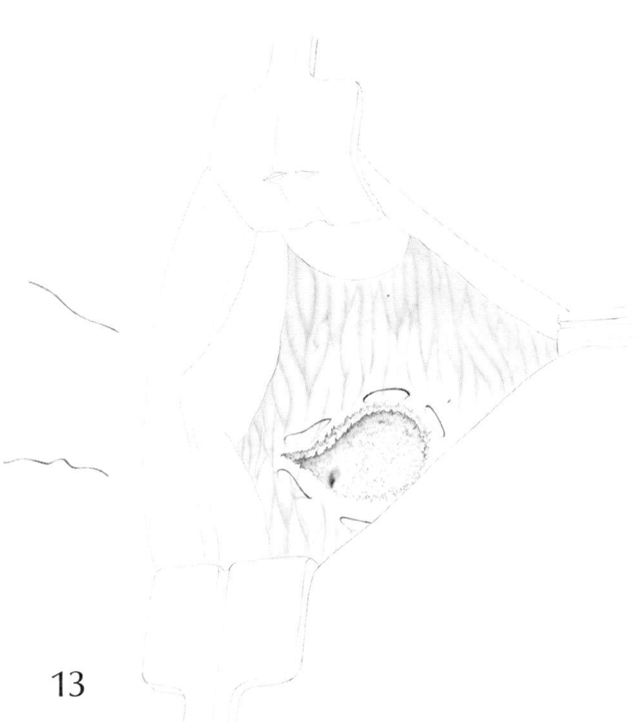

13

13

Malament modification

Malament[8] described purse-string closure of the bladder neck around an indwelling catheter as a method of tamponading the prostatic fossa. This method is undoubtedly effective in many cases and has given good results in experienced hands but may not be practicable when the bladder neck and prostatic fossa are rigid and widely patent. Attempts to close such a bladder neck may result in rupture of the capsule with additional haemorrhage and extravasation of urine.

Postoperative care and complications

In the recovery room, the patient's vital signs are closely monitored and fluid intake adjusted to ensure that blood volume is maintained. Excessive blood loss is replaced. Diuresis is promoted by intravenous fluids, supplemented if necessary by mannitol or frusemide.

The urethral catheter must drain freely at all times. If continuous saline irrigation through the three-way indwelling retention catheter is used, free drainage should be ensured by frequent small washouts with a bulb or Toomey syringe with aseptic technique. The washouts have no therapeutic effect but serve to break up and dislodge clot and debris which may accumulate about the inflated bag and over the bladder base.

If bleeding is excessive, tension on the catheter may be increased to tamponade the prostatic fossa for up to 6 hours postoperatively. In the rare case of uncommonly severe bleeding, ribbon gauze may be packed about the catheter in the prostatic fossa and brought out suprapubically so that tamponade may be made more effective. The gauze packing may be removed without disturbing the urethral catheter after 24 or 36 hours. If clot retention ensues, evacuation of the bladder is best effected *per urethram* using the cystoscope sheath and the Toomey syringe. When there is doubt as to whether the bladder is distending postoperatively, bimanual rectal examination may give useful information. The extravesical suction drain is usually removed after 24 hours.

Policy on the use of chemotherapy in the postoperative period should be flexible. When there is postoperative infection of the urine, appropriate chemotherapy or antibiotics should be given with recourse to a cephalosporin or aminoglycoside if Gram-negative septicaemia is suspected. While there may be objections to routine postoperative chemotherapy in clean cases, many urologists give suppressive doses of co-trimoxazole which may also help prevent chest infections and reduce the incidence of epididymo-orchitis. It is not unusual to give a 10–day course of suppressive chemotherapy on discharge from hospital. Symptomless pyuria and low-grade urinary tract infection may persist until healing of the prostatic fossa is complete after some weeks.

Breathing exercises and active muscle movements are supervised postoperatively. The patient should stand out of bed 12 hours after operation and walk progressively longer distances each day thereafter. Free fluids are given initially and a full diet is usually accepted a day after operation.

Continuous closed, dependent catheter drainage is maintained for 48–72 hours. The bag or plastic container should have a non-return valve and be capable of being emptied without contaminating the contents. Adherent blood clot or urethral discharge at the external meatus should be gently removed and a swab soaked in 1 per cent chlorhexidine solution placed *in situ* to reduce ascending infection.

Painful bladder spasms may be controlled by analgesics and the use of belladonna and morphine rectal suppositories. A mild laxative or suppository is given to ensure a bowel action before the catheter is removed. It is important to prevent faecal impaction at all times.

When the catheter is removed, voiding is usually frequent and painful due to urethritis and bladder spasms associated with a low-grade cystitis. On occasion, the catheter may have to be reinserted for retention, delayed bleeding or suprapubic fistula. If there is difficulty in negotiating the prostatic fossa due to a trigonal shelf, a flexible curved introducer should be used.

On discharge from hospital, the patient is encouraged to continue graded physical exercises and he should be able to resume full activity 4–6 weeks postoperatively, depending on his occupation. Fluid intake should be in excess of 2–3 litres daily and the patient should avoid constipation.

Complications

While the mortality rate of suprapubic prostatectomy of about 1.5 per cent may be higher than reported for transurethral resection, the types of cases are not strictly comparable. Death is most often due to coronary occlusion, pulmonary infarction or cerebrovascular accident, commonly seen in the older age group.

Postoperative anterior penile or bulbar urethral strictures may occur in 2–5 per cent of cases and bladder neck stenosis may be seen in about 4 per cent. Incontinence is most unusual after suprapubic prostatectomy. Late secondary haemorrhage is uncommon, but it may be severe enough to warrant readmission to hospital for evacuation of the bladder contents.

Postoperative epididymo-orchitis is also uncommon but may occur even after some weeks. Routine vas ligation does not seem to reduce the incidence of this complication. Provided all subcapsular adenomatous tissue has been removed, obstruction due to recurrent adenoma is uncommon but may be seen after 10–20 years in the younger age group. Carcinoma may develop at any time in the posterior lamella of the gland.

Most patients have some persisting urinary frequency after transvesical prostatectomy, possibly due to changes in the bladder muscle, but there is usually gradual spontaneous improvement. Suprapubic fistula is virtually unknown after one-stage suprapubic prostatectomy with adequate bladder closure. Retrograde ejaculation occurs in most cases postoperatively but there is usually minimal interference with potency. Return of potency cannot be expected in those previously impotent.

References

1. McGill, A. F. Suprapubic prostatectomy. British Medical Journal 1887; 2: 1104–1105

2. Fuller, E. Six successful and successive cases of prostatectomy. Journal of Cutaneous and Genito-urinary Diseases 1895; 13: 229–240

3. Freyer, P. J. A new method of performing prostatectomy. Lancet 1900; 1: 774–775

4. Thomson-Walker, *Sir* J. W. The Lettsomian Lectures on enlarged prostate and prostatectomy. Transactions of the Medical Society of London 1930; 53: 143

5. Harris, S. H. Suprapubic prostatectomy with closure. British Journal of Urology 1929; 1: 285–295

6. Hryntschak, T. Suprapubic transvesical prostatectomy with primary closure of the bladder by an original method; technique and post-operative treatment. Eng. transl. Rev. ed. Illinois: Thomas, 1955

7. Hryntschak, T. Suprapubic transvesical prostatectomy with primary closure of bladder: improved technic and latest results. Journal of the International College of Surgeons 1951; 15: 366–367

8. Malament, M. Maximal hemostasis in suprapubic prostatectomy. Surgery, Gynecology and Obstetrics 1965; 120: 1307–1312

Retropubic prostatectomy

John P. Pryor MS, FRCS
Consultant Urologist, King's College and St Peter's Hospitals, London;
Dean, Institute of Urology, London University, UK

Introduction

Retropubic prostatectomy is the method of choice for removing the larger benign prostate which is causing bladder outflow obstruction. Each surgeon will have his own criteria for carrying out an open operation and this will depend upon the general condition of the patient, the experience of the surgeon and the equipment that is available to him.

The operation was first described in 1908 by Van Stockum[1], but its present popularity stems from the influence of Terence Millin, an Irishman who worked in London. He first exploited the retropubic route in 1945[2] and published his monograph, *Retropubic urinary surgery*, in 1947[3]. Retropubic prostatectomy rapidly became the method of choice for removing the benign prostate, and it 'undoubtedly yielded the most impressive results in larger subcervical adenomas where the ease of enucleation, good access to the prostatic bed and preservation of an intact bladder combined to make the mortality low and convalescence rapid'[4]. The recent development of fibre-optics, surgical diathermy and the rod lens have led to a resurgence in the use of transurethral resection and have led to a decline in the use of retropubic prostatectomy by surgeons in Europe.

Preoperative

Indications

All patients undergoing prostatectomy require preliminary cystourethroscopy and the decision to perform a retro-pubic operation is made at that time in conjunction with the operative findings, the condition of the patient and the bimanual examination of the prostate when the bladder has been emptied. Urologists perform approx-imately 10 per cent of prostatectomies by the retropubic route and reserve the open operation for the larger benign prostate or when it is also desirable to move a large vesical calculus or diverticulum or to repair an inguinal hernia. A retropubic prostatectomy should not be performed if there is a concomitant bladder tumour or for a prostatic carcinoma. The size of the prostate influences the decision to perform an open operation, but other considerations, such as general fitness of the patient and the experience and equipment of the surgeon, are also important. In general, the decision not to proceed with a transuretheral resection is made when the prostate is estimated to be between 40 and 100 g in size. Occasionally heavy bleeding occurs at the commencement of trans-urethral resection – usually in the hypertensive patient – and in these circumstances it may be wiser to proceed with an open operation.

Preoperative measures

Prophylactic antibiotics are unnecessary but any urinary tract infection should be treated with the appropriate antibiotics. A period of catheter drainage is necessary if there is evidence of an obstructive uropathy and the operation should be delayed until the blood urea level approaches normal.

Routine haematological tests should include haemo-globin estimation, blood grouping, the detection of sickle cell disease and the Australian antigen status of the patient. It is safer to have 2 units of blood available for transfusion, but there is a trend to conserve blood and only crossmatch when the blood is required. This necessitates the immediate availability of a full blood transfusion service within the hospital.

Active prophylaxis against pulmonary embolism is advisable when performing a retropubic prostatectomy. Intermittent calf vein compression is effective and can be applied once the decision to proceed by open operation has been made. Low-dose heparin prophylaxis is safe but requires planning before the patient is anaethetized.

Anaesthesia

The services of a skilled anaesthetist are essential and he may choose a general or regional anaesthetic tehnique. Spinal or epidural anaesthetics are particularly useful if the patient suffers with a respiratory tract disorder. Controlled hypotension is unnecessary and is best avoided as it carries a greater risk in the elderly. It is important that the abdominal musculature is relaxed and that there should be no impediment to the venous drainage such as occurs with coughing. It is essential to commence the administra-tion of the intravenous fluids at the start of the operation, as some degree of blood loss is inevitable.

The operation

A preliminary cystoscopy should always be performed to ensure that there is no intravesical pathology and the bladder is left empty. Small papillary carcinomas of the bladder may be resected and the base fulgurated since the operation should not be performed in the presence of a tumour.

Position of patient

The patient is placed supine on the operating table with 10° head-down tilt and the legs may also be flexed at the knee. Such a position facilitates abdominal access and also encourages venous drainage from the prostatic bed, thereby reducing haemorrhage.

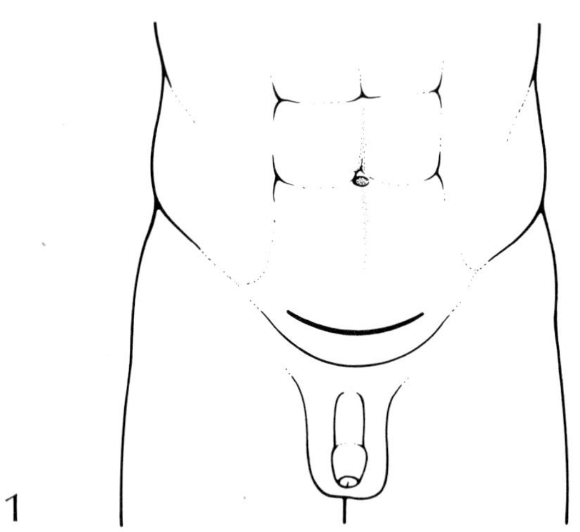

1

1

The incision

The skin is thoroughly cleansed with a 10 per cent povidone-iodine solution and the patient draped in such a way as to allow access to the penis once the prostate has been removed. The operation is performed through a transverse lower abdominal incision situated in the skin crease approximately 3 cm above the symphysis pubis. The incision is 10–15 cm long and depends upon the thickness of the abdominal wall fat. A right-handed surgeon stands on the patient's left, and performs most of the operation facing the patient's feet.

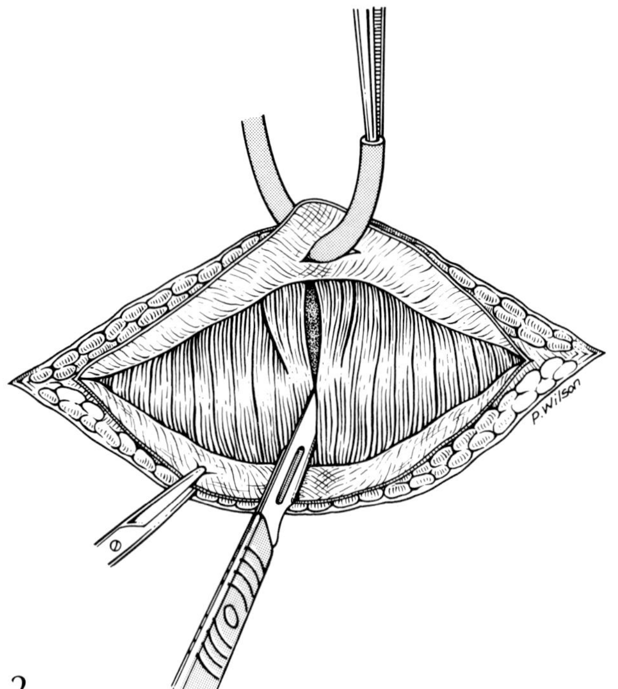

2

2

Separation of rectus muscles

The anterior rectus sheath is incised in the line of the skin incision and is mobilized from the underlying rectus muscles down to the symphysis pubis and upwards towards the umbilicus. It is necessary to coagulate small arteries entering the rectus sheath from the muscles. The rectus and the pyramidalis muscles are widely separated in the lower part of the incision, and it may be necessary to incise the lower part of the linea alba vertically in the upper part of the wound.

It is useful at this stage to insert a tube drain through a small incision in the midline of the lower flap of the anterior rectus sheath midway between the line of incision and the symphysis pubis. The ends of the drainage tube are clamped together with Kocher's forceps and secured to the drapes towards the patient's feet in such a way as to exert traction and obviate any subsequent need for a retractor in the inferior part of the wound.

3

Exposure of anterior surface of prostate

The retropubic fat is gently separated to expose the bladder and prostate and the blades of a Millin self-retaining retractor are inserted. Further separation of the retropubic fat exposes the anterior surface of the prostatic capsule and any haemorrhage is controlled with diathermy. At this stage it is convenient to tuck two 10 cm gauze swabs into the retropubic space just lateral to the prostate. The third blade of the Millin retractor is introduced to retract the bladder, clearly displaying the anterior surface of the prostate and adjacent bladder wall.

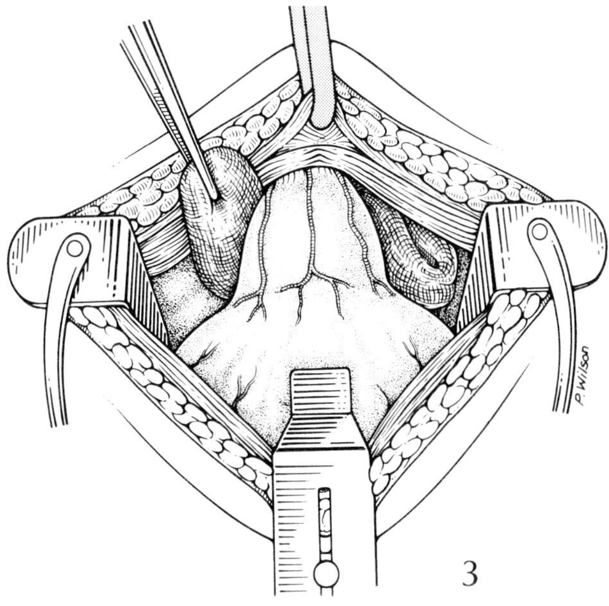

3

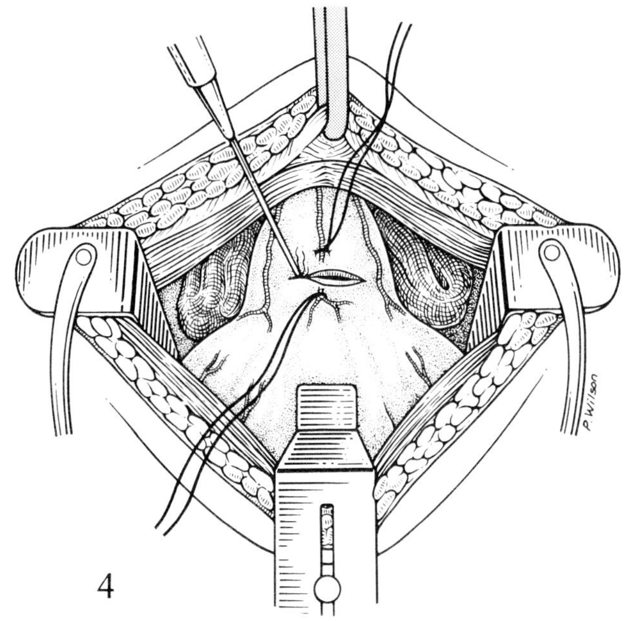

4

4

Incision of prostatic capsule

Two stay sutures (0 chromic catgut on a curved needle) are then placed through the prostatic capsule in such a way as to occlude the vein running longitudinally (a branch of the dorsal vein of the penis). The more proximal of these sutures is placed at the junction of the prostate and bladder neck. The correct situation is recognized by the longitudinal direction of the veins turning to run more laterally. These sutures are left long to facilitate identification of the incision into the prostatic capsule. A 3 cm incision is made in the prostatic capsule between the stay sutures and about 1 cm distal to the bladder neck. The incision is made through the full thickness of the capsule and stops when the white appearance of the prostate is identified. Any bleeding from the prostatic capsule should be controlled at this stage.

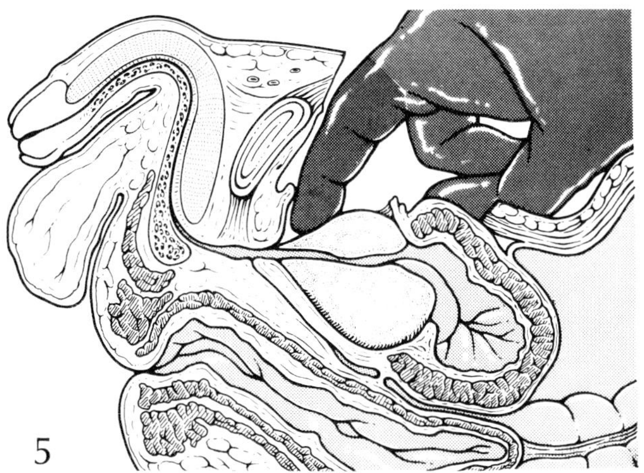
5

5

Plane of enucleation

A pair of scissors is used to commence the distal separation of the anterior surface of the prostatic adenoma from the prostatic capsule. This plane is developed by blind dissection with the pulp of the right index finger. The right lobe is freed first by separating the anterior surface, followed by the lateral and posterior surfaces from the prostatic capsule. The same procedure is repeated for the left lobe but the continuity of the urethra at the apex of the prostate is maintained. The finger dissection may be facilitated by removing the Millin retractor but this is not always necessary and it should be reinserted once the dissection is complete.

6

Division of the urethra

It is possible to insert the index and middle fingers inside the prostatic capsule in such a manner as to straddle the urethra once the lateral lobes of the prostate have been freed. A pair of curved scissors is inserted inside the prostatic capsule and, guided by the position of the fingers, is used to divide the urethra clearly in order to avoid avulsing any of the distal urethra, thereby damaging the sphincter mechanism. It is often difficult to divide the urethra under direct vision but great care is essential at this stage of the operation if postoperative urinary incontinence is to be avoided. The lateral lobes now lie freely within the prostatic capsule

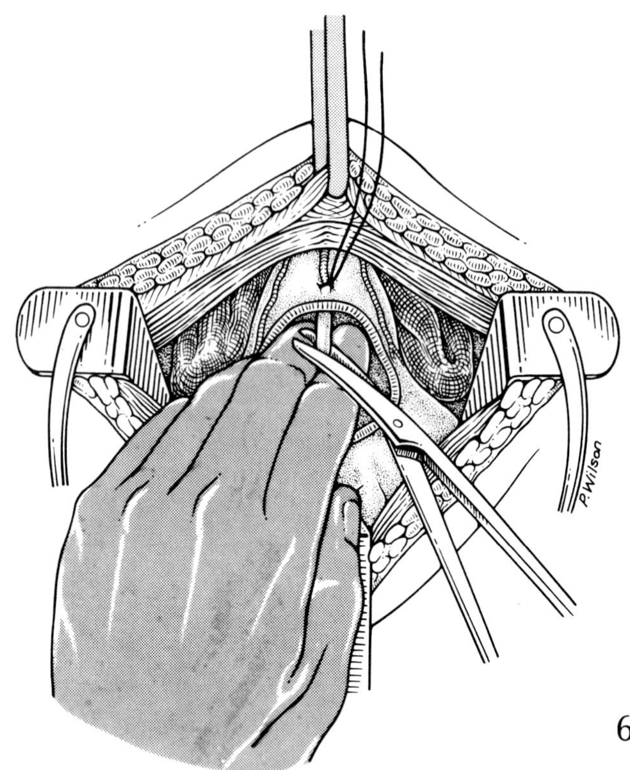

6

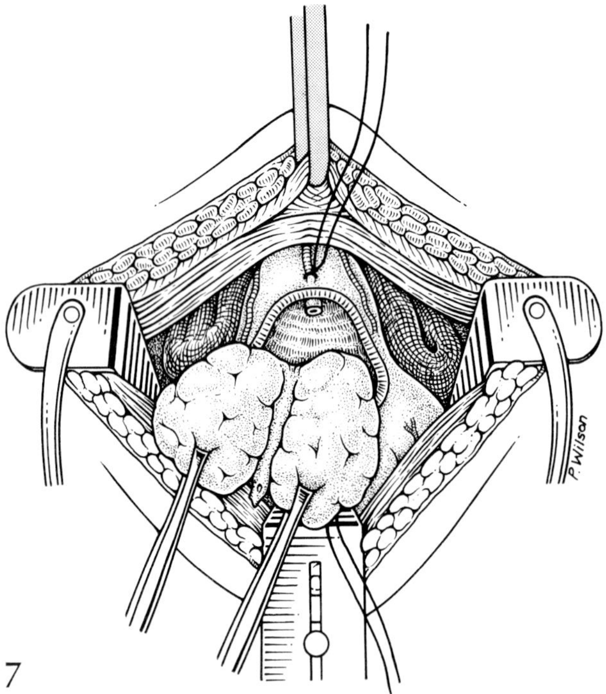

7

7

Dislocation of the adenoma

Each lateral lobe is securely gripped with a pair of volsellum forceps and dislocated anteriorly out of the prostatic cavity. The proximal end of the divided urethra is identified and a pair of scissors placed inside the urethra, which is then divided anteriorly, together with the overlying prostatic tissue, as far as the bladder neck.

8

Removal of the adenoma and control of haemostasis

A pair of bladder neck spreaders are placed inside the bladder to define the bladder neck. The attachment of the prostate to the bladder neck is then divided by sharp dissection with a diathermy point and the prostate removed. Removal of the prostate is always accompanied by bleeding, and on rare occasions this may be profuse. Immediately the adenoma has been removed it is wise to pack the prostatic capsule with gauze swabs and control any bleeding by direct pressure.

The general status of the patient is then assessed and rapid fluid replacement given if required. The packs may then be removed and the prostatic cavity carefully inspected, remnants of prostatic adenoma excised and any bleeding vessels diathermized. It is sometimes difficult to control profuse bleeding from large veins in the prostatic capsule and in these circumstances the cavity is packed and external pressure applied with a swab in a holder for 5 to 10 minutes (timed to avoid impatience). It is neither necessary nor possible to arrest the capillary oozing from the prostatic bed and this will diminish by repacking the prostatic cavity with swabs.

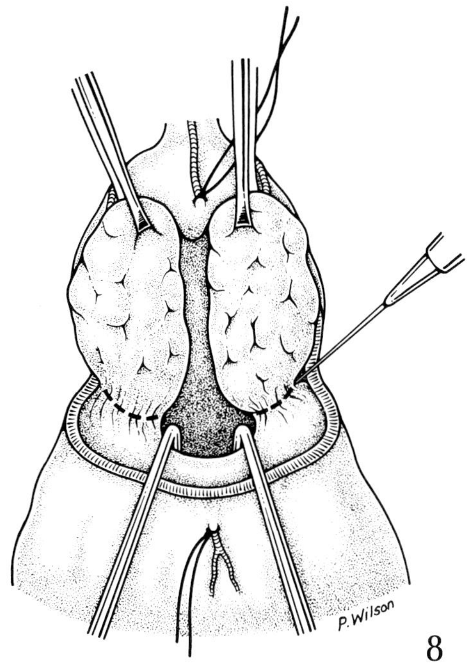

8

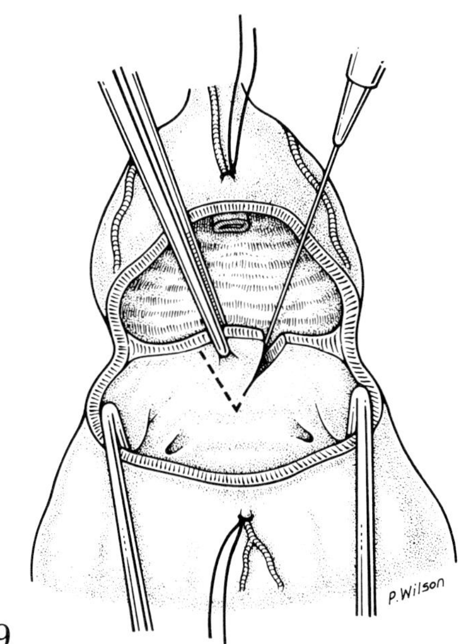

9

9

Excision of a wedge of bladder neck

Attention is next given to the bladder neck which should be sufficiently large easily to admit two fingers. If this is not possible, a wedge is excised from the bladder neck. The ureteric orifices are first identified and the middle of the bladder neck is grasped by a pair of forceps. A V-shaped wedge is then excised as shown.

10

Anchoring the bladder mucosa

It is unnecessary to suture the bladder mucosa to the prostatic bed except in those patients where the prostate extended beneath the trigone. In these circumstances it is useful to anchor the mucosa to the floor of the prostatic cavity with two or three 00 chromic catgut sutures. This technique facilitates catheterization and is of particular benefit should the urethral catheter fall out or require replacement. Persistent haemorrhage from the bladder neck may be controlled by suturing, and in these circumstances the bladder mucosa may be anchored with the same suture.

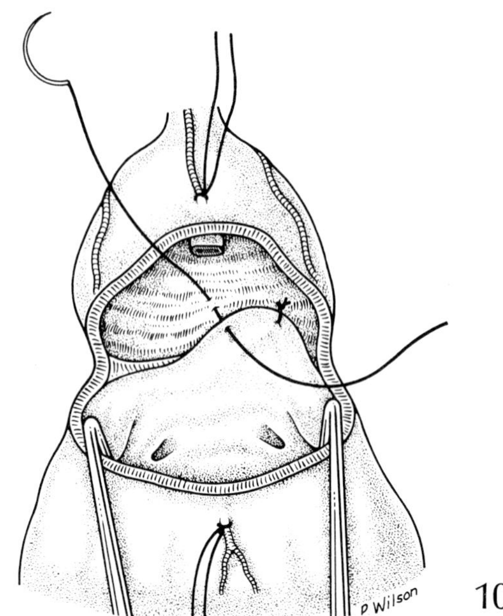

10

11

Insertion of catheter

Any swabs remaining within the prostatic capsule are removed and a marker suture (0 chromic catgut) is placed at each lateral corner of the capsular incision. These sutures act as a guide for the ends of the incision but are also haemostatic. The needle is inserted from without into the cavity of the bladder, then through the bladder mucosa and bladder neck into the prostatic cavity and finally through the prostatic capsule. Each of these sutures is tied and left long and a 20 Fr three-way Foley-type catheter is passed into the bladder. It is preferable that the catheter should be fairly rigid and have large eyes. It is seldom necessary to insert a suprapubic catheter into the bladder.

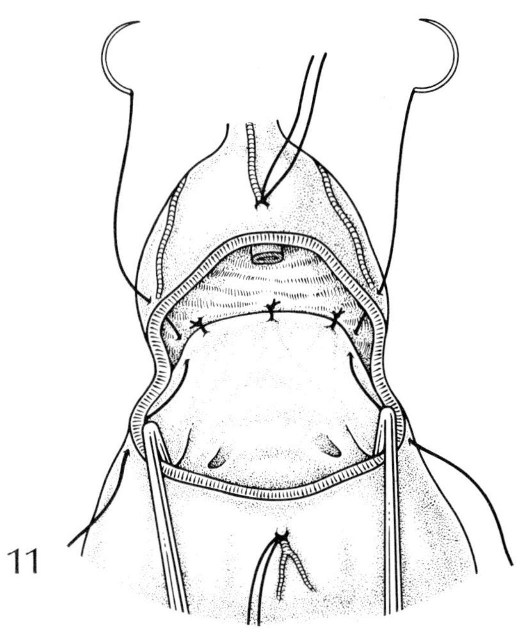
11

12

Closure of prostatic capsule

The prostatic capsule is closed with a continuous 0 chromic catgut suture which arrests any bleeding from the prostatic capsule and also ensures a watertight closure. It is easier to insert this suture by taking each edge of the capsule with separate bites of the needle. There may be some leakage through the prostatic capsule but it is seldom worthwhile attempting to insert any further sutures.

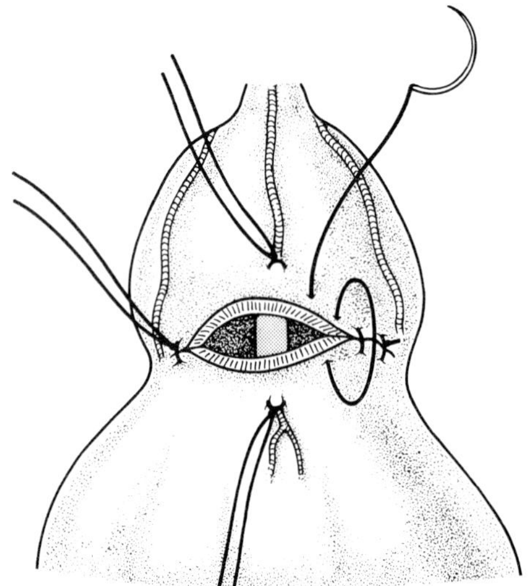
12

13

Final stages

At this stage it is useful to tie together the two initial stay sutures which were placed into the prostatic capsule. The bladder is then washed out to ensure that there is free catheter drainage. The two swabs which were placed on either side of the prostate at the start of the operation are removed and a final check is made for any bleeding from the vessels in the retropubic fat.

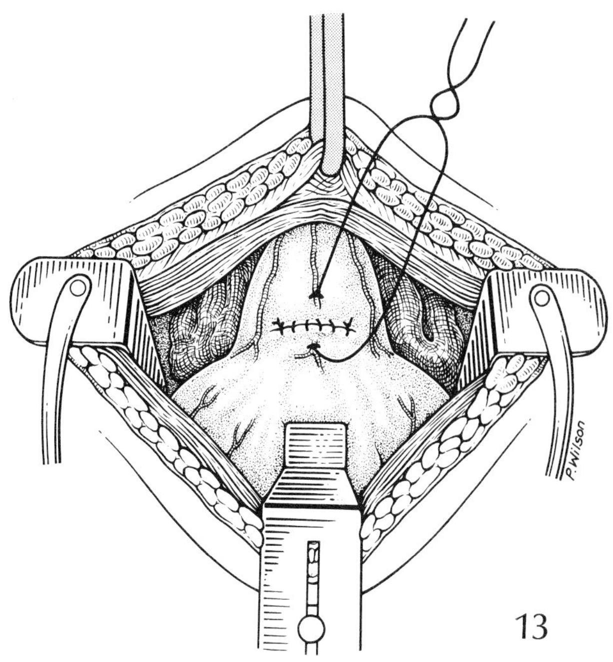

13

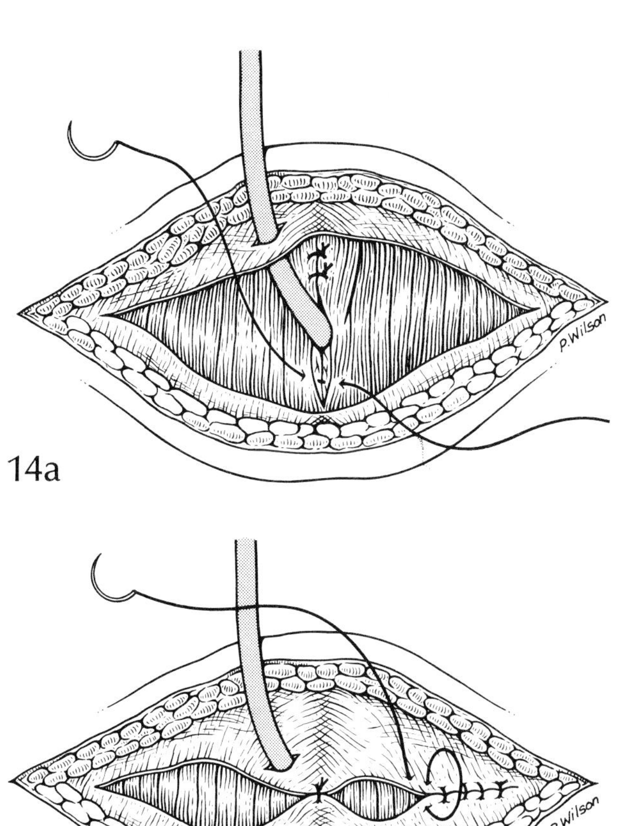

14a

14b

14a & b

Wound closure

The tubular wound drain, which, inserted at the commencement of the procedure, has acted as a retractor throughout, is then unclipped and placed down to the suture line in the prostatic capsule. The rectus muscles are approximated with interrupted 0 chromic catgut sutures and the anterior rectus sheath is closed with a similar suture material. This may conveniently be a continuous suture line. The subcutaneous tissues are loosely approximated with plain catgut sutures and the skin closed with well-spaced interrupted sutures. At the conclusion of the operation the catheter is once again checked to make sure that it is draining freely and is then connected to a closed urine collection apparatus. The retropubic drain is also connected to a closed collection bag.

ADDITIONAL PROCEDURES

It is often convenient to repair an inguinal hernia at the time of a retropubic prostatectomy but this should be deferred until the prostatectomy has been completed safely. Vasectomy is no longer performed in order to reduce the risk of epididymitis.

Postoperative care

Blood transfusion is not usually necessary except in the very large gland (greater than 250 g). Any fluid loss during the course of the operation should have been replaced by intravenous fluids and these are usually given to ensure a high urine output. In elderly patients, or in those with cardiac abnormalities, it is often wise to give furosemide 40 mg by intramuscular injection every 12 hours to minimize the risk of cardiac failure and to prevent the occurrence of clot retention. This technique is particularly useful when there has been profuse bleeding at the time of operation and the use of a three-way catheter will also help obviate the need for a bladder washout. The urine should always be collected in a closed drainage system as this is helpful in lessening the risk of urinary infection. Careful attention should be given to cleansing the penis around the catheter in the postoperative period.

The patient is encouraged to drink at an early stage and intravenous fluids are unnecessary after the first 24 hours. Early mobilization and physiotherapy are important in the prevention of pulmonary embolism and the retropubic drain is usually removed 48 hours after the operation. The urethral catheter is removed when there is no longer any risk of clot retention – usually between the 4th and 7th day.

Complications

The general risk of myocardial ischaemia, chest infection and pulmonary embolism are ever-present with an elderly group of patients undergoing surgery. These risks may be minimized by the skills of the supporting team of anaesthetists, nurses and physiotherapists. The risk of a urinary tract infection may be lessened if preoperative catheterization is avoided, and by the judicious use of antibiotics.

Prostatorectal fistulae have been reported following retropubic prostatectomy but tend to occur when the operation has been performed for an unsuspected carcinoma of the prostate. Urethral strictures are relatively uncommon after a retropubic prostatectomy but bladder neck stenosis occurs in 1 per cent of patients. Regrowth of the prostate may occur but patients rarely present in less than 10 years after the retropubic operation. The regrowth may be due to the occurrence of a prostatic cancer even though the histology of the original gland showed benign prostatic hyperplasia.

Urinary incontinence is common immediately following the removal of the urethral catheter but fortunately this only persists in approximately 1 per cent of patients.

References

1. Van Stockum, W. J. Prostatectomia suprapubica extravesicalis. Zentralblatt für Chirurgie 1909; 36: 41–43

2. Millin, T. Retropubic prostatectomy: a new extravesical technique, report on 20 cases. Lancet 1945; 2: 693–696

3. Millin, T. Retropubic urinary surgery. Edinburgh: E. & S. Livingstone, 1947

4. Sandrey, J. G. Retropubic prostatectomy. In: Innes Williams, D., ed. Operative surgery: Urology. London: Butterworths, 1977: 253–261

Transurethral prostatectomy

Herbert Brendler MD
Professor, Department of Urology, The Mount Sinai Medical Center, New York, USA

Preoperative

Indications

In the past, the transurethral route, as opposed to one or another of the open operations, i.e. retropubic, suprapubic (transvesical) or perineal, has, except in a few specialized centres, usually been reserved for glands estimated to be 40 g or less. The present trend, however, is in favour of transurethral resection for glands of virtually any size, so that at least 60–70 per cent of all prostatectomies in the United States are now being performed by this technique. Occasionally, very large glands may require two sittings for completion. Under certain circumstances the transurethral operation may be difficult, even impossible, for example in patients with severe arthritis involving the hip joints which interferes with abduction. Strictures of the anterior urethra do not ordinarily constitute a contraindication because they can be bypassed via a temporary perineal urethrotomy.

Equipment

Instruments

These should always be in perfect repair, and replacements and spare parts must be available. Sheaths include sizes No. 24, 26 and 28 Fr. The type of working element is optional, e.g. Stern-McCarthy, Iglesias, Nesbit, Baumrucker, Storz, etc. Since the cutting wire loops are subject to breakage they should be checked before use. Loops may also need to be adjusted to ensure proper shearing action when drawn back into the sheath. Telescopes include the foreoblique, right angle (either as part of the resectoscope or a separate cystoscope), retrograde and forward-vision (Vest) lenses. Illumination may be by electric bulb or the fibreoptic system. A complete set of sounds should be available, as well as filiforms and followers. Manual irrigators such as the Ellick evacuator and the Toomey piston syringe are essential, with stiff, large-calibre rubber tubing and tight adaptor connections.

Electrosurgical unit

This provides cutting and coagulation currents. The unit should be checked and adjusted periodically.

Irrigating fluids

Non-haemolyzing solutions, such as 1.1 per cent glycine, are generally used, although some urologists still prefer sterile water because of better visibility.

Table

Leg supports should be arranged to permit adequate manoeuvrability for the resectionist. A commodious drainage tray is essential.

Anaesthesia

Spinal anaesthesia is preferred as it permits early detection of abdominal pain and rigidity in the event of perforation and extravasation.

Preoperative management

In cases of impaired renal function, or ureteric reflux, a preliminary suprapubic cystostomy may have to be performed. In addition to protecting the kidneys, this considerably shortens and simplifies subsequent transurethral prostatectomy by allowing continuous run-off of irrigating medium.

The value of prophylactic antibiotic therapy is uncertain. Many urologists prefer to withhold antibacterials unless they are indicated.

An ample supply of matched whole blood should be immediately available.

The operation

1

Inspection of prostatic urethra at the level of the verumontanum shows hypertrophied lateral lobes.

1

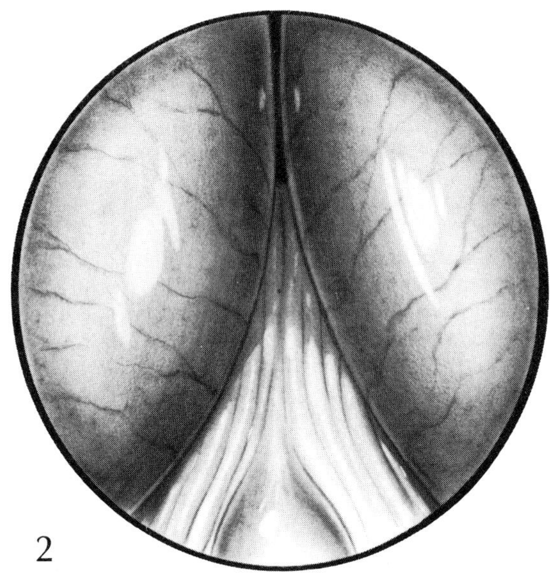

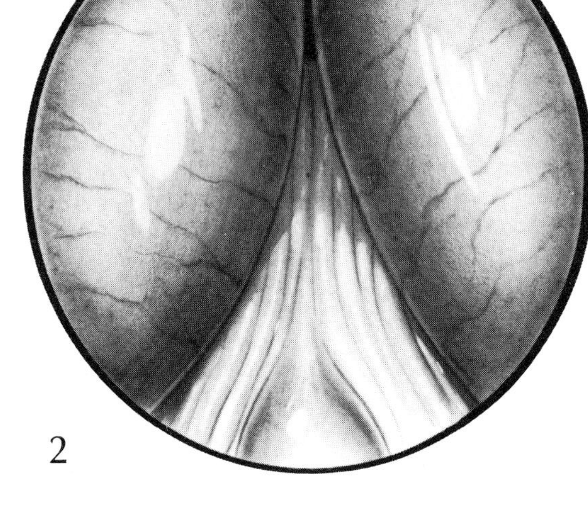

2

2

The resectoscope has now been advanced proximally, permitting the enlarged middle lobe to come into view.

3

As the instrument enters the bladder, the enlarged lateral lobes separate further. Note the vertical markings on the elevated middle lobe – the so-called 'waterfall' appearance.

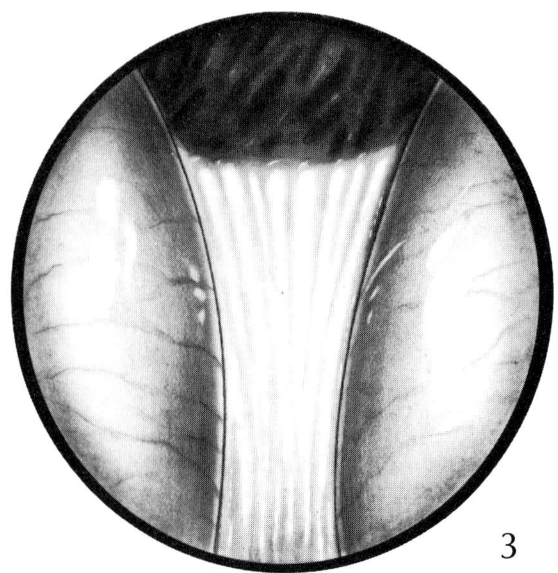

3

4

The bladder neck is resected first. Operation commences on the roof, or anterior aspect, at 11 o'clock and is carried around counter-clockwise until the right side of the bladder neck has been cleared.

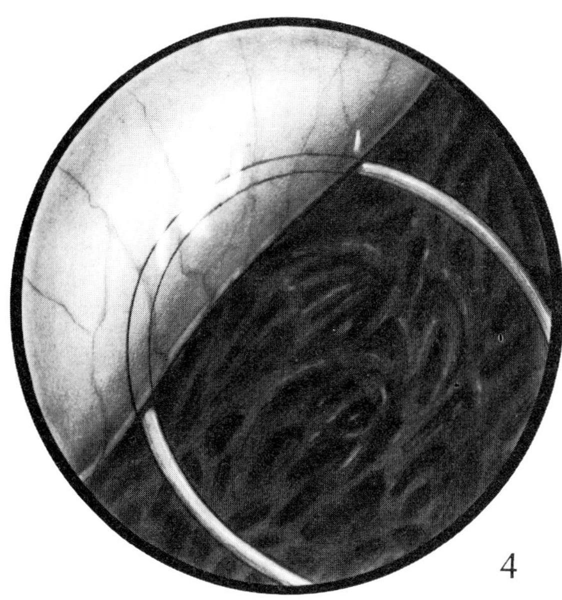

4

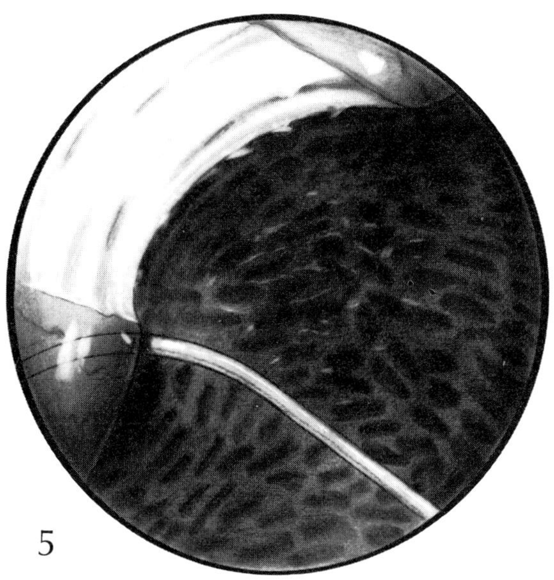

5

5

The first cut has been made, exposing the circular muscle fibres which mark the plane between the hyperplastic portion and the 'surgical capsule', i.e. true prostate. The adenoma is thinnest anteriorly, usually not more than one or two bites deep. Beginning anteriorly enables the resectionist to identify the external limits of the operation early. Using the circular fibres as a landmark, the loop follows the plane of cleavage exactly as the enucleating finger does in open prostatectomy.

6

As resection proceeds, bleeding arterial branches are spot-fulgurated. Generalized searing devitalizes large areas of prostatic tissue and is to be avoided. Resection carried deeply into the circular fibres may cause bleeding from venous sinuses which is often difficult to control. Deep resection may also lead to perforation and extravasation. The appearance of fatty tissue is a danger sign.

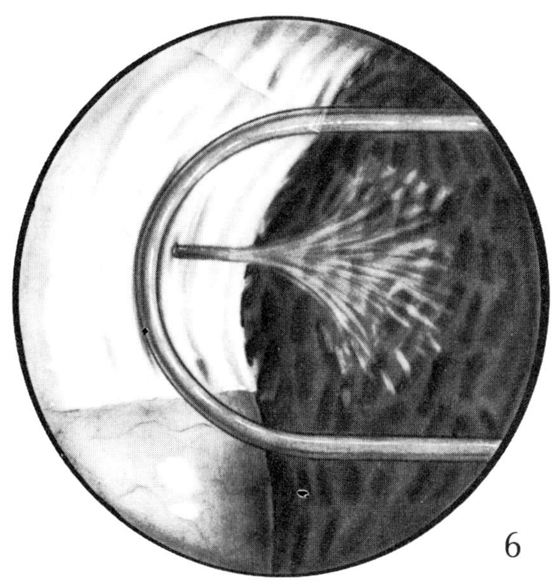

6

7

After the right side of the bladder neck has been resected, the identical procedure is carried out on the left, beginning at 1 o'clock. Midline tissue on the floor between 5 and 7 o'clock is then resected, with the aim of lowering the bladder neck to the level of the trigone. A sizeable middle lobe has to be handled with special care to avoid damaging the ureteric orifices or trigone. It is in this area that the latter may be undermined, leading to perforation and extravasation.

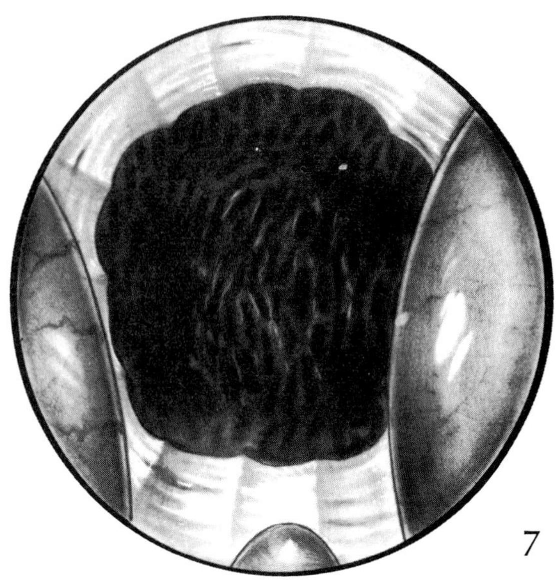

7

8

8

Attention is now turned to the right lateral lobe. If this is large, it is usually advantageous to establish the plane of cleavage peripherally at the outset, again using the loop in a manner similar to the enucleating finger. This speeds up subsequent resection of the lobe and also facilitates control of bleeding. With smaller lobes not more than three to four bites thick, identifying the cleavage plane initially is not always necessary. The verumontanum is an important landmark in avoiding damage to the external sphincter.

9

With the right lobe out of the way, removal of the left one is much easier. Systematic resection is accomplished in the same manner as on the other side.

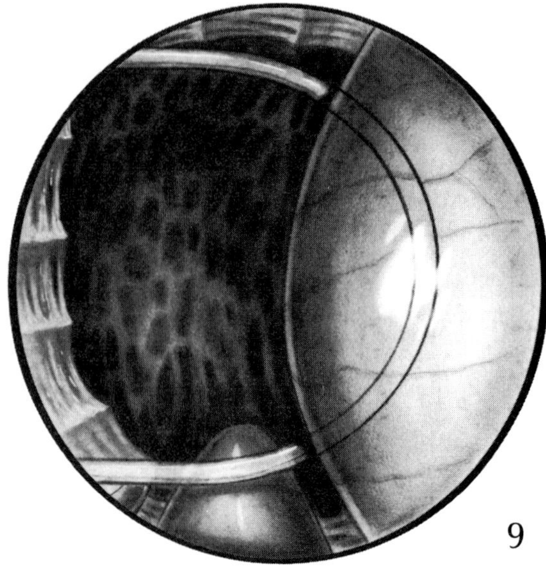

9

10

Following removal of middle and lateral lobes, the remaining tissue at the apex is carefully resected, taking care to preserve the verumontanum. Final trimming is accomplished and bleeding vessels are fulgurated. All loose fragments are evacuated from the bladder. Terminal inspection of the fossa with the resectoscope situated just distal to the verumontanum should present a well coned-out appearance without residual adenoma. A 22 or 24 Fr Foley catheter is inserted and the bag inflated with 20–30 ml, taking care that this is done in the bladder, *not* the prostatic fossa. This will permit the muscular layer of the surgical capsule to contract, thereby minimizing any ooze which may be present. Return irrigations should be clear or pink-tinged at the conclusion of the operation. Approximately 100 ml of irrigant is left indwelling when the patient is sent to the recovery room.

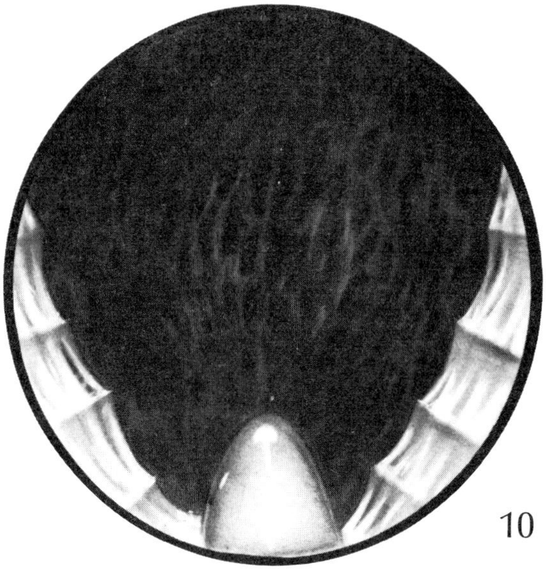

10

Postoperative care

Upon arrival in the recovery room the catheter is attached to straight drainage. Gentle irrigation with 30–60 ml of sterile saline or water at room temperature is carried out at intervals, using a bulb syringe. Frequency of irrigation will depend on the degree of bleeding, but should be kept to a minimum in order to allow blood vessels to seal off. Mannitol is useful in promoting diuresis for purposes of self-irrigation. Catheter traction is usually unnecessary, but may help if bleeding is moderate to severe.

The use of three-way catheters and continuous drip irrigation is favoured by some urologists, but this requires constant monitoring to be certain the bladder does not inadvertently become distended as the result of obstructing clots or tissue debris in the outflow channel.

Severe bleeding in the immediate postoperative period, which cannot be controlled by moderate traction on the catheter requires reinsertion of the resectoscope, evacuation of blood and clots, and a search for bleeding vessels. Sometimes simple bladder decompression will control bleeding by permitting the distended fossa to contract.

In the uncomplicated case the urethral catheter can usually be removed in 48–72 hours. Antibiotic coverage is provided while the catheter is in place and for varying periods after its removal, depending on urine cultures.

The patient is ordinarily discharged one week after surgery, and returns for his first postoperative visit in 3–4 weeks. Further check-ups are scheduled as needed.

Injuries to the urethra

J. P. Mitchell CBE, TD, MS, FRCS, FRCS(Ed)
Honorary Professor of Surgery (Urology), University of Bristol, UK

Introduction

1

For the purposes of diagnosis and treatment, trauma to the urethra should be classified as to whether it is open or closed, whether it involves the male or female and, whether it is located in the anterior or posterior urethra.

The commonest cause of urethral injuries in which many other structures and systems may be involved, is road traffic accident. It should be remembered that 10–15 per cent of injuries of the posterior urethra may also be accompanied by a ruptured bladder. Furthermore, double injuries of both upper and lower urinary tract may occur.

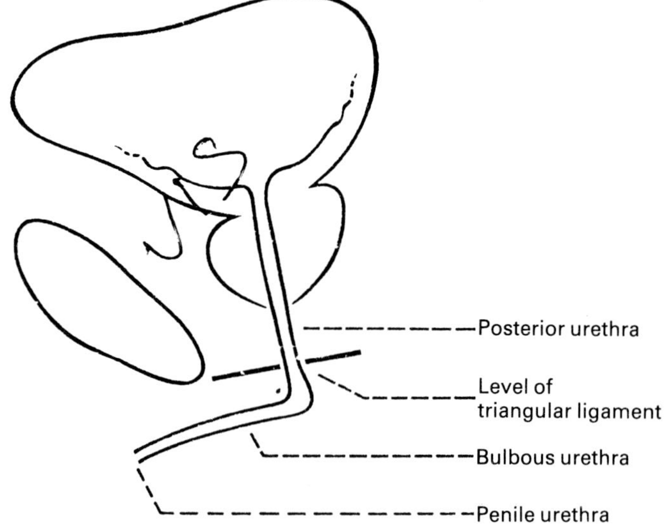

2a, b & c

Injuries of both anterior and posterior urethra are frequently partial ruptures (*b*): part of the wall of the urethra is torn, but the whole circumference of the urethra is not transected. Occasionally the damage to the urethral wall is only a contusion (c). Injuries at the level of the triangular ligament, however, are usually complete transections (*a*). The most important principle in the management of urethral injuries is to ensure that no additional damage is caused by operative or investigative procedures, which can aggravate the extent of a partial rupture or convert a contusion into a partial rupture. Every effort should be made to preserve the remaining strand or bridge of tissue which may exist between the two torn ends of urethra. This bridge of tissue can make the difference between a successful repair and a severe stricture.

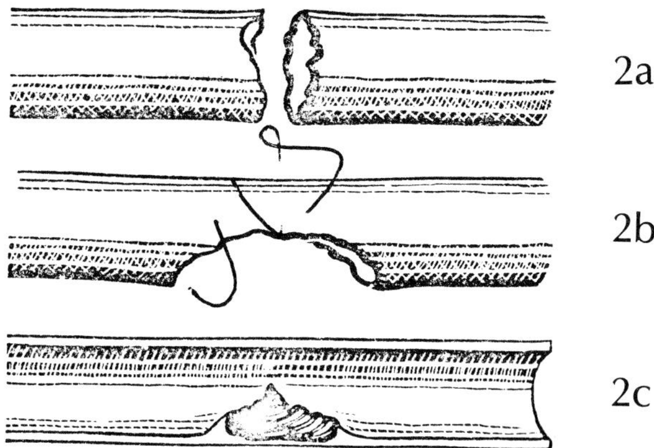

Extravasation of urine is, in fact, unlikely to occur as the bladder neck is usually in spasm. The patient is unable to pass urine, ultimately developing a distended bladder. Even if extravasation does occur, by far the majority of patients will have sterile urine which can cause little harm within the first 24 hours. It is, therefore, safe in closed injuries of the urinary tract to give priority to the treatment of other major injuries.

OPEN INJURIES OF THE URINARY TRACT

Gunshot wounds, penetration of the perineum by sharp objects such as broken glass or being impaled, or any trauma to the penile urethra (which may be caught in machinery or involved in some sexual misadventure) must all be treated by exploration without delay. The wound of entry must be explored. If necessary the urethra can be examined by urethroscopy and the damage repaired by immediate suture over an indwelling silicone catheter, 14 or 16 Fr. The patient should be given a broad-spectrum antibiotic because infection will have been carried into the wound on the penetrating missile. Also, there is bound to be a fairly extensive haematoma and this forms a perfect nidus in which organisms can multiply.

CLOSED INJURIES OF THE URETHRA

Injuries of the perineal part of the urethra (principally bulbous urethra), transections of the urethra at the urogenital diaphragm and closed injuries of the posterior urethra associated with a fracture of the pelvis require careful management to assess the degree of damage and the localization. The diagnosis is suggested by the presence of blood at the external meatus, the inability of the patient to pass any urine and the ultimate development of a distended bladder, easily palpable above the haematoma which rises out of the pelvis. If a distended bladder is not palpable within 24 hours of admission to hospital, the possibility of an associated bladder rupture should be considered.

If an urgent diagnostic answer is required because the patient will be going to the operating theatre for other major trauma, or if he or she develops a distended bladder even though no blood has appeared at the external urinary meatus, then a urethrogram using an aqueous opaque medium will readily confirm the diagnosis and demonstrate the site and extent of the urethral rupture. If the patient's condition is such that he requires urgent surgery, and a urethrogram cannot be performed, suprapubic diversion of the urine is a wise precaution, even if only the physical sign of blood at the external meatus is present.

In no circumstances should a diagnostic catheter be passed *per urethram*: the information obtained can be unreliable. There is a serious risk of contaminating the haematoma at the site of injury by carrying organisms on the catheter from the external meatus: and there is a very real risk of inflicting further damage on the slender bridge of tissue that may constitute only a partial rupture of the urethra. If the diagnostic catheter draws no urine it may mean that the catheter has passed out of the urethra through the rupture. On the other hand, it may have passed into an empty bladder; it may have been obstructed at the bladder neck; the patient may be anuric; or the bladder itself may have been ruptured. Alternatively, if the catheter draws some urine, this does not exclude a partial rupture of the urethra; nor does it exclude a small puncture hole in the anterior wall of the bladder.

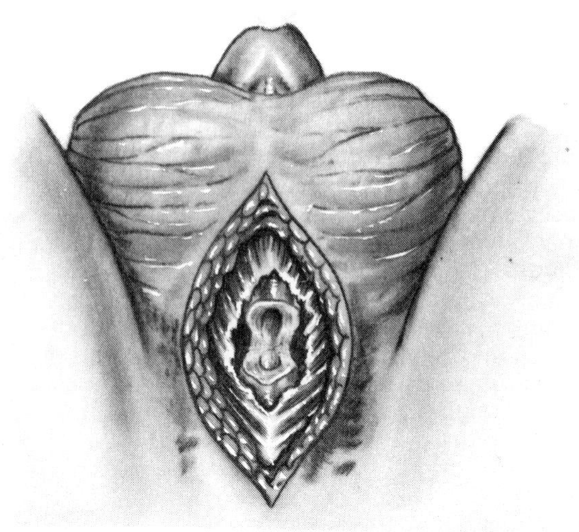

3

The operations

RUPTURE OF THE BULBOUS AND PERINEAL URETHRA

3 & 4

With the patient in the lithotomy position, the extensive haematoma in the perineum is opened. Identification of the urethra will be difficult as the tissues will be discoloured by blood. The bladder is then opened suprapubically by a vertical midline incision and a Harris, or Nelaton, catheter (22 Fr in adults, correspondingly smaller in children), is passed down the posterior urethra from the internal meatus to present in the wound. The tip of this catheter will then identify the proximal end of the ruptured urethra. A smaller sized (16 Fr) Foley catheter, preferably silicone, is then passed from the external urinary meatus, after instillation of chlorhexidine in glycerine as lubricant and antiseptic to identify the distal end of the torn urethra.

If the urethral damage is only a partial tear, a few sutures approximating the rent transversely will help to control bleeding from the corpus spongeosum. No urethral catheter is necessary as this patient may not develop a stricture because part of the circumference of the urethra is still intact. A 26 Fr Foley catheter should be left draining the bladder suprapubically.

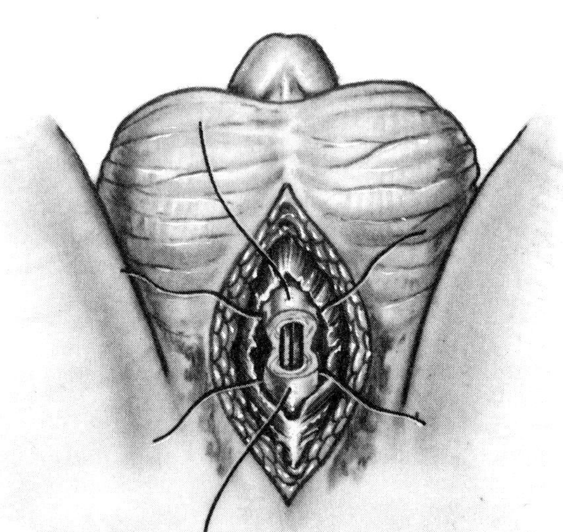

4

5 & 6

If the urethra has been totally transected, then the dorsal aspect of the two torn ends of urethra can be approximated by a few sutures of 4/0 plain catgut (or polyglycolic acid). Again, these sutures will also help to control bleeding from the corpus spongeosum. There should be no attempt at mobilizing either end of the urethra, which should approximate easily. This patient may develop a stricture and correct alignment by an indwelling catheter is essential. The tip of the Harris catheter passed down from the bladder is cut off; the tip of the smaller silicone catheter passed *per urethram* is inserted firmly into the cut end of the Harris catheter which is gently withdrawn back into the bladder, taking particular care to ensure that the mucosa of the proximal end of the urethral rupture is not invaginated. When the smaller gauge Foley catheter has reached the bladder, the balloon is distended in order to anchor it. The bladder is then closed, leaving a suprapubic Foley catheter (22 Fr) draining the bladder by suprapubic cystostomy. The wound is closed in layers with a small perineal drain.

Silicone is a completely inert material and the catheter can, therefore, be left indwelling for 2, 3 or 4 weeks. The patient should be treated with a broad-spectrum antibiotic, and the external urinary meatus should be cleansed by meatal toilet twice a day.

Later, the urethra is inspected by panendoscopy and urethrography and treated initially by endoscopic urethrotomy if a stricture develops. Ultimately the stricture may require some form of urethroplasty.

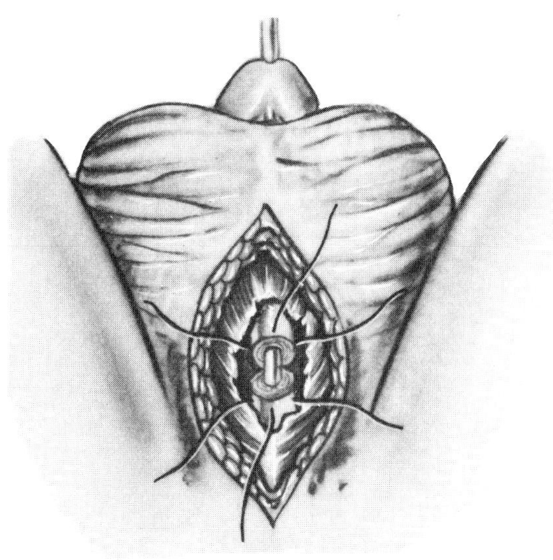

5

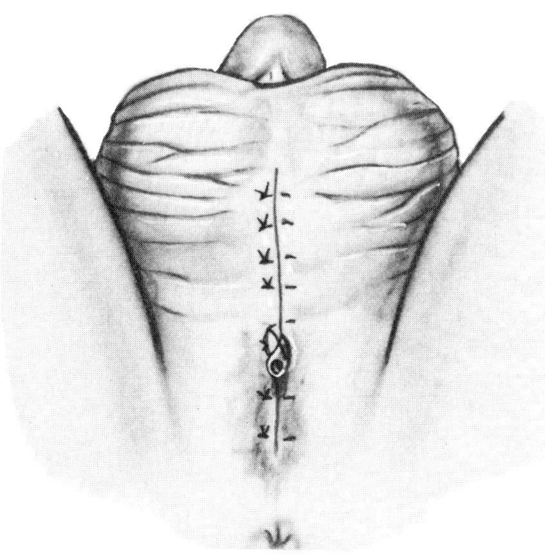

6

RUPTURE OF THE URETHRA AT THE UROGENITAL DIAPHRAGM

This type of injury is usually due to a blow in the perineum. There may be associated damage to the anus, with tearing of the perineal skin, converting the injury into an open injury. Although injury to the urethra at this site is uncommon, it is nearly always a total transection and the torn ends of the urethra retract above and below the urogenital diaphragm respectively.

Immediate repair is difficult. The proximal catheter will present in the pelvis and will then have to be threaded through the triangular ligament, as it does not readily carry the proximal end of the urethra with it. Stricture is inevitable; it is unlikely to respond to endoscopic urethrotomy because its length will probably be more than 2–3 mm. Some form of urethroplasty is usually required. In this type of injury a definitive posterior urethroplasty should be performed as soon as the local tissue reaction following the trauma has subsided i.e. within 2–3 months.

RUPTURE OF THE POSTERIOR URETHRA

This injury is almost always associated with a fracture of the pelvis and in 10–15 per cent of cases there is, in addition, a rupture of the bladder.

The patient is placed on the table in the supine position and draped with towels so that there is access to the external meatus as well as to the lower abdomen. A vertical midline suprapubic incision is made and the extravesical space opened. Blood and urine are aspirated or mopped gently from the prevesical space. It will be difficult to determine the exact site of the lesion because of the bloodstained effusion. If the bladder is distended, the lesion must be situated below the external vesical sphincter. Often the haemorrhage from the depths of the pelvis can only be stopped with packing. This should be done with great care as it is at this stage that the partial rupture can be converted into a total transection. The bladder is then identified by the direction of its muscle fibres, which may be discoloured by suffused blood, and a formal cystostomy is performed.

The damage to the bony pelvis can be felt with a finger inside the bladder and it may be possible to move a central mobile fragment into position. The surgeon then feels for the internal urinary meatus and the prostate gland to assess whether this has been grossly displaced. If the prostate gland is lying high in the pelvis, there is almost certainly a total transection of the membranous urethra and immediate repair should be performed. If the prostate does not appear to be grossly displaced, there is probably a partial rupture of the posterior urethra, in which case it is only necessary to leave a suprapubic drain (Foley catheter 26 Fr).

Immediate repair

If the prostate is lying high in the pelvis and there is no likelihood of any bridge of tissue remaining between the two torn ends of urethra, the procedure is as for open operation on rupture of the bulbous and perineal urethra.

7, 8 & 9

A Harris catheter (22 Fr) is passed from the bladder via the internal urinary meatus to present in the pelvis. This catheter should be of very soft material and should be passed with the greatest gentleness so as not to damage any other structures. After inserting 5 ml of chlorhexidine in glycerine into the external urinary meatus, a silicone catheter (16 Fr) is passed up the urethra and will also present in the depths of the pelvis. The tip of the Harris catheter is then cut off and the tip of the silicone Foley catheter is inserted into the cut end of the Harris catheter. A stitch through both catheters will ensure that they hold together. The proximal Harris catheter is then well lubricated and withdrawn, watching very carefully to see that the proximal torn end of urethra does not retract (invaginate) as the catheter recedes back into the bladder. As the silicone Foley catheter enters the bladder its balloon is inflated.

It is always tempting to try to thread the lower catheter through the proximal end of the urethra using a stilette or guide inside the catheter, all the time feeling with the finger in the bladder. The passage of this catheter may feel successful, but it is very likely to have stripped away some of the urethral mucosa, making a false passage and aggravating the future stricture.

Suturing of the urethra is unlikely to be successful as absorbable sutures will disintegrate too soon; non-absorbable sutures incur the ultimate risk of stone formation. Similarly, traction on the balloon catheter is unlikely to hold the prostate down, due to the reactive swelling of the tissues within the bony pelvis, as well as to the distortion caused by the trauma. Advice should be sought from the orthopaedic surgeon regarding realignment of the bony pelvis, as this can reduce the distortion of the intrapelvic structures. With the passage of time the reactive swelling of the soft tissues will allow the prostate to subside into the pelvis and return nearer to its normal position.

Most of these patients will develop a stricture of the membranous urethra, but with a good result this may take several years. Therefore, any rupture of the urethra should be seen for review regularly for a minimum of 5 years and a mictiograph performed to check the stream. Most of these patients will require either endoscopic urethrotomy or a posterior urethroplasty but, by using a silicone catheter, the severity of the stricture formation will probably be reduced.

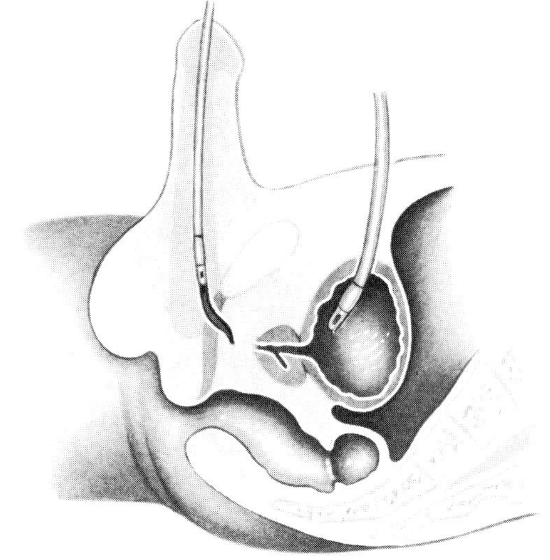

7

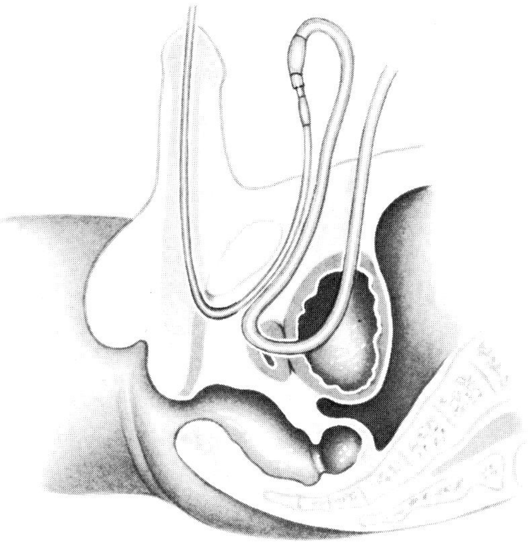

8

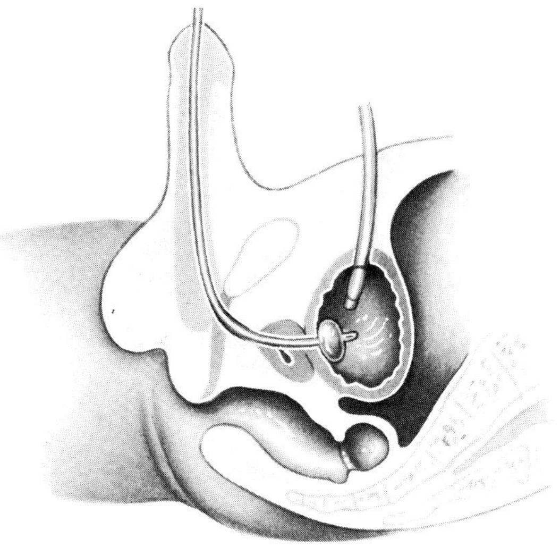

9

Delayed repair

If at the time of the initial suprapubic cystostomy the prostate is found to be almost in its normal position, indicating the probability of partial urethral damage, then a suprapubic catheter, size 22 Fr, is left to drain the bladder via the suprapubic wound. A urethral catheter is not inserted.

Depending on his general condition, the patient is returned to the operating theatre after 3 weeks and the urethra is inspected by urethroscopy. This should be carried out by an experienced endoscopist who will probably be able to find his way past the partial rupture, guided by the intact bridge of mucosa into the bladder. If the endoscopic urethrotome with the catheter guide sheath has been used it is easy to pass a catheter after withdrawing the endoscope and leaving the guide channel *in situ*. Otherwise a ureteric catheter can be left *in situ*. If the endoscopic urethrotome with its catheter guide has not been used and the rupture has been inspected by an ordinary urethroscope, after clearing the blood clot a ureteric is passed via the endoscope sheath into the bladder and left indwelling for 7–10 days. During that time the suprapubic catheter can be removed.

If endoscopy fails to find a route through, the urethra must be explored suprapubically, as for immediate repair.

RUPTURED URETHRA IN THE FEMALE

Damage to the female urethra is much less common than damage to the male posterior urethra. It is usually associated with fracture of the pelvis, but may also be due to penetrating wounds in the perineum, or to a blow to the perineum. Injuries of the female urethra usually also involve the anterior wall of the vagina and will ultimately develop a urethrovaginal fistula. Repair of a high urethrovaginal fistula can be very difficult due to extensive and firm adhesions to the posterior part of the symphysis pubis. Such cases are best treated in the combined approach by the urologist from the suprapubic area and by the gynaecologist from the perineum. Repair of the fistula in layers over a silicone Foley catheter will restore continuity, but may still leave the patient with limited urinary control.

RUPTURED URETHRA IN CHILDREN

Rupture of the urethra can be a very severe injury in children of both sexes under the age of 10. In boys the prostate has not yet developed and rupture is liable to occur just below the neck of the bladder and above the level of the external sphincter. Blood may not be seen at the external urinary meatus, even though the urethra has been torn.

Rupture of the urethra and anterior wall of the vagina seems to occur more often in little girls than in adults. Bleeding from the urethra and vagina can be so severe that the patient may have to be taken to the theatre as an emergency to pack the vagina in order to control the bleeding.

Editor's comment

Posterior membranous urethral disruptions may be treated initially with a suprapubic cystostomy and no manipulation of the urethra. The stricture which develops is repaired by a second procedure performed 4–6 months post injury. The advantage of this form of therapy is reportedly a lower incidence of impotence. The disadvantage is that all patients treated in this manner require a second operation whereas many of those who are approached as the author recommends do not require a second procedure.

Further reading

Blandy, J. P. Injuries of the urethra in the male. Injury 1975; 7: 77–83

Clarke, B. G., Leadbetter, W. F. Management of wounds and injuries of genito-urinary tract: review of reported experience in World War II. Journal of Urology 1952; 67: 719–739

Hunt, A. H., Morgan, C. N. Complete rupture of the membranous urethra. Lancet 1942; 2: 330–331

Hunt, A. H., Morgan, C. N. Complete rupture of the membranous urethra. Lancet 1949; 1: 601–602

Kidd, F. The end-results of treatments of injuries of the urethra. Rapport de la Société Internationale d'Urologie. Paris: Libraire Octave Doin, 1921

Mitchell, J. P. Injuries to the urethra. British Journal of Urology 1968; 40: 649–670

Morehouse, D. D., Belitsky, P., MacKinnon, K. Rupture of the posterior urethra. Journal of Urology 1972; 107: 255

Pasteau, O., Iselin, A. La résection de l'urethre perinéal. Annales des maladies des organes génito-urinaires 1906; 24: 1601–1644

Poole-Wilson, D. S. Injuries of the urethra. Proceedings of the Royal Society of Medicine 1947; 40: 798–804

Poole-Wilson, D. S. Missile injuries of the urethra. British Journal of Surgery 1949; 36: 364–376

Poole-Wilson, D. S., Pointon, R. C. S. The present condition of treatment of epithelial tumours of the bladder. In: Rock-Carling, *Sir* E., Ross, *Sir* J. P. eds. Surgical progress, Vol. II. London: Butterworths 1961: 62–97

Simpson-Smith, A. Traumatic rupture of the urethra. Eight personal cases with a review of 381 recorded ruptures. British Journal of Surgery 1936; 24: 309

Young, H. H. Treatment of complete rupture of posterior urethra, recent or ancient, by anastomosis. Journal of Urology 1929; 21: 417–449

Circumcision, meatotomy and meatoplasty

John P. Blandy MA, DM, MCh, FRCS
Professor of Urology, The London Hospital Medical College;
Consultant Urologist, St Peter's Hospital, London, UK

Circumcision

Indications

Circumcision of newborn babies is a religious rite, not a surgical emergency, but there are very rare instances where the foreskin is provided with a true pinhole meatus and a circumcision may justifiably be performed in order to overcome obstruction. Later on in childhood recurrent balanitis, the development of a secondary meatal stenosis, or an inability to wash behind the foreskin are real indications for circumcision, and it is possible to make a good case for routine circumcision of children who are likely to be brought up in parts of the world where soap and water are rare commodities. Such a policy would prevent the large numbers of penile carcinomas seen in contemporary Africa.

A general anaesthetic is necessary, except perhaps in the newborn. For this reason it is preferable to postpone circumcision if possible until the child is about 3 years of age.

1, 2 & 3

Whatever technique is followed, the first step in circumcision is to make sure that the foreskin has been thoroughly separated from the glans penis. It is still a common error to see boys in whom the corona glandis has been left covered, and smegma has been retained under it. First a probe separates the foreskin from the glans. The foreskin is then stretched and pulled down, any adhesions between its mucosa and the glans being gently broken with a moist dissecting swab until the coronal sulcus is quite clean.

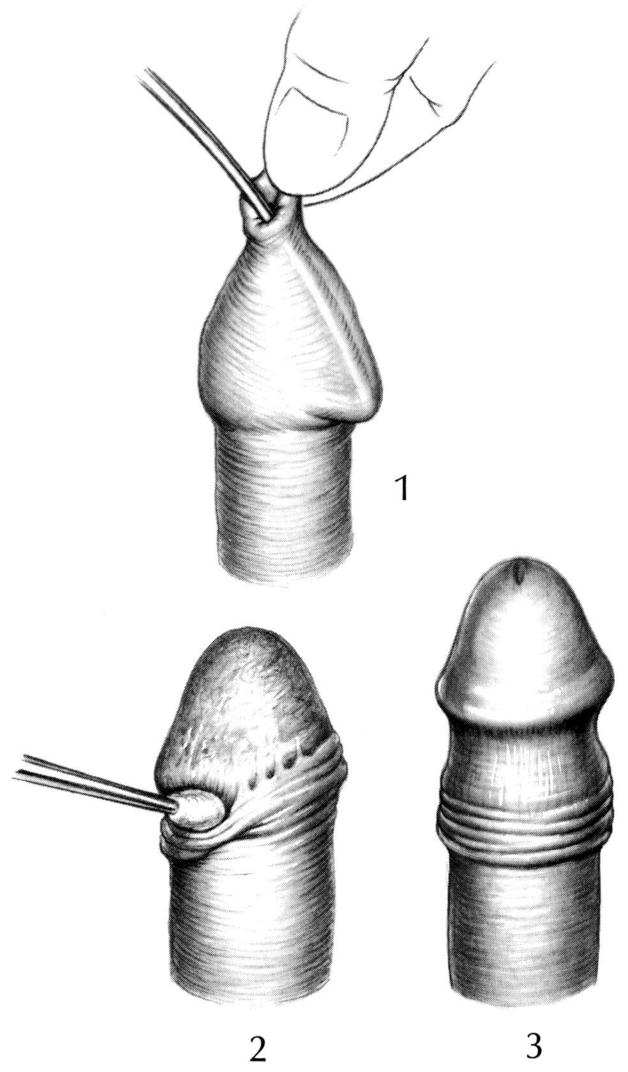

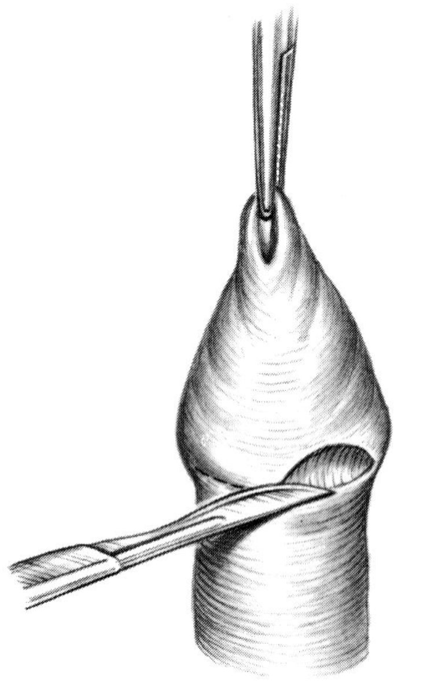

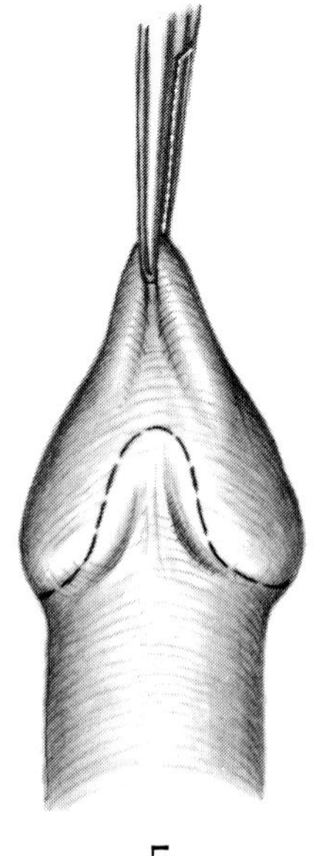

4 & 5

It is very difficult to cut a clean edge with scissors, and preferable to incise the skin and mucosa with a knife. The foreskin is pulled back over the glans, and allowed to lie in a natural position. This will allow the surgeon to choose the right position for the incision through the foreskin, which should coincide with the corona glandis. The knife is carried through skin only, and on the ventral surface of the penis may take the direction shown in order to liberate a frenum which is short.

6–11

The foreskin is now pulled back and, again using a knife, an incision is made some 3 mm away from the coronal sulcus through epidermis and into the underlying areolar tissue. The surplus foreskin is removed with scissors. Small vessels are meticulously caught and ligated with 4/0 catgut. Particular attention is paid to the artery in the frenum which must be carefully ligated. The skin edges are approximated with 5/0 interrupted catgut sutures.

No dressing is necessary. To prevent bedclothes from adhering to the suture line, it may be lightly smeared with sterile Vaseline. Haemostatic dressings should be unnecessary and may give rise to severe skin reactions, even amounting to necrosis.

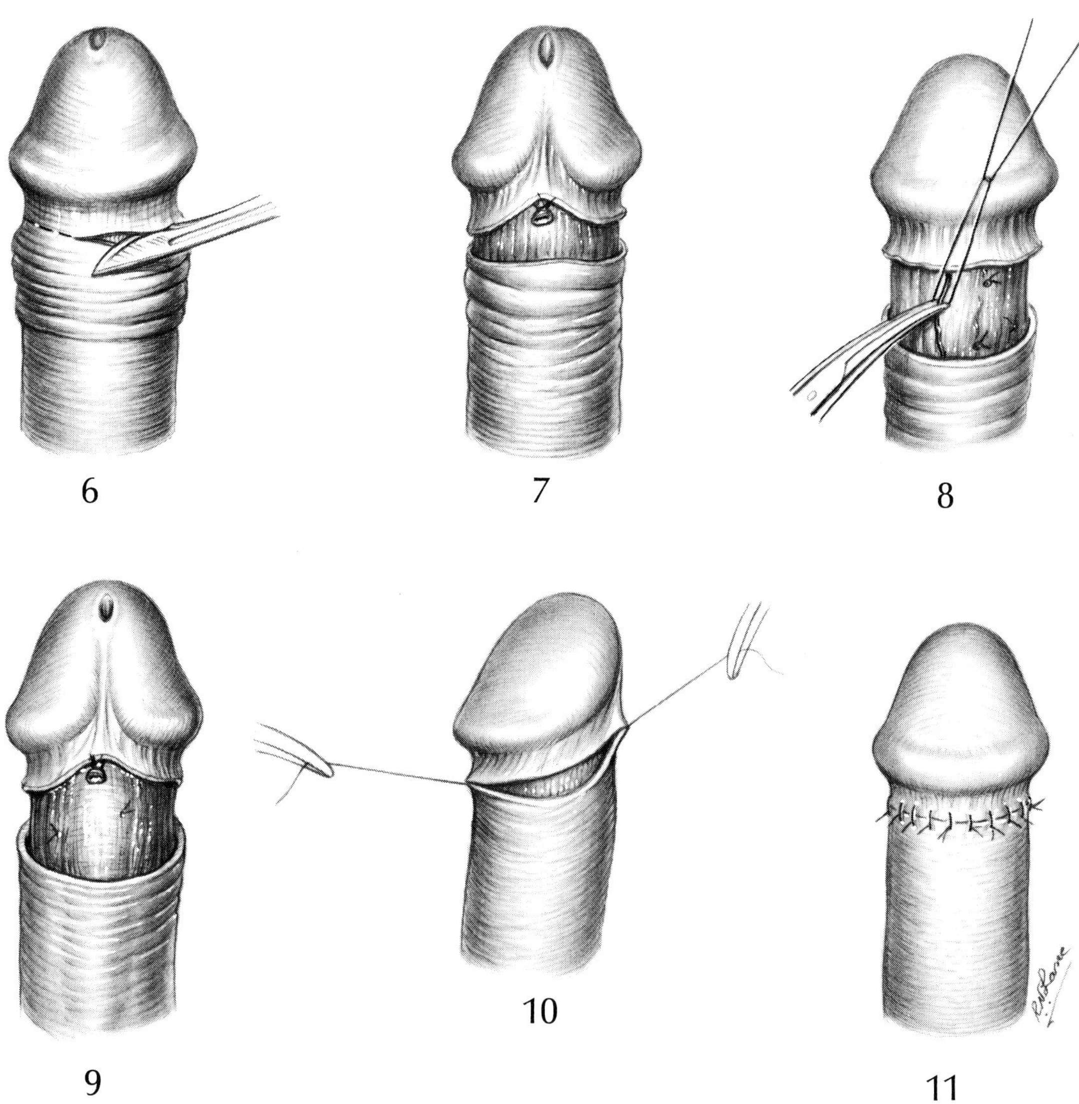

Aftercare

A child may be allowed home at the end of the day of the operation. The mother may bathe it in the usual way and should be instructed to dry the part gently, but not to apply any dressing. Adults will probably need to remain in a little longer in order to become accustomed to the sensitivity of the exposed glans. In those adult patients in whom the two layers of the foreskin have become particularly adherent, and in whom sharp dissection has been necessary in order to remove the foreskin, one must allow a considerable period of time for the glans to epithelialize. It is never necessary to apply skin grafts, for the new glandular skin will completely regenerate in time and give an almost normal appearance.

PLASTIBELL TECHNIQUE

12, 13 & 14

The Hollister Plastibell, and similar devices, are of interest to surgeons obliged to perform circumcision on neonates. The principle is simple: a plastic device is pushed into the cleft between glans penis and foreskin and a ligature (supplied sterile with the device) is tied tightly around the lip of the 'bell'. Surplus foreskin is cut off with scissors and the handle of the plastic bell snapped off. It is essential that the child is examined at intervals until the plastic device has been recovered. The surplus skin separates with a clean line of demarcation, leaving a fine, neat scar. Complications are rare.

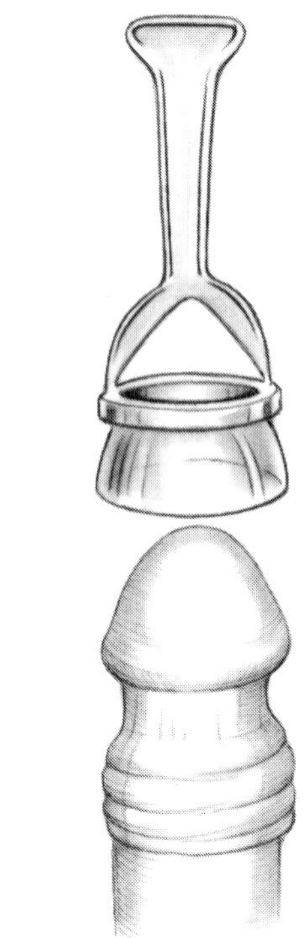

12

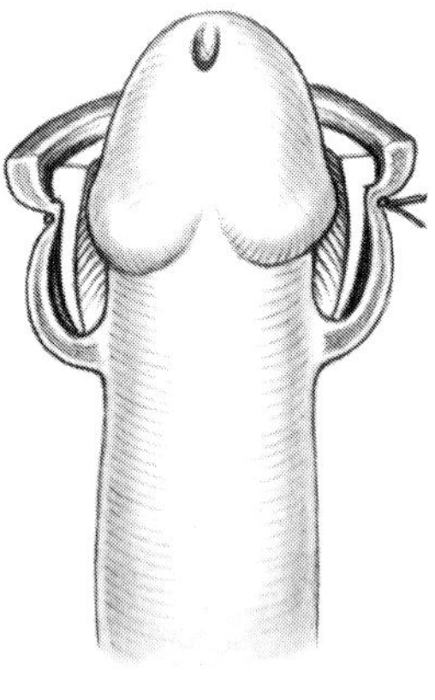

13

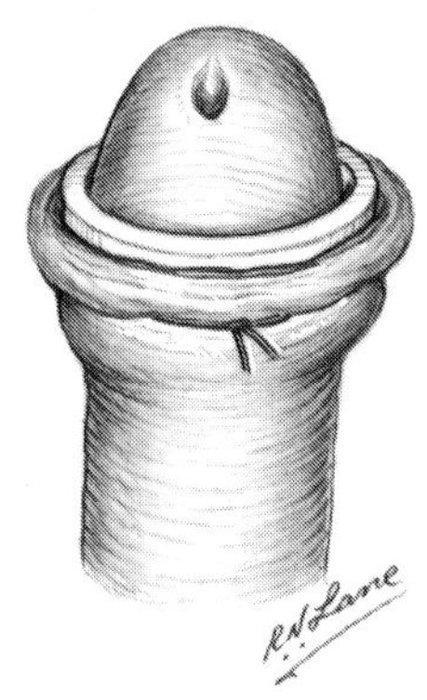

14

Meatotomy

Meatotomy may by itself result in a permanent cure of a meatus narrowed as a result of the trauma of urethral instrumentation. But in most adults it is followed by restenosis, and a meatoplasty is a more certain way of dealing with the problem.

15, 16 & 17

If meatotomy is performed, it should be carried right down into the normal urethra, forming a more generous incision than the circumstances may seem to warrant. However, unless a large incision is made, restenosis is inevitable. A few sutures may be inserted to achieve haemostasis, and the apical suture should attempt to approximate urethral mucosa to skin.

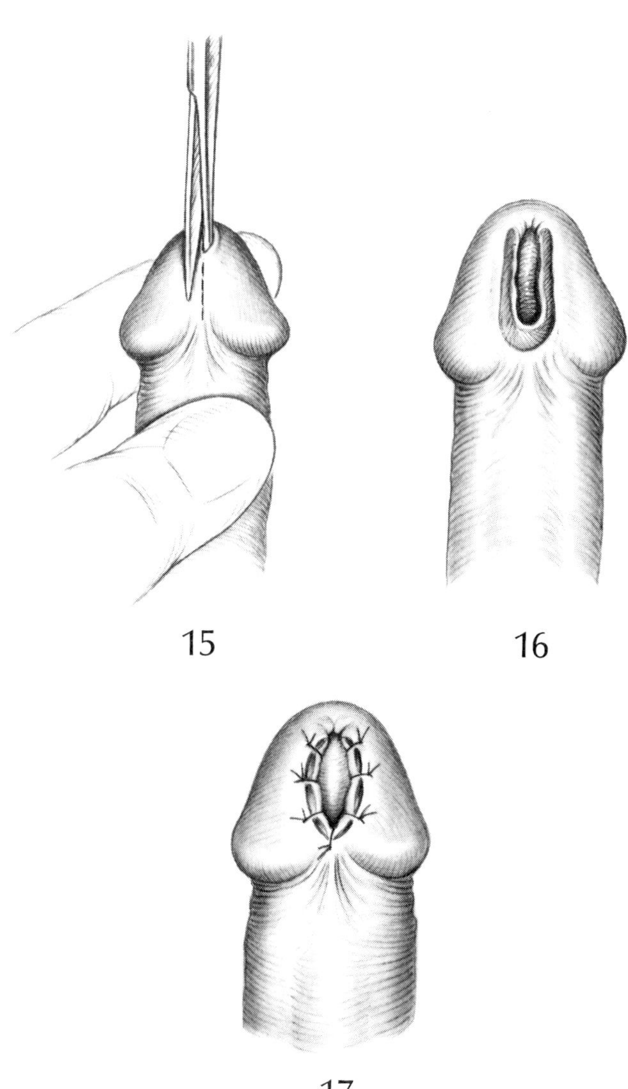

15

16

17

18

Following meatotomy a patient should be provided with a suitable bougie and advised to pass it at increasing intervals until the risk of restenosis has passed.

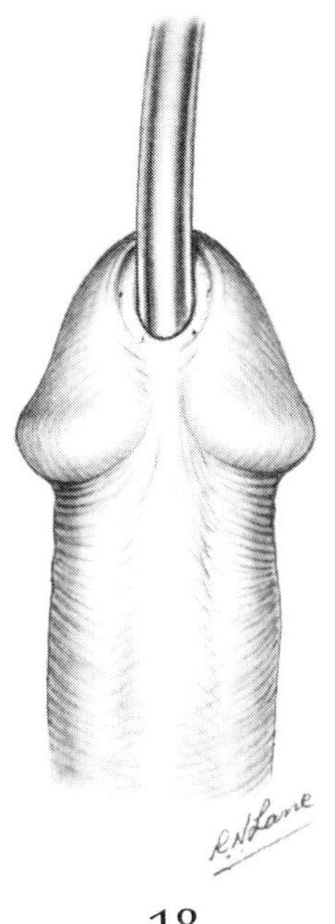

18

Meatoplasty

A more sure way to overcome meatal and submeatal stenosis, as seen after surgical trauma and in cases of balanitis xerotica obliterans, is to insert a ∩-shaped flap of skin into the opened-up urethral meatus.

19–24

A curved ∩-shaped flap is made of the skin on the ventral surface of the penis and this is allowed to drop back. A very generous incision is now made along the ventral midline of the meatus, care being taken that the incision enters healthy urethra and unscarred corpus spongiosum. In many cases of balanitis xerotica obliterans the hard scar tissue extends proximally for 2–3 cm and it is easy to make this incision too short. The ∩-shaped flap of skin is now tucked into the defect. Using 5/0 plain catgut with a double-ended needle, the skin is sewn in position with fine, even bites, making sure that the skin is approximated neatly to the mucosal surface of the urethra. Where the urethra is very scarred at its distal centimetre, the edges should be loosely brought together so that the end-result is like a congenital glandular hypospadias.

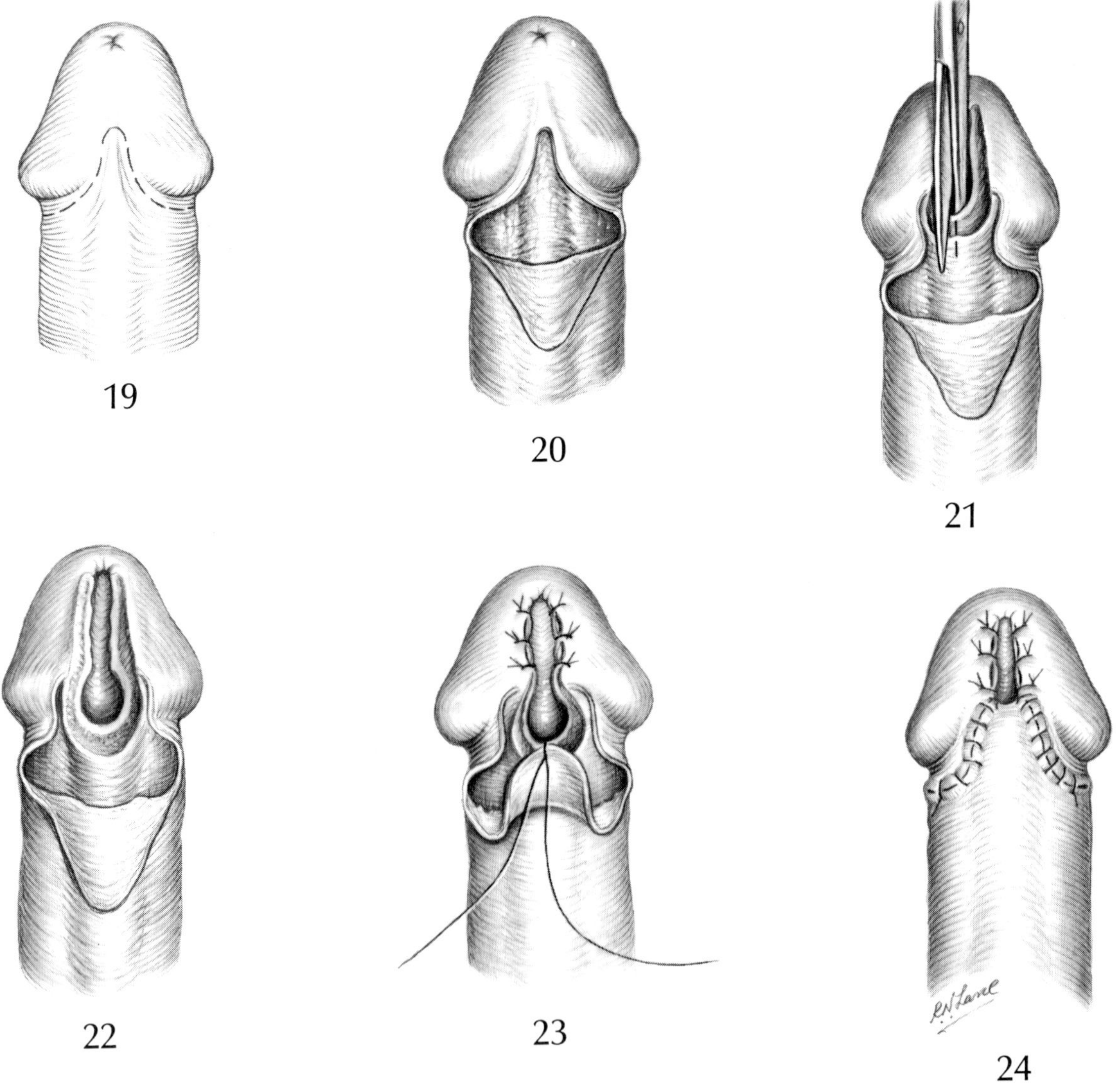

Instrumentation is avoided during the period of follow-up. The author has seen one recurrence in 32 cases – in a patient with balanitis xerotica in whom the original incision was probably not carried far enough proximally, or else the condition recurred. One tiresome complication is mentioned by these patients, namely that on voiding the stream sprays. With a little manipulation and side-to-side compression of the glans, this disability is usually overcome.

Operation for testicular torsion

J. E. A. Wickham MS, BSc, FRCS
Director of the Academic Unit, Institute of Urology, University of London;
Senior Consultant Urological Surgeon, St Bartholomew's Hospital, London;
Consultant Surgeon, St Peter's Hospital Group, London, UK

Introduction

Torsion of the testis or its appendages most commonly occurs in the child or young adolescent. Previous attacks of scrotal pain may have occurred. The definitive attack occurs suddenly, frequently following physical exertion such as riding a bicycle. The scrotum becomes rapidly swollen and exquisitely painful, particularly on palpation, so that it is normally impossible to define the various parts of the scrotal contents with any certainty.

Torsion must be differentiated from the following.

Acute epididymo-orchitis. This develops much less acutely than a torsion. The scrotum, although swollen, is usually reddened and it may be possible to distinguish a normal body of testis from a swollen and tender epididymis. There may also be a history of urinary tract or urethral infection.

Mumps Orchitis. This may simulate a torsion very closely, although the onset of symptoms is usually less acute.

Testicular tumour. Also gives rise to a tender scrotal mass, but again the length of history will normally distinguish a tumour from a torsion.

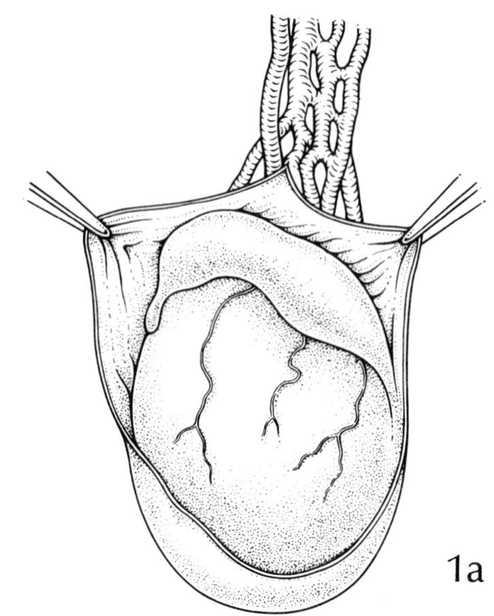

1a

1a & b

Torsion occurs because an abnormal unobliterated prolongation of the tunica vaginalis completely invests the epididymis and distal spermatic cord. (*a*) shows the normal anatomy and (*b*) shows abnormal anatomy with torsion potential. In (*b*) the testis is in effect suspended in the scrotum from a stalk and is free to rotate within the tunica vaginalis. Rotation of the testis twists the spermatic cord, obstructs the contained blood vessels and produces testicular ischaemia with ultimate necrosis.

Torsion is one of the few urological emergencies. There is no place for manipulative management and the treatment is urgent surgical exploration which must be undertaken within 3–4 hours if the testicle is to be saved from ischaemic necrosis.

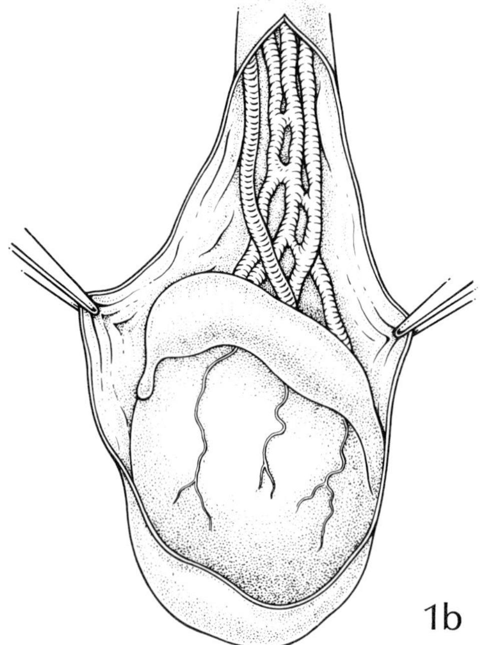

1b

Preoperative preparation

A Ryle's tube should be passed to empty the stomach before anaesthesia. A general anaesthetic should be used, and the patient should be placed supine on the operating table.

The operation

The testicle is delivered from the scrotum by an anterolateral incision. The skin, dartos fascia and tunica vaginalis are all incised in this line.

2

The testicle, frequently surrounded by a secondary hydrocele containing serosanguinous fluid, is delivered gently from the tunica. The epididymis is usually distended and haemorrhagic and the globe of the testis is swollen and cyanotic. The torsion is visualized as the cord comes into view when the direction of twist is usually quite obvious. This is untwisted until the cord lies normally.

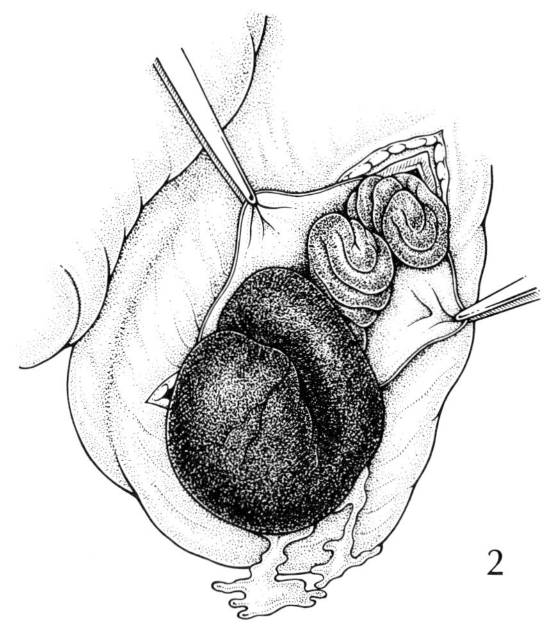

2

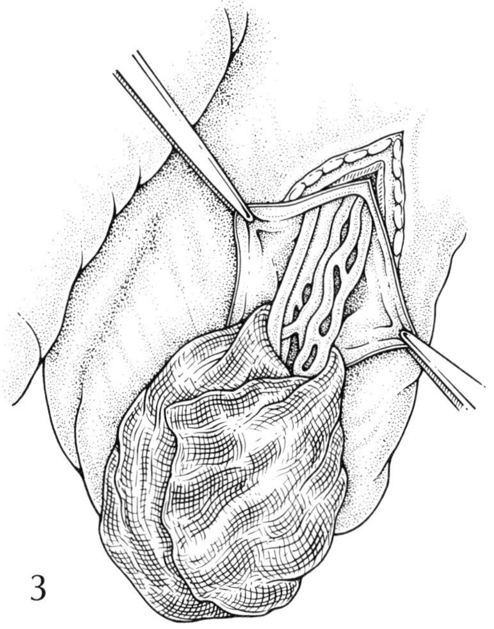

3

3

Conservation or removal of the testicle

The untwisted testicle is wrapped in moist warm swabs for 5–10 minutes and its colour carefully observed. If vascular perfusion has been re-established, with a return to normal, or near normal, colour, the testis is conserved. If the testis is obviously black and necrotic, or the circulation is not re-established on untwisting, then the testicle should be removed. It is better to err on the side of conservation if in doubt. A torted testicle may partially recover and, although small, may function hormonally if not spermatogenically.

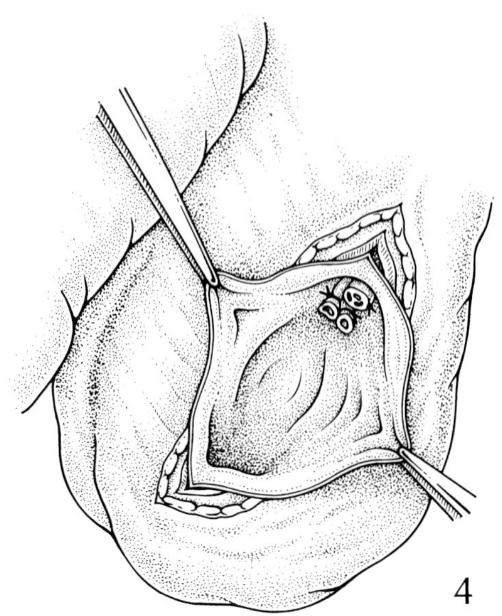

4

Removal of the testicle

The cord should be divided between clamps and ligated with a transfixion ligating stitch of 2/0 chromic catgut.

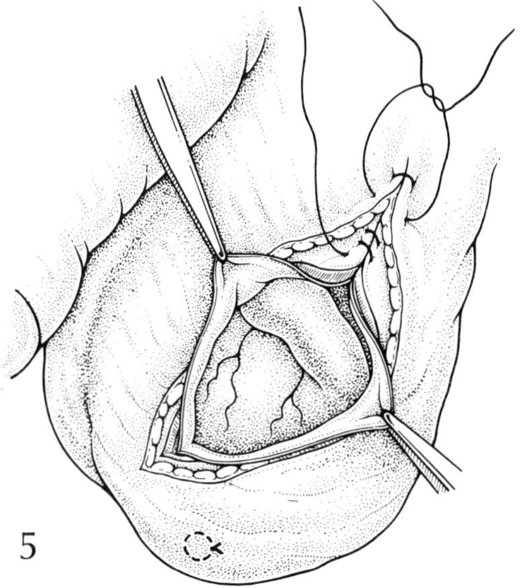

5

Replacement of the testicle

If the testicle is replaced, a small 'tack' suture of 2/0 catgut should be used to attach the lower pole of the testis to the inside of the scrotal cavity to prevent recurrence. The wound is closed with continuous 3/0 chromic catgut suture to the tunica vaginalis and dartos layer, and interrupted sutures of 3/0 chromic catgut or Dexon to the skin.

Fixation of contralateral testicle

The abnormal condition of the tunica vaginalis giving rise to torsion usually occurs bilaterally. Therefore, when the twisted testicle has been dealt with, the contralateral testis should be explored and similarly secured in the scrotum with a 'tack' suture of 2/0 chromic catgut passed between the lower pole of the testis and the tunica vaginalis. This manoeuvre is even more strongly indicated if orchidectomy has been performed for the torsion.

Craniotomy

R. D. Illingworth MB, FRCS
Consultant Neurosurgeon,
Charing Cross and Central Middlesex Hospitals, London;
Honorary Consultant Neurosurgeon, Westminster Hospital, London, UK

Preoperative

Indications and contraindications

Craniotomy is indicated for the diagnosis or treatment of intracranial lesions demonstrated by neuro-radiology, where there is adequate clinical indication. With modern diagnostic facilities, truly exploratory procedures will rarely be needed.

Contraindications may be the nature of the lesion, the speed of progression of symptoms and also the patient's age and fitness. The few absolute contraindications include overwhelming infection or abnormalities of blood coagulation. Poor neurological condition of the patient need not be a contraindication, since surgical treatment of an intracranial mass will usually be required before improvement can occur.

Premedication and anaesthesia

It is customary to use light non-sedative premedication for intracranial operations to allow patients to be assessed immediately prior to operation, and so that recovery of consciousness after operation is not delayed. Dexamethasone 4 mg 6-hourly started 24–48 h before operation will often improve the neurological state of patients with intracranial tumours and appears to reduce the cerebral oedema which may follow operative manipulation of the brain. It may also be helpful in the surgery of intracranial aneurysms to protect the brain from disturbances of local cerebral blood flow.

Endotracheal intubation with hyperventilation, and hypotension if required, is standard practice for most craniotomies. This reduces intracranial pressure and brain bulk and allows easy manipulation of the brain, especially if preoperative dexamethasone has been given. Mannitol can be given to reduce brain bulk during the operation, but has the disadvantage of increasing blood volume and hence bleeding and may mislead the surgeon about the extent of the decompression achieved in partial removal of gliomas. Mannitol will rarely be required where preoperative dexamethasone has been given.

Positioning the patient

The position of the patient is so important in making the planned procedure easier that the surgeon will wish to do this himself. In general:

1. the plane of the craniotomy should be approximately horizontal;
2. the position of the head should allow any dissection at depth to be in the normal line of vision of the surgeon;
3. the airway must be protected and venous drainage from the head not obstructed;
4. vulnerable points on the patient should be protected from pressure, either from the patient's weight or from fittings on the operating table.

Placement of skin incision

This, like the positioning of the patient, is crucial and any operation, however straightforward, may be made infinitely more difficult if the wrong skin incision, and consequently the wrong bone flap, is cut. The skin incision should be planned with three factors in mind:

1. the surgical access to the lesion;
2. the skin blood supply;
3. the cosmetic effect of the scar.

Craniotomy flaps

In general craniotomy flaps fall into five main groups:

1. flaps to expose the surface of the cerebral hemisphere;
2. flaps to expose the base of the brain;
3. flaps to expose the mid-line and medial surface of the cerebral hemisphere;
4. flaps for frontal or occipital lobectomy;
5. flaps for temporal exploration.

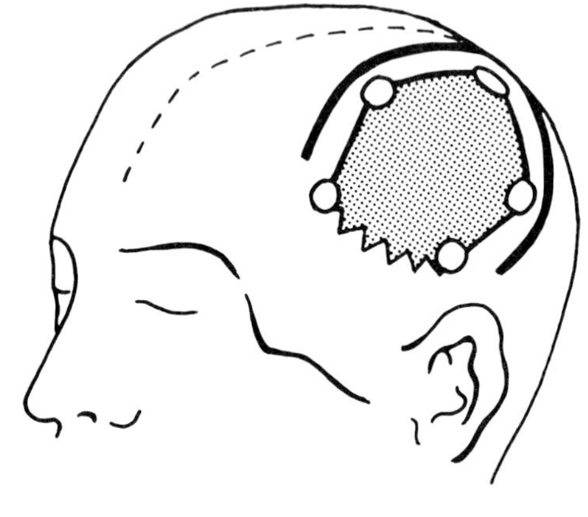

1

1

Flaps to expose the surface of the cerebral hemisphere should be centred on the lesion and made sufficiently large to allow adequate access with some margin for error. A semicircular or rectangular skin incision can be used. The width of the base of the flap should not be narrower than the widest point of the flap and the length of the flap should not exceed the width of the base. These flaps will generally be entirely behind the hair-line, but if exposure anterior to this is required the skin flap should be based anteriorly with one limb of the incision on the mid-line.

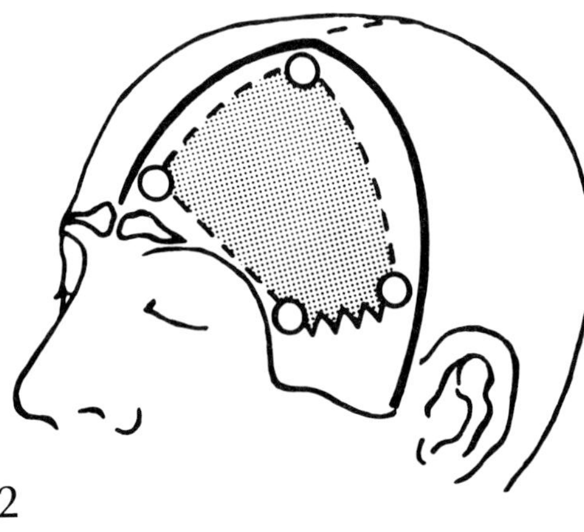

2

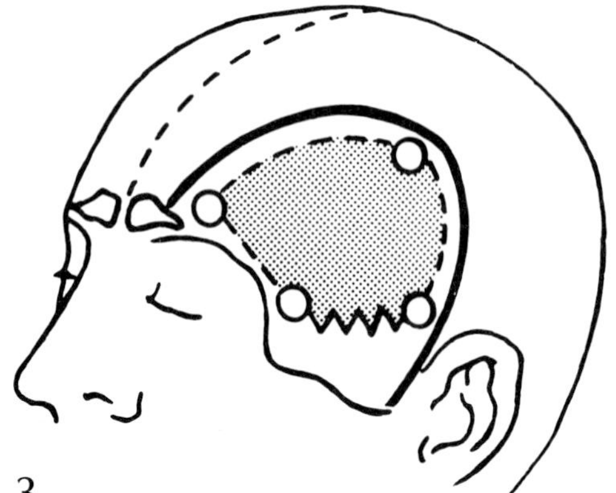

3

2 & 3

Flaps to expose the base of the brain are required for the removal of basal tumours such as meningiomas and pituitary adenomas, and for the treatment of intracranial aneurysms. The skin incision used is generally a frontal (*Illustration 2*) or frontotemporal (*Illustration 3*) flap. The anterior limb of the flap may pass down the mid-line onto the forehead or run obliquely forward on the forehead near the midline. If bifrontal exposure is required a coronal skin incision is used, and this can also be used if a scar on the forehead is to be avoided. The skin flap need not be large but must be taken down to the level of the frontal sinus in the mid-line anteriorly and to the level of the zygomatic arch in the temporal region. The skin flap must be dissected down until the superior orbital margin can be seen, to allow the bone cut above the orbit to be made level with the floor of the anterior cranial fossa. This is essential if brain retraction is to be minimized. The anterior burr hole should be made just above the frontal sinus and a further burr hole made either on the outer end of the sphenoidal wing, as will be described for temporal craniotomy, or immediately anterior to this but level with the floor of the anterior cranial fossa. The bone flap need not include the temporal region unless this additional exposure is required.

4a & b

If large, the frontal sinus may be divided deliberately to improve the access (*a*). If the mucosa is left intact, it need not be disturbed, but if the mucosa of the sinus is opened it must be completely removed from the upper part of the sinus within the bone flap and the hole into the sinus closed with a piece of temporalis fascia held with sutures through dura and pericranium (*b*). It may be advisable in this circumstance not to use high vacuum suction drainage beneath the skin flap to avoid sucking through from the nose. If a burr hole has been made on or posterior to the lesser sphenoidal wing, this may be rongeured away further to improve access.

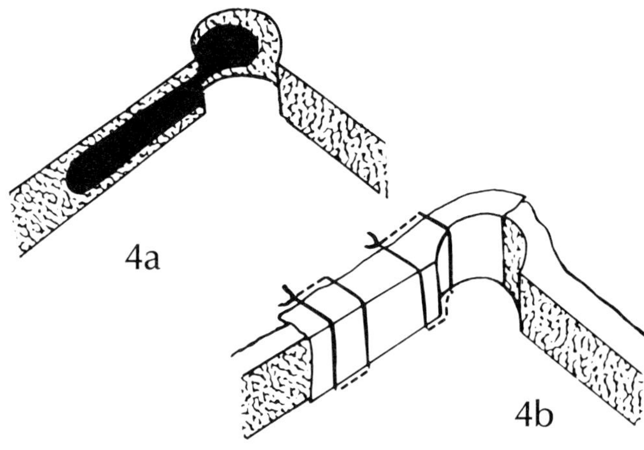

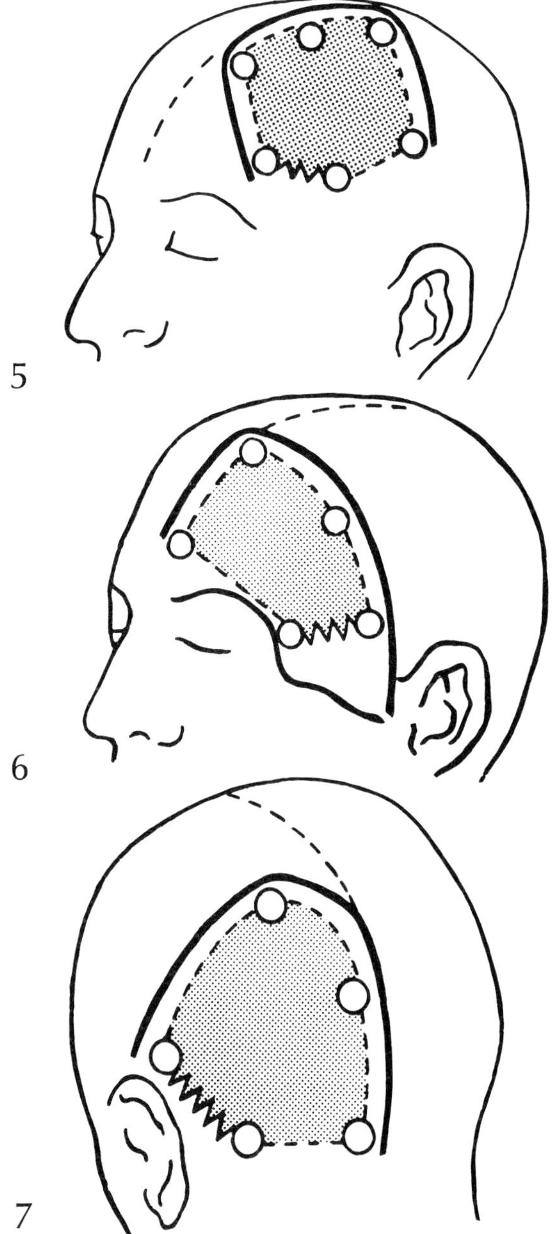

5

Mid-line flaps are used for parasagittal and falx meningiomas and for pericallosal aneurysms. In these situations the mid-line limb of both the skin and bone flaps should be made precisely on the mid-line, since even a small overhang of bone may add considerably to the operative difficulties. There is generally some venous bleeding when the dura is separated from the bone at the mid-line although with modern anaesthesia this is generally not excessive. There may, however, be considerable bleeding if there is a parasagittal or falx meningioma and it is advisable to leave the mid-line bone cuts until last when turning such a flap. Some difficulty may be experienced anteriorly where there may be a sharp ridge of bone continuing up the mid-line from the base of the skull. The dura may be torn if power tools are used at this point and the most anterior frontal burr hole is most conveniently cut by hand.

6 & 7

Flaps for frontal (Illustration 6) and occipital (Illustration 7) lobectomy must extend up to the mid-line and also down to the base of the skull for lobectomy to be easily achieved. Flaps which do not reach the mid-line cause difficulty with the most medial part of the dissection, and flaps which do not reach the base of the skull similarly cause difficulty with the cut across the orbital surface of the frontal lobe or the tentorial surface of the occipital lobe. The skin incision should therefore pass from anteriorly or, in the case of the occipital flap, from posteriorly, up the mid-line and then turn down to the anterior or posterior temporal region. These flaps are a combination of basal and mid-line exposures.

8 & 9

Temporal flaps must be planned to expose as much as possible of the temporal lobe or the exposure will prove to be more parietal than temporal. Two types of incision may be used. In type one, the incision is started on the zygomatic arch, immediately in front of the ear so that the superficial temporal artery is preserved, then curves upwards and forwards and passes obliquely across the forehead near the mid-line (*Illustration 8*). The incision must be made low enough at each end to allow the skin flap to be turned down to expose the outer end of the lesser sphenoidal wing. Type two starts on the zygomatic arch 1 cm in front of the tragus of the ear so that it lies anterior to the superficial temporal artery. The incision runs forward in a low curve to a point no less than 2 cm above the outer end of the eyebrow and then curves upwards and backwards to pass back behind the ear. This incision allows a little anterior flap to be dissected downwards and so improve the exposure anteriorly, and it can be taken as far posteriorly as necessary (*Illustration 9*). If the incision is taken lower than 2 cm above the outer end of the eyebrow the frontal branch of the facial nerve may be cut, with unsightly paralysis of the frontalis muscle. Care must be taken to preserve the superficial temporal artery and not to make the anterior curve of the flap too acute or ischaemic necrosis of the most anterior part of the flap may result. The incision must not go below the zygomatic arch or the facial nerve may be cut.

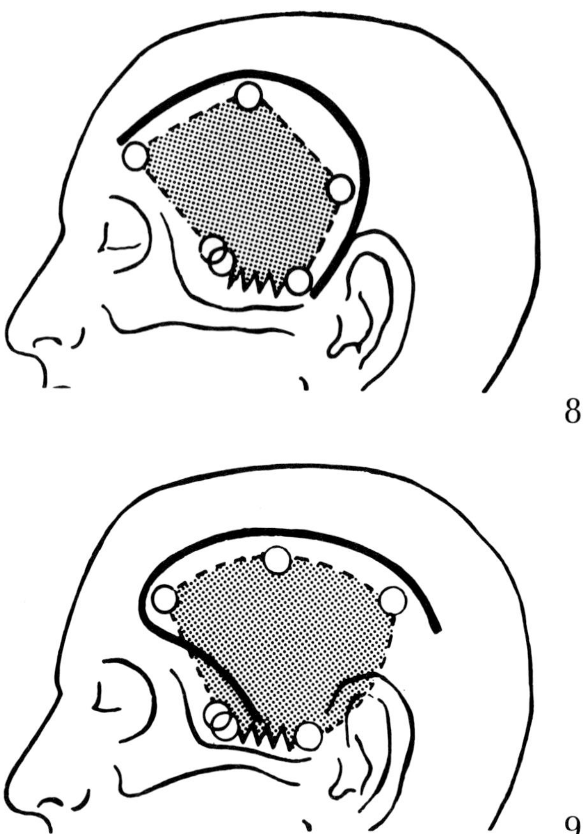

8

9

10

In both these exposures the temporalis muscle is incised, posteriorly down to the level of the zygomatic arch and anteriorly from just above the orbital margin deep into the anterior part of the muscle to expose the external groove on the temporal bone which indicates the position of the lesser sphenoidal wing. The burr holes made at these points are the keys to the exposure. Posteriorly the burr hole must be made as low as possible onto the floor of the middle fossa (*a*). Anteriorly the exposure can be improved if a double burr hole is made on the lesser sphenoidal wing (*b*). The drill is directed anteriorly into the anterior cranial fossa, and posteriorly and inferiorly into the middle cranial fossa. This will often leave a ridge of the lesser sphenoidal wing in between and this may be nibbled through with bone forceps. If the anterior burr hole is made lower, the orbit may easily be entered. The sphenoidal wing may be nibbled away and the exposure generally needs to be extended anteriorly by nibbling bone away from the front and the anterior part of the floor of the middle cranial fossa. The bulky temporalis muscle may obscure the exposure here and the bone flap and muscle can be retracted with a large self-retaining retractor.

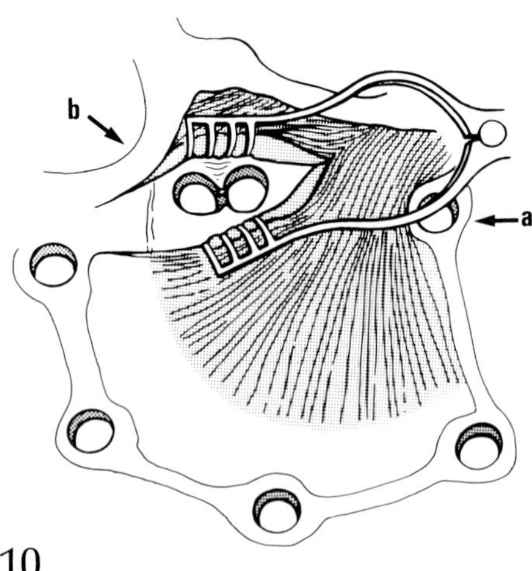

10

The operation

Skin preparation and towelling

The patient having been positioned and the flap planned, the scalp is cleaned, first with a dilute aqueous solution of chlorhexidine and cetrimide and then with chlorhexidine 0.5 per cent in 70 per cent methylated spirit. The skin incision is marked with ink or a skin scratch and the area infiltrated with local anaesthetic with or without adrenaline 1:200000. The head is covered with an adhesive plastic drape or with fabric which may be soaked in antiseptic solution. Towels are placed around and held with towel clips. A table over the patient is useful to place instruments on and to lift the towels off the patient so that the anaesthetist has access. This overtable and the rest of the patient may be covered with a large split towel which leaves only the operative site exposed.

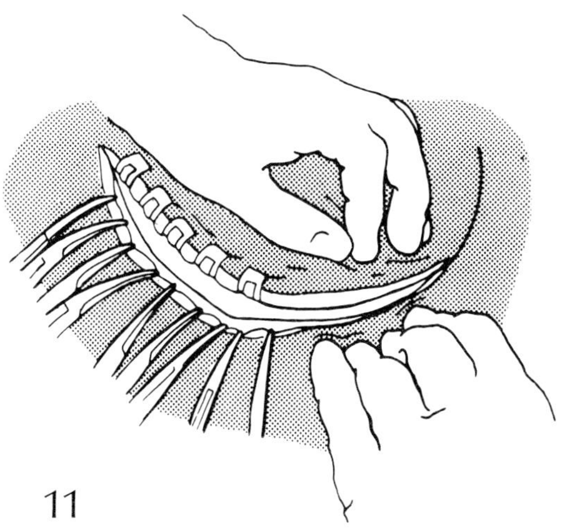

11

11

Skin incisions and haemostasis

The incision is made in short lengths, the bleeding from the scalp being controlled initially by pressure from the surgeon's and assistant's fingers. Bleeding on the side of the flap is stopped with Raney clips and on the side of the scalp by applying curved artery forceps to the galea. The weight of the forceps, which are gathered into groups with rubber bands, is generally sufficient to stop most bleeding. Artery forceps may be applied to the scalp flap instead of Raney clips but the extra bulk tends to be cumbersome. When the incision has been made all round, the scalp flap is elevated from the underlying pericranium by gentle sharp dissection. Bleeding from the deep surface of the scalp or from the pericranium is stopped with diathermy and the flap is then covered with damp gauze.

Cutting the bone flap

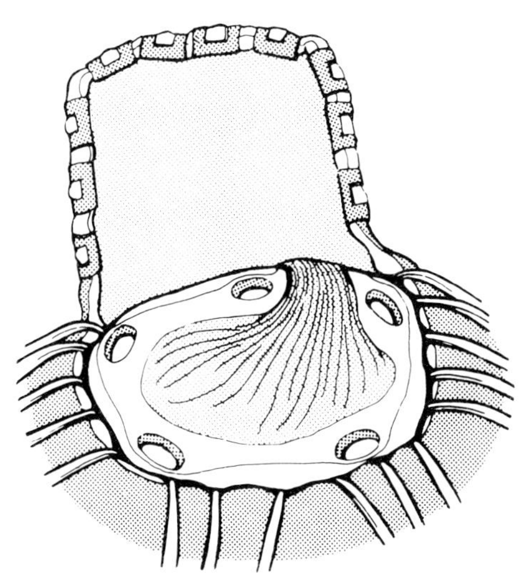

12

12

The pericranium and muscle are incised with cutting diathermy in the line of the intended bone flap except inferiorly where a pedicle of pericranium or temporalis muscle is left uncut to allow some blood supply to the bone to remain. Alternatively, the pericranium and muscle may be detached completely from the intended bone flap but this generally produces little advantage in the exposure and the completely detached bone flap may be absorbed after replacement. The pericranium is reflected with a broad periosteal elevator and the temporalis muscle held back with self-retaining retractors. The bone flap is cut using either hand instruments or power tools.

By hand, the flap is cut by making a series of burr holes about 6 or 7 cm apart. The burr holes will need to be nearer together if the bone is very thick or the dura very adherent. Using gentle dissection with a blunt curved Adson's periosteal elevator, the dura is separated from the bone between the burr holes. Some difficulty may be experienced in this, particularly in older patients and care should be taken to keep the tip of the instrument against the bone to avoid tearing the dura.

13a & b

The cuts between the burr holes are made using a Gigli saw which is passed between the burr holes using the malleable saw guide (*a*). The cuts are made with a steady sawing motion with handles attached to the ends of the saw and the surgeon's hands well separated (*b*). The angle of the cut should be bevelled outwards to allow the bone flap to rest on the surrounding skull when replaced.

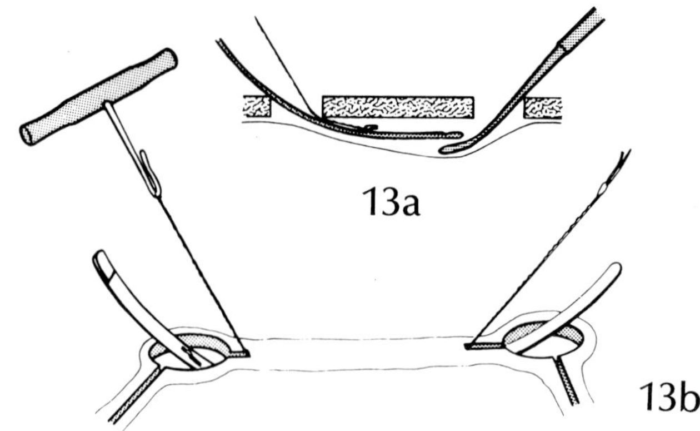

13b

14

At the base of the flap the cut is not made with a saw but by cutting between the burr holes, using the de Vilbis bone forceps until the remaining bridge of bone is weak enough to break easily when the flap is elevated.

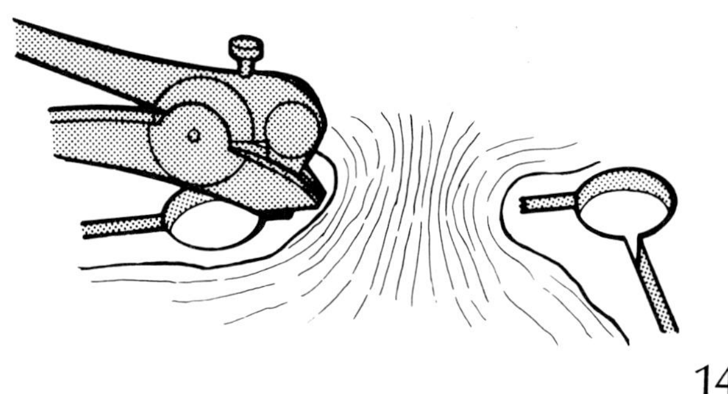

14

15

The flap is elevated by levering it upwards with two Horsley's elevators, carefully separating the dura from the bone as this is done. If the base of the flap has been made thin enough the bone should break straight between the burr holes.

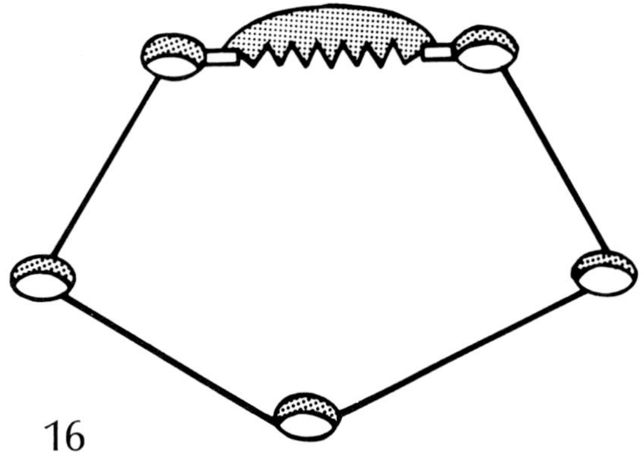

15

16

A little bone must be trimmed from the skull side of the fracture to allow the bone flap to fit when replaced, but subtemporal decompression is rarely required.

The disadvantage of this method is that it may be very slow and laborious if the bone is thick and dense.

16

17

Alternatively, the bone flap may be cut using power tools. Only two burr holes may be necessary at the base of the flap and these are cut using the skull perforator attachment of the drill.

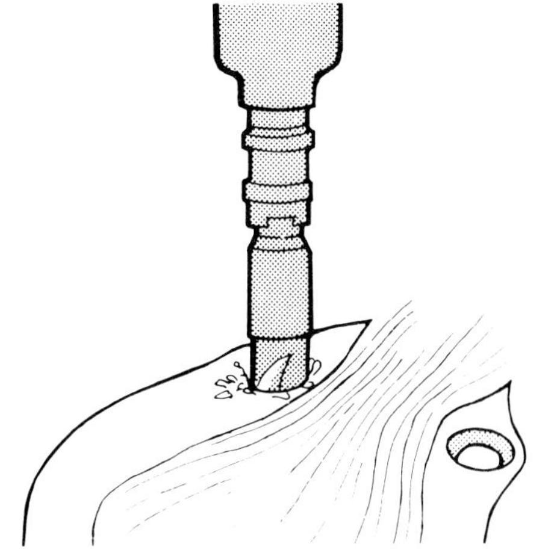

17

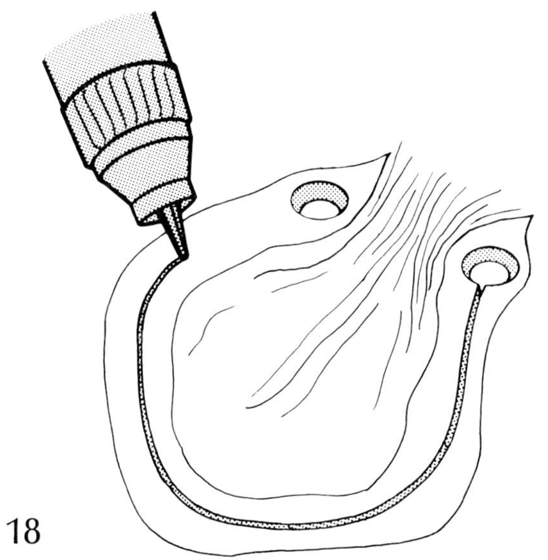

18

18

The dura is then separated from the bone at the burr holes and a large bone flap may then be rapidly cut using the dural guard and the cutting blade.

If the burr holes at the base of the flap have not been made close together, the bony ridge can be narrowed using de Vilbis forceps or the power drill. The technique is a very rapid way of cutting a bone flap, but the dura may be extensively lacerated if it does not separate easily from the inner table and this may cause major difficulties if the sagittal sinus or large veins draining into it are damaged. There may also be difficulty if the bone is irregular as it may be near the base of the skull, and the dural guard may catch. The channel cut by the power drill tends to be rather broad and a small bone flap may need to be held by wire sutures through drill holes if it is not to become depressed. In general the power drill is most suitable for cutting large convexity bone flaps where the dura can be separated easily rather than those near the mid-line or the base of the skull. As a compromise, since cutting the burr holes is the most laborious part of the procedure, these can be made with the power drill and the cuts between made by hand using Gigli's saws.

The bone flap is wrapped in damp gauze and held away from the area with towel clips or a self-retaining retractor.

Extradural haemostasis

Bleeding from the cut edge of the bone is stopped with bone wax. Bleeding vessels on the dura are lightly coagulated with diathermy and venous bleeding which may be troublesome near the mid-line or at the base of the skull is controlled with gelatin sponge which is held in place with gentle pressure.

19

Sutures are inserted all round the edge of the bone to hold the dura up to the inner table of the skull to prevent a postoperative extradural haematoma developing. The sutures, which are placed right against the cut edge of the bone, just pass through the dura so as to avoid piercing the brain, and are tied through the adjacent pericranium or muscle. The sutures are generally not inserted at the mid-line or over the transverse sinus.

Major meningeal vessels may be under-run and tied by the sutures and this will markedly reduce the bleeding from a convexity or parasagittal meningioma. Care should be taken not to detach the dura beyond the edges of the bone flap since this may result in an extradural haematoma developing postoperatively beyond the limits of the exposure. This is a risk where a self-retaining brain retractor is attached to the edge of the bone. Good extradural haemostasis should be achieved before the dura is opened to avoid the field becoming obscured by blood running in from outside. The skin and bone edges are covered with strips of moistened linteen and wound towels are applied before the dura is opened.

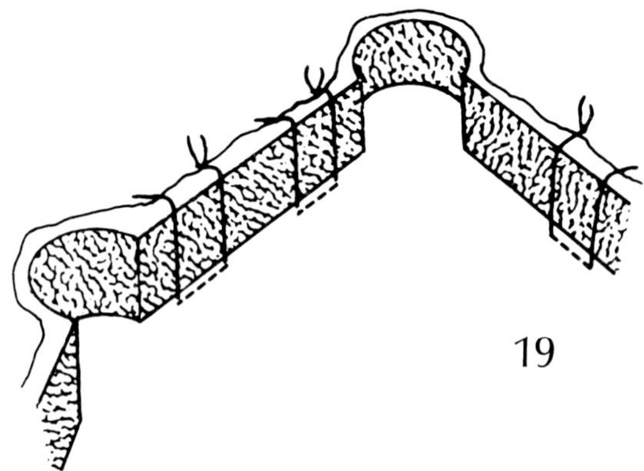

19

20

Opening the dura

The dura is opened by elevating it with a sharp hook and lightly incising it with a scalpel. Care must be taken, particularly when intracranial pressure is raised, to avoid injuring the underlying brain. Once the initial opening is made, the incision may be extended as required using scissors with rounded ends. The dura may be opened with a flap (*a*) or a straight incision which may be extended with side cuts (*b*). Straight incisions have the advantage of being easier to make and close, and when the intracranial pressure is raised the dura may be opened with a straight incision over the tumour to avoid problems with bulging brain. Once sufficient tumour has been removed to lower the pressure, the dura may be opened more widely. This technique has the advantage of allowing inspection of the operative site to check haemostasis until a late stage of the dural closure. Dural flaps are based towards the mid-line to avoid injury to large cortical veins which often run from the brain onto the dura at some distance from the sagittal sinus. Dural incisions should not be taken too near the bone edge since this may cause difficulty with closure. Straight incisions are generally more convenient in the temporal region, where the dura may be opened in a Y-shaped incision with side cuts (*c*), and for basal exploration, where a low curved incision which extends down to the bone edge at each end is adequate (*d*). Bleeding from the edge of the dura is stopped by McKenzie clips. Diathermy should be avoided since it causes the dura to shrink. Once opened, the dura is retracted with sutures weighted with artery forceps to hold it out of the way.

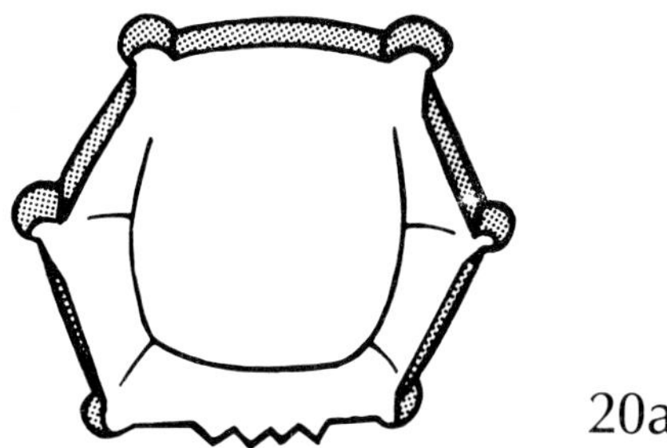

20a

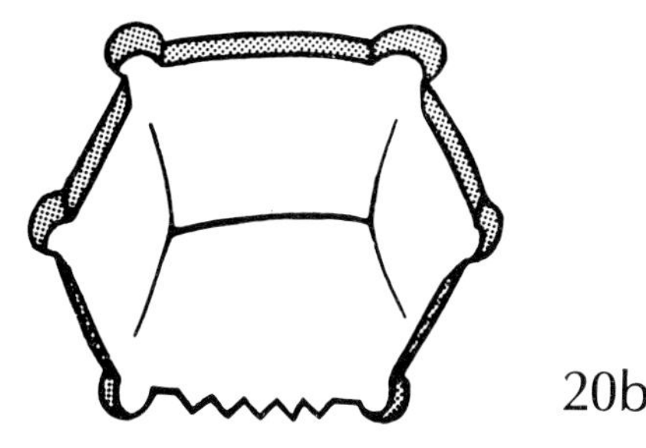

20b

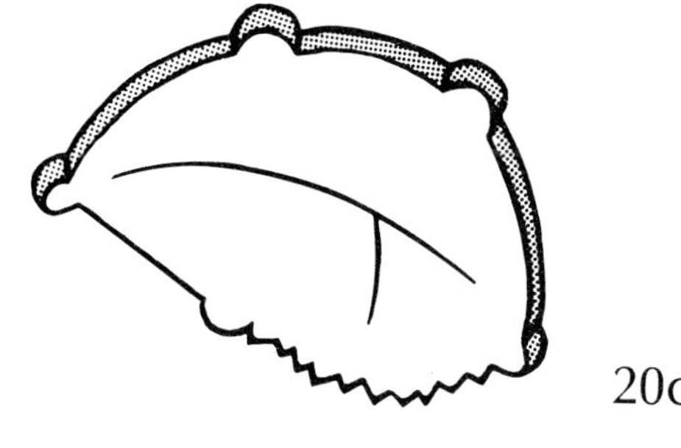

20c

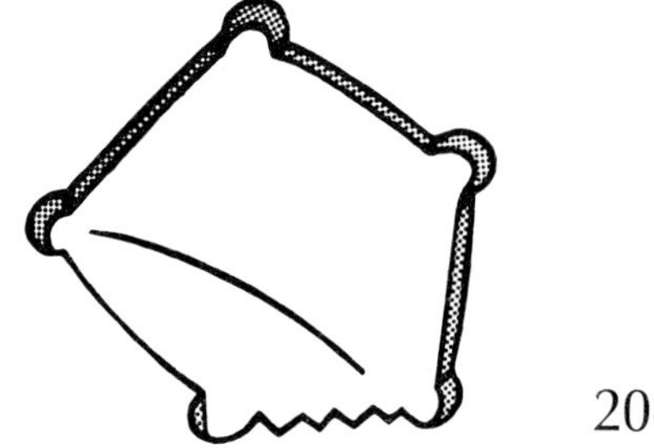

20d

Closing the dura

Before closing the dura it is advisable to confirm absolute haemostasis at the operative site by elevating the blood pressure to at least normal and by returning the patient to spontaneous respiration. The anaesthetist may be asked to compress the jugular veins in the neck to confirm that no veins are open. The dura may be closed with interrupted sutures cut very close to the knots or by a continuous suture. If the dura cannot be closed because of raised intracranial pressure it is advisable to leave it widely open to prevent herniation and strangulation of the brain through a narrow opening. The unsutured dura can be laid back over the brain and the brain covered with sheets of gelatin sponge. Where the dura has been torn while cutting the bone flap, it may be closed as far as possible and any defects covered with sheets of gelatin sponge.

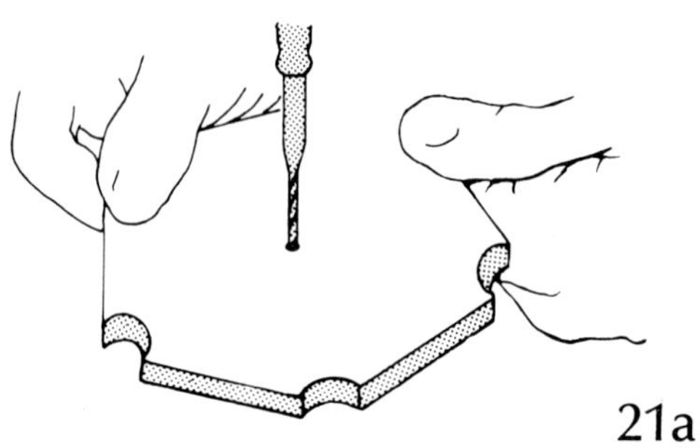

21a

21a, b & c

In addition to the sutures already inserted between the dura and the pericranium, one or more sutures can be used to hold up the dura to the bone flap. These are inserted by making a drill hole in the bone flap (*a*). The bone flap is laid back into the opening and a mark made on the dura with light diathermy by passing a brain needle stilette through the hole in the bone (*b*). A suture is placed through the dura at this point and passed through the drill hole and tied over a straightened McKenzie clip when the bone flap is replaced (*c*). For a small bone flap one such suture is sufficient but if larger, two or more may be required.

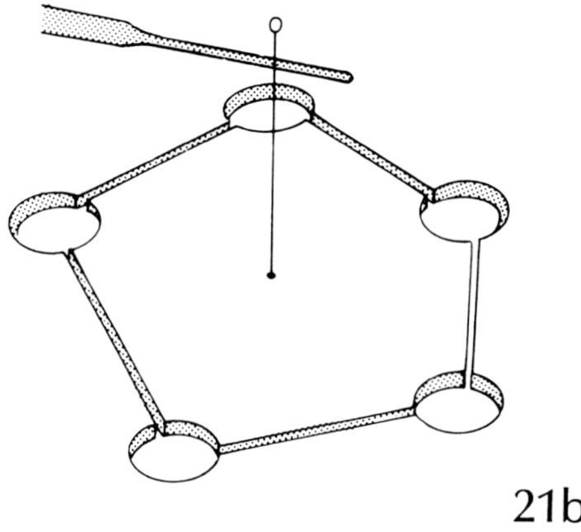

21b

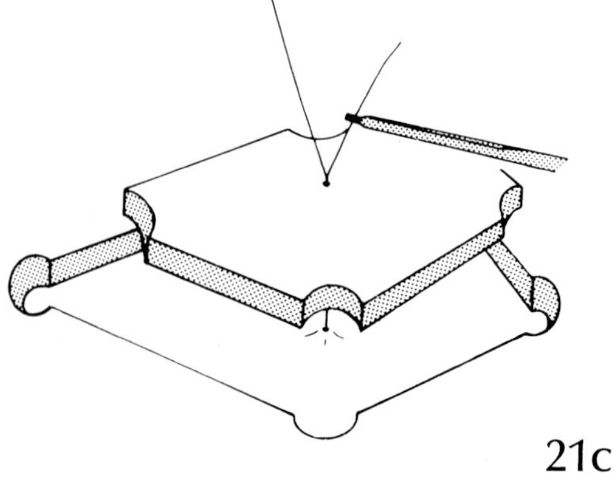

21c

22

The bone flap is held in place by interrupted sutures through the pericardium and muscle.

Alternatively, drill holes may be made and wire sutures used. If the bone flap is partly in front of the hair-line, closure of the pericranium should start anteriorly so that an accurate fit is obtained in an area where any irregularity may be visible. For the same reason any burr holes that lie anterior to the hair-line should be filled with bone dust to prevent insightly dents developing. If the thick muscle in the anterior part of the temporal region has been incised the deep part as well as the superficial part should be closed with a few interrupted sutures to avoid subsequent development of an unsightly groove.

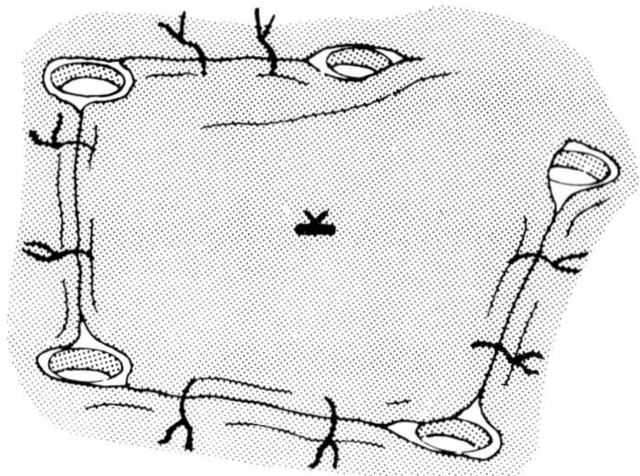

22

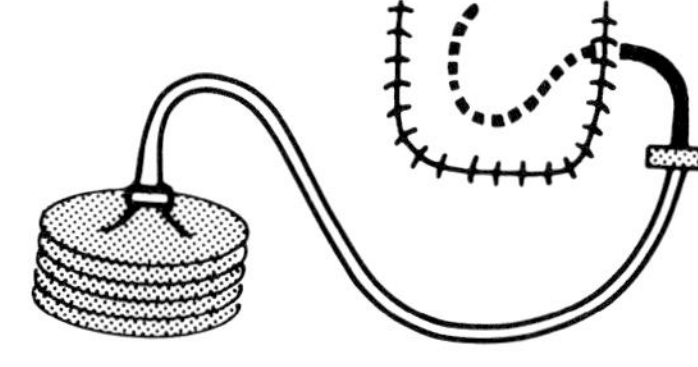

23a

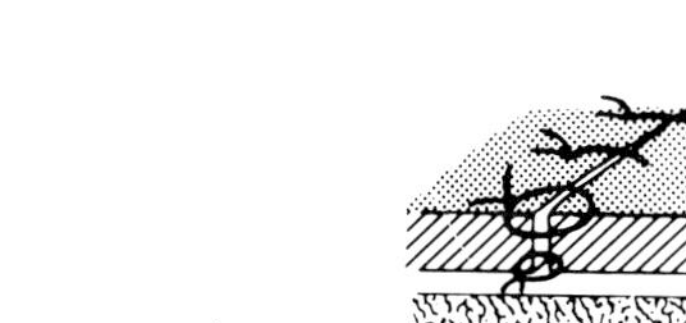

23b

23

A suction drainage tube may be introduced through the skin outside the line of the incision and connected to a vacuum bottle to prevent subcutaneous haematoma developing (*a*). The incision is closed in two layers using interrupted sutures with buried knots through the galea, and interrupted sutures, which do not pass through the galea, for the skin (*b*).

Dressing and wound care

Conventionally the head is covered with many layers of cotton gauze held in place with crêpe bandages, but alternatively narrow strips of gauze held in place with adhesive paper strips to cover just the skin incisions may be used. The suction drainage tube may be removed after 24 h and although this will prevent much of the facial bruising and swelling that occurs after frontal craniotomy, some swelling may develop on the day following removal of the drain. If this drainage is not used blood will tend to collect under the flap and may require aspiration using a wide-bore needle. Even this will generally not prevent marked bruising and swelling of the eyes developing after a frontal or temporal craniotomy. Where the skin incision has been closed in two layers as described, the skin sutures may be removed at between 2 and 5 days postoperatively, according to preference.

Postoperative care

Ideally the patient should be extubated without straining or coughing occurring and yet should rapidly regain consciousness to allow early assessment. Considerable anaesthetic skill is required to achieve this ideal since if patients are allowed to become lightly anaesthetized towards the end of the procedure, they may move when the skin sutures are inserted and cough or strain when the endotracheal tube is removed. In general, patients are nursed supine with the same degree of head-up tilt as was used for the operation. The blood pressure tends to rise as the patients regain consciousness and they may then be sat up further. Observations of pulse, blood pressure, respiration, consciousness level and neurological signs are made at 15 min intervals and recorded during the early postoperative phase. If the patient's postoperative course is satisfactory and the condition stable, the frequency of the observations may be reduced to half-hourly after a few hours, but it is inadvisable to reduce the frequency of the observations further during the first 24 h. The purpose of the observations is to detect any deterioration which may be due to the development of a postoperative intracranial haematoma, although such an event should nowadays be rare if the steps described under extradural haemostasis have been followed and the blood pressure elevated to normal before closure. If deterioration occurs, suggesting the development of a postoperative haematoma, the patient will need to be returned to the operating room promptly for re-exploration, since a haematoma is a serious complication which may result in the patient's death or survival with severe disability. Postoperative sedation is not used lest the assessment of consciousness level is obscured, and strong analgesics are not generally required. There is no evidence that antibiotics are helpful in preventing wound infection in clean uncomplicated operations, although they may be useful where chest infection is anticipated. The state at which the patient gets out of bed depends on the progress and the surgeon's preference. When progress is satisfactory, patients may sit out of bed on the second postoperative day. Dexamethasone, if given to cover the procedure, should be rapidly reduced starting on the first or second postoperative day, and discontinued within one week. If this is not done major gastrointestinal problems, such as perforation or bleeding, may occur.

Burr holes, trephine and ventriculography

R. D. Illingworth MB, FRCS
Consultant Neurosurgeon,
Charing Cross and Central Middlesex Hospitals, London;
Honorary Consultant Neurosurgeon, Westminster Hospital, London, UK

BURR HOLES

Indications

Burr holes may be used for exploration in patients with suspected intracranial haematomas following head injury. Where an extradural haematoma is suspected and there are clear lateralizing signs, a preliminary burr hole is usually made on the point of impact as shown by skin bruising or abrasion, or by a skull fracture, to verify the position of the haematoma before proceeding to craniotomy or craniectomy for evacuation.

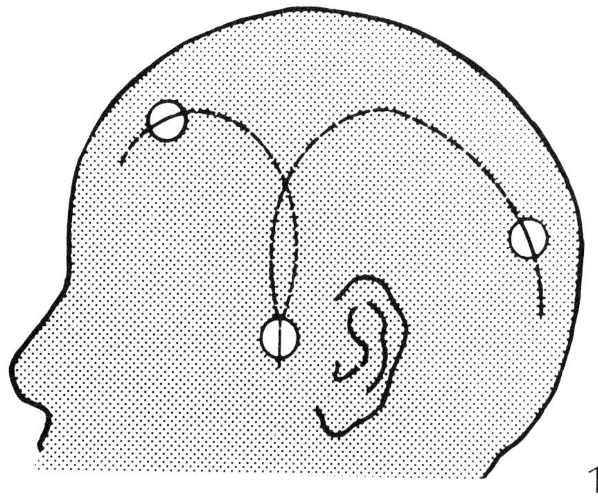

1

1

Burr holes may be made for exploration where clear localizing signs are not present; in these circumstances they are generally made in the frontal, temporal and posterior parietal regions on each side. Incisions near the base of the skull should be made coronally and those near the vertex sagitally to preserve the scalp blood supply and allow extension into a skin flap if required. If no extradural haematoma is found at each burr hole the dura should be opened to exclude subdural bleeding.

Burr holes are also used for the drainage of chronic subdural haematomas, which are generally fluid, and for the aspiration of intracerebral abscesses. Burr hole and needle biopsy of a cerebral tumour is not a completely reliable way of obtaining a histological diagnosis and it may be preferable to explore through a craniotomy or trephine. However, this technique is generally indicated where the tumour lies deep, particularly if it is in the dominant hemisphere and there is no prospect of attempting to remove it. Intracerebral haematomas may also be aspirated through a burr hole, but if clotted, may be easier to remove through a trephine under direct vision.

Anaesthesia

Burr holes may be made under local anaesthetic in conscious, co-operative adult patients and in unconscious patients who are not restless. A little premedication may be given to conscious patients to allay anxiety but heavy sedation should be avoided since the co-operation of the patient is essential.

In all other circumstances general anaesthesia with endotracheal intubation is necessary to prevent movement of the patient and to ensure a good airway. General anaesthesia is also essential if there is any possibility of proceeding from burr hole exploration to craniotomy. In patients under general anaesthetic, spontaneous respiration may be maintained, unless the intracranial pressure is raised, when hyperventilation anaesthesia may be preverable. When local anaesthetic is used, only the skin need be anaesthetized since the bone is insensitive to pain and the dura nearly so. The skin is infiltrated along the line of the incision with 0.5 per cent lignocaine with or without adrenaline 1:2000000.

Position of patient

Burr holes are generally made with the patient supine. In this position there is easy access to the front of the head on both sides. If access to the back of the head is required the operating table must be tilted head-up and the patient's head raised by flexing the neck to bring the back of the head as high as necessary. In this way a patient with head injury can be positioned for exploratory burr holes so that there is access to the whole of the skull vault, except the occipital region and the posterior fossa. To explore the posterior fossa, the patient will need to be repositioned on his side, in the sitting position or prone.

Skin preparation and towelling

Where a single burr hole is to be made the scalp should be shaved for at least 5 cm around the incision. Where exploratory burr holes are being made in patients with head injury, the whole scalp should be shaved to allow as many burr holes as are necessary to be made and to allow burr holes to be converted into a craniotomy. It is advisable to shave and prepare the whole head even if the clinical signs indicate a unilateral lesion, so that both sides may be explored. The skin is cleaned using first an aqueous soapy solution to remove any dirt and skin debris and then with 0.5 per cent chlorhexidine in 70 per cent alcohol. The planned incisions for the burr holes should be marked with ink or by scratching the scalp with a scalpel. The prepared skin can be covered with an adhesive plastic drape or with fabric which may be soaked in antiseptic solution. The rest of the head is covered with sterile towels.

The operation

2

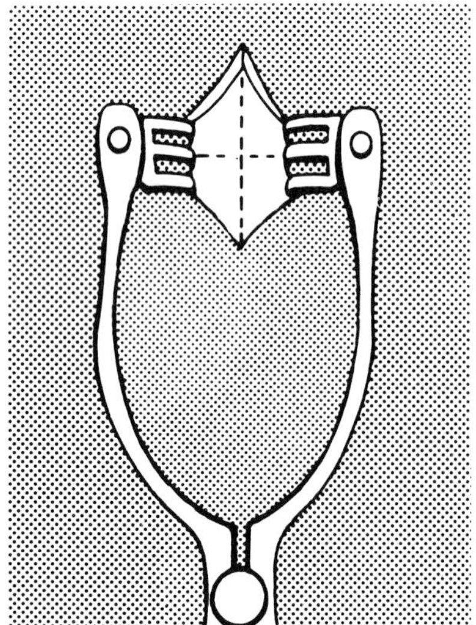

2

The incision

The incision, which need only be about 2 cm long, is made by cutting right down onto the bone. A small self-retaining retractor is inserted and opened widely and this will generally control any skin bleeding. Any persistent bleeding should be controlled with diathermy, but this should be used sparingly near the skin edge. The pericranium is incised and scraped to each side with a small periosteal elevator.

3a, b & c

Cutting a burr hole

The burr hole is cut in two stages using a Hudson's brace. This is fitted first with a skull perforator, which is used until there is a small hole through the inner able (*a*). Care should be taken at this stage since the instrument can penetrate deeply into the brain if the bone gives way; pressure on the instrument should be made from the shoulder rather than with the weight of the body. The progress of the drilling can be checked from time to time and when the inner table is penetrated a slight change in the feel of the drill may be detected. Once the inner table has been penetrated the skull perforator is exchanged for a conical burr (*b*) or Soutar's drill (*c*) and the hole enlarged until it is parallel-sided. Care should be taken to avoid separating the dura from the bone around the burr hole since this may result in troublesome extradural venous bleeding. Bleeding from the bone is controlled with bone wax and extradural bleeding from under the bone may be stopped with oxidized cellulose or gelatin sponge. Bleeding from the dura is controlled with light diathermy.

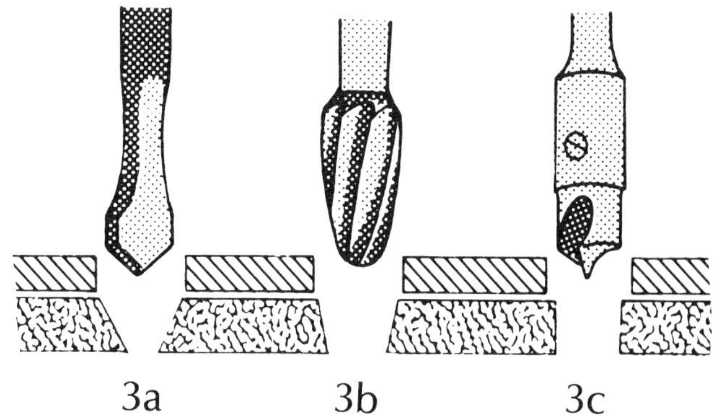

3a 3b 3c

4

Opening the dura

If the dura is to be opened, it is elevated with a sharp hook and gently cut with a small scalpel blade. Care must be taken to avoid injury to the underlying brain and its blood vessels. Once the initial opening is made it can be extended to a cruciate incision with scissors. Any bleeding from the edge of the dura is stopped with diathermy.

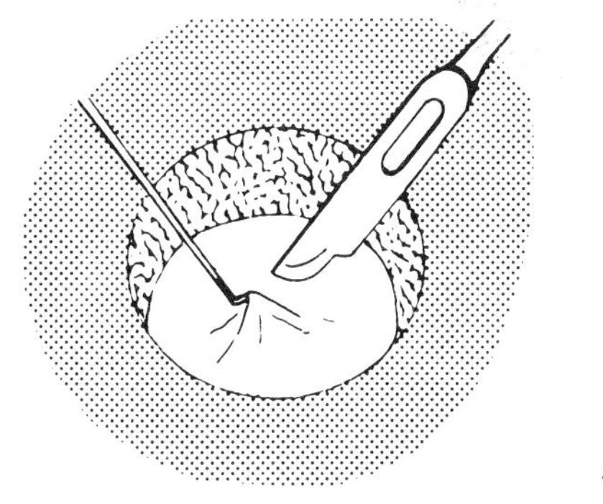

4

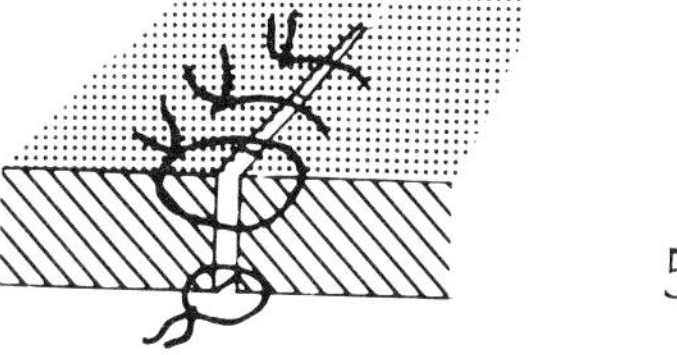

5

5

Closure

When closing, the dura is not sutured but is covered with gelatin sponge. The galea is closed with two or three interrupted sutures, the knots being buried and the ends cut short. The skin is closed with interrupted sutures which will control all but major bleeding. This method is preferable to excessive use of diathermy. The head may be dressed with a thick layer of gauze and wool held with bandages, but a small piece of gauze which just covers the sutures and is held in place with adhesive paper strips serves equally well.

Postoperative care and complications

The sutures can be removed on the fifth day and normally the dressings need not be disturbed until that time. Complications after burr holes are rare. Intracranial haematoma is unusual unless bleeding from the dura or brain has not been stopped. Infection of the wound may have serious consequences if the dura has been opened since this can allow spread into the subdural space with abscess formation. Necrosis of the skin edge may occur if the skin sutures have been inserted too close together and tied too tightly.

TREPHINE

Indications

Generally this technique is used when a burr hole will not provide adequate access and yet the situation does not require the much wider exposure that a craniotomy can afford. Examples are the removal under direct vision of an intracerebral haematoma or the biopsy and removal of a cerebral glioma where the exact location is known and the limited exposure of a trephine can be chosen with confidence that it will be adequate. The procedure can also be used where the approach is necessarily limited to a narrow track in the brain. An example is a tumour in the third ventricle which can be explored through the foramen of Monro by frontal trephine, since a wide exposure of the cerbral cortex is no additional advantage. Trephine should not be used where wide exposure of the cortex may be required, as in the removal of a meningioma.

The operation

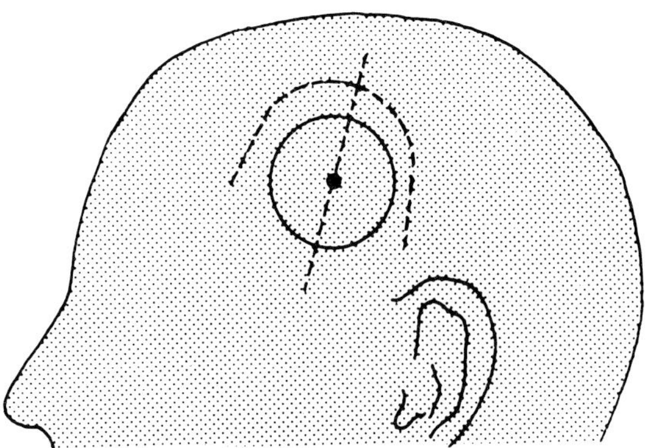

6

6

The incision

The incision may be linear or a small flap. A linear incision will need to be longer than the diameter of the trephine and the skin margins will need to be widely retracted with a self-retaining retractor. Firm retraction will stop most skin bleeding and diathermy should be used sparingly near the skin edge.

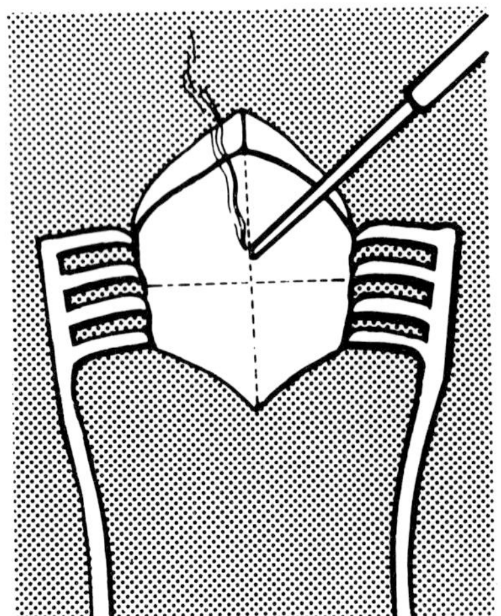

7

7

The pericranium is incised with diathermy and reflected from the skull with a periosteal elevator.

8a, b & c

Trephines come in graduated sizes of between 0.5 and 2 inches (13–51 mm) in diameter, the size used depending on the exposure required. The bone disc is cut in three stages. First a small hole is drilled in the centre of the proposed disc using a guarded drill (*a*). Next the trephine, fitted with a centring pin which engages in the hole, is used to cut a circular groove (*b*). Once the cutting edge of the trephine will remain in the groove, the centring pin is removed, and the skull cut until the dura is exposed in at least part of the circumference, with the remainder of the bone being cut to almost full depth. At this point, the bone disc can be levered out without difficulty using a periosteal elevator (*c*). Bleeding from the bone is stopped with bone wax and any ragged bone edges should be trimmed from the bone disc or from the skull to allow the bone disc to fit when replaced. A small shelf of the inner table can be left to prevent the bone disc sinking in when replaced. Bleeding from the dura is stopped with diathermy.

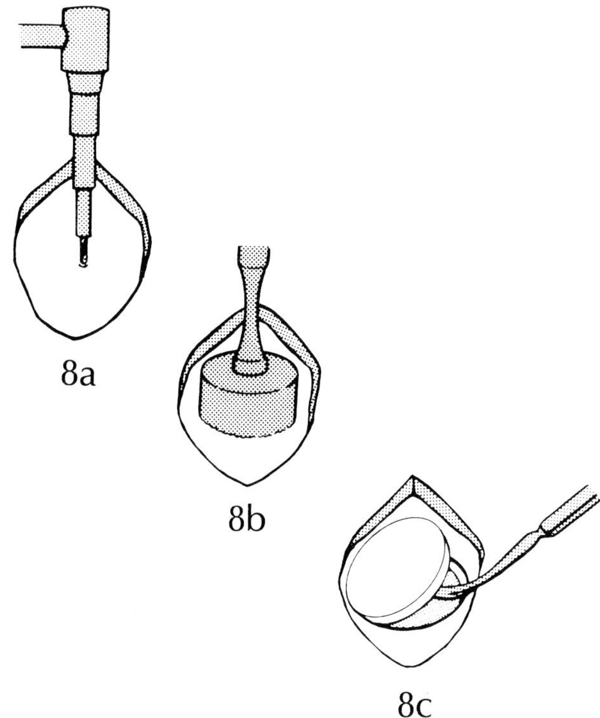

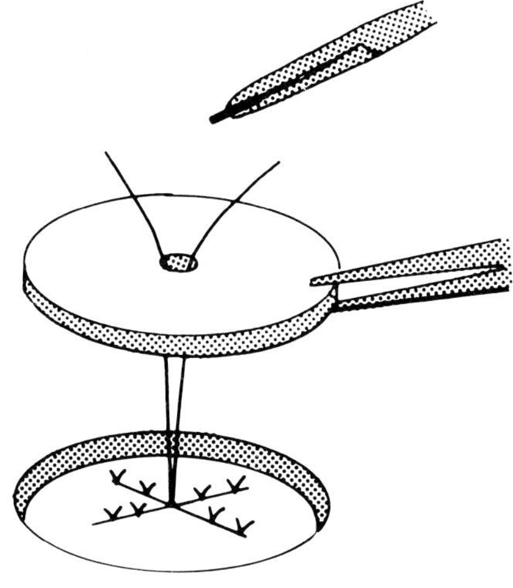

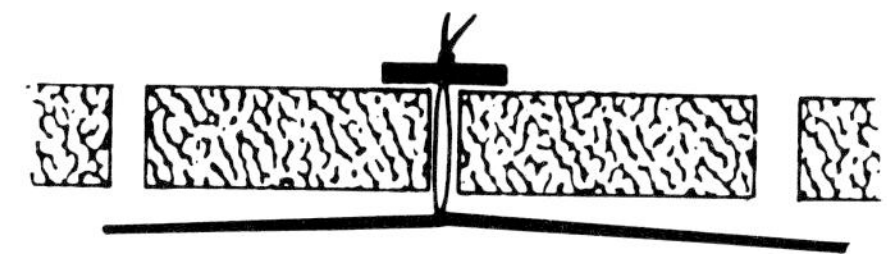

9

9

The dura is opened by elevating the centre with a sharp hook and lightly incising it. The dura can then be opened in a cruciate incision using scissors, taking care not to cut the underlying brain or blood vessels. When closing, the dura should be brought together as far as possible with interrupted sutures and covered with gelatin sponge. The bone disc can be held by a suture from the centre of the dura passed through the drill hole in the bone and tied over a straightened McKenzie clip. The pericranium is drawn back over the bone and the incision closed in layers with interrupted sutures to the galea and to the skin. The dressing and postoperative management are as for a burr hole.

VENTRICULOGRAPHY

Indications

Ventriculography, once the only method of showing uncalcified space-occupying lesions in the brain, has largely been superseded by arteriography and more recently by CT scanning. Before this last procedure became available, ventriculography was used mainly for the localization of masses in the posterior fossa as an alternative to vertebral arteriography. It was also used for the localization of masses in the lateral and third ventricles and those lying deep in the cerebral hemispheres where it may give more information than arteriography.

Arteriography has an advantage over ventriculography in that it may indicate not only the position of a mass but also its nature by showing some characteristic vasularity; and similarly, CT scanning will often indicate the nature of a lesion as well as showing its size and position. However, even when modern methods are available, ventriculography can be useful to show a structural lesion such as aqueduct stenosis, where there is obstruction to the cerebrospinal fluid flow without a mass.

Ventriculography is not recommended as an initial investigation of supratentorial lesions since all that may be found is high intracranial pressure and the ventricles if compressed or displaced may not be located on needling. Multiple attempts to tap the ventricles in this situation may result in the deterioration of the patient.

Anaesthesia

Burr holes for ventriculography can be made under local or general anaesthetic as described under 'Burr holes'. In general, local anaesthetic is to be preferred, especially if the X-ray room is some distance from the operating room and if there will be any delay in proceeding to definite surgery. In anxious patients and in children, it may be possible to make the burr holes under general anaesthetic and introduce a catheter into the lateral ventricle before taking the X-rays on another occasion without anaesthetic. If this is done, it should be remembered that the drainage of cerebrospinal fluid from the lateral ventricles in a patient with raised intracranial pressure may disturb the delicate balance of pressures within the head and result in neurological deterioration.

The operation

Ventriculography may be performed through either posterior parietal or frontal burr holes. The site chosen should avoid important cerebral cortex such as the motor and sensory areas, and in the left hemisphere, the speech areas. If only one burr hole is to be made, the right, normally the non-dominant cerebral hemisphere, should be used.

Posterior parietal burr holes have the advantage of allowing the ventricular system to be filled more completely with air. The patient is positioned supine with the head raised and the neck well flexed. Short incisions are marked symmetrically about 2.5 cm from the mid-line and 7–8 cm above the external occipital protuberance. The position is generally just in front of the lambdoid suture. After the usual cleaning and towelling, the incisions are made and the burr holes cut. The dura is opened and bleeding from the dura stopped with diathermy. A point on the pia free of large blood vessels is coagulated with the diathermy and lightly incised. If the exposed brain has large blood vessels on it, the dural incision is extended to expose a more suitable area. Careful extradural and intradural haemostasis should be achieved before the ventricles are tapped to prevent subsequent subdural or extradural haematoma formation. A blunt-nosed graduated ventricular cannula with stilette and soft rubber connection is passed into the brain on each side, aimed at the centre of the ipsilateral eye. The cannula generally enters the trigone of the lateral centricle about 5 cm from the dura, and with experience a definite alteration in the resistance can be felt at that point. If the ventricles are large, the cerebrospinal fluid may be tapped much nearer to the dura. If the ventricles are not located at the first attempt, the needle should be completely withdrawn and redirected medially and then laterally. Persistent attempts to tap the lateral ventricles may result in hemiparesis or hemi-anopia developing due to cerebral oedema and bleeding in the needle tracks and it is good practice to abandon the attempt if difficulty is experienced. If the cerebrospinal fluid pressure is high, it is gradually reduced since rapid reduction may result in intraventricular bleeding. If a ventricular catheter is to be introduced, it is advisable to insert it before too much cerebrospinal fluid is drained and the ventricles become smaller and harder to locate. A No. 8 Jacques rubber or soft plastic catheter wth side holes cut in the first 2 cm can be used. If a marking suture is placed around the catheter 10 cm from the tip before insertion, the suture can be used to anchor the catheter to the skin and the end of the catheter should lie within the frontal horn. If air ventriculography is to be performed, the aspirated cerebrospinal fluid is replaced by air injected slowly, and this can be continued until the air injected in one side bubbles out through the opposite cannula. If the ventricles are large, the injection of large volumes of air may cause the patient to deteriorate subsequently, and it has been suggested that this is more likely to occur if the patient is under nitrous oxide anaesthesia. In general, if the ventricles are large and an intraventricular mass is not suspected, only a small volume of air need be injected to show ventricular size, and positive contrast can be used to demonstrate lesions in the region of the third ventricle or posterior fossa.

A single frontal burr hole is convenient for performing ventriculography where only positive contrast is to be used. An incision is marked about 2.5 cm from the mid-line just anterior to the coronal suture on the right side thus keeping anterior to the motor cortex. The burr hole is cut and the dura opened as already described. To tap the ventricle, the cannula should be directed slightly medially and also posteriorly towards the plane of the exernal auditory meatus. The ventricle will be tapped at about 5 cm or less from the dura depending on the degree of ventricular dilatation. A ventricular catheter can be introduced into the frontal horn for the injection of contrast or for subsequent ventricular drainage.

When positive contrast ventriculography is to be performed, the contrast medium should be injected after the patient has been moved to the X-ray room. To retap the ventricle or open the ventricular catheter to make the injection at this point risks introducing infection. This can be avoided if the contrast medium to be employed is drawn up into a syringe which is attached to the end of the ventricular catheter in the operating room in place of a spigot. The injection can be made in the X-ray department without compromising sterility by simply depressing the plunger of the syringe.

Iophendylate (Myodil, Pantopaque) is heavier than cerebrospinal fluid and therefore passes downwards. To fill the third ventricle and posterior fossa, the patient is sat up on the X-ray table with the head well tilted forward. Iophendylate, 2 ml, is injected through the catheter and because of the patient's position passes into the frontal horn. With the patient still sitting the head is slightly inclined to the opposite side to bring the contrast into the medial part of the frontal horn. As the head is very slowly extended, the iophendylate should pass through the foramen of Monro into the anterior end of the third ventricle. Once the iophendylate has passed into the third ventricle, the patient is laid down and the contrast will then pass back into the aqueduct and fourth ventricle. If there is no obstruction in the ventricular system, the contrast may pass fairly quickly into the subarachnoid space; and anteroposterior, lateral and Towne's views should be taken quickly. Although X-ray screening can be used for the injection of iophendylate and manipulation of the patient, this can be performed blind if sufficient time is allowed for the contrast to pass through the foramen of Monro.

If meglumine iothalamate (Conray) is used, this can also be injected through a catheter placed via a frontal or posterior parietal burr hole. If a frontal burr hole is used, it may be possible to pass a catheter through the foramen of Monro into the third ventricle. Meglumine, 5 ml, mixed with an equal volume of cerebrospinal fluid is injected. This mixes with the cerebrospinal fluid and will gradually fill the ventricular system without manipulation of the patient. It is considerably easier to demonstrate the third ventricle and posterior fossa structures with positive contrast since the shadow produced is much denser than that of air. If air is to be used to demonstrate posterior fossa structures, the patient must be turned into the prone position. This is somewhat unsatisfacory in both anaesthetized and conscious patients, although simplified by the rotating chair design of modern radiological equipment.

Postoperative care

If a ventricular catheter is not required for subsequent drainage it should be removed soon after the procedure to prevent infection. If ventricular drainage is required, the patient should be placed on antibiotics and the drainage continued for no longer than necessary. If ventricular drainage is continued for more than a few days there is a high risk of ventriculitis developing, with very serious consequences for the patient. The head can be dressed as described under 'Burr holes' and the sutures removed on the fifth day.

Complications

It is not uncommon for a patient's conscious level and neurological state to be disturbed by ventriculography, particularly if large volumes of air are injected in patients with dilated ventricles and raised intracranial pressure. Because of this the surgical treatment of any lesion demonstrated should follow immediately after the ventriculography has been completed.

Intracranial haemorrhage may occur if the intracranial pressure is rapidly reduced, and subdural and extradural haematoma at some distance from the burr hole site have been described as occurring after ventriculography. It should not be assumed that unexpected deterioration of the patient following ventriculography or ventricular drainage is due to haemorrhage into a tumour, and carotid arteriography or CT scanning may be advisable in these circumstances.

Exposure of major blood vessels

H. H. G. Eastcott MS, FRCS
Honorary Consultant Surgeon, St Mary's Hospital, London, UK

A. E. Thompson MS, FRCS
Consultant Surgeon, St Thomas's Hospital, London, UK

Indications

The exposure of the blood vessels is necessary in both emergency and elective surgery. Access to the great vessels is most commonly required in major elective cardiovascular procedures.

Exposure of the peripheral vessels has become more complex as expertise in the surgery of smaller vessels becomes more successful. It is also routinely required for extracorporeal circulation, regional perfusion or rapid blood transfusion.

Contraindications

Surgery on blood vessels carries considerable risk and is best undertaken when adequate support is available: good operating facilities, adequate anaesthetic support and blood replacement. Control of blood loss may be more effectively obtained by exposure of vessels proximal to an infected or scarred area.

Exposure

The use of a wide approach for dealing thoroughly with nerves and vessels needs no defence[1]. When reconstructive surgery is necessary, flexures may be crossed, muscles and tendons divided and the abdomen opened to its fullest extent. Good illumination and effective self-retaining retractors are essential.

The operations

EXPOSURE OF THE ASCENDING AORTA

1

The incision

The incision is made in the midline, extending from the suprasternal notch to just beyond the xiphisternum. The extent is dictated by the need for extracorporeal circulation. A transverse component at the upper end may be added. However, if the upper end of the incision is kept below the level of the sternal notch the transverse component is not needed to achieve a good cosmetic result.

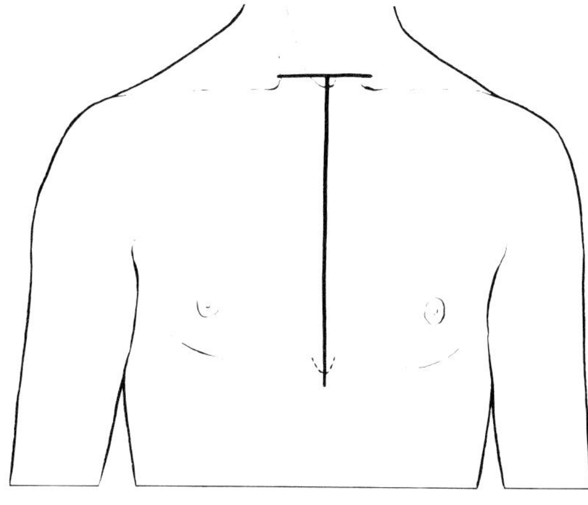

1

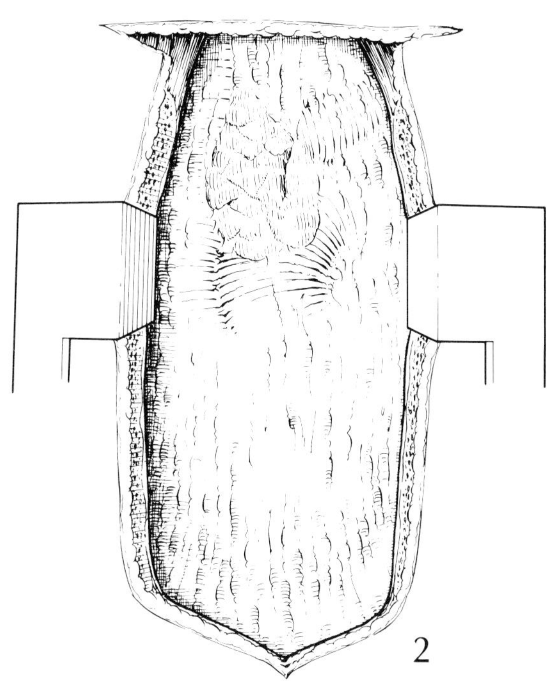

2

2

Entering the mediastinum

The sternum is divided with a power-driven saw. The line of division deviates slightly to the left in its lower half to avoid entering the right pleural cavity.

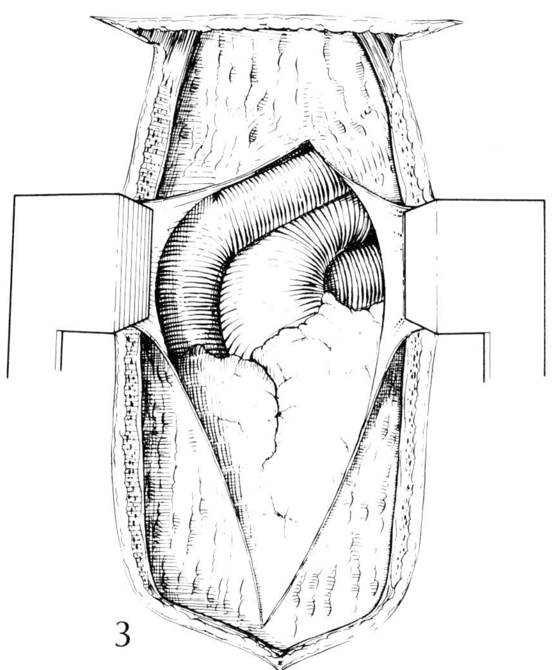

3

3

Deep dissection

The thymic remnant is divided and the innominate vein identified. Final access to the ascending aorta is obtained by opening the pericardium longitudinally.

EXPOSURE OF INNOMINATE ARTERY AND THORACIC PART OF RIGHT SUBCLAVIAN ARTERY

4

The incision

The shoulder girdle is displaced backwards by placing a sandbag between the patient's shoulders. The incision is centred over the right sternoclavicular joint, exposing the medial third of the clavicle, the manubrium and the first two intercostal spaces.

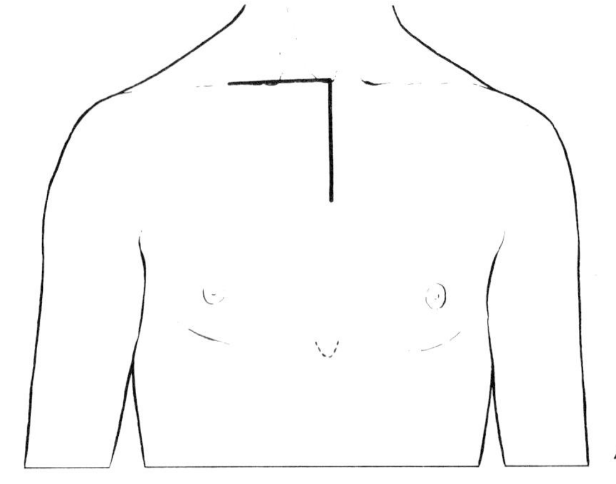

4

5

Splitting the manubrium

The manubrium is divided in the midline with a power-driven saw. The two halves are separated by a self-retaining retractor. Further exposure can then be obtained by transecting the sternum below the manubrium or by dividing the clavicle and anterior ends of the first and second ribs.

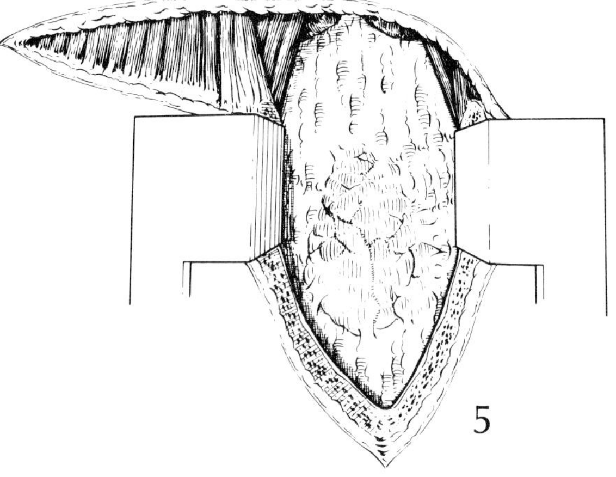

5

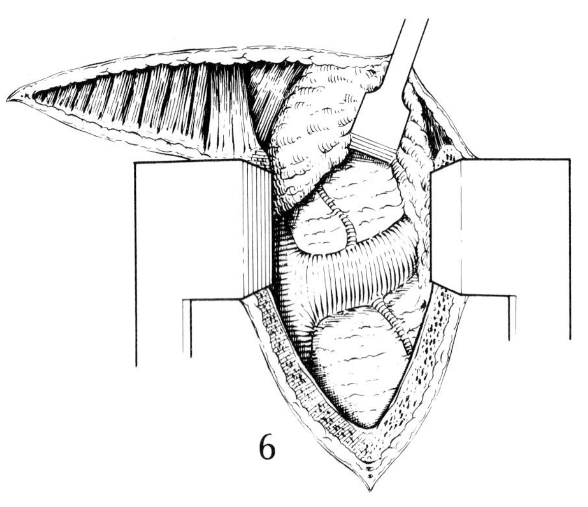

6

6

Deep dissection

The thymic remnant and anterior mediastinal fat are cleared to expose the innominate vein. The anterior borders of the pleural cavities are swept away laterally.

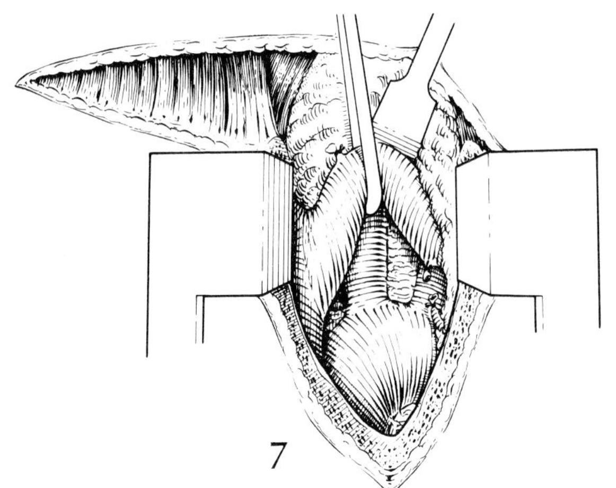

7

7

Exposure of the great vessels

Mobilization of the innominate vein permits it to be retracted upwards, revealing the origins of the great vessels.

EXPOSURE OF THORACIC PART OF LEFT SUBCLAVIAN ARTERY

This can be exposed by modifying the approach for the innominate and right subclavian arteries (above), or by the lateral approach through the 4th left intercostal space.

8

The incision

With the patient in the right lateral position a curved incision is made skirting the angle of the left scapula. Care must be taken to keep the incision inferior to breast tissue anteriorly and to carry it high posteriorly.

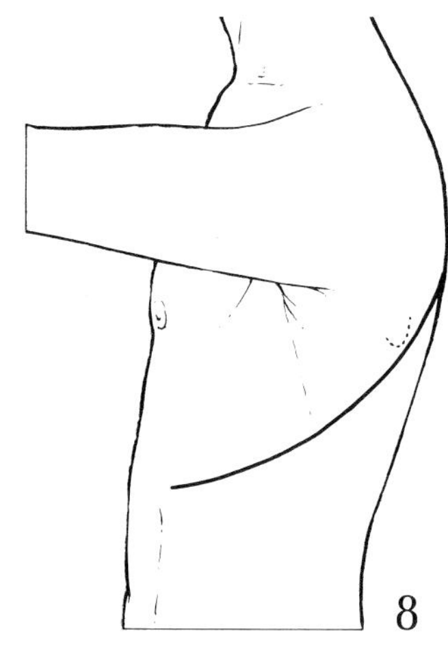
8

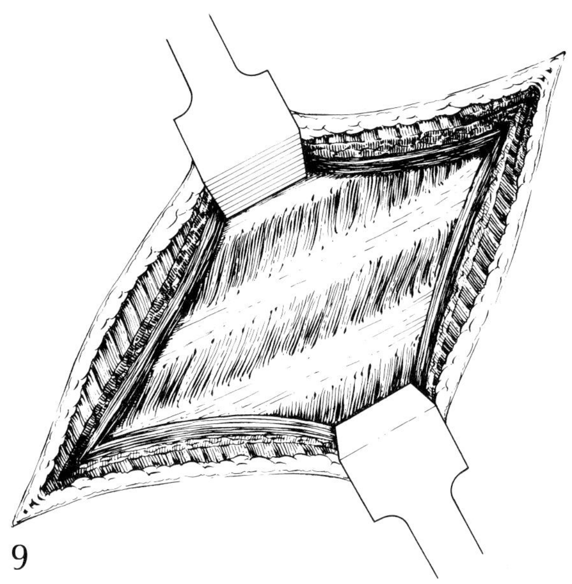
9

9

Deep dissection

The latissimus dorsi and serratus anterior muscles are divided and the chest is entered through an incision along the upper border of the fifth rib. Adequate exposure may require division of the fifth rib (and fourth if necessary) at the posterior end.

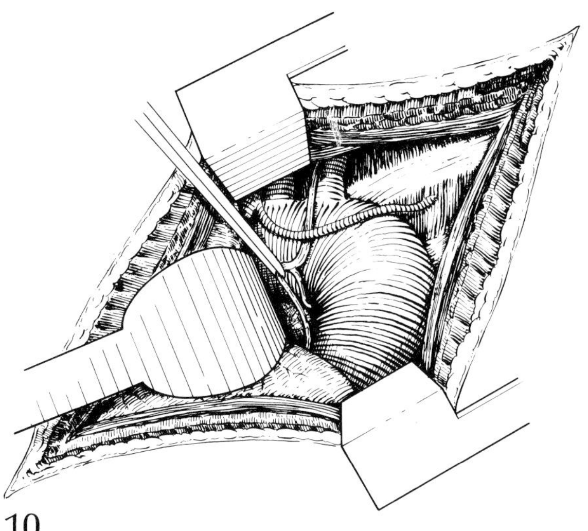
10

10

Intrathoracic exposure

The intrathoracic segment of the left subclavian artery can be exposed by incision of the overlying mediastinal pleura. The left superior intercostal vein is divided during incision of the mediastinal pleura. The vagus nerve is carefully preserved and the thoracic duct lying posterior to the subclavian artery is avoided.

EXPOSURE OF THE AORTIC ARCH

The aortic arch is approached as for the thoracic part of the subclavian artery. Access is improved if the anaesthetist uses a technique allowing deflation of the left lung. The left main bronchus and left pulmonary artery lie beneath the arch, with oesophagus and thoracic duct on the deep aspect.

11

EXPOSURE OF THE DESCENDING THORACIC AORTA

This vessel can be exposed in the same way as the aortic arch, entering the thorax through a lower rib space (*see Illustrations 8–10*).

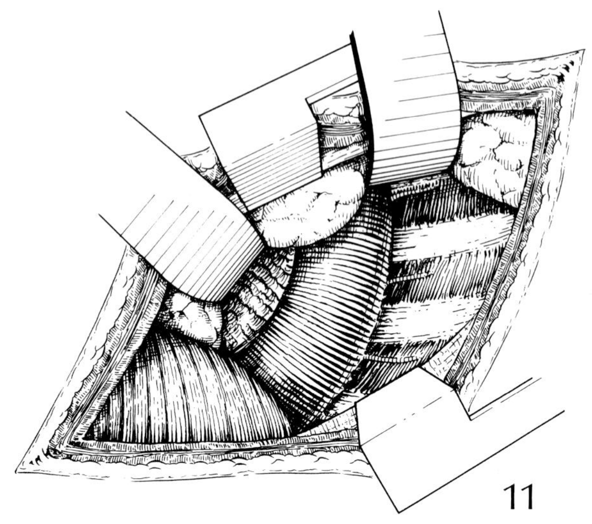

11

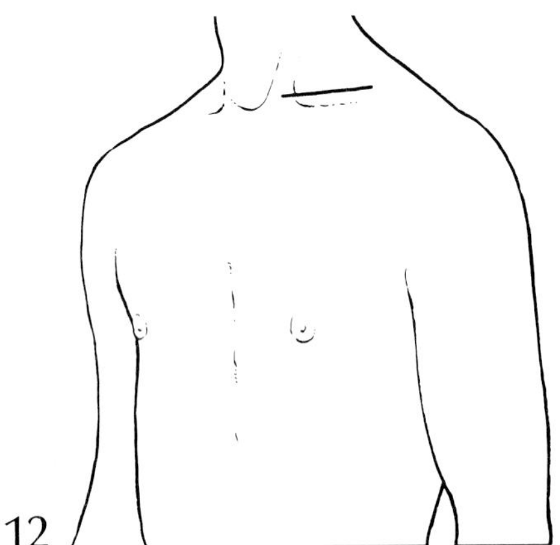

12

EXPOSURE OF CERVICAL PART OF SUBCLAVIAN ARTERY AND ORIGIN OF VERTEBRAL ARTERY

12

The incision

The patient's neck is extended and turned to the opposite side of the planned incision. A skin crease incision is made one fingerbreadth above the middle third of the clavicle. The platysma and the clavicular head of the sternomastoid are divided.

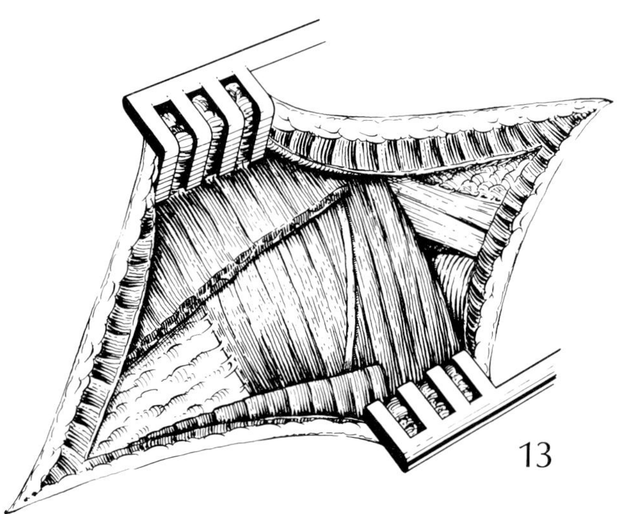

13

13 & 14

Deep dissection

The omohyoid fascia is incised and the scalenus anterior muscle exposed with the phrenic nerve on its surface. The internal jugular vein and the termination of the thoracic duct (on the left side) lie in the medial end of the field. The phrenic nerve is delicately mobilized and retracted medially, before the scalenus anterior muscle is divided piecemeal to avoid damage to the underlying vessel and its branches. The artery is finally exposed by incision of its sheath. The lower trunks of the brachial plexus lie above and lateral to the vessel.

More extensive exposure of the distal part of the vessel and the axillary artery is obtained by subperiosteal excision of the appropriate part of the clavicle.

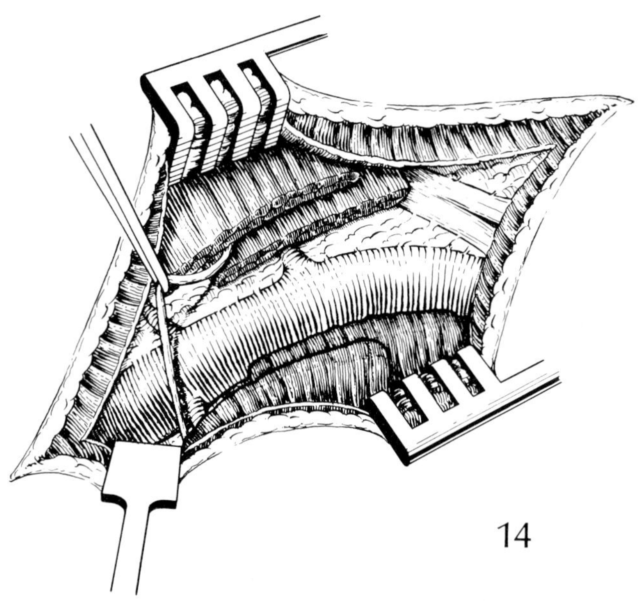

14

EXPOSURE OF AXILLARY ARTERY (FIRST PART)

15

The incision

With the arm abducted to a right angle, the incision is made just below and parallel to the clavicle.

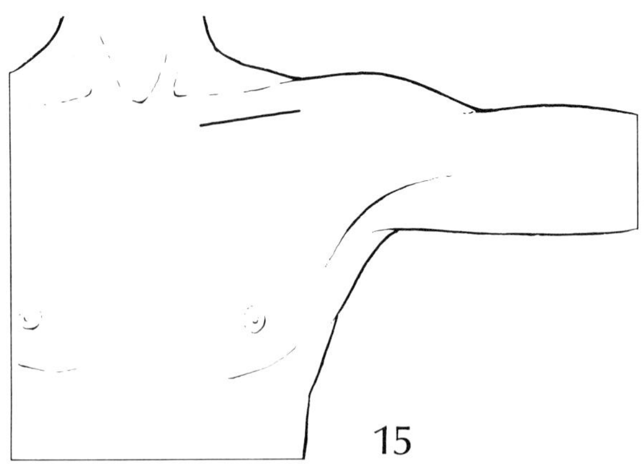
15

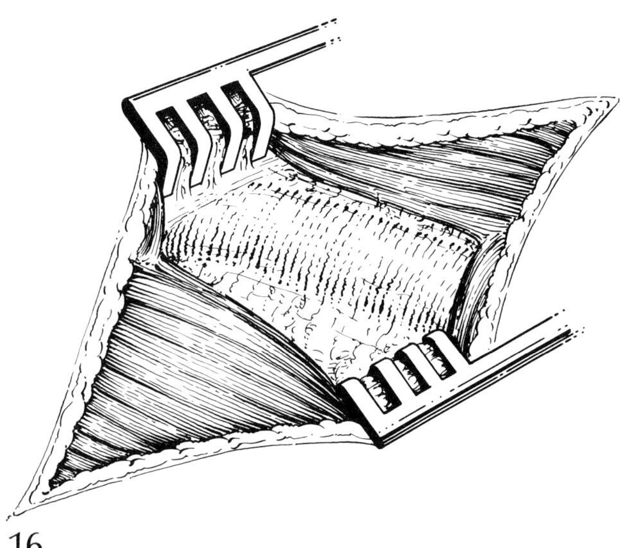
16

16

Dissection

The pectoral fascia is divided along the line of the muscle fibres of the clavicular head of the pectoralis major, which are then split to expose the vascular sheath. The pectoral branch of the acromiothoracic axis may require division.

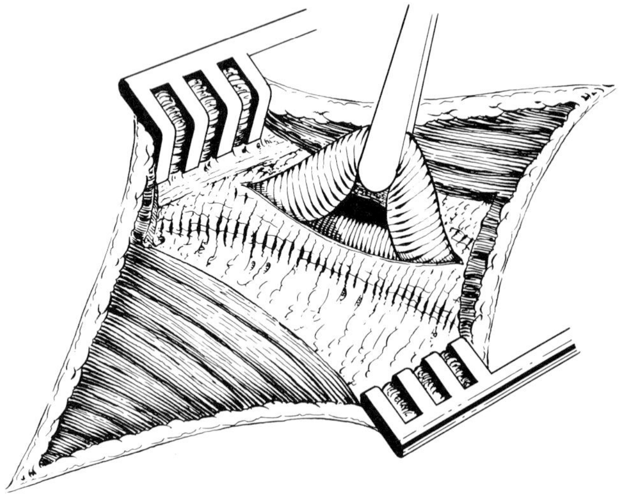
17

17

Division of sheath

The pulsations of the artery are palpated and the vascular sheath is divided along the line thus indicated. Here the only other important structure is the axillary vein. This lies below and medial to the artery from which it is then carefully separated. This is the site for axillofemoral bypass.

EXPOSURE OF AXILLARY ARTERY (SECOND AND THIRD PARTS)

18

The incision

With the arm abducted to a right angle the incision is made along the line of the pulsating artery up to the lower border of the pectoralis major muscle. If the artery is pulseless the groove between the coracobrachialis and triceps is the guide.

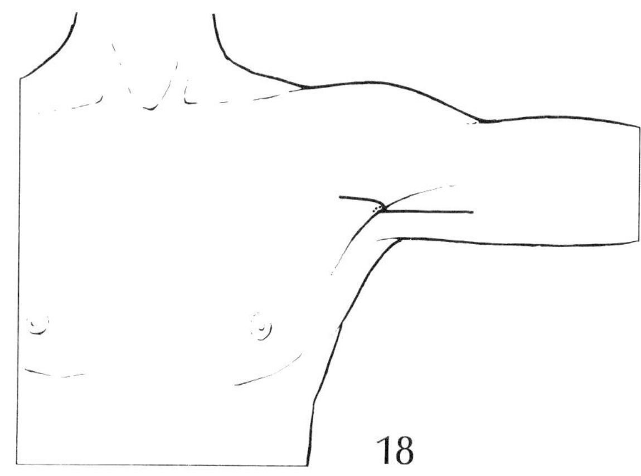

18

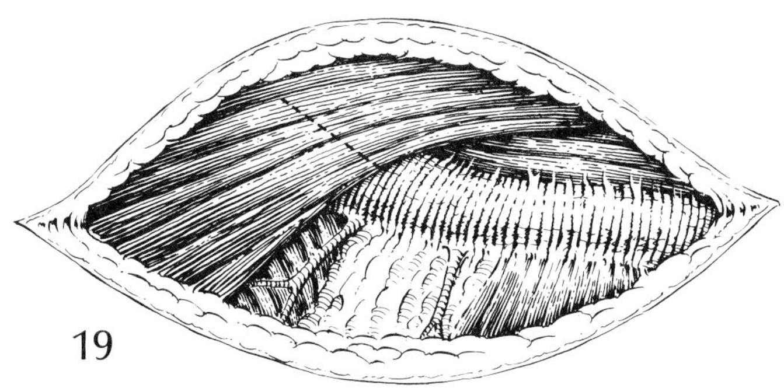

19

19

Dissection

The pectorals are retracted upwards and medially to expose the distal two-thirds of the axillary artery. If necessary, both muscles are divided and a portion of the clavicle resected to gain exposure of the whole length of the subclavian-axillary vessel. Sections of bone need not be replaced[2,3].

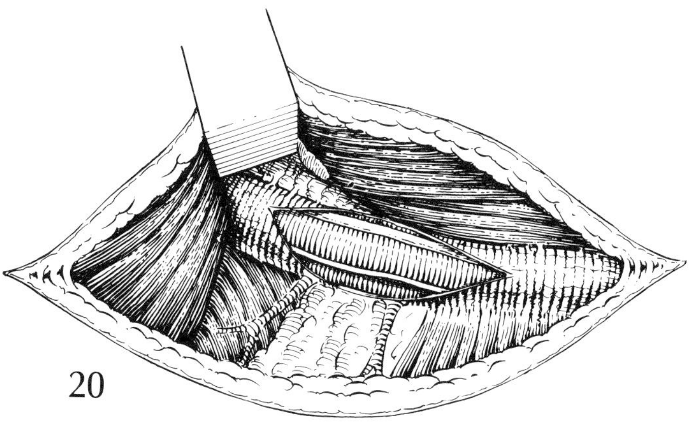

20

20

Exposure of artery

The axillary sheath is opened to reveal the vein medially and the brachial plexus laterally. The artery will be found between these two structures. It can also be identified by following the subscapular artery to its origin.

EXPOSURE OF BRACHIAL ARTERY

21

The incision

The incision is made along the line of the pulsating artery or in the line of the sulcus separating the biceps muscle from the triceps muscle. The length of the incision is governed by the procedure to be performed. In order to facilitate exposure, a sandbag is placed supporting the elbow extension.

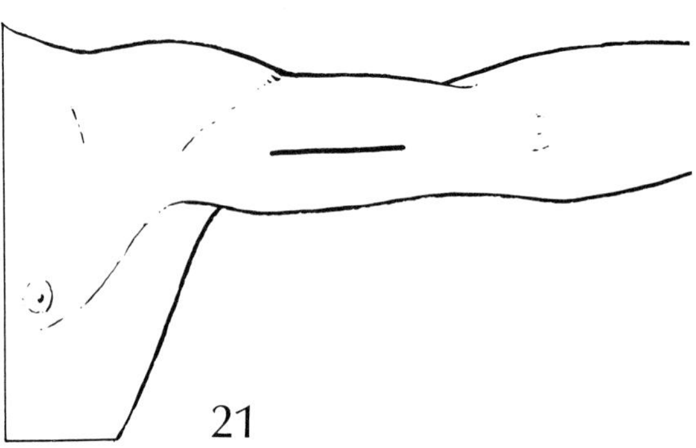
21

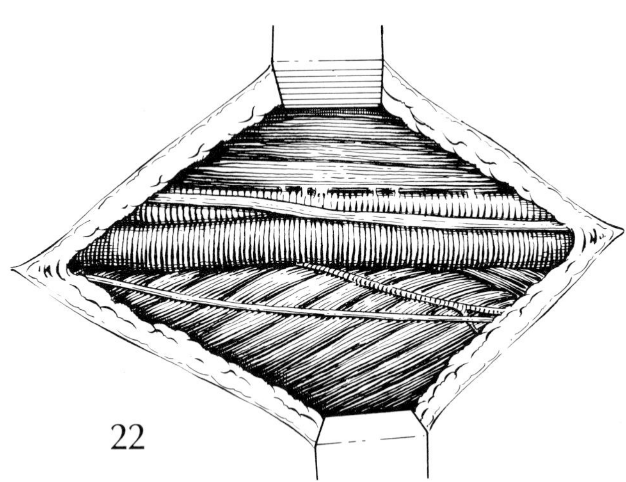
22

22

Dissection

The neurovascular sheath is opened. The veins and the median nerve, which crosses the artery from the lateral to the medial side, are separated from the artery. Care must be taken to recognize a high bifurcation of the vessel. The ulnar collateral artery and medial cutaneous nerve of the forearm lie close to the brachial artery and must not be included in clamps. The dissection is further complicated by the basilic vein which perforates the deep fascia and joins the brachial vein in this region.

EXPOSURE OF BRACHIAL ARTERY AT THE ELBOW

23

The incision

A skin crease incision is made at the elbow with longitudinal extensions along the line of the brachial artery medially and down the brachioradialis laterally. The skin should be marked to allow an accurate closure.

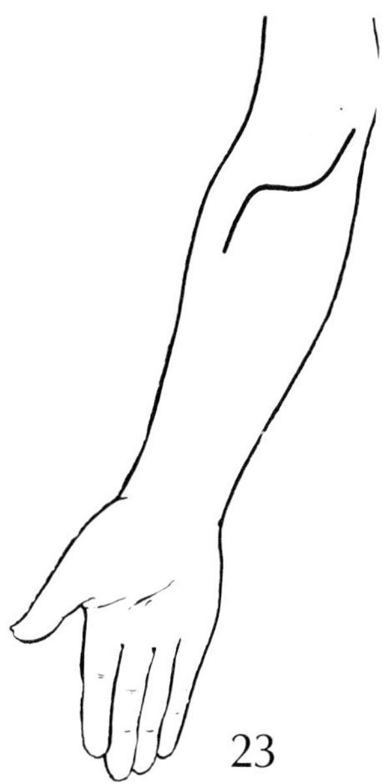
23

24

Superficial dissection

The artery is obscured by the cubital veins, the deep fascia and the bicipital aponeurosis. The two cutaneous nerves to the forearm lie deep to the veins at the medial and lateral ends of this plane of the incision and should be avoided.

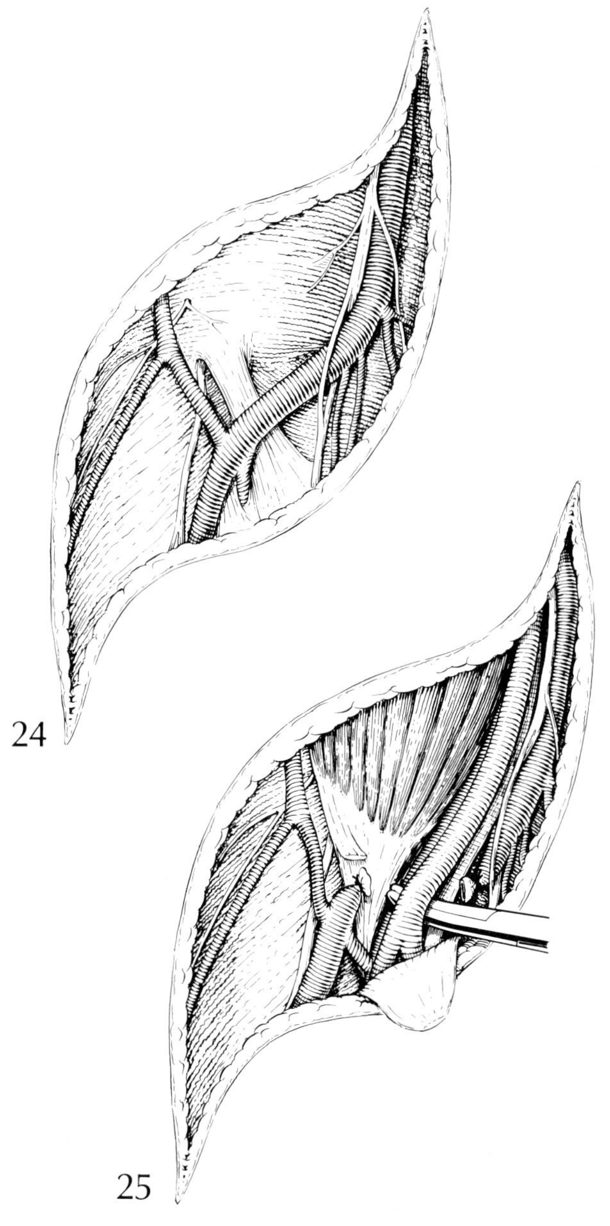
24

25

25

Deep dissection

The overlying superficial veins and the bicipital aponeurosis are divided. This exposes the artery, with its accompanying deep veins, just above the bifurcation which is close to the medial side of the biceps tendon. Opening the sheath allows the vessel to be lifted away from its venae comitantes and from the median nerve, which lies on its medial side. This exposure is most commonly indicated when the brachial artery has been damaged in a supracondylar fracture. Spasm in the intact vessel can be overcome by the injection of saline into the lumen of the affected segment between arterial clamps[4].

EXPOSURE OF RADIAL ARTERY AT THE WRIST

26

The incision

A longitudinal or transverse incision centred 3–4 cm above the radial styloid is used.

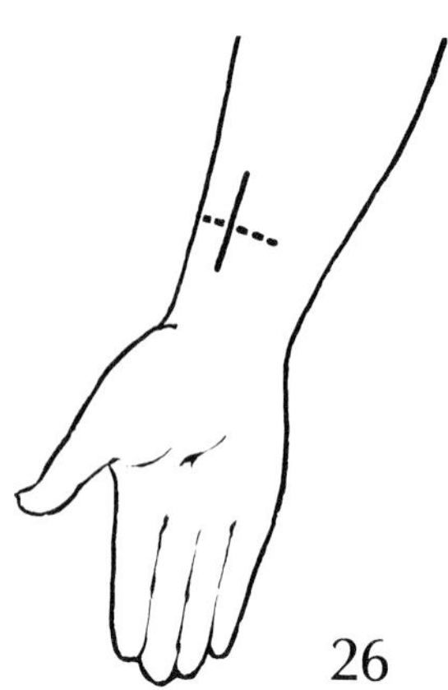

26

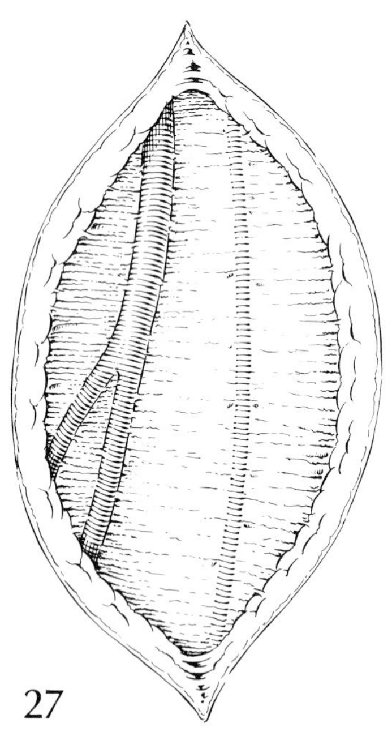

27

27

Dissection

The lower end of the cephalic vein lies in the superficial fascia at the radial side of the wrist. The radial artery lies at a deeper level beneath the deep fascia with its venae comitantes. Both vessels can be mobilized easily and approximated to allow a side-to-side anastomosis, creating an arteriovenous fistula for haemodialysis.

EXPOSURE OF COMMON CAROTID ARTERY

28

The incision

With neck slightly extended, and the head turned to the opposite side, a 6 cm incision is made along the anterior edge of the sternomastoid with its centre three fingerbreadths above the clavicle.

For a wider exposure of the common carotid artery and internal jugular vein the incision is extended along the dotted lines, dividing the origin of the sternomastoid.

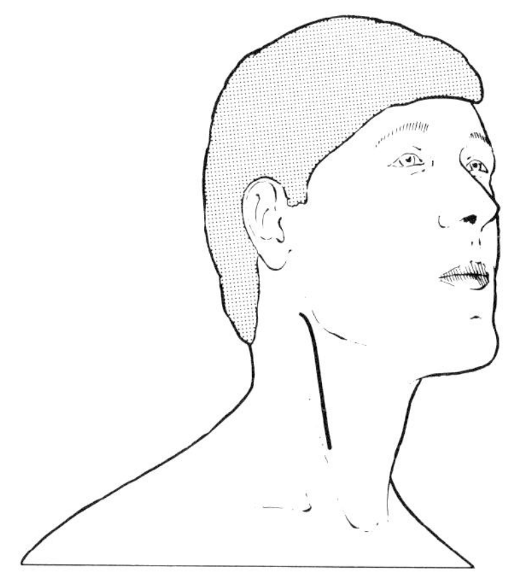

28

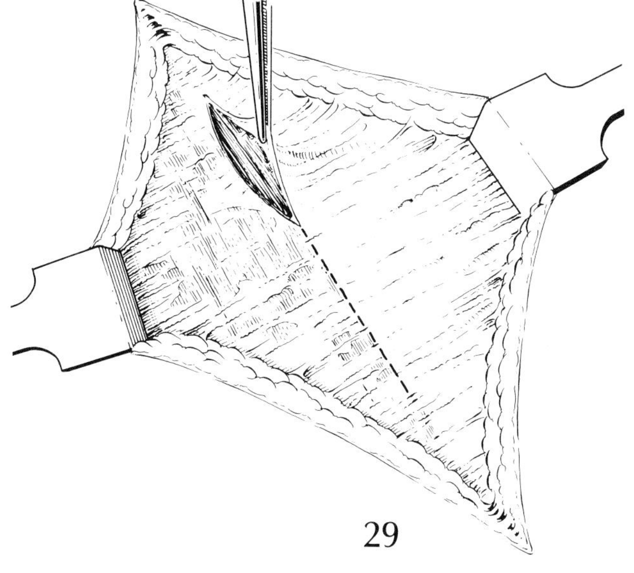

29

29

Dissection

The deep fascia is opened in the same line and the sternomastoid and infrahyoid muscles are separated from the underlying vascular sheath. This plane of dissection is bloodless except for a sternomastoid branch of the superior thyroid artery.

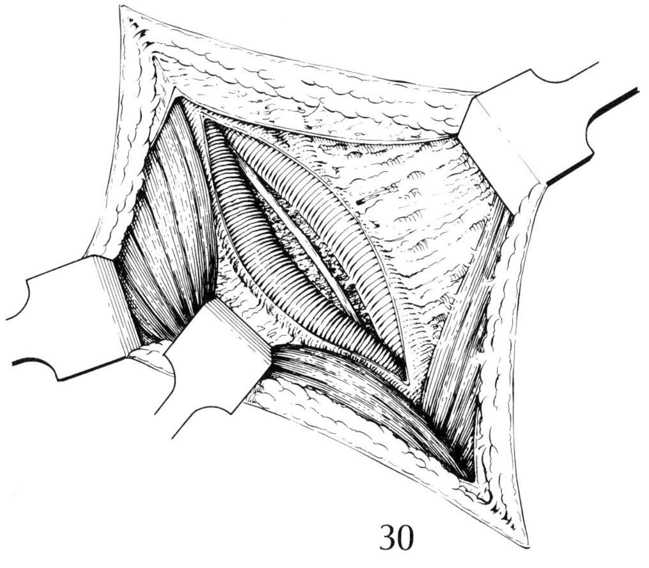

30

30

Exposure

The sheath is opened above the omohyoid. The jugular vein is dissected free and retracted laterally to isolate the artery. The vagus lies well back between the vessels, and the sympathetic trunk back further still and more medially. Lower in the neck the inferior thyroid artery crosses behind the carotid artery.

EXPOSURE OF INTERNAL AND EXTERNAL CAROTID ARTERIES

31

The incision

An incision is made along the anterior border of the sternomastoid from just above the angle of the jaw, passing downwards for 7–9 cm. For simple ligation a shorter skin crease incision may be preferred.

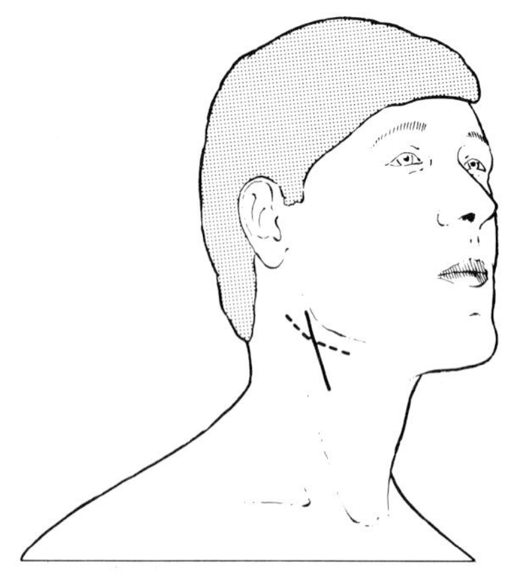

31

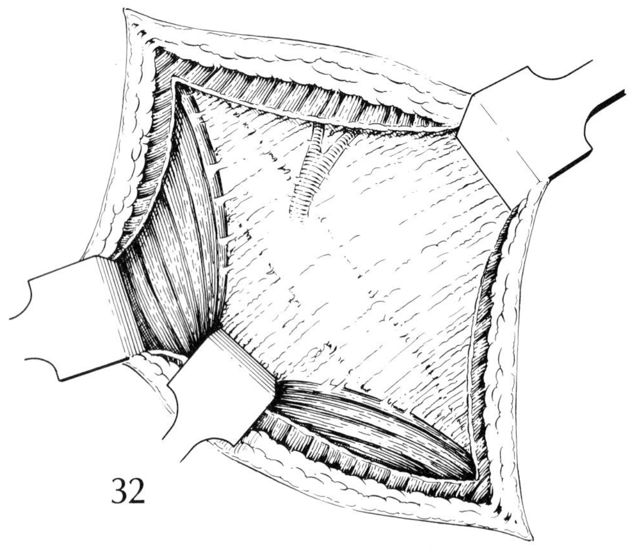

32

32

Dissection

The platysma is divided and the anterior border of the sternomastoid defined to allow retraction of the muscle away from the underlying vessels. The common facial vein is divided at the upper end of the incision and the vascular sheath opened.

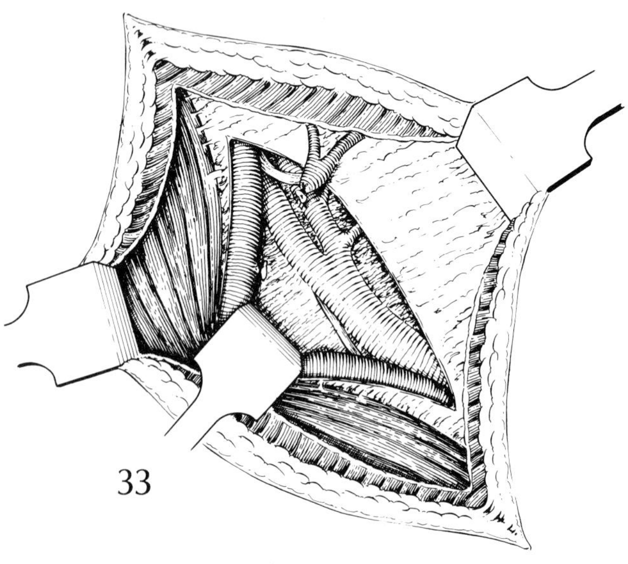

33

33

Exposure

The common carotid bifurcation usually lies much higher in the neck than is supposed. The two arteries lie close together beneath the angle of the jaw. Branches identify the external carotid, which is anterior and deeper. The hypoglossal nerve must be avoided as it crosses the vessels, and the vagus, superior laryngeal and sympathetic nerves which lie behind the bifurcation. The upper part of the internal carotid artery is difficult to expose; it runs deeply and is covered for the most part by the ascending ramus of the mandible. The sternomastoid can be detached from the mastoid process, which may itself be partly removed. The digastric muscle, the occipital artery and the styloid process are divided. This exposes the superficial aspect of the artery to some extent.

EXPOSURE OF THE AORTA ABOVE THE RENAL VESSELS

34

The incision

A thoracoabdominal incision is made along the line of the eighth rib and continued into the abdomen (*see Illustrations 8* and *9*), with the patient inclined backwards from the right lateral position. If only temporary control of the upper abdominal aorta is required during an operation on the distal vessel, a very long paramedian incision will suffice.

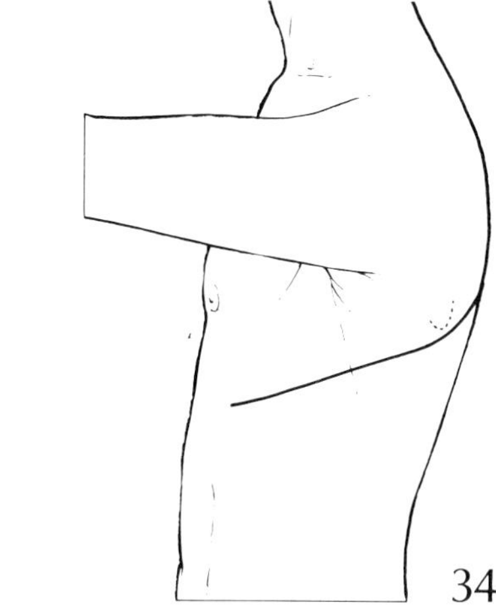

34

35

Deep dissection

The latissimus dorsi is divided. The chest is opened along the upper border of the eighth rib and the costal cartilage divided. The diaphragm is divided peripherally until the incision sweeps up to the aorta. The stomach, spleen and pancreas are swept forwards from the posterior abdominal wall to expose the aorta, the left kidney and the suprarenal gland. The visceral branches can be identified and controlled. Care must be taken in dividing intercostal vessels from which the spinal cord derives its blood supply. Temporary occlusion and hypothermia minimize the risk.

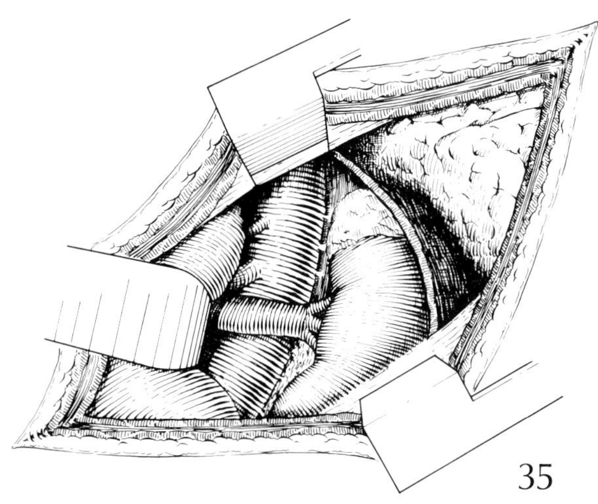

35

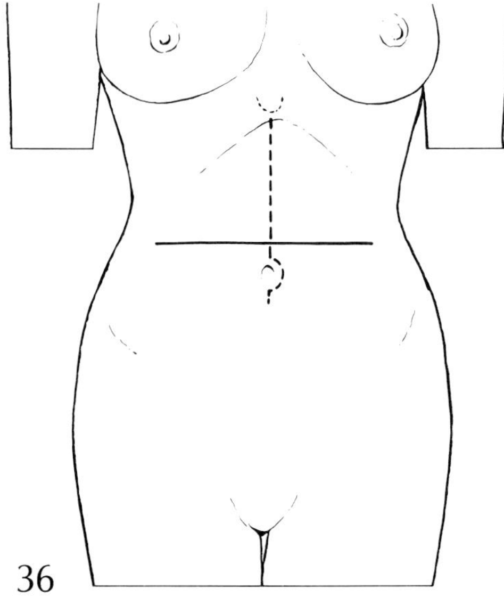

36

EXPOSURE OF RENAL ARTERIES

36

The incision

Either a midline upper abdominal[5] or a transverse incision above the umbilicus[6] gives adequate exposure.

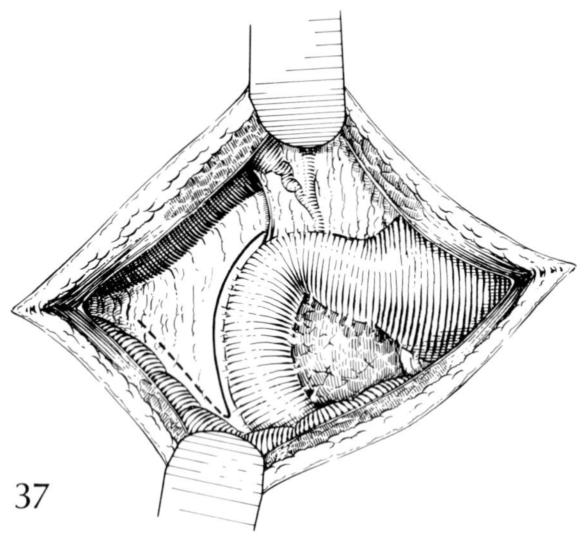
37

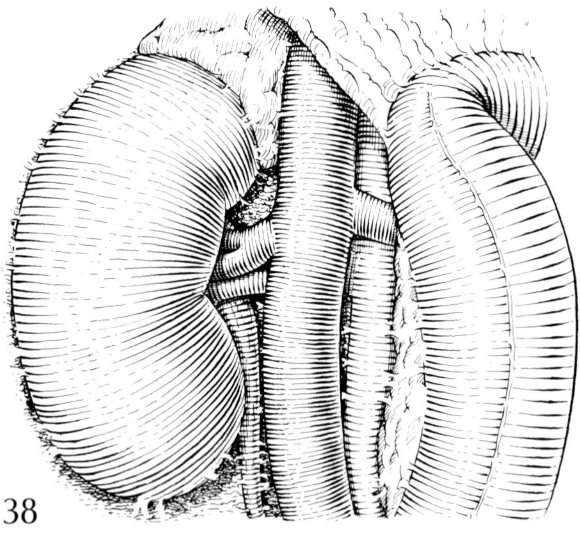
38

37–40

Deep dissection

On the right side, the peritoneum around the hepatic flexure of the colon is incised and the colon displaced downwards. The peritoneum on the right side of the duodenum is incised up to the free border of the lesser omentum. The duodenum can be displaced forwards and to the left, exposing the renal vessels, the vena cava and the aorta.

The left renal vessels are exposed by dividing the peritoneum lateral to the splenic flexure, continuing upwards behind the spleen. The spleen and colon can be displaced forwards and to the right to expose the left kidney and its vessels. The arteries lie behind the larger, more superficial renal veins.

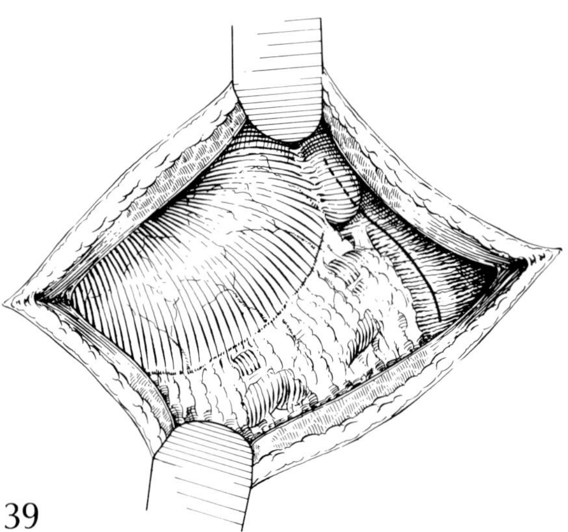
39

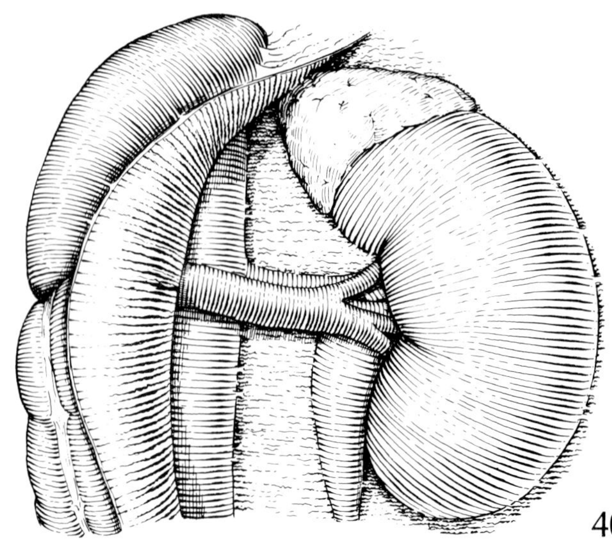
40

EXPOSURE OF SUPERIOR MESENTERIC ARTERY

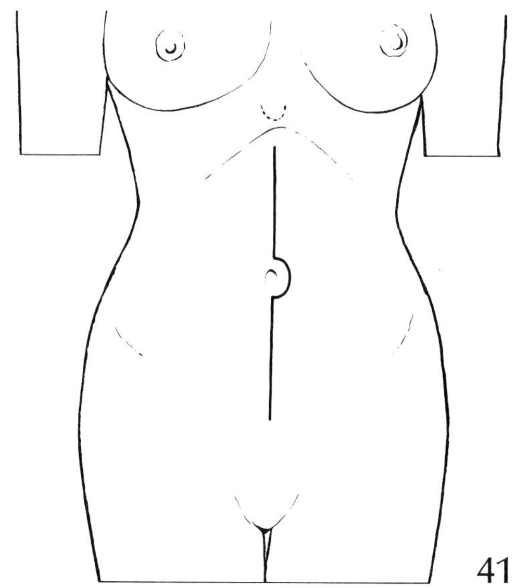
41

41

The incision

A midline or high left paramedian incision is made and the peritoneal cavity opened.

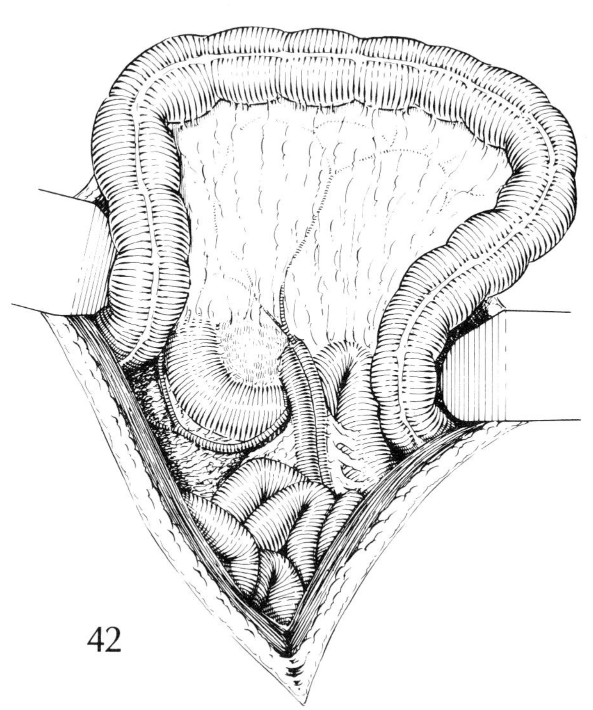
42

42

Deep dissection

The omentum and transverse colon are elevated and the posterior peritoneum incised. The superior mesenteric artery is seen where it emerges below the pancreas. The superior mesenteric vein lies on its right side. The origin of the vessel is exposed by upward dissection and retraction of the pancreas.

EXPOSURE OF INFRARENAL INFERIOR VENA CAVA

43

The incision

A transverse incision is made in the upper part of the right lumbar region.

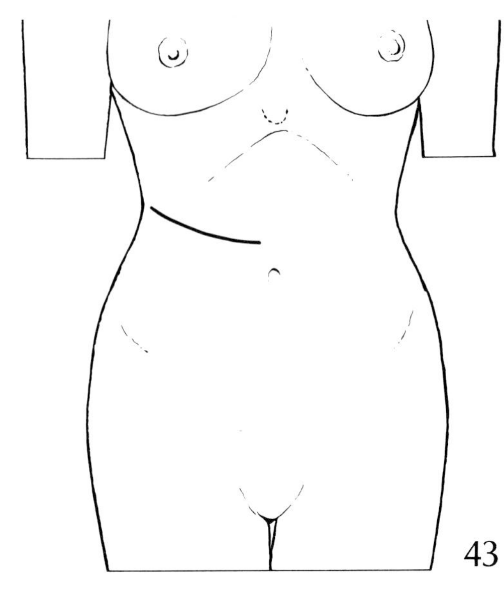

43

44

Deep dissection

The oblique abdominal muscles and transversus are divided in line with the skin incision. The extraperitoneal space is entered and the peritoneum pushed to the left to expose the inferior vena cava. An alternative approach is to enter the peritoneal cavity, perform a Kocher manoeuvre and retract the duodenum medially.

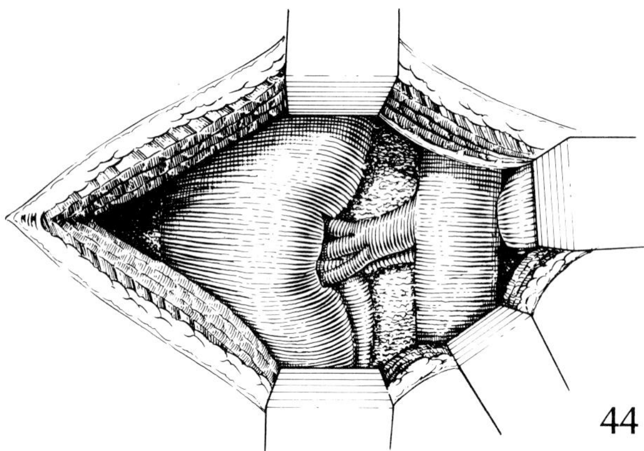

44

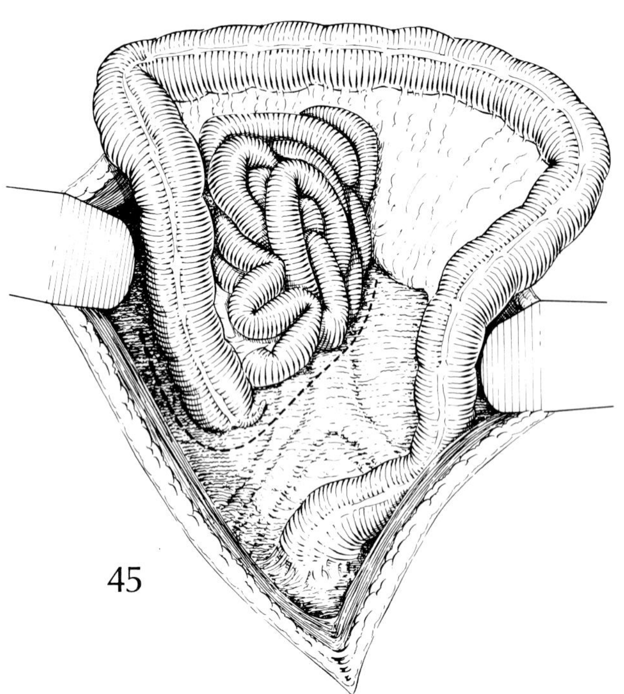

45

EXPOSURE OF ABDOMINAL AORTA BELOW RENAL VESSELS (TRANSPERITONEAL)

45

Incision and dissection

The incision is similar to that used to approach the superior mesenteric artery. Often it is sufficient to turn the small bowel across to the right side of the abdomen and to hold it there under a large abdominal pack with deep retraction. In very obese subjects, or where the aortic lesion is juxtarenal, it is better to mobilize the whole midgut loop by dividing the peritoneal reflection lateral to the right colon, continuing to the left to free the terminal ileum and small bowel mesentery. The intestines are then drawn up out of the abdomen and a plastic bag is placed over them.

EXPOSURE OF ABDOMINAL AORTA BELOW RENAL VESSELS (EXTRAPERITONEAL)

46

The incision

A long J-shaped incision runs along the left linea semilunaris and lateral to its upper half[7]. The patient's left side is lifted up on a sandbag. Alternatively, a transverse or more oblique incision as recommended by Rob[8] may be preferred, running from the tip of the left 12th rib downwards and across the lower abdomen.

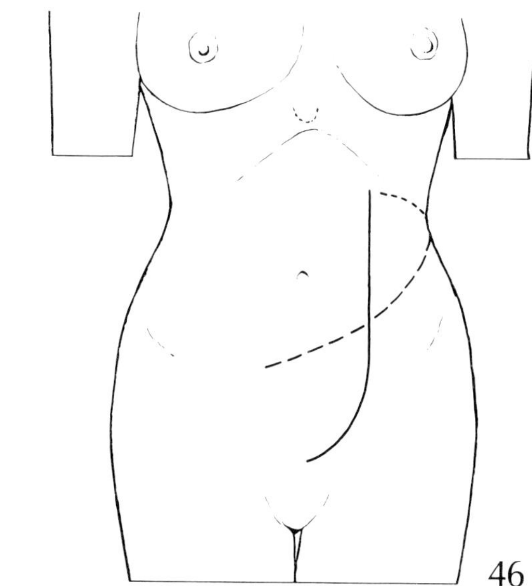

46

47

Dissection

The oblique and transversus muscles are divided in the same line over most of the central part of the incision. They are kept intact with their nerve supply at either end of the incision. The peritoneal sac is then wiped off the muscles. The aortic bifurcation and iliac arteries are exposed. Difficulty is most likely with the lower right iliac and the upper aorta. The inferior mesenteric artery is retracted with the peritoneum across the aorta to the right.

The ureter lies on the left of the aorta and inferior mesenteric artery and must be carefully avoided when extensive pathology is present.

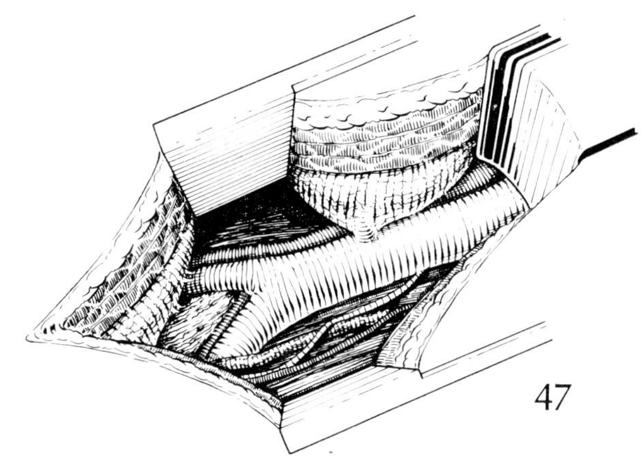

47

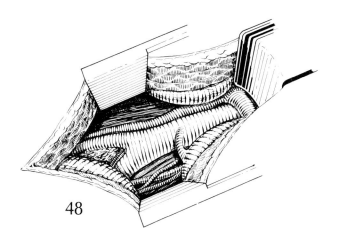

48

48

EXPOSURE OF ABDOMINAL AORTA BELOW RENAL VESSELS (BOTH ROUTES)

Whichever approach has been used the deep dissection is similar. The intestines are displaced to the right with mobilization of the terminal ileum, caecum and ascending colon as required. The aorta can be exposed as high as the left renal vein and the inferior mesenteric vessels displaced to the left. In an extraperitoneal approach these vessels are lifted forwards away from the aorta.

A large self-retaining retractor with deep blades is necessary for adequate exposure.

EXPOSURE OF THE COMMON ILIAC ARTERY (EXTRAPERITONEAL)

49

The incision

An oblique incision crosses the spinoumbilical line in its upper third.

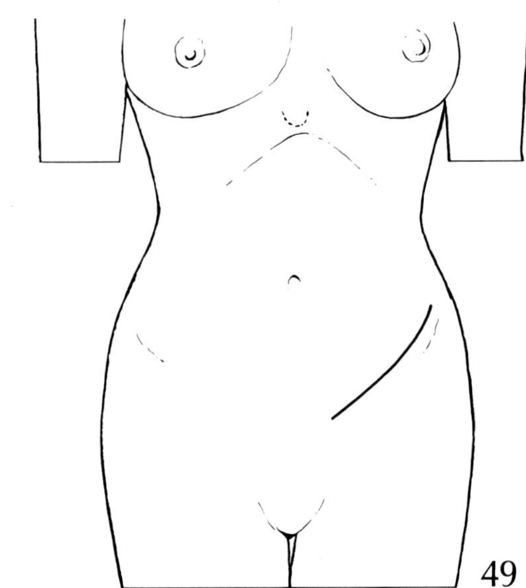

49

50

Dissection

The oblique and transversus muscles are divided in the same line. The peritoneum is carefully separated from beneath the transversus aponeurosis and the plane developed so as to displace the peritoneal sac medially.

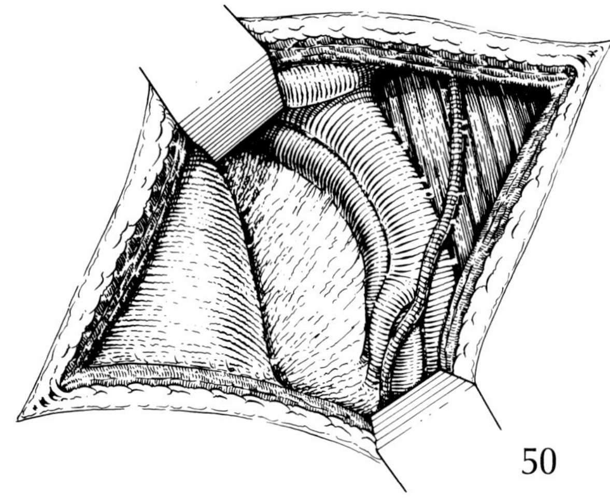

50

51

EXTRAPERITONEAL EXPOSURE OF EXTERNAL ILIAC ARTERY

51

The incision

An oblique incision is made in the iliac fossa extending from the midline to the anterior superior iliac spine.

52

Deep dissection

The posterior parietal peritoneum is pushed up under the medial edge of the incision. The external iliac vessels are found lying on the pelvic brim on the medial side of the psoas muscle. The obturator nerve lies under the vein in its upper part and the genitofemoral nerve on the muscle lateral to the artery. The ureter is seen crossing its origin.

This incision is suitable for renal transplantation, but is also of great value for controlling arterial inflow to the leg.

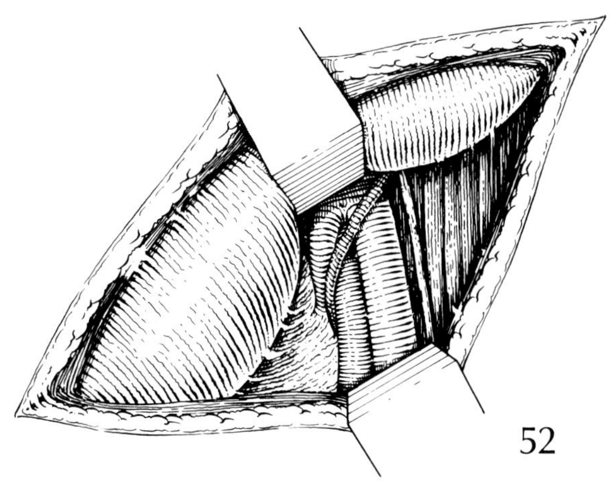

52

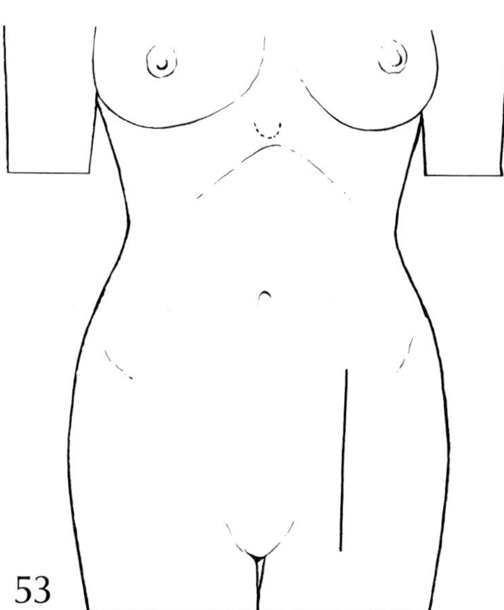

53

EXPOSURE OF COMMON FEMORAL ARTERY

53

The incision

A longitudinal incision allows adequate exposure of the common femoral artery, particularly of its deep branch, and can be extended if necessary. An extension laterally superior to the inguinal ligament allows elevation of the ligament to expose the distal external iliac artery.

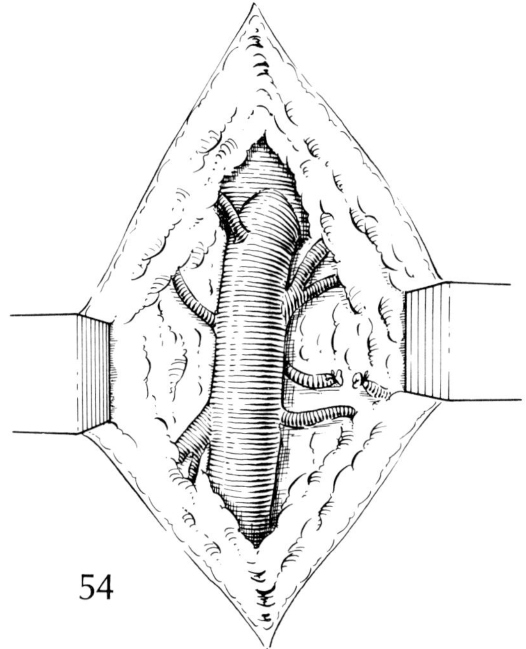

54

54

Superficial dissection

The termination of the long saphenous vein is exposed and retracted medially, dividing tributaries as required. The main vein should be preserved for grafting purposes. The superficial external pudendal artery is ligated as it passes between the saphenous and femoral veins.

55

Deep dissection

The femoral sheath is opened to expose the common femoral vessels. The femoral nerve lies on the lateral side. The profunda femoris artery must be located with care. It arises from the posterior and lateral aspect of the common femoral artery. Its origin is closely related to the termination of the profunda femoris vein. A multiple origin or early branching of the vessel may cause difficulty.

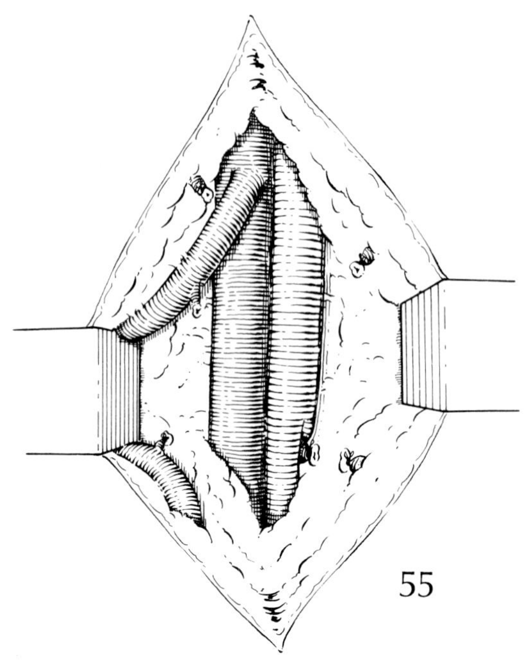
55

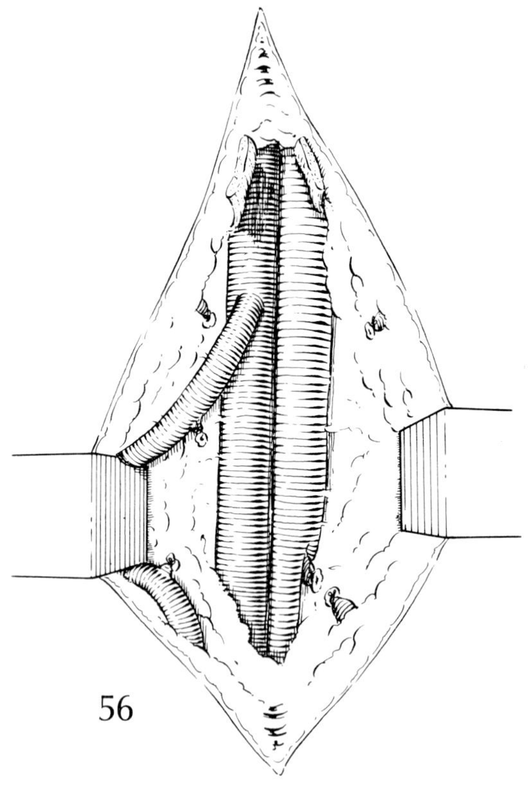
56

56

Iliofemoral junction

This can be exposed by an upward extension of the above dissection, by elevating or dividing the inguinal ligament. The deep epigastric vessels are preserved.

EXPOSURE OF SUPERFICIAL FEMORAL ARTERY IN HUNTER'S CANAL

57

The incision

This is made along the line of the anterior border of the sartorius muscle. The limb is slightly flexed and abducted, with a sandbag placed beneath the knee.

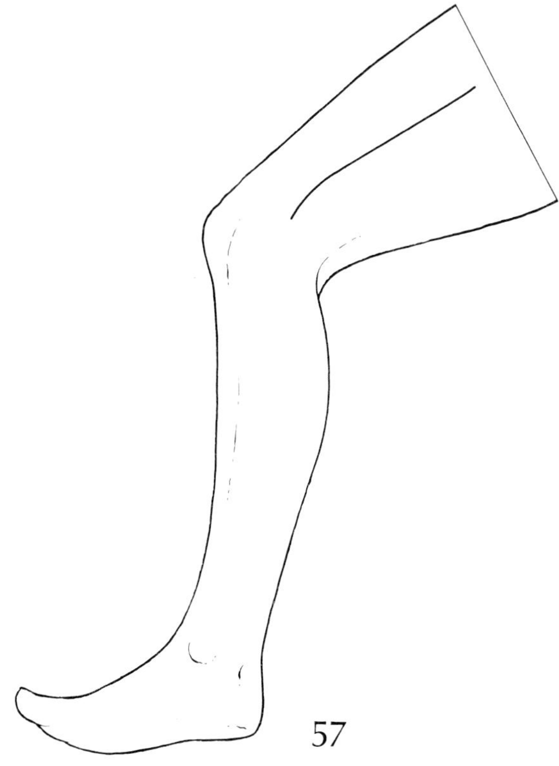

57

58

58

Superficial dissection

The saphenous vein is carefully preserved in the posterior flap. The fascia over the sartorius muscle is incised.

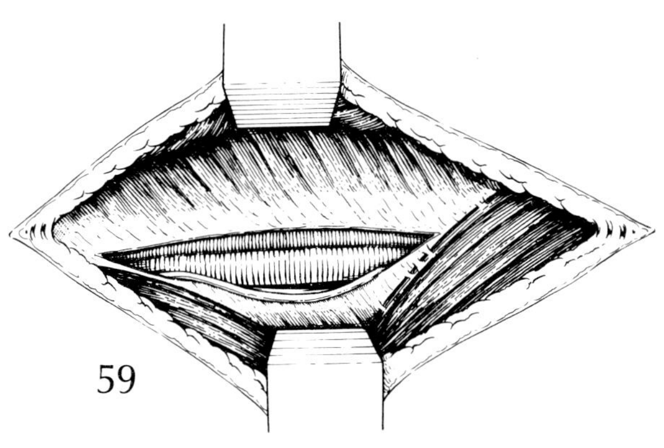

59

59

Deep dissection

The sartorius muscle is retracted backwards. The fascial roof of Hunter's canal is exposed and incised. The saphenous nerve is separated from the artery, which is then dissected from the underlying vein. Care is taken to preserve as many collateral vessels as possible.

EXPOSURE OF POPLITEAL ARTERY

The medial approach is used for most bypass operations, but the posterior approach is better for direct procedures such as the repair of arterial cysts or entrapment.

Medial approach (upper)

60

The incision

The patient is placed supine with the knee flexed over a sandbag. The line of the incision should run from four fingerbreadths above the adductor, opening downwards and backwards to a little behind the medial femoral condyle and avoiding the long saphenous vein.

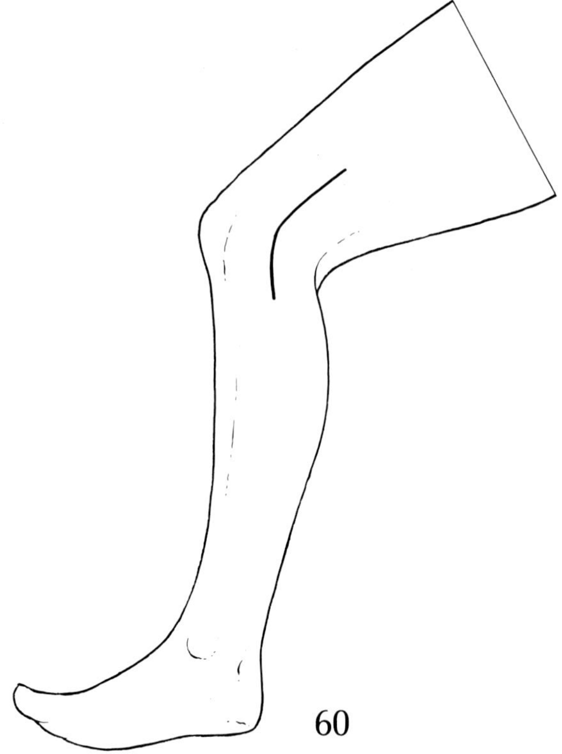

60

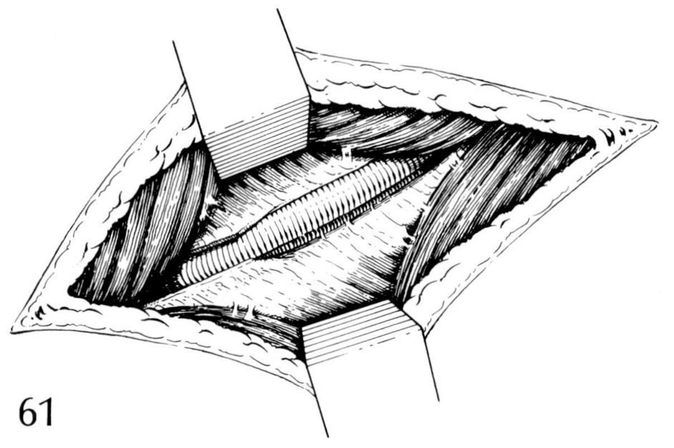

61

61

Dissection

The deep fascia is incised and the anterior border of the sartorius is defined. The muscle is displaced backwards to reveal the thicker aponeurosis of the adductor canal, running into the tendon of the adductor opening. The saphenous nerve leads the dissection to the artery. The fascia is incised to free it and the artery, which can then be followed downwards into the popliteal fat.

Medial approach (lower)

62

The incision

This is made along the posterior tibial border from the lower aspect of the medial condyle, avoiding the long saphenous vein[9].

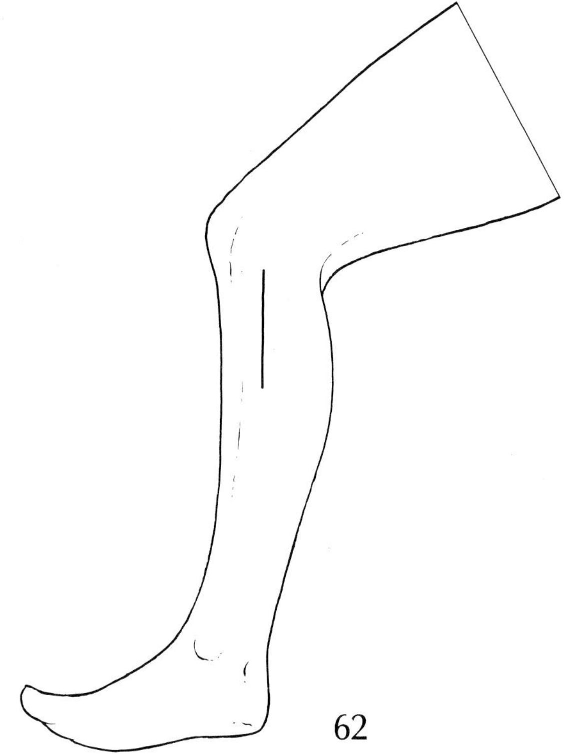

62

63

63

Dissection

The deep fascia, here very thick, is incised and the medial head of the gastrocnemius is displaced backwards. The loose popliteal fat is stroked free from the vascular bundle to reveal the vein, with the artery beneath it. Care should be taken not to damage the medial popliteal nerve. The bifurcation is obscured by the soleus arch and muscular veins, but by division of these the posterior tibial artery can be exposed.

Posterior approach

64

The incision

Recurrent ulceration and contraction often complicate the vertical incision which crosses the flexure at right angles. An S-shaped incision, with its upper limit medial, avoids this. The middle portion should run in the skin crease. A vertical incision is satisfactory, however, for exposing the lower portion of the popliteal vessels. Placed between the two heads of the gastrocnemius, it is commenced below the flexure and can be extended downwards to expose as much of the upper course of the posterior tibial vessels as may be necessary.

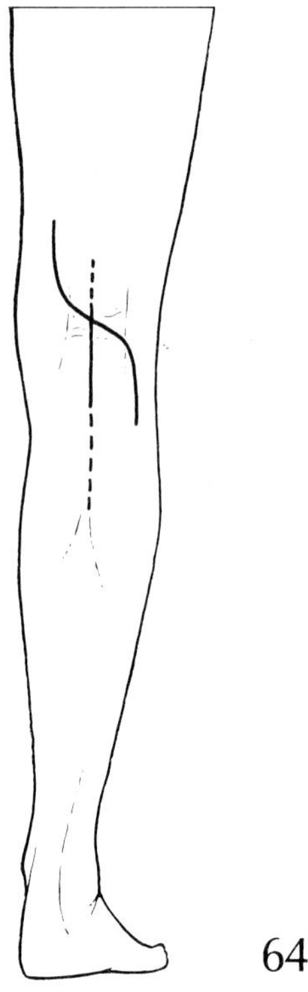

64

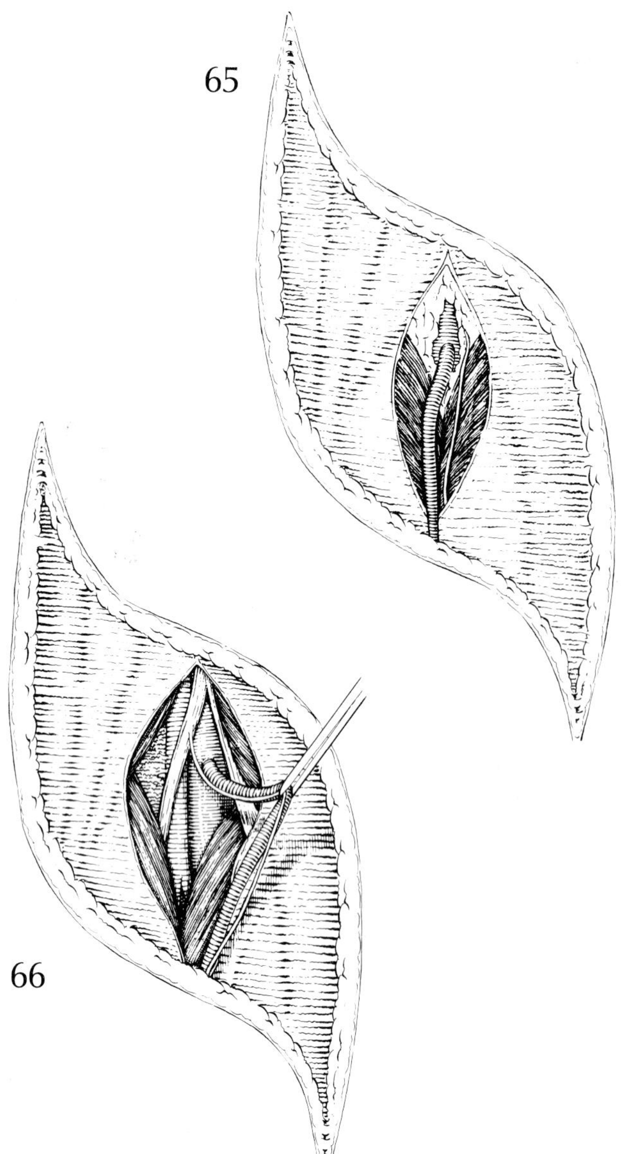

65

66

65

Superficial dissection

The short saphenous vein is followed through the popliteal fascia and the posterior cutaneous nerve is dissected aside. The fascia, the fibres of which run transversely, is split longitudinally to reveal the popliteal fat.

66

Deep dissection

The fat is cleared from the two popliteal nerves. Next the popliteal vein is found, usually via one of its deep tributaries, or perhaps by the short saphenous vein. The artery lies deeper still. It is crossed by a very constant leash of vessels, mainly some large veins from the medial head of the gastrocnemius; these must be divided. The short saphenous vein is preserved if possible.

EXTENSION OF EXPOSURE

Upwards

To reach the femoral vessels, the semimembranosus belly and tendon of semitendinosus are retracted or divided along the line of the artery. The tight hiatus in the adductor magnus is also cut through.

Downwards

The posterior tibial artery is readily exposed by splitting the gastrocnemius and soleus fibres in its line, and also the fascia which covers the vessels as they lie on the long deep flexors. A longitudinal incision through the interosseous membrane in line with the lateral border of the

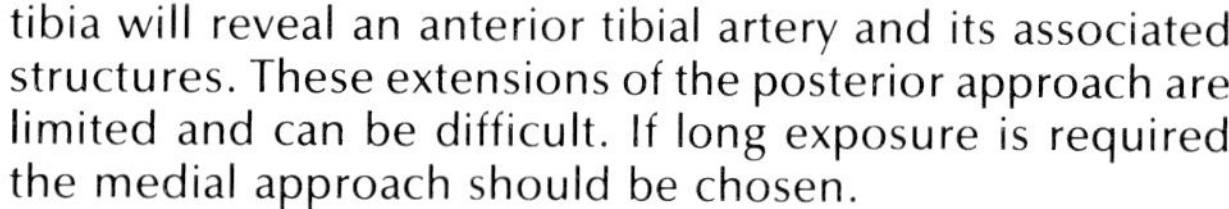

tibia will reveal an anterior tibial artery and its associated structures. These extensions of the posterior approach are limited and can be difficult. If long exposure is required the medial approach should be chosen.

Medial approach

The incision is centred at the site to be exposed, along a line similar to that used for a Scribner shunt. Separation and retraction of the calf muscles will expose the posterior tibial artery which is deep near the knee, becoming more superficial at the ankle[10]. The artery lies on the interosseus membrane near its origin. The anterior tibial artery can be approached through this membrane or from the front of the leg.

THE ARTERIOVENOUS SHUNT

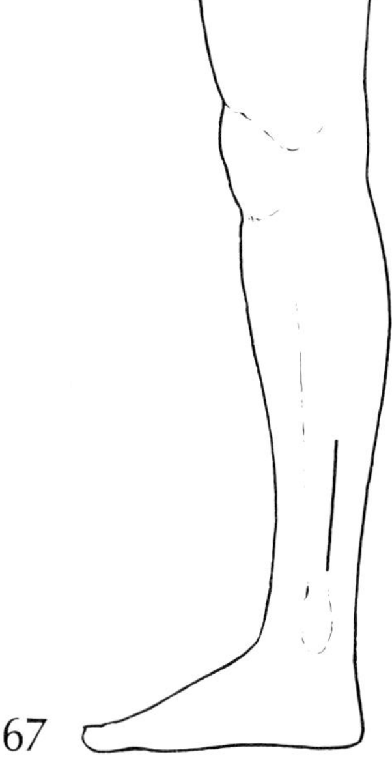

67

The incision

To construct a shunt for access in haemodialysis the incision is centred 4–6 cm above the medial malleolus, 0.5 cm behind the posterior border of the tibia.

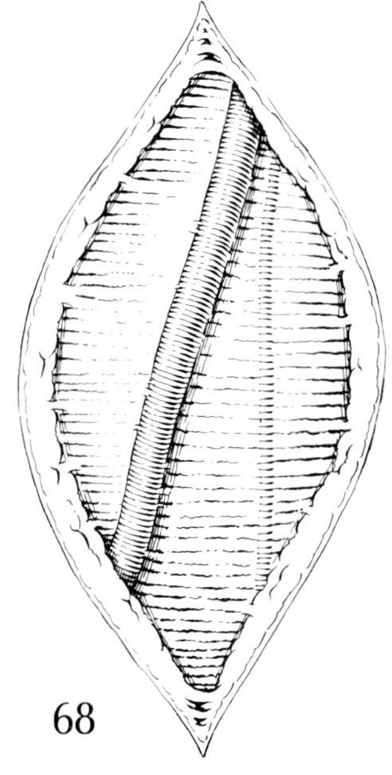

68

Dissection

The origin of the long saphenous vein lies in the superficial tissue in the anterior flap and the posterior tibial artery beneath the deep fascia directly under the incision. Limited mobilization of the vessels permits insertion of the Silastic cannula.

Postoperative care

Postoperative care depends upon the regular, detailed and careful observation of local and general signs. There must be continuity of responsibility to ensure accurate interpretation of the local and general circulation.

In the surgery of atherosclerosis it must be remembered that the disease is generalized. Hypovolaemia and hypotension must be stringently avoided. In all cases of major arterial surgery, postoperative monitoring of central venous pressure and a continuous electrocardiogram are recommended, in addition to the usual observations on pulse, blood pressure and respirations. Oxygen should be administered by mask or catheter to maintain maximal saturation. The urine output is best collected by catheter drainage over the first 24–28 hours.

Posture

The cerebral and coronary circulations take precedence over the peripheral circulation. If postoperative shock is present or the patient has not regained consciousness, head-down tilt is required, When the central circulation is adequate, dependency of an operated extremity promotes the local circulation.

Local signs

Immediately after operation, the state of the distal circulation must be established. In the extremities, the colour of the limb, the skin temperature, filling of the superficial veins and the pulses are all guides to adequate circulation.

Pulses

The distal pulses may not be felt immediately after an operation during which a limb artery has been clamped. They return following improvement in the general circulation and progressive local vasodilation. The latter can be encouraged before the closure of the arteriotomy by the injection of a vasodilator. Intravenous infusion of low molecular weight dextran is favoured by some surgeons to promote capillary circulation in the operated limb.

Skin temperature

After clamping the arterial supply, the distal part of the limb becomes pale and cold. The peripheral veins are collapsed. As recovery progresses the level of transition from warm to cold skin becomes more distal, with improvement in the colour and filling of the peripheral veins.

Sensory impairment

Numbness of the skin is a serious sign, though some skin sensation will often persist in parts of a limb which are on the same level as patches of established necrosis.

Complications

Haemorrhage

The use of heparin during operation and the presence of arterial suture lines require close observation of the operative site. The use of a vacuum drainage system gives an early indication of undue blood loss. The effect of heparin can be reversed at the end of the operation if necessary by the injection of protamine sulphate (protamine 2 mg neutralizes heparin 1 mg). If excessive haemorrhage occurs, re-exploration of the operative site is required.

Ischaemic muscle necrosis

The musculature of a limb is more sensitive to ischaemia than most other tissues. Prolonged ischaemia of the leg may cause necrosis of muscle, particularly in the anterior tibial compartment where the muscles are firmly enclosed by osseous and fascial boundaries. The presence of tenderness over this area and loss of dorsiflexion of the ankle demand early decompression. Delay in diagnosis or deferring active treatment will jeopardize recovery and lead to gangrene, ischaemic muscle contracture and an equinovarus deformity.

Swelling of the leg

Mild oedema of the foot and leg frequently follows operations on the femoral and popliteal vessels even in the presence of normal deep veins[11]. This disappears with increasing activity, and early mobilization should be practised whenever possible.

References

1. Henry, A. K. Extensile exposure applied to limb surgery. Edinburgh: Livingstone, 1945
2. Elkin, D. C. Exposure of blood vessels. Journal of the American Medical Association 1946; 132: 421–424
3. Elkin, D. C., DeBakey, M. E. eds. Vascular surgery in World War II. Washington: Office of the Surgeon General, 1955
4. Mustard, W. T., Bull, C. A reliable method for relief of traumatic vascular spasm. Annals of Surgery 1962; 155: 339–334
5. Morris, G. C., DeBakey, M. F., Cooley, D. A., Crawford, E. S. Autogenous saphenous vein bypass graft in femoropopliteal obliterative arterial disease. Surgery 1962; 51: 62–73
6. Owen, K. The surgery of renal artery stenosis. British Journal of Urology 1964; 36: 7–13
7. Helsby, R., Moossa, A. R., Aorto-iliac reconstruction with special reference to the extraperitoneal approach. British Journal of Surgery 1975; 62: 596–600
8. Rob, C. Extraperitoneal approach to the abdominal aorta. Surgery 1963; 53: 87–89
9. Jarrett, F., Berkoff, H. A., Crummy, A. B., Belzer, F. O. Femorotibial bypass grafts with sequential technique, clinical results. Archives of Surgery 1981; 116: 709–714
10. Hirsch, S. A., Jarret, F. S. Technique of femoropopliteal and femorotibial grafts using umbilical vein. Surgery, Gynecology and Obstetrics 1982; 155 (2): 247–249
11. Husni, E. A. The edema of arterial reconstruction. Circulation 1967; 35 (Suppl. 1): I-169–I-173

Arterial suture and anastomoses

H. H. G. Eastcott MS, FRCS
Honorary Consultant Surgeon, St Mary's Hospital, London, UK

A. E. Thompson MS, FRCS
Consultant Surgeon, St Thomas's Hospital, London, UK

Preoperative

Indications

Repair of a divided or injured major artery is usually preferable to tying its ends. This applies particularly in the lower limb. Trauma, surgical accident and the radical surgery of cancer, as well as the elective treatment of arterial lesions, require the surgeon to be familiar with methods of arterial suture. The methods illustrated will meet the requirements of the arterial operations shown in other sections.

Contraindications

Arteries are best not sutured in the presence of infection. Severe compound or crushing injury with loss of the main artery are indications for amputation, not arterial repair. Simpler procedures are similarly necessary in treating battle casualties when tactical considerations demand early evacuation. Some viscera almost always survive arterial ligation (for example, the left colon). Arterial reconstruction in such circumstances is superfluous.

Suture materials

Fine sutures on atraumatic needles are best for arterial anastomoses. Silk was used for many years but has now been replaced by manmade fibres, which are less traumatic to the vessel walls. Both braided and monofilament sutures are available in varying sizes (2/0 to 10/0). These sutures have the advantage that the anastomosis can be tightened easily by longitudinal tension. Care must be taken to avoid crushing the suture by careless use of instruments. It is necessary to use several throws in each knot to ensure that the knot is secure.

The operations

LATERAL SUTURE

1

This is a simple method of closing a longitudinal incision in the artery wall, such as exists after embolectomy or thromboendarterectomy. A simple continuous stitch is used, taking care that the needle passes through the full thickness of the arterial wall on each side of the anastomosis. Some narrowing of the vessel is always produced and the blood pressure tends to open the repair instead of tightening it, unlike the circumferential suture of an anastomosis.

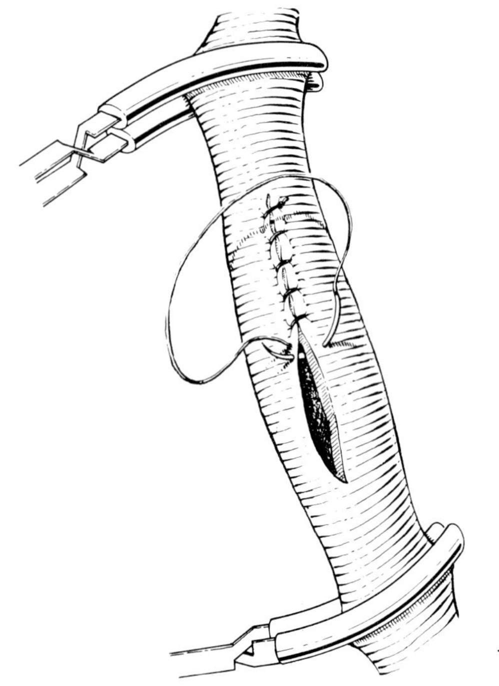

1

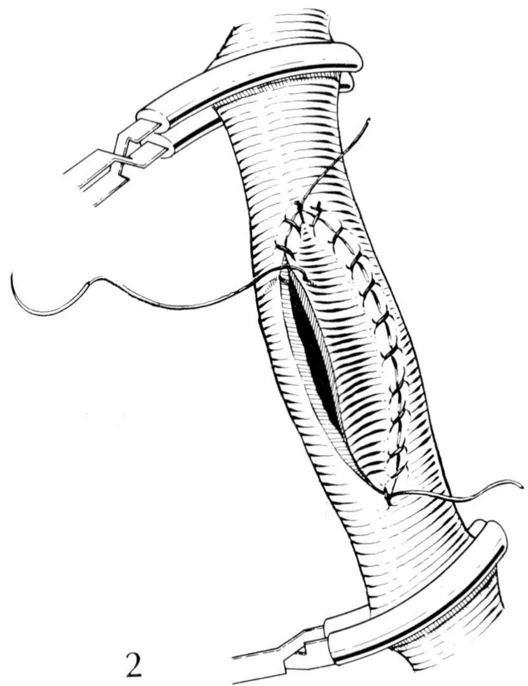

2

2

Where there is loss of substance of the arterial wall, and linear closure may narrow the vessel too greatly, resection and anastomosis or grafting are preferable. A vein patch graft is shown. An ovoid or rectangular patch should be used rather than a sharp-pointed elliptical patch which will narrow the vessel. Four stay sutures are placed and a continuous stitch used between the stays.

END-TO-END ANASTOMOSIS BY MODIFIED CARREL METHOD

3

Stay sutures

The ends of the vessels to be anastomosed are carefully cleared of excess adventitia. Inclusion of adventitia or other extraneous tissue in the suture line may promote thrombus formation. Everting horizontal mattress sutures are used as stay sutures to define the anterior and posterior aspects of the anastomosis.

4

Continuous suture of anterior aspect

A simple continuous suture is placed along the anterior aspect at intervals of 1–2 mm, according to the size of the artery, and a similar distance from the edges which, if the wall is normal, will have already been everted by the stay sutures. These are held apart with sufficient tension to equalize the diameter of the ends of the vessels.

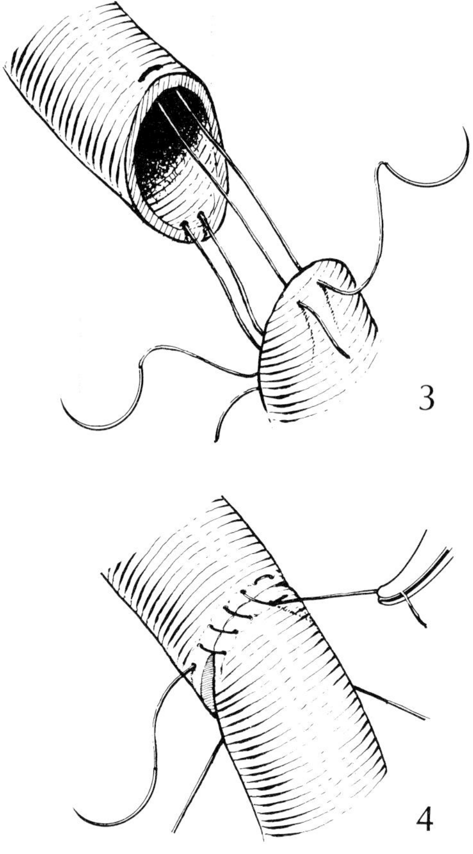

3

4

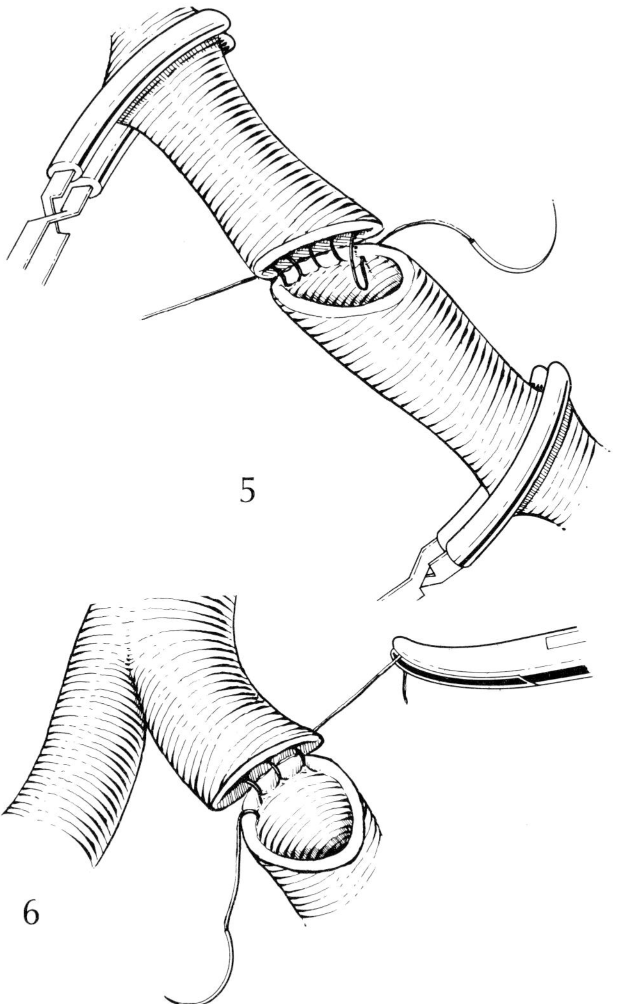

5

6

5

Rotation of anastomosis

The clamps and stay sutures are then used to rotate the anastomosis so that the posterior half can be seen and sutured in the same way. It is often possible to place the clamps in such a position that the anastomosis can be rotated without releasing them.

6

Single stitch method

If difficulty is anticipated in rotating the ends of the artery – near a large bifurcation, for example – a single continuous stitch is used. One supporting suture is placed nearest the operator and this is continued forwards from within the lumen, then back along the front of the anastomosis until the starting point is reached in an accessible position.

This method is particularly useful in diseased arteries which will not allow the smooth pull-up of the Blalock suture.

EVERTING MATTRESS SUTURE

This method still has some place in arterial surgery. It does evert the edges of the vessel and may therefore be chosen in circumstances where a second continuous suture is intended for haemostasis – for example in a healthy aorta. It is also useful in large arteries for ensuring haemostasis and a firm repair when suturing normal to diseased arteries.

Two everting mattress sutures are placed with the loop on the adventitia as shown in *Illustration 3*. Traction is exerted on them to equalize the diameter of the two ends.

7

A continuous everting suture is then placed, first anteriorly, then posteriorly by rotating the anastomosis. One stay suture is passed behind the anastomosis and the ends pulled in opposite directions.

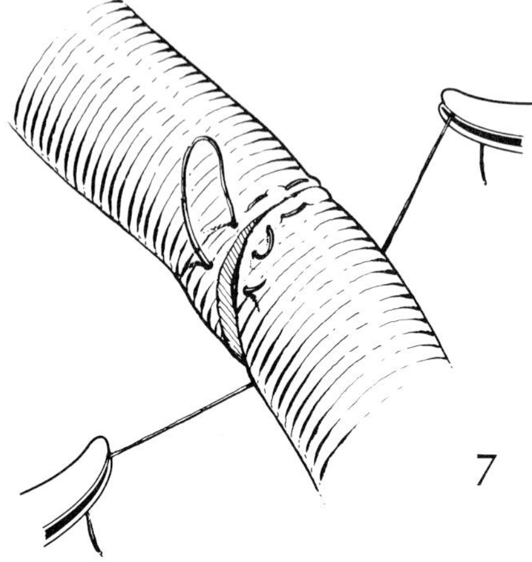

7

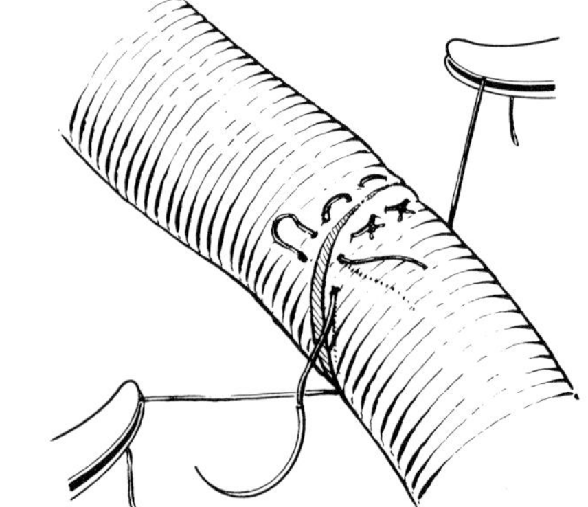

8

8

Use of interrupted sutures

Where growth of the anastomosis must be allowed for, as in coarctation of the aorta in children, interrupted everting mattress sutures may be used.

BLALOCK SUTURE

This is a valuable method of anastomosing normal or thin-walled arteries or veins when access to the posterior aspect of the anastomosis cannot be obtained by rotation. It is used in coarctation, Blalock's and Pott's operations, portacaval anastomoses and in the bypass type of arterial graft.

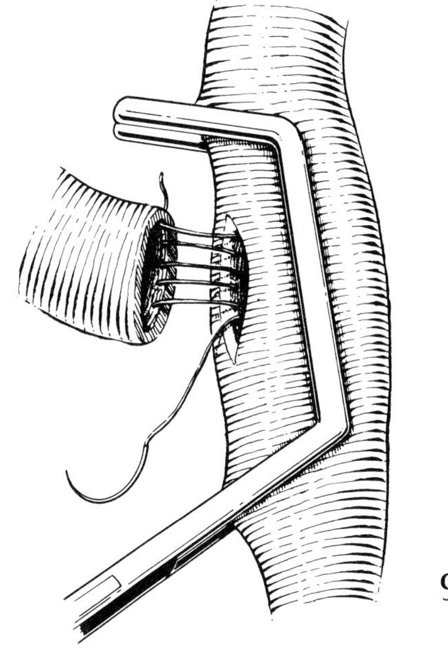

9

9

A continuous everting suture of polypropylene fibre is placed in the posterior half of the anastomosis with the loops on the adventitia. The ends are not tied.

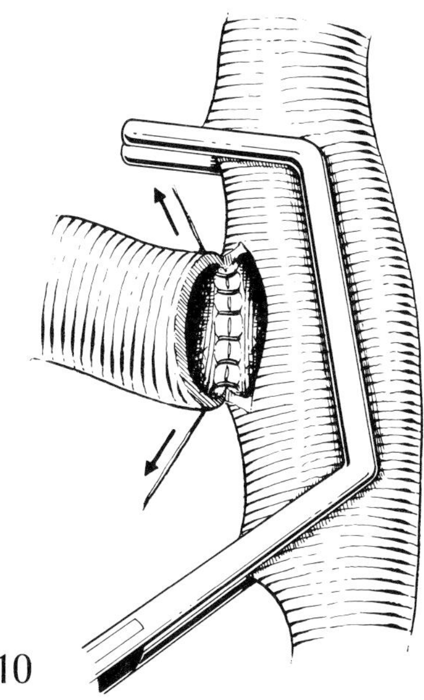

10

10

When this suture line is complete the ends are drawn together with steady traction and the edges are everted. It is then completed as a normal continuous everting stitch, maintaining the tension in the stitch throughout. The suture is finally tied to the free end.

SUTURING THE DISEASED ARTERY

Stronger material (2/0) may be used for suturing densely sclerotic or calcified vessels. Care must be taken so that the suture is not cut by a sharp plaque. A second, finer suture is recommended to ensure haemostasis.

11a & b

Fixation of plaque

If possible the lower limit of an arteriotomy or endarterectomy should be firmly sutured by several mattress sutures through the vessel wall, with the ties on the outer aspect. Unsecured plaques are liable to be dissected free by the subsequent bloodflow and to cause thrombosis.

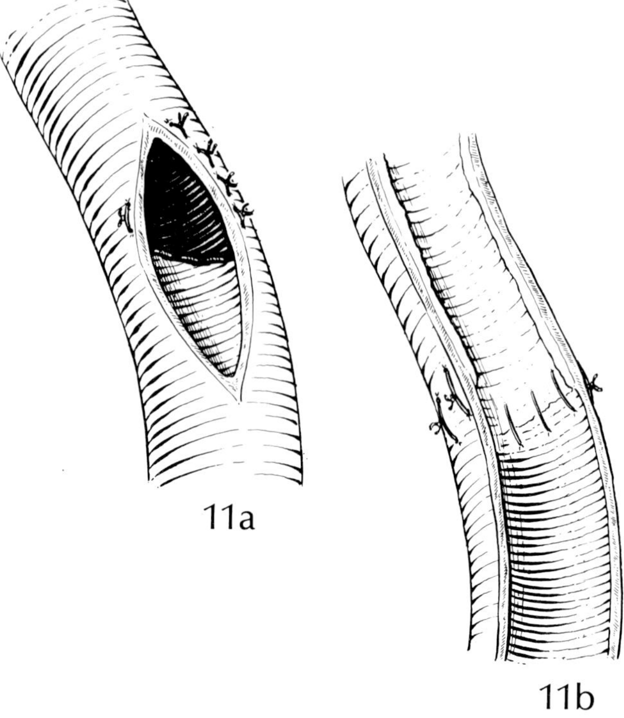

11a

11b

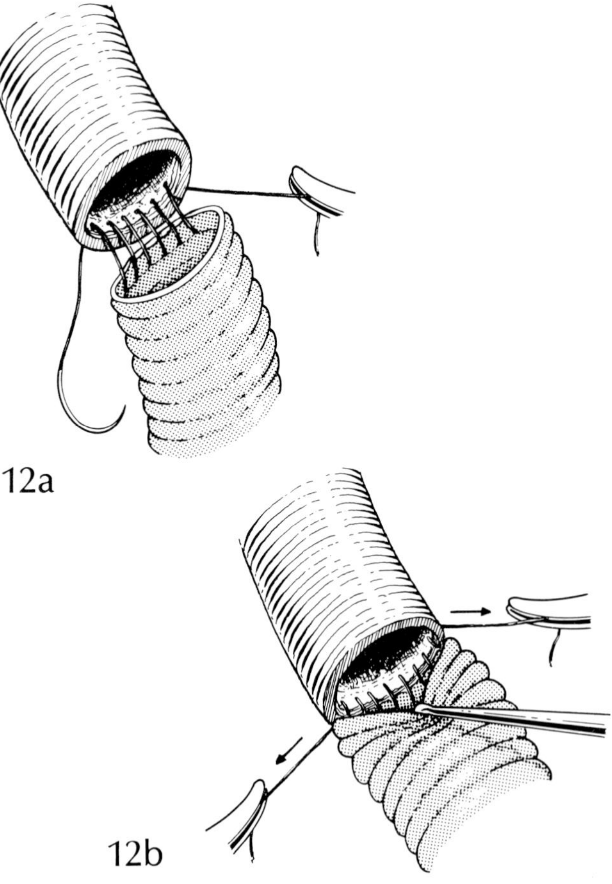

12a

12b

12a & b

Including plaques in end-to-end suture

The anastomosis can sometimes be made to include these plaques in the suture line. The needle should be passed through the plaque from within outwards to avoid loosening the plaques.

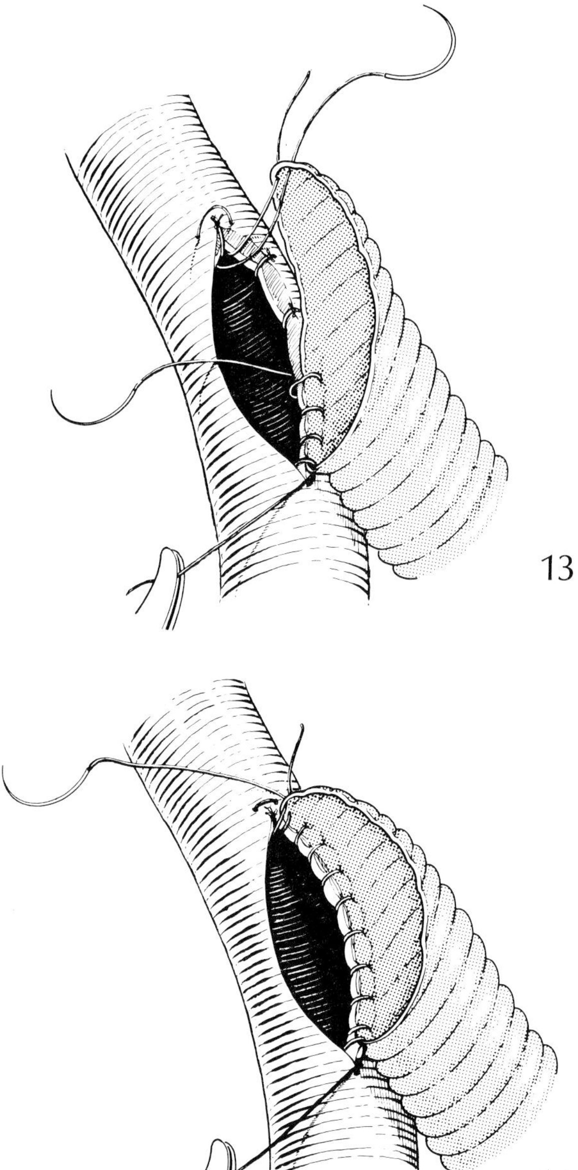

13

Including plaques in lateral suture

Often it is necessary to suture a synthetic graft to the side of a diseased artery, e.g. the femoral. It is particularly important to secure the plaques at its distal end where it may easily become loose. Interrupted sutures hold it well.

14

Completing lateral anastomosis to include plaques

Beginning at the proximal corner of the anastomosis a continuous suture of polypropylene is inserted from within the lumen. This effectively completes the approximation of the plaque to the arterial wall and the graft.

INVAGINATION OF GRAFT

A cloth graft or vein graft also may be sutured within the lumen of a diseased vessel using a continuous everting mattress suture. The bloodflow then tends to dilate the diseased vessel, reducing the tendency to strip plaques by longitudinal pressure.

RELEASE OF CLAMPS

While the artery is clamped the peripheral vessels are constricted. Early recovery of the circulation can be promoted by instillations of a vasodilator into the distal vessel before completing the anastomosis. The lower clamp is released first. This allows the air in the vessel to be expelled and the suture to take up the slack gently. It is customary to have some initial bleeding from the suture lines and the needle holes. This stops after applying steady pressure for 5–6 min over absorbent gauze. An inclination to add supplementary sutures should be resisted until an adequate period of pressure has been tried, as further stitch holes often increase rather than decrease the haemorrhage.

If haemorrhage is persistent, the possibility of the persistence of circulating heparin must be considered. One common practice is to reverse half the dose of heparin originally used with the appropriate amount of protamine sulphate (protamine sulphate 2 mg neutralizes heparin 1 mg). Rarely, a second continuous suture of reinforcement of a suture line with fascia, muscle or a cloth graft may be necessary.

Arterial embolectomy

James A. DeWeese MD, FACS
Professor and Chairman, Division of Cardiothoracic Surgery,
University of Rochester Medical Center, Rochester, New York, USA

Preoperative

Indication

With rare exceptions surgical intervention is indicated whenever the diagnosis of arterial embolism to the upper or lower extremity is suspected. At the present time the risk of the operation itself is practically nil and there is an excellent chance of improving distal circulation in all but the most advanced cases. This more aggressive approach to the problem of arterial embolism is warranted owing to two factors: the increased familiarity of surgeons with the mobilization of major arteries and with the making of and proper closure of an arteriotomy; and the availability of the Fogarty balloon catheter, which allows removal of almost all emboli and thrombi from the arteries of the aorta and lower extremity through an arteriotomy in the femoral artery in the groin made under local anaesthesia. The procedure is also indicated in many patients with embolic obstruction of visceral arteries such as the carotid, renal or mesenteric vessels.

Classically, arterial emboli occur in patients with rheumatic heart disease and atrial fibrillation, or in patients with arteriosclerotic heart disease and atrial fibrillation, or in the patient with a recent myocardial infarction. Patients may embolize for other reasons, and any patient with sudden onset of severe limb-threatening ischaemia should not be denied a groin exploration under local anaesthetic because of age, senility or chronic illness. A patient with a viable limb is always happier and easier to manage, even if he is bedridden.

The symptoms of arterial embolus in order of increasing severity include: sudden onset of claudication, numbness, coldness, rest pain and inability to move the extremity. Similarly, the signs in order of increasing severity include: loss of pulse, coldness, pallor, anaesthesia, paralysis, hard and tender muscles and mottled cyanosis.

The time from onset of symptoms should not determine whether or not an operation should be performed. A patient with an embolus without significant propagation of thrombosis and with good collateral circulation may be seen several days after onset of symptoms and still have a localized problem which can be treated successfully with extraction of the embolus.

Preoperative evaluation

A rapid cardiac evaluation should be obtained and appropriate treatment should be started before surgery. The operation should not be delayed, however, for lengthy evaluations and treatment which can be performed following the operation.

A preoperative trial of conservative care is rarely, if ever, indicated today. But heparin may be commenced as soon as the diagnosis has been made.

The cross-reference in this chapter refers to *Operative Surgery: Vascular Surgery, 4th Edition*

The operation

1

Preoperative preparation

Both groins and entire legs are prepared and draped. Both feet are enclosed in an intestinal bag to allow direct observation of pulses and appearance of the foot. Local anaesthesia is usually sufficient. Almost all emboli of the lower extremity, including those at the aortic bifurcation can now be removed through an arteriotomy in the common femoral artery with the use of the Fogarty catheter.

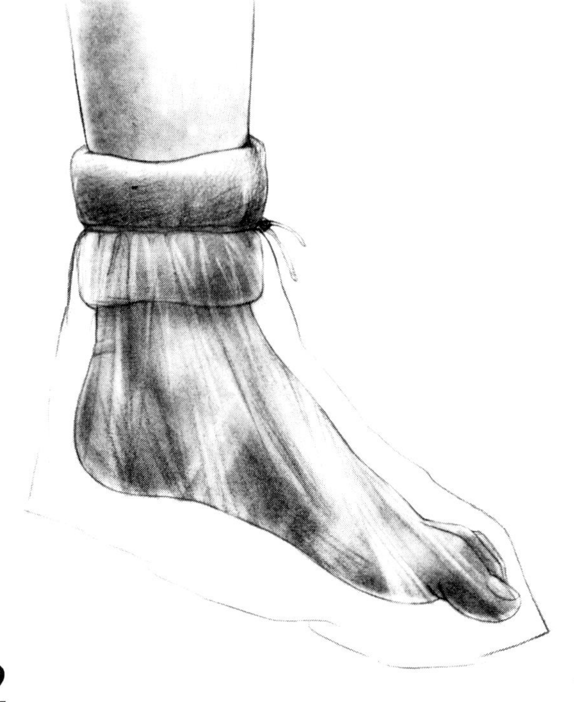

1

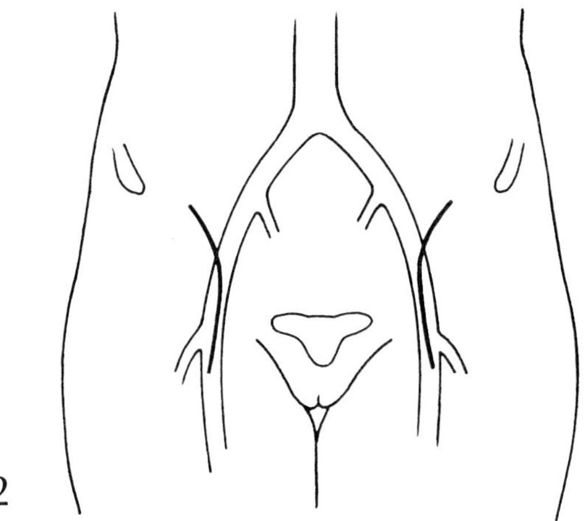

2

2

The incision

The incision begins at the midpoint but one fingerbreadth above the inguinal ligament and is carried medially along the inguinal ligament to a point two fingerbreadths lateral to the pubic tubercle, from which it is extended distally along the course of the femoral artery.

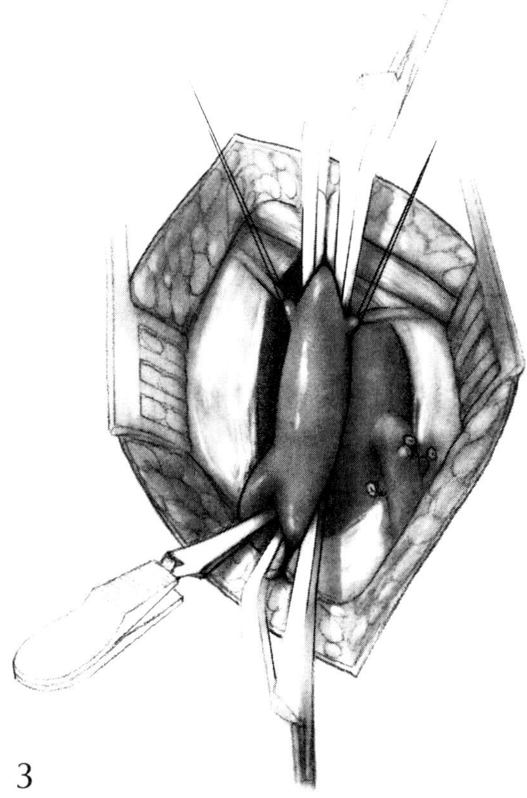

3

3

Exposure of vessels

The lower edge of the inguinal ligament is identified and dissection carried distally along the femoral artery, which can be found two fingerbreadths lateral to the pubic tubercle. Medially, the saphenous vein is seen but only its superior and lateral branches need be divided and ligated. The common femoral artery is mobilized from just distal to the inguinal ligament to its bifurcation into the deep and superficial femoral artery. Tapes are passed around the common, deep and superficial femoral arteries. The superficial circumflex iliac and external pudendal branches can be controlled with an untied suture which has been thrown twice around the vessel.

COMMON FEMORAL EMBOLUS

The iliac and femoral pulse above the embolus may be bounding, but distal pulses are absent and the temperature and colour changes occur at knee level.

4

Embolectomy

A short arteriotomy is made and stay sutures placed in the edges to avoid repeated handling of the vessel with forceps. The arteriotomy incision should be longitudinal. The embolus may be removed quite easily with forceps and flushing. Completeness of the embolectomy cannot be judged by antegrade bloodflow alone. Non-obstructing thrombi may still be present at the iliac or popliteal level. Fogarty catheters should be passed up the common femoral artery and down both deep and superficial femoral arteries.

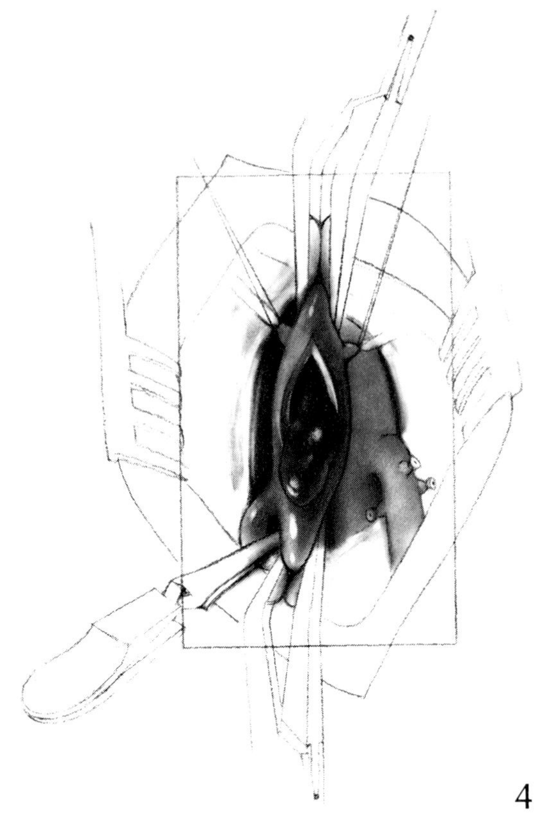

4

AORTIC EMBOLUS

Patients present with no pulses palpable below the aorta. Colour and temperature changes occur in the mid-thigh.

5

Bilateral incisions

It is important to expose the common femoral artery in both groins. Both common femoral arteries are occluded and a Fogarty catheter with the balloon collapsed is passed up one iliac artery.

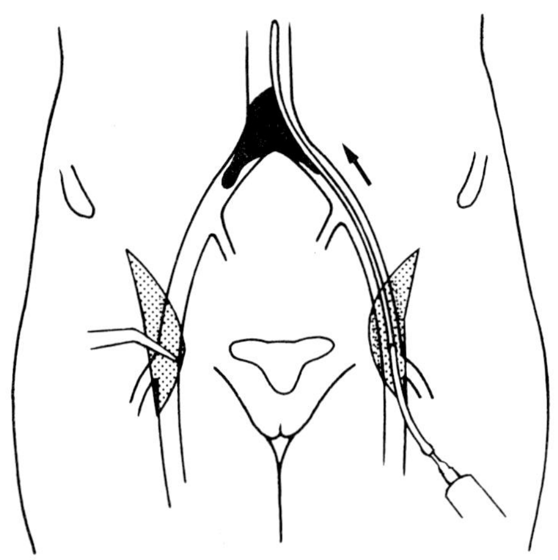

5

Aortic embolectomy

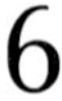

6

The balloon is distended and the catheter removed. Usually the saddle embolus will break into smaller pieces during this manoeuvre and becomes extruded through the arteriotomy incision.

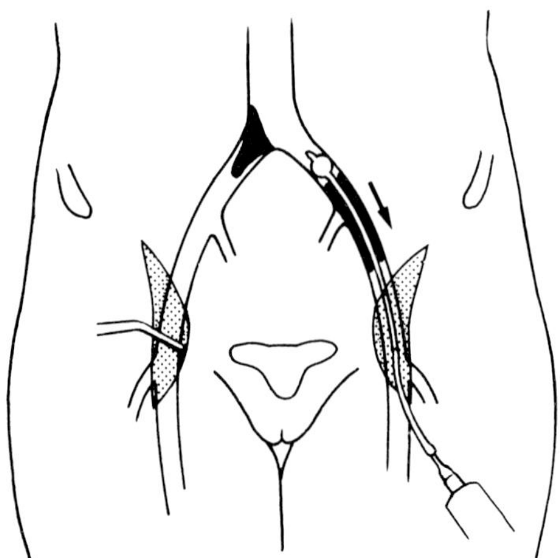

6

7

The catheter is now passed up the opposite iliac artery and further embolus removed. The catheters should be repeatedly passed until no further clot is found. Excessive blood-loss is prevented by occluding the vessel around the catheter with the tape when the catheter is being passed.

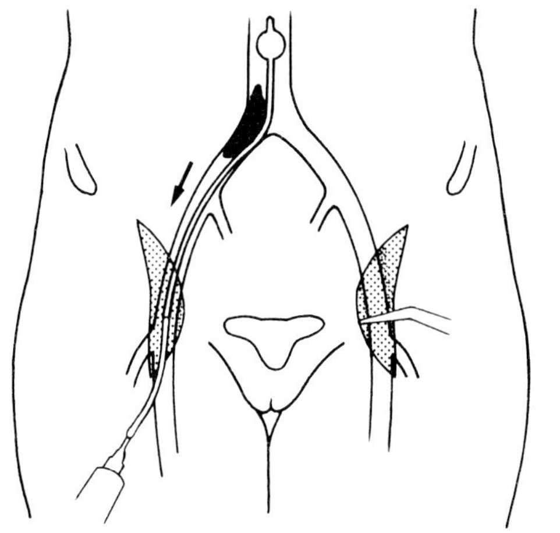

7

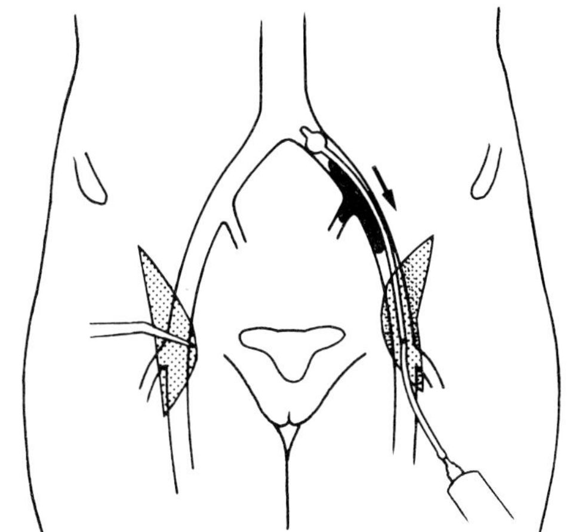

8

ILIAC EMBOLUS

No femoral pulse is present and temperature changes occur at mid-thigh level.

8

Iliac embolectomy

Exposure of the opposite groin is advisable since it is possible to push portions of the embolus into the aorta from whence it could embolize to the opposite leg. The Fogarty catheter is inserted to the common iliac artery, the balloon distended and the catheter removed.

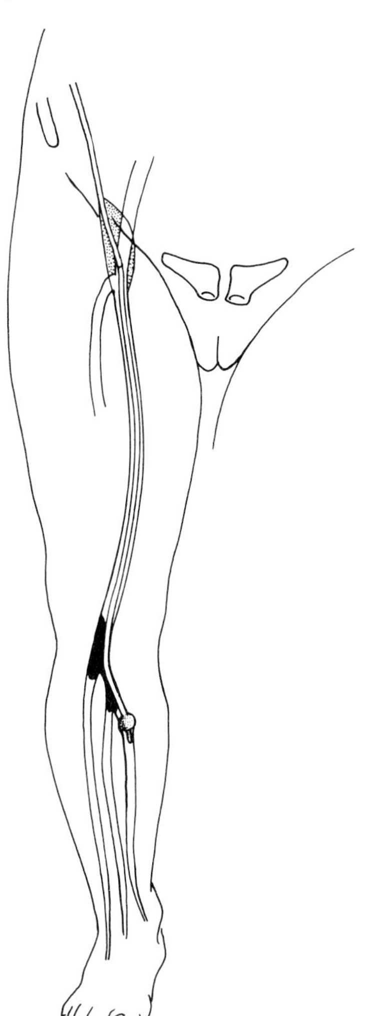

9

POPLITEAL EMBOLUS

The popliteal pulse may be bounding above the embolus. The temperature changes occur at mid-calf level.

9

Popliteal embolectomy

The Fogarty catheter is passed well down the posterior tibial artery, the balloon distended and the catheter removed. The balloon must not be disturbed too much in smaller vessels since plaques may be cracked or the vessel ruptured. The person blowing up the balloon should be the one to remove the catheter, since he can best judge whether the balloon is under- or over-distended.

TIBIAL-PERONEAL EMBOLI

Although popliteal emboli can usually be satisfactorily removed from the groin it may be necessary to approach the popliteal artery and its trifurcation directly. A general or spinal anaesthesia is required.

10

The incision

It is helpful to have the lower leg flexed 90° and externally rotated. The incision begins one fingerbreadth posterior to the medial malleolus and is extended distally parallel to the posterior border of the tibia.

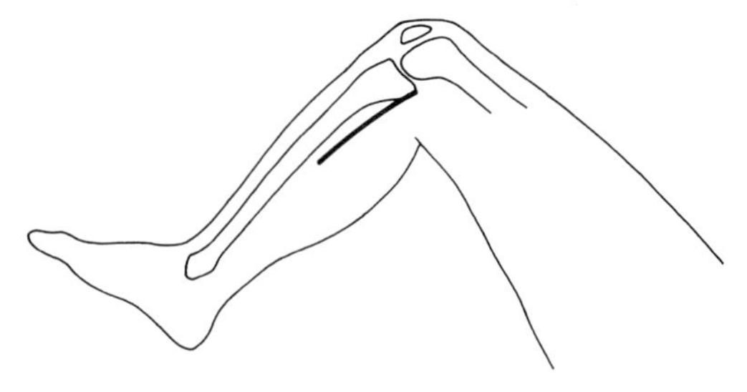

10

11

Exposure

The deep fascia is divided. The gracilis and semitendinosus tendons may be retracted or divided. The medial head of the gastrocnemius muscle is retracted posteriorly.

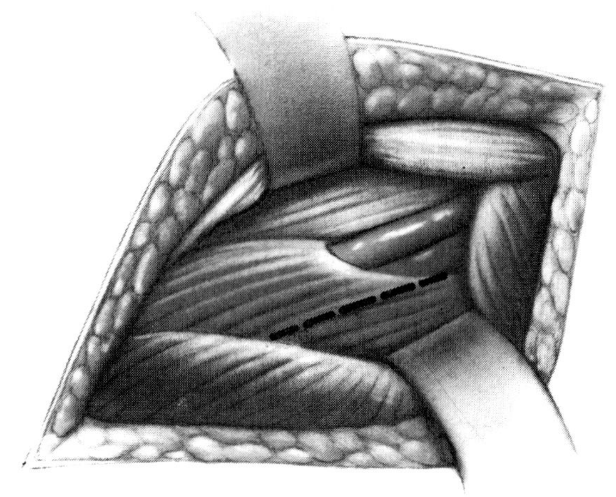

11

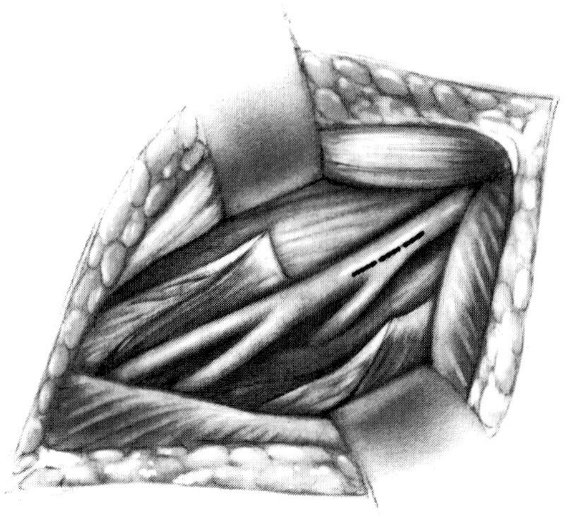

12

12

Embolectomy

The soleus muscle is incised over the popliteal artery which provides exposure of the anterior tibial as well as the posterior tibial and peroneal arteries. Embolectomy from any of the three vessels can be accomplished through an incision in the distal popliteal artery at the level of the anterior tibial vessel.

Intraoperative evaluation

Immediate evaluation of the operative result is possible by visualization of the foot and palpation of the pulses through the intestinal bag. If there is any question as to the patency of the vessels an arteriogram should be obtained (see chapter on 'Arteriography', pp. 15–23).

Postoperative care

Anticoagulation with coumarin drugs is begun the day of surgery. There is a significant in-hospital mortality rate for patients requiring embolectomy. The deaths are usually related to the underlying process responsible for the emboli, such as valvular heart disease and myocardial infarctions, and close medical supervision is required.

Further reading

Darling, R. C., Austen, W. G., Linton, R. R. Arterial embolism. Surgery, Gynecology and Obstetrics 1967; 124: 106–114

Fogarty, T. J., Cranley, J. J. Catheter technique for arterial embolectomy. Annals of Surgery 1965; 161: 325–330

Green, R. M., DeWeese, J. A., Rob, C. G. Arterial embolectomy: before and after the Fogarty catheter. Surgery 1975; 77: 24–33

Gupta, S. K., Samson, R. H., Veith, F. J. Embolectomy of the distal part of the popliteal artery. Surgery, Gynaecology and Obstetrics. 1981; 153: 254–256

Treatment of abdominal aortic aneurysms

James A. DeWeese MD, FACS
Professor and Chairman, Division of Cardiothoracic Surgery,
University of Rochester Medical Center, Rochester, New York, USA

Introduction

Aneurysmal degeneration of major arteries has attracted the attention of physicians for many centuries. The enlargement of some aneurysms with erosion of the chest wall or fistulization into the oesophagus, intestine, or cava dramatizes the lethal nature of the problem. The most common location of aneurysm is in the abdominal aorta beginning below the renal arteries and ending above the bifurcation. The common iliac and internal iliac vessels may also be aneurysmal but the external iliac is usually spared. Aneurysms infrequently involve the proximal abdominal aorta, being even less common here than in the descending thoracic region. Some patients have polyaneurysmal disease with additional involvement of the common femoral and popliteal arteries.

Operative procedures

Dubost is credited with initiating the modern era of management of abdominal aortic aneurysms when in 1951 he resected an aneurysm and replaced it with a homograft[1]. Within a few years significant experiences with resections of aneurysms were reported[2,3,4]. A variety of materials were evaluated but Dacron remains the graft of choice. Alternative methods for the treatment of abdominal aortic aneurysms such as ligation, wrapping or wiring have been abandoned. For the patient with very serious medical problems, ligation of the iliac arteries, thrombosis of the aneurysm and performance of an axillobifemoral graft can be considered[5].

Symptoms

Patients may have aneurysms of considerable size without symptoms. Some patients feel the aneurysm and report that their heart has dropped into the stomach. Others note pulsation when leaning against a firm object, such as a desk top. Some complain of postprandial fullness. Many aneurysms are first discovered on a routine physical examination or at the time of radiological examination for an unrelated problem. Unfortunately the first symptoms may precede frank rupture very closely. These symptoms are usually a deep aching and then sharp abdominal pain frequently radiating to and settling in the flank or back. Depending on the site of the largest retroperitoneal haematoma, the initial diagnosis may be appendicitis, cholecystitis, perforated ulcer, diverticulitis or renal colic. The presence of postural hypotension or shock supports the diagnosis of rupture.

Unless indicated otherwise the cross-references in this chapter refer to *Operative Surgery: Vascular Surgery, 4th Edition*

Preoperative

Indications for operations

Patients with painful symptoms require immediate operation. Asymptomatic patients with proven aneurysms should have an elective operation unless they have significant medical contraindications. There has been an attempt to relate size of aneurysm to risk of rupture. Unfortunately, even small aneurysms may rupture[6]. The mortality rate for patients with ruptured aneurysms who reach the operating room is still 50 per cent in most hospitals. The mortality rate for patients undergoing elective resection is approximately 5 per cent[7]. Therefore, even though an aneurysm is less than 6 cm in diameter, the patient should be evaluated for a possible elective operation. Patients with historical or ECG evidence of coronary artery disease require the most careful evaluation. The postoperative mortality rates as a result of myocardial infarction is significantly higher in patients with known coronary artery disease (2 per cent versus 9 per cent)[8].

Preoperative evaluation

Prior to an elective operation it is advisable to obtain an intravenous pyelogram. It can provide information regarding the relationship of the aneurysm to the renal arteries, reveal a horseshoe kidney and provide baseline evaluation of renal anatomy and function. Ultrasonography may be of help in diagnosing or following the size of an aneurysm but has not been routinely useful to us in evaluating the extent of the aneurysm. Computerized axial tomography may be useful in determining the extent of the aneurysm. CAT and aortography, however, are reserved for patients with associated arterial occlusive disease or suspected suprarenal involvement on the basis of the presence of a palpably high aneurysm or widened descending thoracic aorta on a radiograph of the chest.

Preoperative preparation

Patients undergoing elective operation are hydrated with 1500–2000 ml of a balanced electrolyte solution during the 12 hours prior to surgery. Broad spectrum antibiotics are administered intravenously preoperatively and during the first 4 postoperative days. At least 4 units of whole blood should be available. Patients with ruptured aneurysms are cautiously transfused preoperatively to avoid hypertension and increased bleeding. After the patient has been anaesthetized, a nasogastric tube is inserted and the patient is kept on gastric suction until the bowel regains normal activity, usually 3–5days. A urinary catheter is inserted for constant monitoring of urine flow during the first 48 hours after operation. The radial artery is cannulated for continuous monitoring of blood pressure and intermittent monitoring of blood gases. A central venous pressure line is inserted for constant monitoring of pressures for routine operations. The use of flow-directed, balloon-tipped catheters which allow measurement of both right and left heart pressures and the cardiac output is useful for monitoring high risk patients. Patients with ruptured aneurysms should have preoperative, intraoperative or postoperative placement of these monitoring devices.

Anaesthesia

General anaesthesia with an endotracheal tube is required. It is advisable to prepare and drape patients with ruptured aneurysms prior to induction of anaesthesia. Optimal management of the patient during the operation is dependent on close cooperation between the surgeon and anaesthesiologist. Myocardial depression occurs during anaesthesia and is then aggravated by aortic clamping[9]. Continuous monitoring of systemic arterial pressure, intracardiac pressures and cardiac output permit maintenance of optimal cardiac performance, particularly during the critical periods of clamping, declamping and blood loss. Preload can be increased by infusion of appropriate non-colloidal or colloidal fluids or reduced by appropriate diuretic or drug. Inotropic drugs may be used intelligently, particularly in combination with drugs which decrease after load. Clamping and declamping should be done slowly to allow appropriate pharmacological manipulations[10].

The operations

THE INFRARENAL ABDOMINAL AORTA

Except in the rarest of circumstances, the functional replacement of the abdominal aorta with a plastic graft is the operation of choice for treatment of an abdominal aortic aneurysm. It is not necessary to remove the aneurysm sac itself. Rather, the sac is opened longitudinally and the anastomoses performed from within by suturing the graft to the cuff found at the junction of the aneurysm and aorta. The aorta may or may not be partially or completely transected. This more simplified method of operative management has decreased dissection, blood loss and complications, and has been at least partially responsible for the decreased mortality rate for the operative management of abdominal aortic aneurysms. The operative mortality rates for elective operations now is approximately 5 per cent. On the other hand, mortality rates for patients urgently operated on for symptomatic but unruptured aneurysms is 12–20 per cent in most reported series[7,11].

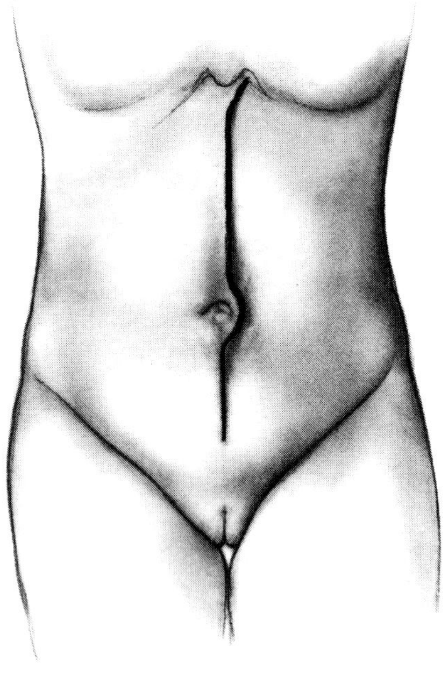

1

1

The incision (midline)

For most aneurysms a long midline incision is made. The supine patient is prepared and draped from the nipples to the midthigh. The incision begins at the base of and to the left of the xiphoid process. It is carried downward and around the umbilicus and ends at the symphysis pubis. Care is taken to make the incision exactly in the midline by following the decussations of the fibres of the rectus sheath.

An extraperitoneal approach should be considered in patients with a history of peritonitis or extensive intra-abdominal operations.

2

High proximal control of aorta

If the aneurysm extends to the renal arteries or if the aneurysm has ruptured, proximal control is best obtained above the level of the renal arteries. The transverse colon and stomach are retracted downward, the lesser omentum incised and the aorta exposed by bluntly separating the right and left crus of the diaphragm. A large vascular clamp is applied, taking care not to injure the coeliac artery. More immediate control can be obtained by compressing the aorta against the lumbar spine with a retractor. Alternatively a large balloon catheter can be introduced through an incision or tear in the aneurysm and positioned in the suprarenal aorta and distended.

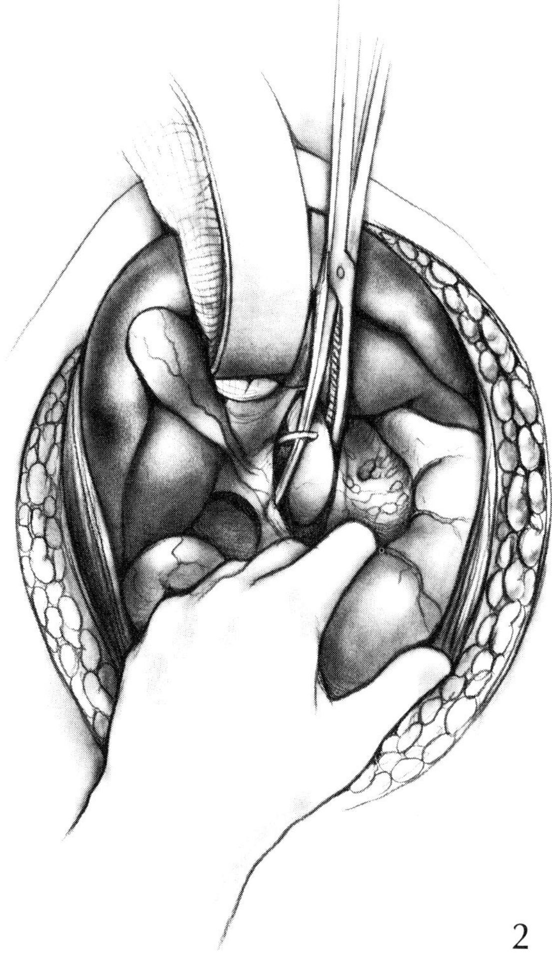

2

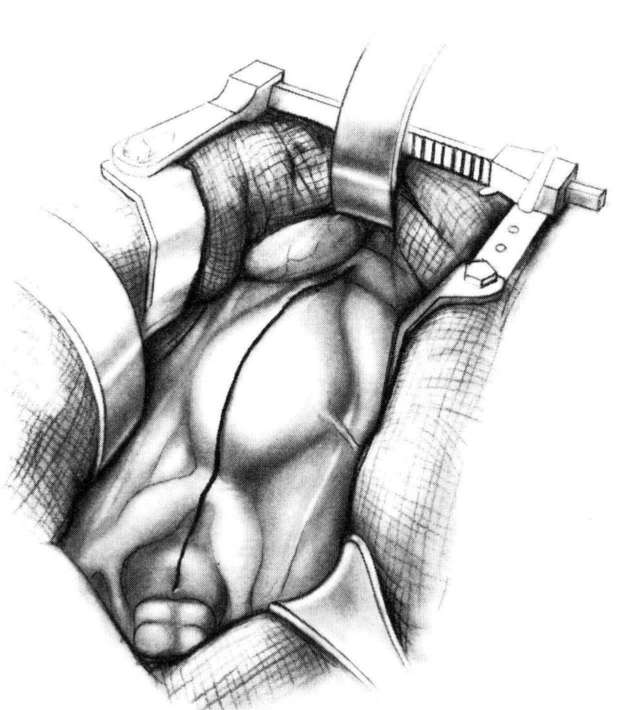

3

3

Exposure of aneurysm

The patient is hyperextended. The small intestine is mobilized superiorly and to the patient's right side and protected by moist pads or within a plastic bag. Moist pads and retractors are used to pack away the duodenum and large bowel. A self-retaining chest retractor with long blades is quite useful. The posterior peritoneum is incised beginning at the ligament of Treitz, carried distally to the right of the midline to avoid the mesenteric artery and vein, and over the sacral promontory in the midline.

4

Infrarenal control of aorta

The ligament of Treitz is incised superiorly to the pancreas, allowing separation of the duodenum from the mesenteric vein. The left renal vein is dissected away from the aorta and the left gonadal vein may be divided. A plane of dissection is established immediately adjacent to the adventitia of the aorta distal to the left renal artery. Using careful sharp and blunt dissection, the aorta is mobilized sufficiently to allow it to be lifted from the lumbar spine. Encircling it with a tape only increases the risk of bleeding from lumbar veins or arteries and is not necessary.

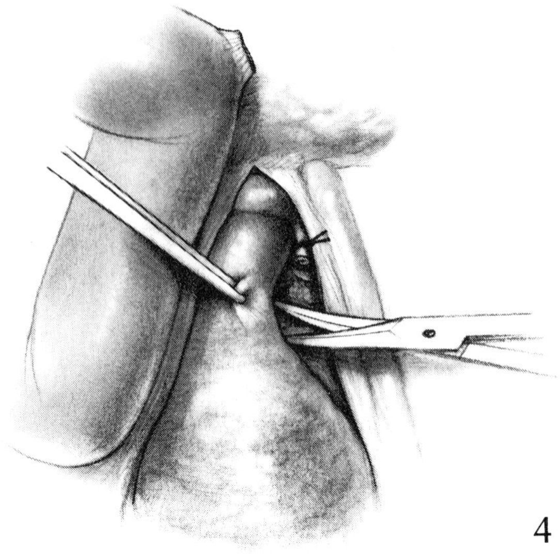

4

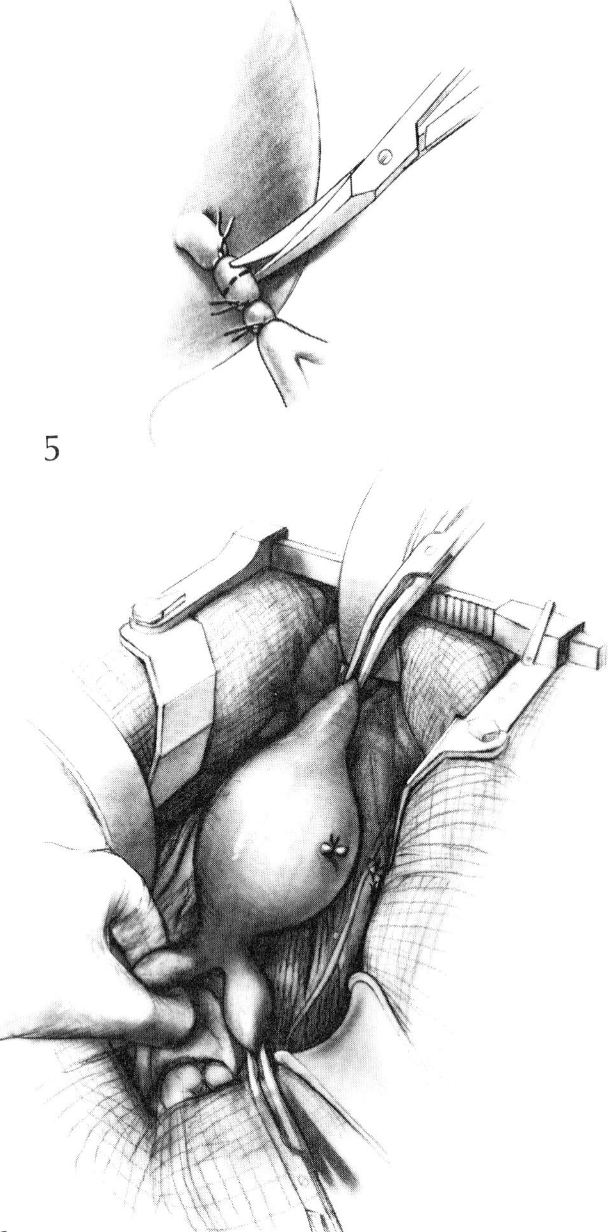

5

6

5

Ligation of inferior mesenteric artery

If the inferior mesenteric artery is immediately visible it is mobilized at its origin. A proximal and two distal ligatures are placed before dividing the artery. It is important that the ligatures do not occlude the first large left colic branch. If no pulsations can be felt in the sigmoid mesentery after ligation of the inferior mesenteric artery, if the vessel is unusually large or if the left colon appears ischaemic, the stump of the vessel should be carefully preserved and implanted into the side of the graft.

6

Clamping of aorta

The granular tissue over the iliac veins is incised and the ureter identified. Using sharp and blunt dissection, the artery and frequently adherent iliac veins are exposed but not separated.

Heparin sodium in 5000–7500 unit amounts is administered intravenously. After 1 minute the aorta and both iliac arteries are occluded with vascular clamps. It is not necessary to encircle the iliac arteries or aorta but it is important that the dissection be extensive enough to allow the vessels to be elevated and the posterior structures pinched by the approximated thumb and index finger.

7

Aortotomy

It is helpful to establish the extent of the aortotomy by cauterizing the adventitia with a broad blade. The final incision will be midline and longitudinal over the bulk of the aneurysm. Superiorly, where the aorta becomes of more normal calibre, there will be a transverse 'T' extension of the incision to encompass 30–50 per cent of the circumference of the aorta. If the iliac arteries are aneurysmal or stenotic, the incision will extend longitudinally along the anterior surface. If the bifurcation of the aorta is relatively normal, a transverse 'T' extension is made at that level. A partial aortotomy is made and a plane of dissection is established either between media and intima or between the intima and old thrombus, which is almost always found within the aneurysm. When the lumen is entered, the remainder of the aortotomy is rapidly completed along the course of the cauterized aorta.

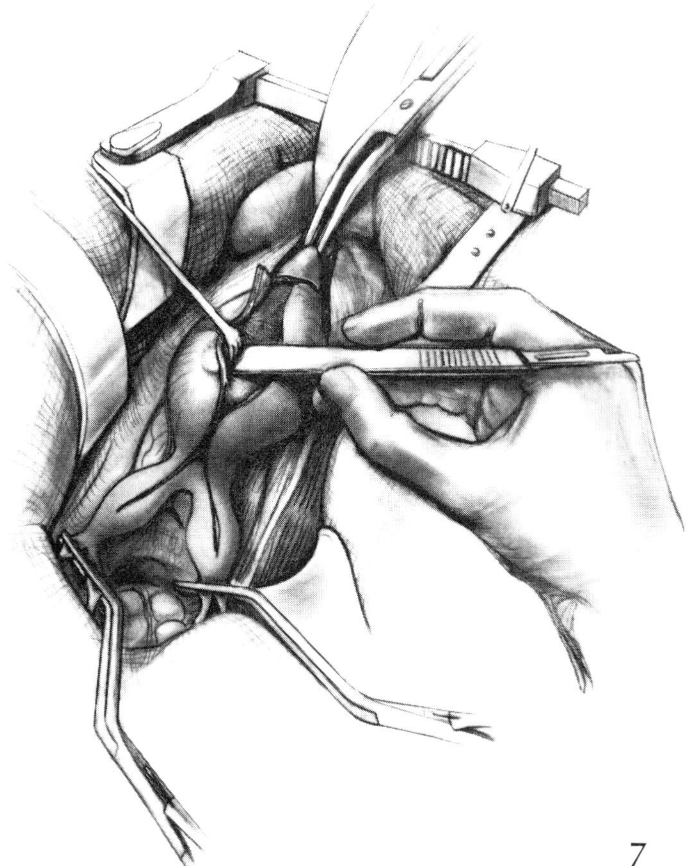

7

8

8

Removal of aneurysm contents and control of lumbar arteries

The thrombus and, if possible, the atherosclerotic intima are removed from within the aneurysm. Most of the lumbar arteries are usually thrombosed. Bleeding from the patent vessels is controlled with mattress or figure-of-eight stitches of 2/0 suture. Atherosclerotic plaques must be debrided away before attempting to suture these vessels. If the inferior mesenteric artery was not previously identified and is patent, it can also be controlled from within the aneurysm.

9

Proximal anastomosis – suturing posterior half

To avoid extensive mobilization of the aorta the posterior half of the proximal anastomosis can be performed from within the aneurysm. The body of the bifurcated woven graft is usually much longer than needed and must be cut before beginning the anastomosis. Usually a distinct ridge can be identified where the aorta becomes aneurysmal. A deep mattress stitch is placed through this ridge and carried through the midpoint of the posterior edge of the graft as an everting stitch, and the suture is tied. The posterior suture is then run around both sides of the graft as a continuous everting over-and-over stitch. It is important that each bite of the stitch be made through the entire thickness of the wall of the aorta.

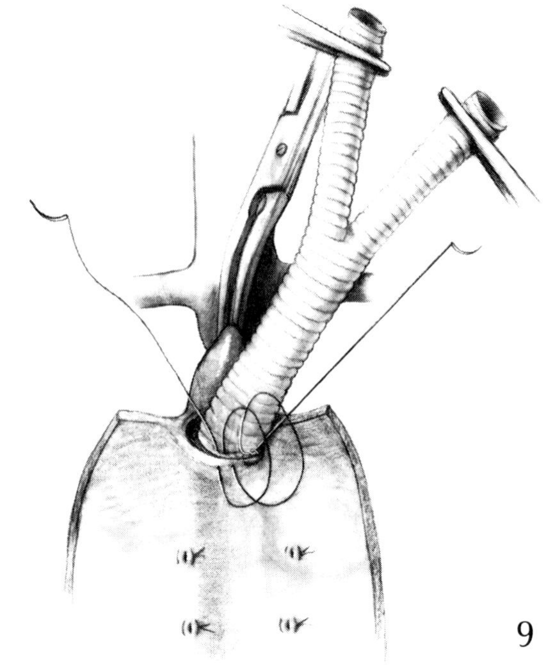

9

10

Proximal anastomosis – suturing anterior half

As the posterior stitch is carried anteriorly it is important to place the sutures under direct vision at the transition zone between the intact and incised aorta to avoid tearing the adventitia. In addition it is frequently necessary to remove calcified arteriosclerotic plaques in order to place stitches, which leaves a thin aortic wall for suturing. It then becomes very important to use smaller needles and stitches of equal depth in the aortic cuff to avoid tearing.

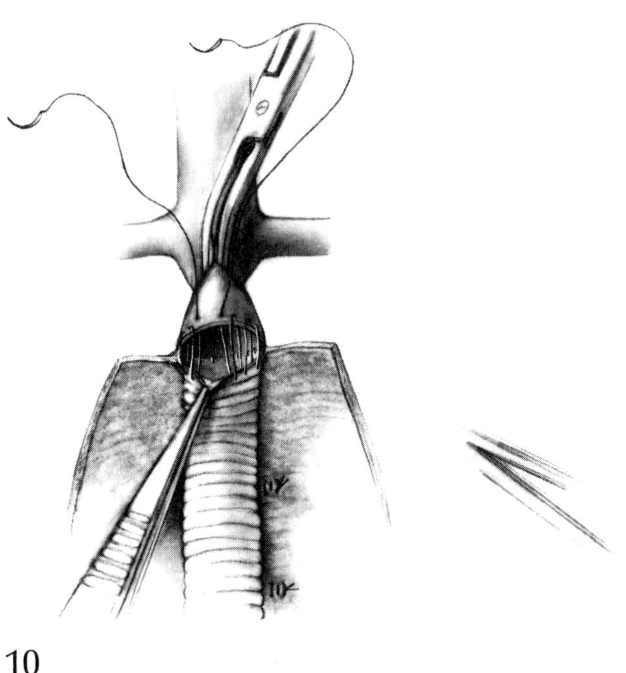

10

11

Testing the proximal anastomosis

Regardless of whether woven or preclotted knitted grafts are used, it is important to test the anastomosis and control bleeding through the graft interstices after completion of the proximal anastomosis. The limbs of the graft are occluded and the proximal clamps slowly released. Any significant bleeding between sutures is controlled with mattress stitches. The graft is then allowed to fill, the clamp occluded and the graft allowed to sit until there is no further bleeding through the interstices.

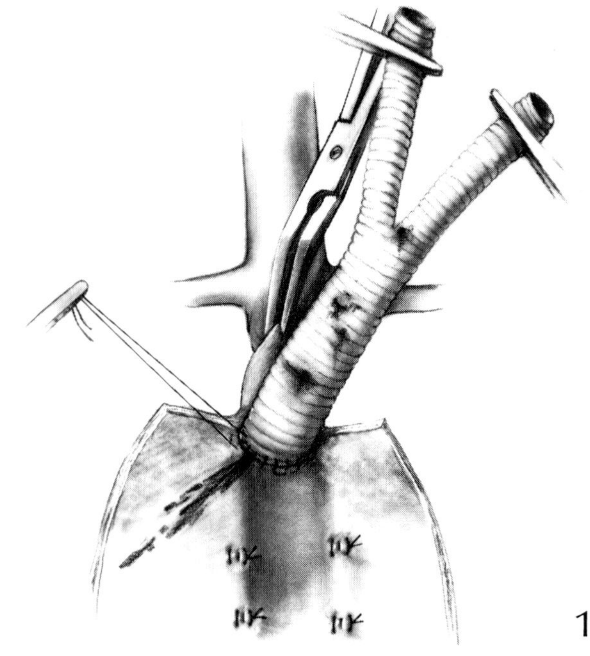

11

12

Distal aortic anastomosis

It is possible to use a tube graft and make the distal anastomosis just proximal to the bifurcation in about 66 per cent of the patients. The anterior wall of the aorta was divided with the original distal transverse 'T' incision. The posterior wall of the aorta is carefully inspected before cutting the bifurcated graft. Calcified arteriosclerotic plaques are debrided and a test stitch passed through the wall of the aorta to be sure that it will be possible to make an anastomosis at that level. The graft is then gently stretched and cut. It is important not to overstretch the graft, since it may be necessary later to elevate it if bleeding occurs from the posterior anastomotic suture line. The posterior part of the anastomosis is begun by placing a deep stitch through the ridge between normal and aneurysmal aorta. The suture is then passed from outside to the inside of the graft and continued as an over-and-over stitch around one-half the circumference of the graft. The original end of the suture is passed from inside to outside of the graft and continued as an over-and-over stitch to join the first suture, and the two ends are tied.

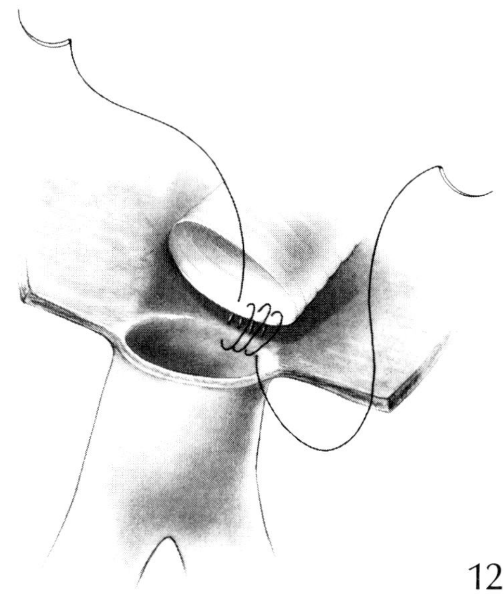

12

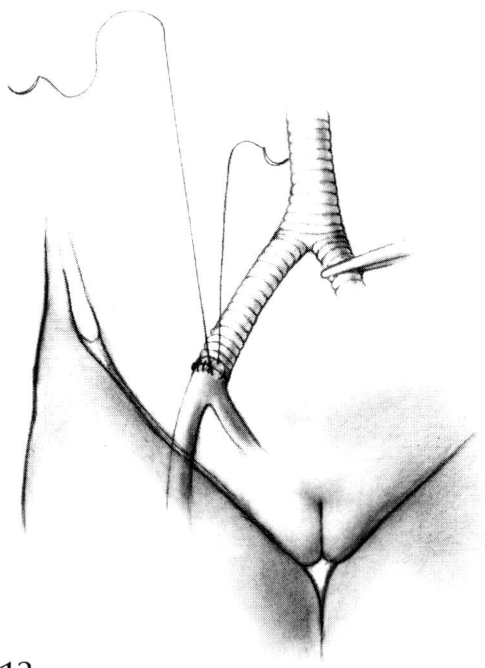

13

13

Anastomosis to the iliac artery

When the proximal iliac arteries are severely diseased, a bifurcation graft is used. One limb of the graft is occluded with a non-crushing vascular clamp. The opposite limb is then cut to the length necessary to reach the site of the distal anastomosis. A suction catheter is introduced into the limb and loose thrombi removed. It is preferable to make the anastomosis to the common iliac artery end-to-end if possible. If the common iliac is severely diseased and the external iliac artery soft-walled, the anastomosis should be made end-to-end to the external iliac artery. The internal iliac artery is divided and the distal end oversewn.

14

End-to-end anastomosis

With any end-to-end anastomosis it is advisable to pass the suture from inside to the outside of the diseased artery to tack loose intima. The suture is passed from outside the graft to inside of the graft at the end of the anastomosis opposite the surgeon. It is then run as an over-and-over stitch from inside the anastomosis. It is continued around the entire circumference of the artery and tied to the original suture. If there is a disparity in the size of the artery and graft it is helpful to place a stay suture through the midpoint of the circumference of both the artery and graft to assist in accurate approximation of the two ends.

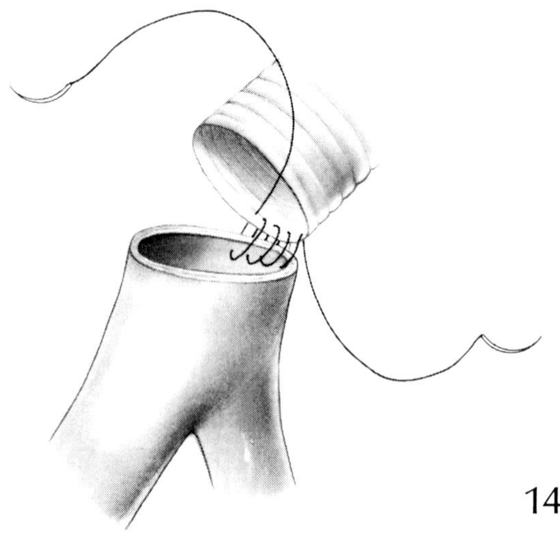

14

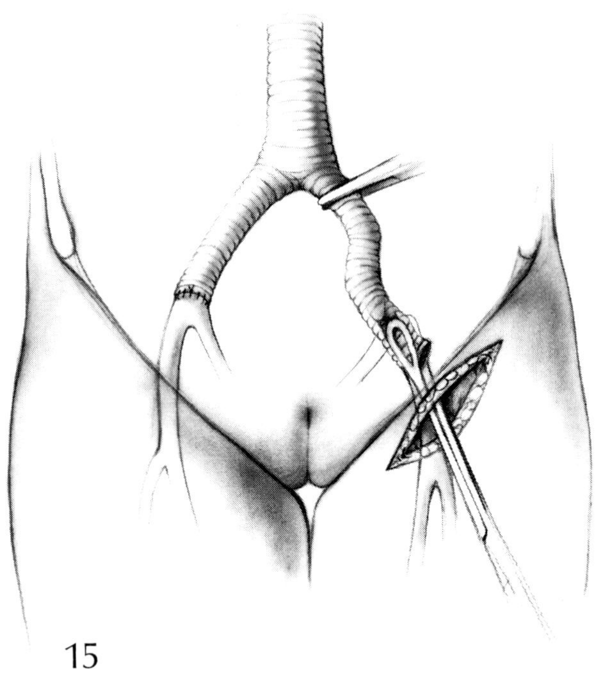

15

15

Preparation for distal anastomosis to common femoral artery

After completing the anastomosis of one limb of the graft, the distal clamp is removed, allowing retrograde filling of the graft. The clamp on the opposite limb is then removed and the limb with the completed anastomosis is occluded as the proximal clamp is removed to flush any debris from the graft. Flow is gradually restored to the leg with the completed anastomosis while carefully monitoring the blood pressure. Sudden drops in blood pressure can be expected unless the clamps are slowly and intermittently removed over a 5–10 minute period. If it is necessary to carry the craft to the groin, a clamp is passed from the groin incision over the femoral artery and retroperitoneally to the sacral promontory. The limb of the graft is carefully orientated and passed to the groin.

16

Oversewing common iliac artery

It is important carefully to oversew the common iliac artery since in the presence of a patent external iliac artery there will be abundant retrograde flow and systemic pressure in the stump of the divided common iliac artery. If there is calcified plaque in the common iliac artery a short endarterectomy is performed. Stay sutures are then placed in opposite sides of the artery about 1 cm from the cut end and tied. A continuous mattress stitch is made from the first stay suture to the other and the suture tied. One end of the tied suture is run as a continuous over-and-over stitch back to the first stay suture and tied.

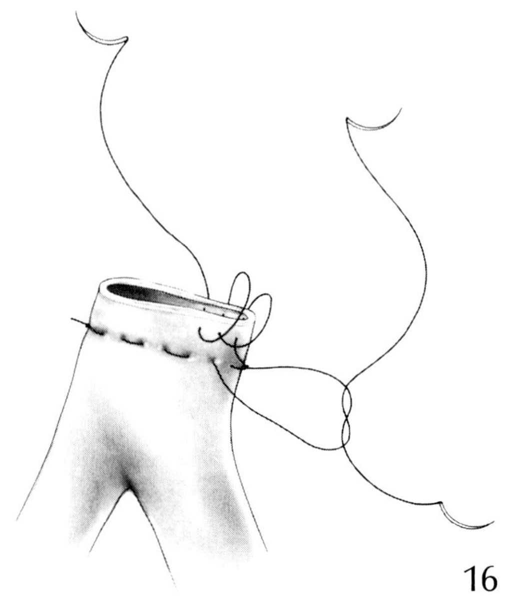

16

17

Distal anastomosis to common femoral artery

The common femoral artery is mobilized from the inguinal ligament to the profunda femoris artery. An end-to-side anastomosis is made to the occluded common femoral artery (*see* chapter on 'Aortoiliac reconstruction', pp.136–151). Backflow from the femoral artery is checked prior to completion of the anastomosis. If the backflow is unsatisfactory, a Fogarty thrombectomy catheter is passed distally and any thrombi removed (*see* chapter on 'Arterial embolectomy', pp. 856–861 in this volume). Flow is also gradually re-established to this limb. Protamine sulphate is then administered intravenously in doses of 1 mg for each 100 units of heparin sodium given when the vessels were clamped.

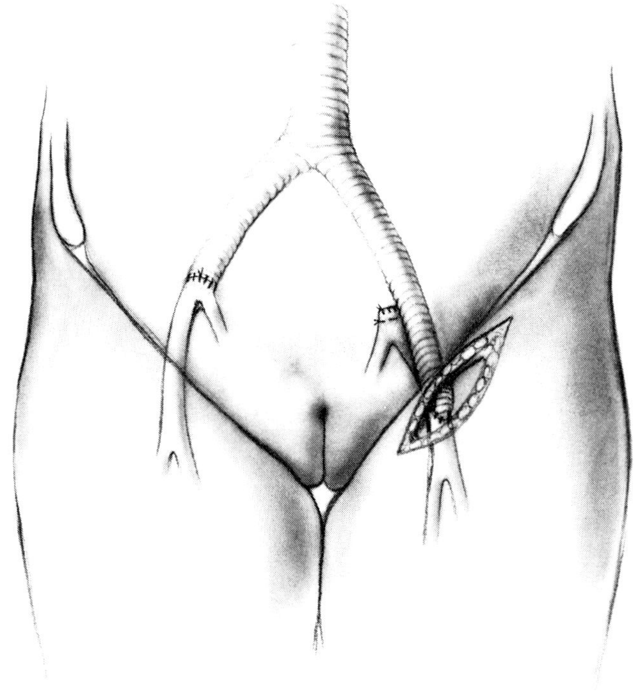

17

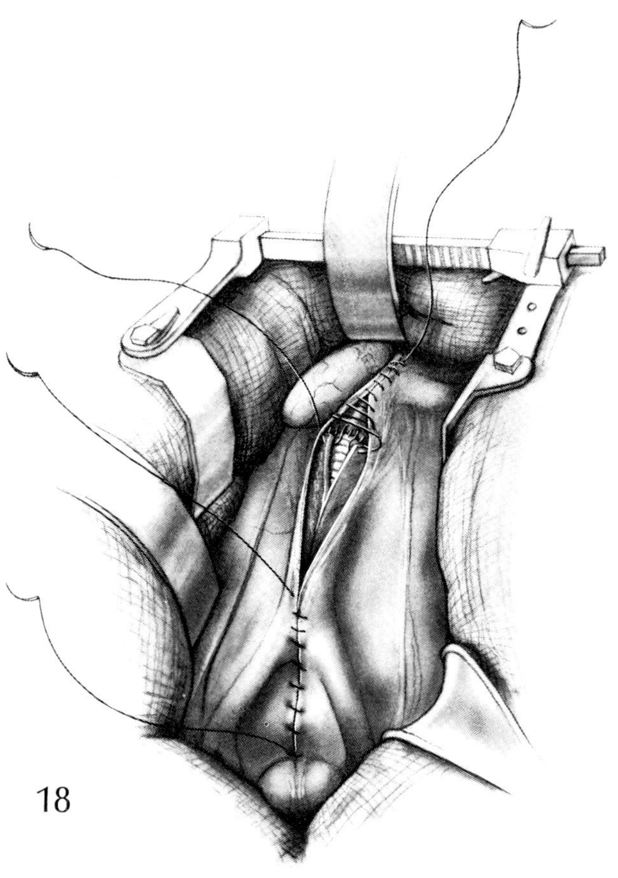

18

18

Closure of peritoneum and aortic wall

In order to avoid aortoenteric fistulae it is important to separate the graft and particularly the anastomoses from direct contact with the duodenum and jejunum. Bleeding from the cut edge of the aneurysm sac is first controlled with cautery and suture ligatures. A stay suture is placed at each end of the incision. The peritoneum and the edge of the aneurysm sac, where appropriate, are then approximated with a single-layer continuous stitch of 0 chromic catgut. As the superior peritoneal stitch reaches the level of the cut aneurysm sac, the tip of the edge of the sac is included in a stitch which is then passed through the adventitia of the aorta, the opposite tip of the edge of the sac and finally the peritoneum. The stitch is continued and tied to the inferior suture.

Suprarenal abdominal aortic aneurysms

Suprarenal aortic aneurysms usually involve the lower thoracic aorta as well but may be confined to the abdominal aorta. These dumb-bell shaped aneurysms may be suspected on the basis of a preoperative aortogram or CAT scan but on occasion are an unexpected finding at operation. If the infrarenal cuff of the aneurysm is narrow and the suprarenal component thick walled, it may be judicious to resect and replace only the infrarenal portion. The suprarenal aneurysm can then be carefully followed and resected through a thoracoabdominal approach if it becomes symptomatic.

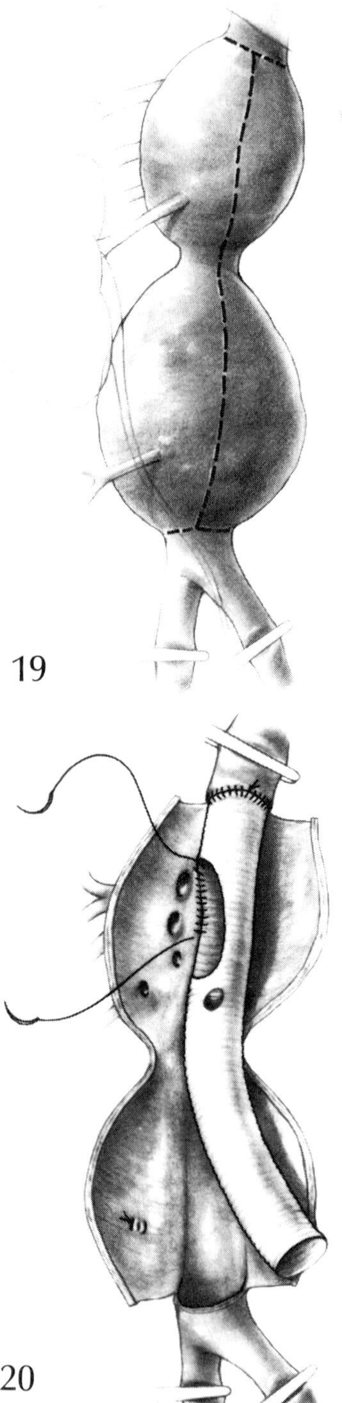

19

20

19

Exposure

The infradiaphragmatic suprarenal aneurysm may be resected through an extended abdominal incision. The left rectus muscle is divided in the epigastrium and the incision carried out through the 9th interspace. The left posterior gutter peritoneum is incised to enter the retroperitoneum. The spleen, stomach, pancreas, left colon and left kidney are retracted medially.

20

Insertion of graft

The aorta is clamped above and below the aneurysm. A longitudinal incision is made 3 cm posterior to the origin of the left renal artery. The clot is removed and any bleeding lumbar arteries are oversewn or included in the anastomosis of the aortic wall to the graft. The proximal aortic anastomosis is performed from the inside as previously described. The origins of two or more of the right renal, coeliac, superior mesenteric and left renal arteries may be close to one another in a relatively thick-walled portion of the aneurysm. The left renal artery is frequently 2–3 cm away. An elliptical button which is large enough to encircle adjacent origins of the arterial branches is cut out of the graft. Back bleeding from the branches may be controlled with balloon catheters if necessary.

21

Anastomosis of aortic wall to graft[12]

The posterior edge of the opening in the graft is sutured from inside the graft to the aorta posterior to the origins of the vessel. The continuous stitch is carried around the anterior edge of the graft opening anterior to the origins of the vessels. It is important to include all layers of the aortic wall in these sutures and to place the suture line close to the origin of the vessels without narrowing the orifices. In this way a minimal amount of the dilated weakened aorta is included in the anastomosis. When all of the anastomoses of the aortic wall to graft are completed the graft is flushed. The proximal aortic clamp is released and the graft clamped distal to the aortic wall anastomoses while the distal anastomosis to the infrarenal aorta is completed.

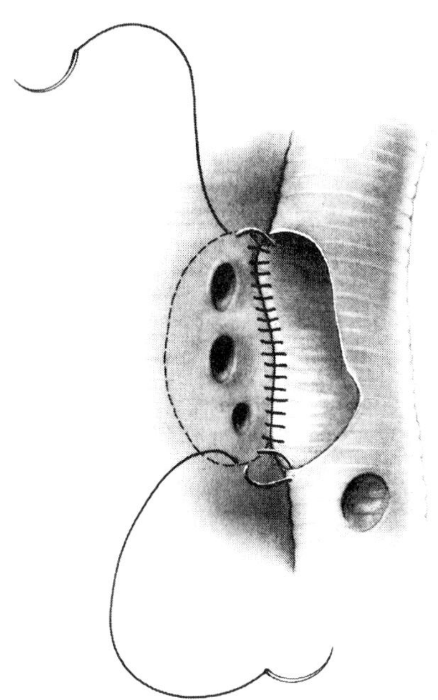

21

Special postoperative care

Monitoring

It is advisable to continue careful continuous monitoring of the patient for at least the first 24–48 hours postoperatively and longer if the patient is unstable. Intra-abdominal bleeding can be recognized by falling central venous, intracardiac or systemic arterial pressures, decreased urinary output and increased girth of the abdomen, which is recorded hourly with a tape measure. It is important to maintain systemic arterial pressures and central pressures within normal limits to prevent decreased cardiac output or left ventricular strain and thereby maintain myocardial oxygenation. In high risk patients endotracheal intubation and assisted respiration is continued for 18 hours to ensure adequate myocardial and cerebral oxygenation and prevent atelectasis. Urinary output is monitored carefully for the first 48 hours and assisted with diuretics or increased fluids as indicated from monitoring devices.

Pulmonary

Vigorous pulmonary therapy is instituted when the patient awakes from anaesthesia. Turning from side-to-side, 'cupping' the chest, deep breathing exercises and assisted coughing are all important. The incision is large and may be painful. Judicious use of narcotics and holding a firm object to the wound makes coughing easier. Early ambulation on the first or second postoperative day also assists the mechanics of respiration.

Paralytic Ileus

This follows nearly every abdominal aortic operation and should be treated by gastric aspiration with an indwelling tube until intestinal mobility has been re-established.

References

1. Dubost, C., Allary, M., Oeconomos, N. Resection of an aneurysm of the abdominal aorta. Archives of Surgery 1952; 64: 405–408

2. DeBakey, M. E., Crawford, E. S., Cooley, D. A., Morris, G. C., Jr, Royster, T. S., Abbott, W. P. Aneurysm of abdominal aorta. Analysis of results of graft replacement therapy one to eleven years after operation. Annals of Surgery 1964; 160: 622–639

3. Rob, C. G., Eastcott, H. H. G., Owen, K. The reconstruction of arteries. British Journal of Surgery 1956; 43: 449–466

4. Vasko, J. S., Spencer, F. C., Bahnson, H. T. Aneurysm of the aorta treated by excision. Review of 237 cases followed up to seven years. American Journal of Surgery 1963; 105: 793–801

5. Leather, R. P., Shah, D., Goldman, M., Rosenberg, M., Karmody, A. M. Nonresective treatment of abdominal aortic aneurysms: use of acute thrombosis and axillofemoral by-pass. Archives of Surgery 1979; 114: 1408–1409

6. Darling, R. C., Messina, C. R., Brewster, D. C., Ottinger, L. W. Autopsy study of unoperated abdominal aortic aneurysms. The case for early resection. Circulation 1977; 56 (Suppl. 2): II,–161–164

7. Hicks, G. L., Eastland, M. W., DeWeese, J. A., May, A. G., Rob, C. G. Survival improvement following aortic aneurysm resection. Annals of Surgery 1975; 181: 863–869

8. Hertzer, N. R. Fatal myocardial infarction following abdominal aortic aneurysm resection. Annals of Surgery 1980; 192: 667–673

9. Bush, H. L., LoGerfo, F. W., Weisel, R. D., Mannick, J. A., Hechtman, H. B. Assessment of myocardial performance and optimal volume loading during elective abdominal aortic aneurysm resection. Archives of Surgery 1977; 112: 1301–1306

10. Babu, S. C., Sharma, P. V. P., Raciti, A., *et al.* Monitor-guided responses. Operability with safety is increased in patients with peripheral vascular disease. Archives of Surgery 1980; 115: 1384–1386

11. McCabe, C. J., Coleman, W. S., Brewster, D. C. The advantage of early operation for abdominal aortic aneurysm. Archives of Surgery 1981; 116: 1025–1029

12. Crawford, E. S. Thoraco-abdominal and abdominal aortic aneurysms involving renal, superior mesenteric, and celiac arteries. Annals of Surgery 1974; 179: 763–772

Management of vascular injuries

Malcolm O. Perry MD
Professor of Surgery, Cornell University Medical College, New York, USA

Aetiology – mechanisms of injury

Although major vascular injuries can be encountered in any civilian setting, the highest incidence is in urban areas where violence is endemic. Penetrating wounds caused by knives and bullets are usually seen, but accidental stab wounds caused by shards of glass or metal also occur. The damage produced by knives or bullets travelling at a low velocity is mainly confined to the wound tract, but high-velocity bullets are associated with blast injury. As the blast cavity collapses, a suction effect is generated which can draw skin, dirt and bits of clothing into the wound. Secondary missiles (bullet fragments or bone splinters) can produce further damage. Such destructive effects may not be suspected from inspection of the skin where, in some cases, rather small wounds are present[1,2].

Motor vehicle accidents are important causes of vascular trauma and victims frequently have multiple injuries. Direct vessel trauma occurs, but often vascular wounds are the result of fractures and dislocations. This is especially likely to occur near joints where the vessels are relatively fixed. Dislocations of the knee, for example, are particularly prone to injure the popliteal artery and similar episodes can damage the brachial or axillary vessels.

Lacerations are seen most often with knife wounds, but contusions, punctures and transections also are encountered. Stretching, angulation and subsequent occlusion are more often seen with fracture dislocations, but the concussive effects of high-velocity missiles can cause such wounds. Immediate vessel disruption and bleeding may not occur, but delayed thrombosis or haemorrhage can lead to ischaemia or false aneurysm formation.

Clinical evaluation

Most arterial injuries can be identified readily because of external haemorrhage or large haematomas. Ischaemia distal to the injury is uncommon with isolated vascular injuries except for wounds of the popliteal and common femoral arteries. Moreover, distal pulses may be intact in up to 20 per cent of patients with acknowledged arterial wounds, although weak or absent distal pulses are important findings[2]. The indications for operative exploration of a suspected vascular wound are summarized as follows:

1. Diminished or absent distal pulse.
2. Persistent arterial bleeding.
3. Large or expanding haematoma.
4. Major haemorrhage with hypotension or shock.
5. Bruit at or distal to suspected site of injury.
6. Injury of anatomically related nerves.

Arteriography can be very useful in the evaluation of potential arterial injuries, especially in patients with multiple pellet wounds, fractures and penetrating injuries of the neck and thoracic outlet. If high-grade, biplane films can be obtained, arteriography presents reliable, although not infallible, evidence regarding the presence or absence of an arterial wound. Moreover, surgical management may be improved by identifying the location and extent of the vascular damage.

Preparation for surgery

Most patients with major vascular wounds require immediate operation, and if haemodynamically unstable they should be taken directly to the operating theatre. If the patient is stable, further diagnostic manoeuvres can be undertaken.

Bleeding is controlled with direct pressure (tourniquets are avoided) and two large-bore intravenous lines secured. Balanced salt solutions are given intravenously while type specific and matched blood is obtained. General anaesthesia is preferred, and special precautions must be taken to avoid extending the damage or dislodging clots in patients with cervical and thoracic wounds. Wide operative fields are prepared since, in patients with wounds in or near the trunk, it may be necessary to enter the abdomen or chest.

General principles

1

Incisions

Vertical incisions are favoured for exposing vascular wounds – they can be extended easily in either direction along the course of the vessel and they are parallel to other neurovascular structures. A vertical incision into the anterior cervical triangle to expose the carotid artery can be extended into a midline sternotomy, for example, or lateral supraclavicular incision as needed. Similarly, a midline abdominal incision can be extended into the sternum or across the costal margin to enter the chest.

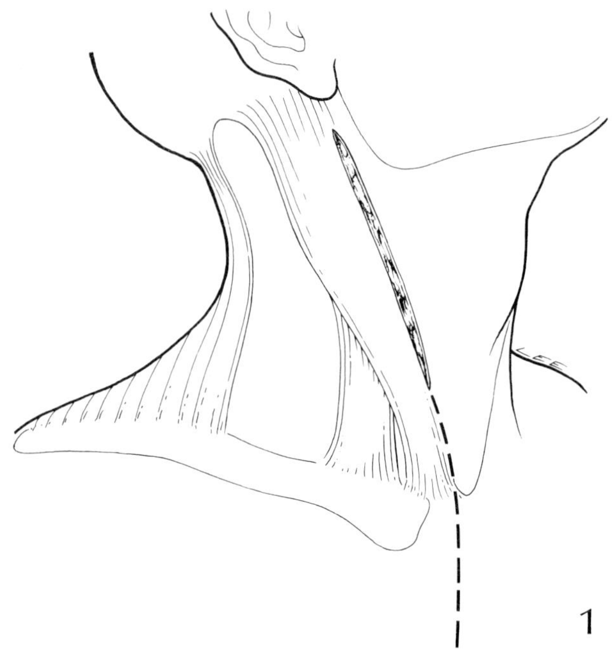
1

Exposure

If the haematoma is large, it is often best to expose the vessels proximally and gain control where the artery is clearly seen. Latex tubing or soft vascular tapes are passed around the vessels and vascular clamps selected. Usually the vascular wound can then be approached safely and the bleeding controlled with direct digital pressure. With multiple injuries, and especially if large veins are involved, temporary proximal and distal vascular occlusion and vigorous suction may be required.

Debridement

Lacerations or punctures of larger vessels can be treated by lateral repair, but it is best not to make a firm decision regarding closure until debridement is concluded. Most civilian wounds are inflicted by knives or low-velocity missiles and wide debridement is unnecessary, but blunt trauma and high-velocity bullets cause more extensive damage.

Graft interposition

Resection and end-to-end anastomosis is usually required, but if this cannot be done without tension, graft interposition is indicated. Autogenous grafts (saphenous vein from the ankle, cephalic vein, autogenous artery) are preferred, but prosthetic grafts have been used successfully, and are required in the large vessels of the aortoiliac system. Dacron has been used more often, but polytetrafluoroethylene is chosen frequently now, and may be more resistant to subsequent infection.

2 & 3

Anastomoses

Continuous suture techniques are satisfactory in most situations, but small vessels (less than 4 mm diameter) are best joined with fine interrupted sutures. A wider suture line in small arteries can be obtained if an oblique or spatulated anastomosis is constructed.

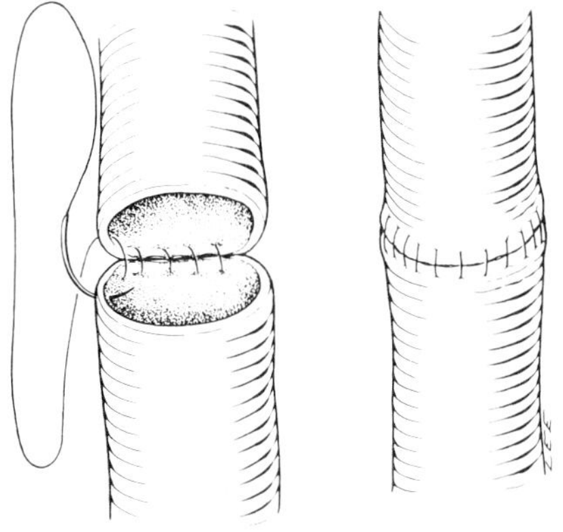

2

Anticoagulants

Systemic heparin is often given to patients with isolated vascular wounds, but many trauma surgeons believe that full doses of heparin are contraindicated in patients with multiple injuries, and in those with damage to the central nervous system and eyes. Local irrigation of the damaged vessels with a solution containing 100 units of heparin per 10 ml saline is helpful in removing debris and retarding local thrombosis. No anticoagulants are used postoperatively.

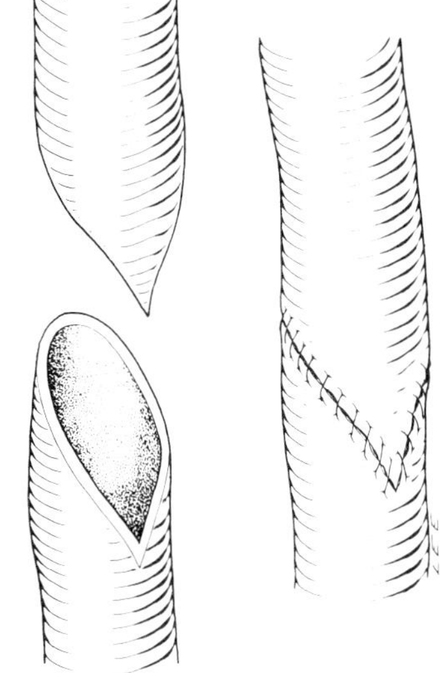

3

Determining patency

A diligent search for distal clots is mandatory, despite what may appear to be adequate backbleeding. Most surgeons routinely pass a Fogarty catheter in both directions prior to completion of the repair. If distal pulses and normal flow are not readily obtained, arteriography is indicated before the operation is terminated.

To illustrate the application of these principles, the management of three of the more common vascular injuries are described: a penetrating wound of the carotid artery, stab wound of the inferior vena cava and a gunshot wound of the femoral artery.

Carotid artery injuries

4

Sites of injury

Penetrating cervical wounds which pierce the platysma muscle usually are explored in the operating theatre. The vessels most often injured are the common carotid artery (CCA) and the jugular vein (usually the vein is ligated). The management of carotid artery injuries is assisted by dividing the neck into three zones: Zone I, above the angle of the mandible; Zone II, between the angle of the mandible and 1 cm above the clavicles; and Zone III, below Zone II (includes the thoracic outlet area).

Preoperative arteriography can be helpful in managing any carotid injury, but those patients with wounds in Zones I and III and those with neurological deficits usually require angiograms to plan the operations[3].

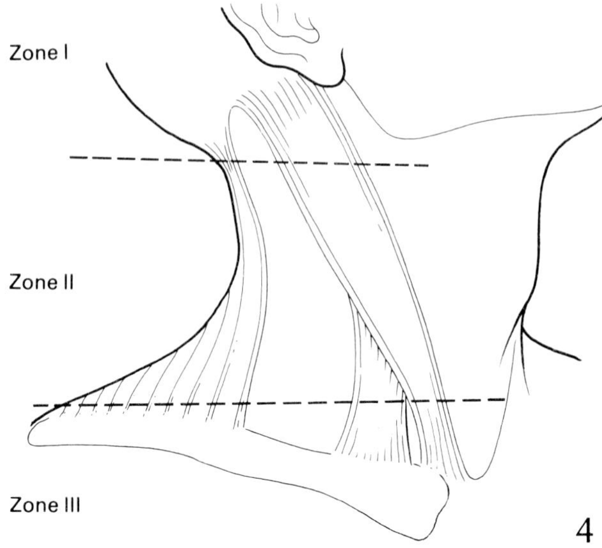

4

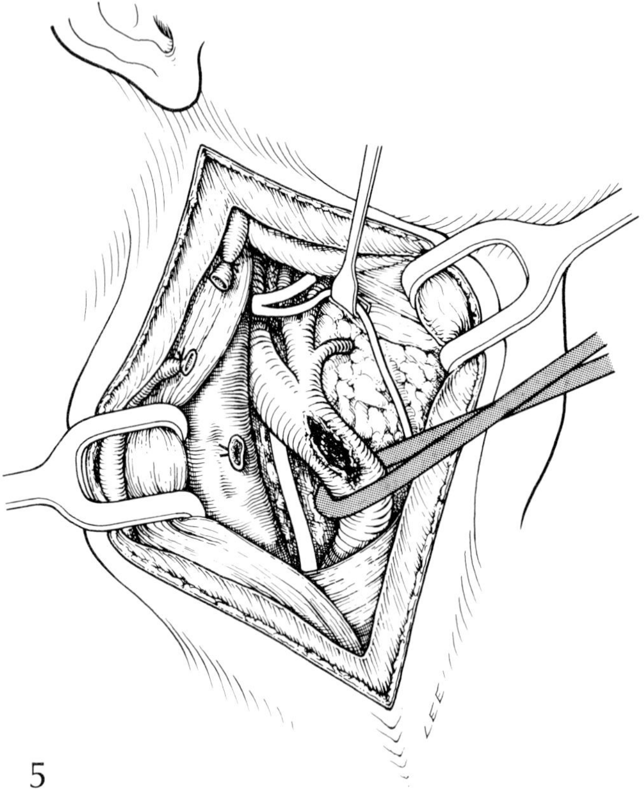

5

5

Zone II injuries (common carotid)

The midcervical carotid artery is exposed through an incision anterior to the sternomastoid muscle. The common carotid artery proximal to the wound is encircled first, then distal control is obtained if feasible. Bleeding initially is controlled with gentle finger pressure, then vascular clamps are applied. If simple suture is impossible, patch graft angioplasty or resection and anastomosis are undertaken.

Zone II injuries (internal carotid)

6

A large proximal wound of the internal carotid artery (ICA) can be repaired by substituting the external carotid. Fine interrupted sutures are used.

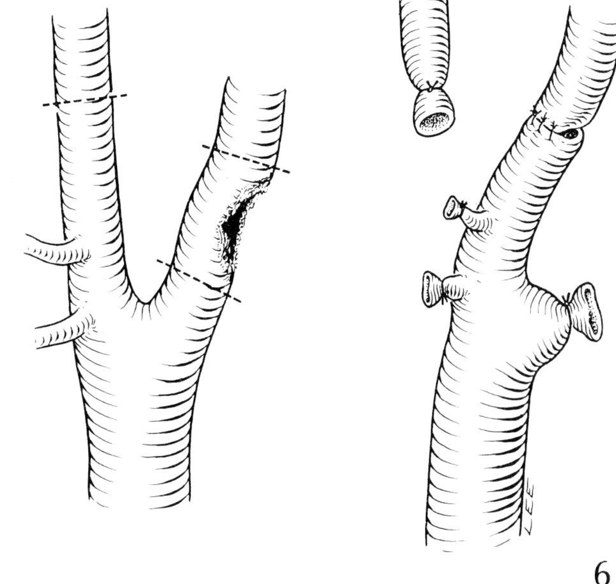

6

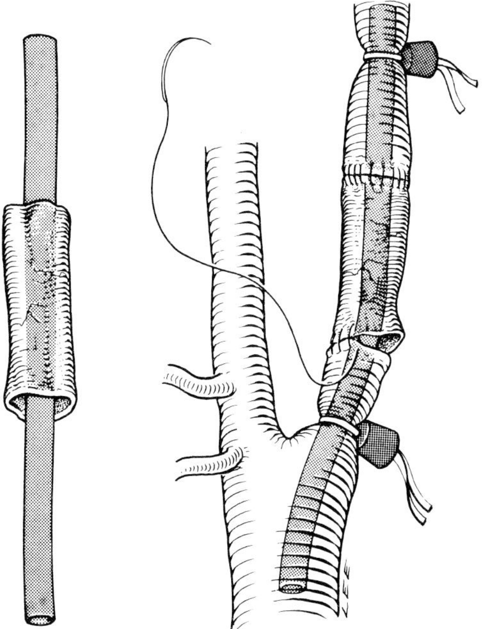

7

7

Graft interposition

If the damage to the ICA is extensive and there is scanty backbleeding from the distal artery, an autogenous saphenous vein graft from the ankle is threaded over a 10 Fr shunt and interposed between the debrided ends of the artery.

Zone III and Zone I injuries

Injuries of the CCA in Zone III may require median sternotomy for control of bleeding before the wound is exposed. ICA wounds at the base of the skull (Zone I) are difficult to expose, and it may be necessary to divide the digastric muscle, excise the styloid process or temporarily dislocate the mandible.

Inferior vena cava injuries

It has been reported that 1 in every 50 gunshot wounds and one in every 300 knife wounds of the abdomen damages the inferior vena cava (IVC). One-third of the victims die before reaching the hospital and half the remainder die during treatment. Multiple wounds of other organs are common – over three-quarters of the patients have damage to other retroperitoneal structures[4].

Most of these patients obviously have a serious injury – usually a bullet wound of the lower chest or abdomen – and shock. There are few laboratory data of diagnostic value and it is best to take unstable patients directly to surgery.

Exposure

The abdomen is opened through a midline incision from xiphoid to pubis, the extent of damage assessed and priorities set. All centrally located retroperitoneal haematomas above the pelvis are explored.

Control of bleeding

8

Initially bleeding is controlled with finger pressure or sponge sticks.

Sometimes small lacerations and punctures can be closed with simple sutures passed beneath an occluding finger or the edges of the IVC can be held together with vascular forceps.

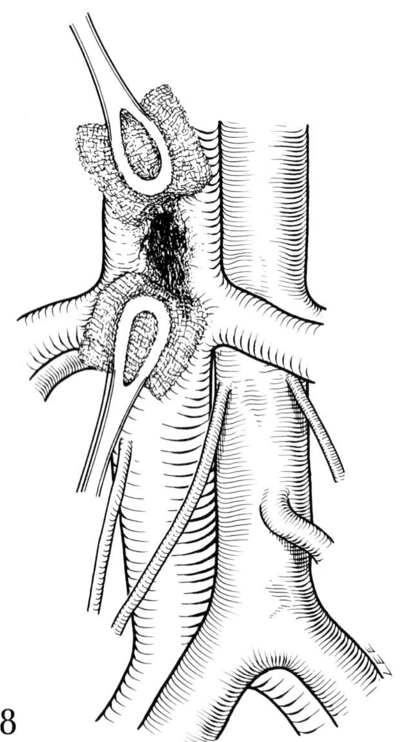

8

9

More often, a partially occluding vascular clamp (Satinsky) is needed to permit accurate repair. Occasionally accurate clamp application may be too difficult and a balloon catheter (Foley or Fogarty) can be inserted to plug the wound and stop the bleeding.

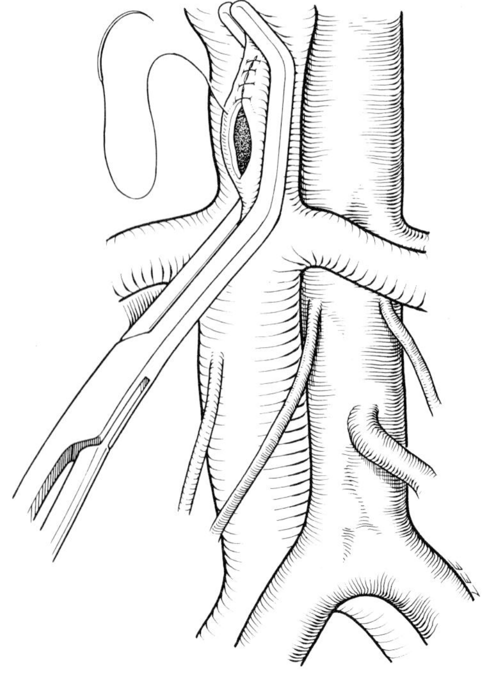

9

10

Through-and-through injuries

Wounds which pierce both anterior and posterior walls of the IVC can be closed by lateral repair after mobilizing the cava by ligating and dividing one or two sets of lumbar veins. Alternatively, the anterior wound can be enlarged and the posterior laceration closed from within the IVC. The anterior wall is then repaired.

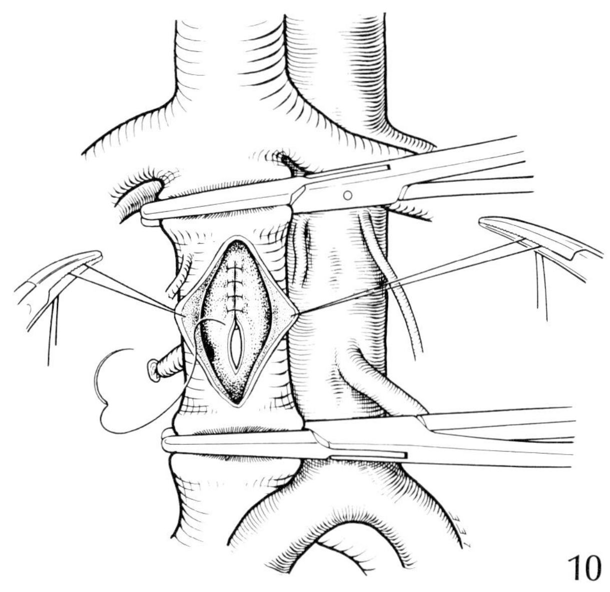

10

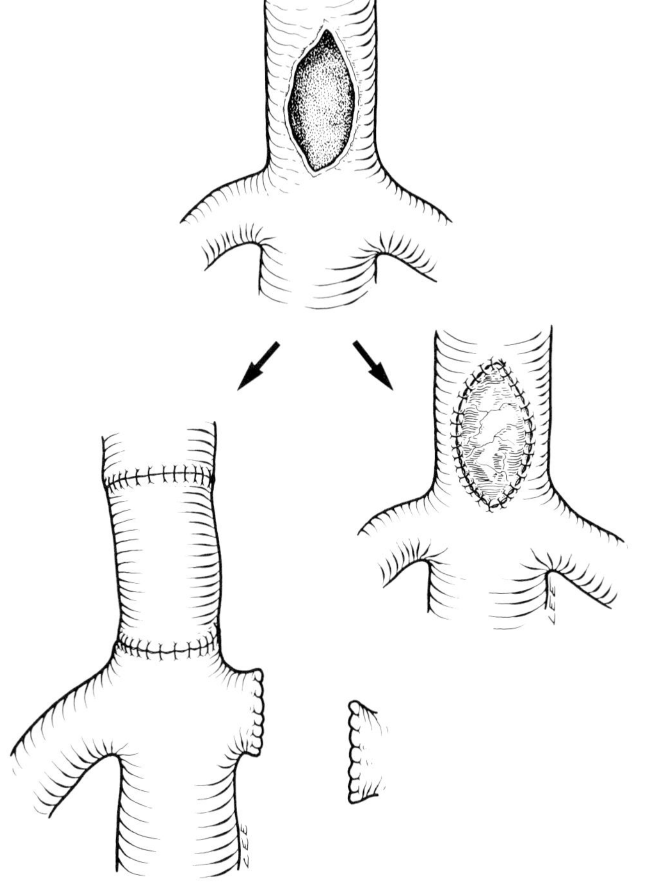

11

Suprarenal cava injuries

11

More extensive suprarenal IVC damage may require a vein graft (the left renal vein or the common iliac vein is preferred) or a patch graft. For the infrarenal cava, especially in unstable patients with multiple injuries, ligation is recommended.

Division of the ligaments and anterior and medial rotation of the right lobe of the liver usually will permit repair of the suprarenal cava and hepatic veins (one major hepatic vein or any small accessory hepatic vein can be ligated safely).

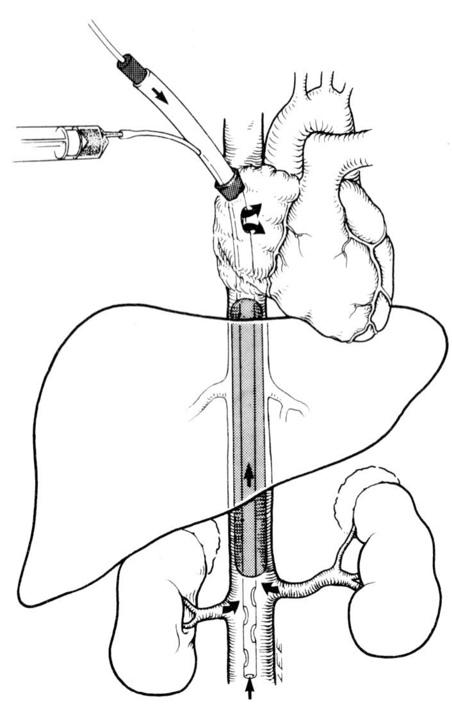

12

12 & 13

If prolonged IVC occlusion is necessary for repair or if bleeding is so brisk as to obscure vision, a transatrial intracaval shunt (Madding-Kennedy) is inserted. The right atrium is reached by extending the abdominal incision into a midline sternotomy. This manoeuvre is not often required, however.

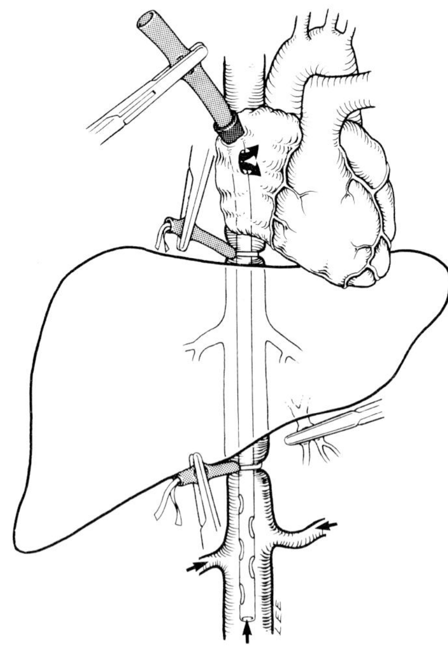

13

Gunshot wound of the femoral artery

Femoral artery wounds comprise approximately 20 per cent of all arterial injuries. These are serious problems. Haemorrhage is often profuse and acute ligation of the common femoral artery results in amputation rates near 50 per cent – only slightly less than that following acute occlusion of the popliteal artery[2].

Most patients with penetrating trauma have severe haemorrhage, or large haematomas: the injury is obvious and immediate surgery is required. If arteriograms are needed to visualize the profunda or popliteal-tibial systems, they can be obtained in theatre.

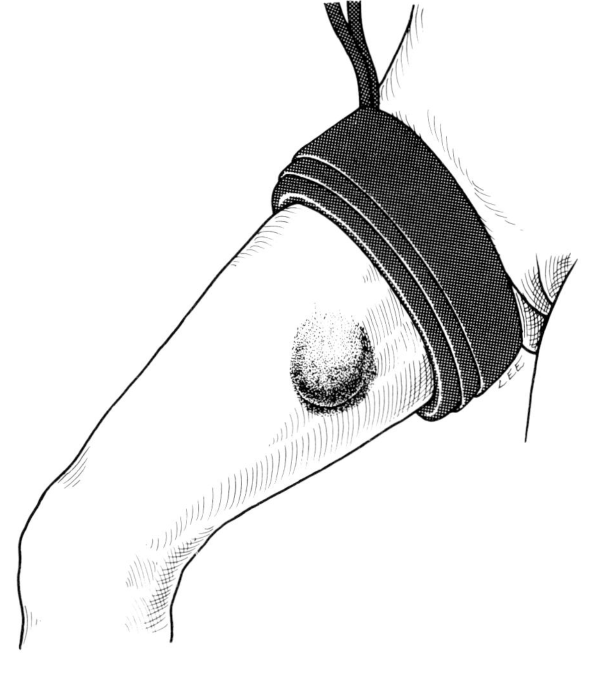

14

14

Compression control

Usually bleeding can be managed at surgery with finger pressure, but if there are multiple wounds, or large haematomas, it is prudent to place an orthopaedic pneumatic cuff proximally before draping the limb. Troublesome bleeding can be arrested quickly by inflating the cuff.

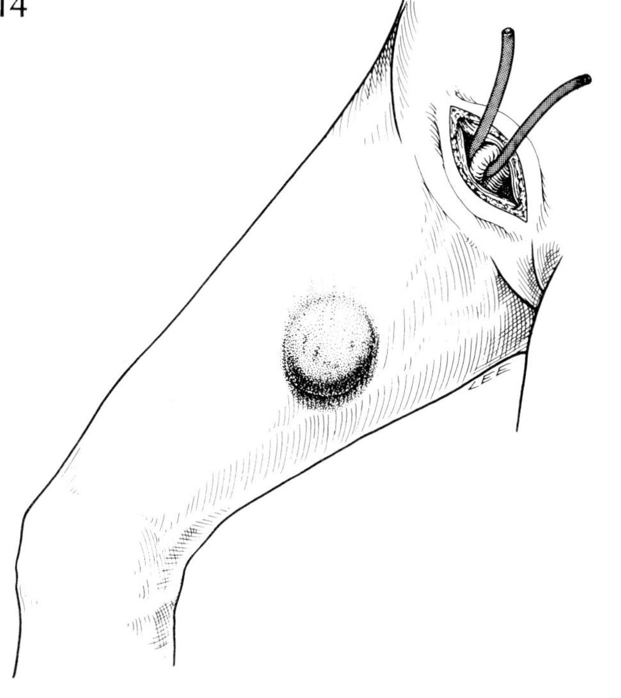

15

15

Proximal control

If there is insufficient room to place a proximal tourniquet, the external iliac artery can be encircled with a vascular tape through a muscle-splitting extraperitoneal incision above the inguinal ligament.

16

Direct control

Once proximal control is secured, the haematoma is evacuated and vascular clamps applied. Although punctures can be repaired with simple sutures, resection and anastomosis is preferred in most situations. If this is not possible without tension a saphenous vein graft is selected.

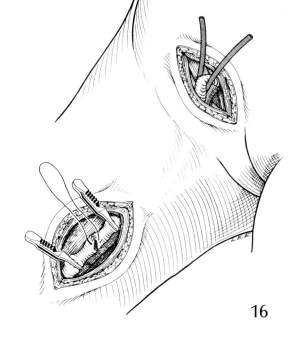

16

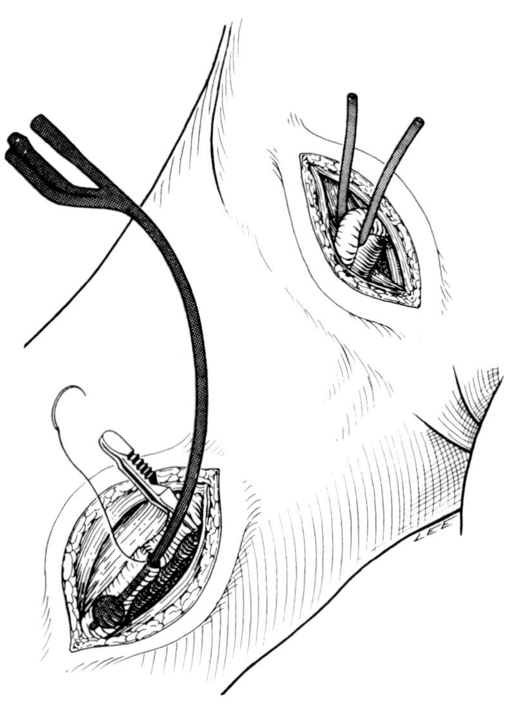

17

17

Determining patency

Prior to completing the repair a Fogarty catheter is passed to ensure a patent system free of clots. Major vein injuries are repaired with simple suture techniques, or resection and anastomosis if this does not prolong the operation unduly. Grafts are needed only on rare occasions (popliteal vein).

Postoperatively the distal pulses and limb blood pressures are followed, but a regular evaluation of neuromuscular function is essential. Any deterioration in the perception of light touch or motor function is a firm indication for further studies – usually arteriography – regardless of skin colour or temperature, distal pulses or limb blood pressure[1].

References

1. Perry, M. O. The Management of acute vascular injuries. Baltimore: Williams and Wilkins, 1980

2. Rich, N. M., Spencer, F. C. Vascular trauma. Philadelphia: W. B. Saunders Co., 1978

3. Thal, E. R., Snyder, W. H., Hays, R. J., Perry, M. O. Management of carotid artery injuries. Surgery 1974; 76: 955–962

4. Perry, M. O. In: Schwartz, S. I., ed. Principles of surgery, 3rd edition. New York: McGraw-Hill, 1979: 273–276

Operations for varicose veins

John T. Hobbs MD, FRCS
Senior Lecturer in Surgery, University of London;
Consultant Surgeon, St Mary's Hospital, London, UK

CLASSIFICATION OF VARICOSE VEINS

The term 'varicose veins' refers to abnormally prominent veins on the lower limb. These can be classified into distinct types as follows.

Dilated venules, venous 'flares', 'bursts' or 'stars', telangiectases

These small vessels are only of cosmetic importance, being related to skin structure and hormonal effects but may be secondary to varicosis, as with the typical 'ankle flare'.

Athlete's hypertrophic veins

In healthy athletes the veins may be prominent but this dilatation is not abnormal being due to high blood volume and increased flow through muscular limbs.

Arteriovenous fistulae

Arterial pressure transmitted to the venous system directly will result in venous dilatation. This may be associated with congenital disorders such as Klippel-Trenaunay syndrome, where grossly dilated veins may be present which are atypical in distribution. Dilated veins are also seen in association with acquired arteriovenous fistula which may follow gunshot, stab wounds or surgical trauma.

1a & b

Internal iliac vein incompetence

This only occurs in women as a complication of pregnancy or, rarely, following pelvic infection and may be a sequel to thrombosis in the pelvic veins. Varices arise from the posterior vulval region and extend down the medial aspect of the upper thigh and over the back of the thigh or across the adductor tendon to join the long saphenous system. These small veins are particularly painful during the premenstrual period and sometimes following coitus.

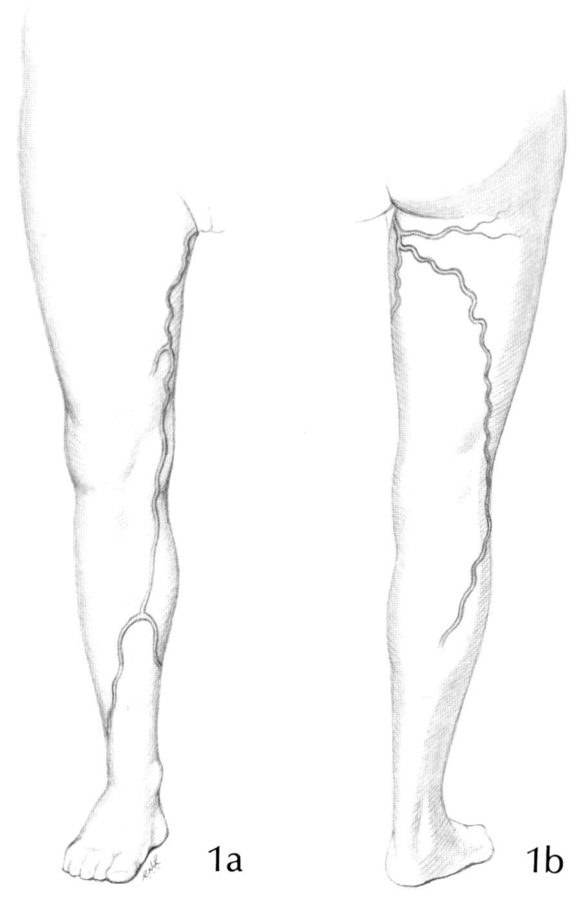

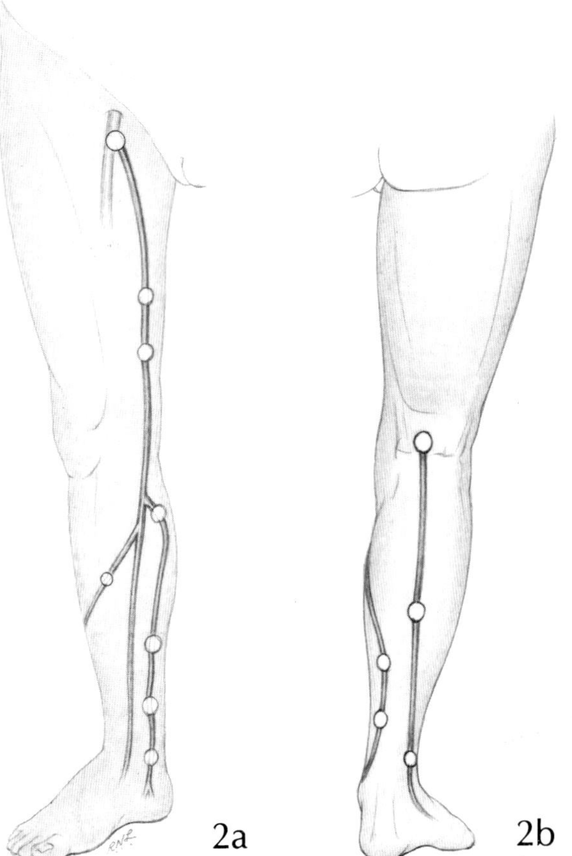

2a & b

Primary varicose veins

This is the most common problem requiring treatment. There is usually a family history and the inherent defect is either a weakness of the vein wall or valvular insufficiency and often a combination of both. The long saphenous system is the most frequently involved vein and the incompetence of the saphenofemoral vein junction may result in dilatation of the long saphenous vein or its anterolateral tributary. Below the knee, the incompetence usually involves the posterior arch tributary, sometimes the anterior tibial vein but rarely the long saphenous vein below the upper third of the calf. Incompetence of the short saphenous system may be associated with incompetence of the long saphenous system or may occur alone. The primary incompetence may also involve the large direct perforating veins.

Secondary varicose veins

The superficial leg veins may become dilated if the venous outflow from the leg is obstructed by extrinsic pressure caused by enlarged lymph nodes, pelvic tumours and bony displacements, or by occlusion of the lumen due to iliac vein thrombosis. Similarly, the superficial veins in the thigh, particularly the long saphenous vein, may become varicose when functioning as collateral pathways to overcome occlusion of the superficial femoral vein in the post-thrombotic syndrome.

In the later stages of the post-thrombotic syndrome with valvular insufficiency of the popliteal vein distal to proximal obstruction or valvular destruction, the perforating veins in the lower leg become grossly incompetent resulting in dilated veins on the lower leg and secondary skin damage. Sometimes the perforating veins become incompetent after local thrombosis without involvement of the deep veins.

Treatment should be confined to eliminating the incompetent perforating veins by sclerotherapy. This protects the skin from the underlying deep vein damage, which cannot be cured.

TREATMENT OF VARICOSE VEINS

It is evident that to treat venous problems effectively each limb must be carefully assessed and an accurate diagnosis established. The correct plan of treatment must then be made and precisely executed. The methods of treatment include reassurance, elastic stockings, sclerotherapy and surgery.

Some patients can be reassured that the veins are not significant and that the symptoms are due to some other cause, such as referred pain from the lumbar spine, arthritis or arterial disease.

Elastic stockings will hide veins and prevent the condition deteriorating but will not cure them.

Venous problems can only be cured by either sclerotherapy or surgery. For sclerotherapy to be effective the vein must be kept occluded after the introduction of a destructive agent until fibrosis is permanent. Therefore injection compression is an effective method whenever the treated veins can be bandaged. The termination of the long and short saphenous veins and the upper thighs cannot be adequately bandaged; therefore venous problems involving these veins and those on the upper thigh are best treated by surgical methods, rather than sclerotherapy.

There is no standard operation for varicose veins–each leg must be carefully assessed, accurately marked and dealt with accordingly. The commonest operations are those on the long saphenous and short saphenous vein systems. Incompetent perforating veins can either be treated surgically whilst dealing with the saphenous systems or they can be treated by sclerotherapy. With the use of effective injection techniques there is now no need for the radical subfascial approach to ligate perforating veins.

Indications for operation

Primary varicosis is progressive and, if untreated, the veins increase in number and size. The condition may often be cured by adequate surgery during the earlier stages. Therefore, progression of the disorder is an indication for active treatment.

The two most common complaints causing patients to seek treatment are aching discomfort in the legs when standing and the cosmetic appearance. Treatment is also indicated for complications, which include superficial thrombophlebitis, acute bleeding, eczema and ulceration.

Operations available

The standard operations are the following.

1. Flush ligation and division of the long saphenous vein at the groin, together with stripping of the main trunks down to the upper calf and removal of the dilated and tortuous tributaries (LSV strip).
2. Flush ligation and division of the short saphenous vein at its termination, which is usually in the popliteal fossa, and stripping of its trunk and major tributaries (SSV strip).
3. Occasional exposure, ligation and division of ankle-perforating veins if they are grossly enlarged and incompetent.

Note: In this context 'flush' refers to ligation and division of the saphenous veins flush with the femoral or popliteal vein, so that the ligature is proximal to all tributaries.

The surgery need not be radical because any residual small tributaries can later be treated by injection if they do not disappear after surgical removal of the proximal incompetent vein. Both legs can be treated together and meticulous care is required to prevent recurrence. Although the operation provides excellent training for the trainee surgeon, supervision is necessary because of the high recurrence rate when the surgery is not accurate.

Preoperative preparation

On admission, a careful physical examination is made and routine investigations include urine examination, chest X-ray, ECG, haemoglobin estimation and other specific tests as indicated. The whole of the leg and adjacent pubic area is shaved.

3a & b

The patient then stands in a good light and the legs are carefully examined to check the venous pathology which is reassessed and compared with the outpatient assessment, previously detailed on the record card.

No.
ST. MARY'S HOSPITAL
LONDON, W.2.
VEIN CLINIC
Mr. JOHN T. HOBBS
HOSPITAL No.

SURNAME | CHRISTIAN NAME | M S W D | AGE | SEX M F | FIRST SEEN | REFERRED BY | COSMETIC PRIMARY RECURRENT

ADDRESS
Telephone
OCCUPATION
Posture
G.P.

SYMPTOMS	R	L	PAST TREATMENT	R	L	FAMILY HISTORY
PAIN			SUPPORT			
			OTHER			
PROMINENT VEINS THIGH			INJECTION			
PROMINENT VEINS CALF						PREGNANCIES
DILATED VENULES						
PIGMENTATION			SURGERY			
ECZEMA			GROIN TIE			THROMBOPHLEBITIS
ULCERATION			LSV STRIP			SUPERFICIAL
OEDEMA			LOCAL TIES			DVT PROXIMAL
NIGHT CRAMPS			SUB FASCIAL			DVT CALF
RESTLESS LEGS			SSV TIE			P. EMBOLUS
LIPOSCLEROSIS			SSV STRIP			ALLERGY SKIN
BLEEDING			SKIN GRAFT			ALLERGY OTHER

GENERAL HEALTH
Weight range
PAST ILLNESS
Photos
Venogram
Isotope venogram
Ultrasound

SKELETAL
BACK
HIP KNEE
FEET
Haemorrhoids
Constipation
Menopause
Hormones
Venous pressure
Impedence plethy.
Photoplethysmography

URINE Sugar Albumin | BP | WEIGHT | HEIGHT

3a

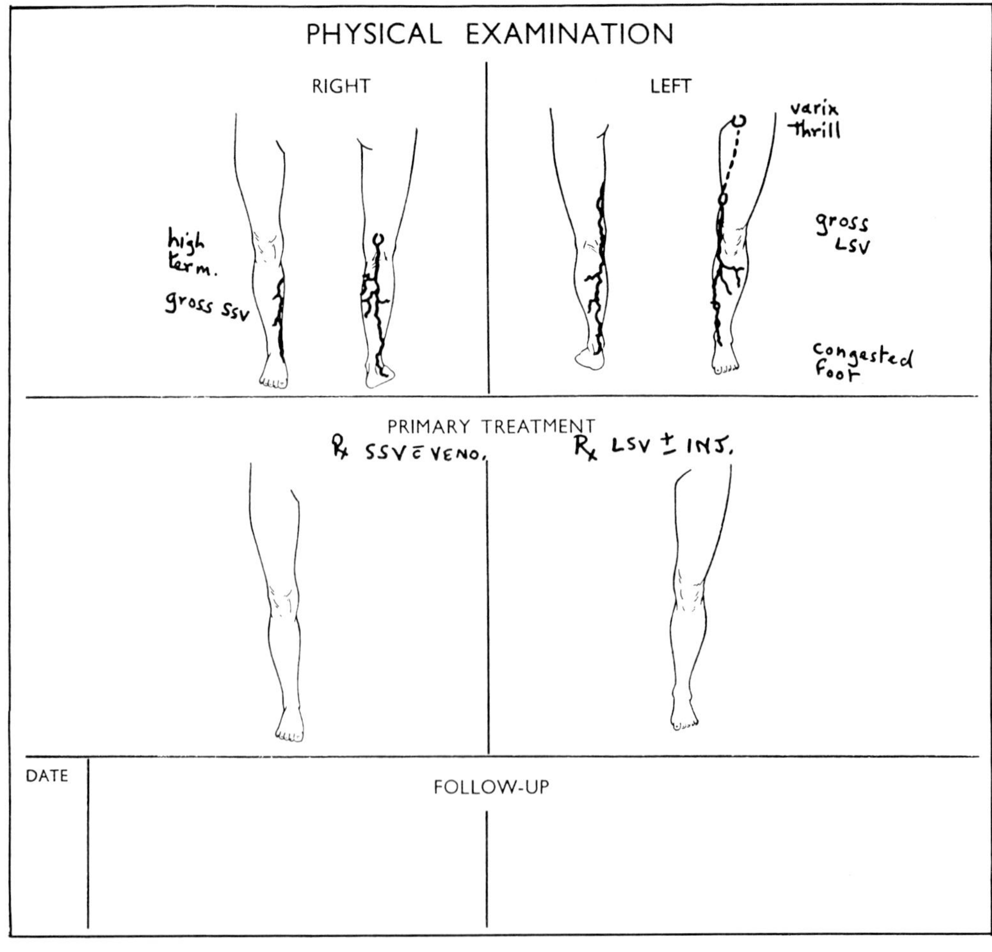

3b

4

The accurate marking of the veins by the surgeon who is to operate is a most important step, because when the legs are elevated many of the veins will no longer be apparent. The superficial veins are outlined between parallel lines which indicate the size of the veins and this is best done with a felt-tipped indelible marker (Pentel, N50).

After the veins have been fully and carefully outlined, the sliding finger method is used to find the points of control from which various sections of vein refill after being emptied, and these points are intended to include the incompetent perforating veins. In the lower leg, in association with incompetence of the long and short saphenous veins there will be a definite perforating vein where the refluxing blood re-enters the deep system but because of gross dilatation this will also show reversed flow during some stages of the walking cycle. There may be further primary and secondary perforating veins which are identified and marked by a circle. Tourniquet tests and examination with Doppler are not necessary at this time.

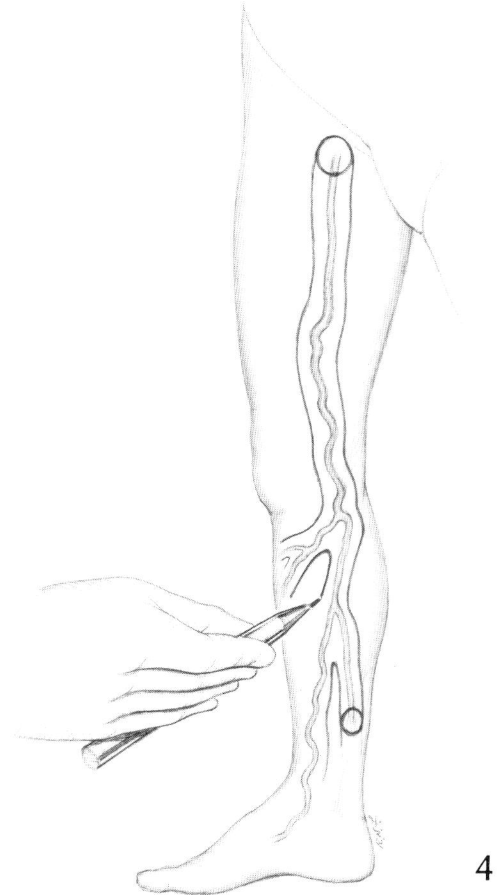

4

Anaesthesia

General anaesthesia is used and endotracheal intubation is only necessary if there is difficulty in maintaining an adequate airway. If general anaesthesia is contraindicated because of cardiac or pulmonary disease the operation may be carried out under lumbar epidural anaesthesia.

Equipment

The following equipment should be available.

Instruments

2 Sponge holders
5 Towel clips
1 Suture scissors
1 Size 3 scalpel handle with No. 10 blade
1 Size 3 scalpel handle with No. 15 blade
1 McIndoe dissecting scissors
1 McIndoe dissecting forceps
2 Small retractors
1 Needle holder
6 Crile artery forceps, 5½ inch, straight
3 Crile artery forceps, 5½ inch, curved
3 Mosquito forceps, 5 inch, straight
3 Mosquito forceps, 5 inch, curved
4 Stripper cables, Bowden with threaded ends
2 Cylindrical stripper tips
2 Olive stripper tips
4 Stripper heads, 9 mm
2 Stripper heads, 12 mm
2 Stripper heads, 6 mm

Sutures

2/0 Plain CGS (W103) for ligature
0 Chromic CGS (W114) for large vessel ligature
3/0 Plain on 25 mm round body curved needle (W438) or 2/0 (W439)
5/0 Ethilon on fine straight skin needle (W624)

Position of patient

5

For operations on the long saphenous vein and front of the legs the patient is placed in the supine position with feet apart but a spreading board or table is not necessary.

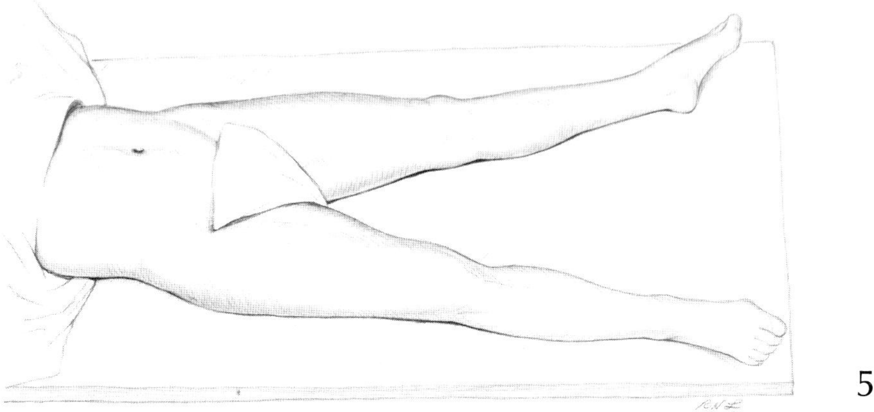

5

6

For operations on the short saphenous vein the patient is placed in the lateral position with the lower leg flexed.

After the proximal part of the operation is complete the table is tilted head down to an angle of more than 10°. This reduces venous pressure to zero and minimizes bleeding. Excessive tilt for a long period may result in oedema of the face, especially the eyelids, and introduces the risk of air entering the circulation if a vein is opened.

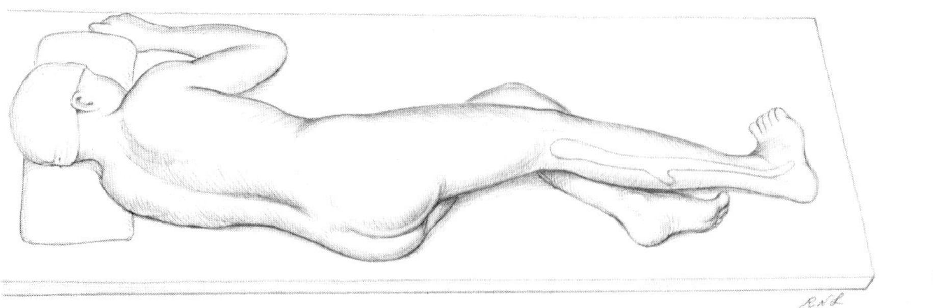

6

Operation for long saphenous vein incompetence

7

The incision

The hip is abducted and the knees slightly flexed so that the tension lines in the upper thigh are parallel to the inguinal ligament.

The saphenofemoral junction is approximately 3 cm below and 4 cm lateral to the pubic tubercle and is located as a slight filling deficiency medial to the femoral artery pulse. A 5 cm incision is centred on this point and made in the line of the skin creases. In case of difficulty the incision should be lengthened. Diathermy is not used.

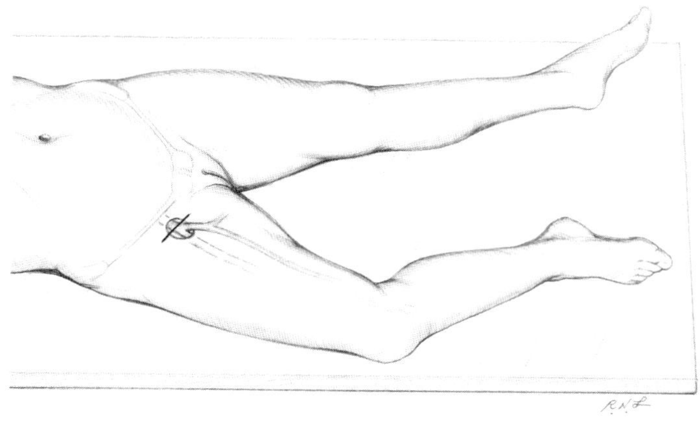

7

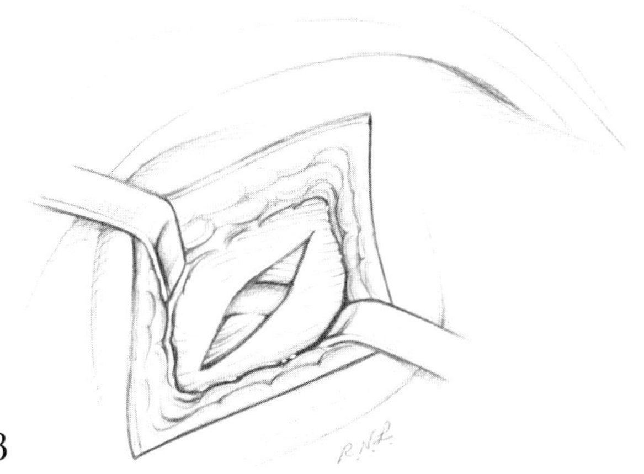

8

8

Division of membranous layer (Scarpa's) of superficial fascia

The superficial tissues are divided in the line of the skin incision, using the scalpel or scissors, until the deep layer of the superficial fascia is exposed. The bluish long saphenous vein can often be seen deep to this fascia. The membranous fascia is then divided in the line of the skin and no other tissues are cut so that there is no risk of damaging lymphatic vessels or nerves. Small skin retractors are manipulated by an assistant to expose the fascia and then the saphenous vein.

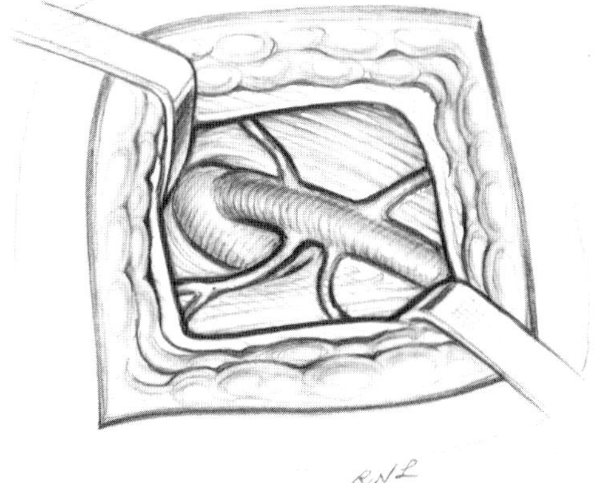

9

9

Exposure of saphenofemoral junction

After exposure, the saphenous vein is then cleaned both distally and proximally using a swab held in non-toothed (McIndoe) dissecting forceps. The tributaries are exposed and the termination of the saphenous vein at the femoral vein is exposed.

10

Division of long saphenous vein

When the saphenofemoral junction has been identified, the long saphenous vein is divided between straight artery forceps, so that the proximal stump can be elevated to aid isolation of the tributaries. If a small artery (superficial external pudendal) passes in front of the saphenous vein, the proximal saphenous vein stump can be passed under the artery, or else the artery is divided. Usually the artery passes through the angle of the saphenofemoral junction along the lower edge of the fossa ovalis.

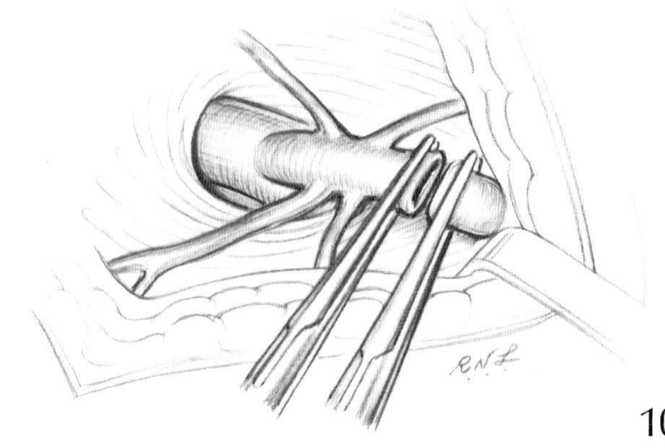

10

Division of tributaries

11

The proximal long saphenous vein stump is then lifted and the tributaries isolated by sweeping off the adjacent tissue using a swab. Although the position and number of tributaries are variable, four groups corresponding to the arterial branches must be identified and divided. On the lateral side the anterolateral tributary and superficial circumflex iliac vein must be found. These are sometimes flattened against the saphenofemoral junction and so overlooked and this is the commonest cause of recurrence.

11

12

If there is a single lateral vessel, it must be followed until it divides, as overlooking this is another possible cause of persistent veins on the front of the thigh.

Proximally, the superficial inferior epigastric vein is easily found and divided. Medially, the superficial external vein is divided. Finally, the posteromedial tributary is found and divided between ligatures to avoid haematoma formation above the bandage. This large medial tributary usually passes down the back of the thigh to join the short saphenous vein and if it is not seen in the surgical field because of a lower termination it must be sought under the distal edge of the wound.

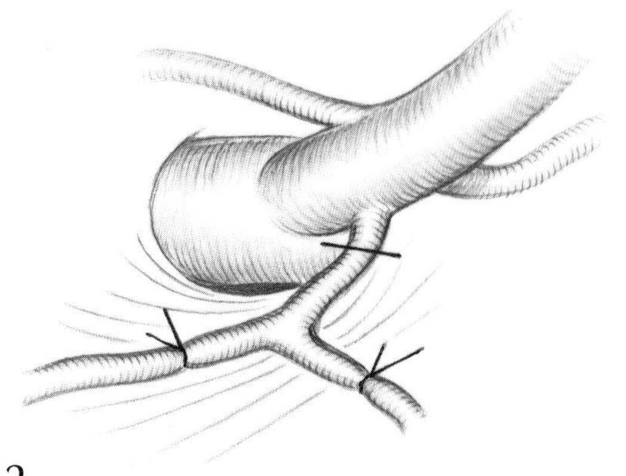

12

13

Exposure of saphenofemoral junction

After dividing all juxtafemoral tributaries, elevation of the long saphenous vein stump reveals the junction with the common femoral vein as a line of demarcation, the colour change being due to the different wall composition. Both the lateral and medial surfaces of the femoral vein must be seen to be clear of tributaries, to ensure a flush ligation. It is not necessary to divide the deep fascia and the deep external pudendal vein needs to be divided only if unusually large.

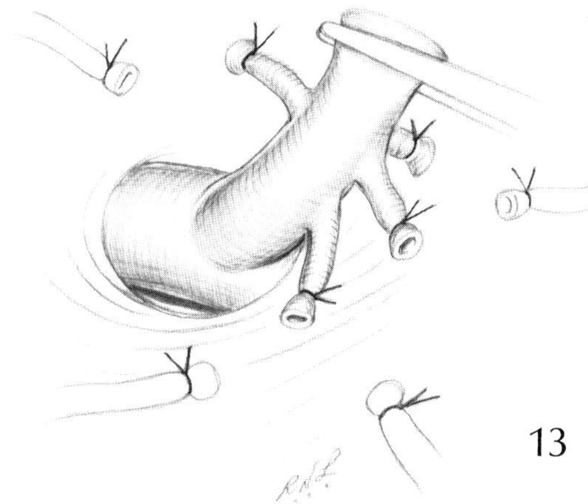

13

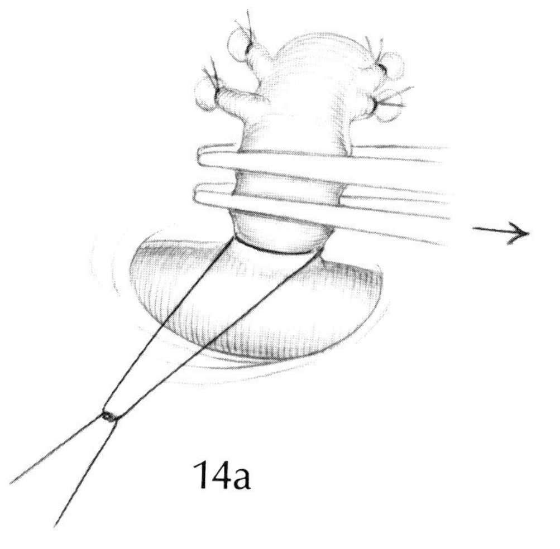

14a

14a & b

Ligation of saphenofemoral junction

Two adjacent forceps are placed on the termination of the long saphenous vein so that the proximal ligature is placed flush on the side of the femoral vein, taking care not to stenose this vein by excessive elevation of the junction. The vessel should not be transfixed because sometimes it is fragile and easily torn. There is no need to use non-absorbable sutures. For the proximal ligature chromic 0 catgut is used; for the second suture on the saphenous vein and for all other vessels and tributaries finer catgut is used (2/0 plain or 3/0 chromic). Once the saphenous vein is isolated the table can be tilted so that the legs are raised to an angle of 10°–20°.

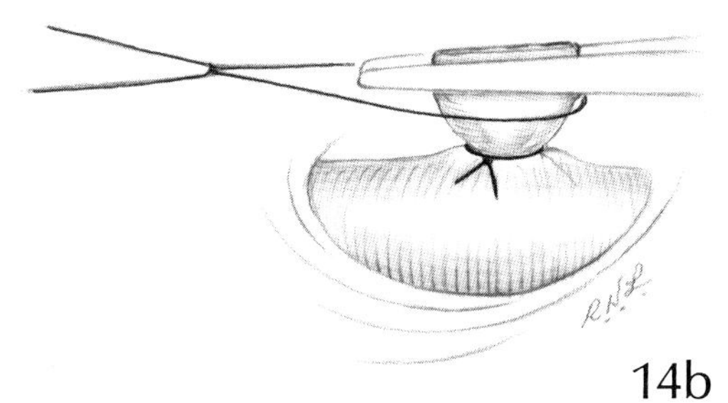

14b

15

Introduction of stripper

The stripper is then introduced into the upper end of the saphenous vein and passed towards the knee. It must be directed down the marked vein by manual manipulation. This is made easier by straightening the leg, and the stripper then passes to the upper calf. Here it often enters an anterior tibial tributary just below the knee and it must therefore be withdrawn and guided into the posterior arch vein tributary or long saphenous vein just below the knee. It is usually possible to pass the stripper down an incompetent saphenous vein and if the vein is duplicated or, rarely, triplicated each vein must be removed after passing strippers distally.

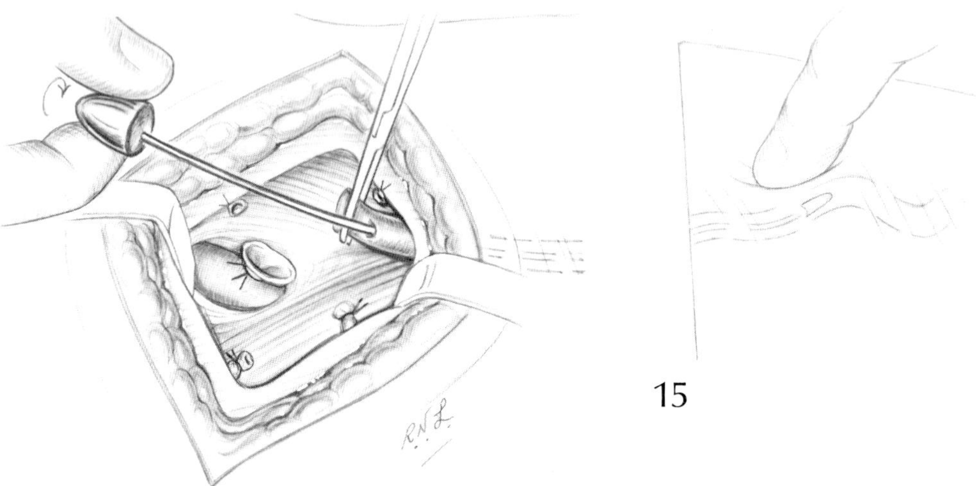

15

16 & 17

Exit of stripper

By twisting and manipulating the stripper with one hand and the vein with the other the tip of the stripper is advanced through the tortuous varicose vein to just below the knee. The perforating vein at the upper tibia must be reached but the long saphenous vein in the lower leg is seldom involved and is protected in a fascial tunnel passing along the tibial border. At this level the saphenous nerve has not joined the saphenous vein and damage to the lymphatic vessels in the lower leg is also avoided by not stripping below the upper calf. A small (1 cm) vertical incision is made over the tip of the stripper using a No. 15 scalpel blade. The vein is then exposed and divided; the distal end is ligated using 3/0 chromic catgut and the stripper brought out.

When the stripper has been pulled down until the head is flush at the upper end of the saphenous vein a ligature is placed around it, to secure the vein to the stripper. Normally a 9 mm head is used, but if the vein is very large a 12 mm head will prevent inversion, as will a double ligature.

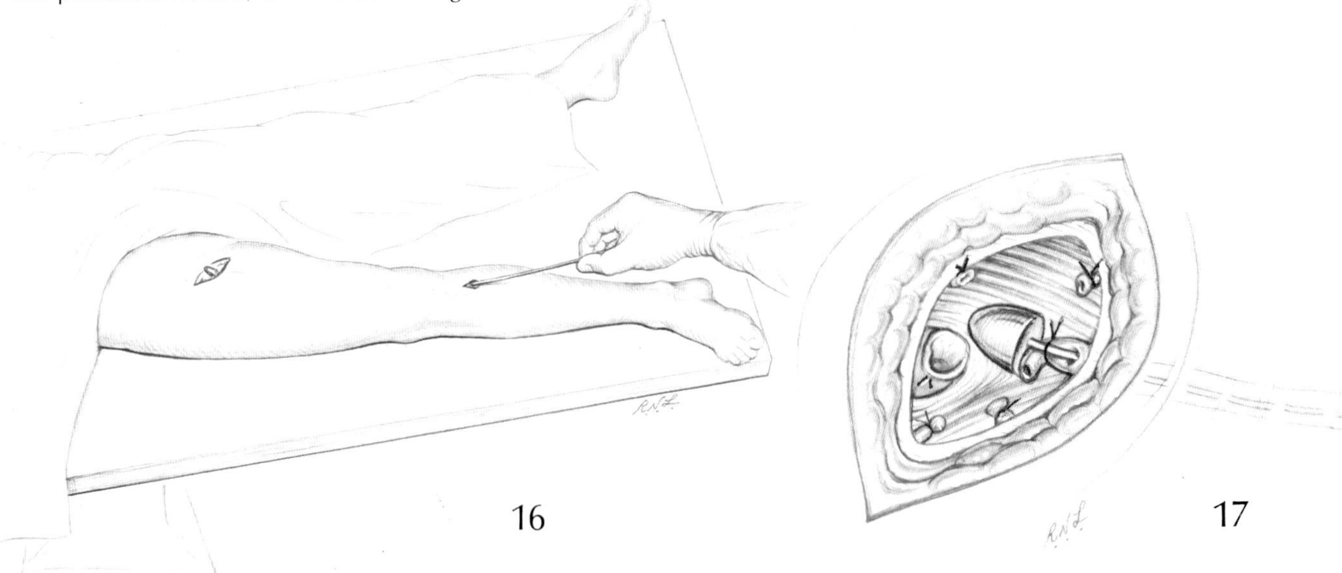

16

17

18

Closure of groin wound

After the head of the stripper has been tied into the vein and buried, the wound is closed in two layers. The membranous layer of superficial fascia is closed with two (occasionally three) interrupted 2/0 chromic catgut sutures which are placed so that the knot is deep.

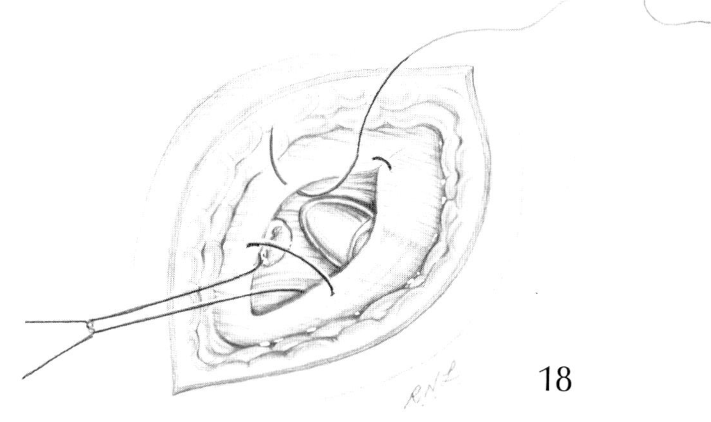

18

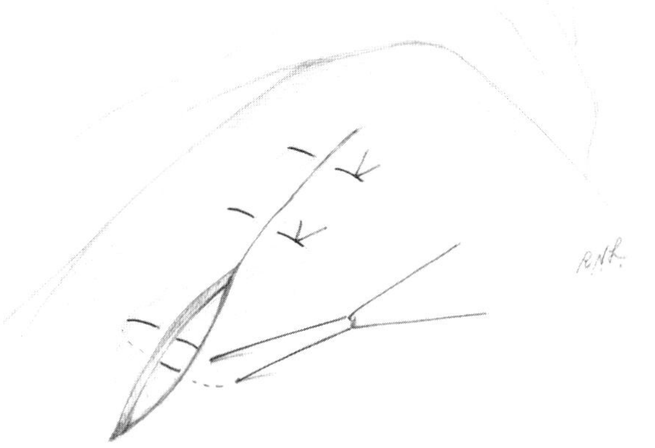

19

19

The skin is closed with three or four interrupted vertical mattress sutures using monofilament nylon, preferably 5/0 or 3/0 mounted on a fine straight needle.

20

Removal of vein and stripper

After the groin wound has been closed, the vein is removed by pulling the stripper from the wound in the upper calf. The stripper is pulled steadily and slowly and if the vein is bulky its removal through a small incision is made easier by pulling the corrugated vein down the stripper and out of the lower wound. Bleeding is usually minimal when the legs are elevated whilst stripping. Bleeding may occur if there is a large incompetent perforating vein in the lower thigh or upper calf, but this is immediately controlled by firm local pressure and further elevation of the leg.

Pulling the stripper downwards facilitates early closure of the groin wound and accurately selects the vein or veins to be removed. By not stripping the long saphenous vein from the lower leg, damage to the saphenous nerve is unlikely and this is further prevented by stripping in a downward direction so that the stripper head will not impact in the divisions of the saphenous nerve.

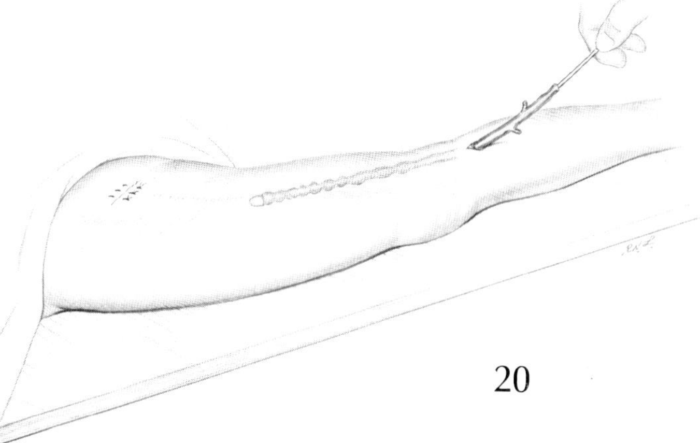

20

Passing the stripper upwards

Rarely is it impossible to pass the stripper in a downward direction and it may be convenient to pass the stripper up from an incision over the vein on the lower leg. Instead of stripping upwards, the head and tip can be removed and reversed, so that the vein is stripped in the usual downward direction. By stripping in a downwards direction much larger lengths of tributaries are removed.

21

Elevation of limb

Immediately after stripping the long saphenous vein and removing any other dilated veins, the table is lowered and the leg elevated. This, plus expression of any blood from the vein tract, controls bleeding and prevents haemotoma formation.

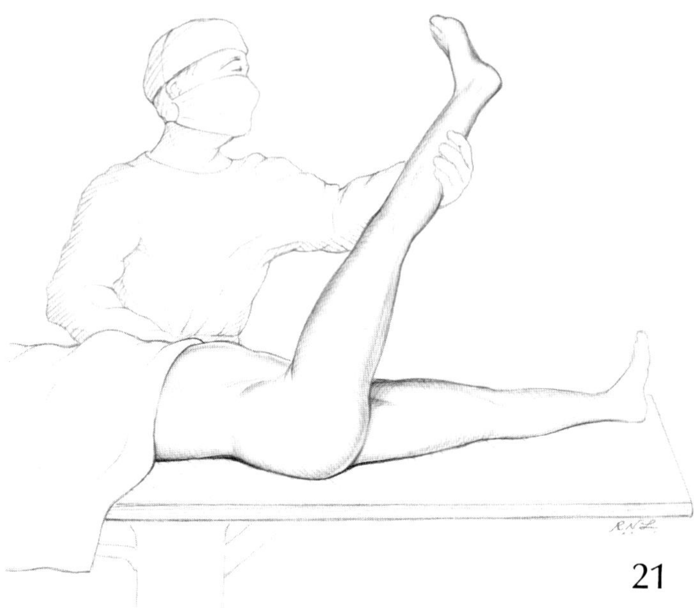

21

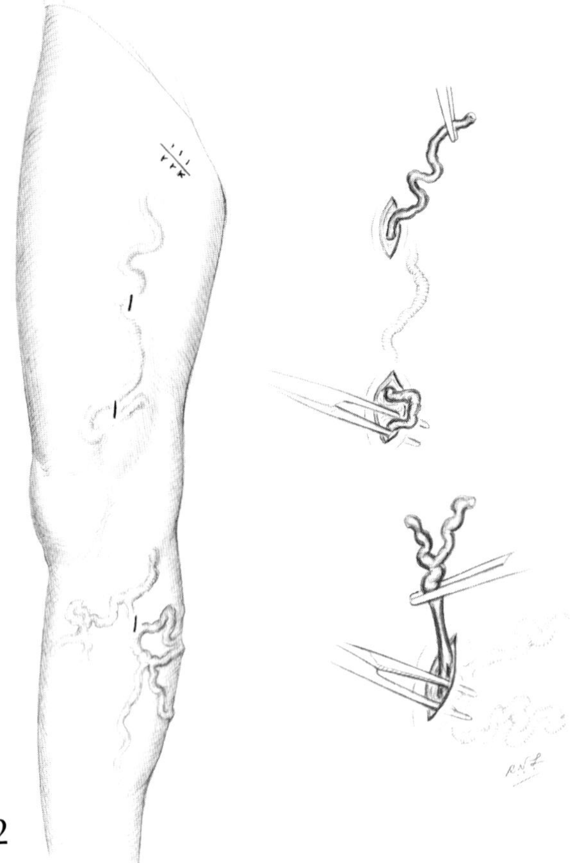

22

22

After the long saphenous vein has been withdrawn on the stripper, the various subsidiary varicose tributaries, which have previously been accurately marked, are withdrawn through a series of small stab wounds. These incisions are vertical, 0.75 cm in length, and made with a No. 15 scalpel blade. The veins are removed using straight artery forceps and care is taken that only veins are removed. Fine artery forceps are opened in each small incision to separate the subcutaneous tissue and isolate the vein. The vein is then grasped firmly and gently eased out; with care long segments of the tortuous veins are removed. The venous tributaries removed in this fashion include the anterolateral tributary on the thigh, the posterior arch vein on the calf and sometimes the anterior tibial tributary. Care is taken to make the small incisions vertical and not in the vicinity of joints.

Ligation of incompetent perforating veins

Incompetent perforating veins may be present as a primary and isolated problem but often they are secondary, either as the re-entry of a large saphenous vein reflux or secondary to deep vein pathology in the post-thrombotic syndrome. When associated with incompetence of the saphenous system, incompetent perforating veins can easily be dealt with during surgical treatment of the saphenous veins. There is no need for extensive subfascial dissections because significant incompetent perforating veins only occur in small numbers and can be ligated through small extrafascial approaches. In the post-thrombotic syndrome the secondary incompetent perforating veins are often associated with pathological changes in the skin and subcutaneous tissue (eczema, ulceration and lipodermatosclerosis) and surgery is best avoided in such tissue, particularly since the underlying problem cannot be cured.

23

When operating on primary varicose veins any grossly incompetent perforating veins are marked by a circle and these fascial defects are also points which control filling of the superficial veins. The typical sites are shown in Illustration 2.

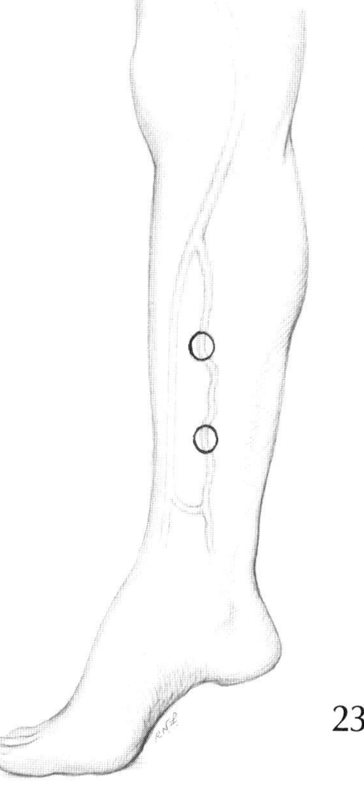

23

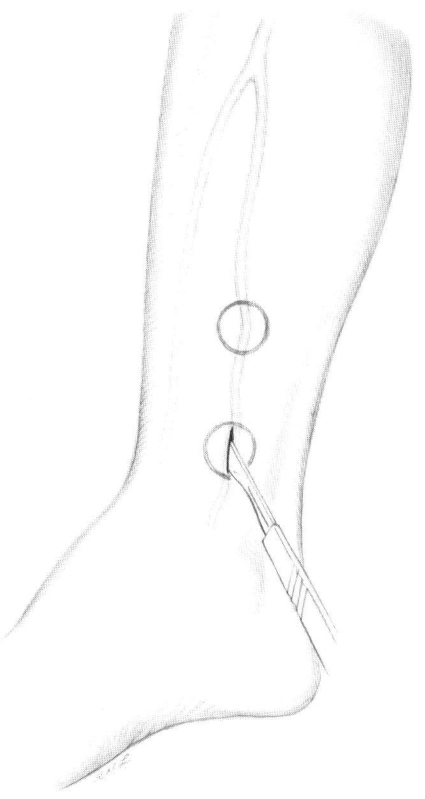

24

24

A 2cm long vertical incision is made over the marked points and the vein isolated.

25

The superficial vein is dissected out proximally and distally until the T-junction with the perforating vein is found and isolated. The vein is divided and ligated on each side and the perforating vein freed down to the deep fascia; often there is an associated artery and when pulling on the vein it is possible to pull the deep vein and posterior tibial artery through the wide fascial defect.

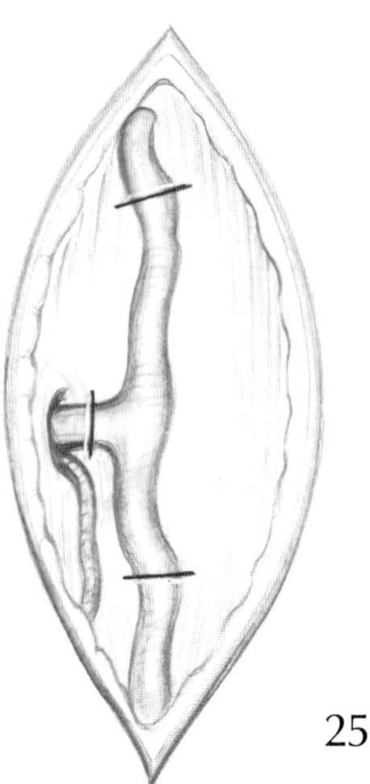

25

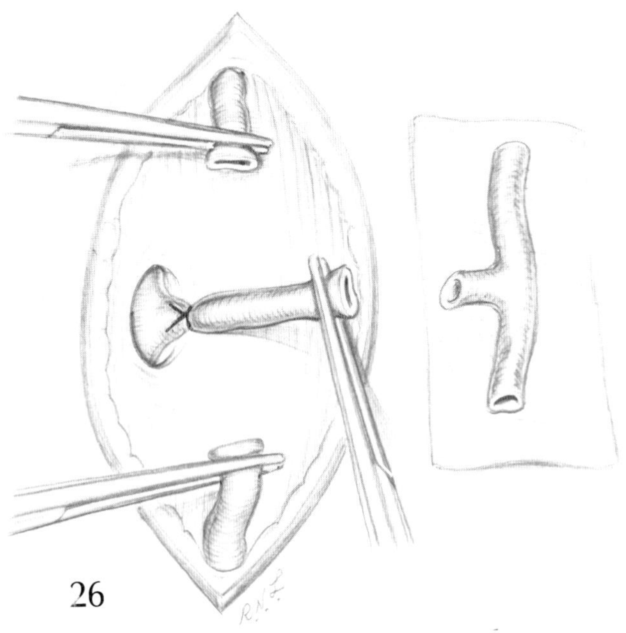

26

26

The perforating vein is ligated at the deep fascia close to its junction with the deep vein. Finally the fascial defect is closed with one or two chromic gut sutures.

27

Closure of wound

After expressing any blood and clots from the wounds the small incisions are closed with one or two interrupted vertical mattress sutures using fine monofilament nylon on a straight needle (3/0 or 5/0). No subcutaneous sutures are used, except for the deep fascia at the groin, popliteal fossa and perforating vein sites.

28

Bandaging

After all free blood has been expressed from the wounds on the elevated leg, the whole limb is covered with a pressure bandage using cotton crêpe bandages of limited stretch (STD Export or S&N Elastocrêpe). Dry dressings are placed over each wound and a 7.5 cm bandage is applied from the metatarsal heads to the upper calf. A 10 cm bandage then overlaps this and continues to the upper thigh.

A small Airstrip dressing is applied to the groin. No pins are used to fix the bandages on an anaesthetized patient. The foot of the bed is elevated 20° until the patient is fully conscious. When conscious the patient is instructed to walk every hour.

29a & b

POSTOPERATIVE CARE

The following morning all bandages and dressings are removed and the wounds covered by short lengths of 2.5 cm Micropore. An elastic stocking is then applied over these and the patient discharged home. The stocking can be removed at night and a bath or shower taken; the Micropore dressings are blotted dry and the patient can sleep without the stocking which is then replaced each morning. The leg should be treated as no more than a bruised leg and normal activities resumed as comfort allows.

On the seventh or eighth day the sutures are removed and the stockings discarded. Excessive bruising can be controlled by the use of bandages or a stronger elastic stocking (Scholl Duoten, Sigvaris).

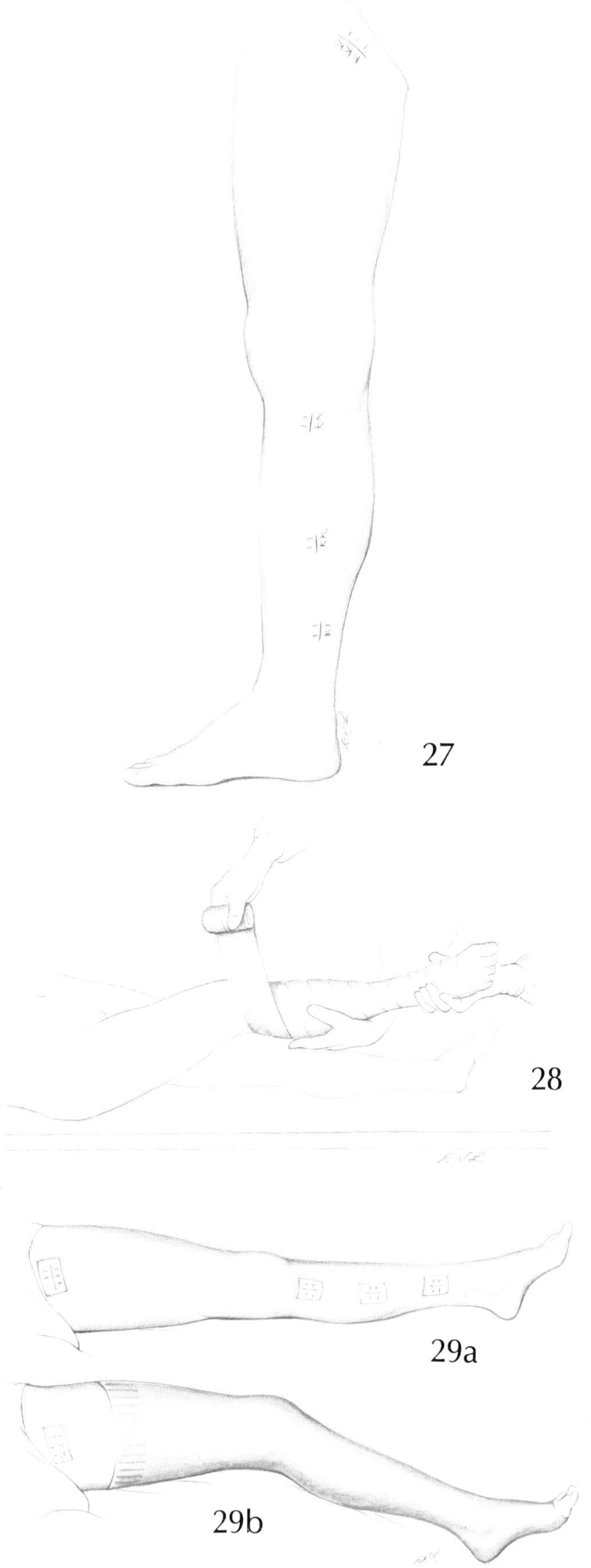

Operation for short saphenous vein incompetence

30

The patient is placed in the lateral position with the lower leg flexed and the upper leg extended; if the incompetence is unilateral the leg for operation is uppermost. A cassette containing a 30 cm × 40 cm X-ray film is placed under the upper leg and the X-ray tube positioned over the leg and centred on the knee joint. Sterile hypodermic needles are used as markers, being inserted intradermally, a 25 gauge needle at the highest point where the short saphenous vein was palpable and a 21 gauge needle at the knee crease (indicated by arrows in *Illustration 31a*).

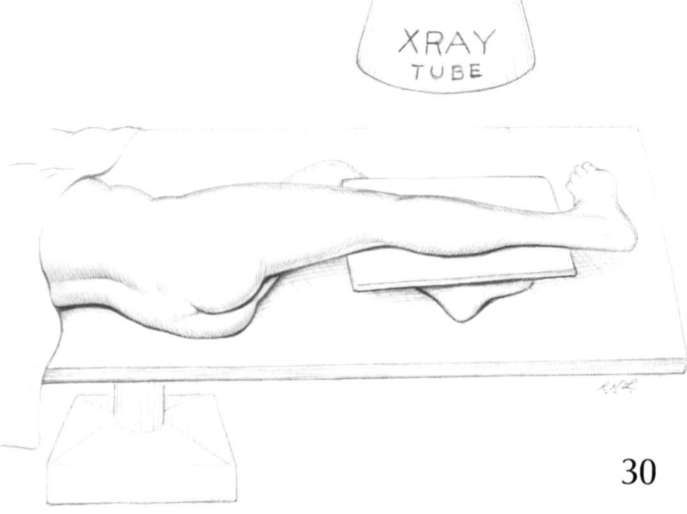

30

31a, b & c

The film is exposed after injecting 10–15 ml of contrast media (Hexabrix is used because of its low osmolality which avoids irritant side-effects); during the second half of the injection of contrast media, central venous pressure is raised by obstructing respiration, so that the valves in the popliteal vein are demonstrated.

The injection of contrast is made directly with a 15 gauge needle if the vein is large or via a butterfly cannula (21 or 23 gauge) if the vein is tortuous. The X-ray film is then processed while the surgeon scrubs and prepares the patient.

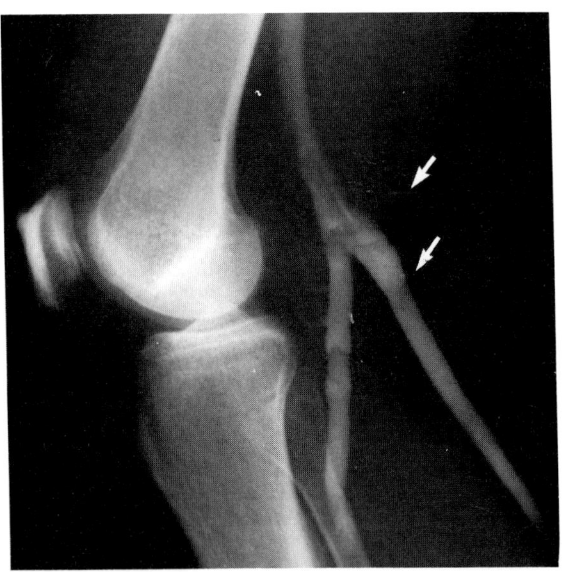

31a

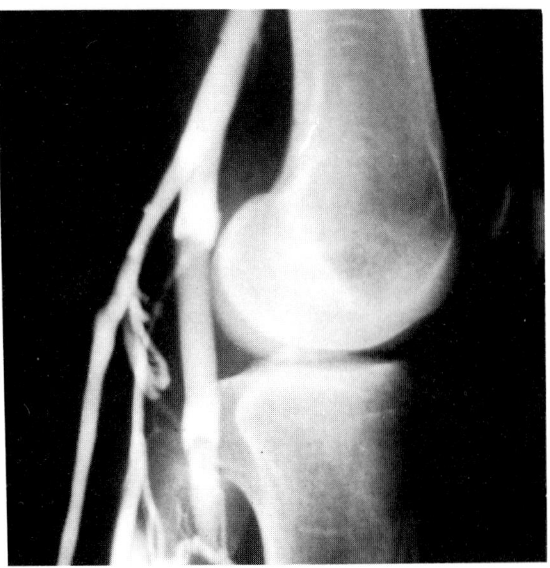

31b

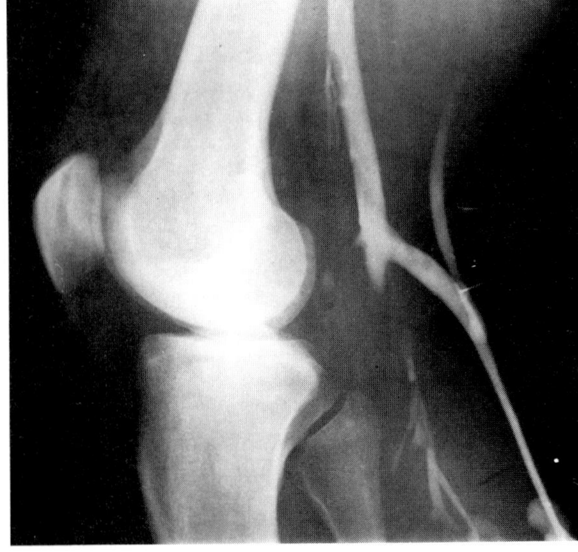

31c

32

The incision

Using the X-ray and skin marking needles as a guide, the surgeon makes a 2.5 cm transverse incision over the saphenopopliteal junction, which is usually on the back of the lower thigh, above the popliteal crease. The X-ray makes possible a small and accurately placed incision which is preferable to larger explorations. The popliteal fascia is exposed and often the underlying vein is visible; the fascia is divided transversely in the line of the skin incision to expose the fat and contents of the popliteal fossa.

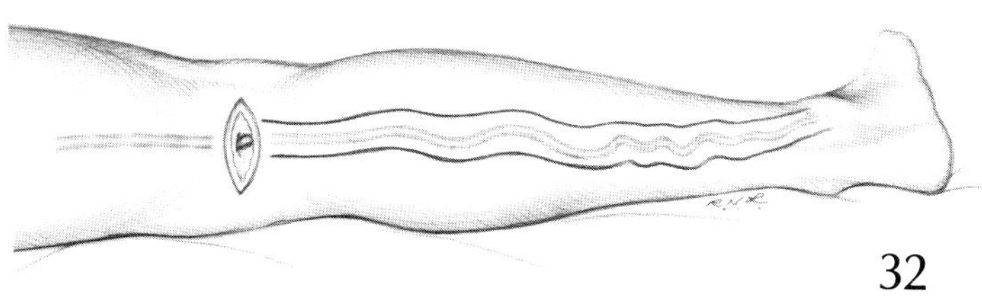

32

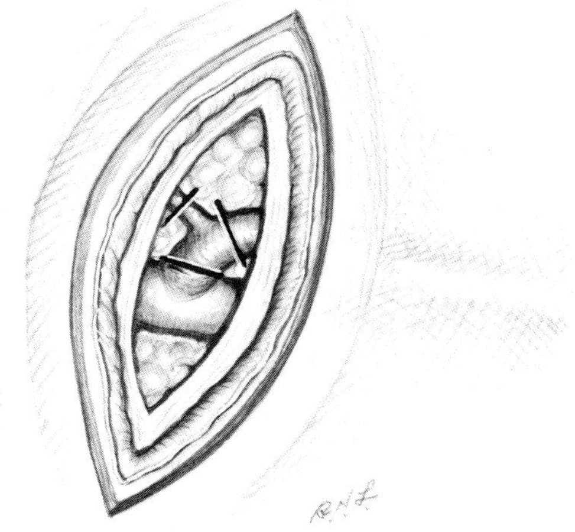

33

Flush ligation and stripping of short saphenous vein

33

The vein is isolated by blunt dissection and carefully separated from the closely applied sural nerve. The vein is lifted up and divided. There is usually a larger superior tributary which passes up the back of the lower thigh to communicate with the posteromedial tributary of the long saphenous vein, the profunda vein or sometimes the tributaries of the internal iliac veins. This vein must be divided to prevent recurrence.

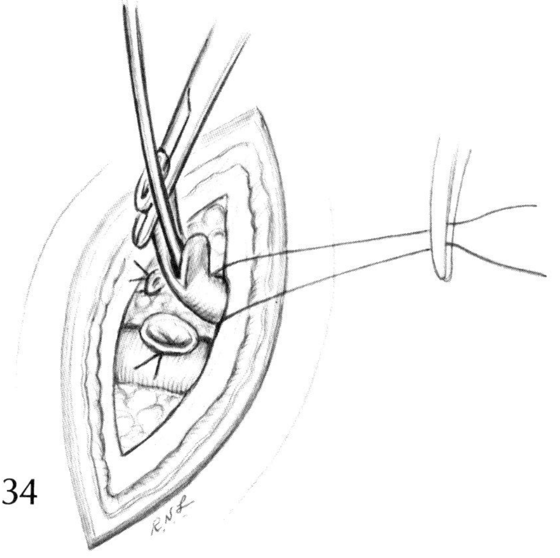

34

34

The termination of the short saphenous vein is located and a flush ligation on the popliteal vein is made using 2/0 chromic gut. A second 3/0 plain ligature is used as a safety measure. A stripper is then passed down the short saphenous vein to just above the lateral malleolus.

35

A small 1 cm vertical incision is made to expose the stripper. After the stripper has been pulled down, the head is tied in the upper end of the vein and the incision at the popliteal fossa closed in two layers: continuous 3/0 chromic gut to the popliteal fascia and three interrupted nylon sutures to skin. Stripping in a downward direction ensures removal of clearly marked veins. The wounds are closed as before.

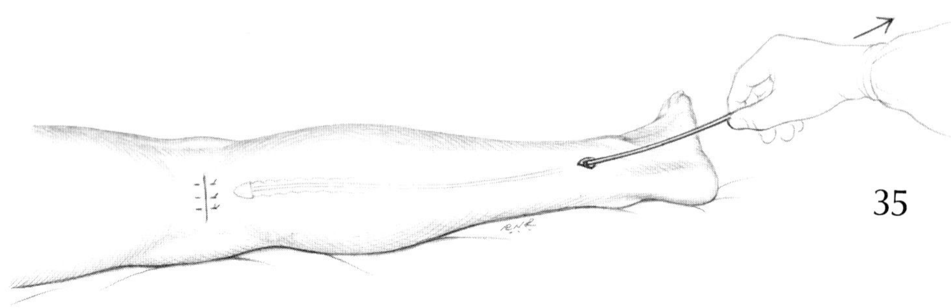

35

36

If the vein does not join the popliteal vein

When the short saphenous vein does not communicate with the popliteal vein, or else this connection is very small, there is no need to expose this area. Instead, the short saphenous vein is exposed above the lateral malleolus and a stripper inserted and passed up into the thigh. The termination may be in the back of the thigh or join the long saphenous vein via the posteromedial tributary. At the highest point a small incision is made over the tip of the stripper which is then brought out of the wound. The ends of the stripper are removed and exchanged. After placing the top end of the stripper (with the vein tied to it) below the deep fascia the wound is closed in two layers, using CGS for the fascia and 5/0 Ethilon for the skin. The stripper is then removed downwards with a gentle pull which avoids damage to the adjacent sural nerve.

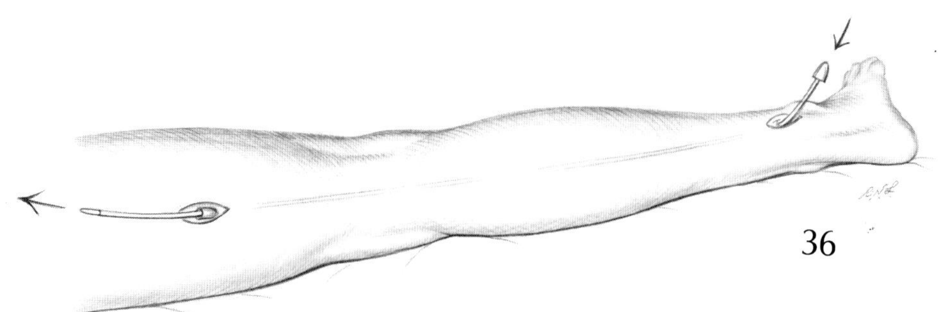

36

Recurrence at the groin

This occurs when a vein is left communicating with the femoral vein. Gross recurrence is immediate when the ligation is not flush and a long stump of saphenous vein with tributaries is present. Sometimes the second part of a double long saphenous vein is missed. Recurrence is most commonly caused by overlooking of the lateral tributaries which may be hidden by fascia during the initial ligation. This results in a tortuous mass of varicosities at the groin surrounded by scar tissue leading to recurrence of irregular varicose veins down the leg.

Because of the friable thin-walled veins, surrounded by dense scar tissue with distorted anatomy, a direct approach is very difficult. Therefore, it may be better to expose the femoral vein, and several approaches have been described. Many surgeons favour a high approach, exposing the femoral artery before the vein[1–4]. A lateral exposing the femoral artery before the vein[1–4]. A lateral vertical incision has been used[5] to expose the artery first and so avoid lymphatic damage. The previous scar was widely excised by Li[6] who also first exposed the femoral artery but recognized the increased risk of lymphatic damage. Foote[7] also reopened the original scar and extended it down medially to expose the femoral vein from below, but when great difficulty was encountered he exposed the femoral vein from above. Dodd and Cockett[8,9] have used a 10 cm long high transverse incision extended down medially for 5 cm as a 'hockey stick' to open the femoral sheath and expose the femoral vein from below. The disadvantage of the medial approach is damage to the important ventromedial bundle of lymphatic vessels[10].

The present author's method is as follows.

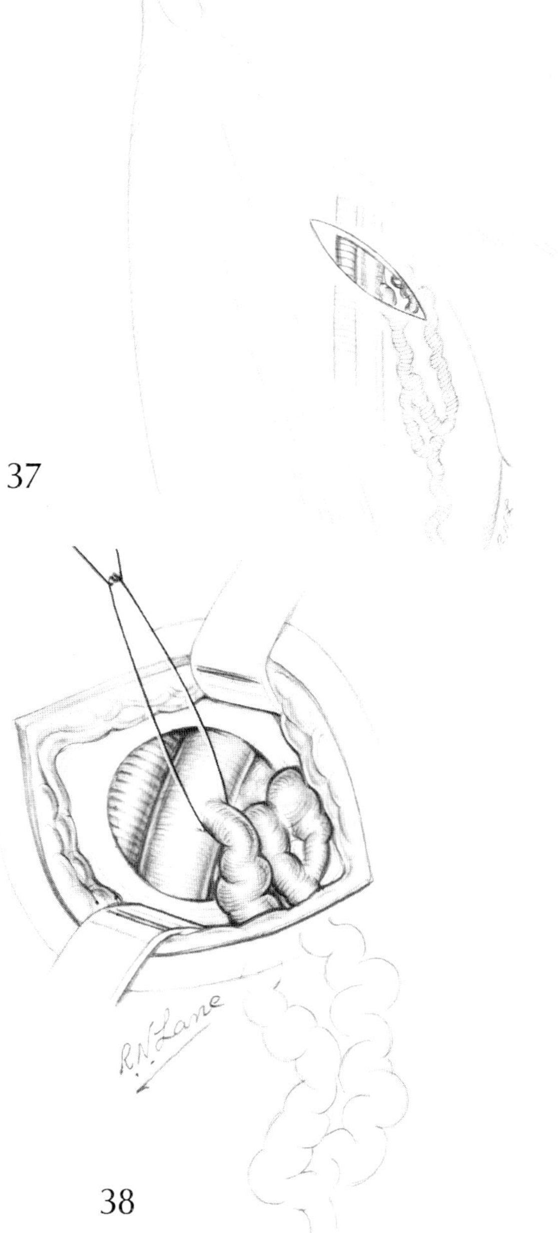

37

Incision for re-exploration at groin

The previous scar is excised, using a longer, 7.5 cm transverse incision placed over the saphenofemoral junction.

The femoral artery is identified by its pulsation lateral to the varicosities. An incision is made in the femoral sheath just medial to the artery, and the femoral vein is exposed below the saphenofemoral junction.

38

Dissection of saphenofemoral junction

The femoral vein is then carefully dissected upwards until the persistent tributaries and saphenofemoral junction are isolated. After ligating and dividing all persistent communications with the femoral vein, the incision is closed in two layers as before and the recurrent veins are removed from the leg through small incisions.

COMPLICATIONS

The most common difficulty, particularly for an inexperienced surgeon, is massive venous bleeding while dissecting out the saphenofemoral junction.

When this occurs, mild finger or swab pressure on the spot will control the haemorrhage while the table is tilted to raise the feet. When the pressure is released after a few minutes the bleeding is usually reduced to a trickle and can be accurately controlled either with an artery forceps or fine suture. Blind clamping should never be done as there is a real risk of further damage to the femoral vein or even the femoral artery.

Occasionally the stripper may pass into the deep vein via a wide short perforating vein. This occurs only when stripping up and it is therefore safer to pass the stripper downwards and always be able to feel the stripper beneath the skin.

Excessive sharp dissection in the groin, especially in large wounds, may disrupt some lymphatics and can occasionally result in the formation of a lymphocele. This should be aspirated.

Slight damage to cutaneous nerves is difficult to avoid completely. Therapy involves explaining to the patient the unavoidability and harmlessness of this small impairment. It will then be forgotten.

Arterial injuries, though serious, are extremely rare. They must be promptly identified and treated. An inexperienced operator must be able to identify them and transfer the patient to a vascular surgeon for urgent repair.

References

1. Luke, J. C. Management of recurrent varicose veins. Surgery 1954; 35: 40–44
2. Lofgren, E. P., Lofgren, K. A. Recurrence of varicose veins after the stripping operation. Archives of Surgery 1971; 102: 111–114
3. Nabatoff, R. A. Technique for operation upon recurrent varicose veins. Surgery, Gynecology and Obstetrics 1976; 143: 463–467
4. May, R. Surgery of the veins of the leg and pelvis. Philadelphia: Saunders, 1979
5. Junod, J. M., Varices et leurs complications: traitement chirurgical des cas difficiles. Helvetica Chirurgica Acta 1971; 38: 167–170
6. Li, A. K. C. A technique for re-exploration of the saphenofemoral junction for recurrent varicose veins. British Journal of Surgery 1975; 62: 745–746
7. Foote, R. R. Varicose veins. 3rd ed. Bristol: Wright, 1960
8. Dodd, H., Cockett, F. B. The pathology and surgery of the veins of the lower limb. Edinburgh: Livingstone, 1956
9. Dodd, H., Cockett, F. B., The pathology and surgery of the veins of the lower limb. 2nd ed. Edinburgh: Churchill Livingstone, 1976
10. Brunner, Phlebologie U. Prokt. 1975; 4: 266

Interruptions of the inferior vena cava and femoral veins

James T. Adams MD
Professor of Surgery, University of Rochester Medical Center, Rochester, New York, USA

Historical background

Since the turn of the century it had been recognized that pulmonary embolism was a cause of death following operations, injuries, severe illnesses and prolonged bed rest. Because autopsy studies demonstrated thrombi in the veins of the lower extremities, Homans[1], in 1934, suggested ligation of the femoral veins for the prevention of pulmonary embolism. In some patients, however, thrombosis extended proximally beyond the femoral vessels or was located in the pelvic venous beds so that ligation at the femoral level was inadequate. This prompted Homans[2], in 1944, to recommend ligation of the inferior vena cava. Subsequently, vein ligation became a frequently performed operation. Yet, although the procedure prevented pulmonary embolism, the ensuing venous obstruction and propagation of the thrombosis distal to the site of ligation resulted in a significant incidence of lower extremity morbidity. This morbidity, referred to as the postphlebitic syndrome and characterized early by leg swelling and pain, and late by pigmentary changes and ulcerations of the skin was appreciable enough after vein ligations to constitute a real disadvantage. In order to prevent or minimize the adverse effects of vein ligation, techniques of partial interruption were devised[3–7]. These techniques consisted of the extraluminal application of sutures or plastic clips which narrowed or compartmentalized the vein sufficiently to prevent passage of potentially fatal pulmonary emboli without interfering significantly with blood flow. More recently, methods of intraluminal partial interruption of the inferior vena cava have been described[8–10]. A major advantage of the intraluminal techniques is that they can be done under local anaesthesia so that a major surgical procedure can be avoided in poor risk patients who require caval interruption.

Indications

Anticoagulation combined with a short period of bed rest and followed by ambulation with elastic support of the legs is the treatment of choice for patients with acute venous thrombosis with pulmonary embolism. Unfortunately, anticoagulation does not always prevent recurrent pulmonary emboli and by far the most frequent indication for vein interruption is recurrent embolism in patients receiving adequate anticoagulation therapy. A second major indication for vein interruption is when anticoagulation therapy is contraindicated in a patient who has suffered a pulmonary embolus. Such patients include those with an ulcerative lesion of the gastrointestinal tract or who have recently had urological or neurosurgical operative procedures. Less frequent indications for vein interruption are: (*1*) in high risk patients during the course of certain surgical procedures such as pelvic or groin lymph node dissection for cancer, resection of abdominal aortic aneurysm, or operations for trauma to the major abdominal veins; (*2*) in cases of suppurative pelvic thrombophlebitis with septic pulmonary emboli; (*3*) in cases of chronic or recurrent multiple small pulmonary emboli causing progressive cor pulmonale; and (*4*) following pulmonary embolectomy.

Site of interruption

The majority (90–95 per cent) of pulmonary emboli come from sites of thrombosis in veins drained by the inferior vena cava with about 65 per cent coming from veins below the inguinal ligaments. Therefore, interruption of the inferior vena cava clearly offers the greatest protection against recurrent pulmonary embolism. However, interruption of the femoral vein in the groin is reasonable when positive identification of thrombi in the deep veins of the lower extremity has been made by phlebography. The advantages of femoral vein over caval interruption include: (*1*) femoral vein procedures can be done safely in poor risk patients under local anaesthesia whereas vena caval procedures require general anaesthesia; (*2*) anticoagulation must be discontinued for a vena caval interruption but can be continued if the femoral vein is interrupted; (*3*) patients with pre-existing cardiac disease do not tolerate sudden interruption of the total venous return from both lower extremities if the cava is ligated or a site of partial interruption becomes occluded by a detached thrombus; (*4*) femoral vein interruption preserves the total venous return from the opposite extremity when unilateral limb thrombosis has been demonstrated on phlebograms. Interruption of the inferior vena cava is indicated when there is clinical or phlebographic evidence of pelvic vein thrombosis, if thrombosis extends above the level of the inguinal ligaments, or if bilateral phlebograms fail to demonstrate any source of venous thrombosis in the lower extremities.

Types of interruptions

Most surgeons now prefer partial interruption of the femoral vein or inferior vena cava rather than ligation because of the reduced incidence of late lower extremity morbidity. The methods of partial interruption include: (*1*) application of an external clip with two serrated edges which divide the vein into channels each measuring 3 mm in diameter[5]; (*2*) application of an external plastic clip with two smooth edges which narrows the lumen of the vessel to a width of 2.5 mm[6]; (*3*) plication of the vein with two or three mattress sutures which divide the lumen into compartments each measuring about 3 mm in diameter[7]; (*4*) creation of a grid-filter by inserting mattress sutures across the lumen of the vein so that strands are 2 or 3 mm apart and tied loosely so that the vein lumen is not constricted[4]; and (*5*) application of a plastic clip with one flat and one serrated edge which divides the vein into compartments measuring 3 mm in diameter[3]. All of the techniques of partial interruption appear equally capable of trapping potential lethal emboli without interfering with venous flow. In general, the methods of partial interruption of the inferior vena cava using external plastic clips are superior to suture techniques because they do not injure the luminal surface, are more reliable in compressing or dividing the vein into channels of appropriate size, and are technically easier to perform.

The Adams–DeWeese clip[3] is preferred for interruption of the vena cava because of its ease of application. The grid-filter suture technique is preferred for partial interruptions of the femoral vein because clips do not seat properly in the narrow femoral space and thus cause angulation and occlusion of the vein. Of the several methods of intraluminal interruption of the inferior vena cava described, the most popular is insertion of a device which has an umbrella design consisting of sharp metallic spokes radiating from a central hub. This is covered by a thin circular sheet of Silastin that has perforations to allow the passage of blood. These three methods of venous interruption will be described although the other methods of partial interruption or ligation can be used if preferred.

Preoperative preparation

Patients with underlying cardiac disease who are in congestive failure as a result of the embolic episode should be fully digitalized and an adequate diureses. If the vena cava is to be interrupted, the bleeding and prothrombin time of patients on anticoagulants achieved should be corrected by the administration of Vitamin K or protamine sulphate intravenously. Anticoagulation can be maintained if interruption is to be carried out at the femoral vein level. In the operating room, the lower extremities should be wrapped with elastic bandages from the toes to below the groin and the legs elevated at least 15° to allow maximal venous return.

Local anaesthesia can be used for femoral vein interruption and for intraluminal interruption of the inferior vena cava. General endotracheal anaesthesia is used for extraluminal interruption of the vena cava.

The operations

EXTRALUMINAL INTERRUPTION OF INFERIOR VENA CAVA

1

The incision

The inferior vena cava can be approached either transperitoneally or extraperitoneally. The transperitoneal approach is preferred because it facilitates exposure of the vena cava at the level of the renal veins, a level which cannot easily be achieved through the standard extraperitoneal approach. Ligation just below the entrance of the renal veins avoids the creation of a cul-de-sac wherein inflow is sluggish and thus conducive to thrombosis should the site of partial interruption be subsequently occluded by thrombosis or a detached clot. The transperitoneal approach also enables simultaneous ligation of the ovarian (or testicular) veins through which emboli may pass from sites of pelvic vein thrombosis.

With the patient in a supine position, either an upper midline or right subcostal incision can be used. With a subcostal incision, the right rectus muscle is transected; with a midline incision the peritoneal cavity is entered through the linea alba.

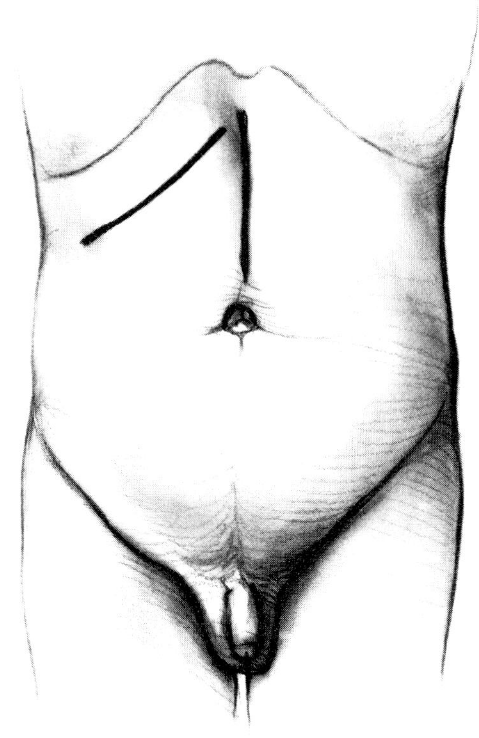

1

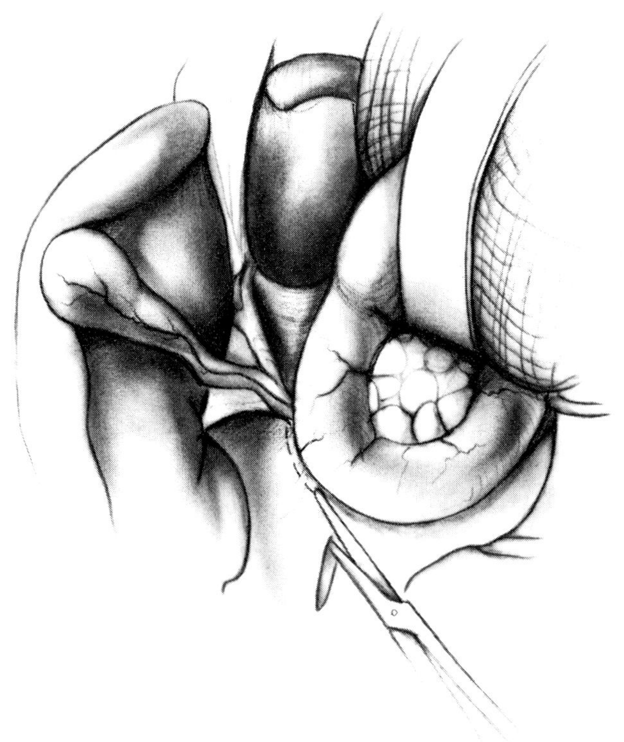

2

2

Exposure of inferior vena cava

The viscera are packed out of the right upper abdomen in a manner similar to that used for a cholecystectomy. The peritoneum lateral to the second portion of the duodenum is incised and the retroperitoneal space entered. By blunt dissection the duodenum and head of the pancreas are then mobilized toward the midline. This manoeuvre exposes the inferior vena cava and both renal veins as they enter the vena cava.

3

Mobilization of inferior vena cava

The fascia over the inferior vena cava is carefully incised, after which a long-limb, right-angle clamp is passed around the cava just below the entrance of the right renal vein. The clamp is passed from the right side of the vena cava and directed behind it by finger palpation to protect the aorta. Care must be taken to avoid injury to the nearby paired upper lumbar veins.

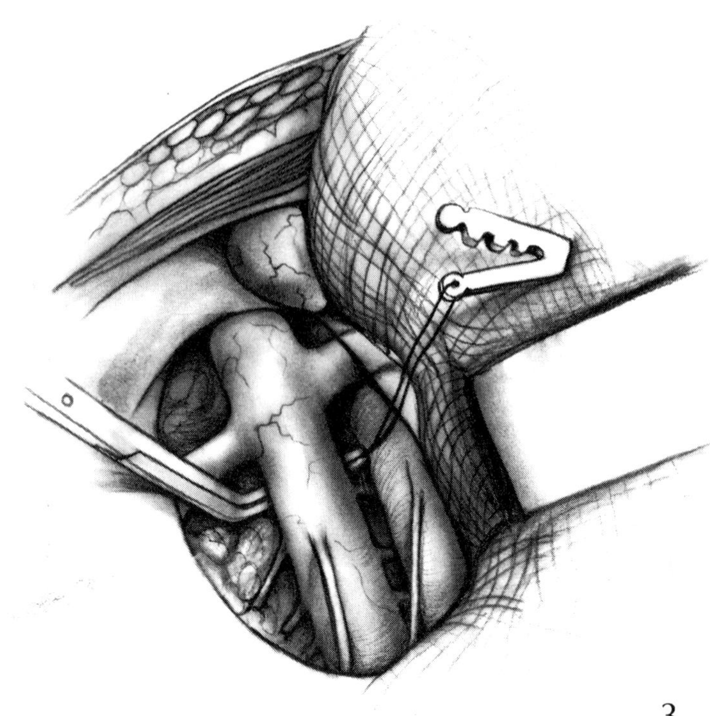

3

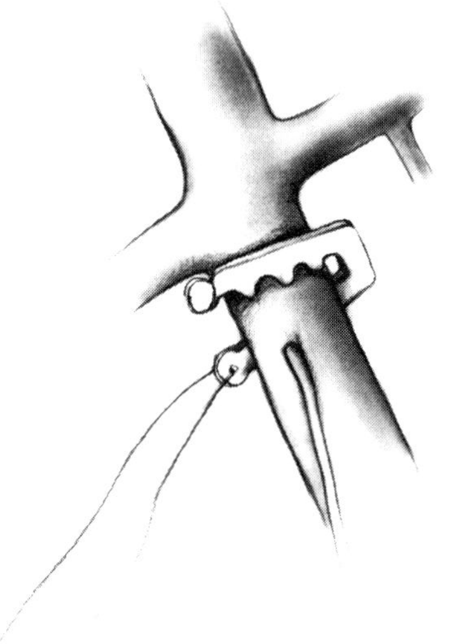

4

4

PASSAGE OF CLIP AROUND THE CAVA

A 4/0 nylon suture threaded through the small perforation in the open end of the smooth limb of the clip is grasped by the clamp and drawn through behind the cava. With traction on the suture, the smooth limb of the open clip is gently guided behind the vena cava.

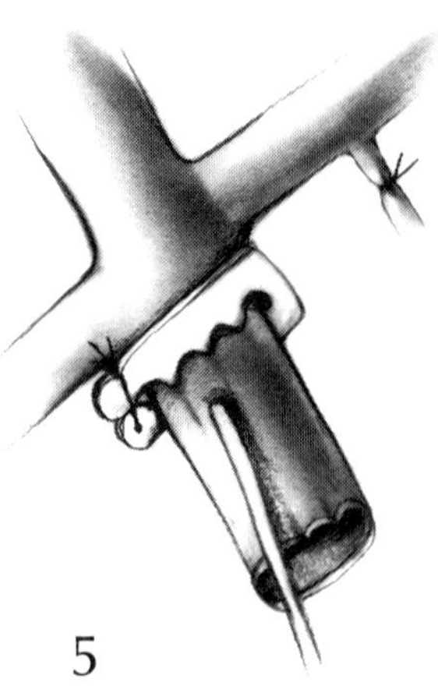

5

5

Securing the clip

The suture is then passed through the perforation in the serrated limb of the clip and, after positioning of the clip just below the entrance of the renal veins, the clip ends are approximated by tying the suture. A second 4/0 nylon suture tie is applied around the end of the clip and seated in opposing grooves on the outer edge of each limb. The interruption procedure is completed by ligating the left ovarian (or testicular) vein as it enters the left renal vein. Since the right ovarian vein enters the vena cava below the level of the clip it does not require ligature. The abdominal incision is then closed in layers, without drainage, to complete the operation.

INTRALUMINAL INTERRUPTION OF INFERIOR VENA CAVA

6

The incision

The patient is placed in a slight Trendelenburg position to protect against accidental air embolism during insertion of the applicator catheter. With the head rotated to the left, an oblique or transverse incision is made on the right side of the neck over the clavicular head of the sternomastoid muscle. Separation of the muscle fibres exposes the internal jugular vein.

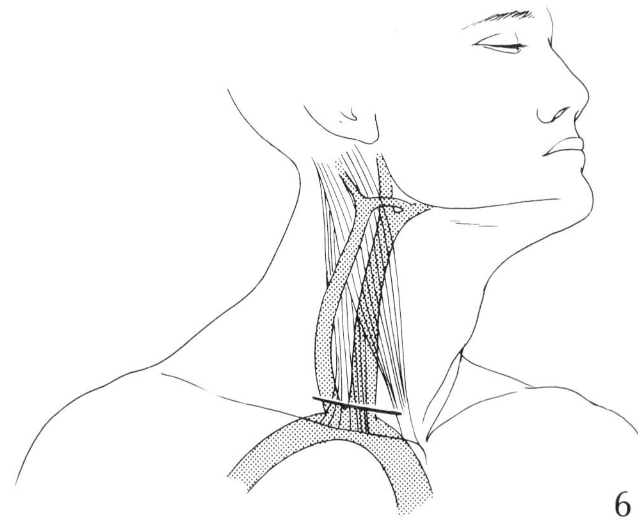

6

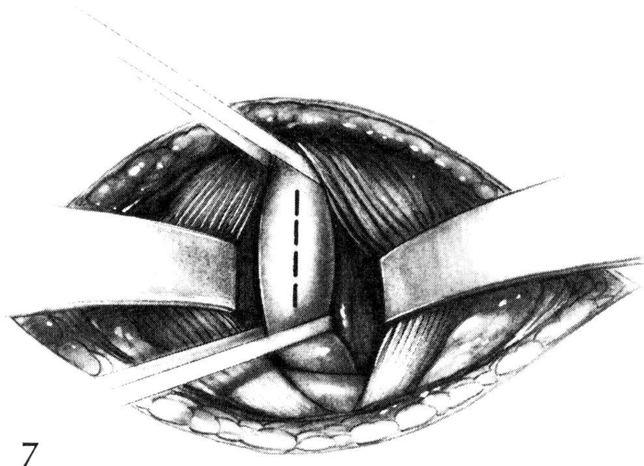

7

7

Isolation of vein

The fascia over the internal jugular vein is incised and about 3 cm of the vein mobilized. Two umbilical tapes are passed around the vein to be retained as keepers to control any subsequent bleeding. A longitudinal incision is then made in the internal jugular vein between the umbilical tapes. The catheter capsule, which contains the folded umbrella filter attached to a guide wire, is inserted into the vein.

8

Passage of catheter

Under fluoroscopic control, the catheter is advanced successively through the superior vena cava and right atrium and into the inferior vena cava. The distal end of the capsule is positioned below the level of the right kidney pelvis. This level is determined by obtaining a preliminary intravenous pyelogram.

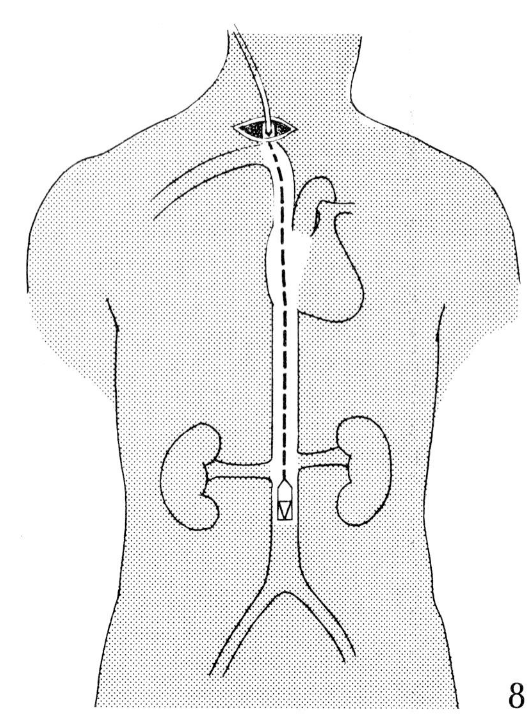

8

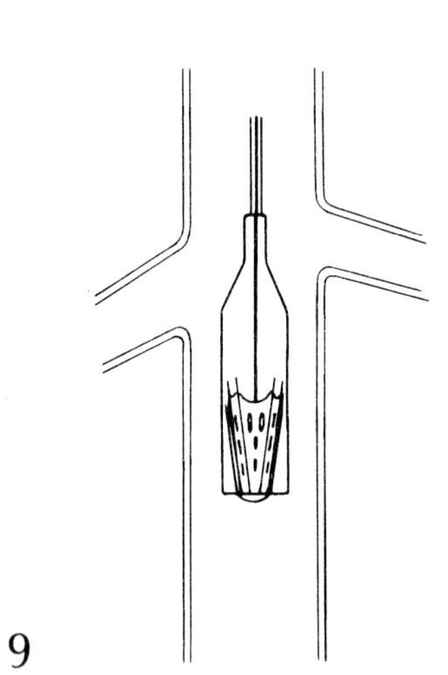

9

9

Insertion of umbrella

The guide wire is then thrust forward through the catheter allowing the umbrella to be ejected from the capsule. When the umbrella springs open its pointed spokes penetrate the wall of the vein.

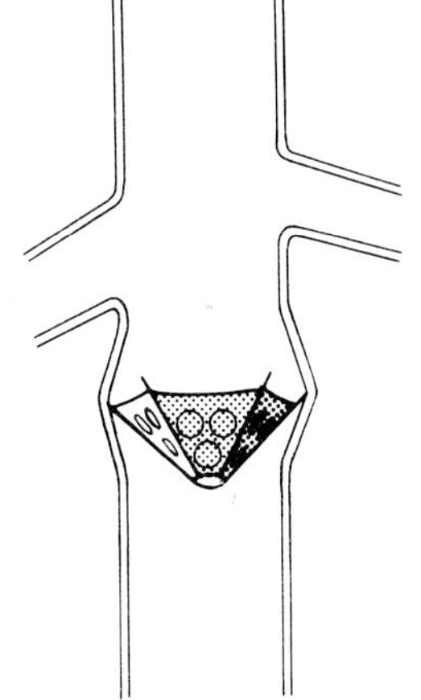

10

10

Fixation of umbrella

The umbrella is fixed in place by slight upward traction on the guide wire. The guide wire is then unscrewed from the umbrella and it, along with the catheter, is removed. The incision in the internal jugular vein is closed with fine plastic vascular suture material and the wound closed in layers without drainage. At the conclusion of the operation, a plain roentgenogram of the abdomen is obtained to verify the position of the umbrella in the inferior vena cava.

PARTIAL INTERRUPTION OF FEMORAL VEIN

11

The incision

An incision is made in the skin crease just below the inguinal ligament and extending medially nearly to the pubic tubercle.

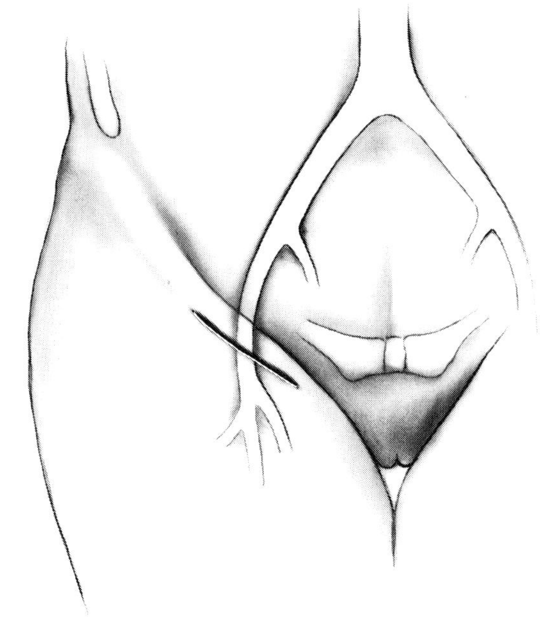

11

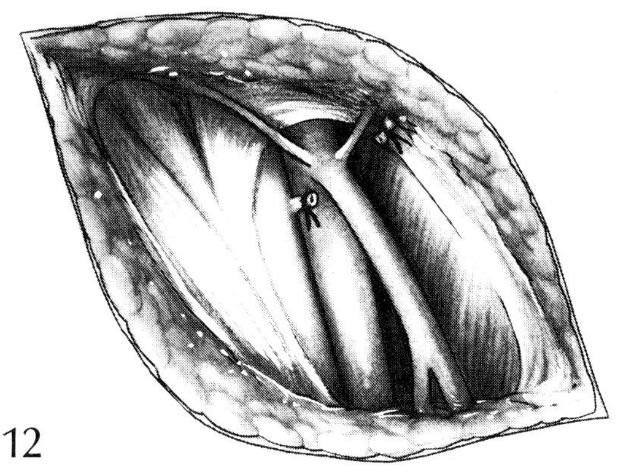

12

12

Exposure of femoral vein

The saphenous vein is identified and followed to the fossa ovalis where it joins the common femoral vein. The small superficial external pudendal artery, lying just beneath the saphenous vein, is ligated and divided. The fascia over the common femoral vein is then incised.

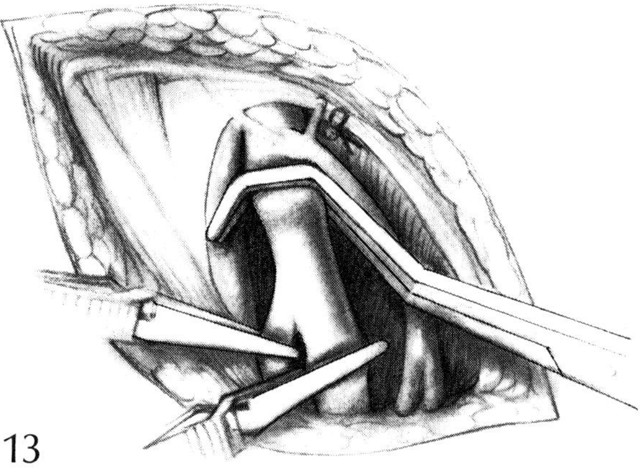

13

13

Isolation of femoral veins

The superficial femoral and deep femoral veins are mobilized and occluded with bulldog clamps. A vascular clamp is then applied across the common femoral vein immediately below the entrance of the greater saphenous vein.

14

Insertion of sutures

Mattress stitches of 4/0 or 5/0 nylon are passed through the common femoral vein just below the occluding vascular clamp. The strands are placed approximately 2 or 3 mm apart. Generally two, and no more than three, sutures are required.

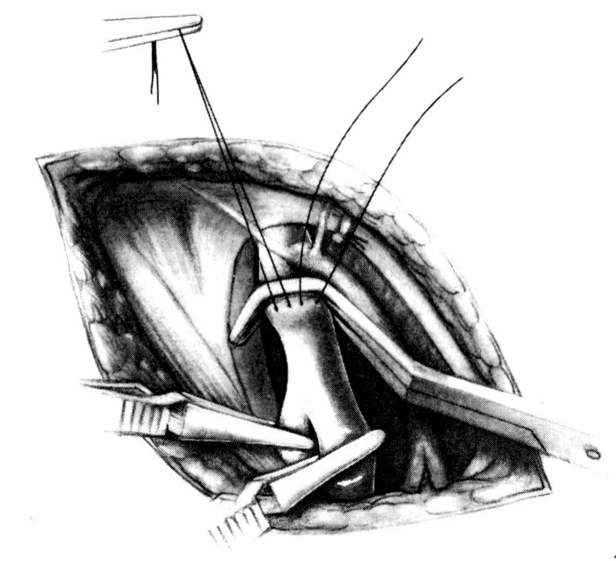

14

15

Tying of sutures

The clamps are removed from the vein and the sutures are individually tied to provide slight tension without significantly compressing the vein. Tying the sutures over a No. 34 hard rubber catheter avoids excessive narrowing of the vein. (The inset indicates the cross-sectional appearance of an ideal filter.) The wound is then closed in layers after meticulous haemostasis has been obtained. If the patient has been maintained on anticoagulants, a small plastic catheter can be brought out of the subcutaneous tissue through a stab incision inferior to the wound and connected to constant low pressure suction for 24–48 hours.

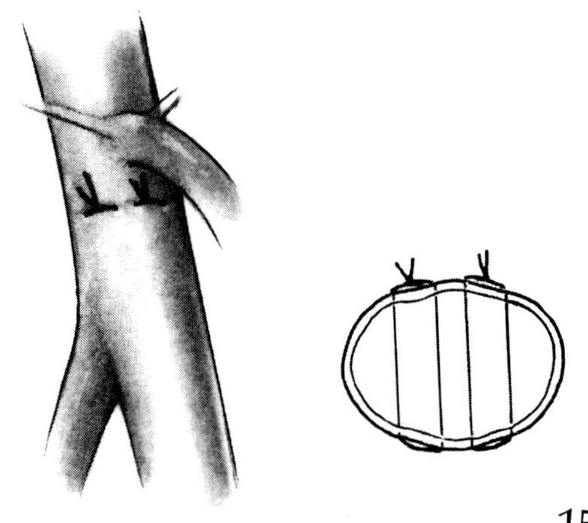

15

Postoperative care

Postoperative management is principally directed towards the prevention of oedema in the lower extremities and the prevention of further thrombosis or new thrombosis. Lower extremity oedema can be minimized by elevation of the lower extremities 15–20° above the heart level and restricting ambulation until all pre-existing leg oedema has disappeared. When the patient becomes ambulatory, support elastic stockings should be worn at all times. The patient should be instructed against prolonged standing or sitting with the legs dependent for 1–4 weeks.

When not contraindicated, anticoagulation therapy should be instituted in the postoperative period. This is initiated using concentrated aqueous heparin given intravenously to achieve a clotting time two or three times above control. The patient is maintained on heparin for 7–10 days and then switched to warfarin sodium for an additional 8–12 weeks. The purpose of postoperative anticoagulation is to prevent progressive thrombosis below the interruption site which will contribute to the postphlebitic syndrome.

Results

Operative mortality

The operative mortality following any type of vein interruption procedure is related primarily to the severity of the underlying cardiac disease and the degree of incapacitation resulting from the episode of pulmonary embolism which led to vein interruption[11,12]. Significant pre-existing cardiac disease has been associated with a 30 per cent mortality rate following inferior vena caval interruption compared to 3–7 per cent mortality rate in patients without cardiac disease. Early mortality as a direct result of or failure of the operative procedure itself is usually from two sources: recurrent pulmonary embolism and fatal shock. Fatal embolism following either ligation or partial interruption of the inferior vena cava is extremely rare and indicates that thrombosis was present or had formed in a vein proximal to the site of interruption or that the interruption site had become disrupted. Fatal shock is almost exclusively a complication of vena caval ligation. This is the result of sudden pooling of blood in the lower extremities causing a critical decrease in venous return to the heart. This complication is rare following partial interruption procedures.

In-hospital mortality following interruption of the femoral vein varies between 5 and 15 per cent and is also related primarily to the severity of underlying myocardial disease[13]. The incidence of recurrent fatal embolism subsequent to interruption at the femoral level is somewhat higher than that following interruption of the inferior vena cava.

Late complications

Recurrent non-fatal pulmonary embolism following either ligation or partial interruption of the inferior vena cava has been reported in between 5 and 15 per cent of patients[11,12]. Recurrent non-fatal embolism after femoral vein interruption occurs in 10–25 per cent of patients[13].

Lower extremity swelling immediately following surgery occurs frequently following vein ligation or when a site of partial interruption becomes suddenly occluded by embolus or thrombosis. Elevation of the lower extremities and early reinstitution of anticoagulation postoperatively will prevent or minimize the development of this early oedema. Significant late extremity morbidity has been reported in up to 30 per cent of patients following femoral or vena caval interruption with a lower incidence in patients undergoing partial interruption procedures[11,12]. Most late morbidity is secondary to pre-existing thrombosis or to progression of this thrombosis. In most large series, 60 to 70 per cent of partial interruption procedures have remained patent by phlebography and in these patients there has been a reduced incidence and severity of the postphlebitic syndrome[12].

References

1. Homans, J. Thrombosis of the deep veins of the lower leg causing pulmonary embolism. New England Journal of Medicine 1934; 211: 993–997
2. Beall, A. C., Fred, H. L., Cooley, D. A. Pulmonary embolism. Current problems in surgery. Chicago: Yearbook Medical Publishers, 1964; February
3. Adams, J. T., DeWeese, J. A. Partial interruption of the inferior vena cava with a new plastic clip. Surgery, Gynecology and Obstetrics 1966; 123: 1087–1088
4. DeWeese, M. S., Hunter, D. C., Jr. A vena cava filter for the prevention of pulmonary embolism: a five-year clinical experience. Archives of Surgery 1963; 86: 852–868
5. Miles, R. M., Chappell, F., Renner, O. A partially occluding vena caval clip for prevention of pulmonary embolism. American Surgeon 1964; 30: 40–47
6. Moretz, W. H., Rhode, C. M., Shepherd, M. H. Prevention of pulmonary emboli by partial occlusion of the inferior vena cava. American Surgeon 1959; 25: 617–626
7. Spencer, F. C., Quattlebaum, J. K., Quattlebaum, J. K., Jr, Sharp, E. H., Jude, J. R. Plication of the inferior vena cava for pulmonary embolism: a report of 20 cases. Annals of Surgery 1962; 155: 827–837
8. Greenfield, L. J., McCurdy, J. R., Brown, P. P., Elkins, R. C. A new intracaval filter permitting continued flow and resolution of emboli. Surgery 1973; 73: 599–606
9. Hunter, J. A., Dye, W. S., Javid, H., Najafi, H., Goldin, M. D., Serry, C. Permanent transvenous balloon occlusion of the inferior vena cava: experience with 60 patients. Annals of Surgery 1977; 186: 491–499
10. Mobin-Uddin, K., McLean, R., Bolooki, H., Jude, J. R. Caval interruption for prevention of pulmonary embolism. Archives of Surgery 1969; 99: 711–715
11. Adams, J. T., Feingold, B. E., DeWeese, J. A. Comparative evaluation of ligation and partial interruption of the inferior vena cava. Archives of Surgery 1971; 103: 272–276
12. Donaldson, M. C., Wirthlin, L. S. Donaldson, G. A. Thirty-year experience with surgical interruption of the inferior vena cava for prevention of pulmonary embolism. Annals of Surgery 1980; 191: 367–372
13. Adams, J. T., DeWeese, J. A. Comparative evaluation of ligation and partial interruption of the femoral vein in the treatment of thromboembolic disease. Annals of Surgery 1970; 172: 795–803

Thyroidectomy

Hugh Dudley ChM, FRCS, FRCS (Ed), FRACS
Professor of Surgery, St Mary's Hospital Medical School, London;
Consultant Surgeon, St Mary's Hospital, London, UK

Introduction

This chapter describes routine thyroidectomy such as would be carried out for a patient with Graves' disease or multinodular goitre. Many modifications are necessary for special circumstances, as are changes in the routine of preoperative preparation and postoperative care. For the euthyroid patient no special preparation is necessary, though the author always has an indirect laryngoscopy performed and determines serum calcium concentration as a base line. A straight X-ray of the neck is useful to establish the degree of tracheal compression, and X-ray of the chest alerts the surgeon to the possibility of an intrathoracic extension which may have escaped his notice on clinical examination.

Preoperative

1

Careful positioning of the patient is essential. The neck is extended to its fullest extent by placing the occiput on a head ring. The neck is thrown forward to make the goitre as prominent as possible. The eyes are protected, and the endotracheal tube is best strapped firmly into position.

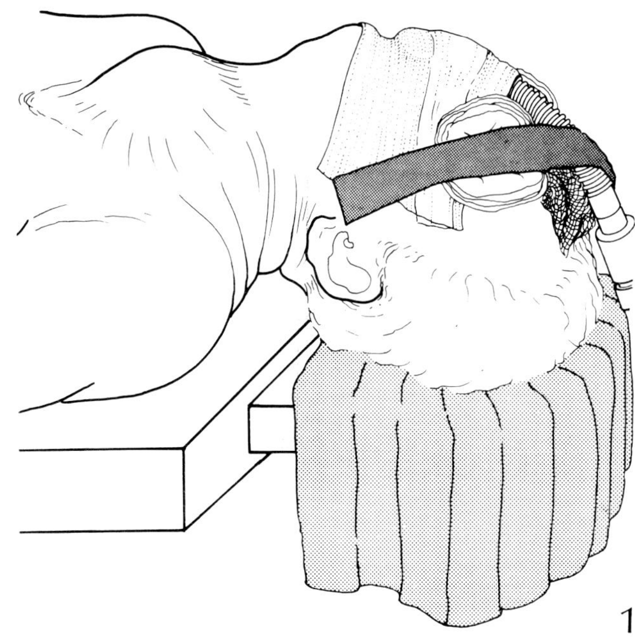

1

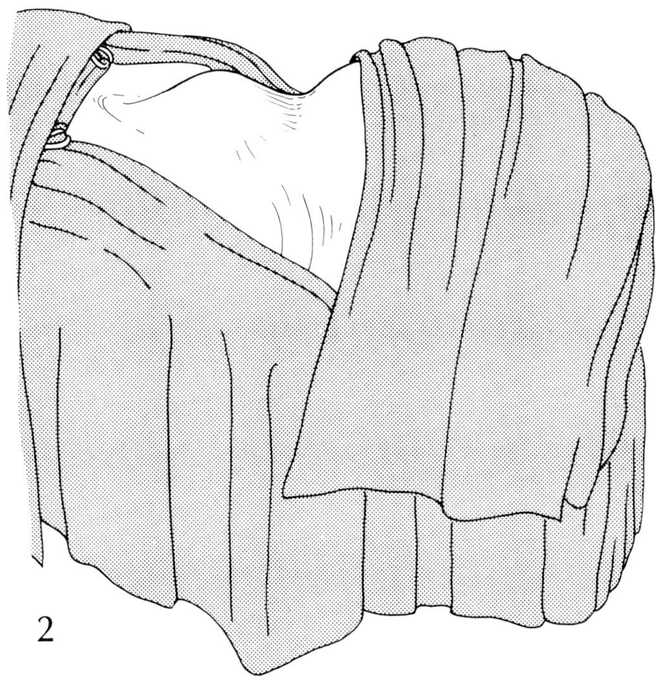

2

2

Draping must leave the surgeon completely free to move around the patient's head, and anaesthetic tubing is led away, outside the plane of the drawing. A wide field is thus available, particularly superiorly above the thyroid process.

3

Many methods of marking the skin are used. The best is to stretch a monofilament suture between two artery forceps pressed firmly across the root of the neck. The suture will conform to the point of maximum convexity of the goitre, and when the neck is brought back to mid-position the line sinks so as to be just above the collar bone and suprasternal notch.

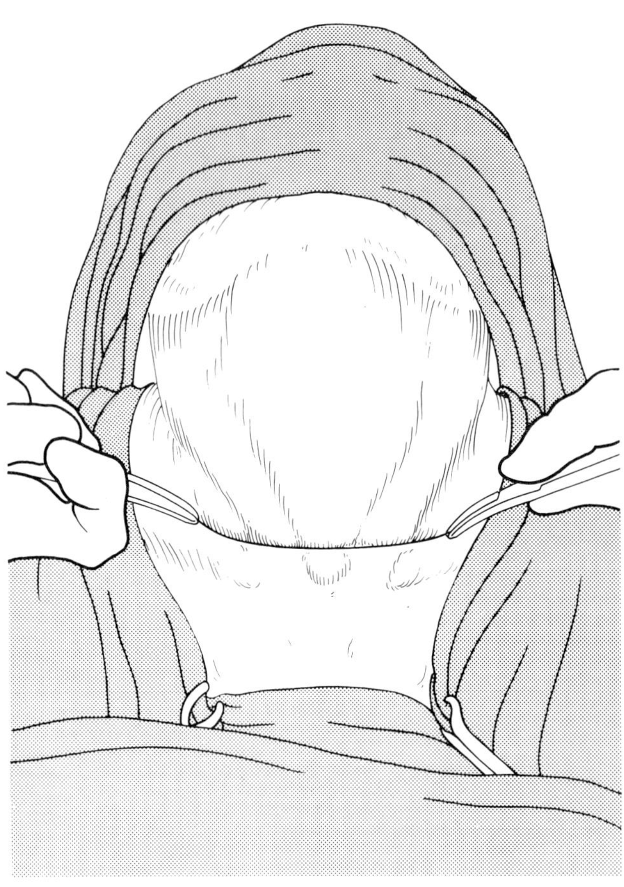

3

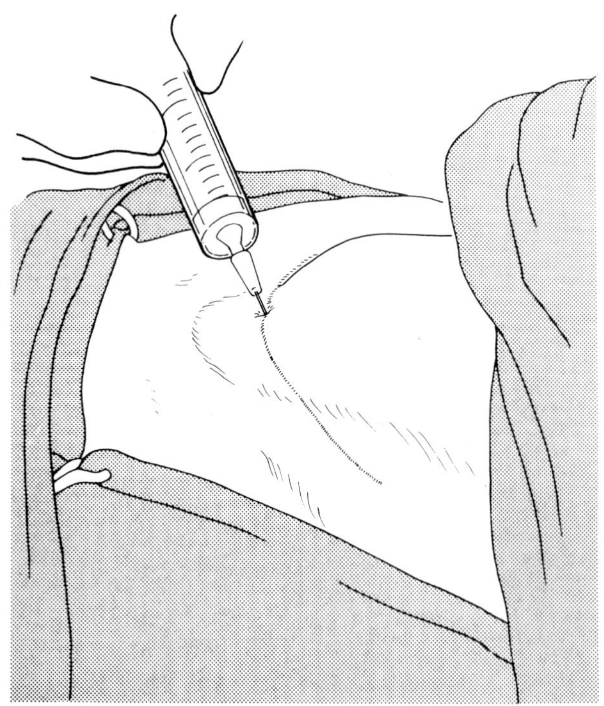

4

4

A fine needle is introduced through the mark, and the subcutaneous tissues up to the thyroid process are infiltrated with 0.9 per cent saline containing 1:500 000 adrenaline. Some surgeons omit this step as there is no direct evidence to support its use.

The operation

5

The skin incision is made down to the subcutaneous layer deep to platysma which is intracutaneous. The knife blade works horizontally across the flap, and small vessels are picked up with fine haemostats and coagulated. The plane is superficial to the anterior jugular veins, but tributaries of these may require attention.

5

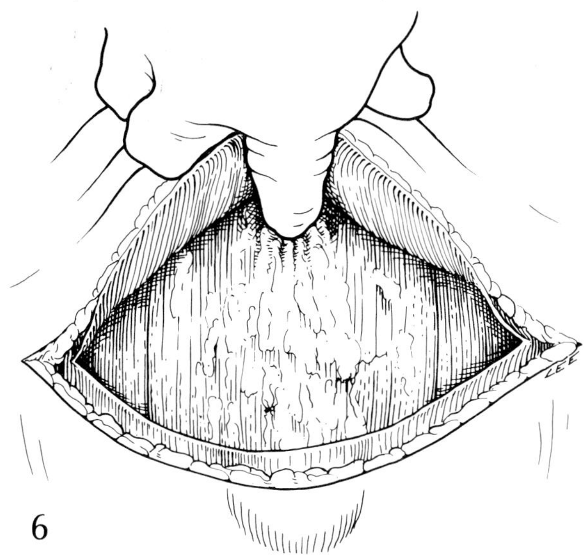

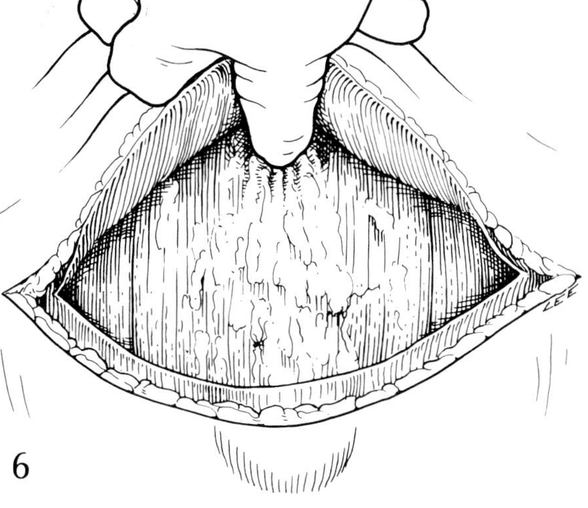

6

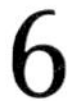

6

The dissection is completed bluntly with finger and gauze, and *must* reach the thyroid prominence.

7

Below a flap is raised down to the suprasternal notch (2–3 cm). Fine catspaw retractors help in this manoeuvre.

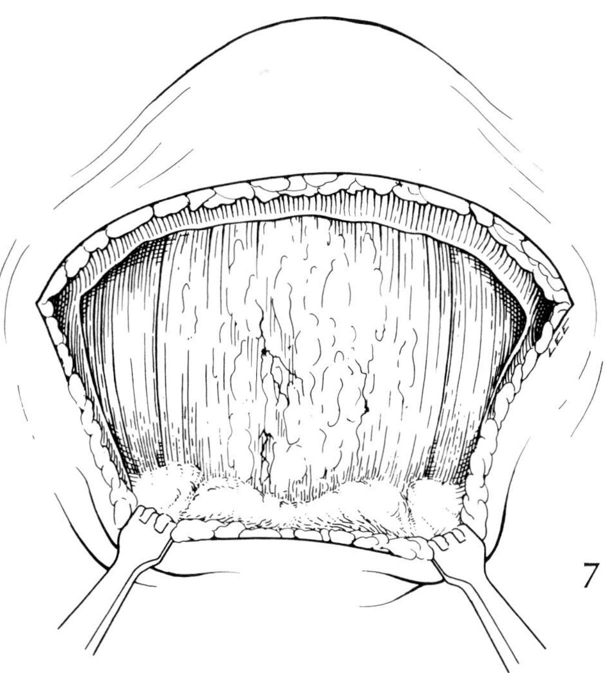

7

8

The edges of the wound are held retracted with a self-retaining retractor, and the neck is then covered with moist gauze which clings to the contours. A vertical incision is made in the mid-line which may or may not exactly define the gap in the strap muscles. It does not matter if a few fibres on one side or the other are misplaced.

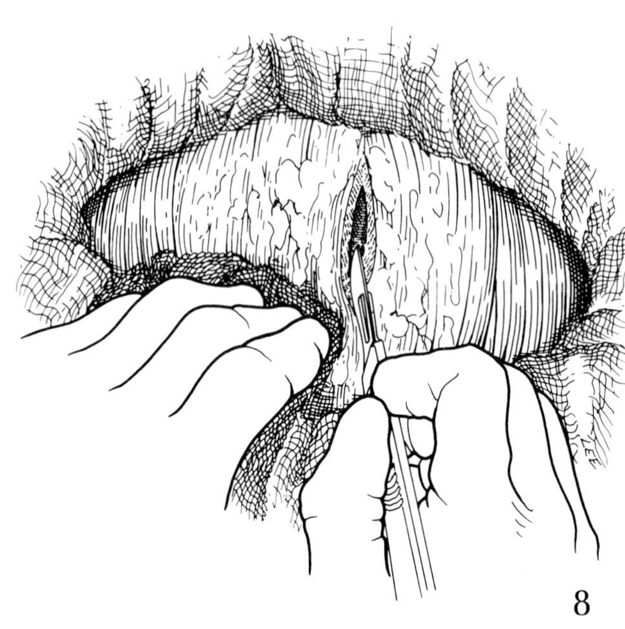

8

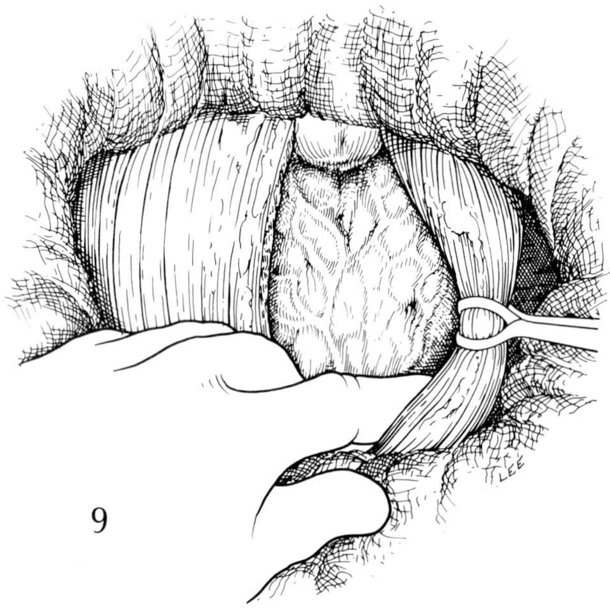

9

9

The incision is caried down to the thyroid and the flap conveniently grasped with a Babcock's forceps and pulled forwards and laterally. The finger or a pledget can then be used to strip the flap away from the convex anterolateral surface of the gland. If this is done in the correct plane bleeding will *not* occur.

10

The gland is now isolated medially, and the inferior thyroid veins are dissected from the areolat fascia. They can be divided between ligatures or, as shown here, between clips. As this is done, the carotid sheath comes into view, and, if the dissection is carried backwards and medially around the lower pole the recurrent nerve may often be seen. Its idealized course is shown in the illustration, but it is rarely so well displayed and, as subsequent illustrations demonstrate, it is initially avoided along with the inferior thyroid artery.

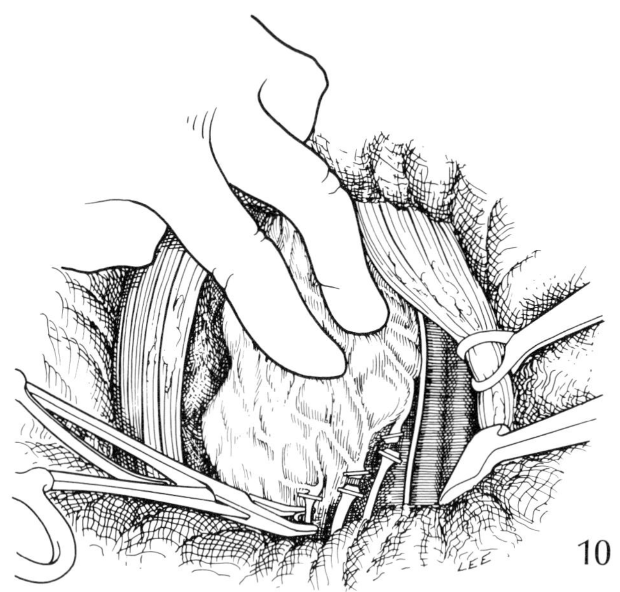

10

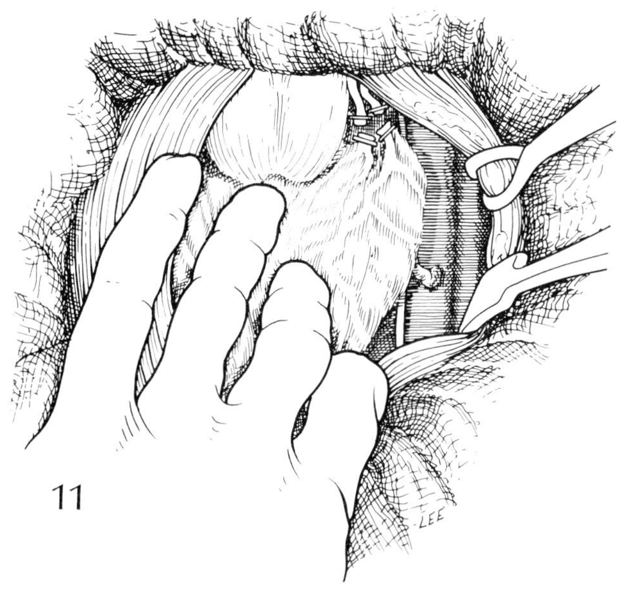

11

11

The superior pole is next mobilized. Dissection is undertaken in the prelaryngeal space superficial to the cricothyroid, thus avoiding the external laryngeal nerve. Once more the vessels may be dealt with by ligature or clipping, depending upon size. Mobilization of the pole downward and forward brings the inferior thyroid artery into view.

12

Safe division of this structure anterior to the recurrent laryngeal nerve is achieved by ligating or clipping *at the gland surface* as shown. The recurrent nerve's position is so variable that each vessel must be clearly seen and ligated separately. The nerve is identified posteriorly if this has not already been achieved.

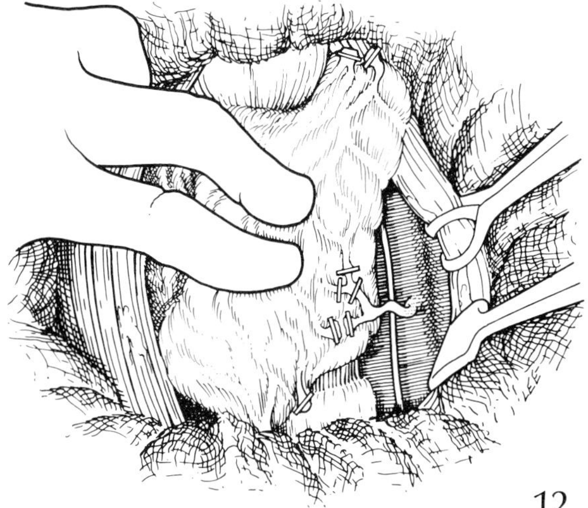

12

13

The contralateral lobe is mobilized as necessary, and it is then possible to divide the isthmus by passing a blunt haemostat up into the pretracheal space. It is usually possible to clamp with a second curved forceps, divide and then turn the lobe laterally.

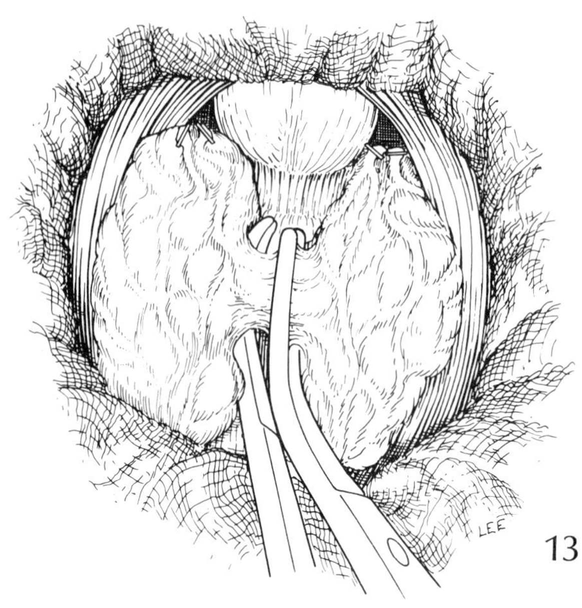

13

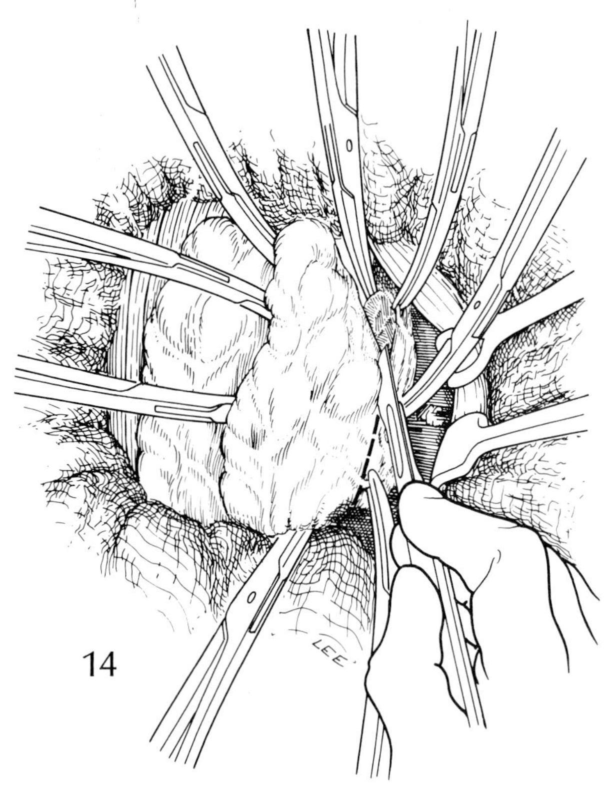

14

14

Fine haemostats are then applied to the margin of the gland, grasping where necessary the veins crossing over the surface. The lobe is then cut across superficial to this point. Some surgeons proceed mediolaterally, others in the reverse direction, but the difference is minimal provided the dissection has been meticulous and the cut is made under direct vision in a dry field.

15

The residual tissue falls back on either side of the trachea. The isthmus is ligated. Clips are applied peripherally and diathermy used on the open mouths of the vessels on the cut surface. Alternatively, bleeding may be staunched with a running suture of polyglycolic acid.

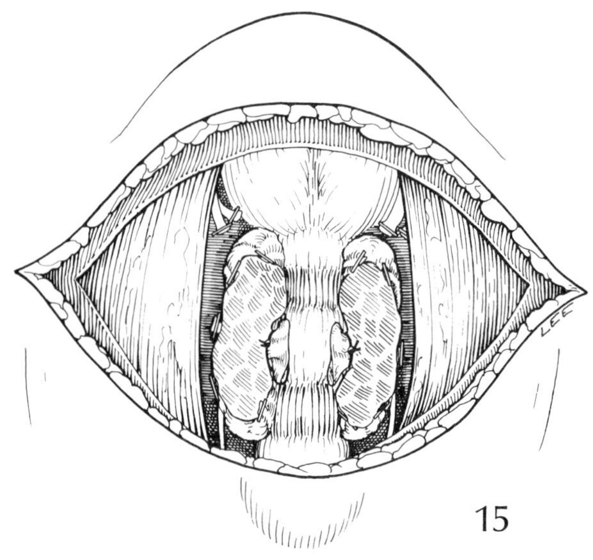

15

16

The vertical incision in the investing fascia is closed with interrupted sutures of the same material and the subcutaneous layer, containing *platysma*, similarly. Although traditionally clips are employed for the skin, the author always uses a running subcuticular prolene suture, which is left in for 10 days until healing is firm.

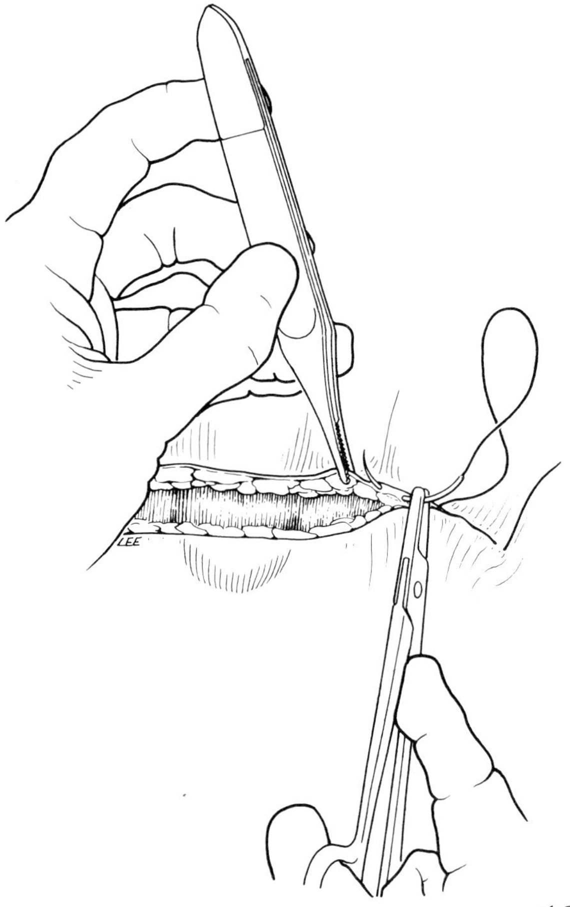

16

Drainage

The author learned thyroidectomy from Keith Patterson Brown, who never used drains. The field should be completely dry before closure, and, given this, drains are nearly always unnecessary. If they appear to be required, it is now the best practice to lead fine suction tubes out laterally at the end of the incision. They are removed at 24–36 h, and the resultant gap closed with a single clip or stitch.

Parathyroid gland exploration

Euan Milroy MB BS, FRCS
Consultant Urologist, The Middlesex Hospital, London

Introduction

Parathyroid exploration is not an operation to be done occasionally. Although many of these operations are not particularly difficult and may be completed in a reasonably short time, the occasional extremely difficult case cannot be predicted in advance. The operations should only be undertaken by surgeons who are familiar with the surgery of the neck and who regularly carry out parathyroid explorations.

Hyperparathyroidism

The only indication for parathyroid surgery is to remove overactive parathyroid tissue in patients in whom it is causing hypercalcaemia, there being no satisfactory long-term drug therapy for hyperparathyroidism. Patients with hypercalcaemia may present in a great variety of ways. The stone, bone and gastrointestinal (peptic ulcers and pancreatitis) symptoms are well known, as are the less common psychological and psychiatric disturbances caused by hypercalcaemia. In a recent personal series of 200 patients with surgically proven hyperparathyroidism 35 per cent presented with stone disease. Of patients presenting with urinary calculi some 10 per cent would be found to have hyperparathyroidism if thoroughly investigated. With a large array of biochemical tests now being carried out on all patients, and with the increasing popularity of regular screening procedures on the healthy population, larger numbers of patients with asymptomatic hyperparathyroidism are being found – 40 per cent of our own series of patients with surgically proven hyperparathyroidism. In fact most of these patients, particularly in the older age groups, will have one or other of a number of rather vague symptoms – lethargy, malaise, polyuria, polydipsia or hypertension – which although not diagnostic of parathyroid disease may be relieved by removing the overactive parathyroid tissue[1].

The incidence of hyperparathyroidism is far higher than was first described and has recently been reported to be approximately 28 new cases per 100000 population per year, both in the USA[2] and in England[3]; the incidence increasing with age, especially in women, to approximately 188 per 100000 among women over the age of 60 years[2]. Seventy per cent of our cases were female.

Diagnosis

The diagnosis of hyperparathyroidism is made by the finding of persistent hypercalcaemia, having ensured that the raised calcium is not the result of a high serum albumen, and having excluded all other causes of hypercalcaemia[4]. It is essential that the surgeon undertaking parathyroid surgery works closely with an experienced endocrinologist as there are many pitfalls to trap the unwary into an incorrect diagnosis. Peripheral venous levels of parathyroid hormone are sometimes but not invariably raised in primary hyperparathyroidism. With the older assay techniques any detectable circulating parathyroid hormone was felt to be an indication of parathyroid overactivity. The more recently developed amino terminal assay is more reliable and gives an excellent correlation of peripheral levels of hormone with parathyroid pathology[5]. The steroid suppression test[6] will help to exclude non-parathyroid causes of hypercalcaemia but again a number of false positive and negative results will be found.

Once a definite diagnosis of hyperparathyroidism has been established, attempts may be made to localize the overactivity to one or other of the parathyroid glands. Unfortunately this is far from easy although many centres are working to improve their ability to localize parathyroid tissue preoperatively. At present we can achieve an 87 per cent chance of predicting the site of a single adenoma using the technique of selective sampling of neck veins for parathyroid hormone[7]. This technique is of particular value in patients in whom previous surgery has failed to find an abnormal gland.

Ultrasound is, in our experience, of some value especially in reoperations on the neck. Computerized axial tomography is of little value in the neck but may find the occasional anterior mediastinal parathyroid adenoma where ultrasound cannot be used. Selective arteriography is effective in expert hands, again particularly in the patient who has been explored previously, but may carry unjustifiable risks in the older patient. Isotope scans of the parathyroids have unfortunately not lived up to their earlier high expectations.

Preoperative localization is therefore at present far from perfect and makes it all the more important that the surgeon has a full knowledge of the various possible pathological abnormalities and anatomical variations of the parathyroid glands and has in his mind a clear plan of the operation he is to undertake to cover all eventualities.

Indications for parathyroid exploration

It is our opinion that all patients with proven hyperparathyroidism should be offered surgery providing they are fit to withstand the anaesthetic and operation. There is of course no argument about the symptomatic patient, but the justification for operating on the many asymptomatic patients is often questioned. It must be remembered that many of these so-called asymptomatic patients have symptoms which may be related to the hypercalcaemia and, although no adequate long-term study of the natural history of mild asymptomatic hyperparathyroidism has been carried out, what evidence there is suggests that some 20 per cent (of 147 patients observed over a 5 year period) will develop complications of the disease which precipitate parathyroid surgery[8]. To have operated on these patients as soon as the diagnosis is made would cure the hyperparathyroidism before more serious and irreversible complications, particularly renal, occur. It is remarkable how frequently these rather vague symptoms improve after surgical correction of the hypercalcaemia, and how the patients feel an improvement in their general health and well-being. It should also not be forgotten that hypercalcaemia is in its own right a lethal condition, particularly in the older patient.

The operation

1

Position of patient and anaesthesia

All patients must have a preoperative inspection of their vocal cords to confirm that both recurrent laryngeal nerves are intact.

The patient is positioned with the neck extended and the head resting on a rubber ring. A small sandbag under the shoulders may help but care must be taken not to overextend the neck. This is not only dangerous in the older patient but may also make the operative exposure less satisfactory. A 20–30° head-up tilt helps to reduce venous bleeding. A general anaesthetic using moderate hypotension down to 70–80 mmHg systolic blood pressure, with the help of an experienced anaesthetist (using a sympathetic blockade, or a sodium nitroprusside technique), is a most useful aid in preventing peroperative bleeding.

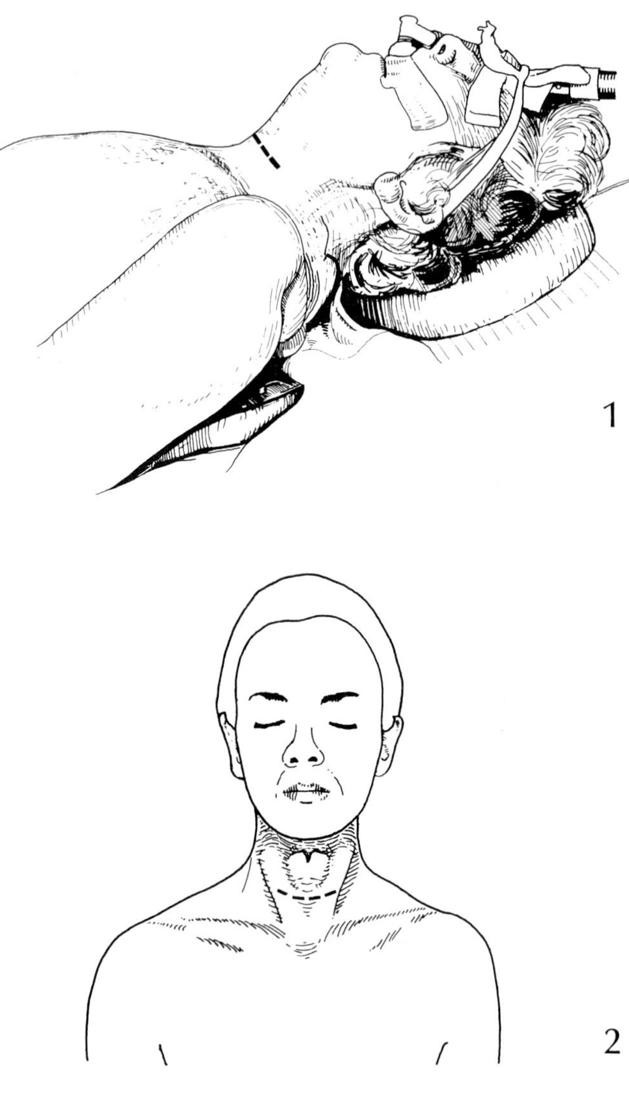

1

2

The two most important factors in the search for the parathyroid glands are adequate exposure and absence of bleeding in the operative field. Vital staining of parathyroid tissue using a preoperative infusion of methylene blue is sometimes suggested. Most surgeons who carry out large numbers of parathyroid explorations find this technique of altering the colour difference between parathyroid and normal tissue unnecessary, unreliable and sometimes even misleading. It is far more important that the surgeon should become confident in recognizing the subtle differences between the reddish brown colour of the normal parathyroid, the somewhat darker abnormal parathyroid, and the various other colours of the adjacent thyroid, lymph nodes and adipose tissues.

Draping and incision

2

The neck is draped as for a thyroidectomy; four single towels will be found to be simpler than a double head towel. An 8–10 cm long transverse skin crease incision is made approximately midway between the notch of the thyroid cartilage and the suprasternal notch. Care should be taken not to curve the incision too much when the neck is well extended; the incision will appear more curved when the head is positioned normally.

3

It may be found helpful in making a symmetrical incision to press a tightly held suture into the skin in order to impress a line to follow with the scalpel. On no account should vertical skin scratches be made across the line of the incision in order to help subsequent wound alignment; these may leave unsightly scars.

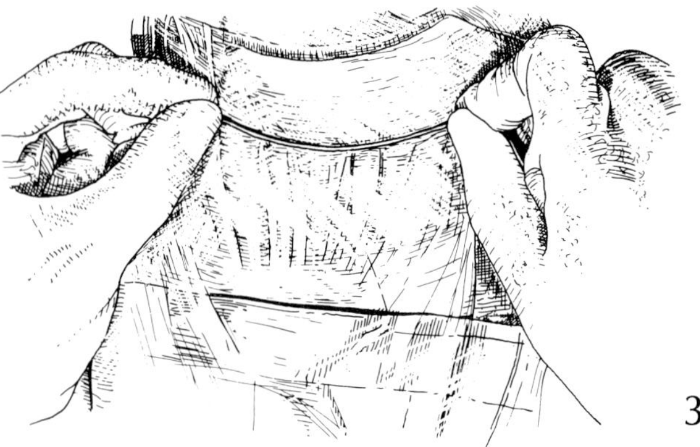

3

4

The incision is taken through subcutaneous fat and, at either end of the incision, the platysma muscle. The skin, fat and muscle are then separated as one layer from the underlying strap muscles. It is most important for adequate exposure to develop this plane as far up as the thyroid and down to the suprasternal notch. Once the correct plane is found this separation is made easier by using blunt dissection with firm but gentle pressure of the fingers of both hands covered by a gauze swab.

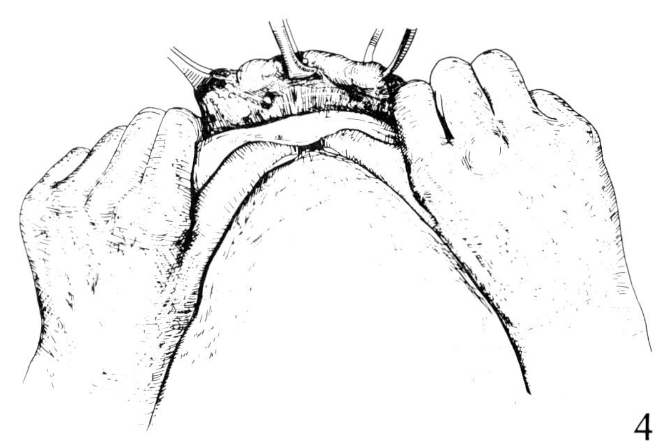

4

5

Exposure of the thyroid and parathyroids

5

A self-retaining ring retractor, bent to lie over the neck, with 4–6 rake blades will be found to be much more satisfactory than other forms of wound retraction. In this and subsequent illustrations the patient's head is on the right.

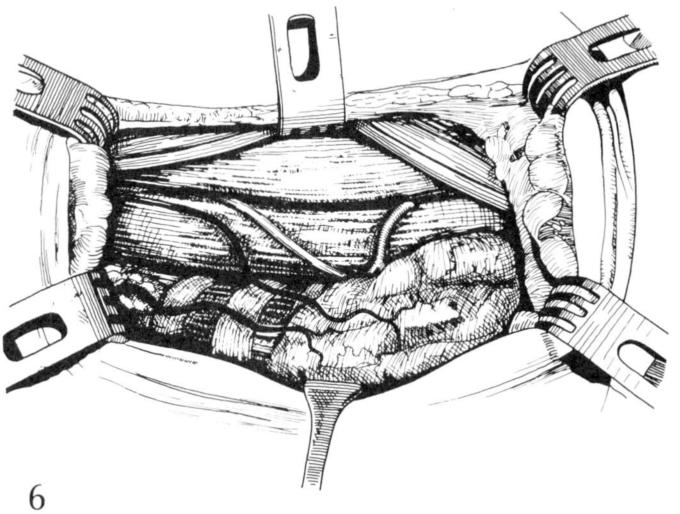

6

6

The strap muscles are separated in the midline. It is never necessary to divide the muscles transversely. These muscles are always thin enough to retract laterally and muscle division causes unnecessary bleeding, which can make adequate parathyroid exploration impossible.

If no gland abnormality has been localized preoperatively each side of the neck must be explored thoroughly in turn. It is the author's practice to start exploring the right side of the neck, standing on the patient's left. The thyroid gland may then be held by one hand while dissection continues with the other, using short fine curved scissors or dissecting forceps. When exploration on one side is complete, the surgeon and assistant change sides to explore the other side of the neck. It must be admitted that some surgeons find this technique awkward and prefer to stand on the same side of the patient's neck they are exploring. The strap muscles are separated from the thyroid gland and the middle thyroid vein ligated and cut.

7 & 8

Finding the parathyroid glands

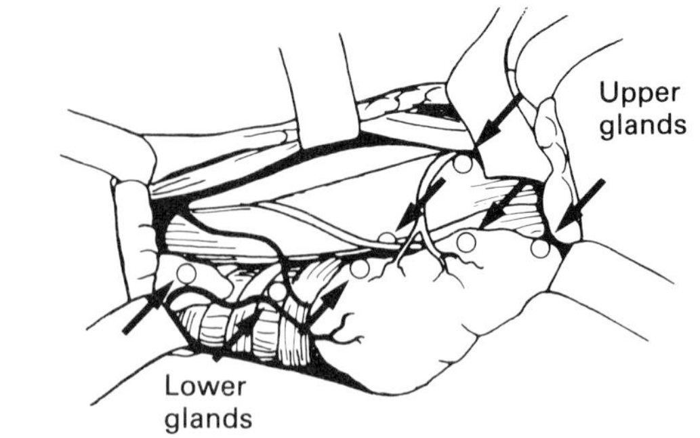

The thyroid gland may now be gently lifted up and the other important landmarks found. These are the inferior thyroid artery and the recurrent laryngeal nerve. The surgeon must be careful not to start looking for parathyroid tissue until this complete exposure of the area has been achieved. *The superior parathyroid* is easier to find than the inferior. It usually lies on the posterior surface of the thyroid gland just cranial to the inferior thyroid artery, always deep to a thin but definite transparent fascial layer under which it can be seen to move, with its associated fatty tissue, when pushed with the scissors or dissecting forceps. It may lie further up the course of the superior thyroid vessels or, if the gland enlarges, may descend deep to the inferior thyroid vessels to lie lateral to, or even behind, the oesophagus. The *mobility* of the gland within its fascial sheath together with its *site*, the typical yellow-brown *colour* and the soft *consistency* of parathyroid tissue compared to the firmer lymph nodes and thyroid gland, are the four all-important factors in the localization of parathyroid glands.

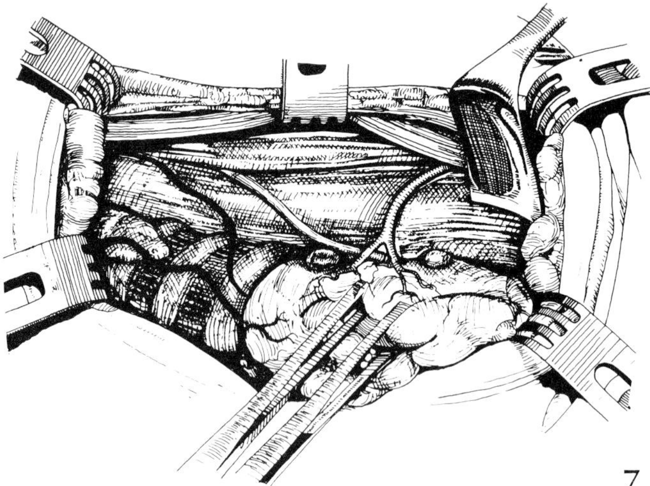

7

The inferior parathyroid is more variable in position and may sometimes be difficult to distinguish from 'brown fat' present in large amounts in the neck of some patients. The normal parathyroid, although varying in size from 1 to 10mm in length, always has a definite structure and vascular supply compared to the more amorphous fatty tissue; it is also not infrequently wrapped, at least in part, in a layer of normal yellow fat. The inferior gland is usually found on the posterolateral surface of the thyroid gland caudad to the inferior thyroid artery. It may however be found anywhere down the course of one of the inferior thyroid veins, along the thymus or in the anterior mediastinum – what is sometimes called the 'thyrothymic axis'. It is important to explore this area and to incise the surface of the thymic lobe as far down as the innominate vein if no inferior gland can be found in the neck. A parathyroid gland may lie within the thymus unseen until the thymic capsule is opened.

Either superior or inferior parathyroid gland may occasionally lie further lateral in the neck but no further out than the carotid sheath. Rarely a gland is completely intrathyroid; most supposed intrathyroid glands are in fact sunk into the surface of the thyroid and may be found by careful dissection of the thyroid surface beneath the fascial covering of the gland. The descent of the glands is also variable; occasionally both parathyroid glands on one side are above or both below the inferior thyroid artery, and occasionally three glands may be on one side of the neck and only one on the other. In approximately 10 per cent of our cases more than four glands were found. Unfortunately the positions of the parathyroid glands are not symmetrical on the left and right sides of the neck.

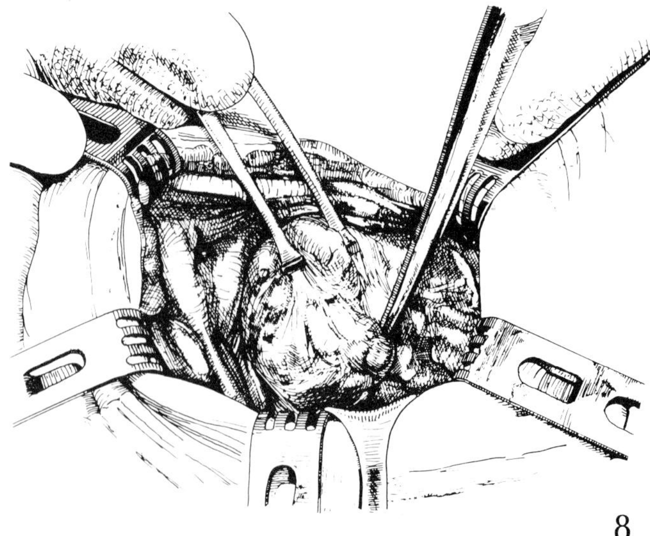

8

It should be noted that the parathyroid glands of children and adolescents are smaller and lighter in colour than adult glands and may be even more difficult to find because of the relatively larger thyroid and thymus glands.

Pathology and surgical plan

Adenoma

Eighty-eight per cent of our patients with hyperparathyroidism were found to have a single parathyroid adenoma; 60 per cent of these were situated in the position of one of the inferior glands. In these patients only the adenoma need be removed although it must be emphasized that care must be taken to remove the adenoma completely. Great difficulty is sometimes encountered in separating a large adenoma in the superior gland position from the recurrent laryngeal nerve which may be completely enclosed by the adenoma as the nerve enters the larynx. One cause for the recurrence of hyperparathyroidism after removal of an adenoma is the further enlargement of a deep fragment of the original adenoma which was not removed at the first operation.

Ten per cent of patients are found to have hyperplasia of all parathyroid tissue. For this reason at least one normal parathyroid gland must be identified in those patients in whom a single adenoma has been found, and a small biopsy taken from the end of the gland furthest from its vascular pedicle and sent for immediate frozen section histological examination in order to confirm the diagnosis.

Hyperplasia

Generalized hyperplasia is usually easy to diagnose because all four glands are large and relatively easy to find. When all the glands have been found and confirmed histologically, three glands are removed completely and the distal two-thirds of the remaining gland are also removed leaving behind the third (approximately 50 mg) adjacent to the vascular pedicle. If possible the remaining fragment should be one of the inferior glands and should be carefully marked with a clip or non-absorbable suture in case further surgical removal becomes necessary. It is our practice to mark all remaining parathyroid tissue, normal or hyperplastic, with one or two vasiular clips placed close to, but not upon, the parathyroid tissue.

Nodular hyperplasia

Patients with nodular hyperplasia of the parathyroid present a difficult problem because the glands, although all histologically abnormal, may vary considerably in size, one or more being enlarged and the others being normal in size but containing nodules of hyperplastic tissue. This diagnosis requires a careful and experienced pathologist and fine surgical judgement as to how much parathyroid tissue needs to be removed[9] – further reasons why this type of surgery should not be undertaken by the inexperienced surgeon. Failure to make this diagnosis is a frequent cause of recurrent hyperparathyroidism. All parathyroid glands must be found in these patients and approximately one-half of the most normal gland should be left and carefully marked. All other parathyroid tissue should be removed.

Nodular hyperplasia is the commonest abnormality found in the parathyroids of patients with hypercalcaemia associated with the rare familial multiple endocrine adenopathy. The type I adenopathy patient usually also has a prolactinoma and gastrinoma. The even rarer type II adenopathy is associated with medullary carcinoma of the thyroid and phaeochromocytoma. Familial hyperparathyroidism may also be found as a single abnormality unrelated to generalized adenopathies.

Carcinoma

Carcinoma of the parathyroid is very rare, accounting for 1–2 per cent of cases of hyperparathyroidism. It is usually diagnosed when a case of recurrent hyperparathyroidism is re-explored and local invasion is found. Parathyroid carcinoma is very difficult to recognize from the histological sections alone. There is no satisfactory treatment for this condition but a surgical attempt should be made to remove as much parathyroid tissue as possible before irradiating the neck, although there is little evidence that radiotherapy is effective.

Frozen sections

Immediate frozen section histological confirmation of parathyroid tissue must always be obtained. If this facility is not available the operation should not be carried out.

Specimens sent for frozen section should be numbered, not given anatomical identities which tend to confuse at this stage. While awaiting the histological results it may be found useful to suture a numbered metal marker adjacent to the biopsy site to aid later identification. If possible, the pathologist should be able to enter the operating room, keep a 'map' of the biopsy sites and be involved in the surgical decisions concerning the patient.

Missing gland

If no abnormal gland can be found and if one of the four glands from normal sites is missing full exploration must be undertaken, up to the angle of the jaw, laterally to include the carotid sheath, posteriorly behind the oesophagus, and caudally to include the removal of all thymic tissue down to the innominate vein. If a gland is still not found a total removal of loose areolar tissue on that side of the neck, and then, after full mobilization and inspection of the thyroid, a total thyroid lobectomy on the side of the missing gland should be carried out. The operation should then be concluded. The same procedure should be followed if four normal glands have been found, but in this case no thyroid tissue should be excised unless one of the localization tests has suggested a definite abnormality. A few lymph nodes should always be taken for biopsy in case a diagnosis of sarcoidosis, causing hypercalcaemia, has been missed.

Mediastinal exploration

If hypercalcaemia persists when no abnormal tissue has been found, the anterior mediastinum should be explored through a full-length median sternotomy. Needless to say this should only be carried out by a surgeon with considerable experience of parathyroid surgery and after a careful review of the evidence for a diagnosis of hyperparathyroidism has been made. The neck should be re-explored no more than one week after the first operation, just before carrying out the sternotomy, and under the same anaesthetic. If carried out at this time no difficulty will be found with adhesions and fibrosis in the neck. After the median sternotomy a complete clearance of all adipose and thymic tissue is made down to the origin of the aorta and laterally to the hilum of each lung. Parathyroid glands in the anterior mediastinum do occur but are rare and most abnormal glands in this position, usually within the capsule of the thymus, can be reached retrosternally from the neck without very much difficulty.

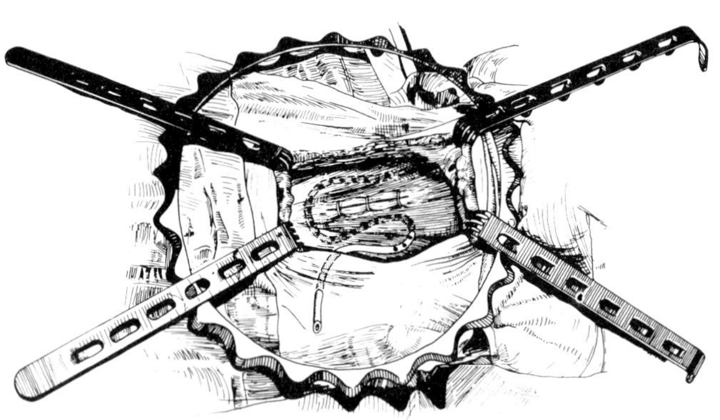

9

9

Closure of incision

Before closing the incision the blood pressure must be allowed gradually to return towards normal; careful haemostasis is then achieved and a fine tube suction drain inserted through the lateral part of the lower skin flap. It is a good idea to allow some of the holes of the drain to lie superficial to the strap muscles in case of bleeding in this plane. The strap muscles are closed with interrupted absorbable sutures. The sandbag under the shoulders is then removed and the head and neck flexed a little to allow the platysma to be closed with interrupted absorbable sutures. Skin clips are used to close the skin. Half of these should be removed at 24 h with the drain, if bleeding has ceased. The remaining skin clips are removed 48 h after the operation.

Postoperative management

The postoperative course of these patients is usually remarkably uneventful. Daily calcium estimations must be carried out to ensure that hypercalcaemia does not persist and to monitor the fall of calcium to within normal limits usually within 2–3 days of the operation. Daily monitoring of calcium levels must continue for at least one week after surgery to make sure that there is no gradual development of hypocalcaemia, and no delayed recurrence of hypercalcaemia. Temporary hypocalcaemia, with associated paraesthesia and possible tetany, may occur if a large abnormal gland has been removed. This can usually be corrected by means of oral calcium supplements. If there is extensive parathyroid bone disease with associated loss of bone calcium the hypocalcaemia will be more profound and may last several months. In these patients oral calcium supplements and 1,25-dihydroxycholecalciferol (Rocaltrol) should be given orally up to 8 μg per day in divided doses until the serum calcium returns to normal levels. The patient is then maintained on approximately 0.5 μg per day, with weekly measurements of serum calcium levels until the bones have recalcified and the residual parathyroid tissue has recovered its normal function. If there is no residual parathyroid or no recovery occurs these supplements may need to be continued indefinitely with careful and regular monitoring of calcium levels in order to prevent iatrogenic hypercalcaemia. Associated magnesium deficiency is also sometimes a problem in patients with severe parathyroid bone disease.

Other postoperative complications are identical with those of thyroid operations (*see* p. 369), haemorrhage with its possible associated tracheal compression being the most serious. Recurrent laryngeal nerve injury should be rare if care is taken always to identify both recurrent laryngeal nerves at operation. Temporary hoarseness is often present after extensive paratracheal and paralaryngeal dissection. Normal function of the vocal cords in these patients can be confirmed postoperatively, as preoperatively, by indirect laryngoscopy.

Recurrent hyperparathyroidism

The surgery for patients with persistent or recurrent hyperparathyroidism after previous exploration is extremely difficult and should only be undertaken at specialist referral centres.

Acknowledgement

I am grateful to Dr Jeffrey O'Riordan for many helpful suggestions during the preparation of this chapter and for providing an invaluable and expert service to our patients.

References

1. Milroy E. J. G., O'Riordan, J. L. H. Investigation and management of urinary calculi of metabolic origin. In: Hadfield, G. J., Hobsley, M., eds. Current surgical practice, Vol. 3, p. 80. London: Arnold, 1981

2. Heath, H., Hodgson, S. F., Kennedy, M. A. Primary hyperparathyroidism. Incidence, morbidity and potential economic impact in a community. New England Journal of Medicine 1980; 302: 189–193

3. Fisken, R. A., Heath, D. A., Somers, S., Bold, A. M. Hypercalcaemia in hospital patients. Clinical and diagnostic aspects. Lancet 1981; 1: 202–207

4. Tomlinson, S., O'Riordan, J. L. H. The parathyroids. British Journal of Hospital Medicine 1978; 19: 40–53

5. Papapoulos, S. E., Hendy, G. N., Manning, R. M., Lewin, I.G., O'Riordan, J. L. H. Amino-terminal labelled antibody assay for human parathyroid hormone. Journal of Endocrinology 1978; 79: 33P–34P

6. Dent, C. E., Watson, L. The hydrocortisone test in primary and tertiary hyperparathyroidism. Lancet 1968; 2: 662–664

7. Dunlop D. A. B., Papapoulos, S. E., Lodge, R. W., Fulton, A. J., Kendall, B. E., O'Riordan, J. L. H. Parathyroid venous sampling: anatomic considerations and results in 95 patients with primary hyperparathyroidism. British Journal of Radiology 1980; 53: 183–191

8. Purnell, D. C., Scholz, D. A., Smith, L. H., Sizemore, G. W., Black, B. M., Goldsmith, R. S., Arnaud, C. D. Treatment of hyperparathyroidism. American Journal of Medicine 1974; 56: 800–809

9. Castleman, B., Roth, S. I. Tumours of the parathyroid glands. Washington D.C.: Armed Forces Institute of Pathology, 1978 (Atlas of tumour pathology, 2nd series, fascicle 14)

Operations on the adrenal glands

R. B. Welbourn MA, MD(Cantab.), HonMD(Karolinska), FRCS, FCS(West Africa), HonMRCS(Denmark)
Professor of Surgical Endocrinology, Royal Postgraduate Medical School and Hammersmith Hospital, London

Introduction

One or both adrenal glands are removed either because they secrete excessive quantitites of hormones, which cause distress, or because they are the sites of tumours, or for both these reasons. Before the advent of cortisone in about 1950 and its use for providing replacement therapy during and after operation[1], radical adrenalectomy and removal of adrenal tumours from patients with Cushing's syndrome were fraught with danger and often proved fatal.

Removal of phaeochromocytomas was similarly hazardous until it was appreciated that many patients were hypovolaemic and before long-acting α-blocking agents and β-blocking drugs were available[2].

Recent developments in the biochemical diagnosis of syndromes and the anatomical localization of tumours have rendered exploratory operations almost obsolete. The surgeon usually knows before operation the nature and site of the lesion that he will find and can plan his approach accordingly.

Operations and indications

Bilateral total adrenalectomy

This is now used mainly for Cushing's syndrome, caused by bilateral adrenal hyperplasia or adenomatous hyperplasia. Several alternative forms of treatment are now available for this condition, including operations on, or irradiation of, the pituitary and the use of drugs. However, they have not yet been shown to be superior to adrenalectomy in the long term. The operation is also required for removal of bilateral phaeochromocytomas. These are particularly common in association with medullary carcinoma of the thyroid (multiple endocrine adenopathy type II). Even if cortical tissue can be preserved to obviate the need for permanent steroid replacement therapy, it is probably wise to remove both glands completely, because any remaining medullary tissue may become tumorous later. In this syndrome the adrenals, if involved, should always be treated before the thyroid so as to prevent vascular accidents, which may be fatal.

Bilateral adrenalectomy was formerly undertaken for primary aldosteronism caused by bilateral hyperplasia, but the results were poor and the operation has been largely superseded by medical treatment with spironolactone. The procedure was also used for treating selected patients with advanced cancer of the breast or prostate, but other forms of endocrine therapy and chemotherapy are now usually preferred.

Subtotal adrenalectomy

This was undertaken formerly for patients with Cushing's syndrome[1] and for those with primary aldosteronism caused by bilateral hyperplasia, in the hope of restoring normal adrenal function. The results, however, were unpredictable and the operation is now rarely used.

Removal of neoplastic glands

Except for about 10 per cent of phaeochromocytomas and a few neuroblastomas, neoplastic glands are nearly always unilateral. Removal is undertaken for the following.

1. *Cortical tumours* (benign or malignant), associated with
   (*a*) Cushing's syndrome;
   (*b*) Conn's syndrome (primary aldosteronism);
   (*c*) virilization;
   (*d*) feminization;
   (*e*) mixed syndromes; or
   (*f*) no endocrine features.

2. *Medullary tumours*
   (*a*) phaeochromocytoma (usually benign);
   (*b*) neuroblastoma (malignant);
   (*c*) ganglioneuroma (benign).

When the tumour is benign and small, non-tumorous cortical tissue is preserved, if possible, except in Conn's syndrome, when it is preferable to remove the whole gland because it may be the site of hyperplasia in addition to neoplasia. When the tumour is malignant, the whole gland is removed as widely as possible, together with adjacent invaded structures, particularly the kidney.

Approaches

Three approaches – posterior, anterior and lateral – are available, and each is ideal in certain circumstances[3]. The posterior route is recommended in most cases for removal of hyperplastic or normal glands or of small tumours. The anterior approach is advised for most patients with phaeochromocytomas and the lateral for all those with large tumours, whether these are cortical or medullary. The lateral approach is also recommended if any special difficulty is anticipated as in reoperations on the adrenal gland.

Special care before, during and after operation

Preoperative

1. Congestive cardiac failure, hypokalaemia, diabetes, infection or psychosis may require emergency treatment in patients with Cushing's syndrome. Metyrapone inhibits the synthesis of cortisol, induces remission and (like antithyroid drugs in toxic goitre) is valuable preoperatively. It is given in a dose of 250 mg 6 hourly, increasing if necessary to 750 mg 6 hourly, until the optimal effect has been achieved. This usually requires 3–6 weeks. Breakdown and infection of wounds were common in Cushing's syndrome, but can be largely prevented by this regimen and also by vitamin A and antibiotics. The former counteracts the adverse effects of cortisol excess on wound healing. Fifty thousand iu per day should be given by mouth for a week before operation, by intramuscular injection until the patient can swallow after operation, and then by mouth again until healing is complete. Appropriate preoperative prophylactic antibiotics should be given. Venous thromboembolism is not uncommon postoperatively, and intermittent pneumatic compression of the legs or other methods should be used to prevent it.
2. In patients with Conn's syndrome, congestive cardiac failure and hypokalaemia may require emergency treatment. Potassium deficiency must always be corrected with spironolactone and potassium supplement before operation.
3. A reliable intravenous infusion must be set up before operation.
4. Bleeding may be profuse in patients with large tumours, and blood must be readily available for transfusion.
5. X-rays showing the lower ribs should be present in the theatre if the posterior or lateral approach is to be used.

Replacement of steroids

The adrenal cortex is essential to life, and death follows within a few hours of bilateral adrenalectomy unless adequate replacement of steroids is provided. Steroids are not usually required in the removal of unilateral tumours, except in patients with Cushing's syndrome. However, if signs of adrenal insufficiency develop, they must be started without delay.

The following schedule is recommended for adults having bilateral total adrenalectomy, except for those with Cushing's syndrome.

Night before operation Cortisone acetate 100 mg by intramuscular injection (50 mg into each buttock).

Day of operation A reliable intravenous infusion is set up shortly before induction of anaesthesia and maintained until the blood pressure has been stable for 48 h after operation. Hydrocortisone succinate is added to the infusion and run in at a rate of 4–5 mg/h, so that 100 mg are given in the first 24 h. If bilateral adrenalectomy was not anticipated (e.g. in patients with bilateral phaeochromocytomas), the hydrocortisone drip may be started and the intramuscular cortisone given during the operation.

First postoperative day Hydrocortisone succinate in the infusion, 100 mg in 24 h.

Second day Hydrocortisone by mouth (or intravenously), 20 mg 6 hourly.

Third to fifth days Hydrocortisone by mouth, 20 mg 8 hourly.

Sixth to ninth days Hydrocortisone by mouth, 20 mg twice daily.

Tenth day and thereafter Hydrocortisone 10 mg thrice daily, and fludrocortisone, 0.1 mg once daily, both by mouth. Some patients need more hydrocortisone and some manage well on less.

If the systolic blood pressure falls below 100 mmHg during the first 48 h (and if bleeding or other causes can be excluded), the rate of infusion of hydrocortisone should be increased. If the pressure falls suddenly, 100 mg of hydrocortisone should be injected intravenously. Within the next few days, if the patient develops anorexia, nausea, abdominal discomfort, tachycardia or slight pyrexia, subacute adrenal insufficiency should be suspected and the dose of hydrocortisone increased.

Replacement of steroids in patients with Cushing's syndrome

The management is similar to that just described, except that larger doses are needed, even if only one hyperplastic gland is removed. The following doses are recommended.

Night before operation Cortisone acetate, 100 mg by intramuscular injection.

Day of operation Hydrocortisone succinate by intravenous infusion, 300 mg in 24 h.

First and second postoperative days Continue infusion at this rate and change to hydrocortisone by mouth, 80 mg 8 hourly, as soon as possible.

Third to fifth days Hydrocortisone acetate by mouth, 60 mg 8 hourly.

Sixth day Hydrocortisone by mouth, 40 mg 8 hourly.

Seventh and eighth days Hydrocortisone by mouth, 40 mg 12 hourly.

Ninth and tenth days Hydrocortisone by mouth, 20 mg 8 hourly.

Twelfth day onwards Hydrocortisone by mouth, 20 mg 12 hourly.

Sometimes a higher dose is needed for a long time, but eventually it can usually be reduced to about 10 mg 8 hourly.

Patients who have undergone unilateral adrenalectomy for tumours eventually recover normal adrenal function in the remaining gland and manage without replacement therapy. Those with carcinomas usually do so in a few weeks, while those with adenomas sometimes require much longer.

Dosage in children

Up to the age of about 5 years the doses should be one-third of those used in adults and up to about 15 years, two-thirds. Older children require adult doses. The maintenance dose of hydrocortisone in those requiring permanent replacement must be adjusted regularly with great care, because any excess stops growth.

Medullary tumours

Patients with phaeochromocytomas and other medullary tumours with hypertension and/or excessive secretion of catecholamines must be prepared for a week or more with the α-blocking agent phenoxybenzamine by mouth to prevent excessive hypertension when the tumour is handled and severe hypotension when it is removed. The β-blocking agent propranolol is used in the presence of tachycardia or cardiac arrhythmias. Labelatol has been used as a combined α- and β-blocking drug, but it is not effective.

During operation the blood pressure is measured continually. Both adrenal glands and any suspicious masses within the abdomen are squeezed gently and the effect on the blood pressure is noted, for squeezing a phaeochromocytoma causes the pressure to rise sharply. Tumours should be handled as gently as possible during removal and their vessels should be controlled as early as convenient. Any excessive rise in blood pressure is controlled with the fast-acting α-blocker phentolamine, or sodium nitroprusside injected into the infusion. Cardiac arrhythmias are treated similarly with propranolol. Any blood which is lost during operation is restored quantitatively. In addition plasma, up to about 2 litres, is usually necessary, as soon as the tumour has been removed, to maintain the systolic blood pressure at about 120 mmHg. The arterial pressure is a better guide to transfusion of the plasma than the central venous pressure. These measures, together with preoperative α-blockade, usually prevent any excessive fall of pressure after operation. When a tumour has been removed, a careful search must be made for another before the abdomen is closed.

Postoperative blood pressure

All patients undergoing adrenalectomy, and especially those with Cushing's syndrome and phaeochromocytoma, should have their blood pressure and pulse rate measured continually, or at least every 15 min, until both have been stable for 48 h. The plasma electrolytes should be estimated daily during this time.

Surgical technique

Although exploratory operations are rarely needed, it may be necessary to inspect both glands or to examine the whole abdomen before either adrenal is removed. The posterior and anterior approaches allow both glands to be assessed before removal of either, but only the anterior approach permits examination of the whole abdomen. The lateral approach gives the best exposure, but allows one gland only to be examined fully.

General anaesthesia is essential.

1

Identification of adrenals

The adrenal glands lie in the perinephric fat above the kidneys. They have close and important relationships to the lower ribs, the pleura and the great vessels. The amount of perinephric fact varies greatly. In patients with Cushing's syndrome, it is usually excessive, sometimes gross, and has a firm consistency, like suet. Some of it may be removed by hand to provide access.

The right adrenal sits like a cap on the upper pole of the kidney and is closely applied medially and anteriorly to the inferior vena cava. Its vein is very short and runs directly into the vena cava. Occasionally there are two, or even three, veins.

The left adrenal lies over the upper pole of the kidney and extends down its medial side, almost to the hilum. Medially, it is separated from the aorta by the crus of the diaphragm. Its vein is longer than that on the right and runs from the lower pole of the gland to join the left renal vein.

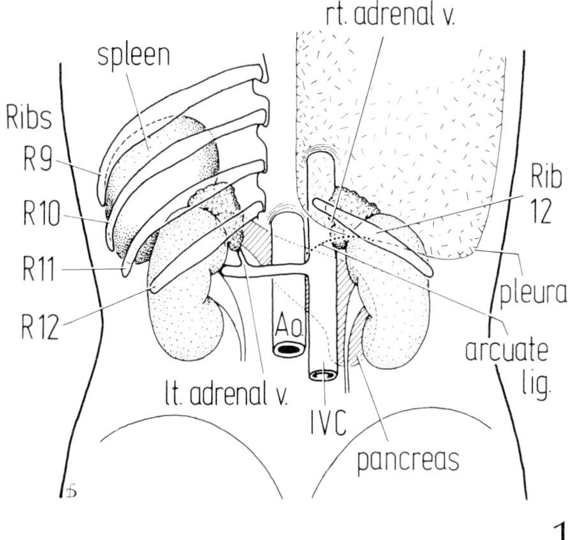

1

Recognition of pathological states

Normal adrenals weigh 5–6g each, and have smooth surfaces. Single *cortical adenomas* or *carcinomas* whose colour is the same as that of the normal cortex and *adrenal medullary* tumours are usually recognized without difficulty. Small tumours (up to about 3cm in diameter) arise from normal-looking glands, while larger ones usually replace all the normal tissue. Carcinomas are often 10cm or more in diameter, are very vascular, often invade adjacent structures, including the kidney or inferior vena cava, and may involve the liver by direct invasion or by metastasis.

In *Cushing's syndrome*, hyperplastic glands are often twice, and occasionally up to five times, as large as normal. The two glands are usually, but not always, about the same size. They often contain micronodules, up to 2 or 3mm in diameter, and occasionally larger nodules, which may be single or multiple (adenomatous hyperplasia). Benign adenomas are single, usually 2–3cm in diameter, and occasionally larger. The non-tumorous parts of the adrenals are atrophic.

In *primary aldosteronism* one, or sometimes more, adenomas, 1–3cm in diameter, and occasionally smaller, are usually found (Conn's syndrome). A small one, which has been demonstrated preoperatively, may not be apparent until the gland has been removed.

POSTERIOR APPROACH

Bilateral posterior incisions, with the patient face-downwards, allow both adrenals to be examined before either is removed. Normal and hyperplastic glands and tumours up to about 5 cm in diameter can be excised readily. The postoperative course is much smoother than that following the other two approaches and, if wounds become infected, any abscess drains readily. This route is advised for bilateral total adrenalectomy unless there are special reasons for entering the abdomen, and for removal of small cortical tumours.

2

Position of patient

The patient is laid face down on the table with the break under the twelfth rib. Firm pillows are placed under the chest and pelvis, so that there is no pressure on the abdomen, and a soft pillow is put under the shins to bend the knees slightly and raise the feet. A strap is fastened round the pelvis. The table is broken to abolish the lumbar lordosis.

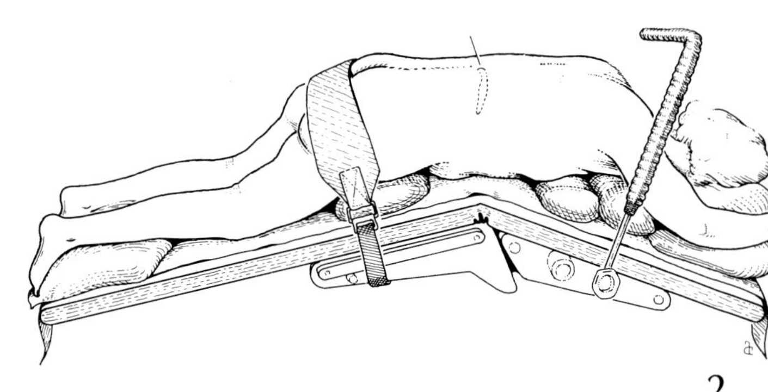

2

One or both glands may be explored and either or both removed. The approach to each side is identical, but the techniques of removal are different. The surgeon stands on the side on which he is operating.

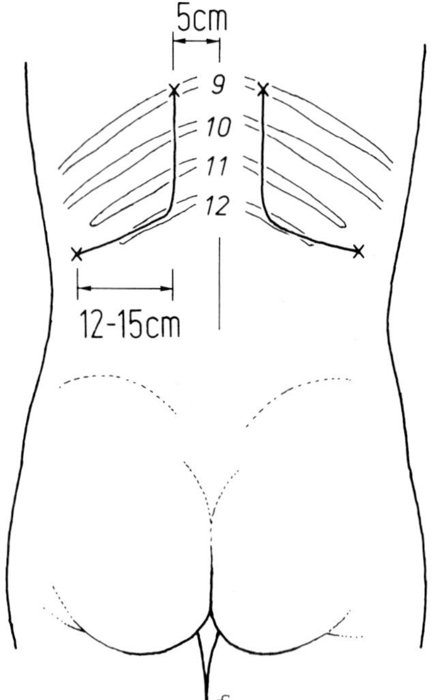

3

3

The incision

The skin incision starts at the level of the ninth rib, about 5 cm from the midline, runs vertically (for 12–15 cm) to the twelfth rib, then takes a sharp turn, running obliquely (for 12–15 cm) along the rib to its tip and finally laterally onto the abdominal muscles. In fat patients the incision must be extended at both ends. The subcutaneous fat is divided and the latissimus dorsi muscle and the sacrospinalis fascia are exposed.

Resection of rib

The twelfth rib is palpated and the incision is deepened through the muscles and fascia, down to the periosteum, and to the lumbar fascia and external oblique muscle. (If the twelfth rib is rudimentary, better access is obtained by resection of the eleventh rib.)

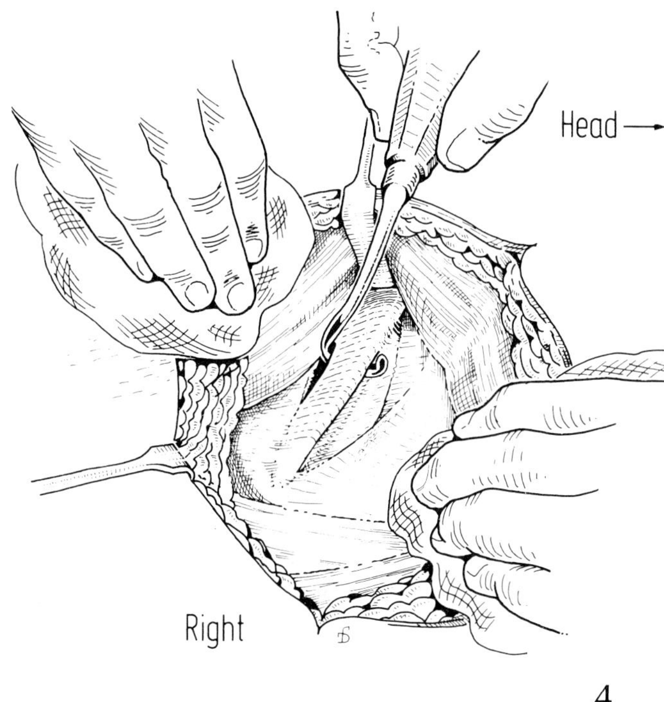

4

4

The sacrospinalis muscle is retracted medially, and the periosteum is incised and then cleared totally from the rib with raspatories. In Cushing's syndrome fractures and callus are often found and the ribs may be extremely friable. The rib is cut with shears, close to the vertebral body, and removed, its lateral attachments being divided with scissors.

The deep layer of periosteum and the renal fascia are then incised together, exposing the perinephric fat. Care is taken to preserve the subcostal neurovascular bundle.

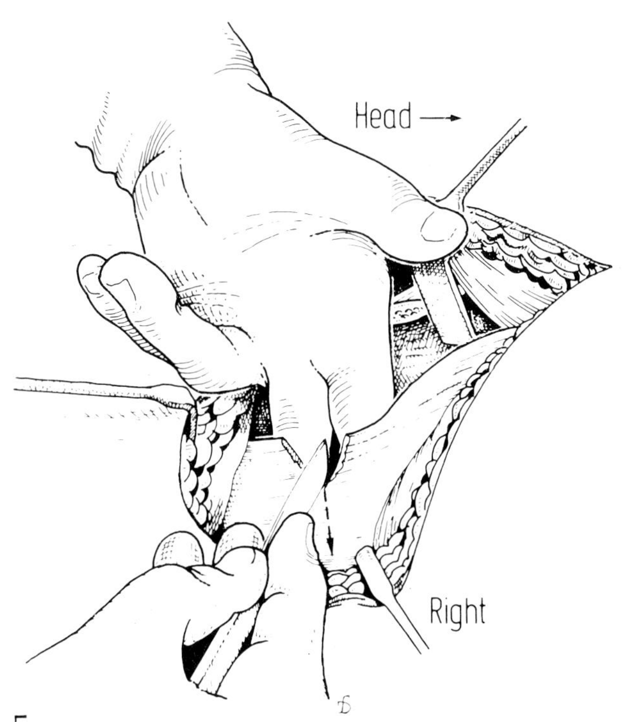

5

5

Incision of flank muscles

Two fingers are then inserted, beyond the tip of the rib, between the lumbar fascia and abdominal muscles superficially and the peritoneum deeply, and the muscles and fascia are divided transversely.

6 & 7

Incision of diaphragm

Retraction upwards of the eleventh rib now exposes the reflection of the pleura and the lateral arcuate ligament of the diaphragm, which are joined by loose connective tissue. The pleura is freed and reflected upwards, partly with scissors and partly by gauze dissection, and the diaphragm is incised vertically up to the eleventh rib. If the pleura is opened, no harm is done, but the lung must be expanded and the pleura sutured before closure of the wound.

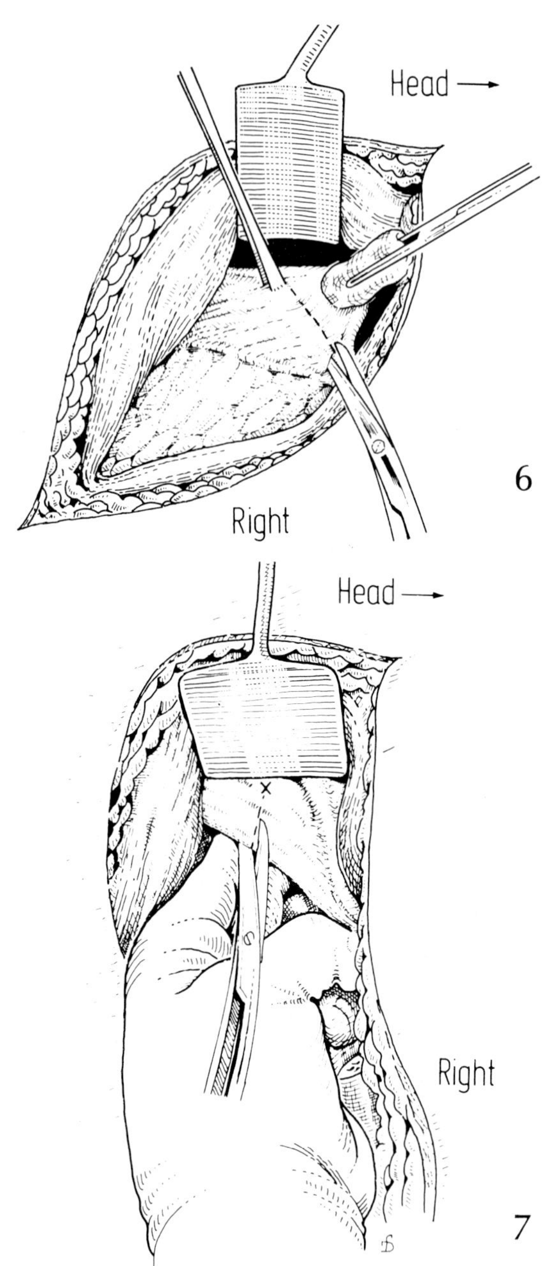

6

7

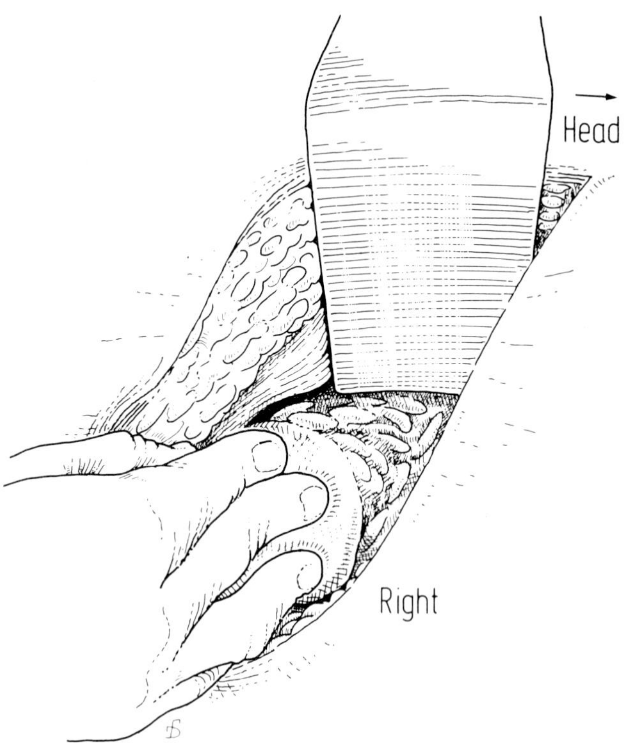

8

Exposure and examination of adrenal

8

The upper pole of the kidney can be felt with the fingers through the perinephric fat. Dissection soon exposes it, and it is cleared and retracted downwards by the assistant's hand. The eleventh rib, pleura, diaphragm and underlying abdominal viscera are now retracted upwards in the costovertebral angle, exposing the perinephric fat above the kidney.

Usually the exposure is adequate, but occasionally the eleventh rib obscures the gland and renders adrenalectomy difficult. If so, the periosteum is cleared from its posterior end, 1 or 2 cm of bone are resected with shears, the rib is retracted further upwards, and the diaphragm is divided a little higher.

9, 10 & 11

The adrenal is found by dissection with scissors and forceps in the perirenal fat. It is readily distinguished by its orange-yellow colour and firm, compact structure. It is mobilized partly by sharp and blunt dissection with scissors and partly by blunt dissection with the fingers. The small vessels which enter the periphery of a normal or hyperplastic gland rarely bleed much and can be controlled with diathermy. The main vein, however, is relatively large and must be preserved until it has been mobilized. The gland is inspected and palpated carefully between fingers and thumb.

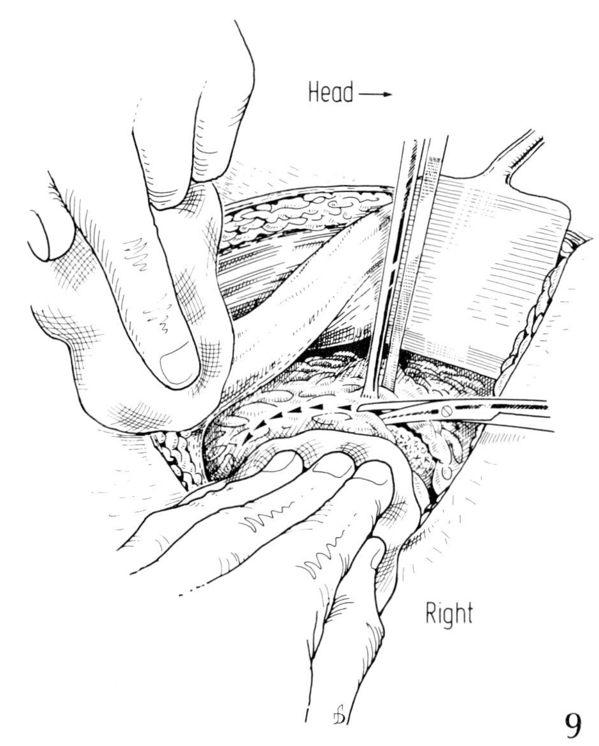

9

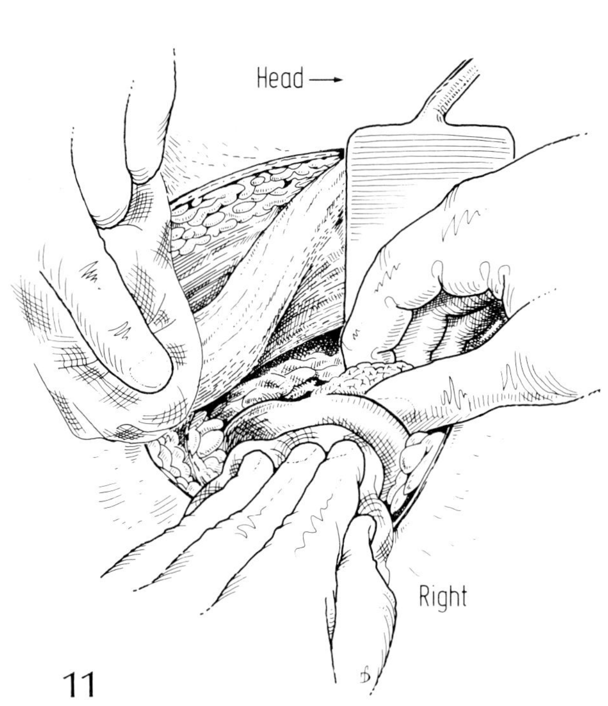

11

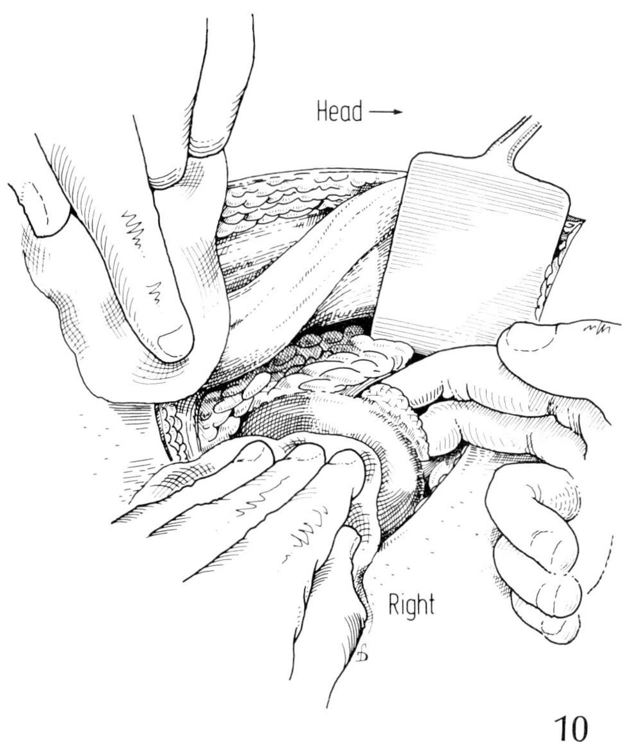

10

Removal of the adrenal

12, 13 & 14

The adrenal is grasped with modified Duval's lung forceps (whose jaws are 6 mm apart when the first teeth of the ratchets engage) and dissection is continued all round the periphery. The main vein is divided with care between ligatures or clips. If, as may happen occasionally on the right, a hole is torn in the vena cava, bleeding is profuse and the hole must be grasped quickly with sponge-holding forceps. If this does not control the bleeding at once, a large pack is inserted firmly and left for 5 min before the forceps is applied again. A Cooley or De Bakey clamp is then applied to the vena cava and the hole is sutured.

When all the surrounding fat and vessels have been divided, the gland is free and can be removed. There are sometimes ectopic nodules of adrenocortical tissue near the glands. If adrenalectomy is to be total, they must be looked for and removed. In hypertensive states (Cushing's and Conn's syndromes and phaeochromocytoma) renal biopsies may be taken. The adrenal beds are usually dry and fill with fat when the retractors are removed.

Closure of incision

The table is straightened and the wound closed. If the pleural cavity has been opened, the lung must be expanded before it is sutured, and an underwater chest drain may be desirable for a day or two.

Drainage of the adrenal bed is rarely necessary.

The wound is sutured in three layers:

1. medially, the intercostal muscles above and the lumbar fascia and quadratus lumborum below; and, laterally, the external oblique muscle and lumbar fascia above and below;
2. latissimus dorsi muscle and the sacrospinalis fascia;
3. skin and subcutaneous tissue.

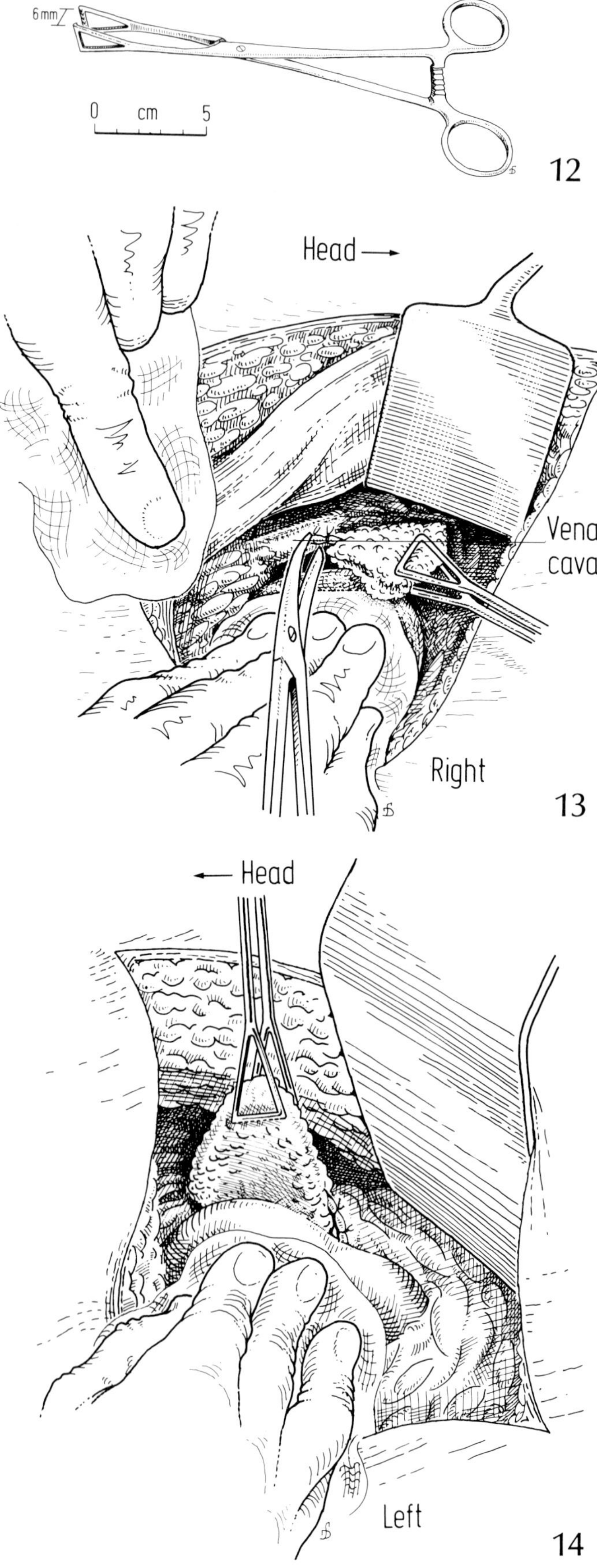

ANTERIOR APPROACH

An anterior abdominal incision allows both glands to be palpated, inspected and removed and the whole of the para-aortic region to be explored. Great difficulty may be experienced on the right side if the patient is very fat or deep-chested or if the liver is enlarged. A tumour more than about 5 cm in diameter on the *right* also presents difficulties because of its relationship (and that of its vein) to the inferior vena cava. This route is advised mainly in patients with phaeochromocytoma. It may be used in those with Conn's syndrome, but the posterior approach is preferable. It is not advised in patients with Cushing's syndrome, unless a primary or secondary ectopic ACTH-secreting tumour is suspected within the abdomen, because postoperative infection may result in the formation of a subphrenic abscess. Nor is it advised in those who have had previous upper abdominal operations or inflammatory disease, because of the likelihood of adhesions.

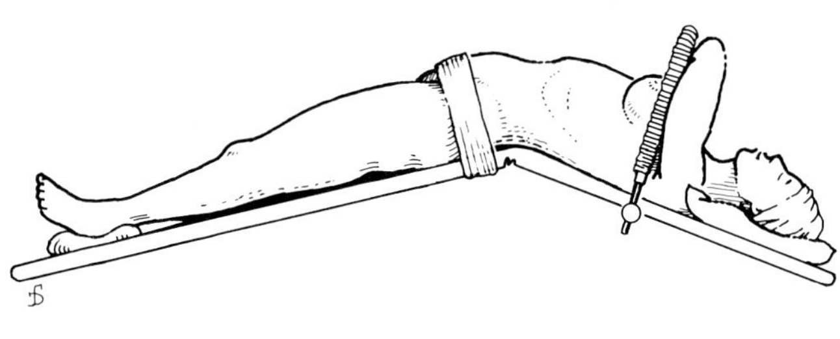

15

15

Position of patient

The patient lies supine with the twelfth thoracic vertebra overlying the bridge or the break in the table. A strap should secure the pelvis so that the table can be tilted to either side. The operation starts with the bridge up or the table broken and with the patient flat.

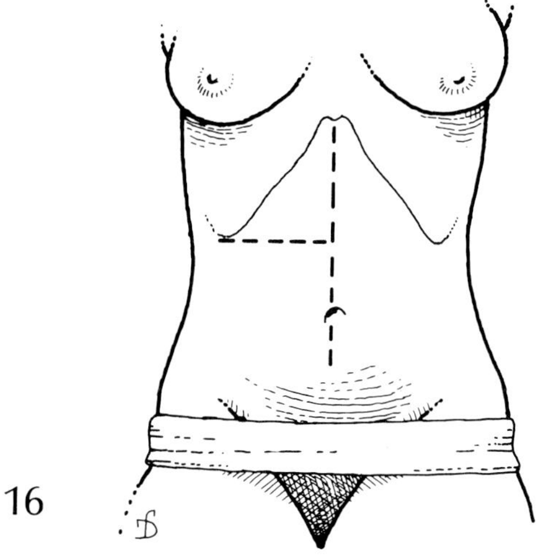

16

The incisions

16

Midline

Usually, and particularly if the subcostal angle is narrow or the patient thin, a midline incision is made from the xiphisternum to 2 cm or so below the umbilicus. If access to either or both glands is inadequate, the incisions may be extended laterally (in either or both direction), at the level of the costal margins.

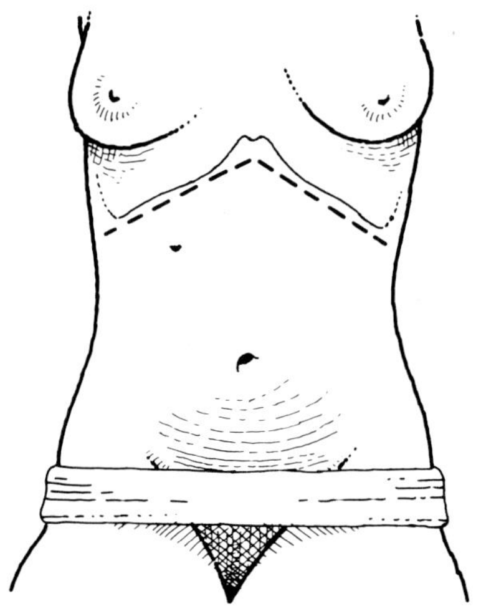

17

17

Roof top

If the subcostal angle is wide and the patient is fat, two long subcostal incisions are made and joined in the centre by a curve to make a 'roof top'. They are made one finger's breadth below the costal margins and extend to the tips of the tenth ribs laterally.

The incision is deepened through the subcutaneous fat and then through the muscles of the abdominal wall. The superior epigastric vessels are secured deep to the rectus muscles. The peritoneum is incised and the falciform ligament divided between ligatures. This incision gives the best possible access from the front, but takes a long time to close.

Abdominal exploration

The abdominal contents are explored. In patients with phaeochromocytomas the whole para-aortic region and pelvis are examined carefully for tumours.

Exposure of left adrenal

18

The surgeon stands on the patient's right. It is sometimes helpful for the table to be tilted about 30° towards him. The viscera are controlled with packs.

The spleen is grasped with the left hand, and the peritoneum behind it is divided with scissors so that it can be mobilized and drawn forwards and to the right, together with the tail of the pancreas, the splenic vessels and the greater curvature of the stomach. (Alternative routes to the left adrenal, through the lesser omentum or the gastrocolic omentum, are much less satisfactory.)

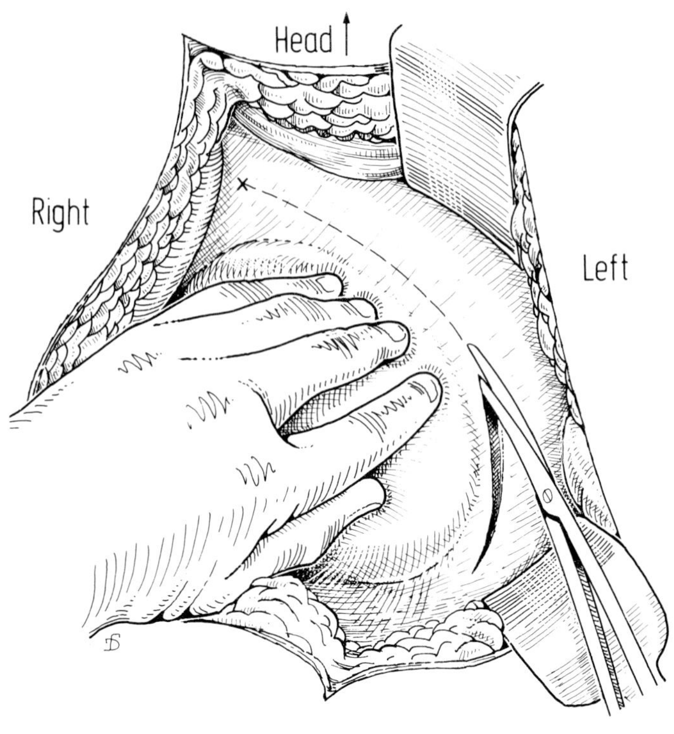

18

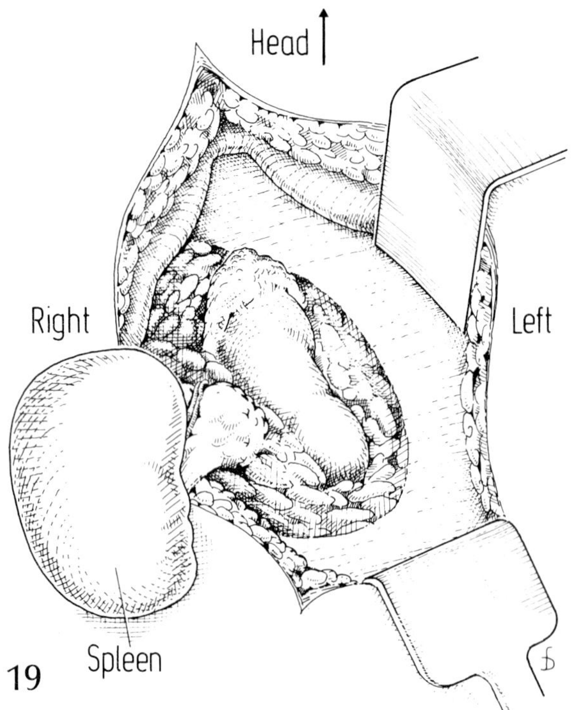

19

19

The spleen is retracted by an assistant's hand over a gauze pack. In a thin patient the adrenal is seen clearly just above the kidney and deep to the renal fascia, lying in front of the left crus of the diaphragm. If there is much fat, the kidney must be felt through it and the adrenal found by dissection in the perinephric fat at its superomedial border.

Removal of left adrenal

Dissection, palpation and removal of the gland have been described already. Ligation and division of the vein may be left to the end, so that it forms a pedicle for the gland.

20

Exposure of right adrenal

The surgeon remains on the patient's right side and, if necessary, the table is tilted about 30° towards the left. The liver is retracted gently upwards and the hepatic flexure of the colon downwards. The duodenum is retracted downwards and to the left, while the peritoneum above it is incised. There is no need to mobilize the duodenum by incision of the peritoneum around it.

21

The inferior vena cava is now exposed and the adrenal is seen, or found, lying close to its right side, behind the renal fascia, above the kidney and below the liver.

Removal of right adrenal

The kidney is retracted downwards by an assistant's hand over a gauze pack, and the adrenal comes down with it.

The adrenal vein should be sought immediately, between the gland and the vena cava. This vein, which is short and runs directly into the cava, may be torn and cause serious bleeding unless it is controlled at this stage. Rotation of the vena cava to the left with a small gauze dab, held in long forceps, aids this manoeuvre.

22

The upper pole of the gland is sited very deeply and may be difficult to expose behind the liver. It is attached closely to the vena cava by a tough bundle of connective tissues which must be cut very carefully with scissors.

Change of approach

If removal of a gland or tumour is impracticable from the front, the incision should be closed and the operation completed by the posterior or lateral route, either at once or later.

Closure of incision

The table is straightened and flattened and the abdomen closed in three layers:

1. peritoneum, posterior rectus sheath (and deep lateral muscles);
2. anterior rectus sheath (and external oblique);
3. skin and subcutaneous fat.

(The structures mentioned in brackets are sutured when the roof top incision is used or when a vertical incision is extended laterally.)

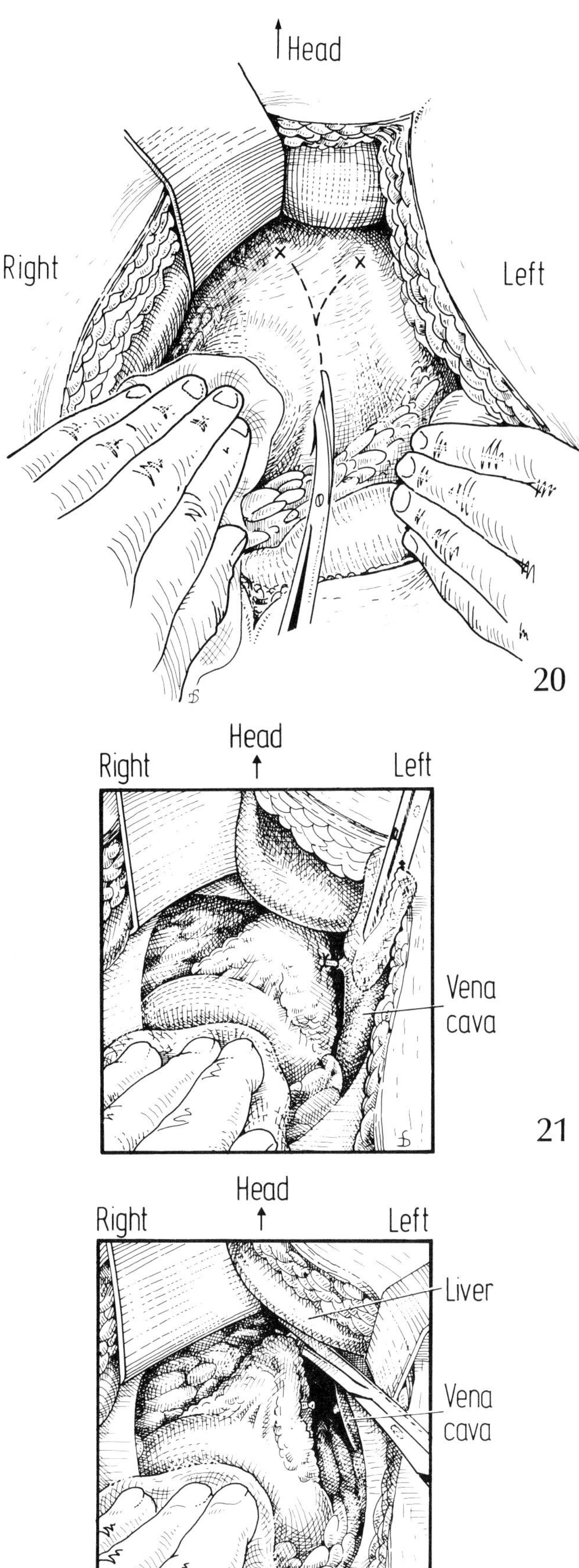

LATERAL APPROACH

An oblique thoracoabdominal incision with resection of a rib gives the best possible exposure of one adrenal. With both the other routes the adrenal is exposed by downward retraction of the kidney, while with this one the gland lies in the middle of the operative field. The opposite gland and ectopic phaeochromocytomas can be palpated *via* the peritoneal cavity, but they cannot be seen or removed.

This route is recommended for nearly all tumours larger than about 5 cm in diameter. The only exception is a left-sided phaeochromocytoma up to about 10 cm, which may be removed from the front. It is also recommended for reoperation for local recurrence of a tumour or for removal of an enlarged adrenal remnant after subtotal adrenalectomy for Cushing's or Conn's syndromes.

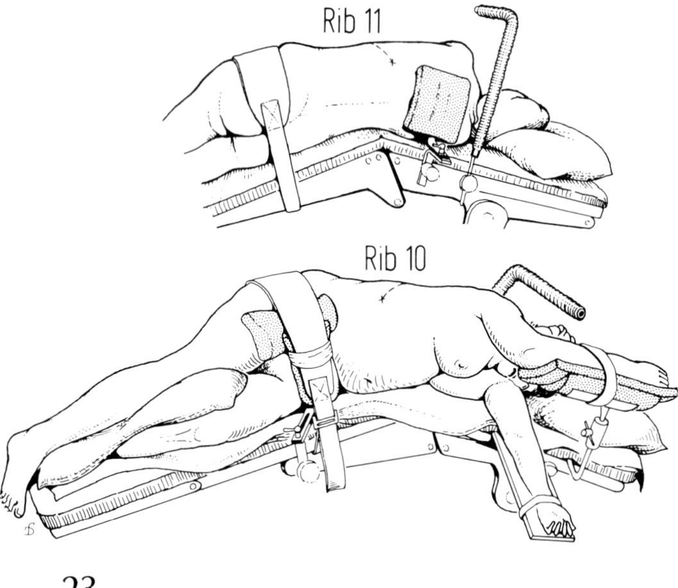

23

23

Position of patient

The patient is placed in the lateral position (without any tilt forwards or backwards) with the side to be explored uppermost and the tenth and eleventh ribs lying over the break in the table. The table is broken to expand the lower chest. Great care should be taken with this manoeuvre, since vertebrae and ribs are often fragile in Cushing's syndrome. The surgeon stands behind the patient.

Left adrenalectomy

The incision

The eleventh rib is found by palpation and a straight incision is started where it emerges from the lateral border of the sacrospinalis. The incision is extended along the line of the rib well into the abdominal wall. The rib and abdominal muscles are exposed and the rib is resected subperiosteally as far back as its angle.

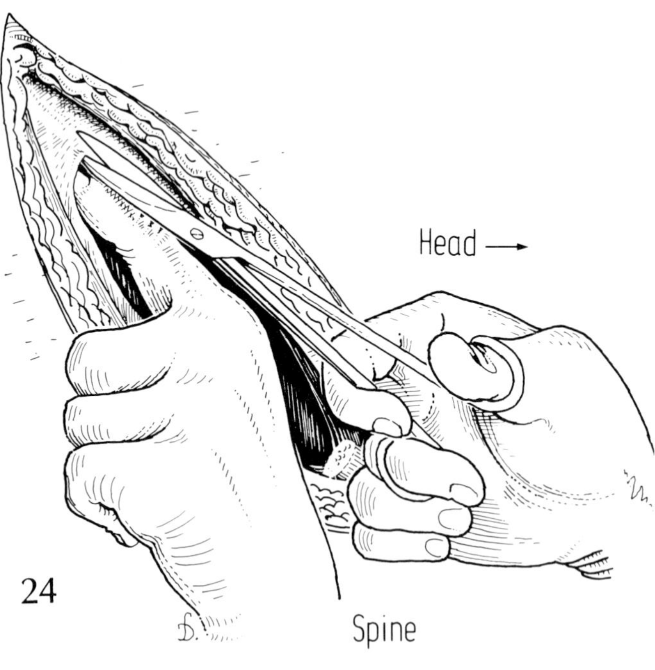

24

24

Incision of abdominal muscles and lumbar fascia

A finger is burrowed between the abdominal wall and the peritoneum, and the abdominal muscles and lumbar fascia are incised in the line of the incision. The intercostal nerve and vessels are preserved carefully. The colon, which lies anteriorly, must not be damaged. The bed of the rib is incised, the pleura is retracted upwards with care and the diaphragm is divided in line with the incision. No harm is done if the pleural cavity is opened inadvertently.

25

Exposure and removal of adrenal

Retractors are inserted, the kidney is found by palpation and the renal fascia is incised widely to expose it. The kidney is retracted downwards and the adrenal is identified. The tail of the pancreas, which lies anterior and inferior to the adrenal, must not be mistaken for it. If the abdominal cavity is to be explored, the peritoneum is incised in front of the colon and a hand is inserted. Dissection and removal of the gland have been described already. Ligation and division of the vein may be left to the end, as in the anterior approach.

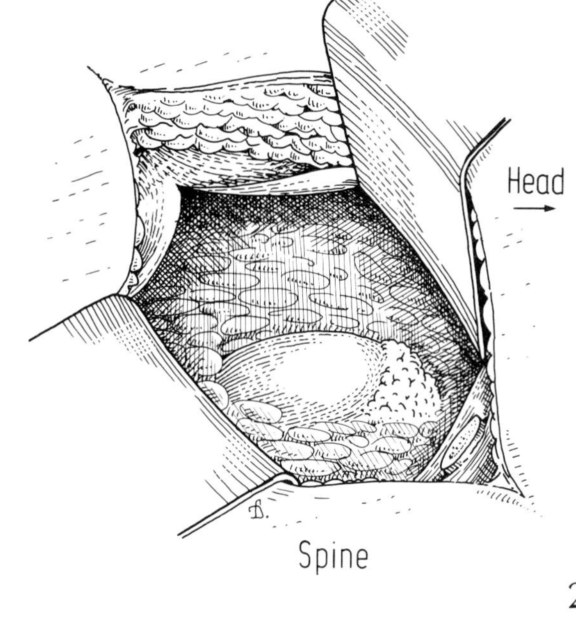

25

Closure of incision

The table is straightened and the incision closed. If the pleura has been opened, care is taken to expand the lung fully before closure. The peritoneum is sutured with continuous catgut, if it has been opened. The wound is closed in three layers:

1. rib bed behind and the lumbar fascia in front;
2. superficial muscles;
3. skin and subcutaneous fat.

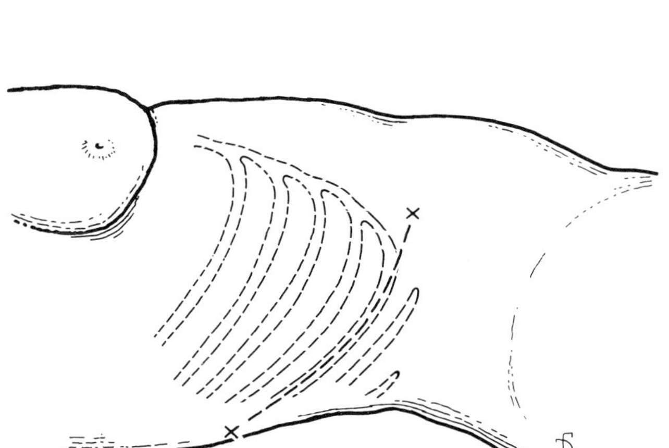

26

Right adrenalectomy

26

The incision

The tenth rib is palpated and an incision made along it from the point where it emerges from the lateral border of the sacrospinalis muscle to 2 or 3 cm beyond the costal margin.

27

Incision of diaphragm

The ribs are held apart by a self-retaining retractor and the kidney is palpated through the diaphragm. An incision about 10 cm long is made *posteriorly* in the diaphragm, approximately at right angles to the skin incision and over the upper pole of the kidney. It should be about 1 cm from the insertion of the diaphragm so that there is sufficient tissue posteriorly to hold stitches when the diaphragm is repaired. Bleeding points in the cut edge of the muscle are sealed with diathermy or ligated.

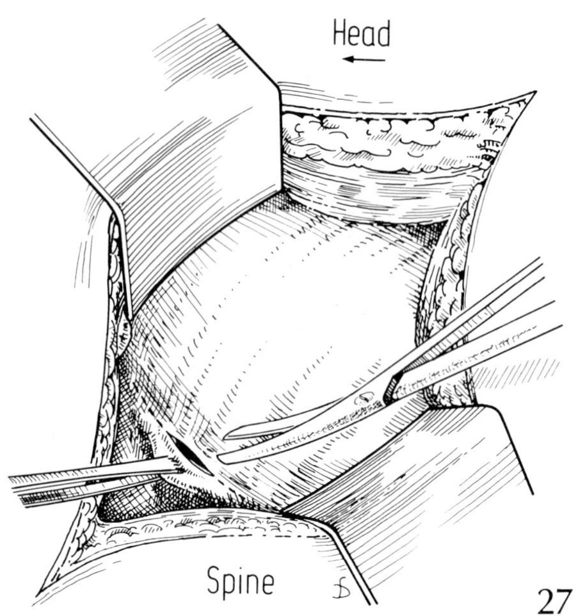

27

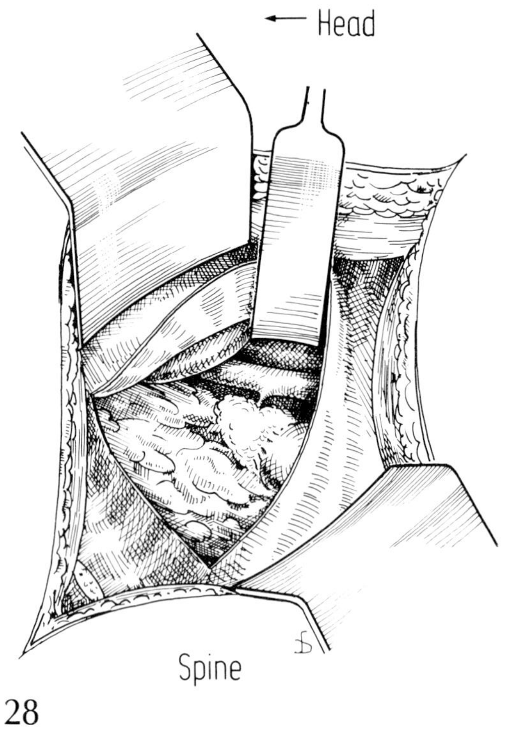

28

28

Exposure and removal of adrenal

The lung is retracted upwards and the liver forwards. The renal fascia is incised widely and the adrenal, which lies in the centre of the field, is located in the perirenal fat at the upper pole of the kidney, close to the inferior vena cava. The peritoneal cavity may be explored, if necessary, through an incision in front of the colon, as on the left side. The gland is removed, as described already.

Closure of incision

The table is straightened and the peritoneum (if it has been opened) and the diaphragm are closed with continuous catgut sutures. An underwater, intercostal drain (through the seventh or eighth space in the mid-axillary line) is advisable for 1 or 2 days. The incision is closed in three layers:

1. rib bed;
2. superficial muscles; and
3. skin and subcutaneous fat.

29

REMOVAL OF SMALL BENIGN TUMOURS

Small tumours can be removed by any route. However, the posterior approach is advised for cortical adenomas and the anterior for phaeochromocytomas. They are removed in the same way as non-tumorous glands, except that more vessels may require ligation. In Cushing's syndrome as much normal adrenal tissue as possible should be left behind, but in other conditions the gland should be removed completely.

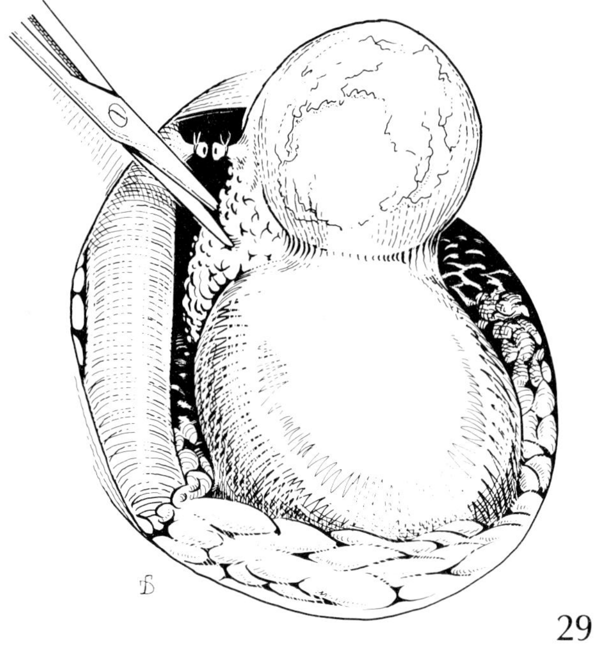

29

REMOVAL OF LARGE TUMOURS

30

The lateral approach gives the best exposure, but the incision must be enlarged forwards and downwards as far as necessary.

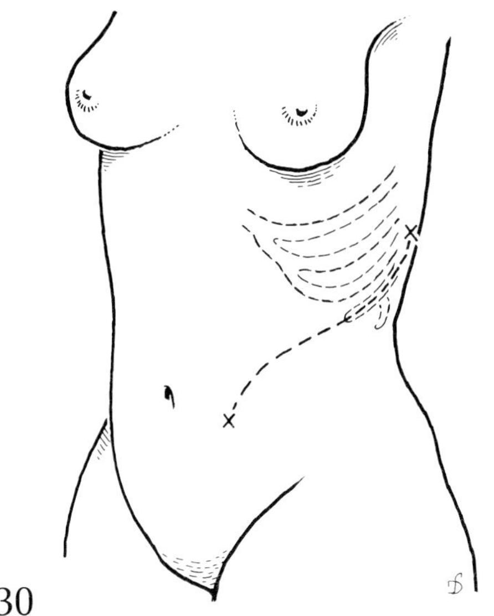

30

31

Direct invasion of surrounding tissues may preclude complete or even subtotal removal, but very large malignant tumours are often resectable. If the kidney alone is invaded, it is removed together with the tumour. A plane of cleavage is found outside the capsule of the tumour, and dissection is made on each side in turn until the main vessels are reached. Bleeding, which may be severe, is best controlled by pressure with abdominal packs. There are often several arteries supplying the tumour, but only one vein (the enlarged adrenal vein) draining it. These vessels are divided and ligated as soon as they are found. Tumour may pack the vein and extend into the vena cava. In this case the cava may be clamped below and above, opened and the tumour withdrawn. It is then closed with a fine arterial suture.

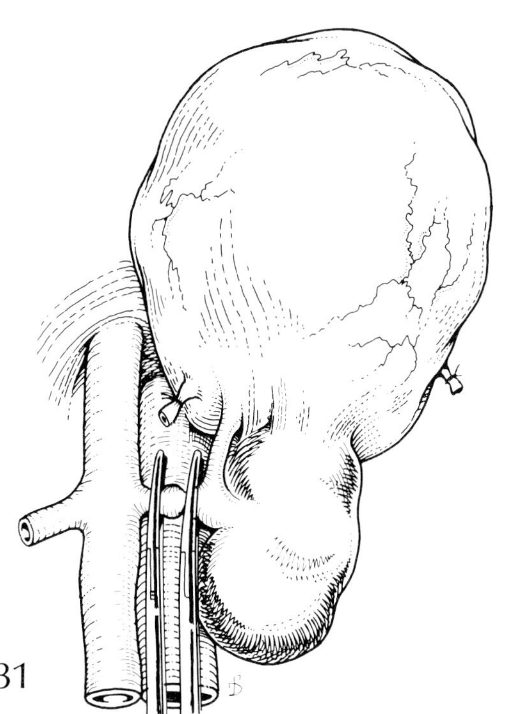

31

ADRENALECTOMY IN CHILDREN

The indications are the same as those in adults, but malignant tumours are relatively more common. Operations for neuroblastoma are described in the *Paediatric Surgery* volume.

Tumours are best approached by a lateral incision and that through the bed of the eleventh rib gives good access on each side. For bilateral adrenalectomy the posterior and anterior approaches may provide inadequate access, even in teenagers, and the bilateral eleventh rib approach is advised. The two operations can usually be undertaken on one occasion, the child being turned from one side to the other.

The smaller doses of steroids required for replacement during and after operation have been described already.

Results

With suitable preparation and care, the operative mortality for removal of benign lesions of the adrenals is now about 1 or 2 per cent. That for patients with large malignant lesions of the cortex or the medulla is appreciably higher.

Survival figures

These are approximately as follows.

Cortical lesions

1. Benign
   (*a*) Cushing's syndrome[4]
   10 years 66 per cent
   20 years 50 per cent
   (*b*) Conn's syndrome[5]
   Good, but no long-term details of large series have been published
2. Malignant[4]
   Almost all patients die within 5 years

Medullary lesions

1. Phaeochromocytoma[6,7]
   10–20 years 66 per cent
2. Neuroblastoma[8]
   (*a*) Infants (<1 year old)
   (i) Stages I, II and IVS
   2 years 90 per cent
   5 years 80 per cent
   (ii) Stages III and IV
   2 years 30 per cent
   (*b*) Children (>1 year old)
   2 years 15 per cent

References

1. Priestley, J. T., Sprague, R. G., Walters, W., Salassa, R. M. Subtotal adrenalectomy for Cushing's syndrome. A preliminary report of 29 cases. Annals of Surgery 1951; 134: 464–475
2. Ross, E. J., Prichard, B. N. C., Kaufman, L., Robertson, A. I. G., Harries, B. J. Preoperative and operative management of patients with phaeochromocytoma. British Medical Journal 1967; 1: 191–198
3. Edis, A. J., Ayala, L. A., Egdahl, R. H. Manual of endocrine surgery. Berlin: Springer-Verlag, 1975
4. Welbourn, R. B. Some aspects of adrenal surgery. British Journal of Surgery 1980; 67: 723–727
5. Ferriss, J. B., Beevers, D. G., Boddy, K. *et al.* The treatment of low-renin ('primary') hyperaldosteronism. American Heart Journal 1978; 96: 97–109
6. Modlin, I. M., Farndon, J. R., Shepherd, A. *et al.* Phaeochromocytomas in 72 patients: clinical and diagnostic features, treatment and long term results. British Journal of Surgery 1979; 66: 456–465
7. Remine, W. H., Chong, G. C., Van Heerden, J. A., Sheps, S. G., Harrison, E. G. Current management of pheochromocytoma. Annals of Surgery 1974; 179: 740–748
8. Grosfeld, J. L., Schatzlein, M., Ballantine, T. V. N., Weetman, R. M., Baehner, R. L. Metastatic neuroblastoma: factors influencing survival. Journal of Pediatric Surgery 1978; 13: 59–65

Operations for benign breast disease

L. E. Hughes DS, FRCS, FRACS
Professor of Surgery, Welsh National School of Medicine, Cardiff

Operations for benign breast disease fall into two broad groups: those necessary to allow a definitive tissue diagnosis to be made, and those necessary to control inflammatory conditions of the breast. Diagnostic procedures are dealt with first.

DIAGNOSTIC PROCEDURES FOR BREAST LUMPS

Plans of action are required for three clinical situations: a palpable breast lump, a subclinical lesion diagnosed on mammography and nipple discharge. For a palpable mass, the diagnostic process recommended is a sequence of needle aspiration (to exclude a cyst), needle biopsy and open biopsy.

Treatment of breast cysts

Simple cysts account for the majority of well-defined breast lumps in women of the 35–55 year age group, and most are satisfactorily dealt with by aspiration. There are two cardinal rules: the lump must disappear completely on aspiration, and the fluid must not contain blood. If either of these situations exist biopsy is mandatory: for a persistent mass because cysts and cancer are both common disorders and may coexist by chance; and for blood-stained fluid because this usually signifies the presence of a papillary tumour in the wall of the cyst. Most of these are benign, but a significant proportion, especially in older women, will be papillary carcinomas.

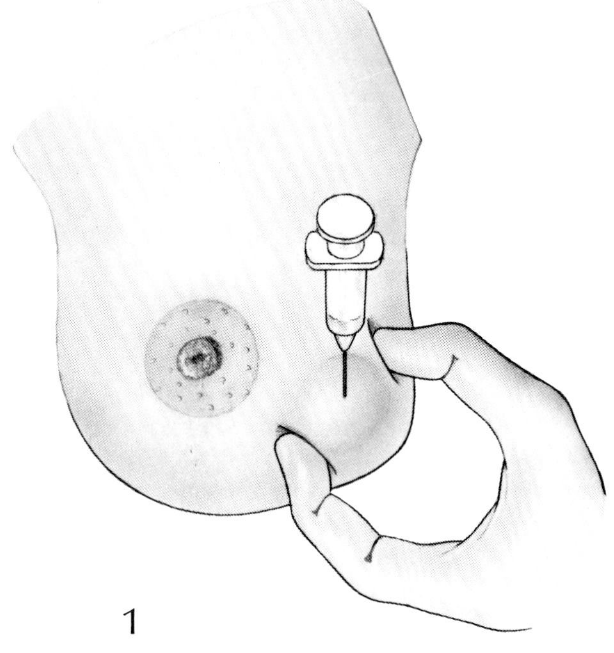

1

Technique of aspiration

The cyst should be steadied between two fingers, which also direct it towards the surface. A sharp 21 gauge needle is inserted (local anaesthetic is unnecessary), and there is a distinctive feel as the needle traverses the fibrous cyst wall and then suddenly penetrates into the cyst. The cyst may be deeper in the breast than appears on clinical examination, so deeper needling should be tried if no result is obtained from aspiration, before concluding that the mass is solid. Recurrence after aspiration is not infrequent, but a second or even third aspiration will usually give prolonged relief.

Pneumocystography

The procedure of pneumocystography is useful when the cyst fluid is found to be blood-stained or when a cyst recurs after two or three aspirations. The fluid is aspirated from the cyst and replaced with an equal volume of air. The patient then undergoes conventional mammography or xeromammography. The outline of the cyst is shown and any tumour in its wall is well demonstrated. We also have a strong clinical impression that persistent cysts are more likely to resolve after this procedure than after simple aspiration.

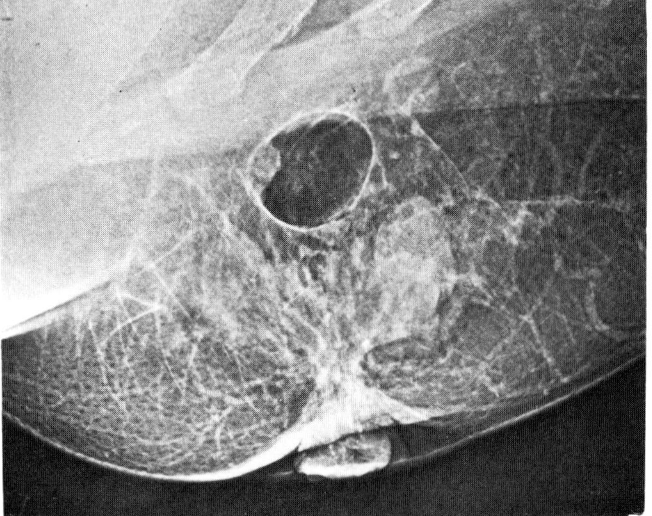

2

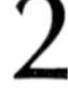

This pneumocystogram is from a patient whose cyst aspirate was blood-stained. It shows a benign papillary tumour in its wall. (The subareolar distortion is the result of an earlier biopsy.)

Needle biopsy

A definitive preoperative diagnosis of cancer is of great advantage both to the surgeon – in planning management and saving operating time – and to the patient by minimizing the psychological strain of going to theatre not knowing whether or not a mastectomy will be necessary. Three techniques are currently in use. Cytology from needle aspiration is favoured by some, but interpretation requires special expertise and the technique does not allow differentiation of preinvasive cytological malignancy from invasive cancer (*see* chapter on 'Fine needle aspiration of solid tumours of the breast', pp. 254–261). Drill biopsy is highly effective in skilled hands, but requires apparatus better suited to a specialized unit. Needle biopsy using the Tru-cut needle (Travenol) will provide definitive histology in most cancers greater than 2 cm in diameter and in a substantial proportion of smaller cancers. Because of the rubbery nature of fibrocystic disease, the technique is less satisfactory for benign masses. The benefit lies only in obtaining a positive diagnosis of malignancy and it is wise to proceed to open biopsy in all cases where the needle biopsy report from a distinct mass is benign, because of possible sampling errors with this technique.

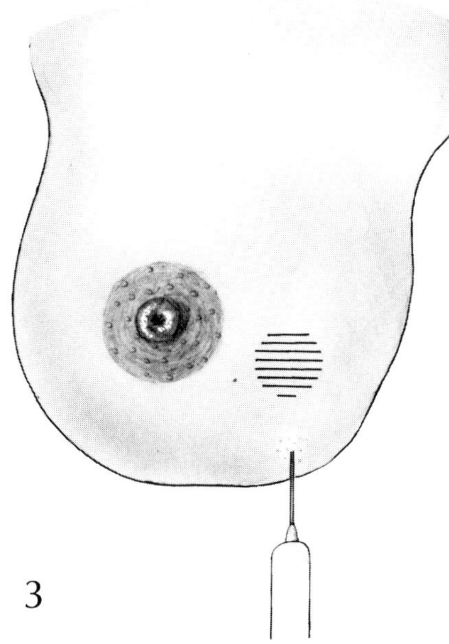

3

3, 4 & 5

Technique of needle biopsy

An intradermal weal of local anaesthetic is raised, avoiding any obvious subcutaneous veins. A stab incision is made with a disposable pointed scalpel blade and a 7.5 cm (3 inch) biopsy needle inserted into the breast in the closed position. The central needle is advanced into the mass and the cutting sheath then closed over it against gentle counterpressure from the opposite aspect of the breast. The closed needle is removed and any bleeding controlled by digital pressure. With practise the manipulation of the needle during insertion can be done with one hand, allowing the other hand to give direction and stability by holding the mass. The final cutting manoeuvre should be rapid, using both hands. It is helpful if an assistant steadies the mass and gives counterpressure at this time.

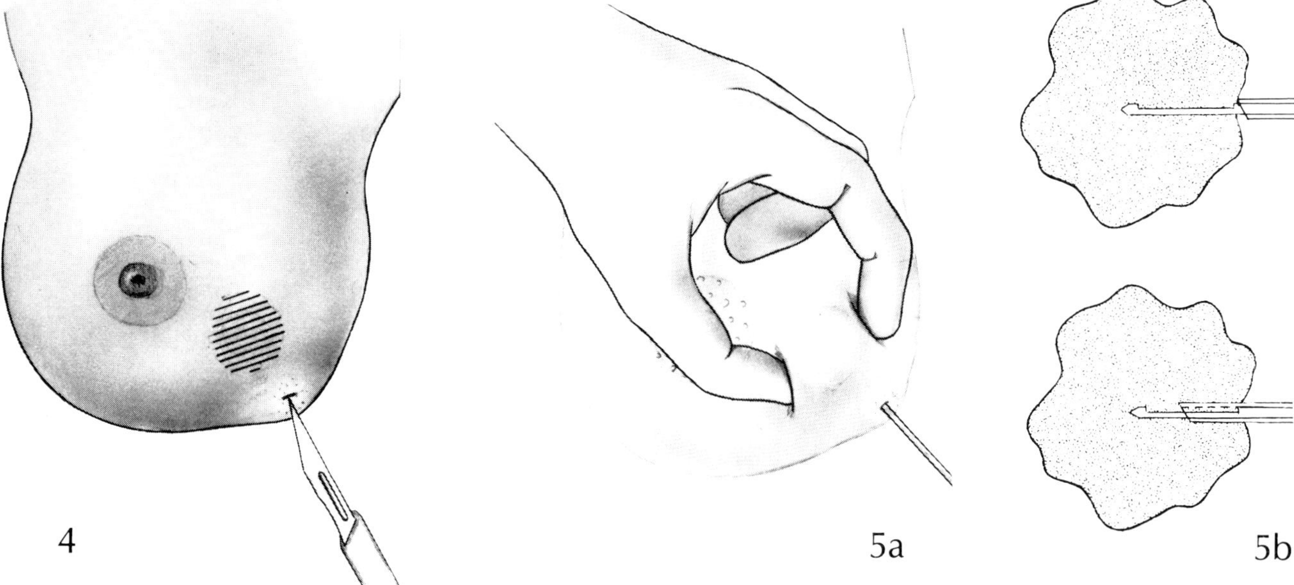

4 5a 5b

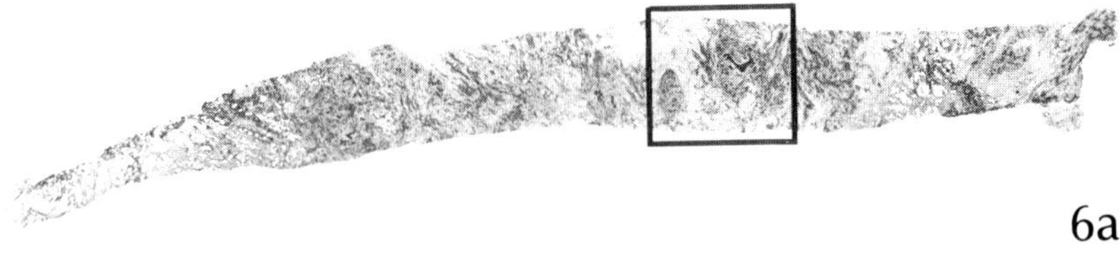

6a

6a & b

Typical biopsy specimens showing the quality of histological material provided.

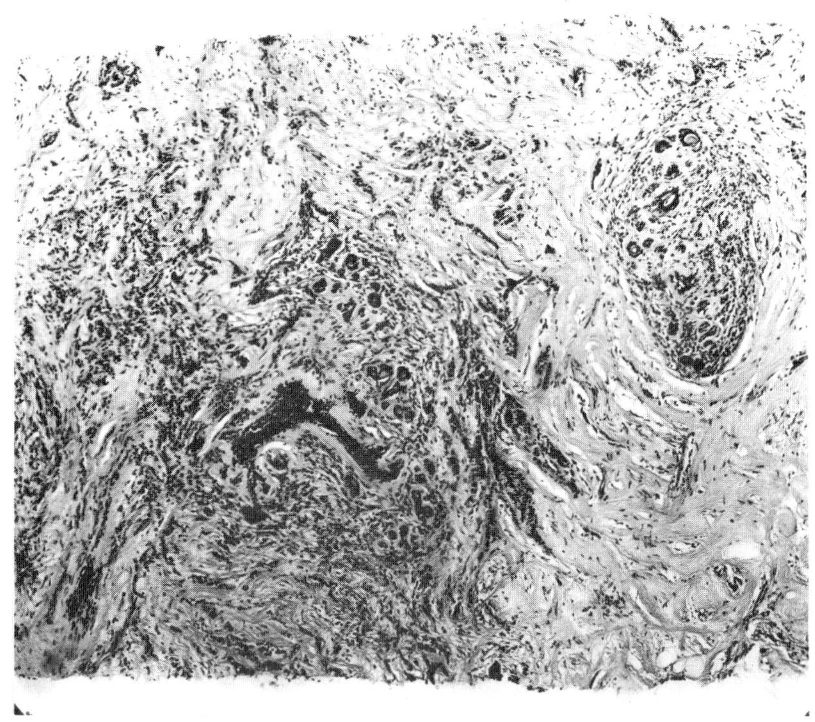

6b

Biopsy excision

Indications

There are four main indications for biopsy excision in benign breast disease: fibroadenoma, a discrete mass in the fibroadenosis/hyperplastic cystic disease complex, a subclinical lesion demonstrated on mammography, and for ductal discharge. Each requires a different technique. A simple cyst should always be excluded by needle aspiration as described above before subjecting a patient to open biopsy under anaesthesia.

Anaesthesia

General anaesthesia is recommended unless there is some special contraindication. Local anaesthesia for breast biopsy should not be undertaken lightly. Masses often lie deeper in the breast than they appear clinically, bleeding may be difficult to control and local tissue infiltration by the anaesthetic agent may obscure the mass that is being sought.

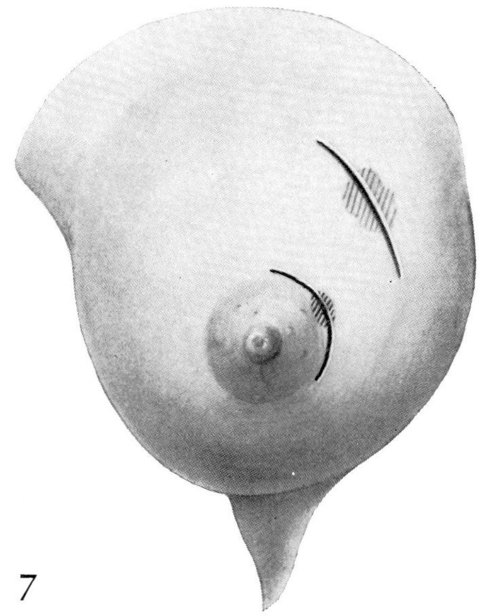

7

The incisions

7

For lesions within about 5 cm of the nipple, a periareolar incision, extending no further than half the circumference, gives good access and an excellent scar. Otherwise, a curved incision sited over the mass and parallel to the areola is satisfactory. Cross-hatching helps accurate suturing of these curved incisions.

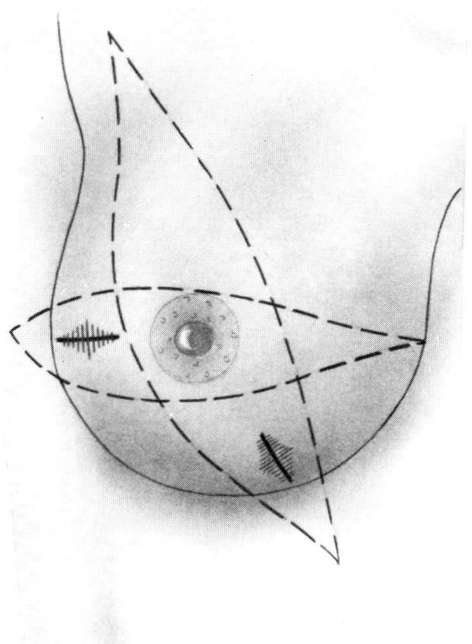

8

8

Radial incisions give a less satisfactory cosmetic result and a higher incidence of painful scars. However, where the mass may be malignant, the biopsy incision should be planned in relation to the possible mastectomy incision, so that the biopsy incision can be completely re-excised with a wide margin at mastectomy. This means that, for some peripheral masses, a radial incision lying in the line of the proposed mastectomy incision may be most suitable.

Excision of a fibroadenoma

Because fibroadenomas are usually found in young women a good cosmetic result is particularly desirable. Most are freely mobile and superficial and can be removed through a small incision lying in a skin crease. An occasional fibroadenoma is multifocal and merges with the surrounding breast tissue – this resembles fibroadenosis in its physical signs and should be removed as described for biopsy of this condition. 'Giant' fibroadenomas call for a special technique.

9

Surgical pathology of a fibroadenoma

The tumour is attached to the capsule by a stalk carrying its blood supply, and sometimes the adenomatous tissue extends into the capsule in the region of the stalk attachment.

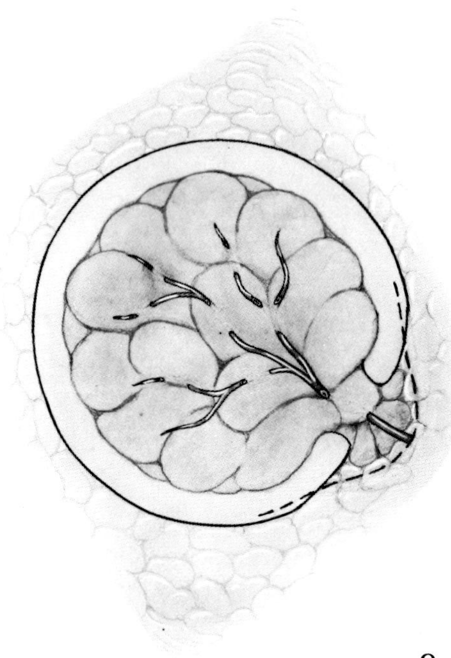

9

10

Technique

After incision through the skin and subcutaneous fat, the lesion is palpated and pushed into the incision, the capsule is opened and the fibroadenoma is shelled out. A piece of the capsule in the region of the stalk attachment should be removed to lessen the risk of recurrence, carefully securing the entering blood vessel, if necessary with a transfixion suture. The dissection should encounter few other vessels, so, if the wound is quite dry, it may be closed without drainage with a 4/0 chromic catgut suture to the subcutaneous tissue and 4/0 silk to the skin. If there is any tendency to oozing, the wound should be drained by a fine suction catheter, ensuring that the catheter lumen is not occluded by blood clot while the wound is being closed and before suction can be applied.

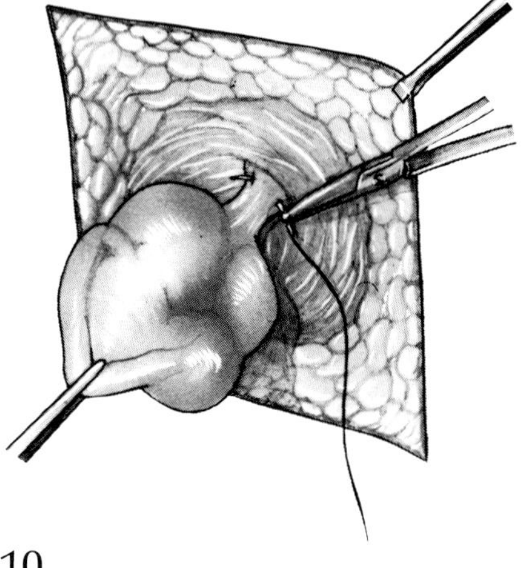

10

'GIANT' FIBROADENOMA

When a fibroadenoma is large, that is, more than 5 cm in diameter, it is likely to be deeper in the breast than is clinically apparent, and is best approached from behind. Such lesions are almost always benign, but histological examination will occasionally show them to be of borderline or even frank malignancy.

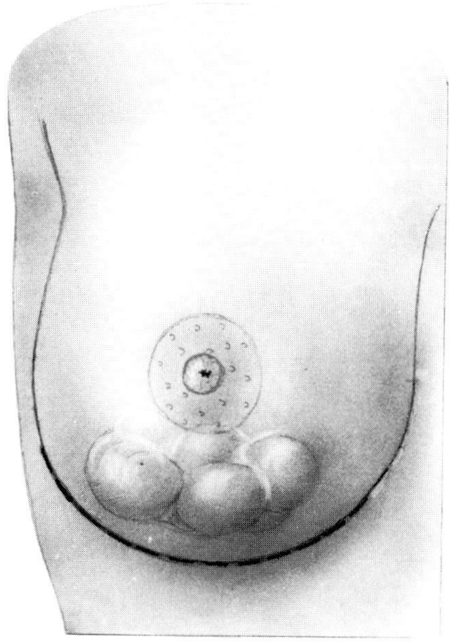

11

11 & 12

An appropriate circumferential incision at the edge of the breast disc, and usually in the submammary fold, is deepened to the fascia overlying pectoralis major or serratus anterior. Blunt dissection is readily developed in this almost bloodless plane between breast tissue and fascia. The fibroadenoma is then pushed into the wound and removed as described earlier. Suction drainage is used routinely, and the wound closed with 4/0 chromic catgut to the subcutaneous tissues and 4/0 silk to the skin.

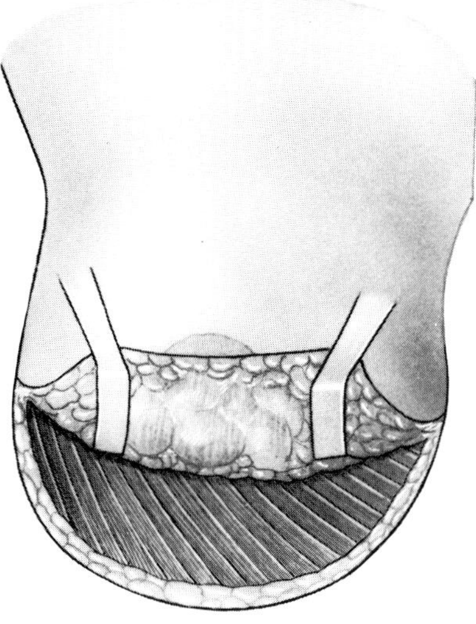

12

Biopsy excision of a discrete mass of fibroadenosis

Biopsy of a dominant mass in a fibroadenotic breast differs considerably from removal of a fibroadenoma for a number of reasons. First, the possibility that the mass will prove to be malignant must be considered from the outset. Second, the lump under suspicion may be more difficult to detect at operation than to palpate before operation. Third, control of bleeding is much more difficult because the blood vessels lie in the tough rubbery stroma of fibroadenosis, into which they tend to retract on division.

The incision

The incision should be more generous than with fibroadenoma, to ensure that the lump in question is completely excised and to facilitate control of bleeding points. A direction parallel to the areola is suitable in most cases, with the proviso related to a possible mastectomy incision discussed earlier.

Localizing the mass

It is helpful to mark the site of the lesion preoperatively, with the arm abducted in the position it will occupy on the operating table. When the patient has been prepared and towelled up in theatre, if the mass is not very obvious, it is useful to insert a needle through the skin into the mass leaving it there as a guide while the incision is deepened through the breast tissue.

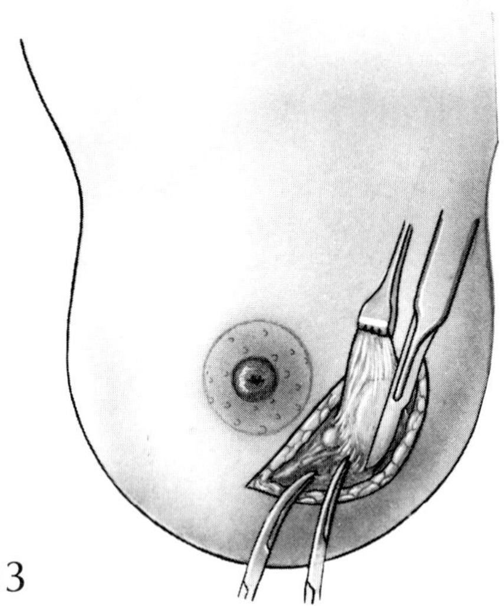

13

13

Removing the mass

After dividing the skin and ligating any subcutaneous veins, the lump is located by palpation and held with an Allis tissue forceps, which is used to draw the mass to the surface. The extent of the lump is then defined by palpation and that area of tissue excised by a scalpel. In the markedly fibroadenotic breast the appearance of the tissue cannot be used to define the extent of the lesion in that fibroadenosis is a diffuse disease with a uniform macroscopic appearance. Any attempt to remove all the macroscopically abnormal tissue must be resisted, because this will lead to an excessively large excision and even to inadvertent simple mastectomy in a small breast. As each vessel is divided, it must be caught with a fine mosquito forceps before it retracts into the rubbery tissue. It may be cauterized, ligated or under-run with fine chromic catgut on a stout needle.

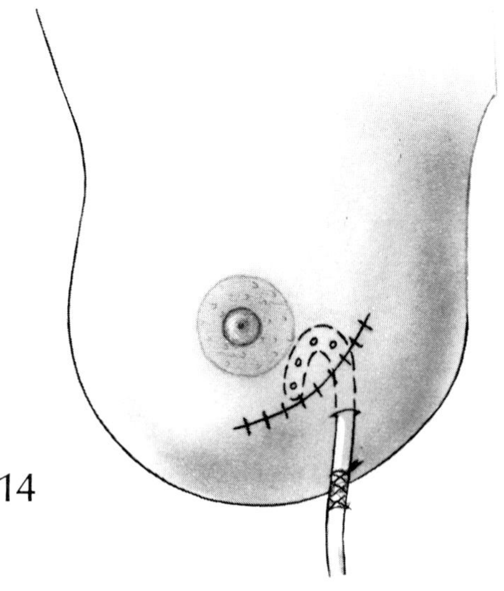

14

14

Drainage and closure

If the incision has been made as large as the underlying cavity and the vessels caught as they have been divided, there should be no major bleeding at the end of the procedure, but small bleeding points ooze from the fibrous tissue and attempts to stop these tend to be unproductive. The cavity may be obliterated but the tough fibrous tissue can only be sewn with a stout trocar pointed needle and strong catgut, and such manoeuvres tend to exacerbate bleeding. Once the major bleeding points are secured it is best to ignore the cavity and to insert a suction drain, suturing skin and subcutaneous tissues only. The drain can be removed at 24 h.

Biopsy of a subclinical lesion

Mammography may demonstrate a lesion suggestive of malignancy in a region where no abnormality can be detected clinically. Such lesions are likely to prove to be either invasive cancer, intraduct cancer or sclerosing adenosis[1]. A particular area of the breast may change its position relative to external markers when the patient assumes different positions, especially abnormal positions such as those used for mammography and surgery. This makes localization of a mammographic lesion difficult at operation. Since at least half these lesions will prove to be benign, a technique should be used which allows definite excision of the radiological abnormality while removing a minimal amount of normal breast tissue.

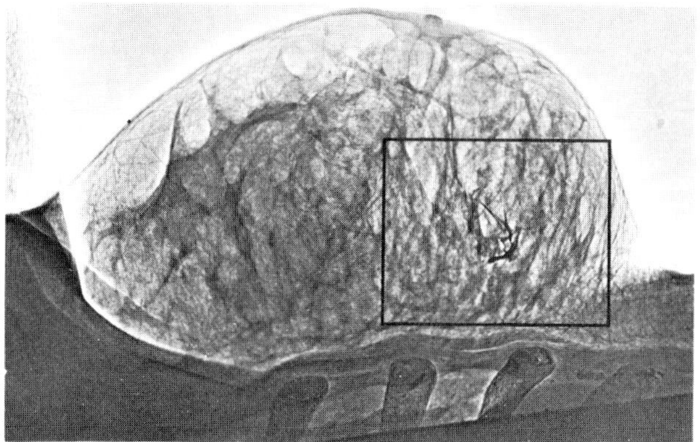

15a

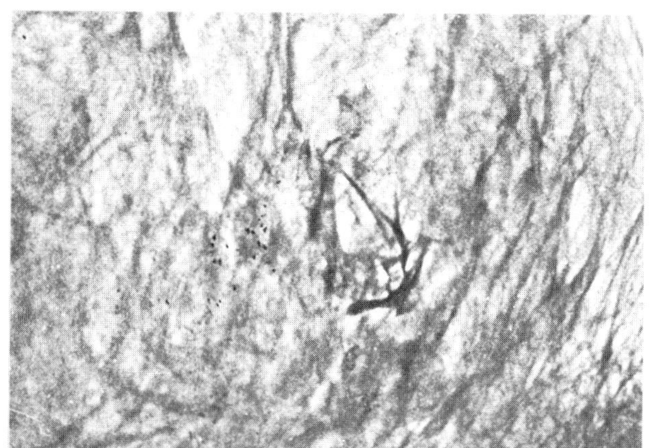

15b

15a & b

Radiological localization

On the morning of operation the patient is taken to the X-ray department and placed on the X-ray table in the position of the lateral film. After consideration of the mammograms, the radiologist injects 0.5 ml of a dye mixture into the site at which he considers the mass to be. The mixture contains 1 ml of 25 per cent Hypaque (to give radiological localization) and two drops of patent blue violet (to allow recognition at operation). Repeat mammograms are then taken in the two conventional planes and the radiologist reports the relationship of the radiological abnormality to the dye. An alternative practice is to leave the needle *in situ*.

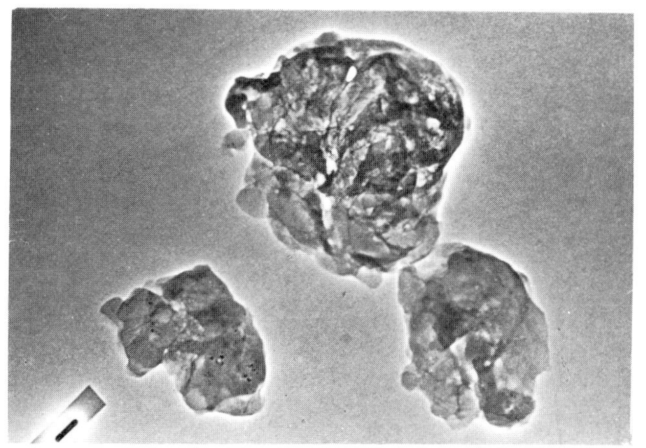

16

16

Operative procedure

The patient is taken to theatre, the site of the dye is exposed and the appropriate area excised. While the patient remains anaesthetized, the specimen is returned to X-ray for specimen radiography to ensure that the radiological abnormality is included and to localize the exact site under suspicion for the pathologist. (Specimen radiography is less certain in the absence of microcalcification.) The specimen radiograph illustrated here shows the microcalcification to be confined to the smallest of the three specimens.

If the specimen removed has classic macroscopic features of a carcinoma it is submitted to frozen section, proceeding to mastectomy if indicated. Otherwise, and in the majority of cases, the author prefers to await urgent paraffin section so that the management can proceed after full evaluation.

Biopsy procedures for nipple discharge

General management of nipple discharge

A blood-stained or clear serous nipple discharge is most frequently caused by benign papilloma, single or multiple. The commonest entity is a solitary papilloma giving discharge from a single duct and this is treated by microdochotomy (excision of a single duct and its drainage system). Occasionally papillomatosis leads to discharge from multiple ducts, usually in women near the menopause and total duct excision is the preferred operation. Rarely a duct carcinoma will be found on histology. (Blood discharge from multiple ducts, and commonly from both nipples, may also be seen during pregnancy when it is due to a physiological hyperplasia of the duct epithelium.)

Discharges other than blood-stained or serous are causally associated with cancer so rarely that operation is not necessary as a diagnostic procedure. But such discharges (usually yellowish or green and due to duct ectasia) may be sufficiently profuse for inconvenience to indicate the operation of total duct excision.

The presence of dilated ducts, as detected on mammography, is not in itself an indication for total duct excision. Likewise, when some duct dilatation is seen during biopsy of a mass behind the nipple, the mass should be removed in the usual way and the ducts left undisturbed. Healing is usually uneventful despite the transected dilated ducts, and it should be remembered that some duct dilatation is present in a majority of women at or near the menopause. Total duct excision is associated with higher morbidity and a less satisfactory cosmetic result than simple biopsy.

MICRODOCHOTOMY

This operation is indicated for blood-stained or serous discharge from a single duct whose orifice can be identified. Where the discharge has ceased by the time the patient is seen, so that the duct cannot be identified, the patient may be observed if she is under the age of 40 years since duct papillomas commonly slough spontaneously. In all patients over this age we would carry out a total duct excision operation because of an increased risk of multiple papillomas or intraduct cancer.

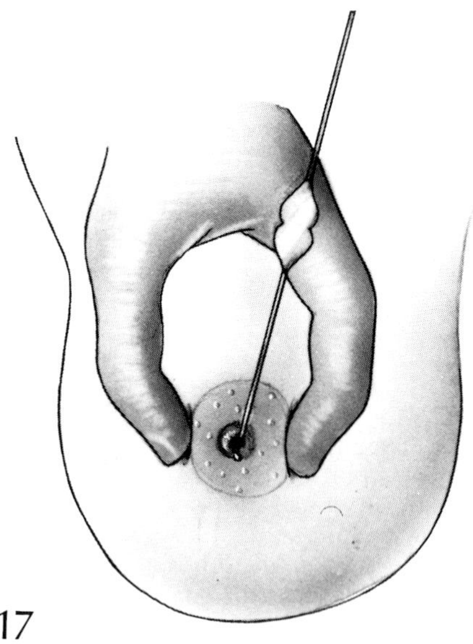

17

17

Technique

The nipple is first squeezed to produce some discharge to identify the affected duct. A lacrimal probe is then gently inserted as far as possible, without forming a false passage. Frequently this is only for 1 or 2 cm because dilated ducts may be tortuous or blocked by papillomas which form little pockets in their walls, but the probe can be passed far enough to show the general direction of the duct and indicate in which direction the excision should be made.

18 & 19

A radial incision is made in a racquet shape to include the terminal part of the duct, then crosses the areola to extend into the breast for about 5 cm. The two flaps are dissected in the level between the deep fascia and the breast lobules – this plane is easiest to develop in the region of the margin of the areola. In the central portion of the duct the incision should be kept as close to the probe as possible, to avoid removing adjacent ducts. The duct system is then dissected peripherally for about 5 cm; this is normally sufficient to remove all the major duct system of the affected segment. Haemostasis is ensured and a suction drain is inserted before closing the wound with 4/0 chromic catgut to the deep fascia and 4/0 silk to the skin. This radial incision heals with a surprisingly good cosmetic result. Where the duct to be removed opens on to the central portion of the nipple, some trauma to adjacent ducts is inevitable, but this does not give long-term problems.

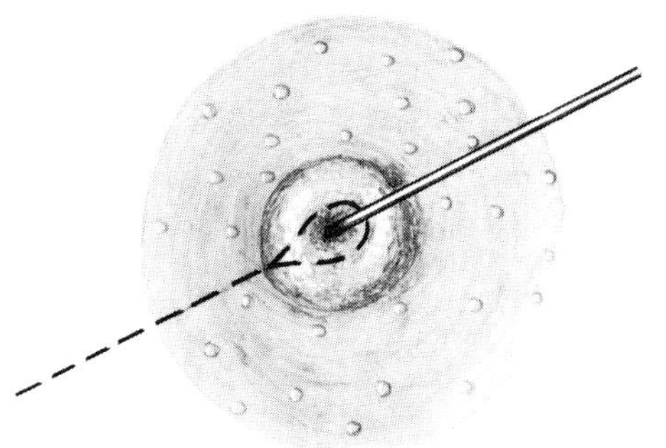

18

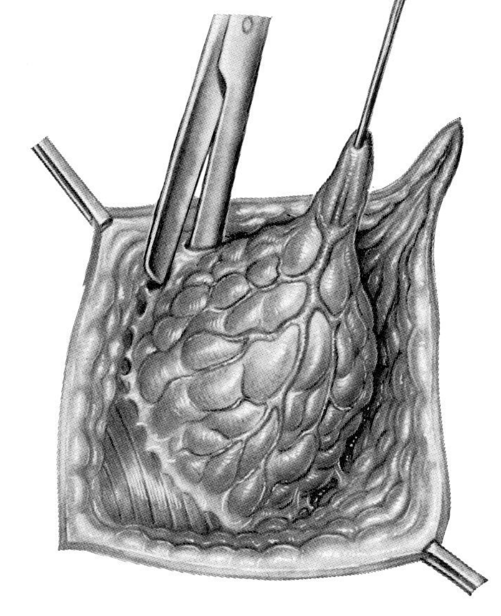

19

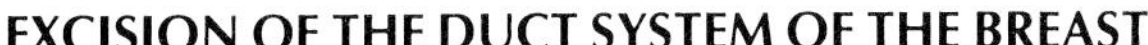

EXCISION OF THE DUCT SYSTEM OF THE BREAST

This operation is indicated for blood-stained or serous discharge from one or more ducts in women over the age of 40; and for nipple discharge from duct ectasia sufficient to embarrass or seriously inconvenience the patient[2]. With milky discharges, galactorrhoea of pituitary origin should be excluded before proceeding to duct excision.

20

The incision

The ducts may be approached by periareolar or radial incisions. The former has the advantages of a better cosmetic result, and of allowing easier access to the correct plane for dissection of the ducts. The incision is deepened through the skin and the subcutaneous fascia until the subcutaneous veins are reached. These are carefully ligated with 4/0 chromic catgut and serve as a guide to the plane of dissection which lies immediately deep to them. This plane is between the fat lobules of the breast and the fascia underlying the areola and preserves the subdermal vascular plexus of the areola, and with it the viability of the nipple.

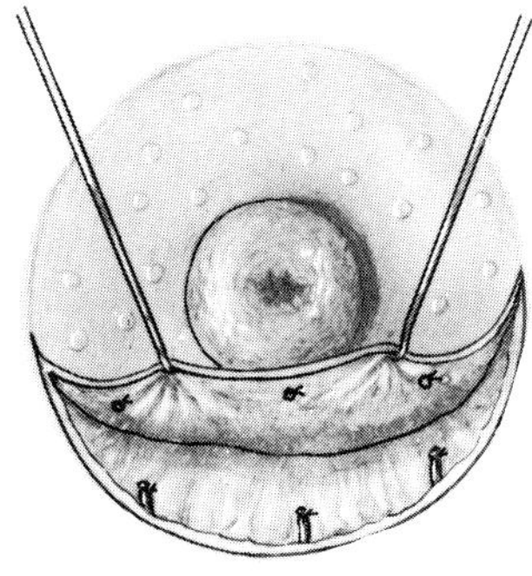

20

21 & 22

The nipple is elevated with hooks and mobilized until the main duct system has been exposed. Keeping in the same plane, further dissection of the areola is carried out on both sides, using blunt curved artery forceps such as Kelly-Halsted. In this way, a subareolar tunnel is produced in the subcutaneous plane right around the ducts, which are then grasped at their termination by a small Kocher forceps and the ducts divided just below the nipple. The duct system is dissected back into the breast for a distance of 2–3 cm and again divided with a scalpel. Bleeding vessels are immediately caught with mosquito forceps and ligated with 4/0 chromic catgut before they are lost through retraction into the breast tissue. In most cases dilated ducts are not detectable more than 2–3 cm into the breast tissue. When they are still dilated at the point of transection, an attempt should be made to catch them with forceps and ligate them with fine catgut, although this is not always possible, and failure to do so seems to cause no trouble.

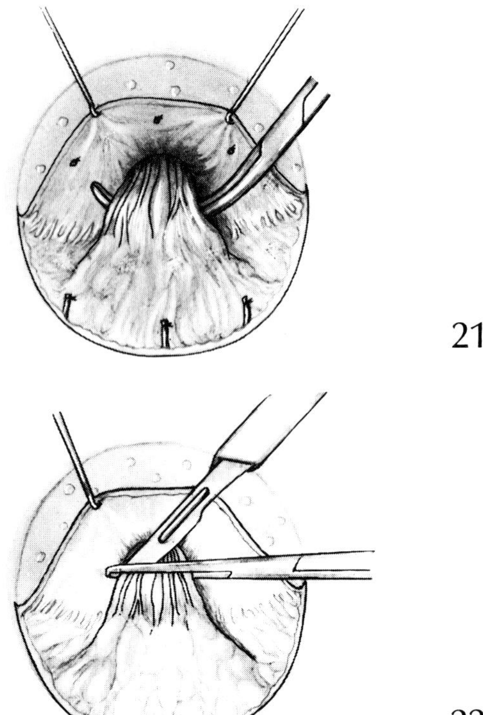

21

22

23

The completeness of excision of the terminal ducts is checked by inverting the nipple and trimming any residual duct with scissors and, second, by ensuring that the subareolar dissection has encompassed the complete duct system.

The nipple will usually remain everted after excision of the duct system, but if it tends to reinvert, a fine catgut suture can be placed in the deep fascia to maintain eversion.

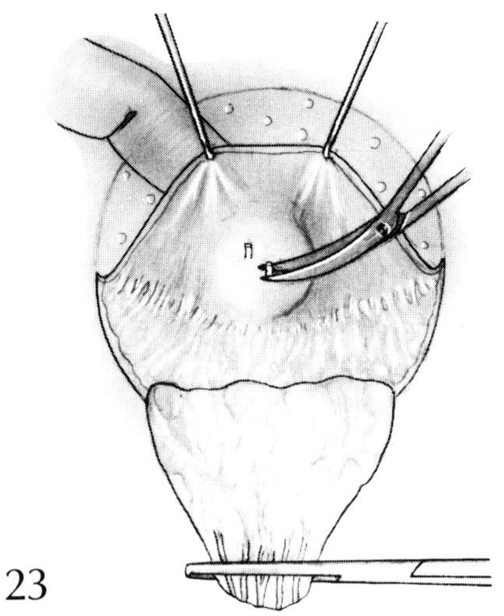

23

24

Closure

Provided there is no evidence of active infection, the skin is closed with 4/0 silk and suction drainage instituted. Some epidermal necrosis of the lower flap may be seen if dissection too superficially has compromised the subdermal plexus, but this usually separates spontaneously.

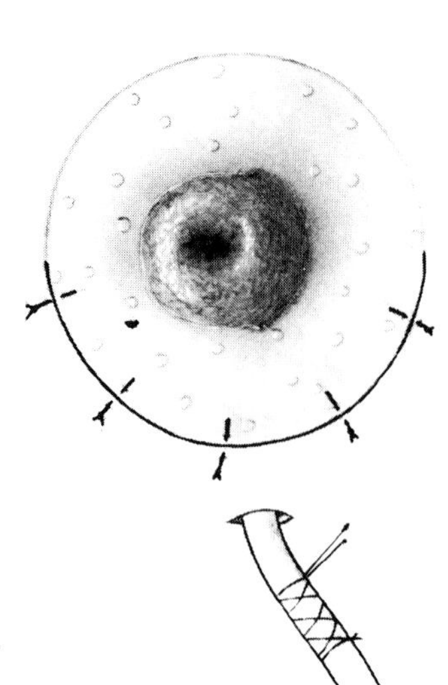

24

PROCEDURES FOR INFLAMMATORY LESIONS OF THE BREAST

Operations for inflammatory conditions fall into two broad groups: the well-defined breast abscess associated with lactation, and a much less well-defined group of conditions of subacute chronic suppuration of the breast.

Drainage of a lactational breast abscess

Acute mastitis in the lactation period is usually the result of a staphylococcal infection associated with a cracked nipple and can sometimes be obviated by control of breast engorgement and antibiotics. But unless resolution is clearly rapid and complete within 48 h, drainage should be undertaken early, because excessive destruction of breast tissue will occur by the time the abscess shows obvious fluctuation or skin involvement. Where the patient is afebrile and throbbing pain absent, the possibility of inflammatory carcinoma should be considered; needle biopsy rather than open biopsy is preferred in this situation.

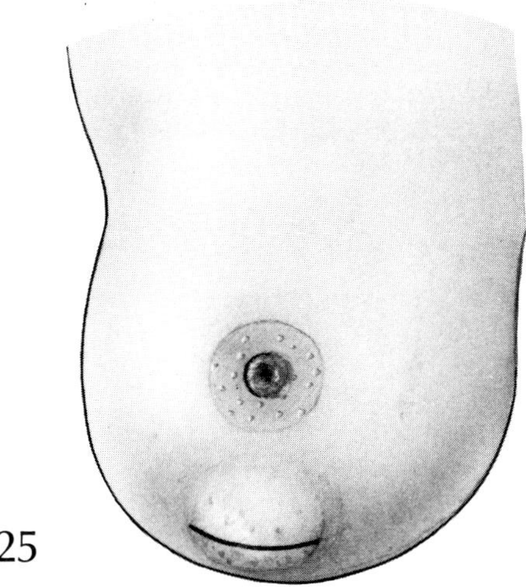

25

25 – 28

Technique

A skin-crease incision is used, slightly below the point of maximal swelling and tenderness.

A finger is then inserted into the cavity to ensure that all loculations are broken down, so that no undrained areas persist. If the resulting cavity is found to be centred behind the incision, counterdrainage is not necessary.

The incision should extend to at least three-quarters of the diameter of the cavity, which is then gently packed – gauze soaked in acriflavine emulsion is suitable.

Where the cavity is obviously dependent in relation to the incision, it is best to use counterdrainage at the lowest point, inserting a wide plastic corrugated drain. The initial incision should be loosely sutured only if the margins are healthy. Where the abscess cavity has already reached the surface, primary healing of the edges will not occur.

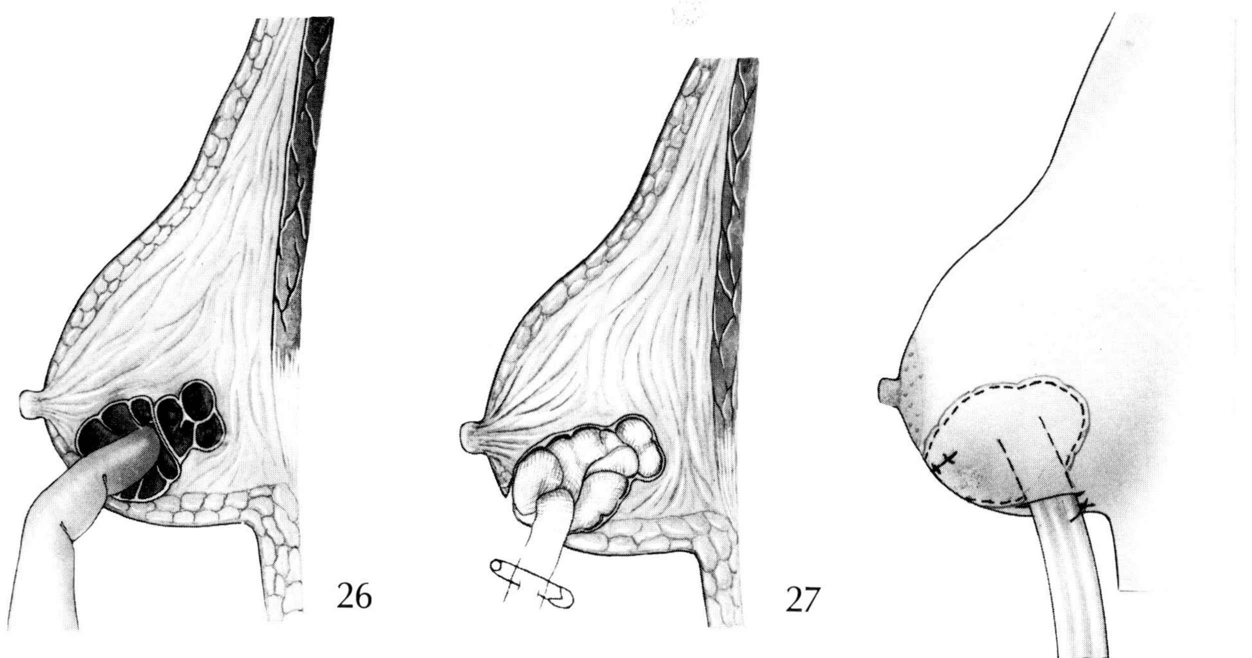

26 27 28

Subacute and recurrent abscesses of the breast

Most breast abscesses unrelated to lactation are associated with duct ectasia and its complication, periductal mastitis. This is a reaction to irritating duct contents which have escaped into periductal tissues and is initially sterile, although secondary bacterial invasion, especially with anaerobic organisms, may occur later or after drainage. The hallmarks of these abscesses are their periareolar location, frequent association with nipple inversion, relatively chronic or relapsing course and a lesser degree of pain than is seen with lactational abscesses. In addition it is not rare for both breasts to be affected, with an interval of several years between the two sides. Patients with these abscesses tend to fall into two main groups which are associated with a single or with multiple duct involvement. This distinction is clinical rather than pathological, since the 'single duct' variety may show a number of dilated ducts. Hence it is not surprising that the distinction is sometimes blurred. However, most cases fall clearly into one or other clinical pattern and are managed satisfactorily by the appropriate surgical approach.

The single duct entity, the mammillary duct fistula of Atkins, is diagnosed when recurrent abscesses always appear at the one site, usually a point on the medial edge of the areola, and when a fistula can be demonstrated in between acute episodes by passing a probe from the site of the abscess discharge through to the nipple. It is satisfactorily treated by the fistula excision operation first described by Atkins[3].

The multiple duct entity, when retroareolar infection is less well localized, is seen more commonly close to the menopause but may on occasions be found even in young nulliparous girls. Where there is extensive and poorly localized retroareolar infection, excision of the whole duct system is necessary to control the infection. This type also differs from the first group in that some cases show dilatation of ducts extending well out into the peripheral breast tissue, the ducts being filled with toothpaste-like material. Recurrent subareolar abscess from a single duct mammillary fistula is not associated with peripheral dilatation.

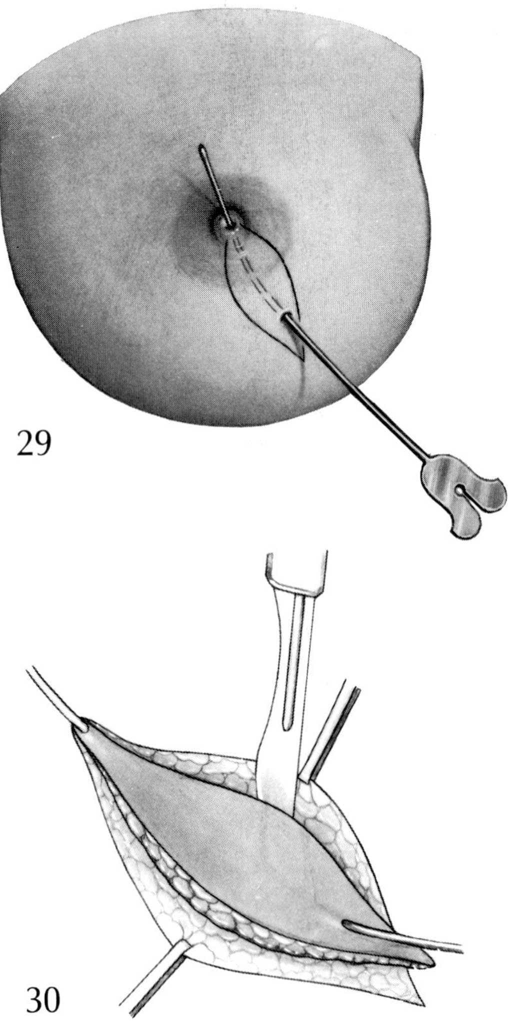

EXCISION OF MAMMILLARY DUCT FISTULA

29 & 30

A probe is passed through the opening and will be found to emerge from the nipple through the affected duct, which is always dilated. The skin incision encompasses the fistulous track, encircles the affected duct and is continued for 2 cm distal to the opening of a fistula. It is unnecessary to remove more than 0.5 cm of skin on either side of the track. The incision is deepened to expose the underlying tissues, and the fistula excised as a formal operation. It is essential to excise the central portion of the duct; if it is left behind recurrence is certain.

31

The wound is best left open and packed to allow healing by granulation. Primary closure is followed by wound breakdown in a considerable number of cases, and may lead to further chronic infection.

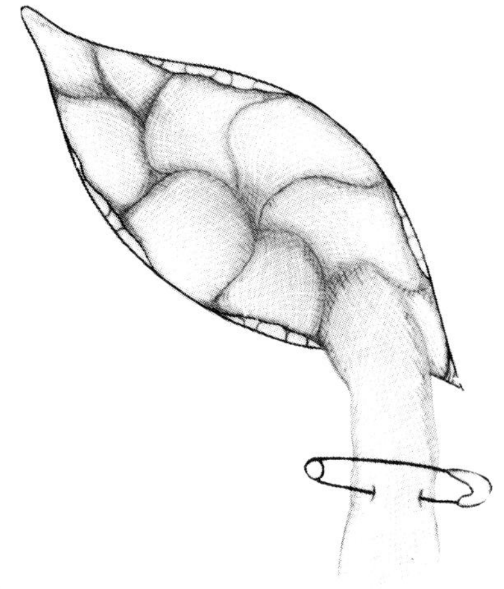

31

TOTAL DUCT EXCISION FOR SUBAREOLAR SEPSIS

This follows the same general principles as described under 'Total duct excision for discharge'. Development of the correct plane may be difficult if persistent inflammation is present. It may then be better to use a radial incision as first described by Urban[4] to excise the most badly affected skin.

If dilated ducts containing cheesy contents are found to extend into the breast tissue beyond the 3 cm normally removed, an attempt should be made to catch the transected ducts with artery forceps and ligate them with fine chromic catgut. The wound is packed and allowed to heal by granulation. Attempts at primary closure, even with drainage, are likely to be followed by persistent sepsis and possible necrosis of the overlying nipple.

Most patients will have no further trouble, but in some, more peripheral inflammation will subsequently develop. This will usually localize to a segment of the breast, so that subsequent excision of perhaps one-third of the breast is necessary. Less commonly, inflammation is so extensive that the condition will only be eradicated by total subcutaneous mastectomy. Perioperative use of an agent active against anaerobic organisms, such as metronidazole, may reduce the incidence of postoperative or recurrent sepsis, but clear evidence to support this is not available at present.

References

1. Preece, P. E., Gravelle, I. H., Hughes, L. E., Baum, M., Fortt, R. W., Leopold, J. G. The operative management of subclinical breast cancer. Clinical Oncology 1977; 3: 165–169

2. Hadfield, G. J. The pathological lesions underlying discharges from the nipple in women. Annals of the Royal College of Surgeons of England 1969; 44: 323–333

3. Atkins, H. B. Mammillary fistula. British Medical Journal 1955; 2: 1473–1474

4. Urban, J. A. Excision of the major duct system of the breast. Cancer 1963; 16: 516–520

Total mastectomy and axillary node sample

A. P. M. Forrest MD, ChM, DSc, FRCS, HonFACS
Regius Professor of Clinical Surgery, University of Edinburgh

Preoperative

Indications and objectives

Histological staging of the axillary lymph nodes is now an accepted part of the treatment of breast cancer. The objective of the operation of total mastectomy and axillary node sample is to remove all breast tissue including the axillary tail of the breast and its contained nodes and to identify and excise, for histological examination, one or more of the lymph nodes of the pectoral group which lie close to the upper medial aspect of the tail. This can be regarded as one of the standard operations for treating the disease.

In all cases a histopathological diagnosis is made preoperatively either by Trucut biopsy (*see* p. 241) or, if the tumour is small (<1 cm), by local excision (*see* p. 243). Preliminary frozen section examination (*see* p. 247) is now rarely used.

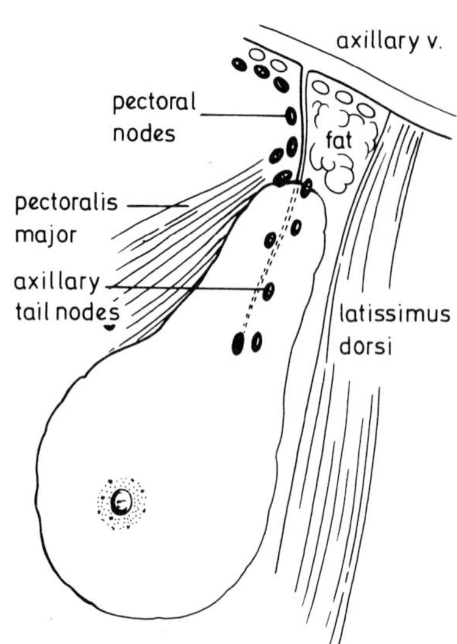

1

Diagram of relationships.

The operation

2

Position of patient

A general anaesthetic is used and the patient lies supine with the arm outstretched. A long rubber wedge placed on an arm board supports the arm forward of horizontal and slightly raises the scapula. A 'terry towel' or pack is placed on the operating table alongside the posterior axillary fold and the affected side is towelled off.

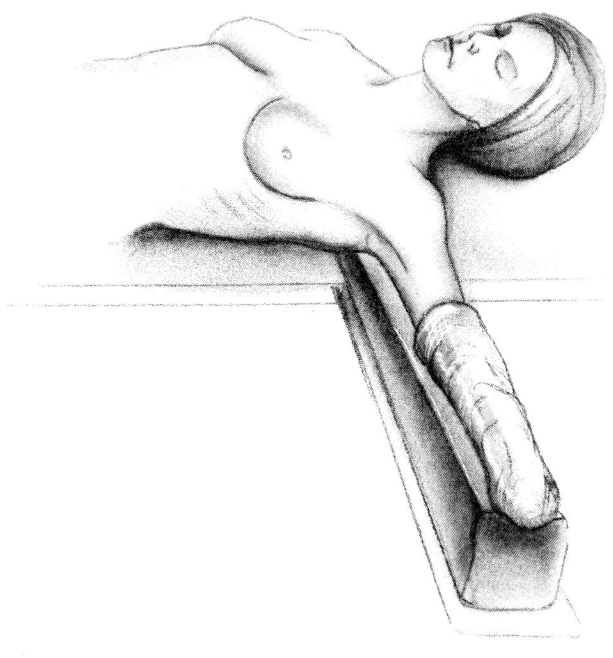

2

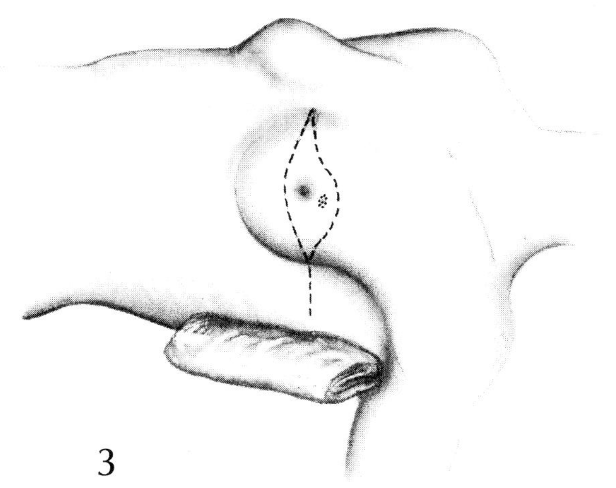

3

3

The incisions

Elliptical incisions to include the nipple and the tumour are planned to leave a scar which will lie as nearly transverse as possible. The margin of skin around the tumour is variable and depends on its size compared to that of the breast. In general, it should not be less than 3 cm from the outer border of the tumour in any direction. The incision should not extend further than the midline anteriorly or posterior to the anterior axillary fold.

Upper skin flap

4

Raising of upper flap

The upper incision is made first and the upper flap mobilized to the level of the second rib. The raising of the flap is started with a knife, but as the dissection extends upwards, curved scissors allow easier definition of the plane of separation of the skin flap which is between the superficial fascia of the breast and the subdermal fat. This plane is wider and easier to define in a stout patient.

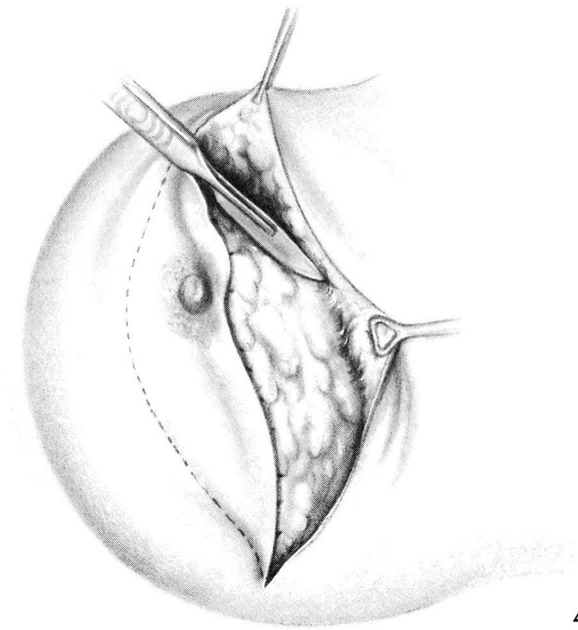

4

(Courtesy of British Journal of Surgery; 73: 569)

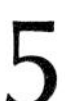

5

Dissection at upper margin of breast

As the upper limits of the flap dissection are reached, the scissors are used to divide the superficial fascia at the upper margin of the breast and to define the underlying pectoral fascia.

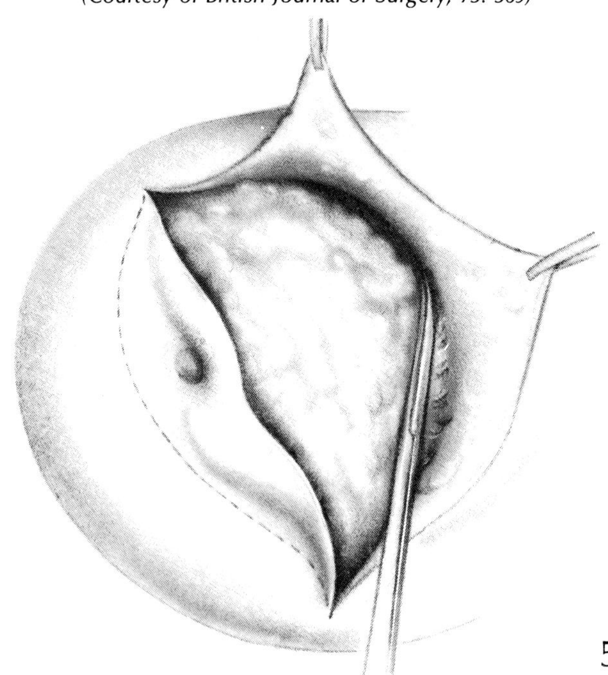

5

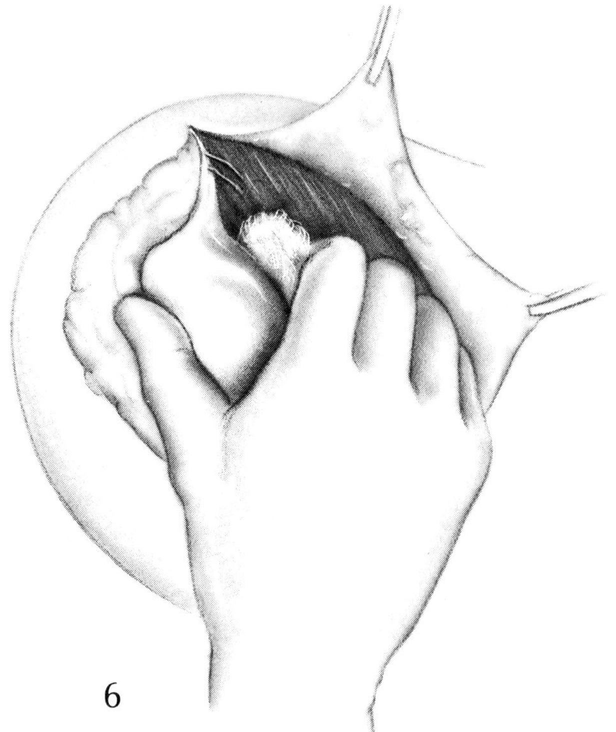

6

(Courtesy of British Journal of Surgery; 73: 569)

6

Mobilization of breast

The breast is mobilized from the pectoral fascia and underlying muscle and chest wall by burrowing from above downwards between the breast and the pectoral fascia using the fingers or a gauze swab. This separates the medial two-thirds of the breast from the chest wall except for its medial attachment to the sternum and its inferior attachment to the pectoral fascia. By pulling the breast forwards and downwards, the perforating branches of the internal mammary vessels may be seen and can be ligated and divided before they enter the deep surface of the breast.

Lower skin flap

7

Completion of incision and mobilization of lower skin flap

The lower skin incision is now made and the lower flap separated from underlying breast tissue first with the knife and then with scissors.

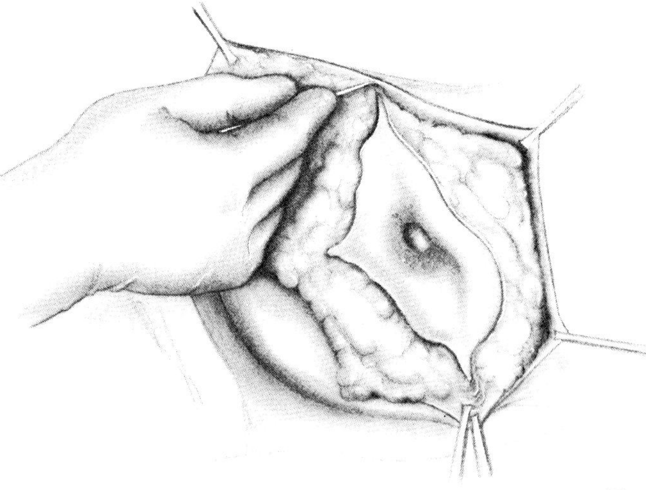

7

(Courtesy of British Journal of Surgery; 73: 569)

8

Completion of mobilization of breast from chest wall

In a thin person, the breast parenchyma may be close to the skin from which it must carefully be dissected.

The medial border of the breast is dissected from the sternum and costal cartilages, the remaining perforating vessels being ligated and divided in turn. The breast is drawn medially and its remaining attachment to the pectoral fascia divided from medial to lateral so that the breast is completely mobilized as far as the outer border of the pectoralis major muscle.

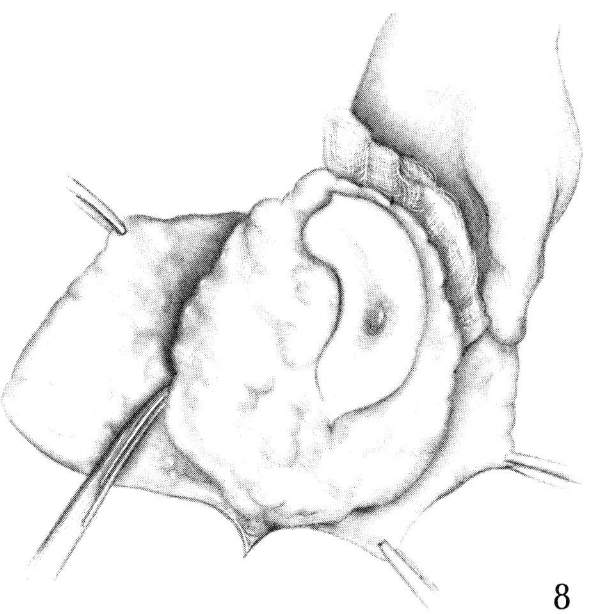

8

(Courtesy of British Journal of Surgery; 73: 569)

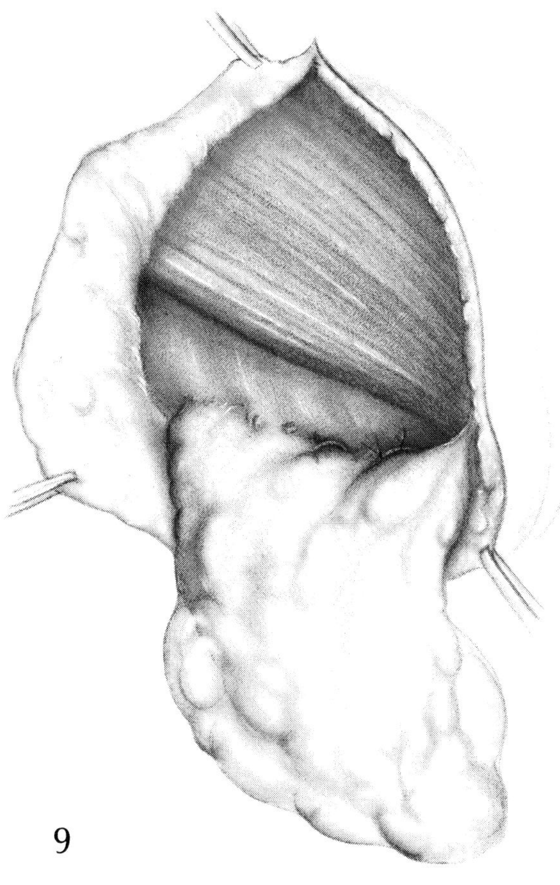

9

Lateral dissection

9

The lateral skin flap is undermined for 2.5 cm to facilitate lateral retraction of the breast. The outer border of the pectoralis major muscle is exposed by sharp dissection and the deep aspect of the breast swept laterally from the fascia overlying the serratus anterior muscle on the lateral chest wall by gauze dissection. The external mammary branches of the lateral thoracic artery and the lateral perforating branches of the intercostal vessels are put on the stretch and can be ligated and divided. Small lymph nodes may be associated with these vessels and should be removed for histological examination.

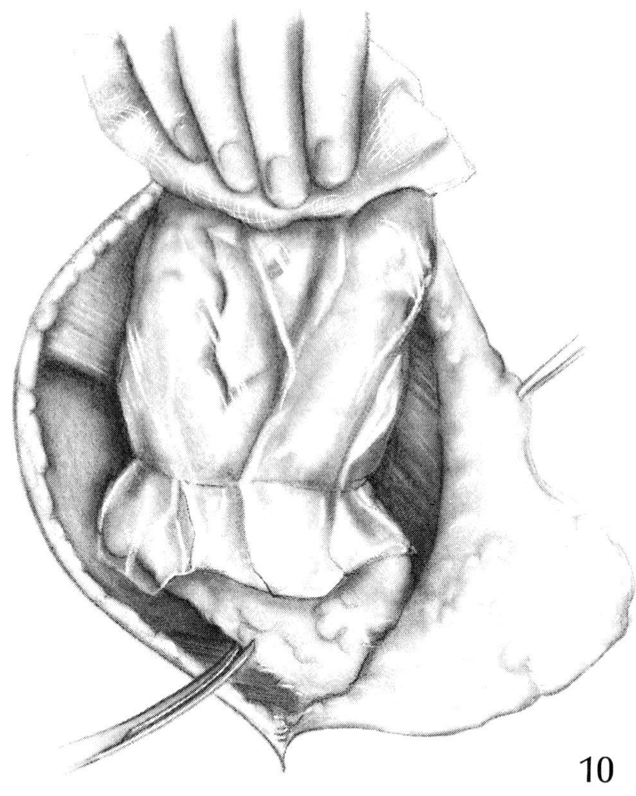

10

10 & 11

The fascia overlying the breast is attached laterally to the latissimus dorsi. The breast is drawn medially and the skin flaps elevated laterally until the anterolateral border of this muscle is reached. The fascial connections of the breast are divided from below upwards. The breast is completely mobilized except for its axillary tail.

The breast is enclosed in a polythene bag secured by a ligature. This facilitates its handling and protects the wound from contamination with fat and shed cells.

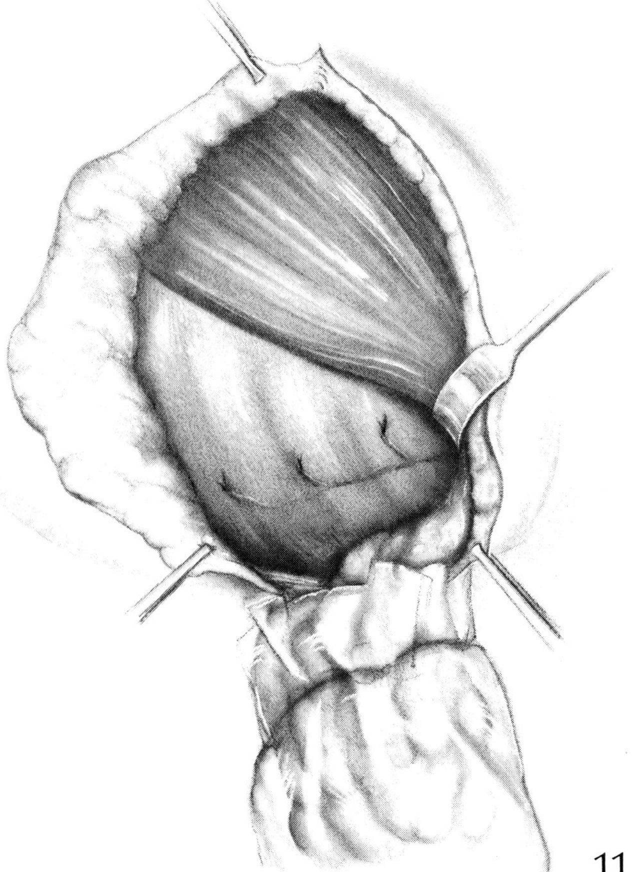

11

Dissection of axillary tail

12

Reflection of skin off tail

The skin and subcutaneous fat of the upper flap is elevated off the anterior surface of the axillary tail of the breast using curved scissors. The dissection is kept close to the breast tissue, particularly as one approaches the axilla, so that the skin is not penetrated.

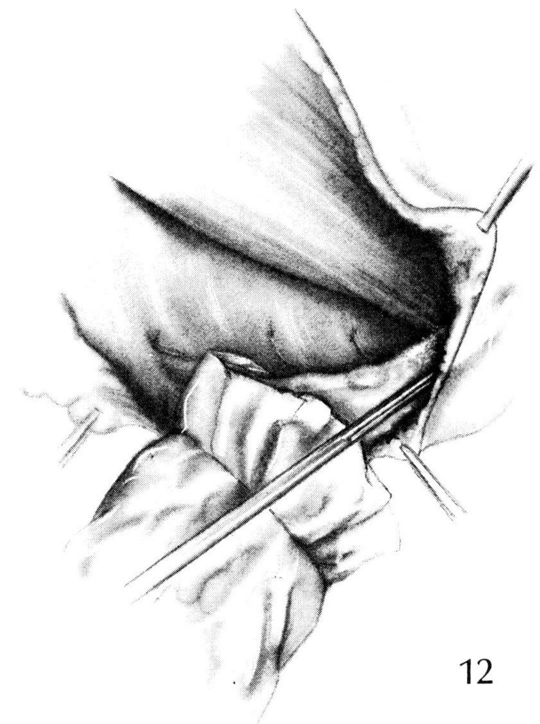

12

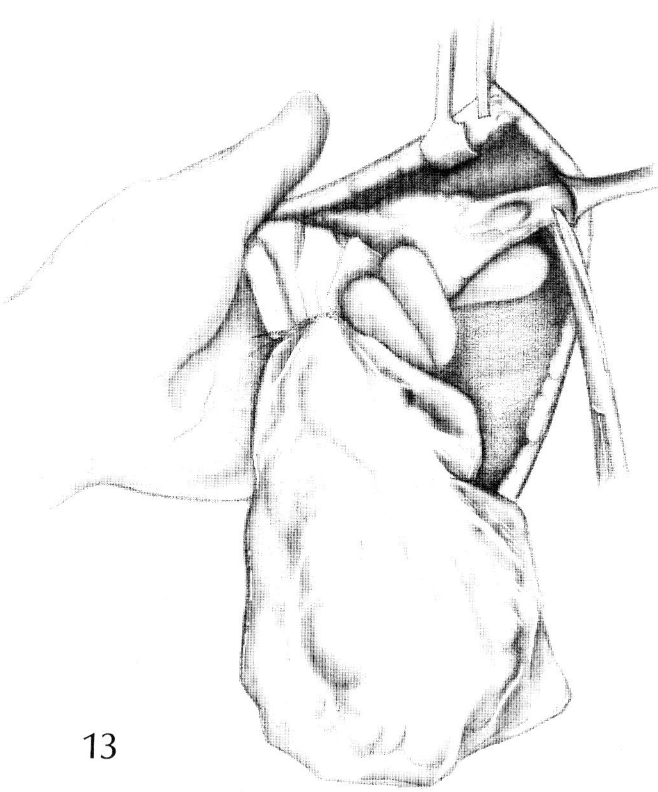

13

13

Final separation of tail

The axillary tail is then separated in front from the pectoralis major and behind from the latissimus dorsi and stripped upwards towards the axilla.

The anterior layer of the axillary fascia is divided with scissors to expose the axillary fat. The level at which the parenchymatous tissue of the axillary tail merges into this fat can be felt between finger and thumb.

It is at this point that lymph nodes of the pectoral group may be seen or felt and three or four nodes should be teased out for histological examination. Separation of the axillary tail from the axillary fat is best performed with scissors. The 'axillary tail' vein which runs into the axillary fat towards the axillary vein and is constantly present requires ligation before it is divided. The intercostobrachial nerve may run in close apposition to the top of the tail and may also be divided.

Careful palpation of the axilla is now performed. The axillary vein may be seen shining through the axillary fat but is not exposed. The fingers should be run up the line of the vein under the pectoral muscles and the findings recorded.

14

Examination of specimen

The surgeon must ensure that three to four lymph nodes have been removed with the specimen and should dissect these out and place them in fixative. Should no nodes be present he should repalpate the axilla and, if necessary, remove a block of axillary fat from the subscapularis medial to the subscapular vessels and nerve to the latissimus dorsi, in which nodes are always present. It cannot be sufficiently stressed that it is the *surgeon's* responsibility to provide the pathologist with nodes for histological examination.

At this stage it is a simple matter to extend the operation into a formal total axillary clearance (*see* p. 270) by retracting the pectoralis major, detaching the pectoralis minor from the coracoid process, defining the axillary vein and dissecting lymph nodes and fat from above down. If this is contemplated the arm must be separately towelled so that it can be elevated during the dissection (*see* p. 267).

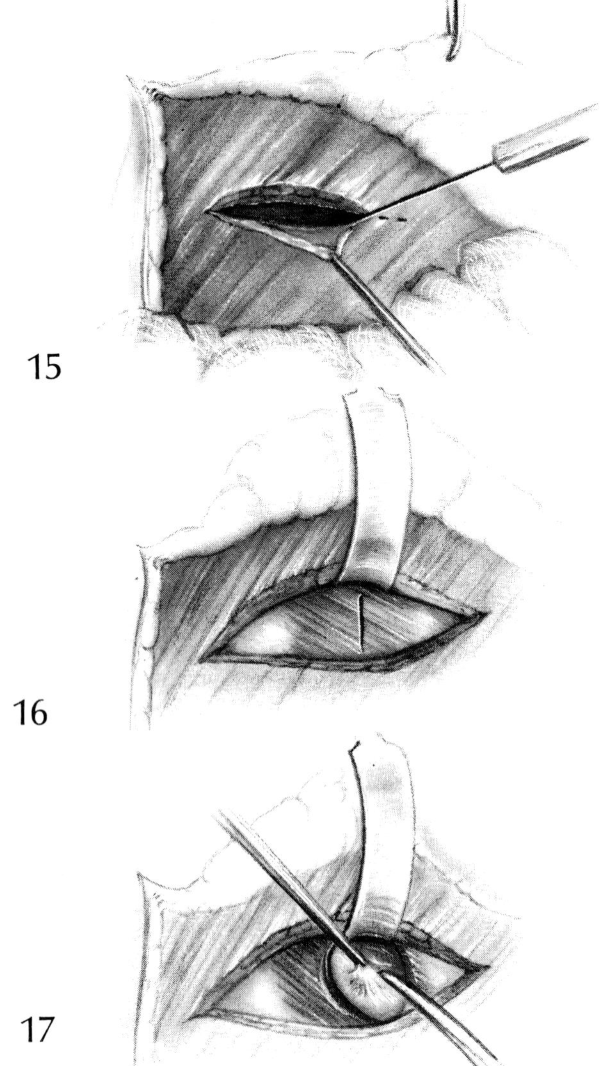

15

16

17

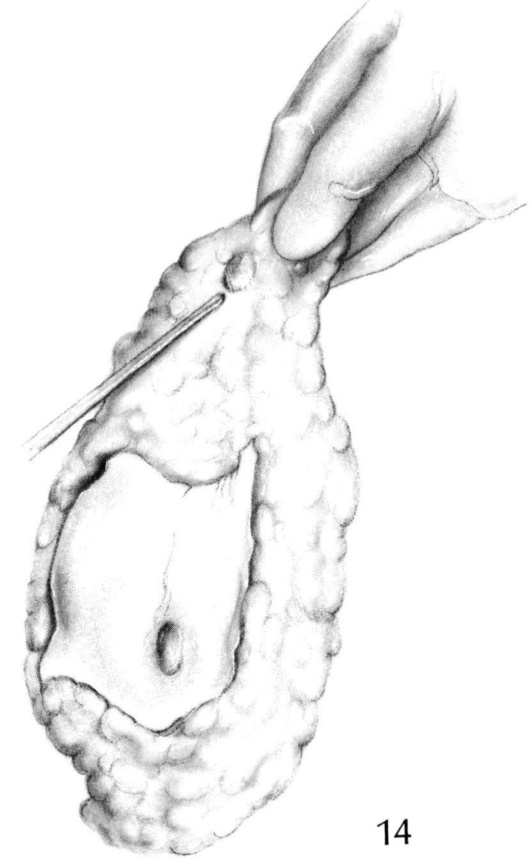

14

15–18

Internal mammary node biopsy

If the tumour is medially placed, the internal mammary vessels can be exposed through the medial aspect of the second, third or fourth intercostal spaces. The pectoralis major muscle is divided in the line of the sternum and the intercostal muscle, parallel to the ribs. A thin layer of fascia roofs over the fatty tissue in which the internal mammary vessels and the lymph trunks and nodes lie and this is divided with fine scissors. The nodes, which may be tiny, lie on the lateral side of the vessels.

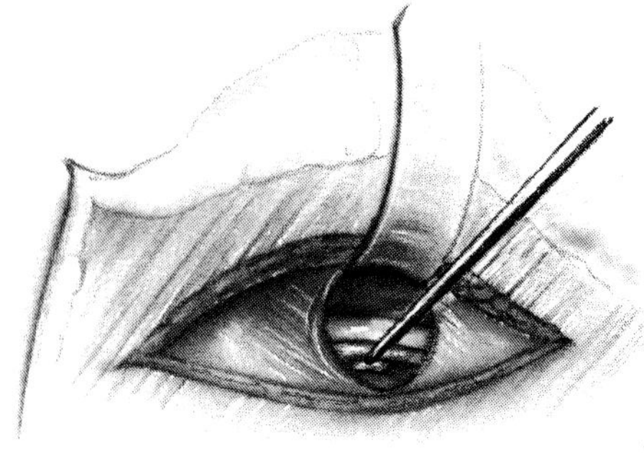

18

Insertion of prosthesis

19

If the patient wishes it, a silicone-containing prosthesis can be inserted. This is best placed in a subpectoral pocket so that healing of the skin wound is undisturbed and encapsulation of the prosthesis avoided. Access to the subpectoral region is by an incision in the serratus anterior and a tunnel under the muscle.

Alternatively, insertion may be from above, splitting the pectoralis over the second interspace in the line of its fibres.

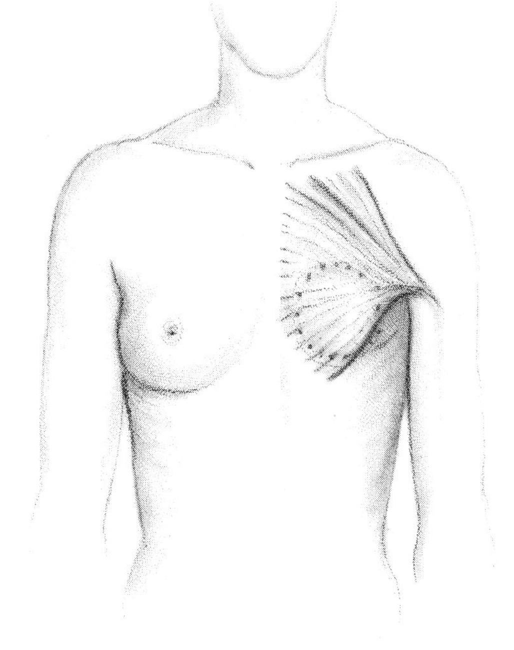

19

Formation of pocket

20

The incision in the serratus anterior is over the sixth or seventh rib and 3–5 cm in length. A finger is used to tunnel forwards under the serratus detaching its fibres from the ribs with scissors and entering the subpectoral space.

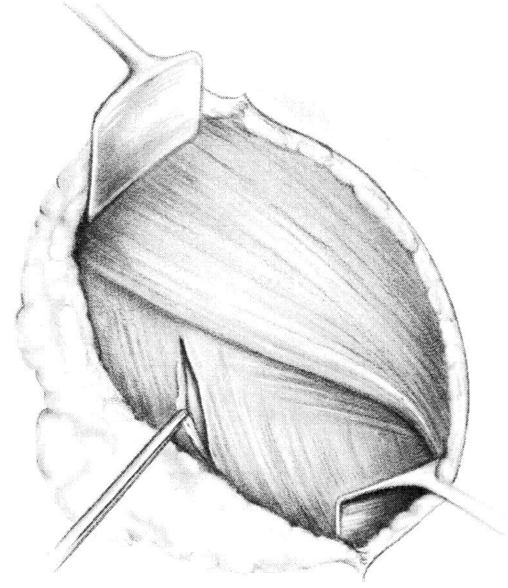

20

21

A pocket is formed under the pectoralis major by sweeping a finger between it and the chest wall and between the pectoralis major and minor muscles superiorly.

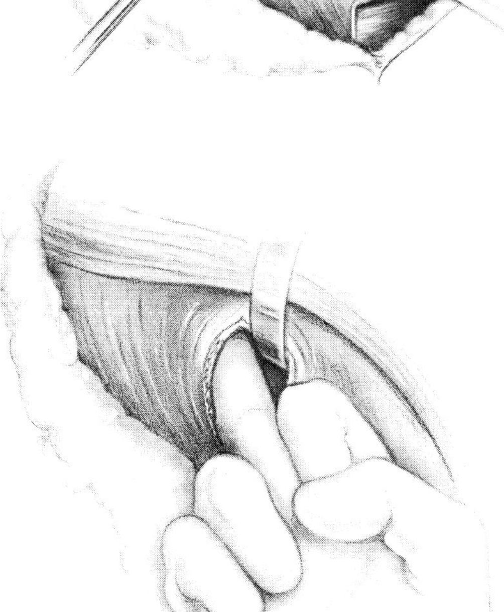

21

22

As the pectoralis major is attached to the anterior rectus sheath and/or ribs at a higher level than the inframammary fold it may be necessary to extend the pocket inferiorly. This can be done by burrowing under the rectus sheath from the lateral to the medial side. In some patients it is necessary to detach the lower medial fibres of the pectoralis major from the ribs and suture these to the anterior rectus sheath or the undersurface of the skin flap.

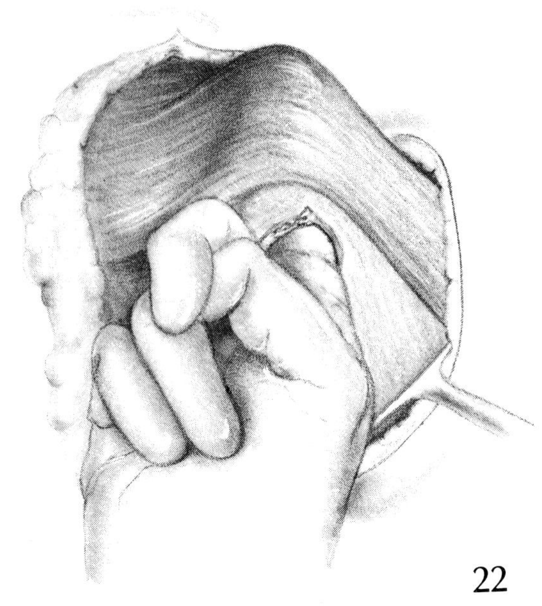

22

23

Placement of prosthesis in pocket

The prosthesis is inserted into the pocket and flattened out onto the chest wall. A 'sizing set' of prostheses is convenient as it allows a better estimate of the most suitable size. Normally a prosthesis of 150–250 ml is used.

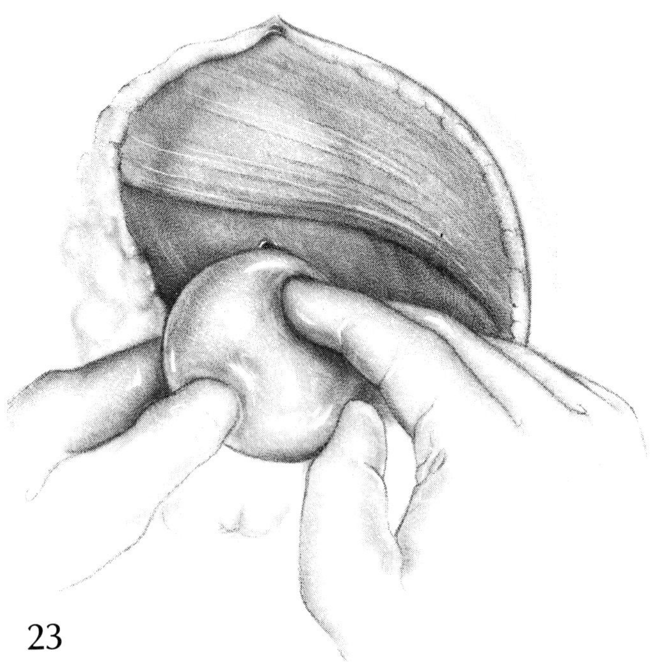

23

24

Closure of serratus anterior

The serratus anterior is closed with interrupted 2/0 Dexon sutures.

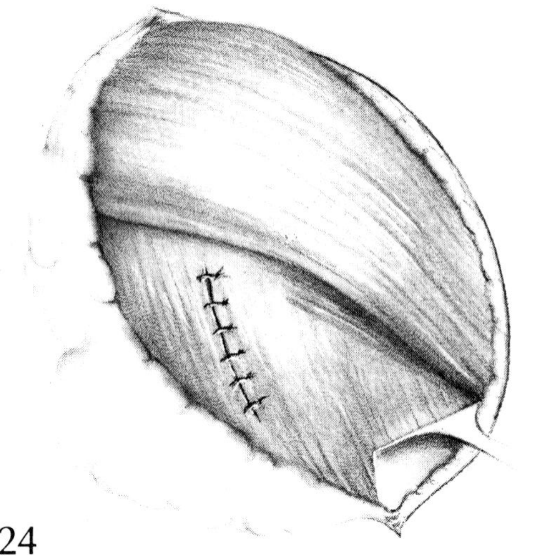

24

25

Wound drainage and closure

The wound is irrigated with 600 ml 1:120 cetrimide (prepared by diluting 100 ml 1:20 solution with 500 ml saline) and two suction drains of small diameter are inserted.

The wound is closed in two layers: a subcutaneous suture of interrupted 2/0 Dexon and a continuous subcuticular suture of Prolene, fixed at either end with a bead and cuff.

Suction drainage bottles (Redivac or Steritex) are attached to the drains and the wound dressed with a strip of gauze fixed with skin adhesive (Nobecutane). No bandages or other dressings are used.

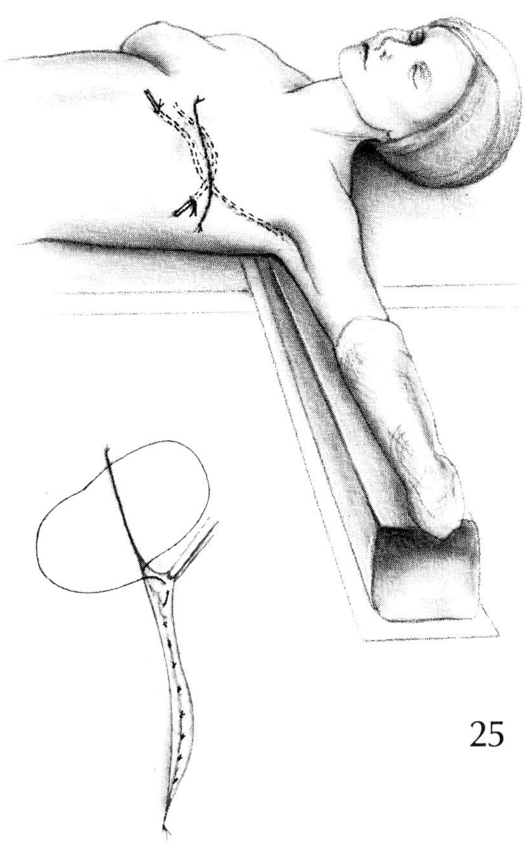

25

Postoperative care and complications

If a silicone prosthesis has been inserted penicillin therapy (penicillin V 250 mg and flucloxacillin 250 mg four times a day) is given for 5 days, starting preoperatively.

The small suction drains are removed when drainage ceases, usually after 2–3 days. Full mobility is encouraged from the day after operation and the patient should wear her normal brassiere as soon as possible. If a silicone prosthesis has been inserted a soft wool pad may be required as a filler. If a subpectoral prosthesis has not been inserted a soft external prosthesis is used.

A collection of serum, most common laterally, may complicate the operation but this is rare. Aspiration is performed. The subcuticular suture is removed in 7–10 days.

A decision regarding additional postoperative treatment, either locally with radiotherapy or systemically with chemotherapy or endocrine means, is dependent upon the results of the node biopsy. Provided nodes have been examined and shown to be free of metastases local recurrence rates are low and it is safe to withhold radiotherapy.

Index